Family Nurse Practitioner Certification Review

FAMILY NURSE PRACTITIONER
CERTIFICATION REVIEW

Pamela S. Kidd, RN, ARNP, CEN, PhD
Professor
University of Kentucky College of Nursing
Kentucky Injury Prevention and Research Center
Lexington, Kentucky

Denise L. Robinson, RN, ARNP, PhD
Professor
Northern Kentucky University
Director, MSN Programs
Northern Kentucky Family Health Centers, Inc.
Highland Heights, Kentucky

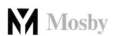 Mosby

St. Louis Baltimore Boston Carlsbad Chicago Minneapolis New York Philadelphia Portland
London Milan Sydney Tokyo Toronto

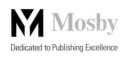
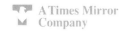

Publisher: Nancy L. Coon
Developmental Editor: Nancy L. O'Brien
Project Manager: Dana Peick
Production Editor: Catherine Albright
Manufacturing Manager: Don Carlisle
Design Manager: Amy Buxton

A NOTE TO THE READER

The authors and publisher have made every attempt to check dosages and nursing content for accuracy. Because the science of pharmacology is continually advancing, our knowledge base continues to expand. Therefore we recommend that the reader always check product information for changes in dosage or administration before administering any medication. This is particularly important with new or rarely used drugs.

Printed in the United States of America
Composition, editing, and production by Top Graphics
Printing/binding by R.R. Donnelley & Sons Company

Mosby, Inc.
11830 Westline Industrial Drive
St. Louis, Missouri 63146

Library of Congress Cataloging in Publication Data

Family nurse practitioner certification review / [edited by] Pamela S. Kidd, Denise L. Robinson.
    p.   cm.
   Includes bibliographical references and index.
   ISBN 0-8151-5581-6
   1. Family nursing—Examinations, questions, etc.   2. Nurse practitioners—Examinations, questions, etc.   I. Kidd, Pamela Stinson.   II. Robinson, Denise L.
   [DNLM: 1. Nurse Practitioners examination questions.   2. Family Practice nurses' instruction examination questions.   WY 18.2 F198 1998]
RT120.F34F353   1998
610.738076—dc21
DNLM/DLC
for Library of Congress   98-23492
                                           CIP

98 99 00 01 02 / 9 8 7 6 5 4 3 2 1

Contributors

Elizabeth Abel, RNC-ANP, PhD
Assistant Professor
School of Nursing
University of Texas at Austin
Austin, Texas
Diverticulosis, Irritable Bowel Syndrome,
Gastroesophageal Reflux Disease

Karen D. Agricola, BSN, MSN, RNCS, FNP
Wyoming Family Practice
Cincinnati, Ohio
Well Male

Cindy M. Allison, RN, MSN, CNP
Certified Pediatric Nurse Practitioner
Northeast Pediatrics
Mason, Ohio
Well Child

Janet L. Andrews, RNC, WHP, PhD
Assistant Professor
School of Health Sciences, Division of Nursing
Georgia College and State University
Milledgeville, Georgia
Dysfunctional Uterine Bleeding

Alanna Conrad Andrus, RNC, MSN, PNP, FNP
Redwood City, California
Congenital Heart Disease, Developmental Dysplasia
of Hip, Pediatric Antibiotics (Appendix J)

Ellen L. Bailey, MSN, CFNP
Bluegrass Regional Primary Care Center
Waddy, Kentucky
Bell's Palsy, Gout

Dorothy R. Baker, RN, MSN, ARNP
Associates in Primary Care
Covington, Kentucky
Seizures

Mavis Bechtle, RN, MSN, ARNP
Administrator, Skilled Nursing
Director, Senior Services
St. Luke Hospital
Fort Thomas, Kentucky
Herpes, Warts

Patricia C. Birchfield, DSD, ARNP, DNSc
Adult Nurse Practitioner
Gerontologic Nurse Practitioner
Associate Professor, College of Nursing
Eastern Kentucky University
Richmond, Kentucky
Arthritis, Low Back Pain, Prostate Disease

Suzanne B. Black, RN, CS, MSN, FNP
Family Nurse Practitioner
Hematology/Oncology Pediatric Outpatient
Children's Hospital Medical Center
Cincinnati, Ohio
Clinical Instructor/Preceptor
Family Nurse Practitioner Program
Northern Kentucky University
Highland Heights, Kentucky
Leukemia

Julie Mead Bogguss, RN, MSN, CFNP
Certified Family Nurse Practitioner
Randolph Pediatric Associates–PHA
Charlotte, North Carolina
Pelvic Inflammatory Disease

Robert Brautigan, RN, CS, MSN
Clinical Specialist in Adult Psychiatric and
  Mental Health Nursing
Assistant Professor, Department of Nursing
Northern Kentucky University
Highland Heights, Kentucky
  Anxiety, Communication, Depression

Audricia Brooks, MSN, CS, FNP
Family Nurse Practitioner
Primary Care and Women's Health
Veterans Administration Medical Center
Cincinnati, Ohio
  Abdominal Pain, Appendicitis

Katherine L. Bushong, RN, BSN, MSN, FNP
Riverhills Healthcare (Neurology)
Independence, Kentucky
  Tinea Infections

Paula Cuthrell, MSN, FNP
Family Nurse Practitioner
Hematology–Oncology Division
Children's Hospital Medical Center
Cincinnati, Ohio
  Anemia

Rita A. Dello-Stritto, RN, MSN, CEN, CNS, ENP
Emergency Nurse Practitioner
Kelsey-Seybold Urgent Care Clinic
Houston, Texas
  Dental Problems, Wound Care

Ann M. Dollins, MPH, MSN, CNM, PhD
Assistant Professor
Northern Kentucky University
Highland Heights, Kentucky
  Pregnancy, Well Woman

Bernice "Bunny" Eades, RN, CS, MSN, ARNP
Family Nurse Practitioner
Clinical Instructor
College of Nursing
University of Kentucky
Lexington, Kentucky
  Lyme Disease

Diane M. Enzweiler, RN, MSN, CS, ANP
Nurse Practitioner–Cardiology Associates
Crestview Hills, Kentucky
Adjunct Faculty, Clinical Nursing
Northern Kentucky University
Highland Heights, Kentucky
  Congestive Heart Failure, Myocardial Infection

Holly V. Fox, RN, MSN, ANP-CS, COHN-S
Occupational Health Adult Nurse Practitioner
Cincinnati, Ohio
  Carpal Tunnel Syndrome

Pamela Gale, RN, MSN, CFNP
Family Nurse Practitioner
Foothills Primary Care
Fort Collins, Colorado
  *Allergic Rhinitis, Eczema and Atopic Dermatitis,
  Otitis, Pharyngitis*

Carrie Gordy, MSN, ARNP, CPNP
Instructor
College of Nursing
University of Kentucky
Lexington, Kentucky
  *Constipation, Cystic Fibrosis, Diarrhea, Encopresis,
  Enuresis*

Jane Harley, RN, MSN, CFNP, CDE
Instant Care Center
Richmond, Kentucky
  *Addison's Disease, Cushing's Syndrome, Diabetes
  Mellitus*

Barbara A. Heidt, RN, CS, MSN
Psychiatric Clinical Nurse Specialist
Children's Hospital Medical Center
Cincinnati, Ohio
  Attention-Deficit/Hyperactivity Disorder

Terry Tippett Herrick, MSN, FNP
Associate Professor
School of Nursing and Health Sciences
Spalding University
Louisville, Kentucky
  *Dermatitis and Miscellaneous Skin Conditions,
  Infectious Diseases, Skin Cancer and Sun-Related
  Conditions*

Laura Herald Hoofring, RN, CS, MSN
Clinical Nurse Specialist
Psychiatric Nursing
Children's Hospital Medical Center
Cincinnati, Ohio
    Eating Disorders

Marilyn J. Jacobs, RNC, MSN, WHCNP
Associate Professor
Missouri Southern State College
Joplin, Missouri
    Scabies

Delwin B. Jacoby, MSN, CFNP
Family Nurse Practitioner
Anderson Family Health Center
Lawrenceburg, Kentucky
    Musculoskeletal Injuries

Pamela S. Kidd, RN, ARNP, CEN, PhD
Professor
University of Kentucky College of Nursing
Kentucky Injury Prevention and Research Center
Lexington, Kentucky
    Dermatitis and Miscellaneous Skin Conditions, Fatigue, Infectious Disease, Issues, Skin Cancer and Sun-Related Conditions, Appendixes A-I

Pam King, RN, MSN, ARNP
Instructor
School of Nursing and Health Sciences
Spalding University
Louisville, Kentucky
    Cataracts, Glaucoma

Cheryl Pope Kish, RNC, EdD, WHCNP
Professor and Coordinator
Graduate Programs in Health Science
Director, Family Nurse Practitioner Program
Georgia College and State University
Milledgeville, Georgia
    Breast Lumps, Lice, Ovarian Cysts, Premenstrual Syndrome

Linda M. Kollar, RN, MSN
Director of Nursing
Division of Adolescent Medicine
Children's Hospital Medical Center
Cincinnati, Ohio
    Acne, Well Adolescent

Linda L. Larson, RN, FNPC, CEN, PhD
Nurse Practitioner
Internal Medicine and Geriatrics
Aurora, Colorado
Adjunct Affiliate Faculty
Assistant Clinical Professor
University of Colorado
Denver, Colorado
    Chest Pain, Dizziness, Transient Ischemic Attacks

Robert Leach, RN, MSN, ENP, CEN
Capitol Emergency Associates
Austin, Texas
    Eye: Foreign Body/Corneal Abrasion, Pneumonia, Tuberculosis

Alice B. Loper, BSN, MN, FNP
Assistant Professor of Nursing
Family Nurse Practitioner Program
Georgia College and State University
Milledgeville, Georgia
    Dysmenorrhea

Kathleen K. McGee, RN, MSN, CPNP
Pediatric Nurse Practitioner
Children's Hospital Medical Center
Cincinnati, Ohio
    Conjunctivitis

Christina McGlothlin-Boggs, MSN, ARNP
Family Nurse Practitioner
Primary Care/Urgent Care Clinics
Veterans Administration Medical Center
Lexington, Kentucky
    Acute Bronchitis, Cough, Shortness of Breath

Barbara Mosely, MSN, ARNP
Adult and Geriatric Nurse Practitioner
Veterans Administration Medical Center
  (Formerly)
Lexington, Kentucky
    Fibromyalgia

Eric Newman, MSN, CPNP
Pediatric Nurse Practitioner
Tates Creek Healthy Kids Center
Lexington, Kentucky
    Lead Poisoning, Scoliosis, Strabismus

Kathy Noyes, RN, MSN, FNP
Comprehensive Cardiology Associates
Cincinnati, Ohio
Edema, Hypertension

Carol A. Ormond, RN, MSN, CS, FNP
Assistant Professor
Georgia College and State University
Milledgeville, Georgia
Cholecystitis

Lori McConlogue O'Shaughnessy, RN, MSN, PNP
Women's Health Center
Northern Kentucky Family Health Centers
Covington, Kentucky
Amenorrhea, Chlamydia, Gonorrhea, Vaginitis

Cynthia A. Pastorino, RNC, MSN
Gerontologic Nurse Practitioner
Division of Geriatrics
University of Louisville
Louisville, Kentucky
Confusion

Betty Porter, MSN, ARNP, DNSc
Department Chairperson
School of Nursing
Morehead State University
Morehead, Kentucky
Director
Dr. Orvis Porter Family Practice
Morehead, Kentucky
Headaches

Kathleen Reeve, RN, CS, MSN, CNS, ANP
Assistant Professor, School of Nursing
Houston Health Science Center
University of Texas
Houston, Texas
Multiple Sclerosis, Systemic Lupus Erythematosus

Veronica Weaver Renfrow, RN, CS, MSN
Family Nurse Practitioner
Veterans Administration Medical Center
Cincinnati, Ohio
Substance Abuse

Angela Riley, RN, MSN, ANP
Cardiology Associates
Crestview Hills, Kentucky
Syphilis

Kay T. Roberts, MSN, FNP-C, EdD, FAAN
Professor of Nursing
University of Louisville
Louisville, Kentucky
Alzheimer's Disease, Osteoporosis

Denise L. Robinson, RN, ARNP, PhD
Professor
Northern Kentucky University
Director, MSN Programs
Northern Kentucky Family Health Centers, Inc.
Highland Heights, Kentucky
Burns, Client Wellness, Irritable Bowel Disease, Issues, Lymphoma, Mononucleosis, Thyroid Disorders, Urinary Tract Infection, Urticaria and Anaphylaxis

Karen Mangus Rogers, RNC, MSN
Family Nurse Practitioner
Family Health Centers
Louisville, Kentucky
Voluntary Faculty/Preceptor
University of Kentucky
Lexington, Kentucky
University of Louisville
Louisville, Kentucky
Fever, Infertility

Karen Ruschman, RN, MSN, FNP-C
Nurse Practitioner
Patient First, Inc.
Fort Thomas, Kentucky
Hepatitis, Well Adult 65 Years and Older

Carol M. Satterly, RN, MSN, CPNP
Pediatric Nurse Practitioner
College of Nursing, University of Kentucky
Lexington, Kentucky
Abuse, Asthma, Behavior Problems

Cinda Crawford Simpson, MSN, ARNP
Advanced Registered Nurse Practitioner
Veterans Administration Medical Center
Lexington, Kentucky
Chronic Obstructive Pulmonary Disease, Edema

Denise Sparks, MSN, ARNP
Family Nurse Practitioner
Veterans Administration Medical Center
Lexington, Kentucky
Cellulitis

Ann Stone, RNC, MSN, FNP
Family Nurse Practitioner
Internists of Fairfield
Fairfield, Ohio
  Deep Venous Thrombosis, Sinusitis

Karen L. Webster, BSN, MSN, CNP
Certified Nurse Practitioner
Cincinnati, Ohio
  Parkinson's Disease

Sandra L. Woods, RNC, MSN
Prime-Med and North College Hill Medical
  Group
Cincinnati, Ohio
  AIDS

Sadie Young-Hughes, RN, MSN, ARNP
Adult Nurse Practitioner
Veterans Administration Medical Center
Cincinnati, Ohio
  Peptic Ulcer Disease, Pityriasis Rosea, Psoriasis

REVIEWERS

Ellen L. Bailey, MSN, CFNP
Bluegrass Regional Primary Care Center
Waddy, Kentucky

Denise F. Coppa, PhD candidate
Director, Family Nurse Practitioner Program
University of Rhode Island
Kingston, Rhode Island

Shirley Davidoff, RN, MS, FNP-C
Family Nurse Practitioner
Cardiology and Internal Medicine Associates
Dallas, Texas

Gail Hetterman, MS, RN, CS-FNP
Certified Family Nurse Practitioner
Coleman Clinic, Ltd.
Canton, Illinois

Cheryl McKenzie, RNC, MN, FNP
Associate Professor, Department of Nursing
Northern Kentucky University
Highland Heights, Kentucky

Barbara E. Prescott, RNC, FNP, BS, MA, ND
President, Montana Advanced Practice Registered
  Nurses Association
Board of Directors, Montana Nurses Association
Member, MNA, AANP, ANA, Sigma Theta Tau
Hog Heaven, Montana

Karen M. Rogers, ARNP
Family Health Centers
Louisville, Kentucky

Carol M. Satterly, RN, MSN, CPNP
Pediatric Nurse Practitioner
College of Nursing
University of Kentucky
Lexington, Kentucky

Carolyn Y. Wagner, RN-CS, MS, FNP-C
Family Nurse Practitioner
Taylorville Medical Associates
Taylorville, Illinois

This book is dedicated to Butch, Leigh, and Elliot, who make me smile and remember what is important in life. It is also dedicated to my mother, who always believed in me, even if she didn't always know what it was that I did for a living. Even in death, you are still teaching me lessons. Thank you.

Special thanks to Spalding University, Louisville, Kentucky, for supporting my efforts. **PSK**

This book is dedicated to my family, who, although puzzled by my endeavors, are proud and supportive of my efforts. Their love and belief in my abilities have always helped me to grow throughout the years. Thanks. **DLR**

Preface

This book was developed to meet the needs of family nurse practitioners (FNPs) preparing to take the national certification examinations. As FNPs, we were frustrated as we tried to prepare for the examinations because there was no comprehensive preparation book. We survived by reviewing adult, pediatric, and women's health books. Most review books are not structured to reflect the FNP's approach to practice (context), based on the Subjective, Objective, Assessment, Plan, Evaluate (SOAPE) format. We found the existing review books to be limited in both content and context.

With these two issues in mind, we wrote this review book to provide greater depth (content) and to develop a format that accommodates both the Academy of Nurse Practitioners (Academy) and the test blueprint of the American Nurses Credentialing Center (ANCC). The SOAPE approach used for both the chapter content and the test questions reflects all components of the Academy's domains (assessment, diagnosis, plan, and evaluate) and the ANCC format (history taking, physical examination, diagnosis, management, and evaluation) for acute and chronic illness. Tables are used to cluster wellness content across the lifespan. Anticipatory guidance is addressed as separate information within the book. The table of contents is structured to reflect the problem areas outlined by the ANCC.

At the end of each section are test questions pertaining to the specific content reviewed. In addition to these postsection questions, there are two comprehensive examinations (Sample Examinations) that reflect the actual length of the certification examinations. Taking these tests allows you to time your performance. Twenty-five pretest items are also included to mimic the setup of the actual examination and to allow you to have a better idea of how much time you are taking to complete the examination. Test questions are classified according to the ANCC problem areas and the Academy domains and across the lifespan. This approach allows you to examine the type of item you are having the most difficulty processing and to focus your study efforts. The rationale for each correct answer is provided, and in most cases it is substantiated by reference material. The reference provides you with another source of information in a given area if you should need additional targeted review.

Most test questions presented in this book were piloted with FNP students at the end of their program of study. In most cases the questions have been subjected to item analysis techniques used in the actual examinations to ensure a given difficulty and discriminatory level for the sample examinations. Information about the difficulty and discrimination levels of the national certification examinations is confidential and is not released to the public. We have made every effort to construct sample examinations that reflect the national examination, based on the published information from both testing agencies. However, the actual test blueprints are not published; only information about the testing categories is available. Therefore the exact weight placed on a given problem area or domain is not known. Thus the weight placed on content areas within the sample examinations may not be representative of the actual examinations. However, we are confident that the major areas are addressed here. In addition, conditions within categories may be placed differently from where they may be placed by the

Academy and the ANCC. For example, we included sexually transmitted diseases in the reproductive system; yet one or both of the certifying agencies may consider sexually transmitted diseases as reproductive or infectious disease content. The important point is that the material is covered somewhere in this book.

Now, as you prepare to take the national certification examinations, you can carry one book. But no book—not even this one—can replace confidence in yourself and your abilities. Go for it!

Pamela S. Kidd
Denise L. Robinson

Acknowledgments

We thank our colleagues across the nation who helped to make this book a reality. Family nurse practitioners are busy people who love clinical challenges but generally do not like to write or review chapters. Thank you for taking the time to share your expertise and help others who want to become family nurse practitioners. We trust that all our persistent phone calls, e-mails, and suggestions did not harm our friendships. We hope that you are proud of your contribution. We certainly are. A special note of thanks goes to our internal reviewers, Carol Satterly, Ellen Bailey, and Karen Rogers. Your years of experience as family nurse practitioners helped us separate reality from theory.

Pamela S. Kidd
Denise L. Robinson

Brief Contents

Contents

PART II
CLIENT WELLNESS

PART I

ILLNESS

Head, Eye, Ear, Nose, and Throat

CATARACTS

OVERVIEW
Definition

A *cataract* is an opacification of the crystalline lens of the eye. Cataracts usually lead to functional impairment caused by visual disturbances.

Incidence

- Cataracts are the leading cause of preventable blindness in adults in the United States.
- Incidence increases with age, with an incidence of approximately 50% in persons older than 75 years.
- Senile cataracts are typically bilateral, but progression may vary between eyes.
- Cataracts rarely occur in the pediatric population and are a result of congenital factors.

CONGENITAL CATARACTS. In infants cataracts may occur as a result of inheritance of an autosomal dominant gene for cataracts. Many infants with Down syndrome may have congenital cataracts. Infants may also acquire cataracts as a consequence of prematurity. Intrauterine factors, such as maternal malnutrition, infection (cytomegalovirus or rubella), metabolic disease (diabetes), or medication ingestion (steroids), may lead to congenital cataract development.

TRAUMATIC CATARACTS. Factors such as eye injury, recurrent exposure to ultraviolet rays, foreign bodies (FBs), or scratches to the crystalline lens may hasten or cause cataracts.

SECONDARY CATARACTS. A variety of eye disorders, including retinal dystrophy or detachment, atrophy of the iris, glaucoma, neoplasia, and ischemia, may lead to cataract formation. Medications, including steroids and radiation, also may lead to cataracts.

METABOLIC CATARACTS. Diseases leading to cataract include diabetes mellitus, Wilson's disease, and hypoparathyroidism.

Pathophysiology

The lens is posterior to the iris and is suspended from the ciliary body. It is normally a transparent structure with an elastic capsule. The lens is avascular, is acellular, and lacks innervation. Transparency of the lens depends on active metabolism of the epithelium. If the epithelium becomes traumatized, this may result in opacity of the lens. Density of the lens fibers increases with age, and chemical changes in protein of the lens occur. Both of these factors contribute to cataract formation. Cataracts may be either nuclear (central) or cortical (peripheral sunflower shape). Nuclear cataracts are most common, especially in older adults.

RISK FACTORS. There are a number of contributing factors related to the development of cataracts. Cataracts may occur congenitally; as a result of trauma, eye disease, or drug therapy; or with metabolic diseases such as diabetes. The most common cause of cataracts is the aging process.

ASSESSMENT: SUBJECTIVE/HISTORY
History of Present Illness

The most common symptom of cataract development is the gradual worsening of vision over time. Some clients report a constant fog over their eyes and rings or halos around lights and objects. Many clients note glare, especially affecting vision in bright light situations. In clients with cataracts, vision appears more blue and yellow and distant vision becomes impaired. The location of the cataract determines the extent of visual loss. Persons with central opacities report improved vision in low light as a result of pupillary dilatation, leading to a larger portion of the lens being available for viewing. Pain does not typically occur with this disorder.

Part of the subjective evaluation should include an assessment of the degree of lifestyle impairment as a result of this condition and social isolation because of visual difficulties.

Past Medical History

Assess for history of long-term steroid use, as in clients receiving immunosuppressive therapy for transplants, or frequent steroid use, as in conditions with chronic inflammation. There may be a history of a former eye injury or recurrent eye trauma. Systemic disease, particularly diabetes, may predispose the client toward cataract development. A history of Wilson's disease or hypothyroidism also may lead to cataracts.

Medication History

Ask about use of steroids or radiation therapy.

Family History

With congenital cataracts, ask about family history of cataracts.

Psychosocial History

Recreational or occupational exposure to ultraviolet B rays may predispose persons toward cataract development. Persons at risk include those who are frequently outdoors in the sun or in areas of high reflection, such as snow, beaches, or water.

ASSESSMENT: OBJECTIVE/ PHYSICAL EXAMINATION
Physical Examination

NUCLEAR CATARACT
- Absence of red reflex in children
- Gray-white opacity of the lens on direct lighted visual examination
- Black against the red reflex on ophthalmoscopic examination

PERIPHERAL CORTICAL CATARACT
- Spokelike shadows that point inward
- As above, gray-white on lighted examination and black against red per ophthalmoscope

In both types of cataracts, no redness of the eye is present.

Diagnostic Procedures

- Visual acuity with Snellen chart
- Slit-lamp examination
- Ophthalmology consult

DIAGNOSIS

Differential diagnosis may include the following:

MACULAR DEGENERATION. May result in loss of central vision in older adults. Onset is gradual, with distorted vision sometimes reported. Clients report no improvement of vision despite use of corrective lens. Macular degeneration is accompanied by characteristic physical findings, including neovascularization of the eye, exudates, drusen, and holes in the macula. These findings are visible on funduscopic examination of the macula.

RETINAL DETACHMENT. This results in a sudden impairment of vision in one eye, with a description of symptoms being "a curtain dropping over the eye," as well as loss of a portion of the visual fields. These findings are often preceded by symptoms such as flashing lights and "floaters." Retinal detachment may result from a blow to the head or eye trauma. The detached retina can be seen by ophthalmoscopy.

GLAUCOMA (CHRONIC WIDE-ANGLE). Glaucoma is caused by increased intraocular pressure. It results in loss of peripheral vision, eventually leading to "tunnel vision." Measurement of intraocular pressure may lead to a diagnosis of glaucoma.

PRESBYOPIA, MYOPIA. Worsening changes in the shape of the eye may result in visual distortions.

This generally affects bilateral vision; the visual fields are not affected and may be improved by corrective lens adjustment.

THERAPEUTIC PLAN
Consult

Ophthalmologic evaluation is indicated to help the client determine options for therapy. Standard means of adaptation for the visually impaired should be pursued. Magnification, modification of spectacles, large print, and tactile cues may allow clients to delay or forgo surgery altogether.

Surgical Procedures

Surgery is usually done on an outpatient basis. The most common surgical procedure is extracapsular extraction of opaque lens. Intracapsular extraction removes the lens through a small incision. In phacoemulsification (ultrasonic), the lens is broken up by vibration and removed extracapsularly, generally avoiding the need for sutures. Surgery also usually involves reimplantation of intraocular lens. Aphakic glasses and contact lenses have been used in the past to restore vision but are rarely used today.

Preoperative Evaluation

Evaluation should address stabilization of chronic disease, including hypertension and diabetes, availability of a caregiver after the operation, and an understanding of client expectations of surgery. Anticoagulants are not generally stopped because their benefit in preventing possible surgical complications outweighs the risks of bleeding during this minimally invasive surgery.

Client Education

- The decision to pursue surgery is a highly individual decision, because surgery is not without risk. However, if surgery is indicated, lens extraction improves visual acuity in 95% of cases.
- Discussion of the probability of surgical correction as a means of improving vision includes ruling out other possible causes for visual impairment. Evaluation of the effects of visual impairment on activities of daily living should contribute to the decision of whether to pursue surgical correction.

EVALUATION/FOLLOW-UP

If surgery is undertaken, the client will be primarily followed up by ophthalmology.

Postoperative Complications

Primary care providers should be aware of signs and symptoms of postoperative complications, including altered lens adjustment, red eye or discharge indicating inflammation or infection, and delayed opacification of the posterior capsule (sometimes referred to as "after-cataracts"). Retinal detachment, macular edema, and glaucoma may also occur; screening for these conditions is therefore part of postoperative evaluation.

Postoperative Restrictions

The primary care provider should be aware of restrictions after cataract surgery, including the following:

- Eye shield should be worn at night and glasses during the day to protect the eye.
- Client should avoid bending, stooping, or heavy lifting for 3 to 4 weeks after surgery.
- Client should not shower or wash hair for 2 postoperative weeks.
- Strenuous or excessive physical activity should be avoided for 4 weeks after surgery.
- Client should not fly before full healing; this may increase intraocular pressure.

Continued Management

If surgery is delayed or avoided, continued assessment of the client's functional capacity as related to visual impairment should be assessed. Clients should be advised to wear sunglasses to protect against further cataract development from ultraviolet B radiation. Mydriatics (e.g., atropine) are occasionally used to improve vision.

REFERENCES

Barker, R. (1995). *Principles of ambulatory medicine.* Baltimore: Williams & Wilkins.

Javitt, J. C. (1995). Cataract surgery in one eye or both. *Ophthalmology, 102,* 1583.

Schein, O.D. (1995). Predictors of outcome in patient who underwent cataract surgery. *Ophthalmology, 102,* 817.

U.S. Department of Health and Human Services. (1993). *Clinical practice guideline: Cataract in adults.* AHCPR Publication No. 93-0542. Washington, DC: Author.

REVIEW QUESTIONS

1. You are working in a senior citizen center screening for sensory impairments affecting activities of daily living. Which of the following history information could indicate increased risk for visual impairment?

    a. Daily use of oxygen
    b. Alcohol or tobacco abuse
    c. Reading in low-light conditions
    d. Infrequent sun exposure

2. You are examining a 67-year-old woman for routine health screening. You are having difficulty visualizing the fundus of the eye. Which of the following would be the most helpful in allowing you to conduct the funduscopic examination?

    a. Encourage the client to look directly at the light of the ophthalmoscope.
    b. Instill miotic drops to improve visualization of the optical field.
    c. Examine from an angle to the eye, shifting to positive diopters as you visualize the lens.
    d. Have the client lie flat and examine the eye from above.

3. The nurse practitioner has been monitoring an 88-year-old man for cataracts for several years. In determining the appropriateness of referral for surgery, which of the following factors would be the most important to consider?

    a. Underlying pathology related to the age of the client
    b. Effect of visual defect on activities of daily living
    c. Whether the client is still driving
    d. Ability of the client to perform self-care

4. You are discussing surgical options with an 82-year-old woman who has acquired bilateral cataracts. Which of the following is correct information about surgery for cataracts?

    a. Bilateral cataract removal provides optimal postoperative progress.
    b. After the operation, clients are typically fitted for special aphakic lenses.
    c. Air travel plans may need to be delayed until full recovery occurs.
    d. Intraocular removal is the most commonly performed procedure for cataracts.

5. After the operation, the client experiencing cataract removal should expect which of the following?

    a. Rapid improvement (1 to 2 weeks) in central vision after lens implantation
    b. Need for continuing eyedrop use to prevent recurrence
    c. Some nausea and possible vomiting related to anesthesia
    d. A 1- to 2-day hospitalization for optimal recovery

6. You are seeing a 4-week-old infant who was born at 38 weeks' gestation. The infant's mother consults the nurse practitioner about normal growth and development. She says she does not know what to expect in growth and development of a normal infant, because her other child was several weeks premature and developed slowly. Which of the following points in a history given by the mother would lead the nurse practitioner to be concerned about possible visual problems?

    a. History of cataract development in the preterm sibling
    b. Family history of visual astigmatism
    c. Infant's failure to track mother when she walks across the room
    d. Maternal exposure to cytomegalovirus

7. While examining a 58-year-old diabetic client for retinopathy, the nurse practitioner notes some cloudiness of the lens. Which of the following techniques would be most helpful in determining whether a cataract is present?

    a. Additional visualization with the aid of a slit lamp
    b. Fluorescein stain to determine degree of opacity
    c. Measurement of eye pressure by tonometry
    d. Determination of visual acuity on a Jaeger chart

8. In making the differential diagnosis of cataracts, the nurse practitioner should rule out other causes of visual loss. Which of the following is true regarding symptomatology of the eyes?

    a. The older the client, the greater is the likelihood that decreased vision is due to cataracts.

    b. Increased intraocular pressure often results in flashes of light in the visual fields and should be treated promptly.

    c. Blood in the anterior chamber of the eye is a benign finding that typically resolves on its own.

    d. Macular degeneration tends to occur abruptly, resulting in exudates, cysts, and holes in the macula.

9. The nurse practitioner is caring for an 80-year-old grandmother who has cataracts. Which of the following is true in planning for the care of this client related to her cataracts?

    a. Use of cholinergic eyedrops may help delay the necessity of surgery.

    b. The cataract will need to develop fully (ripen) before surgery is an option.

    c. Care for this woman will need to be managed by an ophthalmologist.

    d. Appropriate time for surgery may be guided by visual acuity measurement.

10. You see an 80-year-old man who had cataract surgery on his right eye 2 years ago. He reports decreased visual acuity recently. In evaluating this man for this problem, which of the following is true?

    a. This may be the result of a posterior lens opacity in the right eye.

    b. This is likely to be a result of a cataract in the left eye.

    c. This is a normal consequence of aging.

    d. He is not a candidate for repeat cataract surgery.

ANSWERS AND RATIONALES

1. *Answer:* b (assessment: history/HEENT/aging adult)

    Rationale: Alcohol or tobacco abuse has been correlated with increased risk of cataracts.

2. *Answer:* c (assessment: objective/physical examination/HEENT/aging adult)

    Rationale: Positive diopters are helpful in looking at visual lenses whose shapes have changed in response to cataracts.

3. *Answer:* b (diagnosis/HEENT/aging adult)

    Rationale: Quality of life related to degree of sensory deprivation from visual defects is an important consideration in determining whether surgery is indicated.

4. *Answer:* c (plan/management/client education/HEENT/NAS)

    Rationale: Flying before full healing has taken place may result in increased intraocular pressure and may disrupt surgical healing.

5. *Answer:* a (evaluation/HEENT/NAS)

    Rationale: Little adjustment is required for the intraocular implant to improve vision.

6. *Answer:* d (assessment/history/HEENT/child)

    Rationale: Maternal infection may result in congenital cataracts.

7. *Answer:* a (assessment/physical examination/HEENT/adult)

    Rationale: The slit lamp will be of most benefit in allowing the examiner to view the extent of the opacity of the lens.

8. *Answer:* a (diagnosis/HEENT/NAS)

    Rationale: Cataracts tend to occur in older adults as a result of buildup of eye fibers and because of cumulative trauma from such sources as the sun and foreign bodies.

9. *Answer:* d (plan/management/diagnostics/HEENT/aging adult)

    Rationale: Visual acuity measurements will help evaluate the degree of visual impairment and show when surgery is indicated.

10. *Answer:* a (evaluation/HEENT/aging adult)

    Rationale: After-cataracts may occur after intraocular removal and require laser surgery.

CONJUNCTIVITIS

OVERVIEW
Definition

Conjunctivitis is an inflammation of the conjunctiva. *Ophthalmia neonatorum* is a type of conjunctivitis that occurs in the first month of life.

Incidence

- A common infection in children, conjunctivitis is less common in the adult population.
- Children are at increased risk as a result of physical contact with large groups of other children, inadequate handwashing, and increased incidences of upper respiratory tract infections (URIs) and acute otitis media.
- Several studies have concluded that bacteria is the most frequent cause of conjunctivitis and the next is viruses.

Pathophysiology

The conjunctiva is a thin, transparent mucous membrane covering the globe of the eye and inner surface of the eyelids. Irritants, including bacteria, viruses, chemicals, allergens, and FBs, can result in inflammation of this tissue.

PROTECTIVE FACTORS. Tears continually wash the eye, inhibiting colonization and diluting and flushing irritants.

FACTORS INCREASING SUSCEPTIBILITY
- Poor handwashing
- Exposure to someone with conjunctivitis
- Exposure to impetigo
- Presence of URI
- Presence of allergens
- Lack of tears or moisture in eye

Pathogenesis

BACTERIAL CAUSES
- *Streptococcus pneumoniae*
- *Haemophilus influenzae:* Often concurrent with acute otitis media
- *Moraxella catarrhalis*
- *Staphylococcus aureus*
- *Pneumococcus*
- *Proteus*
- *Neisseria gonorrhoeae*
- *Chlamydia trachomatis*

VIRAL CAUSES
- Adenovirus—most common
- Enterovirus
- Coxsackievirus
- Herpes simplex: Complications, optic neuritis

OPHTHALMIA NEONATORUM
- *Neisseria gonorrhoeae:* Complication, destruction and/or perforation of the cornea
- *Chlamydia trachomatis* (leading cause of ophthalmia neonatorum): Complication, conjunctival scarring
- Herpes simplex: Complications, cataracts, keratitis, optic neuritis
- Other listed bacteria
- Antibiotics: Primarily silver nitrate and erythromycin

ALLERGIC/VERNAL CAUSES
- Irritant chemicals
- Medications, antibiotics: Gentamicin, neomycin, tobramycin atropine, and eyedrop preservatives

ASSESSMENT: SUBJECTIVE/HISTORY
Bacterial Conjunctivitis

Ask about presence of mucopurulent discharge, eyes matted on wakening, itching of the affected eye, mild pain, injection of conjunctival vessels, unilateral involvement that often becomes bilateral after 48 hours, and, less frequently, mild photophobia.

CHLAMYDIA TRACHOMATIS. Discharge is thinner, more mucoid. Photophobia is pronounced. Not self-limited, it can persist for months.

Viral Conjunctivitis

Ask about watery discharge, eyes matted on wakening, presence of URI, and bilateral eye involvement.

HERPES SIMPLEX. Look for possible presence of fever blister, vesicles on eyelids.

Allergic/Vernal Causes

Ask about mild to moderate inflammation of conjunctiva, severe itching, marked burning, rhinorrhea, watery drainage, bilateral involvement, seasonal presentation. Conjunctiva of the eyelids may have cobblestone appearance; symptoms are often reported as more severe than clinical presentation.

Chemical Causes

Ask about watery discharge, injected conjunctiva, photophobia, marked burning, and history of exposure to irritant.

Trauma/Corneal Abrasion

Ask about watery discharge (usually unilateral), photophobia of infected eye, and exposure to trauma or FB.

Ophthalmia Neonatorum

GONOCOCCAL INFECTION. Presentation is 24 to 48 hours after birth, with dramatic symptoms: erythemic, edematous conjunctiva and profuse purulent discharge, usually bilateral.

CHLAMYDIA TRACHOMATIS. Presentation is 5 to 12 days after birth. It may be bilateral or unilateral, with moderate inflammation and mucopurulent discharge.

HERPES SIMPLEX. Presentation is 48 hours to 14 days after birth; with marked inflammation, mucoid drainage, and herpetic vesicles.

CHEMICAL CAUSES. Presentation is within the first 24 hours of life. It is usually related to instillation of silver nitrate and, to a lesser extent, erythromycin, both used as chlamydial and gonococcal prophylaxis. There is mild injection and mucopurulent discharge. Self-limited, the condition usually resolves in 24 to 48 hours.

ASSOCIATED SYMPTOMS. URI, fever, ear pain, acute otitis media, and throat pain may be associated.

Past Medical History

Ask about history of previous ear infection, eye diseases, recent illness, concurrent illness, allergies, recent herpes simplex infection, exposure to someone with conjunctivitis, exposure to someone with impetigo, use of contact lenses, history of sexually transmitted disease (STD) of self or partner(s), and recent eye trauma.

INFANTS. Ask mothers about treatment for STD during pregnancy.

Medication History

- Ask about recent use of antibiotics or any eye preparations.
- If corneal abrasion or trauma is suspected, inquire about tetanus immunity status.

Family History

Ask about family history of eye diseases.

ASSESSMENT: OBJECTIVE/ PHYSICAL EXAMINATION
Physical Examination

Use a problem-oriented approach to the physical examination.

VITAL SIGNS. Check temperature, heart rate, respiratory rate, and blood pressure in everyone older than 3 years.

SKIN. Assess color, character.

HEART SOUNDS. Assess and record.

BREATH SOUNDS. Assess and record.

EAR, NOSE, AND THROAT. Look for concurrent URI and acute otitis media.

EYES. Determine visual activity in school-age and older clients. Assess visual fields, extraocular movements, and pupillary functions. Examine sclera and conjunctiva for inflammation, edema, and discharge. Examine cornea for clarity and ulceration. Examine eyelid margins. Perform funduscopic examination on all clients, though this may not be possible for infants and small children.

LYMPHATICS. Focus on head and neck. Enlarged preauricular nodes are often present in viral and chlamydial conjunctivitis.

Diagnostic Procedures

- Culture and Gram stain are not usually necessary, unless infection is recurring or resistant to routine treatment.
- Cultures should always be done on infants younger than 1 month. Cultures of the eye and nasopharynx should be done concurrently. Culture should be done for *Chlamydial trachomatis, Neisseria gonorrhoeae,* and bacteria. If a child has gonococcal or chlamydial ophthalmia neonatorum, both parents need to be screened for gonococcal and chlamydial infection (Baker, 1996).
- Perform flourescein stain with examination under cobalt-blue light source for corneal abrasion or trauma. Epithelial abrasion is brilliant green; deeper injuries are darker.

DIAGNOSIS

Differential diagnosis may include the following:
- Bacterial conjunctivitis

- Viral conjunctivitis
- Allergic conjunctivitis
- Chemical conjunctivitis
- Corneal abrasion or trauma
- Iritis
- Glaucoma
- Herpes simplex blepharitis

THERAPEUTIC PLAN
Pharmacologic Treatment

BACTERIAL CONJUNCTIVITIS

Sulfacetamide Sodium 10%. Ointment 0.5 to 1 cm ribbon in conjunctival sac qid for 7 days or 10% solution 2 gtts every 2 to 3 hours while client is awake. This medicine is effective, well tolerated, and inexpensive.

Bacitracin, Polymyxin. Ointment 0.5 to 1 cm in conjunctival sac qid for 7 days.

Alternative Treatments. Tobramycin ointment or solution, erythromycin ointment or solution. Gentamicin and neomycin preparations are options for use but have higher incidence of allergic reaction (Merenstein, Kaplan, & Rosenberg, 1994).

Children. If concurrent acute otitis media is present, the child can be treated with systemic antibiotic therapy. It is best to use a beta-lactamase–resistant drug, such as sulfamethoxazole (Bactrim) or amoxicillin (Augmentin). You do not need to use topical antibiotics concurrently (Uphold & Graham, 1994). Bactrim should not be given to children younger than 2 months.

OPHTHALMIA NEONATORUM

Gonococcal Conjunctivitis. Ceftriaxone 50 mg/kg/day IM as single dose. If organism is sensitive to penicillin, give aqueous penicillin G 100,000 u/kg/day (Baker, 1996).

The infant may need frequent eye irrigation with sterile normal saline solution to clear discharge.

Chlamydia Trachomatis. Erythromycin suspension 30 to 40 mg/kg/day PO in 3 divided doses.

CORNEAL ABRASION (UNCOMPLICATED)

School-Age Children to Adults. Apply antibiotic ointment and patch eye for 24 hours. Reexamine cornea in 24 hours. Apply antibiotic drops or ointment for 3 days (Ruppert, 1996).

Children Younger Than 6 Years. Do not patch eye.

All Ages. Do not prescribe topical anesthetics or ophthalmic steroids.

ALLERGIC CONJUNCTIVITIS. Administer systemic antihistamines:

Children. Diphenhydramine 5 mg/kg/day for 4 days in 4 divided doses. Be alert for drowsiness.

Adults. Diphenhydramine 25 to 50 mg tid for 4 days.

Children Older Than 4 Years and Adults. Cromolyn sodium ophthalmic solution 4%. 1 to 2 gtts 4 to 6 times per day.

All Ages. Do not prescribe ophthalmic steroids. They are associated with increased incidence of cataracts and glaucoma.

Client Education

MEDICATION ADMINISTRATION

- Clean eye before any medication administration.
- To apply or instill, gently separate eyelids, pulling lower lid down toward the center of the eye. Place the drops or a thin line of ointment in pocket that is formed (Boynton, Dunn, & Stephens, 1994).
- Infection should respond to treatment in 2 to 3 days. Client or parent should call if poor response to medication after 48 hours. Instruct client or parent to call if symptoms worsen or vision decreases.

COMFORT MEASURES

- Wet compresses, cool or warm per client's preference. Use cotton balls.
- Children may need distraction to keep from rubbing eyes.

INFECTION CONTROL

- Encourage good handwashing with client and family.
- Client should keep hands away from face and eyes.
- Client's face cloths and towels should be kept separate from others. These linens should be used one time only.
- Monitor other family members, especially siblings, for symptoms of conjunctivitis.
- Client should refrain from wearing contact lenses for 24 hours.
- Clean contact lenses and storage case with appropriate disinfectant.
- Children should stay home from school or day care until inflammation and discharge

are gone, 24 to 48 hours after treatment begins.

Referral/Consult

CHILDREN

Infants younger than 1 month will need referral.

ALL AGES

- Corneal ulcer
- Extensive corneal defect
- Corneal inflammation
- Suspected gonococcal infection
- Suspected herpes simplex infection
- Any irregularities in pupil size or reaction
- No improvement after 48 hours of treatment
- Client reports any of the following: Moderate to severe pain, severe photophobia, decreased visual acuity

EVALUATION/FOLLOW-UP

Bacterial Infection

- No follow-up is necessary if client responds to treatment.
- Practitioner may want to follow up with severe cases.

Viral Infection

Follow-up is done for persistent symptoms.

Allergic Conjunctivitis

Follow-up is done for persistent symptoms. Referral to allergist or ophthalmologist may be necessary.

Corneal Abrasion or Trauma

Follow-up is done as needed.

Ophthalmia Neonatorum

Follow-up is done as advised by referred physician.

REFERENCES

Baker, R. C. (1996). *Handbook of pediatric primary care.* Boston: Little, Brown.

Barker, L. R., Burton, J., & Zieve, P. (1995). *Principles of ambulatory medicine.* Baltimore: Williams & Wilkins.

Boynton, R. W., Dunn, E. S, & Stephens, G. R. (1994). *Manual of ambulatory pediatrics.* Philadelphia: J. B. Lippincott.

Dambro, M. (1996). *Griffith's 5-minute clinical consult.* Baltimore: Williams & Wilkins.

Merenstein, G. B., Kaplan, D. W., & Rosenberg, A. A. (1994). *Handbook of pediatrics.* Norwalk, CT: Appleton & Lange.

Pellerano, R. A., Bishop, V., & Silber, T. J. (1994). Gonococcal conjunctivitis in adolescents: Recognition and management. *Clinical Pediatrics, 33*(2), 114-116.

Ruppert, S. D. (1996). Differential diagnosis of pediatric conjunctivitis. *Nurse Practitioner, 21*(7), 12-26.

Uphold, C. R., & Graham, M. V. (1994). *Clinical guidelines in family practice.* Gainesville, FL: Barmarrae Books.

Weiss, A. (1994). Acute conjunctivitis in childhood. *Current Problems in Pediatrics, 24*(1), 4-11.

Weiss, A., Brinser, J. H., & Nazar-Stewart, V. (1993). Acute conjunctivitis in childhood. *Journal of Pediatrics, 24*(1), 10-14.

REVIEW QUESTIONS

1. You are taking a history for a 2-week-old infant. The mother has reported an infection in the right eye. In your history it is important to ascertain which of the following?

- a. Mother's history of STD or STD treatment during pregnancy
- b. Day of life when onset of symptoms occurred
- c. Description of drainage
- d. All of the above

2. Which of the following symptoms would **not** usually be identified by a client with a corneal abrasion?

- a. Photophobia
- b. Mild to moderate pain
- c. Mucopurulent discharge
- d. Hyperemia

3. You diagnose your client, a 2-year-old girl, with acute otitis media and bacterial conjunctivitis. The pathogen is unknown. Your treatment choice would be:

- a. Sulfacetamide sodium 10% ophthalmic ointment
- b. Bactrim suspension
- c. Amoxicillin suspension
- d. Augmentin suspension and sodium sulfacetamide ophthalmic solution 10%

4. An infant with ophthalmia neonatorum caused by *Neisseria gonorrhoeae* would probably exhibit all the following symptoms **except:**

   a. Profuse purulent discharge
   b. Edematous conjunctiva
   c. Profuse watery discharge
   d. Hyperemia

5. Your client, a 22-year-old man, has a diagnosis of chlamydial conjunctivitis. All the following findings would have helped you come to this conclusion **except:**

   a. Photophobia
   b. Profuse purulent discharge
   c. Condition present for 1 month
   d. Enlarged tender preauricular nodes

6. All the following statements are true regarding follow-up for bacterial conjunctivitis **except:**

   a. Usually no follow-up is necessary.
   b. Practitioner may want to follow up severe cases.
   c. Follow-up is necessary if symptoms persist after 48 hours of treatment.
   d. All cases of bacterial conjunctivitis require a follow-up visit.

7. Which statement is true regarding diagnostic cultures in conjunctivitis?

   a. All cases of suspected bacterial conjunctivitis require culture and sensitivities.
   b. Culture and sensitivity testing are necessary when conjunctivitis is recurring or resistant to routine treatment.
   c. All infants younger than 3 months should have culture testing, Gram stain, and cultures for chlamydia and gonorrhea.
   d. All teenagers should have culture testing for bacteria, chlamydia, and gonorrhea.

8. The following are all reasons that you would refer your client to an ophthalmologist for care **except:**

   a. Corneal ulcer
   b. Pupil unequal, left pupil slow to react
   c. Suspected gonococcal infection
   d. Client is 10 weeks old

9. You have concluded that your client, a 25-year-old woman, has allergic conjunctivitis. Which of the following findings led you to this diagnosis?

   a. Marked itching, mild to moderate injection, eyelids with cobblestone appearance
   b. Marked itching, purulent discharge, eyelids with cobblestone appearance
   c. Watery discharge, rhinorrhea, severe pain
   d. Rhinorrhea, seasonal presentation, mucopurulent discharge

ANSWERS AND RATIONALES

1. *Answer:* d (assessment/history/HEENT/infant)
   Rationale: The infection is possibly due to the STD of gonorrhea, chlamydia, trachomatis, or herpes simplex. Obtaining a history of STD, onset of symptoms, and description of drainage will help narrow the practitioner's differential diagnosis. (Baker, 1996)

2. *Answer:* c (assessment/history/HEENT/NAS)
   Rationale: Photophobia, mild to moderate pain, and hyperemia are all associated with corneal abrasion. Mucopurulent drainage is associated with bacterial conjunctivitis. (Ruppert, 1996)

3. *Answer:* b (plan/management/pharmacologic/HEENT/child)
   Rationale: A beta-lactamose–resistant systemic antibiotic is the drug of choice. Augmentin is an appropriate treatment, but concurrent treatment with topical antibiotic therapy is not necessary. (Uphold, 1994)

4. *Answer:* c (assessment/physical examination/HEENT/infant)
   Rationale: Gonococcal ophthalmia neonatorum involves a profuse purulent discharge at presentation. (Baker, 1996)

5. *Answer:* b (diagnosis/HEENT/adult)
   Rationale: Profuse purulent discharge is associated with gonococcal conjunctivitis. The discharge seen in chlamydial conjunctivitis is thin and mucoid. (Pellarano, Bishop, & Silber, 1994)

6. *Answer:* d (evaluation/HEENT/NAS)

Rationale: Usually no follow-up is necessary for bacterial conjunctivitis. Follow-up is needed when symptoms persist or client is unresponsive to treatment. (Uphold, 1994)

7. *Answer:* b (assessment/history/HEENT/NAS)

Rationale: Culture and sensitivity testing should be done when the conjunctivitis is recurring or resistant to treatment, with all infants younger than 1 month, and in suspected cases of gonorrhea or chlamydial conjunctivitis. (Baker, 1996; Ruppert, 1996)

8. *Answer:* d (management/consult/referral/HEENT/NAS)

Rationale: A 10-week-old with new-onset conjunctivitis can be treated by a practitioner. All infants younger than 1 month should be referred because of the risk of ophthalmia neonatorum and the potential injury to sight. (Boynton, Dunn, & Stephens, 1994)

9. *Answer:* a (assessment/physical examination/HEENT/NAS)

Rationale: Marked itching, mild to moderate injection, and eyelids with a cobblestone appearance are likely to occur with allergic conjunctivitis. (Uphold, 1994)

DENTAL PROBLEMS

Candidiasis, Gingivitis, Acute Necrotizing Ulcerative Gingivitis, Aphthous Ulcers, and Tooth Fracture Injury

Candidiasis (Thrush)

OVERVIEW
Definition

An oral pharyngeal infection of the mucous membranes, *candidiasis* is most commonly caused by the yeast like fungus *Candida albicans.*

Incidence

- From 50,000 to 100,000 cases per year are recorded in the United States.
- It may occur in any age group.
- It is commonly seen in infants during the first weeks of life.
- In older children it is most commonly associated with antibiotic use.
- In the asthmatic child it is often related to the use of steroids.
- It is seen most commonly in clients with debilitating diseases, diabetes, and cancer diseases. Frequently occurs in clients receiving antibiotics, steroid therapy, radiation therapy, and immunosuppressive drugs.
- It is very common in clients with HIV.

Pathophysiology

PROTECTIVE FACTORS
- Good oral hygiene
- Good nutrition

FACTORS INCREASING SUSCEPTIBILITY
- Poor oral hygiene
- Poor nutrition
- Radiation therapy to head and neck
- Steroid use
- Antibiotic use
- Immunosuppressive drug therapy

COMMON PATHOGENS. *Candida albicans* is the most common cause of candidiasis.

ASSESSMENT: SUBJECTIVE/HISTORY
Symptoms

- White "spots" in mouth
- Mouth pain
- Difficulty eating
- Weight loss
- Infants: Increased irritability; difficulty feeding; mother with possible history of vaginal candidiasis

Past Medical History

- Is there a history of diabetes, cancer, HIV, or other chronic disease states?
- When was the last dental examination, or dental examination pattern?
- What are dental care and oral hygiene practices?
- Does the female client have a vaginal discharge?
- Did the male client have intimate oral sexual contact with a woman with a vaginal discharge?
- Is there a report of recent diaper rash in the infant?
- Are there any allergies?
- When was the last menstrual period (LMP)?

Medication History

- Antibiotics
- Chemotherapy agents
- Steroids: Oral and inhaled
- Radiation therapy

Family History

- Others in household with the same symptoms
- Diabetes
- HIV

Psychosocial History

Consider the possibility of sexual abuse in young children without predisposing factors.

Dietary History

Ask about nutritional status because poor nutritional intake can be a contributing factor.

ASSESSMENT: OBJECTIVE/ PHYSICAL EXAMINATION

Physical Examination

A problem-oriented examination should be conducted with particular attention to the following:

GENERAL APPEARANCE. Does the client appear healthy or ill?

HYDRATION STATUS. Client may become dehydrated because of decreased oral intake.

ORAL MEMBRANES. White plaques scrape off easily with a tongue blade to reveal erythematous areas.

GENITAL/RECTAL AREA

- Female clients with a complaint of vaginal discharge should have a complete pelvic examination.
- Children with suspected sexual abuse should be examined.
- Infants should be evaluated for diaper rash.

Diagnostic Procedures

- None are indicated for typical oral candidiasis.
- Potassium hydroxide (KOH) preparation of the scraping demonstrates budding yeast without hyphae.

DIAGNOSIS

Differential diagnosis may include the following:
- Leukoplakia: Geographic tongue
- Stomatitis: Milk products left on tongue

THERAPEUTIC PLAN

Pharmacologic Treatment

ORAL ANTIFUNGAL AGENTS

- Nystatin (Mycostatin) oral suspension 100,000 U/ml
  - *Infants:* Place 1 ml in each cheek every 6 hours for 7 to 10 days. May also paint lesions with a cotton swab.
  - *Older children and adults:* Place 2 to 3 ml in each cheek; then swish and swallow every 6 hours for 7 to 10 days.
  - *Adolescents and adults:* Nystatin troches (Mycostatin Pastilles) 200,000 U/ml. Slowly dissolve 1 to 2 troches in mouth every 5 to 6 hours for 7 to 10 days.
- Clotrimazole (Lotrimin) buccal troches, 10 mg. Slowly dissolve 1 troche in mouth every 5 hours for 14 days.
- Ketoconazole 200 to 400 mg PO every AM with breakfast for 7 to 14 days. For better absorption of this medicine, the stomach must be acidic.
- Fluconazole 100 mg PO every AM for 7 to 14 days

NOTE: A troche is a lozenge-like tablet that is dissolved in the mouth.

DENTURE WEARERS

Clients who wear dentures must add nystatin powder, 100,000 U/g, applied to dentures every 6 to 8 hours for several weeks.

Client Education

- Rinse mouth with small amount of water before using medication.
- Remove large plaques gently with cotton swabs moistened with water.
- Wash hands thoroughly after changing infants' diapers.
- Wash hands thoroughly after using the bathroom.
- Infants and small children:
  —Caregiver needs to wash toys and sterilize nipples and pacifiers to prevent reinfection.
  —Breast-feeding mother should wash her nipples with mild soap and water, then allow them to air dry.

Referral

- If condition is persistent or recurrent, or if no improvement occurs in 5 days, the client should be referred to immunology to evaluate immunologic status.
- Infants and small children should be referred to a pediatrician if failure to thrive develops.

EVALUATION/FOLLOW-UP

- Older children and adults should return in 5 to 7 days if no improvement.
- Infants should be reevaluated if:
  —They refuse liquids, bottle, or breast.
  —Symptoms do not improve or worsen.

Gingivitis

OVERVIEW
Definition

Inflammation of the gingiva, called *gingivitis*, is caused by tooth-borne bacteria (plaque) buildup, which causes lymphocyte proliferation and the activation of cytokines. This results in the destruction of the periodontal ligament and the alveolar bone, the supporting structures of the teeth.

Incidence

- Pandemic; occurs in 90% of the population.
- Occurs in up to 50% of children; increases in severity with age.
- May lead to tooth and bone loss if untreated.

Pathophysiology

PROTECTIVE FACTORS
- Good oral hygiene
- Good nutrition

FACTORS INCREASING SUSCEPTIBILITY
- Increased bacterial plaque buildup with an acute inflammatory response at the junctional epithelium (attachment of gingiva to enamel surface of tooth)
- Systemic factors
  —Drugs that may cause hyperplasia:
        Phenytoin (Dilantin)
        Calcium-channel blockers
        Cyclosporine
  —Pregnancy, leading to exaggerated inflammatory response, especially in the third trimester
  —Vitamin C deficiency
  —Diabetes mellitus
- Local Factors
  —Food impaction
  —Trauma
  —Smoking
  —Mouth breathing, leading to drying of the gingiva

COMMON PATHOGENS
- Gram-positive filamentous rods
- Actinomyces most common

ASSESSMENT: SUBJECTIVE/HISTORY
Symptoms

EARLY
Bleeding gums after brushing or flossing
"Bad breath"
Red gum
Painless gum swelling
LATE
Sensitivity to sweets and hot and cold
Dull throbbing pain after eating and when awakening

Past Medical History

- Mouth breather
- Dental hygiene habits

- Treatment for malocclusion
- Poor dental restorations; poorly done or deteriorated
- Diabetes
- Pregnancy
- LMP
- HIV exposure
- Access to dental care; last dental examination or pattern for dental examinations
- Smoking history

Medication History

- Antibiotics
- Oral contraceptives
- Dilantin
- Steroids, oral and inhaled
- Insulin
- Chemotherapy

Family History

- Diabetes
- Periodontal disease

Psychosocial History

Economic status: Low economic status often is associated with less access to dental care.

Dietary History

Poor nutritional intake may be a contributing factor.

ASSESSMENT: OBJECTIVE/ PHYSICAL EXAMINATION

Physical Examination

A problem-oriented examination should be conducted with particular attention to the following:

- General appearance: Does the client look healthy or ill?
- Gingiva: Look for inflammation and redness surrounding the neck of the tooth, erosion, presence of plaque, and hyperplasia or recession of gums.

Diagnostic Procedures

No diagnostic procedures are indicated.

DIAGNOSIS

Differential diagnosis may include the following:

- Dental abscess
- Pericoronitis

- Periodontitis
- Stomatitis
- Drug reaction
- Impacted food particles

THERAPEUTIC PLAN

Pharmacologic Treatment

No pharmacologic treatment is recommended.

Nonpharmacologic Treatment

- Removal of plaque and other irritants
- Warm saline and water rinses 2 to 3 times a day

Client Education

- Brush and floss teeth between each meal.
- Rinse mouth with antibacterial mouthwash.
- Have regular dental and hygienist check-ups.
- Improve dietary nutrition, especially vitamin C.
- Stop smoking.

Referral

- Clients must be referred to the dentist for treatment and further education.
- Step above usually results in the return of healthy gingiva.

EVALUATION/FOLLOW-UP

- Close follow-up by the dentist and oral hygienist is essential for continued health of gingiva. Seeing the oral hygienist every 6 months is recommended.
- During pregnancy, visiting the oral hygienist every 3 months is recommended.
- Children should have their first dental examination between 12 and 18 months.

Acute Necrotizing Ulcerative Gingivitis (Trench Mouth, Vincent's Infection)

OVERVIEW

Definition

Acute necrotizing ulcerative gingivitis is a bacterial infection of the gingival tissue that usually begins between the teeth and then spreads in a lateral direction. It may lead to tooth and bone loss.

Incidence

- This condition is most common in adolescents and young adults, who are usually under physical or psychologic stress.
- It was first described by the early Romans.
- During World War I this inflammation was referred to as "trench mouth."

Pathophysiology

PROTECTIVE FACTORS. Good oral hygiene should be practiced, especially when client is under severe stress.

FACTORS INCREASING SUSCEPTIBILITY
- Stress: Physical and psychologic
- Systemic diseases
- Poor oral hygiene

COMMON PATHOGENS. It is believed that both of the following pathogens are present:
- Fusospirochetal complex: (forms are *Fusobacterium fusiforme*, vibrios, streptococci, diplococci, and filamentous)
- Spirochete: *Borrelia vincentii*

ASSESSMENT: SUBJECTIVE/HISTORY
Symptoms

- Sudden onset of acute gingival pain
- Bleeding gums with minimal stimulation
- "Bad" taste: foul, metallic
- Breath odor
- Increased salivation
- Fever
- Malaise
- Loss of appetite

Past Medical History

- Recent emotional or physical stressors
- Diabetes
- HIV
- Dental hygiene habits; date of last dental examination

Medication History

- Steroids: Oral or inhaled
- Chemotherapy agents
- Immunosuppressive therapy

Family History

- Others in household with same condition
- Diabetes
- HIV infection

Psychosocial History

- Recent stressors, such as major life-change events
- Lower socioeconomic status: Client is less likely to receive regular dental care.

Dietary History

- Poor nutritional status, especially lack of vitamin C
- Recent decrease in oral intake related to pain in mouth

ASSESSMENT: OBJECTIVE/ PHYSICAL EXAMINATION
Physical Examination

A problem-oriented examination should be conducted with particular attention to:
- General appearance: Does the client look ill?
- Hydration status: Client may become dehydrated because of decreased oral intake related to pain.
- Gingiva: Classic triad
  —Intense pain
  —"Punched-out" interdental papillae covered with a white pseudomembrane (gray membrane that can be removed with gentle pressure)
  —Foul mouth odor
- Vital signs: Fever, tachycardia
- Neck: Lymphadenopathy

Diagnostic Procedures

- If elevated fever and lymphadenopathy are present, obtain CBC.
- If client is dehydrated, check electrolytes.
- If client has high fever, consider obtaining blood cultures to rule out systemic infection.

DIAGNOSIS

Differential diagnosis may include the following:
- Acute viral or bacterial infections
- Herpetic gingivostomatitis
- Leukemic gingivitis

THERAPEUTIC PLAN
Pharmacologic Treatment

- Penicillin V
  Adults: 250 to 500 every 6 hours for 10 days
  Children: 25 to 50 mg/kg/24 hours in 4 divided doses

- Erythromycin
  Adults: 250 mg every 6 hours for 10 days
  Children: 30 to 40 mg/kg/day in 4 divided doses
- Chlorhexidine gluconate 0.12% and warm water to rinse mouth
- Topical anesthetic
- Hydrogen peroxide 3% soaked into cotton pellets to débride lesions 3 to 4 times a day

Client Education

- Good oral hygiene
- Smoking cessation
- Improvement in dietary intake, especially vitamin C
- Regular dental hygienist and dentist visits
- Stress-relieving exercises

Referral

- If client appears ill (i.e., fever, dehydrated, or experiencing severe pain), he or she should be admitted for IV antibiotic and rehydration.
- Client must be seen by a dentist immediately for definitive care.

EVALUATION/FOLLOW-UP

- Client must be followed up closely by the dentist for continued care (usually two to four visits until healthy gingiva is restored).
- Nutritional status must be monitored.

Aphthous Ulcers (Canker Sores)

OVERVIEW
Definition

An *aphthous ulcer* is a superficial ulceration of the mucous membranes of the mouth and lips.

OCCASIONAL APHTHAE. Single lesions occur at intervals of months or years. They usually heal without complications.

ACUTE MULTIPLE APHTHAE. These are associated with gastrointestinal disorders. An acute episode may last for weeks. Lesions develop sequentially at different sites in the mouth.

CHRONIC RECURRENT APHTHAE. One or more lesions are always present for years.

Incidence

- 20% to 50% of adults affected
- More common in females than males
- Familial tendencies
- More common during the winter and spring months

Pathophysiology

PROTECTIVE FACTORS
- Good oral hygiene
- Avoidance of oral exposure to others with same

COMMON PATHOGENS. These ulcers were once thought to be caused by the herpes simplex virus, but the actual cause is not known.

ASSESSMENT: SUBJECTIVE/HISTORY
Symptoms

- Burning sensation 1 to 48 hours before eruption of ulcer
- Pain
- Swelling
- Redness

Past Medical History

- Allergies to chocolate, nuts, tomatoes, or other foods
- Autoimmune disease
- Recent trauma
- Drugs: Possible reaction
- Stressors: Physical or emotional

Medication History

- Antibiotics
- Steroids: Especially inhaled

Family History

- History of the same
- Autoimmune diseases

Psychosocial History

Inquire about recent life stressors.

Dietary History

Ask about possible recent decrease in oral intake as a result of pain.

ASSESSMENT: OBJECTIVE/ PHYSICAL EXAMINATION

Physical Examination

A problem-oriented examination should be conducted with particular attention to the following:

- General appearance: Does the client look ill?
- Hydration status: May become dehydrated because of decreased oral intake.
- Oral membrane characteristic lesions (lesions found on buccal or labial mucosa, pharynx or lateral tongue):
  —One or more lesions
  —Small size: <10 mm
  —Superficial, shallow, and oval
  —Light yellow to gray fibrinoid center
  —Red ridges

Diagnostic Procedures

Perform incisional biopsy of the lesion if (1) unsure of the cause of the lesion or (2) the lesion becomes larger or changes to a color that is inconsistent with previous aphthous ulcers.

DIAGNOSIS

Differential diagnosis may include the following:

- Herpes simplex virus
- Drug allergies
- Behçet's disease
- Inflammatory bowel disease
- Squamous cell carcinoma

THERAPEUTIC PLAN

Pharmacologic Treatment

- Topical steroids
  —Triamcinolone acetonide 0.1%
  —Fluocinonide ointment 0.05% in an adhesive base (Orbase Plain) applied to lesions 3 times a day
- Mouth coating
  —Mixture of diphenhydramine (Benadryl) suspension (5 mg/ml) and Maalox or Mylanta in equal parts
  —Viscous lidocaine (Xylocaine) 15 ml swished in mouth every 4 hours for clients older than 12 years; 3 to 5 ml for children 5 to 12 years old
- Mouth rinse
  —Tetracycline 250 mg capsule opened and the powder mixed in 30 to 50 ml of water, 3 to 4 times a day for 5 to 7 days. Tetracycline tends to abort the lesions and prevent secondary infections. This should not be used during pregnancy.
  —Chloraseptic mouthwash every 2 hours for children older than 6 years

Client Education

- A topical steroid should be used at first sign of tingling to abort the aphthous eruption.
- Topical anesthetics should be applied directly to a lesion that has been dried.
- Nothing should be eaten within 1 hour of using anesthetic.
- A bland, soft diet should be followed during lesion eruptions.
- Intake of clear liquids should be increased.
- Lesions can recur.

Referral

- If a client, especially a child, becomes dehydrated, he or she may require hospitalization.
- Infants with multiple lesions should be referred to a pediatrician.

EVALUATION/FOLLOW-UP

- Children should be reevaluated within 24 to 48 hours, especially if multiple lesions are present, to ensure that client does not become dehydrated.
- Routine follow-up is not always indicated.

Tooth Fracture Injury

OVERVIEW

Definition

A *tooth fracture injury* is a fracture caused by blunt trauma. Classification of anterior tooth fractures is shown in Figure 1-1.

ELLIS I FRACTURE. Fracture of the enamel resulting in a rough edge to the tooth.

ELLIS II FRACTURE. Fracture that penetrates the dentin. This leads to exposure of the pulp.

ELLIS III FRACTURE. Full-thickness fracture of the tooth. It involves the enamel, dentin, and pulp. Pink tissue or blood will be seen in the fracture.

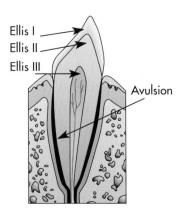

Figure 1-1   Ellis classification of tooth fractures.

AVULSION FRACTURE. Tooth is removed from the socket. It may have bone involvement.

Protective Factors

- Use of protective mouth equipment during contact sporting activity
- Keeping environment safe from falls

ASSESSMENT: SUBJECTIVE/HISTORY
Symptoms

- Tooth pain
- Bleeding gum line
- Swelling to gum line
- Paresthesia
- Jaw pain
- Difficulty opening or closing mouth

Past Medical History

- Recent mouth trauma
- Dental work (e.g., caps, dentures, partials)
- Tetanus status, especially if laceration is noted to lips, tongue, or gums
- Allergies to medications
- Chronic diseases, such as diabetes and HIV infection
- LMP
- Oral hygiene status

Medication History

- Aspirin products: increased bleeding tendencies
- Steroids (especially inhaled): associated with gum disease, which increases risk of tooth loss to trauma

Family History

Family history is noncontributory.

Psychosocial History

- Activities the client is involved in, especially contact sports
- Use of safety equipment, such as mouthguards

Dietary History

Ask about nutritional status.

ASSESSMENT: OBJECTIVE/ PHYSICAL EXAMINATION
Physical Examination

A problem-oriented examination should be conducted with particular attention to the following:

- Neurologic examination: Rule out possible head injury from trauma.
- Oral cavity: Evaluate possible laceration to tongue or gum line and inspect for pieces of broken tooth.
- Cervical spine: Ensure that no injury to C-spine has occurred as a result of trauma to the mouth.
- Airway: Ensure that tooth fragments have not been aspirated or are blocking airway.
- Assess for loose teeth.
- Assess for instability of maxillary bone.

Diagnostic Procedures

X-ray examination:

- Facial, C-spine, mandibular: As indicated to rule out fractures of the bones
- Chest: To rule out aspiration of missing tooth fragments

DIAGNOSIS

Differential diagnosis may include the following:

- Fracture of mandible
- Le Fort's fractures
- Malocclusion injuries
- Closed head injury
- Newly erupting tooth
- Dental infection

THERAPEUTIC PLAN
Pharmacologic Treatment
- Narcotic pain medications if no head injury
- Nonnarcotic pain medications if head injury is suspected

Nonpharmacologic Treatment
- Ice to area
- Pressure dressing to bleeding socket
- Placement of dislodged tooth in saline solution

Client Education
- Use of proper safety equipment (correctly fitted mouth-guard) during contact sports
- Close follow-up by dentist (essential)
- Soft diet until injury resolved
- Good oral hygiene
- Avoidance of injury (home safety evaluation to prevent falls)

Referral
All tooth fractures must have follow-up with a dentist.

ELLIS I FRACTURE. Needs referral to a dentist within 24 hours to have crown filed to remove rough edges.

ELLIS II FRACTURE. Needs urgent referral to dentist within 24 hours to have crown placed to prevent bacterial contamination of the pulp.

ELLIS III FRACTURE. Needs urgent referral to an oral surgeon for probable tooth extraction or root canal.

AVULSION FRACTURE. Needs emergency referral to an oral surgeon within 2 hours for possible tooth reimplantation and root canal.

EVALUATION/FOLLOW-UP

Close follow-up by an oral surgeon or a dentist is essential.

REFERENCES

Abrams, R. B., & Mueller, W. A. (1995). Oral medicine and dentistry. In *Current pediatric diagnosis and treatment* (12th ed., pp. 444-453). Norwalk, CT: Appleton & Lange.

Belanger, G. K., & Casamassimo, P. A. (1994). Dental injuries. In R. M. Barkin & P. Rosen. (Eds.) *Emergency pediatrics: A guide to ambulatory care* (4th ed., pp. 412-417) St. Louis: Mosby.

Belanger, G. K., & Casamassimo, P. A. (1994). Ear, nose, and throat disorders. In R.M. Barkin, & P. Rosen, *Emergency pediatrics: A guide to ambulatory care* (4th ed., pp. 539-560). St. Louis: Mosby.

Boynton, R. W., Dunn, E. S., & Stephens, G. R. (1994). *Manual of ambulatory pediatrics* (3rd ed., pp. 362-363). Philadelphia: J. B. Lippincott.

Dambro, M. R., Griffith, J., & Cann, C. (1997). *Griffith's 5-minute clinical consult* (pp. 164-163, 424-425). Baltimore: Williams & Wilkins.

Hoole, A. J., Pickard, C. G., Ouimette, R. M., Lohr, J. A., & Greenberg, R. A. (1995). *Patient care guidelines for nurse practitioners* (4th ed., pp. 112-113, 150-151). Philadelphia: J. B. Lippincott.

Jackler, R. K., & Kaplan, M. J. (1996). Ears, nose, and throat. In L. M. Tierney, S. J. McPhee, & M. A. Papdakis. *Current medical diagnosis and treatment* (pp. 181-214). Norwalk, CT: Appleton & Lange.

Komaroff, A. L. (1994). Disease of the respiratory tract: Pharyngitis, coryza, and related infections in adults. In W. T. Branch. *Office practice of medicine* (3rd ed., pp. 148-163). Philadelphia: W. B. Saunders.

MacLeod, D. K. (1995). Common problems of the teeth and oral cavity. In L. R. Baker, J. R. Burton, & P. D. Zieve. *Principles of ambulatory medicine* (4th ed., pp. 1479-1492). Philadelphia: Williams & Wilkins.

Rund, D. A. (1996) Facial and oral trauma. In D. A. Rund, R. M. Barkin, P. Rosen, & G. L. Sternbach. *Essentials of emergency medicine* (2nd ed., pp. 231-242). St. Louis: Mosby.

Sonis, S. T. (1994). Lesions of the mouth. In W. T. Branch. *Office practice of medicine* (3rd ed., pp. 164-173). Philadelphia: W. B. Saunders.

Uphold, C. R., & Graham, M. V. (1994). *Clinical guidelines in family practice* (2nd ed., pp. 358-367). Gainesville, FL: Barmarrae Books.

REVIEW QUESTIONS

Situation: *J.R. complains of "white patches" in his mouth. He states that the patches are painful. After you complete your evaluation, you suspect oral candidiasis. (Questions 1-3)*

1. Which of the following laboratory studies can be used to definitively diagnose candidiasis?

   a. Culture and sensitivity of scrapings
   b. Chocolate agar culture of scrapings
   c. KOH preparation of scrapings
   d. Tzank smear of scrapings

2. J.R.'s most significant medical history should include:

   a. Family history of diabetes
   b. Recent emotional stressors
   c. History of IV drug use
   d. Allergies to antibiotics

3. J.R. should be treated with the following:

   a. Penicillin V 250 mg PO every 6 hours for 10 days
   b. Ceftriaxone 250 mg IM 1-time dose
   c. Nystatin troches 200,000 U/ml 1 to 2 dissolved in mouth every 5 to 6 hours for 7 days
   d. Hydrogen peroxide 3% soaks every 5 to 6 hours for 7 days

4. F.C. comes to your clinic with acute gingivitis. He asks you, "What is the most common cause of gingivitis?" You would explain to him:

   a. No one really knows the exact cause of gingivitis, but good dental care is important for its prevention.
   b. Gingivitis is caused by both *Fusobacterium fusiforme* and *Borrelia vincentii*.
   c. Gingivitis is caused by plaque bacteria that builds up below the gum line.
   d. Gingivitis is caused by the trauma related to a hard-bristled toothbrush.

Situation: *P.D. is a 15-year-old boy who states that he fell from his bicycle, striking his face on the ground. He is reporting severe tooth pain. During your evaluation, you note that P.D. has a fracture of his eighth and ninth teeth (upper central incisors). On further evaluation of the tooth, you note pink tissue within the teeth, and it appears to have penetrated the enamel and dentin also. (Questions 5-7)*

5. On the basis of the Ellis classification for fractures of the anterior teeth, you would classify these fractures as: [evaluation]

   a. Ellis I fracture
   b. Ellis II fracture
   c. Ellis III fracture
   d. Ellis IV fracture

6. P.D. states that he is not sure where the remainder of the tooth is. During your evaluation of his mouth, you do not see teeth fragments. Your next step in the evaluation of this client should include:

   a. Chest x-ray
   b. CBC and urinalysis
   c. Skull series
   d. There is no indication for radiologic or laboratory analysis

7. The referral for this client would be:

   a. Client needs an emergency referral to an oral surgeon within 2 hours for a possible reimplantation of the tooth.
   b. Client needs an urgent referral to an oral surgeon for possible tooth extraction or root canal.
   c. Client needs an urgent referral to a dentist within 24 hours for crown placement and reduction of the risk of bacterial contamination.
   d. Client needs a referral to the dentist to have the crown of the tooth filed to remove the rough edges.

ANSWERS AND RATIONALES

1. *Answer:* c (assessment/diagnostics/HEENT/NAS)

   Rationale: KOH preparation demonstrates budding yeast without hyphae, consistent with the fungus *Candidia albicans.* Answer *a:* Culture and sensitivity is used to test for bacterial growth and only needs to be obtained when the diagnosis is in doubt. Answer *b:* Chocolate agars are used to culture out gonorrhea. Answer *d:* Tzank smears are used to diagnosis herpes. (Hoole, Pickard, Ouimette, Lohr, & Greenberg, 1995)

2. *Answer:* c (assessment/history/HEENT/NAS)

   Rationale: History of IV drug abuse is an indicator of possible HIV infections. Oral candidiasis may be an early sign of AIDS. Answer *a:* A family history of diabetes does not increase the risk of oral candidiasis, although a personal history of diabetes puts the client at a higher risk for oral candidiasis. Answer *b:* Emotional stress does not have a role in the development of oral candidiasis. Answer *d:* Oral candidiasis is not a result of allergic reaction to antibiotics, but more likely the result of using antibiotics. (Komaroff, 1994; Uphold & Graham, 1994)

3. *Answer:* c (plan/management/therapeutics/pharmacologic/HEENT/NAS)

Rationale: Nystatin is an antifungal agent used in the treatment of oral candidiasis. Pencillin V and hydrogen peroxide are used in the treatment of acute necrotizing ulcerative gingivitis. Celtriaxone is used in the treatment of gonorrhea. (Komaroff, 1994; Uphold & Graham, 1994)

4. *Answer:* c (physiology/pathophysiology/HEENT/NAS)

Rationale: Gingivitis is caused by the buildup of plaque at the dentogingival junction. The bacteria, if not removed by brushing, will proliferate and lead to this inflammatory process. Answer *b:* Acute necrotizing ulcerative gingivitis is caused by these microorganisms. (MacLeod, 1995)

5. *Answer:* c (diagnosis/HEENT/NAS)

Rationale: This is an Ellis III fracture. An Ellis I fracture is a fracture of the enamel resulting in a rough edge to the tooth. An Ellis II fracture is a fracture that penetrates the dentin. This leads to exposure of the pulp. An Ellis III fracture is a full-thickness fracture of the tooth. It involves the enamel, dentin, and pulp. Pink tissue or blood will be seen in the fracture. An avulsion fracture is a tooth removed from the socket; it may have bone involvement. There is no such classification as an Ellis IV fracture. (Rund, 1996)

6. *Answer:* a (plan/management/diagnostics/HEENT/NAS)

Rationale: It is essential to account for missing tooth fragments. If you are unable to account for the missing fragments, a chest x-ray is indicated to rule out possible aspiration of the tooth fragments. There is no indication for the remainder of the studies, unless you suspect kidney injury or skull fracture in this bicycle crash. (Rund, 1996)

7. *Answer:* b (plan/management/consultation and referral/NAS)

Rationale: This is the correct referral for an Ellis III fracture. Answer *a:* An avulsion of the tooth. Answer *c:* Ellis II fracture. Answer *d:* Ellis I fracture. (Rund, 1996)

EPISTAXIS

OVERVIEW
Definition

Epistaxis, or nosebleed, is a hemorrhage from the nose.

Incidence

Epistaxis is the most common ENT emergency.

Pathophysiology

Ninety-five percent of nosebleeds are caused by rupture of small vessels that overlie anterior nasal septum, usually self-limiting; 5% originate in posterior cavity and can be life-threatening. The condition is often accompanied by hypertension, which is not thought to be the cause but is probably an anxiety reaction.

Etiology
- Nasal trauma such as FB, forceful blowing, blunt trauma, penetrating trauma (a finger)
- URI
- Irritants (OTC nose sprays, cocaine)
- Mucosal drying in low humidity
- Septal deviation
- Vascular abnormalities
- Children: Usually FB
- Older adults: Usually spontaneous from dry or thinned mucosa

ASSESSMENT: SUBJECTIVE/HISTORY
History of Present Illness

Ask about time of onset, spontaneous onset or trauma, which nostril it started in, whether blood ran out of the nose or down throat. Any bleeding in gums, urine, stool?

Past Medical History

Ask about previous epistaxis (if so, what controlled it?) or bleeding diathesis.

Past Surgical History

Inquire about any previous ENT procedures.

Medication History

- Anticoagulants, including aspirin use
- Nasal sprays

ASSESSMENT: OBJECTIVE/ PHYSICAL EXAMINATION

Physical Examination

Focused physical examination is appropriate.

GENERAL. Signs of anxiety, fear, hypovolemia, shock.

VITAL SIGNS. Include orthostatics and oxygen saturation.

HEENT. Typical examination including examination of anterior septum with nasal speculum. Client should be sitting upright with head in "sniffing" position, not with neck extension. Remove all clots and look for bleeding site, signs of septal erosion (cocaine), trauma, color of mucosa. Check posterior pharynx for signs of bloody drainage. Check buccal mucosa for bleeding.

CHILDREN. Look for FB.

Diagnostic Procedures

- CBC if bleeding is prolonged or if orthostatic vital signs changes are present
- Coagulation studies if taking anticoagulants, prolonged bleeding, orthostatic changes
- Urinalysis and stool guaiac if history of bleeding
- Type and cross-match packed RBCs if necessary

DIAGNOSIS

Differential diagnosis may include the following:
- Anterior epistaxis (primary vs secondary)
- Posterior epistaxis
- Clotting abnormality
- Septal perforation
- Children: Nosebleed is usually secondary to trauma or FB.
- Older adults: Usually primary epistaxis is from dry mucosa, but it may indicate a vascular problem.

THERAPEUTIC PLAN

- Reassure client.
- Treat definitively.

- If bleeding, try instilling 1 or 2 sprays of phenylephrine (Neo-Synephrine).
- If bleeding continues, topical 4% cocaine or cauterization (silver nitrate) is indicated.
- If bleeding persists, nostril must be packed with ½-inch iodoform gauze lubricated with petroleum jelly or bacitracin or with commercial nose packs.

Antibiotics

If packing is used, place client on short course of prophylactic antibiotics.

Client Education

- Avoid vigorous exercise and blowing nose for several days.
- Avoid hot or spicy foods and tobacco (may cause vasodilatation).
- Avoid chronic use of nasal sprays; use petroleum jelly or bacitracin for dry mucosa.
- Children: Instruct parents to keep small objects out of reach. If children are old enough, instruct them not to put anything smaller than their elbow in their nose.

Referral

- Return to clinic or emergency department if epistaxis recurs or signs of infection appear.
- If anterior packing is used, return to clinic in 2 to 4 days for removal.
- If posterior packing is used, return to clinic in 3 to 5 days for removal.

EVALUATION/FOLLOW-UP

- Reassess vital signs and check for hemostasis before dismissing.
- Any recurrence of epistaxis is an indication for ENT referral.

REFERENCES

Jackler, R., & Kaplan, M. (1996). Ear, nose and throat. In L. Tierney, Jr., S. McPhee, & M. Papadakis (Eds.). *Current medical diagnosis and treatment* (pp. 198-199). Norwalk, CT: Appleton & Lange.

Roberts, J., & Hedges, J. (1991). Otolaryngologic procedures. In *Clinical procedures in emergency medicine* (2nd ed., pp. 1029-1037). Philadelphia: W. B. Saunders.

REVIEW QUESTIONS

1. The proper way to examine a client with epistaxis is with the client:

    a. Sitting upright in sniffing position
    b. With the neck fully extended
    c. Lying supine
    d. With one naris occluded, and then the opposite naris occluded

2. When assessing a client with epistaxis, the nurse practitioner should ask about:

    a. Family history
    b. Medication history
    c. Immunizations
    d. Sexual history

3. When caring for a child with epistaxis, the nurse practitioner should assess:

    a. Growth patterns
    b. For presence of an FB
    c. Blood pressure
    d. For signs of abuse

4. A client returns for a second episode of epistaxis in a week period. The nurse practitioner should do all the following **except:**

    a. Refer the client to a specialist.
    b. Perform a hematocrit and hemoglobin test.
    c. Increase the dose of topical cocaine used.
    d. Repack the nose.

5. Evidence of effective client education for a client successfully treated for epistaxis is:

    a. The client states that he will avoid cold beverages.
    b. The client states that he will not play racquetball for 3 days.
    c. The client states that he will use saline nose drops faithfully.
    d. The client states that he will avoid caffeine.

ANSWERS AND RATIONALES

1. *Answer:* a (assessment/physical examination/HEENT/NAS)

    Rationale: Supine or with the neck fully extended could occlude the airway. Having one naris occluded while examining the other naris would also diminish air intake. (Jackler & Kaplan, 1996)

2. *Answer:* b (assessment/history/HEENT/NAS)

    Rationale: The use of aspirin or aspirin products increases one's risk for epistaxis. The other information would be less relevant. (Jackler & Kaplan, 1996)

3. *Answer:* b (assessment/physical examination/HEENT/child)

    Rationale: Children usually experience epistaxis from nose picking, traumatic injury (e.g., fall), or placement of an FB. The abused child rarely has a nose injury. Hypertension may produce epistaxis in the adult. (Jackler & Kaplan, 1996)

4. *Answer:* c (plan/management/therapeutics/non-pharmacologic/HEENT/NAS)

    Rationale: The client should be referred to an ENT specialist. A hemoglobin and hematocrit or CBC should be performed to determine blood loss. The nose may need to be repacked. The dose of cocaine used for vasoconstriction remains the same. (Jackler & Kaplan, 1996)

5. *Answer:* b (evaluation/HEENT/NAS)

    Rationale: Vigorous exercise should be avoided. Hot, spicy foods should be avoided. Nasal sprays should not be used. Caffeine is not significant. (Jackler & Kaplan, 1996)

EYE: FOREIGN BODY/CORNEAL ABRASION

OVERVIEW
Definition

Ocular *foreign bodies (FBs)* may be extraocular or intraocular. (This chapter discusses extraocular FBs.) A *corneal abrasion* is a defect in the bulbar conjunctiva that extends through one or more layers of the conjunctiva.

Incidence

Corneal abrasion caused by an FB is the most common ocular emergency.

Etiology

FOREIGN BODY. Wood, metal, sand, dust. May be imbedded in bulbar conjunctiva (white surface of eye), under lid (palpebral conjunctiva), or removed with continued FB sensation.

TRAUMA. Tree or bush limbs, mascara brush, paper, infant fingernail.

CONTACT LENS. Improper wear or inadequate cleaning.

ASSESSMENT: SUBJECTIVE/HISTORY
History of Present Illness

Ask about time of onset, activity at time of injury, whether FB sensation persists, problems with visual acuity or photophobia, drainage or bleeding from eye. Was FB from explosion, pounding metal, or other high-velocity projectile?

Past Medical History

- Diabetes
- Eye disease including glaucoma
- Hypertension
- Last tetanus inoculation
- Contact lenses

Past Surgical History

Ask about corneal implants.

Medication History

Inquire about drops for glaucoma.

Allergies

- Local anesthetics
- Fluorescein stain
- Antibiotics

ASSESSMENT: OBJECTIVE/ PHYSICAL EXAMINATION
Physical Examination

A focused examination is indicated.

GENERAL: Signs of anxiety, fear, pain

HEENT: Assess visual acuity. Inspect eye for globe penetration, corneal FB, hyphema, injected conjunctiva. Instill topical anesthetic and fluorescein stain. Examine eye with slit lamp, Wood's lamp, or other cobalt-blue light for abrasions. Abrasions will show as pooling of stain under cobalt-blue light. Inspect the cornea, bulbar, and palpebral conjunctiva (underside of eyelids) for retained FB. Vertical linear abrasions are usually sign of FB under upper lid.

Diagnostic Procedures

No diagnostic procedures are indicated.

DIAGNOSIS

- Intraocular FB
- Chemical injury (acid, alkali, solvents, etc.)
- Thermal burn
- Ultraviolet keratitis (welders, sunlamp, high-altitude snow)
- Extraocular FB
- Corneal abrasion (mechanical)

THERAPEUTIC PLAN

- Instill topical anesthetic (if client is not allergic). (These FBs *really* hurt.)
- Perform fluorescein examination.
- Remove FB from cornea or bulbar conjunctiva with eye spud or 22- to 25-gauge needle used as spud.
- Remove FB from under eyelids with moist cotton swab.
- If FB is metallic and rust ring has formed, refer to ophthalmologist for removal of ring with corneal bur.
- Instill broad-spectrum antibiotic ointment (erythromycin, gentamicin, or sulfacetamide) in eye.
- Do not patch affected eye unless abrasion is extensive. If patching is used, the affected eye should be double-patched, with possible referral to ophthalmologist.

- Prescribe pain medication (Vicodin is not too strong).
- Caution: Topical anesthetics should *never* be prescribed.

Client Education

- Patch will affect depth perception, so no driving, operating machinery, or reading.
- Client must wear patch for 24 hours.

Referral

- Ophthalmologic consult should be considered if there are multiple FBs, rust rings, if FB is in lens or iris (visual axis), or if mechanism is high velocity.
- Ophthalmologic follow-up if pain persists or if visual acuity is decreased after 24 hours with removal of patch.

EVALUATION/FOLLOW-UP

- Client should be pain free before discharge.
- Visual acuity should be normal and client should be pain free 24 hours after treatment.

REFERENCES

Ghezi, K., & Renner, G. (1992). Ophthalmologic disorders. In P. Rosen (Ed.), *Emergency medicine concepts and clinical practice* (pp. 2434-2439). St. Louis: Mosby.

Roberts, J., & Hedges, J. (1991). Ophthalmologic procedures. *Clinical procedures in emergency medicine* (2nd ed., pp. 1002-1007). Philadelphia: W. B. Saunders.

REVIEW QUESTIONS

1. When examining a client for a possible FB in the eye, the nurse practitioner notices vertical linear abrasions under the cobalt-blue light after using fluorescein stain. This may indicate:

    a. Allergic reaction to the stain
    b. Removal of FB
    c. Overwearing of contact lens
    d. Retained FB under upper lid

2. When discharging a client treated for a corneal abrasion, the nurse practitioner should:

    a. Refer the client to an ophthalmologist.
    b. Warn the client that pain may be present as long as 48 hours after treatment.

    c. Tell the client to wear an eyepatch over the affected eye for 48 hours.
    d. Inform the client about impaired depth perception.

3. The nurse practitioner should prescribe which of the following for the client with a corneal abrasion?

    a. Topical anesthetic agent
    b. Systemic antibiotic
    c. Glaucoma medication
    d. Oral pain medication

4. Which of the following should be assessed in a client with a potential corneal abrasion?

    a. Visual acuity
    b. Extraocular movements
    c. Color acuity
    d. Amblyopia

ANSWERS AND RATIONALES

1. *Answer:* d (assessment/physical examination/HEENT/NAS)

    Rationale: Vertical lines indicate a repeated rubbing of the conjunctiva by a foreign object.

2. *Answer:* d (plan/management/client education/HEENT/NAS)

    Rationale: Ophthalmologist referral is needed only if there are multiple FBs, rust ring formed, FB in the lens, or an abrasion from a high-velocity mechanism. Both pain and the eyepatch should disappear or be discontinued in 24 hours.

3. *Answer:* d (plan/management/pharmacologic/HEENT/NAS)

    Rationale: Topical anesthetic and antibiotic ointment may be used during the client visit. Although topical antibiotics may be useful in some cases, systemic antibiotics are not normally used. Topical anesthetics may prevent the client from feeling and seeking treatment for an acute change in the eye. Oral pain medication is necessary.

4. *Answer:* a (assessment/physical examination/HEENT/NAS)

    Rationale: Visual acuity should be checked and compared with that before injury. Extraocular movements are associated with a blow directly to the eye or with a neurologic condition. Color acuity and double vision are not associated with FBs.

GLAUCOMA

OVERVIEW
Definition
Glaucoma is a condition in which the intraocular pressure becomes increased and the optic nerve becomes cupped, leading to visual field loss. *Elevated intraocular pressure* is defined as a pressure >21 mm Hg. However, higher pressures leave some clients unaffected, and some persons with normal pressures have optic nerve and visual field changes. Acute glaucoma is *narrow-angle glaucoma*. Chronic glaucoma is *wide-angle glaucoma*.

Incidence
- Glaucoma is the second most common cause of permanent blindness (after macular degeneration).
- There are an estimated 3 million persons in the United States with elevated intraocular pressure.
- It occurs in as many as 15% of the older adult population.

Pathophysiology
Aqueous humor fills the posterior chamber of the eye, flows through the pupil and the anterior chamber, and leaves the eye through the trabecular meshwork, a connective tissue filter at the angle between the iris and the cornea. The aqueous humor passes out of the trabecular meshwork into Schlemm's canal. Intraocular pressure is maintained by a balance between inflow and outflow of aqueous humor. Increased intraocular pressure is related to improper aqueous humor flow. Elevated intraocular pressure results in optic nerve damage. The exact mechanism of this damage is unknown but probably relates to ischemia.

TYPES OF GLAUCOMA
- Primary *open-angle* glaucoma occurs from obstruction at the microscopic level in the trabecular meshwork or from overproduction of aqueous humor in 90% of all cases.
- Acute *closed-angle* glaucoma results from obstruction of trabecular network by the iris, by a narrow angle between the anterior iris and the posterior corneal surface, shallow anterior chambers, or a thickened or bulging iris.

- *Congenital* glaucoma occurs rarely as a result of an autosomal recessive gene.

RISK FACTORS
- Increasing age (prevalence 0.7% after age 40 years, 20% after age 60 years)
- Blacks older than 40 years (five times more likely than whites)
- Diabetes
- Hypertension
- Familial history of glaucoma
- Eye injury

FACTORS INCREASING SUSCEPTIBILITY
- Eye inflammation or trauma
- Neoplasm
- Neovascularization
- Corticosteroid therapy
- In closed-angle glaucoma:
  —Pharmacologic mydriasis
  —Anticholinergics

ASSESSMENT: SUBJECTIVE/HISTORY
Open-Angle Glaucoma
- Bilateral symptoms
- No symptoms in early stages
- Slow loss of peripheral vision
- Tunnel vision
- Eventual loss of central vision
- Mild, dull ache in the eyes
- Halos around lights, blurred vision
- Headache

Closed-Angle Glaucoma
- Unilateral symptoms
- Acute pain and pressure over one eye
- Decreased visual acuity
- Photophobia
- Halos around light
- Nausea and vomiting

Past Medical History
- Trauma to the eye
- Intraocular surgery
- Hypertension
- Diabetes
- Sarcoidosis

- Herpes zoster
- Myopia
- Migraine headache

Medication History

OPEN-ANGLE GLAUCOMA. Steroid use may predispose the client to glaucoma.

CLOSED-ANGLE GLAUCOMA. In certain cases glaucoma may be precipitated by the following:

- Antihistamines
- Stimulants
- Vasodilators
- Sympathomimetics
- Cocaine
- Clonidine

Family History

Persons with a first-degree relative with glaucoma are five times more likely to have glaucoma develop than the general population.

Psychosocial History

Closed-angle glaucoma may be precipitated by the following:

- Sitting in a darkened movie theater
- Stress leading to epinephrine excretion

ASSESSMENT: OBJECTIVE/ PHYSICAL EXAMINATION
Physical Examination

BOTH TYPES
- Diminished fields of vision
- Funduscopic examination may reveal:
  —Increased cup-to-disk ratio (>1:3)
  —Large optic cup
- Tonometry reading
  —>24 mm Hg (not always present)
  —Increasing tonometry readings

OPEN-ANGLE GLAUCOMA
- Bilateral symptoms
- Asymmetry of cup between eyes

CLOSED-ANGLE GLAUCOMA
- Unilateral symptoms
- Pupil dilated, nonreactive to light
- Cloudy cornea
- Decreased visual acuity
- Unilateral red eye

Diagnostic Procedures

- Tonometry (pressure measurement in anesthetized eyes)

—Schiøtz: Sits on eye surface, often undermeasures pressures in early disease
—Applanation: More accurate but slightly difficult to use
—Air puff: Per ophthalmologist, no anesthesia necessary
—Hand-held Tonopen: New, easy to use
- Central visual field testing (difficult to perform accurately)

DIAGNOSIS

Differential diagnoses may include the following:
- Open-angle glaucoma (mostly symptom free): Presbyopia may be one of the few differential diagnoses.
- Closed-angle glaucoma
  —Conjunctivitis—usually bilateral, rare pain, no nausea, vomiting, AM matting
  —Uveitis
  —Corneal disorders

THERAPEUTIC PLAN

Prevention is a better option than treatment. There is no cure for glaucoma. The primary care provider must be able to recognize early stages of optic nerve damage, symptoms of increased intraocular pressure, and especially acute, closed-angle glaucoma. Also, primary care providers need to be familiar with glaucoma medications and their possible impact on other chronic disease management.

Open-Angle Glaucoma

Medical management includes the following:
- Eyedrops
  —Beta-blocker eyedrops (timolol, betaxolol) given bid
  —Sympathomimetics (epinephrine)
  —Miotics (pilocarpine) given qid
- Systemic medications
  —Carbonic anhydrase inhibitors (acetazolamide)
  —Beta-blockers
- Surgery
  —Argon laser trabeculoplasty
  —Surgical trabeculectomy

Closed-Angle Glaucoma

CAUTION: *This is a medical emergency.*
- Immediate referral to ophthalmologist is es-

sential. Untreated acute glaucoma results in severe and permanent visual loss within 2 to 5 days after onset of symptoms.

- Surgery is almost always indicated.
- Medications may be instituted to reduce intraocular pressure while preparing for surgery.
- Miotic drugs: 4% pilocarpine solution, 1 drop every 20 minutes.
- Acetazolamide, a carbonic anhydrase inhibitor, is given 500 mg IV, followed by 250 mg qid.
- Osmotic diuretics such as urea or mannitol may be used.
- Iridectomy (laser or surgical) is often done prophylactically for the unaffected eye.

Postoperative Care

- Give cycloplegic drops to relax ciliary muscle.
- Encourage early ambulation.
- Observe unaffected eye for symptoms.
- Avoid activities that increase intraocular pressure—straining, coughing, stooping, or lifting.

EVALUATION/FOLLOW-UP

- Follow-up of intraocular pressure and visual field changes should be done weekly at first, then monthly.
- Compliance with medical regimen is often difficult, requiring eyedrop use as often as qid.
- Monitor for side effects of drugs, especially with noncardioselective beta-blocker use. Even with topical use, bronchoconstriction may be a side effect of these drugs.

REFERENCES

Everitt, D. E., & Avorn, J. (1990). Systemic effects of medications used to treat glaucoma. *Annals of Internal Medicine, 112,* 120.

Hahn, M. (1996). Common eye problems in primary care. *Advance for Nurse Practitioners, 4,* 3.

Leske, C. (1995). Risk factors for open-angle glaucoma: The Barbados Eye Study. *Archives of Ophthalmology, 113,* 918.

Margolis, K. L. (1989). Physician recognition of ophthalmoscopic signs of open angle glaucoma. *Journal of General Internal Medicine, 4:* 296.

Rosenberg, L. (1995) Glaucoma: Early detection and therapy for prevention of vision loss. *American Family Physician, 52,* 8.

Vaughan, D., Asbury, T., & Riordan-Eva, P. (Eds.). (1992). *General ophthalmology.* Norwalk, CT: Appleton & Lange.

REVIEW QUESTIONS

1. Untreated or uncontrolled glaucoma damages the optic nerve. Which of the following symptoms is associated with optic nerve damage?

   a. Improved vision in low light
   b. Dull ache behind the eyes
   c. Decreased pigmentation of the iris
   d. Floaters and scotomata

2. A 50-year-old man with wide-angle glaucoma comes in for care. Which of the following symptoms might this client have reported when his condition was first diagnosed?

   a. Redness and tearing of the eye
   b. Extreme pain in one eye
   c. Decreased peripheral vision
   d. Worsening near vision

3. Which of the following is a typical finding in narrow-angle glaucoma?

   a. Cloudy cornea
   b. Pupillary constriction
   c. Excessive tearing
   d. Altered extraocular movements

4. During the eye examination, the nurse practitioner should attempt to visualize the physiologic cup. Which of the following is true about the physiologic cup?

   a. It lies medial to the retinal vessels.
   b. It appears light colored in dark-skinned clients.
   c. It is best visualized with the blue light of the ophthalmoscope.
   d. Blurring of the nasal outline is normal.

5. Tonometry readings are often used to screen for glaucoma. Which of the following is true regarding tonometry readings?

   a. Schiøtz tonometry readings are often falsely low.
   b. Applanation tonometry readings are usually done by the ophthalmologist.
   c. Glaucoma may be ruled out if the tonometry reading is <21 mm Hg.
   d. Accurate measurement of optic pressure is impractical in primary care settings.

6. Carbonic anhydrase inhibitors are sometimes used in the treatment of glaucoma because they:

   a. Reduce aqueous humor production
   b. Diminish pupillary dilatation
   c. Promote diuresis
   d. Constrict the pupil

7. A 72-year-old man has a 1-day history of eye pain. He reports no visual disturbances. Eye examination reveals an injected conjunctiva, cup-to-disk ratio of 2:3, tonometry readings of 20 mm Hg, and visual acuity of 20/30. Which of the following should the nurse practitioner do next?

   a. Refer for ophthalmology evaluation.
   b. Evert the eyelid to look for FBs.
   c. Instill anesthetic ophthalmic drops.
   d. Correlate findings with vital signs.

8. When following up a client who has a family history of glaucoma, client education and evaluation should include:

   a. Yearly eye examination by primary care provider
   b. Review of symptoms of wide-angle glaucoma
   c. Annual dilated pupil examination by an ophthalmologist
   d. Measurement of intraocular pressure of family members

9. Which of the following would be indicative of the need for surgery in a client with a history of wide-angle glaucoma treated medically?

   a. Elevated tonometry readings despite use of miotic drops
   b. Poor compliance in following the medical regimen for treatment
   c. Evidence of gradual visual field loss
   d. Increased aqueous humor production

10. An 88-year-old man with a history of hypertension and hyperlipidemia comes in for evaluation. You note that he seems to be in some respiratory distress, and he tells you that he has been having increasing problems with shortness of breath. A review of his medications reveals that he is using eyedrops prescribed by the ophthalmologist to treat glaucoma and a variety of nonprescription drugs. Use of which of the following medications may be related to his symptoms?

   a. Pseudoephedrine (Sudafed)
   b. Timolol (Timoptic) eyedrops

   c. Acetazolamide (Diamox)
   d. Ibuprofen (Advil)

ANSWERS AND RATIONALES

1. *Answer:* b (assessment/history/HEENT/NAS)
Rationale: A dull ache in the eyes is not an uncommon finding in glaucoma, probably related to optic nerve ischemia.

2. *Answer:* c (assessment/history/HEENT/adult)
Rationale: Narrowing of the visual fields is the hallmark of wide-angle glaucoma. Narrow-angle glaucoma is characterized by pain and a red eye.

3. *Answer:* a (assessment/physical examination/ HEENT/NAS)
Rationale: A steamy cornea is a classic finding in acute glaucoma. Pupillary dilation is common.

4. *Answer:* d (assessment/physical examination/ NAS)
Rationale: The nasal outline of the cup is normally somewhat blurred.

5. *Answer:* a (diagnosis/HEENT/NAS)
Rationale: Schiøtz tonometry measurements may err toward low readings. There are several simple-to-use devices that may help detect changes in ocular pressure. Glaucoma has been found in clients with normal tonometry readings.

6. *Answer:* a (plan/management/therapeutic/pharmacologic/HEENT/NAS)
Rationale: Acetazolamide results in decreased aqueous humor production.

7. *Answer:* a (plan/management/consult/HEENT/ aging adult)
Rationale: The increased cup-to-disk ratio in the presence of a red eye and eye pain is a clear indicator of acute glaucoma, which is a medical emergency. The ophthalmologist will most likely recommend immediate surgery.

8. *Answer:* a (evaluation/HEENT/NAS)
Rationale: The primary care provider can be very effective in detecting early glaucoma by a funduscopic examination. Dilating the pupils may itself precipitate acute glaucoma in selected individuals.

9. *Answer:* c (evaluation/HEENT/NAS)

Rationale: Visual field loss despite treatment indicates optic nerve damage. Surgery would be recommended to prevent further damage once pharmacologic measures have been proved ineffective in managing the glaucoma.

10. *Answer:* b (evaluation/HEENT/aging adult)

Rationale: The most commonly prescribed eyedrops include noncardioselective beta-blockers such as timolol. Systemic absorption of this drug could cause exacerbation of respiratory problems and other side effects common to beta-blockers.

PHARYNGITIS: INFECTIOUS AND NONINFECTIOUS

OVERVIEW
Definition

Pharyngitis is an inflammation of the throat and surrounding structures, most often the tonsils *(tonsillopharyngitis)*.

Incidence

The third most common cause of visits to a health care professional for adults, pharyngitis is more common in children than in adults. It is infrequent in children younger than 2 years and most frequent in school-age children. Most cases in children occur during "strep season" (September through May); fewer cases occur during the summer months.

Pathophysiology

BACTERIAL PATHOGENS

- *Streptococcus pyogenes* is the most common agent (accounts for 5% to 38% of sore throats). It is rare in children younger than 3 years and most common in children 5 to 12 years old. A major concern is that it can lead to rheumatic fever.
- Beta-hemolytic streptococci group C and G are becoming more common but are not associated with rheumatic fever or glomerulonephritis.
- *Neisseria gonorrhoeae*
- *Chlamydia pneumoniae*
- *Haemophilus influenzae* type B
- *Mycoplasma pneumoniae*

VIRAL PATHOGENS

- Adenoviruses most common
- Influenza, parainfluenza, respiratory syncytial virus (RSV), rhinovirus, and cytomegalovirus
- Enteroviruses, including herpangina and coxsackievirus

- Epstein-Barr virus
- *Candida albicans*
- Kawasaki disease
- Herpesvirus

NONINFECTIOUS CAUSES

- Blood dyscrasias
- Gastroesophageal reflux disease (more common in adults)
- Mouth breathing
- Allergic rhinitis
- Postnasal drip
- Inhalation of irritant gases
- Trauma

ASSESSMENT: SUBJECTIVE/HISTORY

- No single symptom is diagnostic of group A beta-hemolytic streptococci
- Description of most common symptoms is given in the next two sections:

Streptococcal Pharyngitis

- All ages: Pharyngeal pain for more than 24 hours, temperature 101.5° F (>38.5°C), fever and chills, myalgias, headaches, swollen glands, nausea, and, in children, emesis
- Infants: Rare to see diagnosis of streptococcus
- Children younger than 3 years: May not complain of sore throat but may have diminished appetite and fluid intake; may see scarletina rash
- Adults and older adults: Fever less common, primary complaint of pharyngeal pain

Viral Pharyngitis

ADENOVIRUSES

- All ages: Sore throat, fever, headache, cough, runny nose, cervical adenopathy, exanthem (skin eruption or rash), and gastrointestinal symptoms

- Infants and toddlers: May have more severe pulmonary infection

ENTEROVIRUSES
- Sudden onset of fever, malaise, headache, and mild gastrointestinal symptoms; may see viral exanthems

EPSTEIN-BARR VIRUS
- Fever, exudative pharyngitis, cervical adenopathy, and mild gastrointestinal symptoms
- Infants and preschool-age children: May be fairly asymptomatic
- Adolescents: Prolonged course with residual fatigue

OTHERS
- RSV and rhinoviruses: Typically more upper respiratory symptoms, including nonexudative pharyngitis, rhinorrhea, and significant cough

Past Medical History

- Recent exposures (children at day care or school, occupational exposures for adults)
- History of frequent episodes of streptococcal pharyngitis, especially within the past year
- History of previous rheumatic fever
- History of orogenital sexual contact, concurrent steroid or immunosuppressive therapy

Medication History

Ask about recent use of antibiotics or any other medications.

Family History

Inquire about recent exposure or carrier status of any family member or close contact.

Psychosocial History

Ask about frequent absences from school.

ASSESSMENT: OBJECTIVE/ PHYSICAL EXAMINATION
Physical Examination

Include vital signs (including weight for children for drug dosing purposes). Perform thorough examination of head, eyes, ears, nose, throat, heart, lungs, and skin.

- Findings consistent with group A beta-hemolytic streptococci include tonsillar exudate, anterior cervical adenopathy, temperature >101° F, and petechiae of the palate. NOTE: A sandpaper-like rash on the trunk is consistent with scarlet fever in a client with pharyngitis and should be considered a sign of group A beta-hemolytic streptococci until proved otherwise.
- In addition to the symptoms above, generalized adenopathy, scleral icterus, and hepatosplenomegaly are more consistent with infectious mononucleosis.
- URI usually has cough and coryza as primary findings.
- Examination of pharynx may lead to other diagnoses—if epiglottitis is suspected, do not examine airway or insert any instruments such as tongue depressor.
- If ulcerative pharyngitis seen, you must suspect viral etiology, such as coxsackievirus.

Diagnostic Procedures

- Rapid streptococcal test is 50% to 90% accurate, with accuracy depending greatly on user technique.
- Overnight throat culture (retropharyngeal swab) takes as long as 48 hours for results; used as backup when rapid culture result is negative.
- WBC count may be elevated but is not commonly used for routine cases of pharyngitis. Only done if systemic symptoms or streptococcus result is negative and further workup is needed.
- Do Monospot test if symptoms suggestive of mononucleosis; results may remain negative in young children even if they do have mononucleosis.

DIAGNOSIS

Differential diagnosis includes the following:
- Streptococcal pharyngitis
- Viral pharyngitis
- Mononucleosis
- *Chlamydia*
- *Mycoplasma*
- Epiglottitis
- Acute rheumatic fever
- Toxic shock syndrome
- Sepsis
- Meningitis
- Retropharyngeal abscess

- Palatal cellulitis
- Diphtheria
- Tularemia
- Gonococcal pharyngitis
- Herpangina thrush

THERAPEUTIC PLAN
Pharmacologic Treatment

- Antibiotic treatment if culture positive for streptococcus as follows:
  —Initial treatment. *Children:* Administer 10-day course of amoxicillin (if allergic to penicillin, may use erythromycin or cephalosporin antibiotic). *Adults:* Follow 10-day course of penicillin VK (use erythromycin or cephalosporin if allergic to penicillin).
NOTE: In both children and adults, IM injection of benzathine penicillin may be used for 1 dose. This is not usually recommended for children younger than 5 years.
  Trimethoprim-sulfamethoxazole is *not* effective against streptococci.
  —Reinfection. *Children and adults:* Use a second-line antibiotic such as cephalosporin or amoxicillin clavulanate for 10 days. Consider taking culture after antibiotic course is completed to ensure eradication of bacteria (this is controversial).
- Viral infections: Symptomatic treatment includes acetaminophen, humidification, OTC products for comfort, and saline gargles qid (¼ teaspoon salt in 8 ounces of water).
- Pharyngeal candidiasis: Nystatin oral suspension (100,000 U/ml), 15 ml swish and swallow 4 to 6 times per day or 10 mg clotrimazole troche (tablet that dissolves in the mouth) for 15 to 30 minutes tid.
- Epiglottitis: Hospitalization is needed.
- Gonococcal pharyngitis: Ceftriaxone, amoxicillin, penicillin, or tetracycline regimens are effective.

Client Education

- Explain proper use of antibiotics:
  —Antibiotics are not needed if condition is not caused by *Streptococcus pyogenes.*
  —If it is streptococcus or other bacterial cause, client needs to complete the entire 10-day course to prevent recurrent infection and progression to rheumatic fever or other serious complication.
- Emphasize need for at least rapid antigen testing if symptoms are suggestive of streptococci.
- Discuss prevention of spreading of pharyngitis through measures such as good handwashing, avoidance of close contact (contagious for 24 hours after beginning antibiotic therapy for streptococci), and not sharing utensils or glasses in the home.
- Clients with recurrent pharyngitis will ask about tonsillectomy; review risks and benefits to help them make a decision.

Referral

CHILDREN. Complicated streptococcal pharyngitis, recurrent symptomatic pharyngitis, children in whom symptoms of rheumatic fever or glomerulonephritis develop.

ADULTS. Recurrent streptococcal pharyngitis may lead you to consider referral to ENT specialist. Referral to appropriate physician if complications develop.

PREGNANT WOMEN. Need to be referred to OB/GYN if culture is positive for streptococcal pharyngitis.

EVALUATION/FOLLOW-UP

- Recurrent streptococcal pharyngitis is defined as three cases in 6 months or six cases in 1 year.
- No follow-up is required if, after appropriate treatment, client has no symptoms.
- If client still has symptoms after 10-day course of antibiotics, reculture and treat appropriately.
- If streptococcal pharyngitis recurs, consider referral to ENT specialist for tonsillectomy.
- If client is carrier of streptococci but has no symptoms, consider eradication treatment in the following cases:
  —Family has a history of rheumatic fever.
  —Family has been passing streptococci back and forth to each other.
  —Family has high level of anxiety regarding streptococcal infection.
  —Outbreaks of streptococci have occurred or are occurring in closed or semiclosed communities.

—Tonsillectomy is being considered only because of carrier status of streptococcus.

NOTE: Eradication treatment is defined as complete eradication of the streptococcal bacteria. This is diagnosed by a negative throat culture result.

REFERENCES

Feldman, W. (1993). Pharyngitis in children. *Postgraduate Medicine, 93*(3), 141-145.

Gerber, M., Markowitz, M. (1992). Streptococcal pharyngitis: Clearing up the controversies. *Contemporary Pediatrics, 9*(9), 118-131.

Goroll, A., May, L., & Mulley, A., Jr. (1995). *Primary care medicine: Office evaluation and management the adult patient.* Philadelphia: J. B. Lippincott.

Hoelkelman, R. (1992). *Primary pediatric care:* St. Louis: Mosby.

Perkins, A. (1997). An approach to diagnosing the acute sore throat. *American Family Physician, 55*(1), 131-138.

Peter, J., & Haney, H. M. (1996). Infections of the oral cavity. *Pediatric Annals, 25*(10), 572-576.

Rakel, R. (1995). *Conn's current therapy.* Philadelphia: W. B. Saunders.

Ruoff, G. (1996). Recurrent streptococcal pharyngitis: Using practical treatment options to interrupt the cycle. *Postgraduate Medicine, 99*(2), 211-222.

REVIEW QUESTIONS

1. Which of the following clients would most likely have streptococcal pharyngitis?

   a. A 9-month-old infant with a decreased appetite and fever of 102° F
   b. A 7-year-old child with nausea and vomiting for 6 hours and fever of 102.5° F
   c. An adult with a fever of 102° F and complains of sore throat
   d. An older adult with no fever, enlarged cervical lymph nodes, but no sore throat

2. Which of the following statements is true regarding pharyngitis?

   a. A sore throat always requires antibiotic treatment.
   b. Streptococcal pharyngitis has a high likelihood of developing into rheumatic fever if left untreated.

   c. Bacterial pharyngitis is usually more painful and symptomatic than viral pharyngitis.
   d. The standard of treatment with pharyngitis is to do a throat culture to determine whether *Streptococcus pyogenes* is present.

3. When assessing a client with a complaint of a sore throat, the nurse practitioner would **not** include which of the following in the differential diagnosis?

   a. Mononucleosis, *Chlamydia,* and *Haemophilus influenzae*
   b. *Streptococcus pyogenes,* adenovirus, and herpes
   c. *Streptococcus* groups C and G, *Staphylococcus*
   d. Kawasaki disease, *Candida albicans,* and allergic rhinitis

4. A 27-year-old client comes to the clinic with a sore throat and tender cervical glands. She has a diagnosis of streptococcal pharyngitis and is given a prescription for amoxicillin 500 mg PO tid. Instructions given to the client include which of the following?

   a. She is contagious for 72 hours while taking the medication.
   b. Salt water gargles are not necessary because the antibiotic will alleviate the symptoms.
   c. She will feel immediate relief from the antibiotics (within 10 to 12 hours).
   d. She must take necessary precautions, such as good handwashing, to prevent the spread of the infection even though she is receiving antibiotics.

5. Eradication therapy for streptococcal pharyngitis is necessary if:

   a. The client has a history of frequent sore throats.
   b. There is a family history of rheumatic fever.
   c. The culture is positive for streptococci and the client has symptoms.
   d. The client has had a tonsillectomy.

ANSWERS AND RATIONALES

1. *Answer:* c (assessment/history/HEENT/NAS)

   Rationale: Infants rarely get streptococcal pharyngitis. Children often have presenting symptoms of nausea and vomiting and high fever. Adults most frequently experience significant pharyngeal pain, as do older adults (although they may not exhibit a fever).

2. *Answer:* d (assessment/physical examination/HEENT/NAS)

   Rationale: Many sore throats are caused by viruses, and very few cases of untreated streptococcal pharyngitis actually progress to rheumatic fever. Often the virus-induced sore throats are more painful than streptococcal pharyngitis, and a culture is necessary to determine whether antibiotic treatment is needed.

3. *Answer:* c (diagnosis/HEENT/NAS)

   Rationale: All the other diagnoses are appropriate in diagnosing pharyngitis. *Streptococcus* groups C and G are not concerns because they do not preclude rheumatic fever. *Staphylococcus* is not a common pathogen of pharyngitis.

4. *Answer:* d (plan/therapeutic management/HEENT/NAS)

   Rationale: The client is considered contagious for 24 hours after starting the antibiotic. Salt water gargles are beneficial to soothe inflamed pharyngeal tissue and can decrease the duration of the discomfort. It often takes 48 to 72 hours for the client to experience relief of symptoms after starting antibiotics. Handwashing is always important to prevent the spread of infectious illness.

5. *Answer:* b (evaluation/HEENT/NAS)

   Rationale: History of frequent sore throats does not mean it was streptococcal pharyngitis; it may have been caused by allergies, or other factors. Typically, a client who is a carrier of streptococci has no symptoms. Although the client may still have streptococcal pharyngitis develop after a tonsillectomy, the carrier state is rare after the surgery.

OTITIS

Otitis Media

OVERVIEW
Definition

Otitis media is an inflammation of the middle ear. Specifically, the middle ear becomes filled with fluid and pus, causing inflammation and bulging of the tympanic membrane. This condition is most often painful.

Incidence

Second only to URIs for largest number of office visits for children, otitis media accounts for 24.5 million pediatric visits per year. Peak incidence is 6 to 36 months; it is least frequent in the 4 to 7 year age group. Risk is greater for boys, children in day care, those whose parents smoke, and children who have not been breast-fed. Peak occurrence is October through April, with a decline in summer.

Classification

ACUTE OTITIS MEDIA. Lasts approximately 3 weeks. Typically rapid onset, but may be subtle or insidious. Tympanic membrane bulges and is erythematous, injected, and opaque. An effusion develops in the middle ear, causing poor tympanic membrane mobility.

SUBACUTE OTITIS MEDIA. Defined as acute otitis media that lasts 4 to 8 weeks. The tympanic membrane may remain purulent or have a serous appearance. The drum may continue to bulge slightly, retract, or even return to its normal position. Tympanic mobility is decreased as a result of effusion.

CHRONIC OTITIS MEDIA. Present longer than 8 weeks. Tympanic membrane is usually in retracted position. Effusion becomes thick and mucoid. Effusion may be clear or dark. Air bubbles signify a higher likelihood that the effusion will resolve; otherwise, referral to an ENT specialist for ventilation tube placement may be appropriate.

Pathophysiology

Otitis media typically follows a URI. The most accepted theory is that the eustachian tubes become blocked from chronic negative pressure. This leads to formulation of fluid or effusions in the middle ear.

RISK FACTORS
- Anatomic anomalies of the midface
- Eskimo, Latino, or Native American ethnicity
- Sibling or parent with chronic otitis
- Allergies, such as atopic dermatitis or asthma
- Day care attendance

COMMON PATHOGENS

Most Common
- *Streptococcus pneumoniae* (35%)
- *Haemophilus influenzae* (23%)
- *Moraxella catarrhalis* (14%)

Less Common
- *Pseudomonas aeruginosa*
- Group A and B streptococci
- *Staphylococcus aureus*
- *Escherichia coli*

ASSESSMENT: SUBJECTIVE/HISTORY

Symptoms

- Usually preceded by upper respiratory symptoms
- Otalgia: Often worse at night
- Otorrhea: Usually signifies rupture of the tympanic membrane
- Hearing loss corrected once the effusion resolves
- Fever absent in ⅓ of cases
- Diminished appetite
- Restless or little sleep
- Diarrhea or vomiting
- Tinnitus
- Infants: May pull at ears, although this is not a reliable sign because it can be habitual. Often will not suck on bottle or breast.
- Toddlers: Can often talk about ear pain.
- School-age children and adults: Primary symptom is ear pain.

- Older adults: Less common, but may not exhibit fever.

Past Medical History

Ask about infants who drink bottle while lying down, exposure to smoke, allergies (including atopic dermatitis and asthma), and any craniofacial abnormalities.

Medication History

Ask about recent use of antibiotics and any other medications.

Family History

Inquire about siblings or parents with frequent otitis, family history of allergies, or exposure to smoke.

Psychosocial History

Ask about frequent absences from school.

Dietary History

Otitis media may be associated with food allergies.

ASSESSMENT: OBJECTIVE/ PHYSICAL EXAMINATION

Physical Examination

- Vital signs (weight is needed for children for drug dosing purposes)
- Thorough examination of head, eyes, ears, nose, throat, heart, lungs, and skin
- Check tympanic membrane:
  —Acute otitis media: Membrane usually is erythematous, and the middle ear may contain fluid that is pink, red, or yellow (indicating pus). Membrane may be bulging and opaque and can perforate, leaving purulent drainage in the external canal.
  —Otitis media with effusion: Membrane may appear slightly thickened but without redness. Mobility is poor and fluid is clear. Air bubbles may also be seen.
  —Chronic otitis media: Drum often has a yellowish appearance (from pus). Membrane may or may not return to its normal position; mobility is poor.

Diagnostic Procedures

- Visual examination is primary diagnostic tool. Pneumatic otoscopy is an extremely valuable and simple procedure (eardrum will have poor mobility).
- Tympanometry can be helpful when used as adjunct to physical examination.
- CBC may show an increased WBC count, as with any illness, but usually it is not diagnostic and does not correlate with severity of illness.
- Culture of ear drainage is not routinely done because most common organisms can be predicted and result does not change treatment plan. If culture comes back showing no organism but client has symptoms and visual examination shows otitis, client still requires treatment.

DIAGNOSIS

Differential diagnosis includes the following:
- External otitis
- Cellulitis
- Malignant otitis
- Sinusitis
- Pharyngitis
- Tumor
- Older adults: Assess for problems caused by wearing hearing aid.

THERAPEUTIC PLAN
Pharmacologic Treatment

- Antibiotic therapy (10-day course)
  —First-line: Amoxicillin
  —Second-line: Trimethoprim-sulfamethoxazole, erythromycin-sulfisoxazole, amoxicillin-clavulanate, cefaclor, cefuroxime axetil, or cefixime. Indicated for resistant organisms, allergy to penicillins, treatment failure with amoxicillin, persistent otitis, and for prophylaxis when amoxicillin has been ineffective.
  —Prophylaxis: Amoxicillin or trimethoprim-sulfamethoxazole preferred. Dose is half of therapeutic dose given in single dose at bedtime. May be continued as long as 6 months. Need to recheck every month.
- Analgesic therapy:
  —Auralgan Otic Suspension
  —Acetaminophen or ibuprofen
  —Acetaminophen with codeine (if severe pain)

Client Education

- Complete full course of antibiotic.
- Side effects of medication may include upset stomach, allergic reactions, and others.
- Especially important to educate parents of nonverbal children.
- Recheck when antibiotic course is completed if nonverbal client or verbal client is still having symptoms.
- Avoid smoke exposure.
- For infants, avoid having them drink from bottle while lying down.
- Reassurance to parents that episodes of otitis diminish with time (as the eustachian tubes lengthen).
- Avoidance of water entering the ear for 7 days if perforated eardrum is present.

Referral

CHILDREN. Chronic otitis not relieved after antibiotic therapy; unresolved effusions; hearing loss; glue ear; delayed speech.

ADULTS. Persistent tinnitus or hearing loss; recurrent otitis.

EVALUATION/FOLLOW-UP

- Recurrent otitis is defined as six episodes by 6 years of age, five episodes in 1 year, or three episodes in 6 months.
- Recheck in office:
  —Acute/chronic otitis media—every 10 days while receiving antibiotics
  —Prophylaxis—every month while receiving antibiotics

External Otitis

OVERVIEW
Definition

External otitis is an infection of the external auditory canal. It can be local or diffuse.

Incidence

Affects all ages; occurs after swimming, aggressive cleaning of the canal, or trauma.

Pathophysiology

External otitis is usually caused by *Staphylococcus aureus*. Occasionally it is caused by *Pseudomonas aeruginosa*.

ASSESSMENT: SUBJECTIVE/HISTORY
Most Common Symptoms

- Otalgia
- Ear swelling
- Occasional hearing loss
- Severe tenderness when outer ear (pinna and tragus) is touched

Associated Symptoms

Usually localized to ear discomfort, but fever and nausea are also possible.

Past Medical History

- Previous occurrences of external otitis
- Hearing loss
- Hearing aids (can add to retention of moisture in canal)
- Use of steroids

Medication History

Inquire about recent use of antibiotics or any other medications.

Family History

This information is not usually significant.

ASSESSMENT: OBJECTIVE/ PHYSICAL EXAMINATION
Physical Examination

Include vital signs. Do thorough examination of head, eyes, nose, throat, heart, lungs, and skin. Focus on the ear:

- There is exquisite tenderness when pressure is placed on tragus or when pinna is moved.
- Ear canal is erythematous and inflamed, with moist debris present.
- May see furuncle.
- Tympanic membrane is usually normal (unless accompanied by otitis media).

Diagnostic Procedures

Diagnosis is based on the physical examination.

DIAGNOSIS

Differential diagnosis includes the following:
- Otitis media
- Malignant otitis externa
- Folliculitis

THERAPEUTIC PLAN
Pharmacologic Treatment

- Eardrops containing combinations of polymyxin, neomycin, hydrocortisone, and propylene glycol (Cortisporin Otic Suspension)
- Inserting a cotton wick into ear may facilitate contact of medication with the skin

Nonpharmacologic Treatment

- If furuncle is present, may require incision and drainage.
- If diffuse debris is present, may require cleaning of debris by manual removal or suctioning.

Prophylaxis

- Instillation of 2% acetic acid into external auditory canal twice daily and after each contact with water
- Thorough drying of external auditory canal after washing or wearing hearing aids can be helpful

Client Education

- Proper technique to clean ears and minimal use of cotton swabs or instruments to clean ears (to prevent trauma)
- Proper technique for instilling eardrops
- Avoidance of water in the ear for 7 days after infection

Referral

- Persistent otitis externa
- Hearing loss

EVALUATION/FOLLOW-UP

Follow-up is needed only if symptoms persist.

REFERENCES

Eden, A. N., Fireman, P., & Stook, S. E. (1996). Managing acute otitis: A fresh look at a familiar problem. *Contemporary Pediatrics, 13*(3), 64-93.

Facione, N. (1990). Otitis media: An overview of acute and chronic disease. *Nurse Practitioner, 15*(10), 11-22.

Goroll, A., May, L., & Mulley, A., Jr. (1995). *Primary care medicine: Office evaluation and management of the adult patient.* Philadelphia: J. B. Lippincott.

Hanson, M. J. (1996). Acute otitis media in children. *Nurse Practitioner, 21*(5), 72-80.

Hoekelman, R. (1992). *Primary pediatric care.* St. Louis: Mosby.

Rakel, R. (1995). *Conn's current therapy.* Philadelphia: W. B. Saunders.

Stevenson, L., & Brooke, D. S. (1995). Managing otitis media with effusion in young children. *Journal of Pediatric Health Care, 9*(1), 36-39.

Zenk, K. E., & Ma, H. (1990). Pharmacologic treatment of otitis media and sinusitis in pediatrics. *Journal of Pediatric Health Care, 4*(6), 297-303.

REVIEW QUESTIONS

1. A 6-year-old girl is brought in by her mother for treatment of an earache. The child's past medical history is negative except for 1 episode of streptococcal sore throat. The parents smoke in the home. Which of the following increases the likelihood that the child has otitis media?

a. Gender of the child
b. Exposure to secondhand smoke
c. Age of the child
d. Previous episode of streptococcal sore throat

2. Which of the following physical examination data would best help discriminate otitis media from otitis externa?

a. Hearing loss
b. Drainage, material in ear canal
c. Pain on examination of the ear
d. Decreased tympanic membrane motility

3. A parent asks the nurse practitioner whether her child should avoid water in the ear canal after a diagnosis of otitis media. The best response is:

a. This is not necessary, unless your child's eardrum perforates.
b. Your child should avoid water in the ear canal for 7 days.
c. Water in the ear canal may cause the infection to last longer.
d. Use ear plugs during bathing.

4. A child with recurrent otitis media should be placed on a prophylactic regimen. The drug of choice is:

a. Erythromycin
b. Trimethoprim-sulfamethoxazole (Bactrim)
c. Biaxin
d. Augmentin

5. Clients with which of the following should be referred?

a. Otitis media with initial effusion
b. Speech delay
c. Acute otitis externa
d. Prophylactic therapy for otitis media

ANSWERS AND RATIONALES

1. *Answer:* b (assessment/history/HEENT/child)
Rationale: Boys have shorter eustachian tubes than girls do and are at a higher risk for otitis media. The incidence decreases at age 4 years. A previous episode of streptococcal sore throat would not be relevant unless it was recent (within 1 month). (Facione, 1990)

2. *Answer:* d (assessment/physical examination/ HEENT/child)
Rationale: Both conditions can result in hearing loss. If the tympanic membrane ruptures in otitis media, material may be in the ear canal. Although pain on manipulation of the tragus is classic for otitis externa, pain on manipulation of the ear can be present in both conditions. In otitis externa the tympanic membrane is normal. (Goroll, May, & Mulley, 1995)

3. *Answer:* a (plan/nonpharmacologic/HEENT/child)
Rationale: Only in otitis externa and otitis media with perforation is water in the ear canal avoided for at least 7 days. (Eden, Fireman, & Stook, 1996)

4. *Answer:* b (plan/pharmacologic/HEENT/child)
Rationale: Bactrim and amoxicillin are the preferred drugs for prophylaxis. (Rakel, 1995)

5. *Answer:* b (plan/nonpharmacologic/HEENT/ child)
Rationale: Recurrent ear infections can produce scarring and hearing loss, which leads to speech delays. The other situations do not require referral. Clients undergoing prophylactic therapy need monthly rechecks. (Hoekelman, 1992)

SINUSITIS: ACUTE AND CHRONIC

OVERVIEW
Definition

Sinusitis is defined as inflammation of the mucous lining of the paranasal sinuses.

Acute sinusitis is a symptomatic sinus infection lasting up to 3 weeks. *Chronic sinusitis* is a symptomatic sinus infection that persists for longer than 3 weeks, despite adequate treatment.

Incidence

This common health problem is prevalent in *all ages* and equally prevalent in both sexes. In fall, winter, and spring, it usually follows a viral URI; in summer, it is often associated with swimming and diving or allergic rhinitis.

Pathophysiology

PROTECTIVE FACTORS. A protective mucous blanket traps bacteria and other irritants, covers the respiratory cilia, and is most consistent along predetermined pathways to the sinus ostia.

FACTORS INCREASING SUSCEPTIBILITY. Any interference with the normal cleansing of the mucosal cilia. Causes include the following:
- Response to a virus, bacterium, or allergen
- Fungal infestation
- Mechanical obstruction
- Trauma
- Air pollution, tobacco smoke, or low humidity

COMMON PATHOGENS. Similar pathogens occur in adults and children.
- *Streptococcus pneumoniae* (35%) and *Haemophilus influenzae* (35%)
- *Moraxella catarrhalis* (5%), a common cause in children
- *Streptococcus pyogenes* and α-hemolytic streptococcus (10%)
- Viruses (9%)
- Chronic: Anaerobic bacteria; *Staphylococcus aureus;* pathogens often opportunistic

ASSESSMENT: SUBJECTIVE/HISTORY
Most Common Symptoms

Persistent symptoms of URI for more than 10 days that have not begun to abate:

ACUTE SYMPTOMS. Nasal discharge (serous, mucous mucopurulent), cough, tooth or facial pain, pain with chewing, sore throat, decreased or loss of sense of smell, a metallic taste in the mouth, and headaches often worse at night and early in the morning.

CHRONIC SYMPTOMS. Same as acute sinusitis, but lasting longer than 30 days.

CHILDREN. Often have more nonspecific complaints than adults. Suspect sinusitis if URI symptoms persist beyond 10 days without improvement, especially with persistent cough; the child with URI seems sicker than usual with high fever and has purulent nasal drainage and periorbital swelling; the allergic child has an acute exacerbation of respiratory symptoms.

Associated Symptoms

Early morning periorbital edema; fever; malaise; increased pain while coughing, bending forward, and making sudden head movement.

Past Medical History

Ask about history of diabetes, asthma, or immunosuppression; a seasonal relationship with symptoms; allergies; recent nose trauma, dental work or URI; and past sinusitis episodes and treatments.

Medication History

Inquire about recent use of antibiotics, steroids, decongestants, nasal sprays, or antihistamines.

Family History

Ask about a family history of asthma, allergies, and chronic sinusitis.

Psychosocial History

CHILDREN. Inquire whether a smoker resides in the household; ask about household pets.

ADULTS. Ask whether client is a smoker or whether a smoker resides in the household; ask about household pets.

ASSESSMENT: OBJECTIVE/ PHYSICAL EXAMINATION

Physical Examination

A problem-oriented physical examination should be conducted with particular attention to the following:

VITAL SIGNS. Include temperature.

EYES. Look for allergic shiners or periorbital edema.

NASAL MUCOSA. Assess for color, edema, and mucopurulent discharge. Look for polyps and patency of both nares. Examine structures of the nasal septum.

EARS, THROAT, AND MOUTH. Look for signs of inflammation.

FRONTAL AND MAXILLARY SINUSES. Look for pain on percussion and inability to transilluminate.

MAXILLARY TEETH. Percuss to check for a dental source of maxillary sinusitis.

NECK AND JAW. Assess for lymphadenopathy.

HEART AND LUNGS. Auscultate.

Diagnostic Procedures

- None are indicated for typical presentation.
- Sinus x-rays for refractory cases—a Waters plain radiographic view: Air-fluid level or complete opacification of the sinuses and thickening of the mucosal lining are most diagnostic.
- CT scan is indicated for chronic sinusitis.
- Allergy testing may be indicated.

DIAGNOSIS

Differential diagnosis includes the following:
- Rhinitis: Allergic, vasomotor, or viral
- Dental abnormality, abscesses, or peridontitis
- URI
- Cluster or migraine headaches
- Nasal polyps
- Foreign body (especially children)
- Tumor
- Temporal arteritis

THERAPEUTIC PLAN

Goals are management of infection, establishment of drainage, and relief of pain.

Pharmacologic Treatment

- Antimicrobial agents
  —For chronic sinusitis, use the same antibiotics but extend the therapy for 3 to 4 weeks.
  —Choice of antibiotics, first considerations: Amoxicillin-clavulanate, erythromycin-sulfisoxazole, cefuroxime, cefpodoxime proxetil, and loracarbef.
- Decongestants
  —Topical decongestants (Afrin or Neo-Synephrine spray) should not be used for more than 3 or 4 days.
  —Oral decongestants are used in combination with mucolytics (Humibid, Zephrex, Entex).
- Analgesics and antipyretics

Client Education

- Humidify the air. Increase fluid intake.
- Use steam inhalation and apply warm compresses to the face.
- Avoid swimming and diving during the acute phase.
- Encourage smoking cessation.
- Avoid allergens.

Referral

ENT referral is indicated for recurrent sinusitis or complications of acute sinusitis.

EVALUATION/FOLLOW-UP

- Instruct client to return if no improvement within 48 hours or swelling develops in the periorbital area.
- Schedule return visit in 10 to 14 days.

REFERENCES

Baker, R. (1996). *Handbook of pediatric primary care.* Boston: Little, Brown.

Evans, K. (1994). Diagnosis and management of sinusitis. *British Medical Journal, 300,* 1415-1422.

Schwartz, R. (1994). The diagnosis and management of sinusitis. *Nurse Practitioner, 19*(12), 58-63.

Uphold, C., Graham, M. (1994). *Clinical guidelines in family practice.* Gainesville, FL: Barmarrae Books.

Wilder, B. (1996). Management of sinusitis. *Journal of the American Academy of Nurse Practitioners, 8*(11), 525-529.

REVIEW QUESTIONS

1. Risk factors for the development of acute sinusitis include:

    a. A family history of diabetes
    b. Recent antibiotic therapy
    c. Allergic rhinitis
    d. A history of migraine headaches

Situation: *A 20-year-old male college student reports having had a "cold" for 3 weeks. His symptoms are yellow nasal discharge, facial pain increased with bending over, and a low-grade fever. He has no known allergies. Family history shows a sister with asthma and a father with chronic sinusitis. Vital signs and ears are normal. Nasal mucosa are erythematous with yellow discharge. Pharynx appears benign. Sinuses are tender to percussion.*

2. Your tentative diagnosis is acute sinusitis. What additional information would be helpful in confirming your diagnosis?

    a. Time of the year
    b. Client's eating habits
    c. Client's smoking history
    d. Impaired light transmission of maxillary sinuses

3. Major signs and symptoms for a diagnosis of sinusitis include:

    a. Purulent nasal discharge
    b. Facial pain
    c. URI symptoms beyond 10 days
    d. All of the above

4. In addition to antibiotics, which other medications are necessary for the treatment of acute sinusitis?

    a. Antifungals
    b. Antihistamines
    c. Decongestants
    d. Antihistamine-decongestant combinations

5. Sue, a 33-year-old woman, returns 1 week after being seen for sinusitis with complications of acute sinusitis. Her treatment should include:

    a. Antifungal medication
    b. Antihistamines
    c. EENT referral
    d. Nasal irrigation

6. Which of the following symptoms are more indicative of acute sinusitis?

    a. Maxillary sinus pain, vomiting, and diarrhea
    b. Cluster headaches, clear nasal discharge, and diffuse wheezes
    c. Periorbital edema, purulent nasal discharge, and cough
    d. Productive cough, chest congestion, and rhonchi

7. To confirm your suspicions of sinusitis in a refractory case, which of the following tests is most reliable?

    a. CBC with differential
    b. Sinus x-rays, Waters view
    c. Sedimentation rate
    d. Serum complement

8. Client education for a 23-year-old client with acute sinusitis should include all the following **except:**

    a. Smoking cessation
    b. Warm compresses to the face
    c. Humidify the air
    d. Antihistamines

ANSWERS AND RATIONALES

1. *Answer:* c (assessment/history/HEENT/NAS)
    Rationale: Allergic rhinitis is a risk factor for the development of sinusitis because it interferes with the normal cleansing of the mucosal cilia. Diabetes, recent antibiotic therapy, and migraine headaches do not. (Wilder, 1996)

2. *Answer:* d (assessment/physical examination/HEENT/adult)
    Rationale: Impaired light transmission of maxillary sinuses is diagnostic for maxillary sinusitis. The other choices are not. (Uphold & Graham, 1994)

3. *Answer:* d (diagnosis/HEENT/NAS)
    Rationale: All choices are major signs and symptoms of sinusitis. (Uphold & Graham, 1994)

4. *Answer:* c (plan/management/therapeutics/pharmacologic/HEENT/NAS)
    Rationale: Decongestants are considered a necessary part of the treatment plan because they thin secretions; thus sinus drainage is enhanced. (Wilder, 1996)

5. *Answer:* c (evaluation/HEENT/adult)

Rationale: EENT referral is indicated for complications of acute sinusitis. (Uphold & Graham, 1994; Wilder, 1996)

6. *Answer:* c (assessment/history/HEENT/NAS)

Rationale: Periorbital edema, purulent nasal discharge, and cough are frequently seen in both acute and chronic sinusitis. Vomiting, diarrhea, diffuse wheezes, and rhonchi may or may not. (Baker, 1996; Uphold & Graham, 1994)

7. *Answer:* b (diagnosis/HEENT/NAS)

Rationale: Sinus x-rays in the Waters view are specific for sinusitis. The others are not. (Evans, 1994)

8. *Answer:* d (plan/management/client education/NAS)

Rationale: All are client education recommendations except for antihistamines, which dry out the secretions and are not recommended in the treatment of sinusitis. (Uphold & Graham, 1994)

STRABISMUS

OVERVIEW
Definition

Strabismus is a deviation of one or both of the eyes. The eyes fail to stay in alignment. Strabismus may be *manifest* (occurs under binocular conditions) or *latent* (occurs only under monocular conditions). Manifest deviations can be intermittent, constant, alternating, or unilateral.

Incidence

Five percent of children have strabismus.

Pathophysiology

Healthy neonates often have intermittent and/or alternating strabismus. Proper alignment is not established until approximately the first month of age. An intermittent exotropia ("walleye") can be normal until 6 months of age. Esotropia ("cross-eye") is more often a sign of a pathologic condition and would be significant if noted after 2 months of age. If the condition persists, a loss of vision (amblyopia) can result from suppression of the image in the deviating eye.

Etiology

Strabismus can be caused by a blow to the head, disease, heredity, or a malfunction of the muscles that move the eyes.

ASSESSMENT: SUBJECTIVE/HISTORY

- Parental report of deviation of the eye
- Complaint of squinting
- Complaint of visual difficulties
- Parental report of school problems

ASSESSMENT: OBJECTIVE/PHYSICAL EXAMINATION
Physical Examination

ESOTROPIA OR EXOTROPIA. If either condition is found on examination, note whether it is intermittent, constant, or alternating (i.e., asymmetrical light reflex).

ABNORMAL RESULT OF HIRSCHBERG TEST. This corneal reflex test is performed by projecting a light source onto the cornea of both eyes at the same time that the child looks straight ahead. The positions of the light reflex in each eye are compared. If the eyes are in proper alignment, the light reflex will be in the same location on the cornea of each eye. If they are not, the test result is positive for strabismus.

ABNORMAL RESULT OF COVER/UNCOVER TEST. This is the only test for latent strabismus. To perform the cover/uncover test, have the child look at a distant object. Cover one eye and watch for movement of the uncovered eye (movement of the uncovered eye when alternate eye is covered). If no movement occurs, there is no apparent misalignment of that eye. Repeat test with the other eye.

ABNORMAL RESULT OF SNELLEN OR OTHER VISUAL ACUITY TEST. Record this information.

DIAGNOSIS

Differential diagnosis is pseudostrabismus (can easily be ruled out by the Hirschberg test).

THERAPEUTIC PLAN

Immediate referral to an ophthalmologist is necessary for the following:

- A child of any age with a constant or fixed deviation
- A child 6 months of age or older with intermittent exotropia
- A child 2 months of age or older with intermittent esotropia.

Treatment by the ophthalmologist depends on the etiology of the strabismus but may involve patching, corrective lens, and/or surgery. Speed of intervention helps to increase changes of an optimal outcome with full restoration of vision.

EVALUATION/FOLLOW-UP

Assess parent's and child's compliance and understanding of treatment and follow-up treatment recommended by the ophthalmologist.

REFERENCES

Burns, C., Barber, N., Brady, M., & Dunn, A. (1996). *Pediatric primary care: A handbook for nurse practitioners.* Philadelphia: W. B. Saunders.

Essman, S., & Essman, T. (1992). Screening for pediatric eye disease. *American Family Physician, 46*(4), 1243-1252.

Nelson, W. (1996) *Textbook of Pediatrics.* Philadelphia: W. B. Saunders.

REVIEW QUESTIONS

1. A deviation of one or both of the eyes in which the eyes fail to stay in alignment is:

   a. Myopia
   b. Conjunctivitis
   c. Strabismus
   d. Ptosis

2. Latent strabismus:

   a. Occurs under binocular conditions
   b. Occurs under monocular conditions
   c. Can be intermittent or constant
   d. Can be alternating or unilateral

3. Esotropia is:

   a. Cross-eye
   b. Walleye
   c. Eyes deviated outward
   d. Eyes deviated downward

4. Eyes deviated outward is:

   a. Hyperopia
   b. Exotropia
   c. Esotropia
   d. Myopia

5. Loss of vision from suppression of the image in the deviating eye in strabismus is:

   a. Corneal abrasion
   b. Astigmatism
   c. Amblyopia
   d. Ocular trauma

6. Consider strabismus if the parents report:

   a. A droopy eyelid
   b. A lazy eye or wandering eye
   c. A cloudy lens
   d. Staring spells

7. To screen for latent strabismus perform the:

   a. Hirschberg test
   b. Snellen test
   c. Cover/uncover test
   d. Bruckner test

8. To rule out pseudostrabismus, perform the:

   a. Hirschberg test
   b. Snellen test
   c. Cover/uncover test
   d. Bruckner test

9. Immediate referral to an ophthalmologist is necessary for a child:

   a. Of any age with a constant or fixed deviation
   b. Younger than 6 months with intermittent exotropia
   c. Younger than 2 months with intermittent esotropia
   d. Of any age with alternating deviation

10. A child 3 months of age with intermittent esotropia should be managed as follows:

   a. Continue to observe until 6 months of age.
   b. Immediate referral is necessary.
   c. Ask parents to call if it becomes fixed.
   d. Reassure the parents that this is normal.

ANSWERS AND RATIONALES

1. Answer: c (diagnosis/HEENT/NAS)
Rationale: The definition of strabismus is a deviation of one or both eyes in which the eyes fail to stay in alignment. (Burns, 1996)

2. Answer: b (diagnosis/HEENT/NAS)
Rationale: Latent strabismus occurs under monocular conditions only. (Burns, 1996)

3. Answer: a (diagnosis/HEENT/NAS)
Rationale: The definition of esotropia is cross-eye, or the deviation of the eyes inward. (Burns, 1996)

4. Answer: b (diagnosis/HEENT/NAS)
Rationale: Eyes deviating outward (walleye) is exotropia. (Burns, 1996)

5. Answer: c (diagnosis/HEENT/NAS)
Rationale: The loss of vision from suppression of the image in the deviating eye in strabismus is called *amblyopia.* (Essman, 1992)

6. Answer: b (assessment/history/HEENT/NAS)
Rationale: The report of a lazy or wandering eye is often an indication of strabismus. (Essman, 1992)

7. Answer: c (assessment/physical examination/HEENT/NAS)
Rationale: The cover/uncover test is one of the few tests for strabismus that reveals latent strabismus. (Nelson, 1996)

8. Answer: a (assessment/physical examination/HEENT/NAS)
Rationale: Pseudostrabismus can be ruled out with the Hirschberg test. With pseudostrabismus, the light reflex will be in the same location on the cornea of each eye. (Nelson, 1996)

9. Answer: a (plan/management/therapeutic/HEENT/child)
Rationale: A child of any age with fixed or constant strabismus needs immediate referral to an ophthalmologist. This would be indicative of a more problematic form of strabismus. (Essman, 1992)

10. Answer: b (plan/management/therapeutic/HEENT/infant)
Rationale: A child 3-months old with intermittent esotropia should receive an immediate referral to an ophthalmologist because of the increased complication rate with esotropia. (Essman, 1992)

UPPER RESPIRATORY TRACT INFECTIONS

Common Cold, Pharyngitis, Epiglottitis and Croup

Common Cold

OVERVIEW
Definition

A *cold* is a mild, self-limited viral syndrome involving the upper respiratory tract mucosa.

Incidence

The most common acute illness in the industrialized world, a cold is highly contagious. It is a common cause for seeking medical attention and for absences from work and school. The number of colds per year tends to decrease with age:

- Infants and preschool children: 4 to 8 per year
- School-age children: 2 to 6 per year
- Adults: 2 to 4 per year
- In households with children, adults tend to have higher rates, with the mother having more than the father.

Pathophysiology

The source of the common cold is viral.
TRANSMISSION
- Direct physical contact: Nasal mucosa to hand to another person's hand to eyes or nasal membranes
- Large and small droplets produced by cough or sneeze
COMMON PATHOGENS
- Most common

—Rhinoviruses: Fall, mid-spring to summer
—Coronaviruses: Winter
- Common
  —Parainfluenza: Fall, spring
  —Respiratory syncytial virus: Winter to early spring
  —Influenza: Winter
- Infants
  —RSV
  —Rhinovirus

ASSESSMENT: SUBJECTIVE/HISTORY
Symptoms

24-78 HOURS
- Dry, scratchy throat
- Clear nasal discharge
- Malaise
- Sneezing
- Loss of taste and smell
- Low-grade fever
- Redness and inflammation of nasal and pharyngeal membranes

4-7 DAYS
- Cough
- Hoarseness
- Thickening of nasal drainage

NEONATES. Minimal respiratory signs and symptoms; nonspecific signs: poor feeding and lethargy; severe sign: unexpected apnea episodes.

INFANTS. Anorexia, vomiting, and diarrhea.

CHILDREN. Filling of eustachian tubes, causing obstruction and ear pain.

SMOKERS. Symptoms usually worse with same outcome.

Past Medical History
This history is usually noncontributory.

Psychosocial History
- Day care or school attendance
- Children in the home
- Smoker, or exposure to secondhand smoke
- Recent exposure to others with cold symptoms

ASSESSMENT: OBJECTIVE/ PHYSICAL EXAMINATION
Physical Examination
A problem-oriented examination should be performed with special emphasis on the following:

- Tympanic membranes
- Mucous membranes
- Lymph nodes
- Breath sounds

Infants and Children
Look for signs and symptoms of dehydration.

Diagnostic Procedures
- Sputum culture is done if copious amount of sputum; consider acid-fast bacilli (AFB) if tuberculosis is in the differential diagnosis.
- CBC is measured if temperature is elevated.
- Sinus x-rays are taken if increased nasal congestion with sinus tenderness is present.
- It is difficult and unnecessary to identify the causative virus for management of the common cold.

DIAGNOSIS
Differential diagnosis may include the following:
- Pharyngitis
- Influenza
- Allergic rhinitis
- Lactose intolerance leads to URI symptoms in infants.

Complications
NEWBORN TO 3 YEARS. Otitis media is associated 29% of the time.

INFANTS. Sudden infant death syndrome (SIDS): 90% of the infants dead of SIDS had cold symptoms reported before death.

ADULTS AND CHILDREN. Exacerbation of obstructive sleep apnea, disturbed sleep patterns, and bronchospasms are possible.

THERAPEUTIC PLAN
Pharmacologic Treatment
ASPIRIN, IBUPROFEN, OR ACETAMINOPHEN. Relieves body aches and fever.
- Aspirin and acetaminophen have been shown to excrete the virus more quickly from the mucous membranes.
- Aspirin products are not recommended in children younger than 16 years.
- Tylenol is the only recommended medication in pregnancy.

ANTIHISTAMINES
- Chlorpheniramine
  —Action: Reduces sneezing, nasal mucous production.
  —Side effects: Drowsiness
- Diphenhydramine (Benadryl)
  —Action: Does not differ from placebo effect.
  —Side effects: Drowsiness
- Triprolidine (Actifed)
  —Action: Does not differ from placebo effect.
  —Side effects: None
- Astemizole (Hismanal)
  —Action: Treats seasonal allergic rhinitis.
  —Side effects: Weight gain

DECONGESTANTS
- Pseudoephedrine/phenylephrine spray or oral preparations
  —Action: Reduces congestion, sneezing.
  —Side effects: Tachycardia, palpitations, elevated diastolic blood pressure, fatigue, dizziness, bladder outlet obstruction
- Oxymetazoline spray (Dristan, Afrin)
  —Action: Improves nasal symptoms.
  —Side effects: Rebound nasal congestion

EXPECTORANTS
- Guaifenesin
  —Action: Thins sputum; does not reduce cough.
  —Side effects: None

ANTICHOLINERGICS
- Ipratropium spray (Atrovent aerosol)
  —Action: Reduces sneezing and nasal discharge.
  —Side effects: Dry throat

COMBINATIONS
- Decongestant-antihistamine
  —Action: Decreases congestion, postnasal drip, rhinorrhea.
  —Side effects: Dry mouth, nervousness, insomnia

STEROIDS
- Steroids (Medrol Dose Pack)
  —Action: Reduces inflammation (e.g., vocal cords).
  —Side effects: Weight gain, mood alteration

Nonpharmacologic Treatment

- Bed rest is not necessary for a more rapid recovery.
- Steam or cool mist: Liquefies nasal secretions.
- Chicken noodle soup: Studies have shown that chicken soup helps to clear nasal secretions.
- Voice rest: Helps to decrease inflammation of vocal cords, which decreases hoarseness.

Client Education

- Avoid touching nasal or eye membranes.
- Wash hands after sneezing, coughing, or blowing nose.
- Throw tissues away.
- Cover nose and mouth during sneeze or cough.
- Avoid crowds.
- Do not use nasal preparations for longer than 5 days to avoid rebound congestion.
- Clean toothbrushes or purchase new ones.
- Clean pillow linens.
- Use well-dried pillows (viruses may remain in humid droplets).

Referral

INFANTS. Infants with apnea episodes should be admitted for observation and evaluation and treatment of RSV.

CHILDREN AND OLDER ADULTS. Hospitalization may be required if pneumonia develops.

EVALUATION/FOLLOW-UP

- Worsening of symptoms
- Increase in fever
- Difficulty breathing, wheezing
- Color change of nasal drainage or sputum

Pharyngitis

OVERVIEW
Definition

Pharyngitis is an inflammation and pain within the oropharynx area.

Incidence

Pharyngitis tends to be one of the most common diseases treated by primary care providers in the

United States. It is the fourth most common symptom seen and accounts for nearly 40 million primary care visits each year.

Pathophysiology

- Bacterial and viral pathogens
- Spread by person-to person contact by droplets of oral, respiratory, and nasal secretions

COMMON PATHOGENS

Adults

- Most common
  - —Beta-hemolytic streptococci groups A (10% to 15%)
  - —*Mycoplasma pneumoniae*
  - —*Chlamydia pneumoniae*
  - —Influenza type A and B
  - —Parainfluenza
  - —Epstein-Barr virus
  - —Adenovirus
  - —Herpes simplex virus
  - —Enteroviruses
- Less common
  - —Beta-hemolytic streptococci groups (groups C and G)
  - —*Corynebacterium diphtheriae*
  - —*Neisseria gonorrhoeae*
  - —*Neisseria meningitidis*
  - —*Haemophilus influenzae*
  - —RSV

Children

- Most common
  - —Beta-hemolytic streptococci , group A
    Age younger than 2 years, 3%
    Age 5 to 10 years, most common cause
  - —Influenza A and B
  - —Parainfluenza
  - —Adenoviruses
  - —Herpes simplex virus
  - —Epstein-Barr virus
- Less common
  - —RSV
  - —Rhinovirus
  - —Coronaviruses
  - —Cytomegalovirus
  - —Rubeola
  - —Rubella
  - —*Candida* species
  - —*Toxoplasma gondii*

ASSESSMENT: SUBJECTIVE/HISTORY

Most Common Symptoms

- Generally clients have complaints of fever, sore throat, tender cervical nodes, cough, and general malaise.
- Children may have abdominal pain, nausea, and vomiting.
- Infants may have excoriated nares.

Associated Symptoms

GROUP A STREPTOCOCCUS. Tonsillar exudate (yellow or creamy white).

GROUP C STREPTOCOCCUS. Fever >101° F (38.3° C).

MYCOPLASMA PNEUMONIAE. Nonproductive cough, fever, alveolar infiltrates of the lower lobes.

HAEMOPHILUS INFLUENZAE. Associated with otitis media, epiglottitis, meningitis; usually seen in children.

CORYNEBACTERIUM DIPHTHERIAE. Blue-white or grayish pharyngeal membranes, cervical lymphadenopathy, peripheral neuritis.

NEISSERIA GONORRHOEAE. Urethritis, vaginal itching and/or discharge.

INFLUENZA VIRUS. Headache, myalgia.

EPSTEIN-BARR VIRUS. Mononucleosis syndrome.

CYTOMEGALOVIRUS. Splenomegaly, hepatitis, and aseptic meningitis.

Past Medical History

- Previous streptococcal infections
- Autoimmune disease
- STDs
- Rheumatic fever
- Diabetes

Medication History

- Recent use of antibiotics and other medications
- Drug allergies

Family History

- Recent pharyngeal infections
- History of rheumatic fever

Psychosocial History

- Attendance in school or day care
- Living conditions (crowded)
- Smoking history

- Sexual exposures
- Drug use

Dietary History

Ask about recent decrease in oral intake, especially in young children as a result of pain.

ASSESSMENT: OBJECTIVE/ PHYSICAL EXAMINATION

Physical Examination

A problem-oriented physical examination should be conducted with special attention paid to the following:

- Vital signs
- Respiratory effort
- General appearance
- Hydration

THROAT. Erythema, color of exudate, breath odor.

NECK. Cervical and submandibular nodes.

EARS. External otitis, otitis media.

NOSE. Drainage, excoriated nares (infants).

SKIN. Rashes, lesions.

Diagnostic Procedures

- Rapid streptococcal screen
  —Sensitivity: 95% to 99%
  —Specificity: 70% to 90%
  If positive, confirms diagnosis; if negative, do throat culture
- Chocolate agar culture: Suspected gonorrhea
- Tzank smear: Ulcer base scraping for suspected herpes
- Monospot: Suspected mononucleosis
- CBC with differential if elevated fever
- Electrolytes with BUN and creatinine if decrease in oral intake or urine output

DIAGNOSIS

Differential diagnosis may include the following:

- Streptococcal infection
- Common cold
- Influenza
- Infectious mononucleosis
- Herpangina
- Herpetic pharyngitis
- *Mycoplasma*
- Acute HIV infection
- Diphtheria

- *Yersinia*
- *Candida*
- Synthetic lupus erythematosus
- Vincent's angina

THERAPEUTIC PLAN

Pharmacologic Treatment

GENERAL. Acetaminophen or ibuprofen for fever and pain.

VIRAL. Symptomatic and warm salt-water gargle.

STREPTOCOCCAL

- Aim of treatment is to attempt to reduce the risk of rheumatic fever, sinusitis, otitis, and glomerulonephritis.
- Adults
  —Penicillin G benzathine: 1.2 million U IM (if at high risk for rheumatic fever, repeat once a week for 4 weeks)
  —Penicillin V: 125 to 250 mg PO bid for 10 days
  —Sulfadiazine: 250 mg PO qid for 10 days (if allergic to penicillin)
- Children
  —Penicillin VK: 25 to 50 mg/kg/day PO in divided doses every 6 hours for 10 days (250 mg PO bid has also been shown effective)
  —Penicillin G benzathine: IM one time only:
    <30 kg: 300,000 U
    31-60 kg: 600,000 U
    61-90 kg: 900,000 U
    >91 kg: 1,200,000 U
  —Erythromycin: 30 to 50 mg/kg/day PO in divided doses every 8 hours for 10 days (10 mg/kg PO every 12 hours has also been shown effective)
  —Erythromycin estolate (has less gastric upset and covers *Chlamydia*): 30 to 50 mg/kg/day PO in divided doses every 6 to 8 hours for 10 days
  —Cefadroxil (Duricef): 30 mg/kg PO every day for 10 days

GONORRHEA

- Ceftriaxone: 250 mg IM one time
- Erythromycin: 500 mg PO qid for 10 days

MYCOPLASMA OR DIPHTHERIA

- Erythromycin: 500 mg PO qid for 10 days
- Penicillin G: 1 g PO qid for 10 days

Client Education

- Rest.
- Drink fluids to stay hydrated.
- Cover mouth and nose during cough or sneeze.
- Wash hands after cough or sneeze.
- Avoid crowds.
- Dispose of tissues properly.

Referral

OTOLARYNGOLOGY

- Multiple recurrent episodes for possible tonsillectomy
- Severe episode of pharyngitis
- Suspected abscess formation

HOSPITALIZATION

- Inability to maintain hydration
- Risk of sudden airway obstruction
- IV antibiotic therapy if unable to take oral antibiotics because of airway obstruction, difficulty swallowing, or persistent nausea and vomiting
- Surgical intervention (drainage of abscess)

EVALUATION/FOLLOW-UP

- Continued fever
- Inability to swallow medications
- Development of new symptoms
- Recurrent pharyngitis (more than four times in 12 months)

Epiglottitis and Croup

OVERVIEW
Definition

Epiglottitis is a rapidly developing, life-threatening bacterial infection of the supraglottic area. A true medical emergency, it may or may not be proceeded by a URI syndrome.

Croup is an acute viral inflammatory disease of the subglottic mucosa. It is usually proceeded by a viral URI.

Incidence

- Croup is at least 10 times more common than epiglottitis.
- Croup is most common in the fall and winter months, peaking between October and December.
- Croup is the most common cause of stridor in young children.
- Croup rarely occurs in infants younger than 1 month and school-age children.
- The most common age group is 6 months to 3 years; incidence declines with age.
- Boys are at higher risk than girls.
- Croup is generally self-limited; epiglottitis is not.
- Epiglottitis is rare and generally occurs in children aged 2 to 6 years. Adult cases do occur and are most often seen between the second and fourth decade of life.
- Epiglottitis can occur at any time of the year and is most often seen in temperate climates.

Pathophysiology

COMMON PATHOGENS

- Croup
  —Parainfluenza virus, type 1 (most common)
  —Parainfluenza virus, type 3
  —RSV
  —Adenoviruses
  —Rubeola
  —Influenza
- Epiglottitis
  —*Haemophilus influenzae:* The incidence is decreasing in children with the use of the *Haemophilus influenzae* vaccine, whereas the incidence is increasing in adults.

ASSESSMENT: SUBJECTIVE/HISTORY
Most Common Symptoms

CROUP

- Low-grade fever
- Rhinorrhea
- Barking cough, especially during the night

EPIGLOTTITIS

- High fever
- Drooling, difficulty swallowing
- Children: Possible presenting symptoms of URI symptoms, sore throat, and voice change
- Infants: Possible nonclassic presentation with URI symptoms, croupy cough, and low-grade fever

Associated Symptoms

CROUP

- URI symptoms
- Hoarse voice
- Inspiratory and/or expiratory stridor

Table 1-1 Comparison of Signs: Croup and Epiglottitis

	CROUP	EPIGLOTTITIS
Throat	Normal appearing epiglottis	"Cherry red" epiglottis
Appearance	Nontoxic	Toxic
Temperature	<103° F (39.5° C)	High >103° F (39.5° C)
Breath sounds	Good air movement	Decreased air movement
Positioning	Variable	"Tripod" sitting

EPIGLOTTITIS
- Toxic looking
- Muffled voice
- Dysphagia
- Inspiratory stridor
- Sitting position preferred

Past Medical History

- Recent viral infections
- Exposures
- Allergies
- Medications
- Immunization status

Family History

Inquire about any recent illness.

Psychosocial History

- School or day care exposure
- Smoking
- Profession (possible exposure to inhaled irritants such as paints, chemicals, dust particles, and smoke)

Dietary History

Ask about decreased oral intake.

ASSESSMENT: OBJECTIVE/ PHYSICAL EXAMINATION

CAUTION: *Ensure that the airway is not compromised before proceeding with any physical examination.*

Physical Examination

CAUTION: *Have emergency life support equipment available.*

A problem-oriented physical examination should be conducted with particular attention to the following:
- Airway compromise
- Vital signs
- General appearance
- Respiratory status
- Ears
- Nose
- Lymph nodes

Diagnostic Procedures

CAUTION: *Diagnostic procedures should not be attempted until the airway is secured.*

LATERAL NECK X-RAY
- Croup: Normal epiglottis, with narrowing of the subepiglottis area
- Epiglottitis: "Thumbprint" sign consistent with inflammation of the epiglottis (children near C2-3; adults near C5-6)

CBC WITH DIFFERENTIAL
- Croup: Within normal limits
- Epiglottitis: WBC count 10,000 to 25,000 cells/mm³ with elevated bands

ABGS AND PULSE OXIMETRY
- Croup and epiglottitis: Results variable, depending on the degree of respiratory distress

BLOOD CULTURES. Assess results of blood cultures.

DIAGNOSIS

Differential diagnosis may include the following:
- FB
- Traumatic obstruction
- Neoplasm
- Angioneurotic edema
- Laryngitis
- RSV
- Bacterial tracheitis
- Inhalation injury

THERAPEUTIC PLAN
Pharmacologic Treatment

CROUP WITHOUT STRIDOR AT REST. Acetaminophen or ibuprofen to control fever.

CROUP WITH STRIDOR AT REST
- Racemic epinephrine 2.25% solution by nebulizer every 2 hours while stridor continues at rest. (Lasts approximately 4 hours, watch for rebound effect.)
  <20 kg: 0.25 ml in 2.25 ml saline solution
  20-40 kg: 0.50 ml in 2.25 ml saline solution
  >40 kg: 0.75 ml in 2.25 ml saline solution
- Dexamethasone (Decadron): 0.6 mg/kg/dose IV, IM, or PO for 1 to 4 doses every 6 to 12 hours. (Use in handheld nebulized treatments has the same results.)
- Oxygen: requires ICU admission.

EPIGLOTTITIS. Refer/consult immediately.
- Oxygen at 100% followed by intubation.
- Antibiotics: IV for at least 5 days then may switch to oral
  —Cefotaxime: 50 to 150 mg/kg/day divided every 6 to 8 hours
  —Ceftriaxone: 50 to 75 mg/kg/day divided every 12 hours
  —Cefuroxime: 100 mg/kg/day divided every 6 to 8 hours

Nonpharmacologic Treatment
- Oral fluids to maintain hydration
- Cool-mist humidifiers

Client Education
CROUP
- Keep room humidified with cool mist.
- Keep fever under control.
- Encourage intake of oral fluids.
- If stridor begins, take child outside into the cool air for 5 minutes; if it does not resolve, then take child to emergency center.

EPIGLOTTITIS. Explain need for intubation and procedures to family.

Referral
- Epiglottitis
- Croup with stridor at rest
- Dehydration or inability to drink fluids
- Inability to control fever
- Inability to maintain airway

EVALUATION/FOLLOW-UP
- Recurrent croup episodes
- If no improvement in 4 to 5 days

- Increase in stridor
- Stops drinking
- Inability to control fever
- New symptom development

REFERENCES

Bamberger, B. M., & Jackson, M. A. (1994). Upper respiratory tract infections: Pharyngitis, sinusitis, otitis media and epiglottitis. In M. S. Niederman, G. A. Sarosi, & J. Glassroth. *Respiratory infections: A scientific basis for management.* (pp. 77-87). Philadelphia: W. B. Saunders.

Barker, L. R., Burton, J. R., & Zieve, P. D. (1995). *Principles of ambulatory medicine* (4th ed.) Baltimore: Williams & Wilkins.

Barkin, R. M., & Rosen, R. (1994). Pulmonary disorders. In R. M. Barkin & R. Rosen. *Emergency pediatrics: A guide to ambulatory care* (4th ed., pp. 712-720). St. Louis: Mosby.

Berman, S., & Schmitt, B. D. (1995). Ear, nose, and throat. In W. W. Han, J. R. Groothuis, A. R. Hayward, & M. J. Levin. *Current pediatric diagnosis and treatment* (12th ed., pp. 482-483). Norwalk, CT: Appleton & Lange.

Casmmassima, P. S., & Belanger, G. K. (1994). Ear, nose, and throat disorders. In R. M. Barkin & R. Rosen. *Emergency pediatrics: A guide to ambulatory care* (4th ed., pp. 552-555). St. Louis: Mosby.

Hall, C. B., & McBride, J. T. (1994). Upper respiratory tract infections: The common cold, pharyngitis, croup, bacterial tracheitis and epiglottitis. In J. E. Pennington. *Respiratory infections: Diagnosis and management* (3rd ed., pp. 101-119). New York: Raven Press.

Jacoby, D. B. (1995). Adult epiglottitis. *Journal of the American Academy of Nurse Practitioners, 7*(10), 511-512.

Komaroff, A. L. (1994). Disease of the respiratory tract: Pharyngitis, Coryza, and related infections in adults. In W. T. Branch. *Office practice of medicine* (3rd ed., pp. 148-163). Philadelphia: W. B. Saunders.

Koster, F. T., & Barker, L. R. (1995). Respiratory tract infections. In L. R. Barker, J. R. Burton, & P. D. Zieve (1995). *Principles of ambulatory medicine* (4th ed). Baltimore: Williams & Wilkins.

Larsen, G. L., Abman, S. H., Fan, L. L., White, C. W., & Accurso, F. J. (1994). Respiratory tract and mediastinum. In W. W. Hay, J. R. Groothuis, A. R. Hayward, & M. J. Levin. *Current pediatric diagnosis and treatment* (12th ed., pp. 501-503). Norwalk, CT: Appleton & Lange.

Paluzzi, R. G. (1995). Respiratory tract infections: Pharyngitis. In K. R. Epstein. *Manual of office medicine* (pp. 562-567). Boston: Blackwell Science.

REVIEW QUESTIONS

1. Epiglottitis is most commonly caused by the following:

   a. *Staphylococcus aureus*

   b. *Streptococcus* group A

   c. *Haemophilus influenzae*

   d. RSV

2. Which of the following symptoms are more indicative of pharyngitis in an infant?

   a. Cough, fever 101° F, and sore throat

   b. Cough, increased nasal secretions, and vomiting

   c. Rapid onset of fever (101° F), muffled voice, toxic-looking appearance

   d. Excoriated nares

3. Ms. White comes to your clinic with the complaint of sore throat. She denies fever, nausea, vomiting, or diarrhea. During the review of symptoms, Ms. White admits to an itchy vaginal discharge for several weeks. Which of the following diagnostic procedures should be performed?

   a. Throat culture on swab

   b. Throat culture applied to chocolate agar

   c. Throat culture placed in saline solution (wet mount)

   d. Throat culture placed in KOH

4. Which of the following clients would you suspect as having group A streptococcal pharyngitis?

   a. A 6-month-old with fever and barking cough

   b. An 8-year-old with fever and sore throat

   c. A 29-year-old mother of three with sore throat, low-grade fever, without exudate

   d. A 50-year-old man with complaint of sore throat

5. C.W., 2 years old, has a sudden onset of stridor. There is no history of a viral illness, fever, or vomiting. The child's mother states that C.W. was well this morning. What would be of highest suspicion on your differential diagnosis?

   a. Croup

   b. Epiglottitis

   c. Neoplastic tumor

   d. FB aspiration

6. Which of the following clients should be referred to the ENT clinic?

   a. Child with viral pharyngitis for the second time in 1 year

   b. Child with group A streptococcal pharyngitis for the fourth time in 1 year

   c. Adult woman with group A streptococcal pharyngitis for the first time in her life time

   d. Adult man with a sore throat, fever, rhinitis, and productive cough

ANSWERS AND RATIONALES

1. *Answer:* c (diagnosis/HEENT/child)

   Rationale: The most common bacteria associated with epiglottitis is *Haemophilus influenzae*. (Hall & McBride, 1994)

2. *Answer:* d (assessment/history/HEENT/infant)

   Rationale: Infants often have unusual presenting signs and symptoms for pharyngitis; one of the most common signs is excoriated nares. Answer *c* is associated with epiglottitis, which is rare in an infant. Answers *a* and *b* could be associated with the common cold and pharyngitis. (Bamberger & Jackson, 1994)

3. *Answer:* b (plan/HEENT/NAS)

   Rationale: The female client who has a sore throat without symptoms consistent with a bacterial or a viral throat infection and also has a vaginal discharge should be evaluated for the presence of STD. In this case the client should be tested for *Neisseria gonorrhoeae* by application of a throat culture specimen to a chocolate agar. A culture swab is used for culture and sensitivity studies. Wet mount and KOH studies are not generally useful throat culture media. (Koster & Barker, 1995)

4. *Answer:* b (diagnosis/HEENT/NAS)

   Rationale: The most common age group for group A streptococcal pharyngitis is 5 to 10 years of age. Answer *a* is the most common presentation for croup. The 29-year-old woman does not have exudate, which would be suggestive of a streptococcal pharyngitis. The 50-year-old man is out of the population age group consistent with streptococcal pharyngitis. (Hall & McBride, 1994)

5. *Answer:* d (diagnosis/HEENT/child)

Rationale: This child has no other clinical symptoms that suggest croup or epiglottitis, such as fever. Neoplastic tumor would not be associated with a sudden onset of stridor. Two-year-old children often place objects into their mouths; therefore they are at greater risk for accidental aspiration of FBs. In any client who has a sudden onset of stridor, FB aspiration should always be considered. (Barkin & Rosen, 1994)

6. *Answer:* b (plan/HEENT/child)

Rationale: Clients with recurrent group A streptococcal pharyngitis should have an ENT referral for possible tonsillectomy. The others do not need referral unless the present condition persists despite treatment. (Berman & Schmitt, 1995)

2

Respiratory System

ACUTE BRONCHITIS

OVERVIEW
Definition

Acute bronchitis has been defined as a transient infectious inflammatory condition of the trachea, bronchi, and bronchioles characterized by a cough. It is usually a diagnosis of exclusion.

Incidence

- Commonly affects all ages.
- Seven million episodes per year occur in outpatients older than 18.

Factors Increasing Susceptibility

- Smoking
- Secondhand smoke
- Environmental allergies
- Hypertrophied tonsils and adenoids in children
- Immunosuppression
- Chronic sinusitis
- Chronic obstructive pulmonary disease (COPD)

Common Pathogens

Viral pathogens are the most common:
- Cold virus
- Influenza
- Adenovirus
- *Mycoplasma pneumoniae*

Secondary bacterial pathogens include the following:
- *Chlamydia pneumoniae*
- *Moraxella catarrhalis*
- *Streptococcus pneumoniae*
- *Haemophilus influenzae*

ASSESSMENT: SUBJECTIVE/HISTORY
History of Present Illness

- Productive cough is usually the hallmark symptom.
- How long has cough been present?
- Is cough productive or nonproductive?
- Is cough mucoid (clear, white) or purulent (yellow, green)?
- Was cough preceded by upper respiratory symptoms? If so, for how long?
- Do others in the household have similar symptoms?

Symptoms

- Substernal chest discomfort/burning
- Dyspnea
- Wheezing
- Fatigue
- Decreased appetite
- Hemoptysis
- Fever
- Chills

Past Medical History

- Asthma/COPD
- Congestive heart failure (CHF)
- Chronic sinusitis
- Environmental allergies

Medication History

Name, dosage, and amount of recently used medications:

- Antihistamines
- Decongestants
- Antibiotics
- Cough syrups
- Inhaled medications

Family History

- Asthma
- Cystic fibrosis
- Allergies

Psychosocial History

- Smoker or exposure to smoke
- Occupational exposures to bronchial irritants such as dust or toxic fumes

Dietary History

Ask about amount and type of liquids being consumed.

ASSESSMENT: OBJECTIVE/ PHYSICAL EXAMINATION

Physical Examination

- General: Appearance, energy level, hydration status, vital signs
- HEENT: Look for signs of sinusitis/rhinitis/otitis, lymphadenopathy, jugular venous distention
- Heart: Any irregular rhythm, murmurs, rubs, gallops
- Lungs: May find scattered wheezes and rhonchi; should not have any focal areas of crackles, wheezes, or rhonchi (which would be more indicative of pneumonia)
- Abdomen: No hepatomegaly
- Extremities: No edema

Diagnostic Procedures

- Diagnostic procedures are usually not necessary.
- Indications for CBC/chest x-ray examination include the following:
  - Children, adults, or older adults with any co-existing illnesses that could potentiate the seriousness of a pneumonia compared to a healthy client (examples: cancer, diabetes, coronary artery disease, COPD, immunosuppression)
  - Symptoms persistent for longer than 2 weeks
  - Unclear clinical picture (i.e., possible CHF)
- Sputum Gram stains are generally not helpful.

DIAGNOSIS

Differential diagnosis includes the following:

- Pneumonia
- Pertussis (particularly in children younger than 6 months or never immunized)
- Tuberculosis
- Asthma
- CHF
- Postnasal drainage from chronic sinusitis or allergic rhinitis
- Influenza

The diagnosis of acute bronchitis is acceptable after the previously listed conditions have been suspected and ruled out on the basis of history and physical examination, as well as necessary diagnostic testing.

THERAPEUTIC PLAN

Viral Etiology

- Rest
- Fluids
- Humidification of heat or room where sleeping
- Cough suppressants
  - Dextromethorphan
  - Codeine (mostly for nighttime use)
- Acetaminophen
- Bronchodilators to decrease the cough and symptoms of dyspnea/chest tightness
  - *Children 2 to 6 years:* Albuterol syrup 0.1 mg/kg tid
  - *Children older than 6 years to adult:* Albuterol metered dose inhaler (MDI) 2 puffs every 6 hours prn wheezing/chest tightness
- Prednisone taper for children/adults with underlying chronic respiratory disease and significant dyspnea

Bacterial Superinfection

If bacterial superinfection is suspected (purulent sputum in a smoker or sputum that was originally mucoid but is now purulent), treat with antibiotics and implement the previously outlined measures for viral etiology.

Children

Erythromycin 30 to 50 mg/kg/day in divided doses every 6 hours

Amoxicillin 20 to 40 mg/kg/day in divided doses every 8 hours

Adults/Older Adults

Erythromycin 250 to 500 mg qid for 10 days

Trimethoprim-sulfamethoxazole bid for 10 days

Doxycycline 100 mg bid for 10 days

Amoxicillin 500 mg tid for 10 days

EVALUATION/FOLLOW-UP

Instruct client to return immediately if any of the following occur:

- Increase in fever
- Increase in dyspnea
- Dehydration, decreased voiding
- Worsening cardiovascular state

1. Client with co-existing illnesses: Schedule return visit in 7 to 14 days to assess status.
2. Client without co-existing illnesses: Educate to return if no improvement after 7 to 14 days.
3. Client who returns with complaints of continued cough: Dry, hacking cough following acute bronchitis may represent temporary reactive airway disease and should be treated with bronchodilators as necessary for up to 1 month. If symptoms persist after 1 month, consider another cause for the cough (see discussion of cough, next section).
4. Client with more than two episodes per year: Ascertain that bronchitis is the correct diagnosis and not asthma. Bronchial provocation testing can aid in the diagnosis of asthma.

REFERENCES

Cropp, A. J. (1997). Acute bronchitis. In M. R. Dambro (Ed.), *Griffith's 5-minute clinical consult* (pp. 154-155). Baltimore: William & Wilkins.

Davis, A. L., Hahn, D. L., Niederman, M. S., & O'Connell, E. J. (1996, January 15). Acute bronchitis in adults and children. *Patient Care*, pp. 102-124.

Hoole, A. J., Pickard, C. G., Ouimette, R. M., Lohr, J. A., & Greenberg, R. A. (1995). *Patient care guidelines for nurse practitioners.* Philadelphia: J. B. Lippincott.

Leiner, S. (1997). Acute bronchitis in adults: Commonly diagnosed but poorly defined. *Nurse Practitioner, 22,* 104-114.

Mainous, A. G., III, Zoorob, R. J., & Hueston, W. J. (1996). Current management of acute bronchitis in ambulatory care. *Archives of Family Medicine, 5,* 79-85.

Uphold, C., & Graham, M. (1994). *Clinical guidelines in family practice* (p. 331). Gainesville, FL: Barmarrae Books.

REVIEW QUESTIONS

1. Which of the following symptoms are suggestive of bronchitis?

    a. Sudden onset of fever, purulent sputum, shortness of breath

    b. Fever, cough, substernal chest pain following URI

    c. Rhinitis, headache

    d. Pharyngitis, nasal congestion

2. Which physical finding is most suggestive of bronchitis?

    a. Unilateral wheezing or rhonchi

    b. Scattered wheezing or rhonchi

    c. Unilateral decreased breath sounds

    d. Inspiratory crackles

3. A 46-year-old client complains of rhinitis and head congestion, followed by white productive cough and wheezing. Which diagnosis is least likely?

    a. Bacterial pneumonia

    b. Acute bronchitis

    c. Influenza

    d. Environmental allergy

4. A prednisone taper might be indicated for:

    a. A long-distance runner who has a scheduled competition and needs a speedy recovery

    b. A client with COPD and significant dyspnea

    c. A 24-year-old smoker

    d. A 48-year-old farmer

5. A 10-year-old boy is sent home with a diagnosis of viral bronchitis. Symptomatic treatment is prescribed. The mother calls and states that her son is now, 48 hours later, having purulent productive cough, temperature of 103° F, and chills and is not eating. What plan is most appropriate?

    a. Call in a prescription of amoxicillin.
    b. Ask the client to return for a chest x-ray examination to rule out pneumonia.
    c. Encourage the mother to continue giving acetaminophen.
    d. Reassure the mother that symptoms will subside within 24 hours.

6. A 65-year-old client with a history of diabetes, coronary heart disease, and CHF has been diagnosed with bronchitis. What follow-up is appropriate?

    a. Inform the client to return if symptoms do not improve.
    b. Schedule a CBC and chest x-ray examination in 1 week.
    c. Schedule an office visit within 7 to 14 days.
    d. Advise the client to keep the regular 3-month checkup.

ANSWERS AND RATIONALES

1. *Answer:* b (assessment/history/respiratory/NAS)
    Rationale: Fever, cough, and substernal chest burning following URI suggest bronchitis. (Cropp, 1997)

2. *Answer:* b (assessment/physical examination/respiratory/NAS)
    Rationale: Focal findings such as unilateral wheezes, crackles, and unilateral decreased breath sounds are more worrisome for another etiologic factor. (Davis, Hahn, Niederman, & O'Connell, 1996; Hoole, Pickard, Ouimette, Lohr, & Greenberg, 1995)

3. *Answer:* a (diagnosis/respiratory/NAS)
    Rationale: Bacterial pneumonia is least likely because clients usually have high fevers, crackles, and purulent sputum. (Leiner, 1997; Uphold & Graham, 1994)

4. *Answer:* b (plan/respiratory/NAS)
    Rationale: Clients with preexisting lung disease may need systemic corticosteroids to help decrease bronchial hyperreactivity. (Davis et al., 1996)

5. *Answer:* b (plan/respiratory/NAS)
    Rationale: A client who is not improving should return for a chest x-ray examination. (Davis et al., 1996; Mainous, Zoorob, & Hueston, 1996))

6. *Answer:* c (evaluation/respiratory/NAS)
    Rationale: Clients with co-existing illnesses should be evaluated for resolution of bronchitis symptoms. (Davis et al., 1996)

COUGH

OVERVIEW
Definition

Cough can be acute or chronic. *Acute cough* is generally defined as being one that is present less than 3 weeks. *Chronic cough* is one that has lasted longer than 3 weeks. Chronic cough is a physiologic reflex to protect the airways by clearing secretions and foreign particles.

Incidence

Cough is the fifth most common symptom seen in outpatient clinics, resulting in 30 million visits annually.

Pathophysiology

The cough reflex has five components:
    1. Cough receptors
    2. Afferent nerves (vagus, trigeminal, glossopharyngeal, and phrenic)
    3. A cough center located in the medulla and separate from the respiratory center
    4. Efferent nerves (vagus, phrenic, intercostal, lumbar, trigeminal, facial, and hypoglossal)
    5. Effector organs (diaphragm, intercostal, and abdominal muscles; muscles of the larynx, trachea, and bronchi; and upper air-

way and accessory respiratory muscles) (Corrao, 1996)

An effective cough has three components:

1. The rapid inhalation of a large volume of air, followed by closure of the glottis
2. An elevation of intrathoracic pressures caused by the contraction of abdominal and thoracic muscles
3. With increased pressure, a sudden opening of the glottis that expels the trapped air, thus producing the cough

ASSESSMENT: SUBJECTIVE/HISTORY
History of Present Illness

- How long has the cough been present?
- Is it productive or nonproductive?
- If productive, is it clear, mucoid, or purulent?
- Is it harsh, barking, or coarse?
- Was it preceded by upper or lower respiratory tract infection symptoms, allergy exposure, or a choking/feeding episode?
- Is it present during the day, night, or both?
- Are there any other precipitating factors?

Symptoms

Cough is usually accompanied by other symptoms, which can help lead to the diagnosis:

- Dyspnea on exertion or orthopnea (consider CHF)
- Bloody sputum, weight loss (consider tuberculosis or lung cancer)
- Substernal burning, indigestion, regurgitation of digested material, hoarseness, choking, bitter taste in mouth (consider gastroesophageal reflux disease [GERD])
- Paroxysmal dry, hacking cough made worse by cold air, cardiovascular exercise, laughing, or allergy exposure (consider asthma)
- Tickle in throat, sensation of secretions in throat, frequent clearing of throat (consider a postnasal drainage syndrome)
- Cough that disappears with sleep and worsens when attention is drawn to it (consider psychogenic cough [a very rare cause])
- Children with recurrent URIs, poor weight gain, fatty stools (consider cystic fibrosis)
- High fever, dyspnea, productive purulent cough (consider pneumonia)
- Acute onset with upper respiratory tract symptoms (consider bronchitis)
- Dry cough after acute bronchitis (consider hyperreactive airways)

Past Medical History

- Asthma
- COPD
- CHF
- Gastroesophageal reflux
- Postnasal drainage syndromes
  —Allergic rhinitis
  —Acute sinusitis
  —Chronic sinusitis
  —Vasomotor rhinitis
  —Primary nasal polyposis
- Psychiatric illnesses

Medication History

- Recent angiotensin converting enzyme (ACE) inhibitor therapy (may cause cough)
- Frequent use of antacids
- Cough syrups

Family History

- Cystic fibrosis
- Asthma/COPD
- Allergies

Psychosocial History

- Tuberculosis exposure
- Smoker/smoke exposure
- Occupational/environmental irritants

Dietary History

- Food allergies
- Eating late at night or lying down after meals

ASSESSMENT: OBJECTIVE/ PHYSICAL EXAMINATION
Physical Examination

- General appearance: Comfort level, use of accessory muscles, spontaneous coughing, dyspnea, cyanosis
- HEENT: Signs of sinusitis, postnasal drainage, boggy nasal membranes, cobblestone appearance of pharyngeal mucosa, lymphadenopathy, jugular venous distention
- Heart: Murmurs, rubs, gallops, S_3, S_4
- Lungs: Any wheezes, rhonchi, crackles, anteroposterior diameter, decreased breath sounds

- Abdomen: Any organomegaly, epigastric tenderness
- Extremities: Edema

Diagnostic Procedures

The following procedures should be used based on the suspected diagnosis:

- Chest x-ray examination (pneumonia, CHF, tuberculosis, unexplained cough)
- Pulmonary function tests (COPD; often normal results even with diagnosis of asthma)
- Peak expiratory flow (see Chapter 14 for more detail)
- Sputum for AFB (tuberculosis)
- Barium swallow (GERD)
- 24-hour esophageal probe (GERD)
- Nasal smear (postnasal drainage syndromes)
- Sweat test (cystic fibrosis)
- Purified protein derivative (PPD) (tuberculosis)
- Bronchial provocation test (asthma)

DIAGNOSIS

The most common causes of an acute cough are upper and lower respiratory tract infections. Other causes include FB aspiration (especially in children) and allergy/irritant exposure.

The most common differential diagnoses of chronic cough in nonsmokers are postnasal drainage, asthma, and GERD. Other diagnoses include recurrent viral infections, cystic fibrosis, tuberculosis, pneumoconiosis, carcinoma, CHF, psychogenic cough, ACE inhibitor–induced cough, environmental allergies, bronchiectasis, impacted cerumen in external auditory canal, and chronic bronchitis.

Keep in mind that cough can be the sole manifestation of asthma and GERD.

THERAPEUTIC PLAN

General measures for acute cough include the following:

- Smoking cessation
- Avoiding environmental irritants
- Air humidification

- Cough suppressants (should only be used temporarily for acute cough syndromes and be limited to nighttime usage to provide adequate rest)
- Inhaled beta-agonist (if wheezing present with lower respiratory tract infection)

Treatment for chronic cough depends on the suspected diagnosis. Appropriate empiric treatment should be started if there is enough evidence from the client's history and physical examination to suggest one of the three most common causes of chronic cough: GERD, asthma, or postnasal drainage. (See Chapters 4 and 14 for treatment guidelines.)

EVALUATION/FOLLOW-UP

Acute cough syndromes should improve within 3 weeks as the underlying illness resolves. If cough persists for longer than 3 to 4 weeks, begin workup for chronic cough.

If chronic cough is being treated empirically for GERD, asthma, or postnasal drainage and there is no improvement within 4 to 6 weeks, consult with/refer to a collaborating physician and/or pulmonologist.

REFERENCES

Collins, R. D. (1995). *Algorithmic diagnosis of symptoms and signs.* New York: Igaku-Shoin.

Corrao, W. M. (1996). Chronic persistent cough: Diagnosis and treatment update. *Pediatric Annals, 25*(3), 162-168.

Graham, M. V., & Uphold, C. R. (1994). *Clinical guidelines in child health.* Gainesville, FL: Barmarrae Books.

Newman, K. B., & Milgrom, A. C. (1995, October). Chronic cough: A step-by-step diagnostic workup. *Consultant,* pp. 1535-1542.

Porth, C. M. (1990). *Pathophysiology: Concepts of Altered Health States* (3rd ed.). Philadelphia: J. B. Lippincott.

Smith, P. L., Britt, E. J., & Terry, P. B. (1995). Common pulmonary problems: Cough, hemoptysis, dyspnea, chest pain and the abnormal chest x-ray. In L. R. Barker, J. R. Barton, & P. D. Zieve (Eds.), *Principles of ambulatory medicine* (4th ed., pp. 633-649). Baltimore: Williams & Wilkins.

Uphold, C., & Graham, M. (1994). *Clinical guidelines in adult health.* Gainesville, FL: Barmarrae Books.

REVIEW QUESTIONS

1. Which of the following medications may cause a cough?

    a. ACE inhibitors
    b. Dextromethorphan
    c. Sulfonylureas
    d. Ibuprofen

2. Which initial test would be most appropriate for a client with a cough if the history and physical examination have failed to lead the examiner to a diagnosis?

    a. PPD
    b. Pulmonary function tests
    c. Sweat test
    d. Chest radiograph

3. Which test would be most appropriate in the diagnosis of asthma?

    a. Bronchial provocation test
    b. Nasal smear
    c. Sputum for AFB
    d. Sweat test

4. The most common differential diagnosis for chronic cough includes all **except:**

    a. Postnasal drainage
    b. CHF
    c. GERD
    d. Asthma

5. General measures for cough include all **except:**

    a. Smoking cessation
    b. Vitamin and mineral supplementation
    c. Air humidification
    d. Avoidance of environmental irritants

6. When is it most appropriate to use cough suppressants?

    a. When the client has coronary artery disease
    b. When sleep/rest patterns are significantly disrupted
    c. When the client's family members are disturbed by the cough
    d. When chronic cough of unknown cause is present

7. When chronic cough is treated empirically for GERD, asthma, or postnasal drainage, the client should be referred after which of the following?

    a. No improvement within 6 months
    b. No improvement within 4 to 6 weeks
    c. No improvement within 2 weeks
    d. No improvement within 1 year

ANSWERS AND RATIONALES

1. *Answer:* a (assessment/history/respiratory/NAS)
    Rationale: ACE inhibitor therapy causes coughing in about 5% to 20% of persons who are treated with these medications. (Newman & Milgrom, 1995)

2. *Answer:* d (plan/respiratory/NAS)
    Rationale: If no cause can be identified, a chest radiograph should be obtained. (Newman & Milgrom, 1995)

3. *Answer:* a (plan/respiratory/NAS)
    Rationale: If a client has a positive bronchial provocation test and responds to a bronchodilator, the diagnosis of asthma is more certain. (Corrao, 1996)

4. *Answer:* b (diagnosis/respiratory/NAS)
    Rationale: Corrao (1996) describes several studies that show the three most common causes of chronic cough to be postnasal drainage, GERD, and asthma.

5. *Answer:* b (plan/respiratory/NAS)
    Rationale: Smoking cessation, air humidification, and avoiding environmental irritants are more likely to decrease airway irritability. (Smith, Britt, & Terry, 1995)

6. *Answer:* b (plan/respiratory/NAS)
    Rationale: There are few situations in which cough suppressants are necessary; their use should be for the purpose of allowing clients to sleep and to avoid posttussive syncope or stress incontinence. (Smith, Britt, & Terry, 1995)

7. *Answer:* b (evaluation/respiratory/NAS)
    Rationale: After trying empiric treatment for 4 to 6 weeks and the client has shown no improvement, more testing is warranted (Newman & Milgrom, 1995). Further testing includes 24-hour monitoring with an intraesophageal pH probe, fiberoptic laryngoscopy, and fiberoptic bronchoscopy.

CHRONIC OBSTRUCTIVE PULMONARY DISEASE

OVERVIEW

Definition

Chronic obstructive pulmonary disease (COPD), also referred to as chronic airflow limitation, is a complex syndrome of decreased pulmonary function made up of three components (chronic bronchitis, emphysema, and asthma) in various combinations. All three components are caused in part by oxidative and elastase-mediated lung damage of the small airways and alveoli. COPD is characterized by obstruction or limitation of expiratory airflow that fails to reverse completely following the use of bronchodilators.

Chronic Bronchitis. The definition of *chronic bronchitis* is based on clinical criteria (a chronic productive cough for 3 consecutive months in 2 successive years). Chronic mucus hypersecretion by itself with chronic cough does not necessarily result in significant airway obstruction. When the hypersecretion leads to chronic obstructive bronchitis, rapid deterioration of pulmonary function results.

Emphysema. Based on morphologic features, *emphysema* is defined as the irreversible dilation and destruction of alveolar ducts and air spaces distal to the terminal bronchiole. This results in air trapping.

Asthma. *Asthma* is defined as increased responsiveness of the tracheobronchial tree, inflammation, and reversible airway obstruction.

Incidence

- Sixteen million persons are affected by COPD in the United States.
- COPD is the fifth leading cause of death in the United States.
- Mortality from COPD has risen substantially since 1978.
- Men are affected more than women.
- Mortality rates are higher among whites than among other ethnic groups.

Pathophysiology

- There is a 20- to 40-year preclinical period when the client is asymptomatic, but lung damage accumulates and function declines.
- Forced expiratory volume (FEV) is <50% predicted for size:

 —Middle stage: Cough and shortness of breath, FEV <35% to 49%
 —Late stage: Chronic oxygen therapy FEV <35%
 —Predisposing factors: Cigarette smoking, recurrent infections, allergies, exposure to irritants
 —Genetic factor: Congenital homozygous alpha$_1$-antitrypsin (AAT) deficiency

ASSESSMENT: SUBJECTIVE/HISTORY

History of Present Illness

- Risk factors, symptoms, and overall quality of life; ability to perform activities of daily living (ADLs)
- Cough (time of day; onset, duration, and productivity; type, character, and amount of sputum)
- Wheezing
- Hemoptysis
- Dyspnea (onset, duration, and degree)
- Past/present smoking habits
- Exposure to passive smoking
- Lost/gained weight
- Foods
- Daily fluid intake
- Exercise
- Sexual activity
- Exposure to irritants or noxious materials

Symptoms

- Emphysema: Progressive dyspnea/dyspnea on exertion, mild hypoxia, cough with clear sputum, muscle wasting, weight loss
- Chronic bronchitis: Intermittent dyspnea, severe productive cough of mucopurulent sputum, obesity, cyanosis

Past Medical History

- Allergies, previous respiratory diagnosis and recurrent pulmonary disease, hypertension, obesity, CHF, peptic ulcer disease, cor pulmonale, morning headache

Medication History

Ask about current prescription medications and OTC medications.

Family History

Inquire about indications for AAT deficiency.

Psychosocial History

- Passive smoke
- Past/present smoking habits
- Alcohol or drug usage
- Question regarding wishes concerning intubation and resuscitation: Living will, power of attorney

ASSESSMENT: OBJECTIVE/ PHYSICAL EXAMINATION

Physical Examination

- Height, weight, and vital signs: Respirations (tachypnea), pulse (tachycardia), blood pressure (pulsus paradoxus), general appearance (cachexia, diaphoresis)
- HEENT: Pursed-lip breathing, mucous membrane or perioral cyanosis
- Neck: Jugular venous distention
- Chest: Increased anteroposterior diameter, retractions, and accessory muscle use; expect to hear expiratory wheezes; if crackles present, suspect accompanying heart failure
  —Emphysema: Barrel chest, hyperresonance, diminished breath sounds
  —Chronic bronchitis: Wheezes, rhonchi
- Heart: Right ventricular heave, S_3 gallop or premature atrial complexes, atrial fibrillation if cor pulmonale is present
- Abdomen: Palpate for organomegaly, liver engorgement (cor pulmonale)
- Extremities: Note peripheral edema and pulses, cyanosis, clubbing
- Neurologic: Mental status (somnolence, confusion)

Diagnostic Procedures

- Spirometry (perform at least once in every smoker at age 40 and in all clients who wheeze, cough, or have shortness of breath): FEV greater than or less than 3 seconds, decreased vital capacity and expiratory flow rates in COPD, increased respiratory volume and total lung capacity in emphysema
- CBC (polycythemia in advanced stages of chronic bronchitis)
- Chemistry profile
- ECG (advanced COPD, right atrial hypertrophy)

- Chest x-ray examination (hyperinflation, diaphragm flattening)
- ABGs (if forced expiratory volume in 1 second [FEV_1] is <1 L) indicate hypoxemia, respiratory alkalosis (early), acidosis (late), hypoxia
- For mild-to-moderate disease: All tests within normal limits except spirometry
- For severe disease: CBC (erythrocytosis)
  Clients with a positive family history of emphysema and/or who are younger than 45 should be tested for 1-protease inhibitor deficiency.

DIAGNOSIS

Differential diagnosis includes the following:

Cardiac Causes

- CHF
- Infarction
- Arrhythmia

Pulmonary Causes

- Acute bronchitis
- Pulmonary embolus
- Lung cancer
- Pneumothorax
- Atelectasis

Other Causes

- Deconditioning
- Obesity
- Psychogenic factors
- Anemia
- GERD
- Postnasal drip
- Chronic aspiration
- Tuberculosis
- Aspiration
- Anaphylaxis
- Epiglottitis

THERAPEUTIC PLAN

Goals of Therapy

- Prevention of progression of disease, improvement of symptoms, control of infection
- Nurse practitioner functions as care coordinator
- Cessation of smoking
- Prevention of infection
  —Yearly influenza vaccine

—Pneumococcal vaccine polyvalent (Pneumovax) every 6 to 10 years

—Smoking cessation and reduction in exposures to airway irritants

—Avoidance of foods that increase bronchospasm and sputum (alcohol, spicy food, dairy products)

—Avoidance of extremes in temperature (or wear a mask)

—Home humidification and ingestion of 2 to 3 L of water per day for sputum liquefaction

• Reduction of airflow obstruction

Pharmacologic Treatment

• Level 1: All symptomatic clients—Anticholinergic: Ipratropium (Atrovent) maternal-dose inhaler (MDI) plus

• Level 2: Inhaled beta$_2$-selective agonist (albuterol [Ventolin] or metaproterenol [Alupent]) MDI plus

• Level 3: Inhaled corticosteroid (beclomethasone, triamicinolone, or flunicolide) MDI plus

• Level 4: Extended-release theophylline plus

• Level 5: Extended-release oral albuterol plus

• Level 6: Oral corticosteroid (taper) plus
Avoid sedatives, antihistamines, and beta-blockers.

Infection Control (Acute Exacerbation)

• Educate the client regarding factors that contribute to upper respiratory tract infections.

• *S. pneumoniae, H. influenzae, M. pneumoniae,* and *M. catarrhalis* are the most common infection-causing organisms.

SIGNS AND SYMPTOMS

• Increased cough and sputum

• Thick/odorous sputum

• Change of sputum color

• Increased shortness of breath, fatigue, chest congestion, fever/chills

Treatment

Broad-spectrum antibiotics covering common organisms for 7 to 10 days include the following:

• Trimethoprim-sulfamethoxazole (Bactrim DS) 1 tablet PO bid

• Erythromycin 250 mg qid or azithromycin (Zithromax) (if compliance with frequent medication dosing is a problem)

• Amoxicillin 250 to 500 mg PO tid

To treat a cough that is combined with a difficulty in clearing secretions, use mucolytic agents such as benzonatate (Tessalon) or guaifenesin.

ENCOURAGE EXERCISE

• Exercise to increase tolerance at a lower oxygen consumption rate

• Upper extremity training to lessen diaphragmatic work

• Pulmonary rehabilitation program (pursed-lip breathing and diaphragmatic exercises)

OXYGEN THERAPY AND SAFETY ISSUES

• Low flow has been shown to improve survival in clients with COPD.

• Use home oxygen when Pao$_2$ is <55 mm Hg or oxygen saturation is <85%. (Do not use oxygen within 6 feet of open flame.)

• Instruct the client regarding the need for a fire extinguisher and smoke alarms.

Client Education

• Multidisciplinary pulmonary rehabilitation: Instruct the client on coughing (deep breath then cough).

• Effects of COPD on lung function, breathing techniques, and coping skills

—Educate family members.

—Educate clients on the use of an MDI.

—Counsel clients about advance directives.

—Review signs and symptoms of respiratory infections.

Referral

• AAT deficiency: Refer to endocrinologist.

• Cor pulmonale: Refer to pulmonologist.

• Oxygen needed: Refer to pulmonologist.

EVALUATION/FOLLOW-UP

• For acute attacks, phone contact within 24 to 48 hours needs to be made.

• If the client is taking theophylline, measure drug levels 1 to 2 weeks after initiation of therapy. (Desired level is 10 to 20 ng/dl [Gammon & Bailey, 1995].)

• Schedule follow-up visits every 3 to 6 months for stable chronic disease.

• Stress importance of early recognition of respiratory infection or distress.

REFERENCES

Boyars, M. C. (1997, June). COPD: A step-care approach when FEV$_1$ is deteriorating. *Consultant,* pp. 1673-1687.

Celli, R., Costentino, A., Fiel, S., & Petty, T. (1997, January). COPD: Step by step through the workup. *Patient Care,* pp. 20-52.

Chan, P. (1993). *Diagnostic history and physical exam in medicine* (p. 20). Fountain Valley, CA: Current Clinical Strategies Publication International.

Davis, A., Hahn, D., Niederman, M., & O'Connell, E. (1996, January). When chronic bronchitis turns acute. *Patient Care,* pp. 124-127.

Gammon, B., & Bailey, W. C. (1995, July). COPD: Steps to improve pulmonary function and quality of life. *Patient Care,* pp. 939-950.

Hoole, A., Pickard, C., Ouimette, R., Lohr, J., & Greenberg, R. (1995). *Patient care guidelines for nurse practitioners.* Philadelphia: J. B. Lippincott.

Johannsen, J. (1994). Chronic obstructive pulmonary disease: Current comprehensive care for emphysema and bronchitis. *Nurse Practitioner, 19*(1), 59-67.

Uphold, C., & Graham, M. (1994). *Clinical guidelines in family practice.* Gainesville, FL: Barmarrae Books.

Witta, K. (1997, July). COPD in the elderly. *Advance for Nurse Practitioners,* pp. 18-27 & 72.

REVIEW QUESTIONS

1. Which of the following is a risk factor for COPD?

   a. Age
   b. Inhaled irritant and noxious agents
   c. Heredity
   d. Edema

2. COPD is a progressive respiratory disease syndrome associated with varying combinations of all the following **except:**

   a. Asthma
   b. Tuberculosis
   c. Chronic bronchitis
   d. Emphysema

3. Diagnostic testing for a client with COPD would include all the following **except:**

   a. Stress test
   b. Chest x-ray examination
   c. ABGs
   d. Pulmonary function tests

4. A 56-year-old man complains of having a morning cough for the past 5 years that has increased during the last 2 days. He has smoked cigarettes for 30 years and has noticed wheezing lately. He has also experienced dyspnea for several months. What is the most likely diagnosis?

   a. COPD
   b. Lung cancer
   c. GERD
   d. Asthma

5. Which of the following components would **not** be a part of the complex syndrome of decreased pulmonary function?

   a. Emphysema
   b. Asthma
   c. Acute bronchitis
   d. Chronic bronchitis

6. Pharmacologic interventions for a client with COPD include all the following **except:**

   a. Steroids
   b. Bronchodilators
   c. Sedatives
   d. Mucolytics

7. The purpose of beclomethasone in the treatment of asthma would be:

   a. Decongestant
   b. Antitussive
   c. Antiinflammatory
   d. Antibiotic

8. Theophylline was prescribed for Mrs. Crawford at her last office visit. She should have drug levels drawn at which of the following?

   a. 2 weeks
   b. Never
   c. Every 3 to 6 months
   d. Yearly

ANSWERS AND RATIONALES

1. *Answer:* d (assessment/history/respiratory/NAS)
   Rationale: A nonsmoking adult has a yearly decline of 15 to 30 ml in FEV_1. Cigarette smoking and urban/industrial pollution, first-degree relatives with COPD and an AAT deficiency, and airway hyperreactivity are risk factors for COPD. (Hoole, Pickard, Ouimette, Lohr, & Greenberg, 1995)

2. *Answer:* b (diagnosis/respiratory/NAS)
   Rationale: The components of COPD are chronic bronchitis, emphysema, and asthma. They are caused by oxidative and elastase-mediated lung damage of the small airways and alveoli. (Celli, Costentino, Fiel, & Petty, 1997)

3. *Answer:* a (plan/respiratory/NAS)
   Rationale: Spirometry assesses the risk of pulmonary disease in high-risk populations. Chest x-ray examination can confirm the diagnosis with hyperinflation and diaphragm flattening. ABGs can indicate hypoxemia. (Gammon & Bailey, 1995)

4. *Answer:* a (diagnosis/respiratory/NAS)
   Rationale: Nighttime cough might suggest asthma or GERD. With a history of a morning cough and significant smoking and 59 years of age, the most likely diagnosis is COPD. (Celli, Costentino, Fiel, & Petty, 1997)

5. *Answer:* c (diagnosis/respiratory/NAS)
   Rationale: COPD encompasses three disease entities or combinations: chronic bronchitis, emphysema, and asthma. (Celli et al., 1997)

6. *Answer:* c (plan/respiratory/NAS)
   Rationale: Avoid sedatives, antihistamines, and beta-blockers.

7. *Answer:* c (plan/respiratory/NAS)
   Rationale: An antiinflammatory MDI is used to prevent and modify the late asthmatic response and to control persistent symptoms. Beclomethasone is used for maintenance.

8. *Answer:* a (evaluation/respiratory/NAS)
   Rationale: To prevent caffeinelike side effects, theophylline should be started in low dosages and gradually increased to a maintenance level. It is important to monitor the client's serum level 1 to 2 weeks after initiation of the medication, dosage change, or switching brands.

CYSTIC FIBROSIS

OVERVIEW
Definition

Cystic fibrosis is a multisystem disorder characterized by COPD, maldigestion, and excessive sodium chloride excretion in sweat and saliva.

Incidence

- Autosomal recessive inheritance
- Cystic fibrosis gene located on chromosome 7
- Most common genetic disorder of the white population
- Approximately 1 of 3000 white live births and 1 of 17,000 black live births in the United States
- Chronic progressive disease with life expectancy of 30 to 35 years
- Usual presentation before age 1 year (70%)
- Presentation of milder forms often not until childhood and rarely adulthood

Pathophysiology

RESPIRATORY TRACT. Defective chloride ion transport in respiratory epithelial cells leads to cellular dehydration, causing bronchial secretions to become viscous and difficult to clear. Additionally, pH-sensitive enzymes function abnormally, producing epithelial cell composition abnormalities that result in glycoprotein secretions on cell surfaces that adhere to *Pseudomonas* and *Staphylococcus aureus*, increasing the individual's susceptibility to infection.

DIGESTIVE TRACT. Increased viscosity of mucous gland secretions obstruct pancreatic ducts, resulting in pancreatic fibrosis. Pancreatic enzymes are unable to reach the duodenum, and the digestion and absorption of nutrients is impaired. Intrahepatic bile ducts become blocked with viscous secretions, leading to biliary cirrhosis. The disease may first appear as prolonged neonatal jaundice;

however, the condition usually occurs over a more prolonged period.

REPRODUCTIVE SYSTEM. Cervical glands become distended with mucus, and the cervical canal is filled with copious amounts of mucus. Endocervicitis develops in many teenagers and young women. In males the epididymis, vas deferens, and seminal vesicles become occluded.

ASSESSMENT: SUBJECTIVE/HISTORY
Newborn
- Family history of cystic fibrosis
- Meconium ileus (failure to pass meconium within first 48 hours)

Infant
- Chronic cough
- Recurrent URI
- Failure to thrive
- Chronic diarrhea
- Abdominal distention
- Persistent vomiting, especially with cough
- Salty taste when kissed

Child
- Frequent bulky and foul smelling stools that float
- Rectal prolapse
- Wheezing
- Recurrent upper and lower respiratory tract infections
- Poor weight gain
- Exercise intolerance

Adolescent/Adult
- Delayed puberty
- Pansinusitis
- COPD (rarely diagnosed this late)

ASSESSMENT: OBJECTIVE/ PHYSICAL EXAMINATION
Physical Examination
NEWBORN
- Prolonged jaundice
- Intestinal atresia
- Meconium ileus

INFANT
- Recurrent bronchiolitis
- Persistent infiltrates
- Atelectasis
- Chronic cough
- Failure to thrive
- Chronic diarrhea and abdominal distention
- Persistent vomiting (with cough)
- Use of accessory muscles to breath

CHILD
- Hyperinflation
- Infiltrates
- Rales
- Rhonchi
- Wheezes
- Digital clubbing
- Barrel chest
- Rectal prolapse
- Nasal polyps
- Steatorrhea

ADOLESCENT/ADULT
- Delayed puberty
- Growth failure
- Portal hypertension
- Sterility in males
- Nasal polyps
- Persistent sinusitis
- COPD

Diagnostic Procedures
- Sweat test: Quantitative pilocarpine iontophoretic test is done. Sweat chloride values of 60 mEq/L are generally considered diagnostic for cystic fibrosis. Results of 40 mEq/L are considered normal.
- Chest x-ray examination: Early changes include hyperinflation and increased peribronchial markings. Later findings include infiltrates, bronchial thickening, bronchiectasis (tram lines, parallel bronchial markings), and patchy atelectasis.
- Sputum culture: Findings are positive for bacteria.
- Pulmonary function tests: Not reliable until age 6 years. Findings include decreased midmaximal flow rate and increased residual volume and residual capacity.
- Elevated serum glucose levels, elevated serum amylase levels, and vitamin deficiency may be found on blood chemistry profiles.

DIAGNOSIS

Differential diagnosis includes the following:
- Infant: Bronchiolitis, *Chlamydia* pneumonitis, gastroesophageal reflux with aspiration, celiac disease, immune deficiency syndromes, and gastrointestinal allergies
- Child: Asthma, upper and lower respiratory tract allergies, tuberculosis
- Adolescent/Adult: Asthma, upper and lower respiratory tract allergies or infections, AIDS, tuberculosis

THERAPEUTIC PLAN

- Refer to pediatric or adult pulmonary disease specialist for long-term management:
  —Regular, vigorous chest physiotherapy (percussion and postural drainage, vibratory vest)
  —Monitoring of sputum for pathogens and prescription of appropriate antibiotics
  —Bronchodilators by MDI
  —Antiinflammatory agents such as corticosteroids
  —Nutritional supplements: Fat-soluble vitamins A, D, and E; pancreatic enzyme capsules with every meal and snack; high-protein, high-calorie diet
  —Dornase alfa (recombinant DNase) by nebulizer to break down extracellular DNA in sputum

NOTE: The family nurse practitioner or pediatric nurse practitioner may participate in the therapeutic plan as a member of the pulmonary center team. Pulmonary care of these children should always be managed by the pulmonary specialty team, not the family/pediatric care provider.
- Routine health maintenance: Follow the routine health maintenance plan carefully. Stress the importance of immunizations (including influenza and pneumonia vaccines).
  —If the client's weight is not routinely followed by a nutritionist, monthly weight checks will be required.
  —Psychosocial help may be required in dealing with chronic illness. Counsel adolescents regarding sexual maturation, potential reproductive problems (males are usually sterile, females have difficulty becoming pregnant because of thick cervical mucus), and increased risk for STDs.

- Refer to the Cystic Fibrosis Foundation.
- Refer for genetic counseling.

EVALUATION/FOLLOW-UP

Respiratory infections must be treated vigorously. Hospitalize for acute exacerbations. Follow growth and development closely, especially weight gain. Children with cystic fibrosis usually remain at or below the 5th percentile but should not be permitted to lose weight or fail to gain weight for extended periods.

Refer for treatment of atelectasis, persistent or severe hemoptysis, or acute respiratory failure. Evaluate unexplained or persistent gastrointestinal symptoms carefully (increased risk for digestive tract malignancy).

REFERENCES

Arvin, A. M., Behrman, R. E., Kliegman, R. M., & Nelson, W. E. (Eds.). (1996). *Nelson textbook of pediatrics* (15th ed.). Philadelphia: W. B. Saunders.

Bindler, R. M., & Howry, L. B. (1997). *Pediatric drugs and nursing implications* (2nd ed.). Norwalk, CT: Appleton & Lange.

Dershewitz, R. A. (Ed.). (1993). *Ambulatory pediatric care* (2nd ed.). Philadelphia: J. B. Lippincott.

Duffield, R. A. (1996). Cystic fibrosis and the gastrointestinal tract. *Journal of Pediatric Health Care, 10,* 2, 51-57.

Groothuis, J. R., Hay, W. W., Hayward, A. R., & Levin, M. J. (Eds.). (1995). *Current pediatric diagnosis and treatment* (12th ed.). Norwalk, CT: Appleton & Lange.

Neglia, J. P., et al. (1995). The risk of cancer among patients with cystic fibrosis. Cystic fibrosis and cancer study group. *New England Journal of Medicine, 332,* 494-499.

White, K. R., Munro, C. L., & Pickler, R. H. (1997). Therapeutic implications of recent advances in cystic fibrosis. *The American Journal of Maternal Child Nursing, 20,* (6),304-308.

Wilmott, R. W., & Fiedler, M. A. (1994). Recent advances in the treatment of cystic fibrosis. *Pediatric Clinics of North America, 41,* 431-451.

REVIEW QUESTIONS

1. Which of the following symptoms are least suggestive of cystic fibrosis?

    a. Three episodes of bronchiolitis and one episode of pneumonia in the past 8 months

    b. A history of meconium ileus

    c. Abdominal distention with a history of constipation

    d. Failure to gain weight with a steady decline on the growth chart

2. Which of the following findings is considered diagnostic of cystic fibrosis?

    a. Sweat test result of 40 mEq/L

    b. Wheezes and crackles bilaterally on chest auscultation

    c. Digital clubbing and use of accessory muscles with respiration

    d. Sweat test result of 70 mEq/L

3. A 14-year-old girl comes into the clinic because she is concerned about not having started her period. In looking over her records, the family nurse practitioner notes that the client is below the 5th percentile for height and weight and has a history of recurrent respiratory infections. The differential diagnosis for this client would include all the following **except:**

    a. Cystic fibrosis

    b. Asthma

    c. Pneumonia

    d. Turner's syndrome

4. An 18-year-old with cystic fibrosis comes to the clinic with midepigastric pain and recurrent nausea. This is her second visit with the same complaints. The most appropriate action by the family nurse practitioner would be to:

    a. Obtain a careful history and complete physical examination including an upper gastrointestinal tract x-ray examination.

    b. Ask the client to keep a dietary record for the next week and return to the clinic for follow-up.

    c. Question the client regarding compliance with her nutritional supplements.

    d. Reassure the client that these problems go along with cystic fibrosis and help her identify which foods seem to "upset" her stomach.

5. After a diagnosis of cystic fibrosis has been established, appropriate management by the family nurse practitioner would include:

    a. Start a short course of corticosteroids.

    b. Begin antibiotics for any current infection and refer the client for long-term treatment by a pulmonary specialist.

    c. Admit the client to the hospital for further evaluation and development of a long-term treatment plan.

    d. Teach the client and parents how to use the nebulizer to administer dornase alfa at home.

6. The family nurse practitioner knows that teaching regarding pancrelipase administration has been effective when the client's mother states:

    a. I'll make sure he takes his pancrelipase every time he eats.

    b. I'll make a schedule so that I can be sure he gets his pancrelipase 4 times every day.

    c. It embarrasses him to take medicine at school, so I'll make sure he gets in all his doses at home.

    d. I'll make sure he takes his pancrelipase as soon as he wakes up in the morning so that he will be covered for the day.

ANSWERS AND RATIONALES

1. ***Answer:*** c (assessment/history/respiratory/child)

    Rationale: Recurrent respiratory infections, meconium ileus, and poor weight gain are consistent with the diagnosis of cystic fibrosis. Diarrhea is consistent with the diagnosis of cystic fibrosis, whereas constipation is not. (Dershewitz, 1993)

2. ***Answer:*** d (plan/respiratory/child)

    Rationale: The diagnosis of cystic fibrosis is based on a quantitative sweat test result of 60 mEq/L (Arvin, Behrman, Kliegman, & Nelson, 1996). Answers *b* and *c* may be found on physical examination in a child with cystic fibrosis but are not diagnostic.

3. *Answer:* c (diagnosis/respiratory/child)

Rationale: Recurrent respiratory infections and poor weight gain can indicate both asthma and cystic fibrosis. Short stature and delayed puberty are consistent with a diagnosis of Turner's syndrome. A diagnosis of pneumonia is not logical in the absence of current respiratory symptoms. (Groothuis, Hay, Hayward, & Levin, 1995)

4. *Answer:* a (plan/respiratory/child)

Rationale: Unexplained or persistent gastrointestinal symptoms must be evaluated carefully because of the increased risk of digestive tract tumors in individuals with cystic fibrosis. (Neglia et al., 1995)

5. *Answer:* b (plan/respiratory/child)

Rationale: Although the family nurse practitioner can function as a valuable member of the treatment team, all clients with cystic fibrosis should be referred to a cystic fibrosis treatment center where a team approach can be employed. (Duffield, 1996)

6. *Answer:* a (evaluation/respiratory/child)

Rationale: Creon is a pancreatic enzyme replacement that must be taken with all food to aid in the digestion of fats, starches, and proteins. (Bindler & Howry, 1997)

PNEUMONIA

OVERVIEW
Definition

Pneumonia is an infection of the pulmonary parenchyma with consolidation.

Incidence

- Sixth overall cause of death in the United States and leading cause of infectious death
- 500,000 hospital admissions annually

Classifications

- Community-acquired
- Hospital-acquired

Pathophysiology

- Aspirated oropharyngeal secretions
- Infected droplet inhalation from human contacts
- Spread from another site (urinary tract infection, infected IV catheter)
- Direct introduction of organisms iatrogenically or by trauma

Protective Factors

- Cough and gag reflex protect against gross aspiration
- Mucociliary lining of tracheobronchial tree
- Immune response: Leukocytes and phagocytosis

Factors Increasing Susceptibility

- Altered upper respiratory tract flora: Predisposition to more virulent organisms as a result of recent antibiotic therapy, recent hospitalization, diabetes, or alcoholism
- Altered immune status: Diabetes, AIDS, alcoholism, malignancy, chemotherapy, uremia
- Impaired cough and gag reflex: Increased risk of aspiration with altered mental status, alcohol or drug intoxication, anesthetics, cerebrovascular accident, seizure
- Impaired function of natural defense mechanisms: Mucociliary clearance damaged by smoking, inhaled environmental pollutants, COPD, alcohol, viral infection
- Mechanical bypass of normal defenses: Tracheal intubation, chest tube
- Underlying lung pathology: Pulmonary embolus or contusion, foreign body, atelectasis
- Chest wall abnormality: Postoperative pain, chest trauma, myopathy

Common Pathogens

Common community-acquired pathogens include the following:

- *S. pneumoniae* (60% to 75%)
- *Legionella* series (5% to 15%)
- *Moraxella pneumoniae* (5% to 18%)
- *H. influenzae* (2% to 5%)

- *S. aureus* (1% to 5%)
- *M. catarrhalis* (1% to 5%)

ASSESSMENT: OBJECTIVE/ PHYSICAL EXAMINATION

Physical Examination

A problem-oriented physical examination is appropriate, with emphasis on the respiratory system:

- Observe for cyanosis, dyspnea, tachypnea, tachycardia
- Lobar consolidation: Dullness to percussion, crackles/rales, bronchial breath sounds, increased vocal fremitus, bronchophony, egophony, whispered pectoriloquy

  CHILDREN. A respiratory rate of >50 breaths/min in infants and >40 breaths/min in children younger than 3 years old with history of rapid breathing and chest retractions is sensitive and specific for lower respiratory tract infection.

Diagnostic Procedures

- Oxygen saturation measurement is helpful.
- Chest x-ray examination may help with the diagnosis.
- Normal CBC does not mean absence of infection!
- Sputum Gram stain and culture may help isolate the organism.
- ABGs may help with the decision to admit to the hospital.

DIAGNOSIS

When the presenting features are fever and cough, the diagnosis is usually one of the following:

- Lower respiratory tract infection (pneumonia, bronchitis): In children, bronchiolitis is more common than bronchitis.
- Pulmonary embolus (fever, usually low grade)
- Septic pulmonary embolus

When the presenting feature is dyspnea in younger clients (<40), the diagnosis is usually one of the following:

- Pulmonary embolus
- Pneumonia
- Pneumothorax
- Asthma: Wheezing may be reactive airway from pulmonary infection.
- Costochondritis/pleuritis

When the presenting feature is dyspnea in older adults, the diagnosis is one of the following:

- Acute myocardial infarction (AMI)
- Pulmonary embolus
- CHF
- Exacerbation of COPD
- Pneumonia
- Pulmonary abscess
- Rib fracture from fall

THERAPEUTIC PLAN

- Stabilize any respiratory failure; intubation may be required.
- Provide supportive care:
  —Provide supplemental oxygen.
  —Ensure hydration; fever and tachypnea may cause dehydration.
  —Instruct the client regarding nebulizer treatments with bronchodilators.
- Administer antibiotics after collecting cultures:
  —Use broad-spectrum antibiotic until C&S returns.
  —Consider inpatient versus outpatient treatment.

Disposition

The following are factors that may indicate the need for hospitalization:

- Physical findings
  —Respiratory rate >30 breaths/min
  —Diastolic blood pressure ≤60 beats/min or systolic blood pressure ≤90 beats/min
  —Temperature >101° F (38° C)
  —Altered mental status
- Extremes of age
- Failure to respond to outpatient therapy
- Immunocompromised client
- Risk of poor compliance
- Evidence of toxicity
- Comorbid illness (COPD, diabetes, chronic renal failure, CHF, liver disease)
- Multilobar disease

EVALUATION/FOLLOW-UP

- The client should report improvement in symptoms:
  —No dyspnea
  —Decreased fever
  —Improvement in cough (Is the client able to sleep?)

- If the client's condition worsens or there is no improvement, consider hospitalization and/or a change in antibiotics.
- Reevaluate the client's condition after the course of antibiotics.

REFERENCES

Ashbourne, J., & Downey, P. (1993). Pneumonia. In P. Rosen (Ed.), *Emergency medicine: Concepts and clinical practice.* St. Louis: Mosby.

Guidelines for the initial management of adults with community acquired pneumonia: Diagnosis, assessment of severity, and initial antimicrobial therapy. (1993). *American Review of Respiratory Disease, 148,* 1418-1426.

Stauffer, J. (1996). Lung. In L. Tierney Jr., S. McPhee, & M. Papadakis (Eds.), *Current medical diagnosis and treatment* (pp. 238-246). Norwalk, CT: Appleton & Lange.

REVIEW QUESTIONS

1. An alcoholic client is at risk for pneumonia because of all the following **except:**

a. Possible impaired gag reflex and aspiration
b. Impaired immune status
c. Underlying lung pathology
d. Impaired mucociliary clearance

2. The organism most likely responsible for pneumonia in a middle school age child during the fall is:

a. *Pneumocystic*
b. *H. influenzae*
c. *Mycoplasma*
d. Fungus

3. A positive clinical sign on the physical examination indicating pneumonia is:

a. Wheezing
b. Hyperresonance
c. Dullness on percussion
d. Decreased vocal fremitus

4. A client with a temperature of 102° F (38.5° C) and respiratory rate of 36 breaths/min is diagnosed with pneumonia. The nurse practitioner should:

a. Consult with the physician about hospitalization of the client.
b. Prescribe two oral antibiotics.
c. Prescribe a metered-dose inhaler.
d. Treat symptoms, since the pneumonia is most likely viral in nature.

5. A client treated with azithromycin for pneumonia has improved but is not well. The nurse practitioner should:

a. Consult with the physician about hospitalization of the client.
b. Prescribe another antibiotic.
c. Prescribe another round of azithromycin.
d. Suggest the use of a vaporizer.

ANSWERS AND RATIONALES

1. *Answer:* c (pathophysiology/respiratory/NAS)
Rationale: Altered consciousness and elevated blood alcohol levels may impair the gag reflex and decrease leukocyte production and mucociliary action. (Guidelines, 1993)

2. *Answer:* c (diagnosis/respiratory/NAS)
Rationale: Mycoplasma organisms are more common in children and young adults and in enclosed settings during the seasons of fall and winter. (Ashbourne & Downey, 1993)

3. *Answer:* c (assessment/physical examination/respiratory/NAS)
Rationale: Wheezing indicates obstruction. Hyperresonance indicates overinflation. Decreased vocal fremitus may indicate collapsed lung. Dullness indicates fluid and consolidation. (Ashbourne & Downey, 1993)

4. *Answer:* a (plan/management/nonpharmacologic/respiratory/NAS)
Rationale: Indications for hospitalization are a temperature >101° F (38° C), respiratory rate >30 breaths/min, altered mental status, and diastolic blood pressure ≤60 beats/min or systolic blood pressure ≤90 beats/min. (Stauffer, 1996)

5. *Answer:* b (evaluation/respiratory/NAS)
Rationale: There is no information suggesting the need for hospitalization. Another antibiotic may be indicated if the client remains ill after one course. Doubling the use of a single antibiotic increases drug resistance and is not effective. Vaporizers are more helpful in releaving congestion in nasal breathers (infants) or preventing URIs. (Guidelines, 1993)

SHORTNESS OF BREATH (DYSPNEA)

OVERVIEW
Definition

Shortness of breath is correctly termed *dyspnea*. *Dyspnea* is broadly defined as an uncomfortable sensation of breathlessness that is inappropriate or unusual for the client's baseline respiratory status. Dyspnea can be either acute or chronic. The client may also complain of dyspnea only on exertion. *Paroxysmal nocturnal dyspnea* is inappropriate breathlessness at night. *Orthopnea* is dyspnea on recumbency. *Platypnea* is dyspnea in the upright position relieved by recumbency.

Pathophysiology

The cause of dyspnea is uncertain. Four types of mechanisms have been proposed to explain the sensation: (1) stimulation of lung receptors, (2) increased sensitivity to changes in ventilation perceived through central nervous system mechanisms, (3) reduced ventilatory capacity or breathing reserve, and (4) stimulation of neural receptors in the muscle fibers of the intercostals and diaphragm and of receptors in the skeletal joints (Porth, 1990).

ASSESSMENT: SUBJECTIVE/HISTORY
History of Present Illness

- How long has the sensation been present?
- Are there any aggravating or alleviating factors?
- Females: When was the last menstrual period (possible pregnancy)?
- Children: Is there a possibility of the child having swallowed an object?

Symptoms

Dyspnea is often accompanied by other symptoms that can help lead to the diagnosis:

- Fever, chills, purulent sputum (consider pneumonia)
- Orthopnea, crackles, shifted point of maximal impulse, jugular venous distention, hepatomegaly, S_3 or S_4, lower extremity edema (consider CHF)
- Sudden chest pain, recent immobility, hemoptysis (consider pulmonary embolism)
- Wheezing (consider asthma, COPD, foreign body aspiration)
- Chest pain, diaphoresis, nausea (consider MI)
- Amenorrhea, weight gain (consider pregnancy)
- Headache, pale and dusky mucous membranes (consider carbon monoxide intoxication)
- Anxiety, rapid breathing, tingling of hands and feet, circumoral numbness (consider hyperventilation)
- Sharp, stabbing chest pain (consider pneumothorax)

CHILDREN

- Stridor, recent swallowing of object (consider foreign body airway obstruction)
- Gastrointestinal symptoms, weight loss, failure to thrive (consider cystic fibrosis)

Past Medical History

- Anemia
- CHF
- COPD
- Tuberculosis
- Histoplasmosis
- MI
- Coronary artery disease
- Hypothyroidism
- Hyperthyroidism
- Anxiety/depression
- Weight gain
- History of spontaneous pneumothorax
- Environmental allergies and exposures
- Dysphagia or aspiration
- Lung cancer

Medication History

- Recent new medications that could be causing a drug reaction (such as antibiotics)?
- Use of beta-blockers (may cause or worsen bronchospasm)?
- Use of inhaled medications, theophylline, or terbutaline?
- Use of OTC products such as Primatene Mist?
- Any accidental or purposeful drug ingestion/overdose (especially narcotics)?

Family History

- COPD
- Coronary artery disease

Psychosocial History

- Anxiety/increase in stressors
- Exercise/activity patterns
- Illegal drug use
- Alcohol intake
- Smoker

Environmental History

- Exposure to bronchial irritants such as smoke, dust, or toxic fumes
- Heat source (coal, wood, electric, gas)
- Carbon monoxide detectors

Dietary History

- Any food allergies
- Sodium intake (may worsen CHF)

ASSESSMENT: OBJECTIVE/ PHYSICAL EXAMINATION

Physical Examination

- General appearance: Pallor, obvious distress, use of accessory muscles, position of comfort, rate and regularity of breathing
- HEENT: Nasal congestion, trachea deviation, jugular venous distention, tonsillar edema
- Heart: Any murmurs, rubs, gallops, irregularities, extra heart sounds
- Lungs: Any wheezes, crackles, rhonchi, decreased breath sounds, increased anteroposterior diameter
- Extremities: Any edema or clubbing

Diagnostic Procedures

Acute dyspnea should always be evaluated with a chest x-ray examination. Other tests should be selected based on the suspected diagnosis:

- Chest x-ray examination (CHF, pneumonia, pneumothorax, cancer, tuberculosis)
- ABGs (hypoxia or if diagnosis is unclear)
- Echocardiogram (CHF, MI)
- Pulmonary function tests (COPD)
- Ventilation-perfusion ($\dot{V}/\dot{Q}$) scan (pulmonary embolism)
- Complete blood count (anemia, pneumonia)

- PPD (tuberculosis)
- Cardiac isoenzymes (MI)
- Bronchial provocation test (asthma)
- Carboxyhemoglobin (carbon monoxide)
- ECG (suspect arrhythmia, MI)
- Holter monitor (if arrhythmia not captured by ECG is suspected)

DIAGNOSIS

Acute Dyspnea

The differential diagnosis includes pulmonary edema, pulmonary embolism, spontaneous pneumothorax, pneumonia, acute exacerbation of COPD, hyperventilation, and MI.

Chronic Dyspnea

The differential diagnosis includes asthma, COPD, interstitial lung disease, respiratory muscle weakness, deconditioning, pulmonary hypertension, bronchiectasis, pulmonary fibrosis, sarcoidosis, and lung cancer.

THERAPEUTIC PLAN

Acute Dyspnea

- Quickly obtain history, physical examination, and diagnostic procedures.
- If AMI is suspected, arrange immediate transport to the nearest hospital capable of administering thrombolytic therapy.
- If pulmonary embolism is suspected, arrange immediate transport to the nearest hospital for possible anticoagulation.
- If pneumonia is suspected, decide on outpatient versus inpatient treatment (see section on pneumonia in this chapter).
- If acute exacerbation of COPD is suspected, administer bronchodilator per nebulizer and low-flow oxygen per nasal cannula; consider systemic steroid administration and possibly antibiotics. Some clients may require hospitalization during the acute exacerbation.
- If the diagnosis of the condition or treatment of the diagnosed condition is not possible, refer the client immediately to the nearest urgent treatment center or emergency room. Consider calling for emergency transport.

Chronic Dyspnea

- If COPD is suspected, treat with MDIs or bronchodilators, anticholinergics, and corticosteroids (see Chapter 2).
- If asthma is suspected, treat with MDIs or bronchodilators, anticholinergics, corticosteroids, and/or cromolyn as indicated (see Chapter 14).

EVALUATION/FOLLOW-UP

- Clients with acute dyspnea should be contacted by phone or seen for follow-up within 24 to 48 hours to reevaluate/reassess respiratory status.
- Clients with chronic dyspnea should be seen for follow-up according to the diagnosis and the treatments prescribed. Clients with chronic dyspnea should have an etiologic diagnosis that will help guide treatment and follow-up. If no cause can be elicited or if the client does not show satisfactory improvement within the time frame suggested by the diagnosis and treatment initiated, the client should be referred to a consulting/collaborating physician or a pulmonologist for evaluation.

REFERENCES

Barker, L. R. (1995). Hypertension. In L. R. Barker, J. R. Burton, & P. D. Zieve (Eds.), *Principles of ambulatory medicine* (4th ed., pp. 803-845). Baltimore: Williams & Wilkins.

Burki, N. H. (1995, September). Acute dyspnea: Is the cause cardiac or pulmonary—or both. *Consultant,* 1387-1390.

Collins, R. D. (1995). *Algorithmic diagnosis of symptoms and signs* (p. 415). New York: Igaku-Shoin.

Dalen, J. E. (1997). Pulmonary embolism. In M. R. Dambro (Ed.), *Griffith's 5-minute clinical consult* (pp. 882-883). Baltimore: Williams & Wilkins.

Manning, H. L. (1994, June). Acute and chronic dyspnea: Finding the cause of breathlessness. *Emergency Medicine,* 61-69.

Massie, B. M. (1996). Heart. In L. M. Tierney, S. J. McPhee, & M. A. Papadakis (Eds.), *Current Medical diagnosis and treatment* (35th ed., pp. 295-383). Norwalk, CT: Appleton & Lange.

Porth, C. M. (1990). *Pathophysiology—Concepts of altered health states* (3rd ed., p. 427). Philadelphia: J. B. Lippincott.

Smith, P. L., Britt, E. S., & Terry, P. B. (1995). Common pulmonary problems: Cough, hemoptysis, dyspnea, chest pain, and the abnormal chest x-ray. In L. R. Barker, J. R. Burton, & P. D. Zieve (Eds.), *Principles of ambulatory medicine* (4th ed., pp. 638-649). Baltimore: Williams & Wilkins.

Stauffer, J. L. (1996). Lung. In L. M. Tierney, S. J. McPhee, & M. A. Papadakis (Eds.), *Current Medical diagnosis and treatment* (35th ed., pp. 215-294). Norwalk, CT: Appleton & Lange.

Uphold, C. R., & Graham, M. V. (1994). *Clinical guidelines in adult health* (pp. 271-327). Gainesville, FL: Barmarrae Books.

REVIEW QUESTIONS

1. Suspected pneumonia should be evaluated with:

a. ABGs
b. $\dot{V}/\dot{Q}$ scan
c. Pulmonary function tests
d. Chest x-ray examination

2. A tall, thin 21-year-old has sudden sharp pain in the chest and mild dyspnea. What differential diagnosis is most likely?

a. Spontaneous pneumothorax
b. Pulmonary embolism
c. Pneumonia
d. MI

3. A 42-year-old smoker complains of gradually feeling more short of breath. He smokes two packs per day and denies any chest pain, sputum production, or weight loss. After appropriate testing, you suspect early COPD. What initial treatment should be started?

a. Begin a bronchodilator or anticholinergic per MDI.
b. Avoid starting treatment and schedule for a second chest x-ray examination.
c. Send the client to smoking cessation classes.
d. Consult a pulmonologist.

4. After an appropriate diagnostic evaluation, a 20-year-old is treated for suspected asthma. After treatment with bronchodilators, she still shows no improvement. What follow-up is appropriate?

    a. Refer the client to a pulmonologist.

    b. Reevaluate the client's condition in 1 month.

    c. Assure the client that no evaluation is necessary because her symptoms are most likely to be from hyperventilation.

    d. Inform the client to return if her symptoms worsen.

5. Orthopnea is often suggestive of:

    a. Coronary artery disease

    b. Pulmonary embolism

    c. CHF

    d. Hyperventilation

ANSWERS AND RATIONALES

1. *Answer:* d (plan/respiratory/NAS)

    Rationale: A chest radiograph is included in the initial evaluation of a client with symptoms and signs suggestive of pneumonia. (Stauffer, 1996)

2. *Answer:* a (diagnosis/respiratory/NAS)

    Rationale: Spontaneous pneumothorax is characterized by sudden sharp pain and dyspnea. Incidence is highest in young men or in older clients with COPD. (Uphold & Graham, 1994)

3. *Answer:* a (plan/respiratory/NAS)

    Rationale: The best indication of the primary underlying cause is a therapeutic trial. (Burki, 1995)

4. *Answer:* a (plan/respiratory/NAS)

    Rationale: Referral to a specialist is indicated when the client is not responding to therapy. (Uphold & Graham, 1994)

5. *Answer:* c (assessment/history/respiratory/NAS)

    Rationale: This symptom is most characteristic of CHF, especially with left ventricular failure. (Collins, 1995)

TUBERCULOSIS

OVERVIEW
Definition

Tuberculosis is a chronic, infectious, inflammatory, reportable disease. Clients infected with the bacillus are distinguished from those who have disease. Tuberculosis usually infects the lung but may occur in other tissues and organs in the body (extrapulmonary).

Incidence

- The World Health Organization (WHO) estimates one third of the world population is infected with *Mycobacterium tuberculosis.*
- Incidence in reported cases increased between 1985 and 1992; thought to be the result of increased prevalence of HIV-infected persons.
- The period 1992 to 1996 showed a decline of approximately 20%.
- Tuberculosis cases in the United States in 1996 were 8 per 100,000 (lowest since 1953); 37% of cases were in persons born outside the United States.

    OLDER ADULTS. Those older than 65 have the highest case rate (16 per 100,000).

    CHILDREN. From 1988 to 1992, the number of cases of pediatric tuberculosis increased 51%, whereas the number of cases in all ages increased by 19%.

Pathophysiology

- Tuberculosis is transmitted by airborne droplets.
- The infected individual does not develop the disease unless the immune system is compromised.
- Manifestations usually occur in the first 6 to 11 months.

- The disease can be pulmonary or extrapulmonary.
- Extrapulmonary disease can include meningitis and lymphadenitis and renal, bone, and joint involvement.
- Children generally do not transmit the disease to other children and are usually infected by contact with an adult with active tuberculosis.
- Children younger than 4 years with tuberculosis are much more likely to have pulmonary and extrapulmonary disease, and they also have a higher risk for tuberculosis meningitis.

Protective Factors

- Avoidance of exposure to known cases and at-risk populations
- Intact immune system
- Early diagnosis and treatment
  CHILDREN. Identify and treat adults with active tuberculosis who are in close proximity to children.

Factors Increasing Susceptibility

- Contact with high-risk populations (prison guards, health care workers)
- Poor and medically underserved populations, homeless
- Institutionalization
- Alcoholism, IV drug abuse
- Impaired immunity (HIV, AIDS, chemotherapy, radiation therapy)
  CHILDREN
  - Living in household with adult with active tuberculosis
  - Living in household with adult who is at high risk for contracting tuberculosis
  - HIV positive or otherwise immunocompromised
  - Born in country with high prevalence of tuberculosis
  - Living in medically underserved communities

Pathogen

M. tuberculosis is the causative organism.

ASSESSMENT: SUBJECTIVE/HISTORY
History of Present Illness

- Chronic cough (usually with hemoptysis)
- Night sweats

- Unexplained weight loss
- Anorexia
- Fever, chills
- Malaise
  CHILDREN
  - Less likely to have obvious symptoms
  - Difficult to collect sputum samples
  - Usually must rely on C&S of adult source case

ASSESSMENT: OBJECTIVE/ PHYSICAL EXAMINATION
Physical Examination

No specific findings are relevant on examination.

Diagnostic Procedures

- Tuberculin skin test: The test is indicated for persons with signs/symptoms/laboratory abnormalities suggestive of tuberculosis or recent contact with persons known to have or suspected of having active tuberculosis if HIV positive. A positive result usually appears 2 to 10 weeks after exposure.
- Chest x-ray examination
- Sputum for AFB, C&S

DIAGNOSIS

- Tuberculosis
- HIV infection
- Chronic bronchitis
- Pneumonia
- Pulmonary embolus

THERAPEUTIC PLAN

- Treatment varies, but the shortest course (6 months) is with a four-drug regimen: isoniazid, rifampin, pyrazinamide, and ethambutol.
- Rifater is a newly-approved drug that combines isoniazid, rifampin, and pyrazinamide.
  CHILDREN. The drug regimen and length of treatment are the same as for adults, except ethambutol is not used.

EVALUATION/FOLLOW-UP

- Monitor therapy clinically and with cultures where possible.

- A qualitative decrease in AFB on smears is a reliable indicator of response.
- Most clients receiving a four-drug regimen have negative results from smears after 3 months of treatment.
- Consistently positive results from smears indicate noncompliance.
- Noncompliance may cause multidrug-resistant tuberculosis (MDR TB).
- For noncompliant clients, consider directly observed therapy short course (DOTS), where a health care worker observes while the client takes each dose.

REFERENCES

American Lung Association fact sheet: Pediatric tuberculosis (1997). *http://www.brooks.af.mil/ABG/MDS/disease.htm.*

American Lung Association fact sheet: Tuberculosis (1997). *http://www.lungusa.org/noframes/global/news/report/tubercul/tubtfact.html.*

Barkin, R. M., & Rosen, P. (1994). In R. M. Barkin & P. Rosen (Eds.), *Emergency pediatrics: A guide to ambulatory care* (4th ed., pp. 657-658). St. Louis: Mosby.

Chambers, H. (1996). Infectious diseases: Bacterial and chlamydial. In L. Tierney Jr., S. McPhee, & M. Papadakis (Eds.). *Current medical diagnosis and treatment* (pp. 1221-1224). Norwalk, CT: Appleton & Lange.

Markowitz, N., Hansen, N., Hopewell, P., Glassroth, J., Kvale, P., & Mangura, B. (1997). Incidence of tuberculosis in the United States among HIV-infected persons. *Annals of Internal Medicine, 126,* 123-132.

REVIEW QUESTIONS

1. A client with a positive result from a tuberculin skin test is:

   a. Ill with tuberculosis
   b. Infected with the organism
   c. Contagious
   d. Allergic to the vaccine

2. Which of the following symptoms is most indicative of tuberculosis?

   a. Night sweats
   b. Weight loss
   c. Fever
   d. Chronic cough

3. Pneumonia may be mistaken for tuberculosis when a diagnosis is made. Which of the following should help confirm which of the two is present?

   a. Housing situation
   b. Pulmonary examination
   c. Cough characteristics
   d. Chest x-ray examination

4. Treatment for tuberculosis requires:

   a. Isolation
   b. At least 6 months of drug therapy
   c. Penicillin plus isoniazid
   d. Desensitization

5. A client under your care for 12 months for treatment of tuberculosis is still having positive culture results. The best option is to:

   a. Consider the client a carrier and stop treatment.
   b. Refer the client to directly observed therapy (DOT).
   c. Increase the drug dosage.
   d. Refer the client to a pulmonologist.

ANSWERS AND RATIONALES

1. ***Answer:*** b (plan/management/diagnostics/respiratory/NAS)

   Rationale: The only positive finding is that the person has the organism. Active disease (and therefore contagious status) may not be present and is confirmed with a chest film or sputum cultures. (Markowitz et al., 1997)

2. ***Answer:*** d (assessment/history/respiratory/NAS)

   Rationale: All four symptoms may occur with tuberculosis. However, of these only cough is associated with tuberculosis versus other systemic chronic diseases that compromise the immune system. (Chambers, 1996)

3. ***Answer:*** b (diagnosis/respiratory/NAS)

   Rationale: Overcrowding may cause both conditions. Cough may be associated with both conditions. Consolidation may occur with either disease. There are no significant findings on the pulmonary examination of a person with tuberculosis. In pneumonia, increased vocal fremitus, dullness to percussion, crackles, and decreased breath sounds may occur. (American Lung Association, 1997)

4. *Answer:* b (plan/management/pharmacologic/respiratory/NAS)

Rationale: Isolation is not required if the person can and will control droplet spread. Treatment requires isoniazid, rifampin, pyrazinamide, and in adults ethambutol. No one can be desensitized to tuberculosis.

5. *Answer:* b (evaluation/respiratory/NAS)

Rationale: Clients with positive culture results must receive continued treatment. The positive culture result is usually a sign of nonadherence with treatment, and referral to DOT is indicated for public health. Increased dosage is not necessary and contributes to resistance.

3

Cardiovascular System

OVERVIEW

Chest pain is most closely associated with cardiac events, although it may also be associated with pulmonary events. Coronary artery disease (CAD) remains one of the most common causes of death in our society, accounting for about 50%. In 35- to 65-year-olds, coronary artery disease accounts for about 33% of deaths. The most predictive risk factors for CAD include hypertension, smoking, and hyperlipidemia. Other factors that may play a part are diabetes mellitus type II, obesity, sedentary lifestyle, psychosocial factors (e.g., stress), and heavy alcohol consumption. Unmodifiable factors, such as advanced age, genetic predisposition, male gender, race (particularly black and Asian), and diabetes mellitus type I, are those factors that cannot be altered by persons wishing to decrease their risk.

ASSESSMENT: SUBJECTIVE/HISTORY
History of Present Illness

Onset, duration, intensity, aggravating and alleviating factors, location, and quality are critical components to differentiate chest pain.

Symptoms

These can help distinguish the cause of the pain. If a client reports diaphoresis, radiation down the left arm or into the jaw, shortness of breath, midsternal pain with exercise, or shortness of breath with exercise, consider the pain to be cardiac in nature until proved otherwise. Pain with inspiration indicates a pleuritic component.

Past Medical History

- Hypertension
- Diabetes
- Hyperlipidemia
- Cardiovascular or peripheral vascular disease
- Gout
- Angina
- Previous or recent deep venous thrombosis (DVT)
- Cancer (from hypercoagulability)
- Chronic obstructive pulmonary disease (COPD)
- Previous spontaneous pneumothorax
- Previous or recent surgery (particularly orthopedic or trauma)
- Recent delivery

Medication History

- Ask about use of antihypertensive or vasoactive medications and use of oral contraceptives.
- Be sure to include all OTC medications the client may have taken in the past 2 weeks.

Family History

- History of cardiovascular disease
- History of pulmonary disease
- History of hypercoagulability or blood dyscrasias

Psychosocial History

- Smoking
- Increased stress levels
- Increased alcohol intake

Dietary History

Ask about increased or excessive intake of fats.

ASSESSMENT: OBJECTIVE/ PHYSICAL EXAMINATION

Physical Examination

GENERAL APPEARANCE. Obvious pallor, diaphoresis

VITAL SIGNS. Hydration status, orthostatic changes

NECK. Listen to carotid arteries for bruits; check for diminished or absent carotid pulsations.

CARDIOVASCULAR STATUS. Listen for irregular rhythms, S_3 or S_4, murmurs, artificial heart valves. Check extremities for possible signs of DVT.

PULMONARY STATUS. Adventitious diminished or absent breath sounds

Diagnostic Procedures

SPECIAL TESTS. Do ECG and stress testing (graded exercise test [GXT]). Consider doing a thallium or technetium Tc-99m sestamibi (Cardiolite) GXT if the client has bundle-branch block. Consider doing a dipyridamole thallium stress test if the client is unable to walk on the treadmill.

LABORATORY TESTS. Complete blood cell count (CBC), biochemical survey 19, Troponin I if myocardial infarction (MI) must be ruled out (more accurate assessment than cardiac enzymes)

RADIOLOGIC TESTS. Do chest x-ray (CXR). Consider ventilation perfusion (V/Q) scan if possible pulmonary embolus; consultation with physician should occur before this is undertaken.

DIAGNOSIS

Differential diagnosis includes the following:
- Angina
- Myocardial infarction
- Endocarditis
- Pericarditis
- Pulmonary embolus
- Pneumonia
- Pleurisy
- Pneumothorax
- Hemothorax if related trauma
- Gastroesophageal reflux disease (GERD; clients sometimes have difficulty in distinguishing between cardiac and epigastric pain)
- Chest wall pain

THERAPEUTIC PLAN

- The therapeutic plan depends on the selected diagnosis. Acute life-threatening or potentially life-threatening problems should be referred to a physician, or at least a consultation should be obtained.
- A non–life threatening condition may require further workup during the next several days but may not require hospitalization. For example, clients with chest pain that they are not feeling at present but have had several times recently can be worked up for CAD as outpatients. However, if there is a strong indication that the pain is cardiac in nature, the client should be sent home with nitroglycerin tablets and a careful explanation of how and when to use them.
- If all cardiac workup results are negative and pain persists, begin a gastrointestinal (GI) workup for GERD or gastritis.

Pharmacologic Treatment

If cardiac origin is suspected, inhibit platelet aggregation with aspirin 81 mg daily. Enteric-coated aspirin is best in the older adult.

EVALUATION/FOLLOW-UP

Schedule return visit for 1 to 2 weeks, depending on the diagnosis. If indicated, a GXT should be scheduled as soon as possible. Have the client document symptoms and notify about any new symptoms or change in the symptoms.

REFERENCES

McCance, K., & Huether, S. (1994). *Pathophysiology: The biologic basis for disease in adults and children* (2nd ed.). St. Louis, Mosby.

Reuben, D., Yoshikawa, T., & Besdine, R. (Eds.) (1995). *Geriatrics review syllabus.* New York: American Geriatrics Society.

Wilson, J., Braunwald, E., Isselbacher, K., Petersdorf, R., Martin, J., Fauci, A., & Root, R. (Eds.). (1991). *Harrison's principles of internal medicine* (12th ed). New York: McGraw-Hill.

Woodley, M., & Whelan, A. (Eds.). (1992). *Manual of medical therapeutics* (27th ed). Boston: Little, Brown.

REVIEW QUESTIONS

1. Chest pain that lasts for less than 15 minutes and is relieved with rest is considered to be:

    a. COPD
    b. Pulmonary embolus
    c. Angina
    d. MI

2. The presence of an S_3 heart sound in the presence of chest pain may be indicative of:

    a. Pneumonia
    b. Pericarditis
    c. Pulmonary embolus
    d. MI

3. All the following symptoms are associated with chest pain and are likely to represent CAD **except:**

    a. Jaw pain
    b. Shortness of breath
    c. Diaphoresis
    d. Pain with inspiration

4. Chest pain that is reproducible with palpation of the chest is most likely:

    a. MI
    b. Chest wall pain
    c. Pneumonia
    d. Angina

5. Which of the following can be worked up on an outpatient basis?

    a. Pulmonary embolus
    b. MI
    c. Angina
    d. Pneumothorax

6. Clients sent home with SL nitroglycerin should be taught to take this medication as follows:

    a. 1 tablet SL q 5 minutes to a total of 3 tablets
    b. 1 tablet SL q 2 minutes to a total of 6 tablets
    c. 1 tablet SL q 10 minutes to a total of 5 tablets
    d. 1 tablet only; if no relief, call ambulance

ANSWERS AND RATIONALES

1. *Answer:* c (diagnosis/cardiovascular/NAS)
    Rationale: Angina is myocardial ischemia relieved by rest and by definition lasts less than 15 minutes.

2. *Answer:* d (assessment/physical examination/cardiovascular/NAS)
    Rationale: Because the injured myocardium is not functioning normally and part of the left ventricle can become dyskinetic, the S_3 indicates left ventricular function.

3. *Answer:* d (assessment/history/cardiovascular/NAS)
    Rationale: Pain with inspiration indicates a pleuritic component; this indicates a lung rather than cardiac problem.

4. *Answer:* b (assessment/physical examination/cardiovascular/NAS)
    Rationale: Chest wall pain is the inflammation of the joint between the rib, sternum, and cartilage located between the rib and the sternum.

5. *Answer:* c (plan/cardiovascular/NAS)
    Rationale: Although angina may be a precursor of MI, it can be worked up on an outpatient basis unless it is unstable and the client is experiencing ischemic changes on the ECG.

6. *Answer:* a (plan/cardiovascular/NAS)
    Rationale: If pain relief has not been achieved with this regimen, the pain may be indicative of more extensive myocardial ischemia and possible MI.

CONGENITAL HEART DEFECTS

Acyanotic Lesions, Obstructive Lesions: Coarctation, and Cyanotic Congenital Heart Defects

OVERVIEW
Definition

A *congenital heart defect* is a cardiac lesion present in neonates.

Incidence

Approximately 0.8% of all neonates are born with a congenital heart defect. This includes lesions diagnosed later in life.

Types

ACYANOTIC HEART DEFECTS. Congenital heart defects in which *no* deoxygenated or poorly oxygenated blood enters the systemic circulation are *acyanotic*. Types include the following:

- Left-to-right shunting through abnormal opening:
  —Patent ductus arteriosis (PDA)
  —Atrial septal defect (ASD)
  —Ventricular septal defect (VSD)
- Obstructive lesions that restrict ventricular outflow:
  —Aortic valvular lesions
  —Pulmonary artery stenosis
  —Coarctation of the aorta

CYANOTIC HEART DEFECTS. Congenital heart defects in which deoxygenated blood enters the systemic circulation are *cyanotic*. Types include the following:

Right-to-left-shunting:
  Tetrology of Fallot
  Tricuspid atresia
  Transposition of great arteries (TGA)
  Truncus arteriosus
  Hypoplastic left heart syndrome
  Total anomalous pulmonary venous communication

Risk Factors

- Fetal and maternal infection during the first trimester (especially rubella)
- Maternal alcoholism
- Maternal use of other drugs with teratogenic effects
- Maternal age older than 40 years
- Maternal dietary deficiencies
- Maternal insulin-dependent diabetes
- Other congenital defects

NOTE: All children with congenital heart lesions should be closely followed up by cardiology or cardiothoracic specialists. Information is provided to review the lesions, presenting symptoms, and diagnostic findings. Treatment options are briefly discussed as a point of interest; it is not necessary to be familiar with specifics of diagnostics or treatment because most nurse practitioners are not primary caregivers of these clients.

Acyanotic Lesions

❧ *PATENT DUCTUS ARTERIOSUS*

OVERVIEW
Definition

Patent ductus arteriosus is the persistent patency of the fetal structure bridging the pulmonary artery and the descending aorta. Two types of shunting are possible. One is *left-to-right shunting,* in which congestive heart failure is possible depending on the size of the PDA. The other is *right-to-left shunting,* in which oxygenation is a problem.

Incidence

In term infants the ductus arteriosus usually closes at birth. PDA accounts for between 2% and 5% of symptomatic cardiac diseases seen in the first 28 days. Premature infants of less than 34 weeks' gestational age have a significantly higher incidence of PDA in conjunction with respiratory distress syndrome.

Pathophysiology

Factors that influence ductal patency include the following:

- Muscle mass
- Low oxygen tension

- Low pH
- Acetylcholine
- Prostaglandin E_2
- Catecholamines
- Bradykinin

ASSESSMENT: OBJECTIVE/ PHYSICAL EXAMINATION
Physical Examination

A physical examination should be conducted, with particular attention to the following:
- Blood pressure
- Pulse pressure
- Vital signs
- Weight
- General appearance
- Respiratory and cardiac status

CIRCULATORY STATUS. Bounding pulses with wide pulse pressure, hyperactive precordium, enlarged heart, and pulmonary edema can all be signs of decompensation.

CARDIAC STATUS. A continuous, "machinery" grade I to IV/VI murmur may also be audible at the upper left sternal border or left intraclavicular area.

URINARY STATUS. Decreased urinary output may be seen.

Diagnostic Procedures

- Echocardiography with Doppler detects the structural defect.
- CXR findings are dependent on the direction of flow across the PDA and on the degree of the shunt.
- ECG findings may be normal or reveal left ventricular hypertrophy in small to moderate PDAs.

DIAGNOSIS

Differential diagnosis includes the following:
- Noncardiogenic pulmonary edema
- Respiratory distress syndrome
- ASD
- VSD

THERAPEUTIC PLAN

- Client may be free of symptoms and in hemodynamically stable condition with a small PDA; this would require no immediate intervention.
- Client should be closely monitored for any respiratory or hemodynamic instability.

- In clients with symptoms and hemodynamic instability, surgical ligation is the treatment of choice.

❖ ATRIAL SEPTAL DEFECTS

OVERVIEW
Definition

An *atrial septal defect* is an opening between the two atria that permits the shunting or mixing of blood.

Incidence

ASD occurs in approximately 10% of clients with congenital heart disease. It is twice as common in females as in males.

Pathophysiology

There is no pressure differential between the right and left sides of the heart during the first month of life as a result of relatively elevated pulmonary artery pressures. As the right-sided pressures begin to fall, more blood is shunted along the path of least resistance from both atria into the right ventricle and pulmonary vessels. This creates an increased volume load on the right ventricle. Excessive flow passes through the pulmonic valve, creating a relative pulmonic stenosis with a concomitant murmur. It also leads to right-sided heart failure. In addition, through time this may lead to pulmonary hypertension as a result of high blood flow through the pulmonary arteries.

ASSESSMENT: SUBJECTIVE/HISTORY

Client may have no symptoms or may demonstrate varying degrees of right-sided heart failure. Older children are seen with fatigue, shortness of breath, and poor growth and development.

ASSESSMENT: OBJECTIVE/ PHYSICAL EXAMINATION
Physical Examination

A physical examination should be conducted with particular attention to general appearance and cardiac status.

GENERAL APPEARANCE. Failure to thrive; cyanosis only with pulmonary hypertension

CARDIAC STATUS. Arterial pulses are normal and equal; the heart is hyperactive, with heave best felt at left lower sternal border. S_2 is widely split and fixed at pulmonic area, with no thrills. A grade I to III/VI systolic ejection murmur (SEM) is heard best at the left sternal border.

Diagnostic Procedures

- ECG shows right axis deviation, right ventricular hypertrophy, and right atrial enlargement.
- CXR demonstrates cardiac enlargement, with the main pulmonary artery dilated.
- Echocardiography shows paradoxic motion of the ventricular septal wall and a dilated right ventricular cavity.
- Cardiac catheterization reveals a significant increase in oxygen saturation at the atrial level. Pulmonary pressures are normal or elevated.

THERAPEUTIC PLAN

Surgery is recommended for clients with a ratio of pulmonary to systemic blood flow greater than 2:1. Elective surgery is performed in clients between 2 and 4 years. Early surgery is recommended for infants with CHF or critical pulmonary hypertension.

❀ VENTRICULAR SEPTAL DEFECTS

OVERVIEW
Definition

A *ventricular septal defect* is an opening between the two ventricles permitting the shunting or mixing of blood. Defects may occur in the membranous, muscular, or apical portions of the ventricular septum.

Incidence

VSD is the most common form of congenital cardiac heart defect, representing 20% to 25% overall. From 30% to 50% of all VSDs close spontaneously. From 60% to 70% of small defects also close.

Pathophysiology

There is only a slight pressure difference between the right and left ventricles during the first month of life as a result of relatively elevated pulmonary artery pressures. Therefore there is little flow across the VSD and only a slight murmur is heard. As the right-sided pressures begin to fall, more blood is shunted along the path of least resistance from the left ventricle into the right ventricle and pulmonary vessels. As the pressure gradient increases, turbulence of circulation between the two ventricles increases and creates a louder murmur. It also creates an increased volume load on the right ventricle and left atrium. This leads to biventricular failure or right-sided heart failure. In addition, in time this may lead to pulmonary hypertension as a result of high blood flow through the pulmonary arteries.

ASSESSMENT: SUBJECTIVE/HISTORY
Symptoms

- Acyanosis
- Frequent respiratory infections during infancy or early childhood
- Dyspnea
- Exercise or feeding intolerance
- Edema
- Abdominal distention
- Fatigue

Past Medical History

Ask about frequent respiratory infections, as noted above.

Dietary History

Inquire about feeding intolerance and high salt intake if edema is present.

ASSESSMENT: OBJECTIVE/ PHYSICAL EXAMINATION

A problem-oriented physical examination should be conducted with particular attention to vital signs and weight, general appearance, respiratory status, and cardiac status.

GENERAL STATUS. Many children demonstrate failure to thrive, with slow growth and poor weight gain. Some may even demonstrate developmental delay. This is predominantly due to CHF, which develops between 1 to 4 months.

RESPIRATORY STATUS. Signs of respiratory distress include grunting, flaring, retracting, and increased respiratory rate. Inspiratory rales and expiratory wheezing may occur.

CARDIAC STATUS. The degree of symptoms varies depending on the size of the shunt.

- Small left-to-right shunts
  —Grade II or III pansystolic murmur, left sternal border

- Moderate left-to-right shunts
  —Grade III to IV/VI harsh, pansystolic murmur, lower left sternal border at fourth intracostal space
  —No heaves, lifts, or thrills

Diagnostic Procedures

- ECG is normal in most cases.
- CXR may also vary according to the size of the shunt.
- Echocardiography only will identify VSD ≥4 mm
- Angiography shows normal to increased left atrial pressures.
- Pulmonary vascular resistance varies from normal to markedly increased.

DIAGNOSIS

Differential diagnosis may include the following:
- ASD
- Tetralogy of Fallot (the acyanotic type, "pink tet")
- PDA

THERAPEUTIC PLAN

If the client does not respond to selective therapy or has increasing pulmonary hypertension, surgery is indicated. Age at elective surgery ranges from younger than 2 to 5 years.

Obstructive Lesions: Coarctation

OVERVIEW
Definition

Coarctation is a constricture of the aorta, most commonly surrounding the insertion site of the ductus arteriosus into the descending thoracic aorta.

Incidence

Coarctation occurs in 0.2 per 1000 live births, with a male predominance of almost 2:1. As the eighth most common defect among all age groups, it is seen frequently in infancy when collateral circulation is poor.

Pathophysiology

Left ventricular outflow tract obstruction occurs with development of left ventricular hypertrophy and eventually CHF.

Factor Increasing Risk of Recurrence. One parent with coarctation.

OTHER ASSOCIATED DEFECTS OCCURRING WITH COARCTATION
- Bicuspid aortic valve
- VSD
- PDA
- TGA
- Hypoplastic left ventricle

ASSESSMENT: SUBJECTIVE/HISTORY

Most common symptoms include the following:
- Dyspnea
- Tachypnea
- Irritability
- Feeding difficulties
- Tachycardia
- Failure to thrive
- Cool lower extremities with decreased pulses
- Ashen color
- Cyanosis

These symptoms are typically not present until 2 weeks of age. Circulatory shock, as demonstrated by oliguria, anuria, or any of the above symptoms, may not appear until 2 to 6 weeks of age. Relatively symptom-free children may only report leg pains.

ASSESSMENT: OBJECTIVE/ PHYSICAL EXAMINATION
Physical Examination

Attention should focus on four-extremity blood pressure, vital signs, weight, and general appearance.
- *Respiratory:* Pulmonary rales
- *Circulatory:* Mild periorbital edema, dorsum hand and feet edema
- *Cardiac:* SEM most common at left sternal border; frequent hypertension from poor renal perfusion; typically, upper extremity blood pressure higher than that of lower extremities by >10 mm Hg
- *Hepatic:* Hepatosplenomegaly
- *Renal:* Oliguria or anuria

Diagnostic Procedures

- ECG reveals left ventricular hypertrophy for mild cases and right axis deviation with right ventricular hypertrophy in more severe forms.
- CXR shows normal or enlarged heart.

- Two-dimensional (2D) echocardiography shows shelflike narrowing of descending aorta.
- Cardiac catheterization measures an increased pressure gradient or pressure drop across the coarctation.

DIAGNOSIS

Differential diagnosis includes the following:
- Hypoplastic left heart syndrome
- CHF

THERAPEUTIC PLAN

Plan of care depends on whether a client has symptoms or not. Observe for increasing symptoms. In some cases balloon angioplasty may be necessary. The surgical options of choice include resection of the coarctated segment with an end-to-end anastomosis.

Cyanotic Congenital Heart Defects

❋ *TRANSPOSITION OF THE GREAT ARTERIES*

OVERVIEW
Definition

Transposition of the great arteries (TGA) is defined as a switch of the origin of the great arteries from their normal ventricular origins so that the aorta originates from the right ventricle and the pulmonary artery arises from the left ventricle.

Incidence

Prevalence is 2 in 10,000 live births, representing the second most common defect in the first year of life.

Pathophysiology

ASSOCIATED FACTORS
- Male (3:1)
- Normal to slightly increased birth weight
- No maternal or fetal distress
ASSOCIATED DEFECTS
- VSD
- Tricuspid regurgitation
- Pulmonic stenosis

ASSESSMENT: OBJECTIVE/ PHYSICAL EXAMINATION
Physical Examination

GENERAL STATUS. Infant is normal or large at birth; however, a growth and developmental delay is seen if the condition remains undetected.

CIRCULATORY STATUS. Baseline cyanosis increases with crying and has little or no response to increased inspired oxygen. Clubbing of the digits is seen.

CARDIAC STATUS. The S_2 is single and loud. When auscultating, no murmur is audible if ventricular septum is intact. CHF may be present.

Diagnostic Procedures

CXR indicates right axis deviation and right ventricular hypertrophy, "egg on a string" appearance.

ELECTROLYTES. Hypoglycemia, hypocalcemia, and acidosis

DIAGNOSIS

Differential diagnosis includes the following:
- Truncus arteriosus
- Hypoplastic right ventricle syndrome
- Hypoplastic left ventricle syndrome
- Double-outlet right ventricle (DORV)
- Double-outlet left ventricle (DOLV)

THERAPEUTIC PLAN

Before surgical intervention, temporizing measures include infusion of prostaglandin E_1, to maintain patency of the ductus arteriosus, and treatment of CHF.

❋ *TETRALOGY OF FALLOT*

OVERVIEW
Definition

Tetralogy of Fallot is a congenital heart disease consisting of four different abnormalities, including pulmonary stenosis or atresia, VSD, right ventricular hypertrophy, and overriding or dextroposition of aorta.

Incidence

Tetralogy of Fallot accounts for 10% to 15% of all congenital heart disease, representing the most prevalent form of heart disease beyond infancy. Incidence is the same for males and females.

Pathophysiology

Severe right ventricular outflow tract obstruction coupled with a large VSD results in a right-to-left shunt at the ventricular level, with subsequent desaturation of arterial blood. The size of the shunt determines the degree of desaturation and amount of cyanosis. The greater the obstruction, the larger is the VSD; the lower the systemic vascular resistance, the greater the right-to-left shunt noted. Therefore right ventricular pressure cannot surpass left ventricular pressure but they may be equal.

ASSOCIATED DEFECTS
- Right-sided aortic arch, 25%
- ASD, 15%

ASSESSMENT: SUBJECTIVE/HISTORY

Most common symptoms include the following:
- Dyspnea on exertion or squatting
- Cyanosis, especially during vagal maneuvers

ASSESSMENT: OBJECTIVE/ PHYSICAL EXAMINATION
Physical Examination

A physical examination should be conducted with particular attention to vital signs, weight, general appearance, and the following:

RESPIRATORY STATUS. Client may have hypoxic spells, peaking at 2 to 4 months. These begin with rapid and deep respirations, followed by irritability with crying. Cyanosis and heart murmur intensity decrease. An intense spell can lead to limpness, seizures, cerebrovascular accident (CVA), or even death. Death during a cyanotic spell is extremely rare.

CARDIAC STATUS. Thrill at lower left sternal border, aortic ejection click, normal S_1, loud and single S_2, III to V/VI SEM at middle to upper left sternal border

CBC shows polycythemia, iron deficiency anemia with normal hematocrit, coagulopathies.

Diagnostic Procedures

- ECG shows right axis displacement and right ventricular hypertrophy. Rhythm disturbances occasionally occur.

- CXR shows decreased pulmonary vascular markings. Heart size is overall normal, but CHF may be present in acyanotic clients. The classic finding of a boot-shaped heart is due to a normal heart size with significant right ventricular hypertrophy and upturning of the apex of the heart. Right aortic arch may be present in 25%.
- 2D echocardiography reveals a large PDA and overriding of the aorta. Doppler studies confirm antegrade pulmonary flow or continuous or diastolic pulmonary flow. A VSD is also seen.

DIAGNOSIS

Differential diagnosis includes the following:
- Severe valvular pulmonic stenosis with intact ventricular septum
- Truncus arteriosus with decreased pulmonary flow
- Double-outlet right ventricle
- TGA with subpulmonic stenosis, VSD, and tricuspid atresia

THERAPEUTIC PLAN

Diagnose and treat iron deficiency anemia because clients are predisposed toward CVAs.

PALLIATIVE TREATMENT
- Detect and treat hypoxic spells.
- Propranol decreases heart rate and may increase stroke volume.
- Prostaglandin E_1 is indicated with severe cyanosis and ductal dependence in infancy.
- Atrial septostomy is performed by means of cardiac catheterization.
- Surgical procedure is shunt to allow flow to bypass the obstructive lesion to the lungs.

DEFINITIVE TREATMENT. Closure of VSD with removal of ventricular outflow obstruction frequently results in rhythm disturbances.

❧ *TRUNCUS ARTERIOSUS*

OVERVIEW
Definition

Truncus arteriosus is a condition in which the arterial trunk arises out of both ventricles in fetal life and later divides into the aorta and the pulmonary artery with the development of the bulbar septum.

Incidence

Truncus arteriosus accounts for less than 1% of all congenital heart disease. Occurrence is 3 in 100,000 live births, with frequency more in females than in males.

Pathophysiology

Associated defects include the following:
- Large VSD
- Right aortic arch in 50% of cases
- DiGeorge syndrome should be considered in any infant with this defect.

ASSESSMENT: OBJECTIVE/ PHYSICAL EXAMINATION

Physical Examination

A physical examination should be conducted with particular attention to: vital signs, weight, general appearance, and the following:

CIRCULATORY STATUS. Variable degrees of cyanosis may be present after birth.

RESPIRATORY STATUS. Signs of CHF may develop within several weeks.

CARDIAC STATUS. A harsh grade II to IV/VI systolic murmur, similar to VSD, that can go into diastole may be present at the upper left sternal border. An apical diastolic rumble with or without gallop may be present if pulmonary blood flow is large. A constant ejection click, bounding pulses, and wide pulse pressure may be present.

Diagnostic Procedures

- Arterial blood gases (ABGs) shows mild desaturation, with little improvement with hyperoxia.
- ECG shows electrographic signs of CHF in 70% of cases.
- CXR shows cardiomegaly (biventricular and left atrial enlargement), narrow mediastinum, and increased pulmonary blood flow. Right aortic arch is present 50% of the time.
- 2D echocardiography reveals large PDA right under truncal valve.

DIAGNOSIS

Differential diagnosis includes the following:
- TGA
- Hypoplastic right ventricle syndrome
- Hypoplastic left ventricle syndrome
- Double-outlet right ventricle
- Double-outlet left ventricle

THERAPEUTIC PLAN

- Diuretics and digoxin are required to decrease pulmonary congestion.
- Cardiac catheterization demonstrates the abnormal anatomy as well as the hemodynamics and pressures. It can determine the size and branching pattern of the main pulmonary artery. An aortogram rules out truncal insufficiency and major stenosis in pulmonary arteries.
- Early surgical repair is the treatment of choice. Most infants die of CHF between 6 and 12 months unless surgery is performed.

GENERAL CARE STRATEGIES FOR CONGENITAL HEART DEFECTS

Whenever caring for a client with a congenital heart defect in either the preoperative or postoperative period, some simple principles should be followed to ensure optimized care. The three major areas of concern are worsened CHF, increased shunt, and inadequate surgical correction. These can be easily followed up with careful histories and physical examinations. Parents should also be alerted to these same signs so that they can seek the earliest possible care to correct the problem. If an infant is experiencing hypoxic spell, place infant over the shoulder in the knee-chest position.

Assessment: Subjective/History

The history should concentrate on the following:

RESPIRATORY STATUS
- Shortness of breath
- Dyspnea
- Inability to feed
- Cyanosis (at rest or exacerbating factors)
- Cough
- Retractions

- Grunting
- Flaring

CARDIOVASCULAR STATUS

- Sweating
- Cyanosis
- Pallor
- Increased facial ruddiness
- Increasing head size
- Limb discrepancies
- Mottling
- Increasing edema

ABDOMINAL STATUS

- Increased abdominal girth
- Vomiting
- Constipation
- Diarrhea

RENAL STATUS. Decreased wet diapers or decreased urination.

NEUROLOGIC STATUS

- Lethargy
- Irritability
- Seizures
- Disorientation
- Developmental delay (inability to achieve milestones)

Assessment Objective: Physical Examination

The physical examination should concentrate on the following:

VITAL SIGNS/GENERAL STATUS

- Failure to thrive/poor weight and height gain
- Tachypnea
- Tachycardia
- Hypotension
- Hypertension

RESPIRATORY STATUS

- Shortness of breath
- Dyspnea
- Cyanosis (at rest or exacerbating factors)
- Cough
- Retractions
- Grunting
- Flaring
- Inspiratory rales
- Wheezing

CARDIOVASCULAR STATUS

- Murmur changes
- Decreased pulses
- Decreased capillary refill

- Sweating
- Cyanosis
- Pallor
- Increased facial ruddiness
- Increasing head size
- Limb discrepancies, mottling, and edema

ABDOMINAL STATUS. Hepatosplenomegaly.

NEUROLOGIC STATUS

- Lethargy
- Irritability
- Seizures
- Disorientation
- Developmental delay (inability to achieve milestones)

Evaluation/Follow-Up

During follow-up appointments, the client must always be evaluated for recurrence of symptoms.

REFERENCES

Kempe, C. H., Silver, H., O'Brien, D., & Fulginiti, V. (1997). *Current pediatric diagnosis and treatment.* Norwalk, CT: Appleton & Lange.

Korones, S., & Bada-Ellzey, H. (1993). *Neonatal decision making.* St. Louis: Mosby.

Long, W. (1990). *Fetal and neonatal cardiology.* Philadelphia: W. B. Saunders.

Park, M. (1991). *The pediatric cardiology handbook.* St. Louis: Mosby.

REVIEW QUESTIONS

1. All the following are signs of CHF in an infant **except:**

   a   Sweating during feedings
   b. Tachycardia
   c. Failure to thrive
   d. Cyanosis

2. At birth an infant is noted to be cyanotic with respiratory distress. The test most specific for detection of congenital heart disease would be:

   a   Physical examination for a heart murmur
   b. CXR
   c. Echocardiography
   d. ABG analysis

3. A 2-day-old 32-week gestational age female infant who is presently on a mechanical ventilator suddenly needs increased oxygen. She is noted to have a hyperdynamic precordium, bounding femoral pulses, palmar pulses, and a widened pulse pressure. CXR demonstrates bilateral pulmonary edema. The most likely cardiac defect would be:

   a. TGA
   b. PDA
   c. Tetralogy of Fallot
   d. Truncus arteriosus

4. A 5-year-old boy is seen for his preschool physical examination and is noted to have cool lower extremities with weak pulses and hypertension (blood pressure 164/92 mm Hg). Initial tests to examine for possible coarctation of the aorta would include all the following **except:**

   a. Four-extremity blood pressures
   b. ECG
   c. CXR
   d. GXT

5. In evaluation of TGA, the classic CXR would reveal:

   a. A figure of 3
   b. A snowman in a snowstorm
   c. A boot
   d. An egg on a string

6. A term female infant is born cyanotic with an oxygen saturation of 74% on 100% inspired oxygen. The infant is noted to have a loud, harsh heart murmur and a single S_2. The most likely diagnosis is:

   a. Tetralogy of Fallot
   b. TGA
   c. Truncus arteriosus
   d. VSD

7. Physical findings consistent with a clinically significant ASD include all the following **except:**

   a. Hypertension
   b. A murmur consistent with pulmonic stenosis
   c. Failure to thrive
   d. Normal pulses

8. Physical findings of CHF in the presence of congenital heart defects would include all the following **except:**

   a. Failure to gain weight
   b. Hepatosplenomegaly
   c. Dysrhythmia
   d. Increasing head circumference

ANSWERS AND RATIONALES

1. *Answer:* d (assessment/history/cardiovascular/infant)

  Rationale: Although it can be associated with CHF, cyanosis is a sign of shunting of blood from the right to the left side of the heart without oxygenation in the lungs. Signs of CHF in an infant include tachycardia, tachypnea, failure to thrive, sweating, oliguria, edema, lethargy, respiratory distress, pallor, coughing, seizures, developmental delay, and hepatosplenomegaly.

2. *Answer:* c (assessment/physical examination/cardiovascular/infant)

  Rationale: Heart murmurs are very common in the neonatal period and may either represent congenital heart lesions or be simple benign flow murmurs. This is an extremely nonspecific test. Although CXR and ABGs can assist in the assessment of cyanosis and dyspnea, they fail to distinguish between pulmonary and cardiac primary lesions. Echocardiography can be used not only to visualize the heart but also to examine blood flow and to estimate pressures within the chambers and overall ventricular function. This is therefore the most specific of the examinations listed and would be superseded only by the highly invasive procedures of cardiac catheterization and direct observation of the heart for true specificity.

3. *Answer:* b (diagnosis/cardiovascular/infant)

  Rationale: Failure of the ductus arteriosus to close results in progressive heart failure in the first days of life. It is significantly more common in premature infants and is especially characterized by widened pulse pressures as a result of diastolic shunting of blood to the pulmonary circulation. The other lesions would all be characterized by cyanosis and would benefit from ductal patency.

4. *Answer:* d (assessment/physical examination/cardiovascular/child)

Rationale: Coarctation of the aorta can be essentially diagnosed with simple tests that can be performed in the office, such as four-extremity blood pressures to examine for significant blood pressure discrepancies between the upper and lower extremities. ECG and CXR add evidence of left-sided heart failure with this obstructive lesion. GXT would not be appropriate unless there were evidence of myocardial ischemia.

5. *Answer:* d (assessment/physical examination/cardiovascular/child)

Rationale: Although CXR frequently does not demonstrate clear-cut findings, they do demonstrate many features of the classic picture. A figure of 3 is seen with coarctation of the aorta as the stricture narrows the aorta at a single fixed location. The snowman in the snowstorm represents the extreme heart failure and pulmonary edema seen in total anomalous pulmonary venous return. The boot is the right ventricular hypertrophy and lack of pulmonary blood flow in tetralogy of Fallot. The egg on the string in TGA represents significant CHF with a narrowed mediastinum as a result of alignment of the great vessels in the midline.

6. Answer: c (diagnosis/cardiovascular/infant)

Rationale: A VSD would not result in cyanosis in an infant. Although tetralogy of Fallot, TGA, and truncus arteriosus are all characterized by cyanosis, only truncus arteriosus features a single S_2 because there is only a single heart valve that exits from the two ventricles.

7. *Answer:* a (assessment/physical examination/child)

Rationale: Initially, ASDs can go undetected until pulmonic pressures decrease. As right ventricular overload occurs, the client has increased flow across the pulmonic valve and a murmur of relative stenosis. Left ventricular output remains within normal limits until extremely late in the disease process. Therefore pulses and blood pressure remain normal. As ventricular failure progresses, clients have failure to thrive as they expend increased energy to maintain normal metabolism.

8. *Answer:* c (assessment/physical examination/child)

Rationale: Although dysrhythmias can be heard on auscultation and seen on ECG with some congenital heart lesions, this is not secondary to the CHF. Dysrhythmias are due to electrolyte abnormalities, such as hypomagnesemia, hypocalcemia, and hypokalemia, or to structural defects that interrupt the normal paths of conduction. For historical and physical findings of CHF in congenital heart disease, see the section on general education and care strategies.

CONGESTIVE HEART FAILURE

OVERVIEW
Definition

Congestive heart failure occurs when the heart is unable to maintain an output adequate to meet the metabolic demands of the body.

Incidence

- In the United States, 2 million people have CHF.
- Each year 400,000 new cases are diagnosed.
- The 5-year mortality is greater than 50%.
- Persons with CHF are six to nine times more likely than those without it to die of sudden cardiac death (Konstam & Dracup, 1994).
- CHF is the most common inpatient diagnosis.

Pathophysiology

Symptoms occur as a result of organ hypoperfusion and inadequate tissue oxygen delivery caused by a decreased cardiac output and decreased cardiac reserve; pulmonary and venous congestion.

SYSTOLIC DYSFUNCTION
- Inotropic abnormalities
- Decreased systolic emptying

DIASTOLIC DYSFUNCTION. Impaired ability of ventricle to accept blood

COMPENSATORY MECHANISMS
- Left ventricular dilatation and hypertrophy
- Increase in systemic vascular resistance related to activation of the sympathetic ner-

vous system and an increase in catechol-amines
- Activation of the renin-angiotensin system

CHILDREN. Primary cause of CHF in first 3 years of life is congenital heart disease.

RISK FACTORS
- CAD
- Hypertension
- Valvular disorder
- Anemia (severe)
- Thyroid disease
- Cardiomyopathy
- Arrhythmias
- Infection
- Pregnancy
- Volume overload
- Medications (e.g., beta-blockers, nonster-oidal antiinflammatory drugs (NSAIDs)
- Decreased client compliance with medications
- Congenital heart disease

ASSESSMENT: SUBJECTIVE/HISTORY

Symptoms

- Dyspnea on exertion
- Orthopnea with paroxysmal nocturnal dyspnea (PND)
- Edema
- Decreased exercise capacity
- Dry, hacky cough
- Fatigue
- Recent weight gain
- Bloating or abdominal fullness
- Change in mental status (mainly in older adults)
  CHILDREN
  - Feeding difficulties
  - Failure to thrive

Past Medical History

Ask about listed risk factors. Assess for the following:
- CAD
- COPD
- Renal disease
- Diabetes
- Hypertension
- Previous MI
- Valvular disease

Medication History

Look for recent use of the following:
- Beta-blockers
- NSAIDs
- Calcium-channel blockers

Family History

Ask about family history of the following:
- Heart disease
- Hypertension
- Diabetes mellitus

Dietary History

- Inquire about recent increase in use of sodium.
- Ask about increased consumption of fluids in clients with previous decompensated heart failure and known left ventricular dysfunction.

ASSESSMENT: OBJECTIVE/ PHYSICAL EXAMINATION

Physical Examination

A problem-oriented examination should be performed with attention to the following areas:

VITAL SIGNS, WEIGHT, GENERAL APPEARANCE
- Client may be hypotensive, normotensive, or hypertensive.
- Pulse rate may be tachycardic.
- Weight may be increased (it is important to assess the time span in which the weight gain occurred).

NECK. Jugular venous distention.

CHEST
- Basilar rales that do not clear with cough
- Wheezes
- Cough
- Respiratory distress in children

CARDIAC STATUS
- S_3 gallop
- Laterally displaced point of maximal impulse (PMI)
- Murmur

ABDOMEN
- Hepatomegaly
- Hepatojugular reflex

EXTREMITIES. Peripheral edema

SPECIFIC FINDINGS. The most specific diagnostic physical findings in a client with symptoms include elevated jugular venous pressure, S_3, and displaced PMI (Konstam & Dracup, 1994).

Diagnostic Procedures

- CXR: Cardiomegaly, pulmonary venous congestion
- ECG: Ischemia, arrhythmias, conduction abnormalities, left ventricular hypertrophy
- CBC: Anemia
- Electrolytes
- Serum creatinine
- Thyroid function tests: Thyroxine and thyroid-stimulating hormone should be checked in all clients 65 years old and older who have heart failure of no obvious etiology.
- Serum albumin: There may be increase in extravascular volume as a result of hypoalbuminemia.
- Urinalysis: Presence of proteinuria, RBCs
- Echocardiography or radionuclide ventriculography to measure left ventricular ejection fraction

DIAGNOSIS

- List New York Heart Association (NYHA) functional class (I through IV).
  Class I: No dyspnea with exertion
  Class II: Dyspnea with maximal exertion
  Class III: Dyspnea with minimal exertion
  Class IV: Dyspnea at rest
- Differential diagnosis includes the following: pulmonary disease, pneumonia, MI, arrhythmias, cirrhosis, nephrotic syndrome

THERAPEUTIC PLAN

The goal is to improve the quality of life; treatment is aimed at the underlying etiology and symptom control. Refer clients to physician in cases of new-onset heart failure or heart failure refractory to conventional therapy; refer children.

Nonpharmacologic Treatment

- Client and family education includes explanation of the diagnosis, prognosis, and symptoms of worsening heart failure and resultant interventions.
- Dietary restrictions: 2 g sodium diet, fluid restriction if appropriate, decrease in ethanol consumption
- Obtain and record daily weights. Weight gain of 2 to 4 pounds in a 2- to 3-day period should be reported.
- Regular exercise and activity to improve functional capacity
- Smoking cessation
- Medications and compliance: Include rationale for medications and side effects. (Konstam & Dracup, 1994; Miller, 1994)

Pharmacologic Treatment

- *Angiotensin-converting enzyme (ACE) inhibitors:* These decrease mortality and prolong survival in clients with CHF. They should be prescribed for all clients with systolic dysfunction unless contraindicated.
  —Contraindications include intolerance or side effects, potassium level >5.5 mEq, signs and symptoms of hypotension.
  —Starting doses may need to be adjusted in the older adult.
- *Diuretics:* These decrease preload, dyspnea on exertion, orthopnea with PND, and edema.
  —Increased doses may be needed in clients with renal failure, and decreased doses may be necessary in older adults.
  —Use loop diuretics when a rapid response is needed (acute presentation of CHF). CAUTION: Overdiuresis may lead to renal insufficiency or hypotension.
  —Complications of diuretic use include electrolyte imbalances and carbohydrate intolerances.
- *Digoxin:* This increases the force of ventricular contraction in clients with left ventricular systolic dysfunction. It should be used in conjunction with diuretics and ACE inhibitors in clients with severe heart failure.
- If ACE inhibitors are contraindicated, an alternative may be the combination of hydralazine and isosorbide. (Konstam & Dracup, 1994)

EVALUATION/FOLLOW-UP

- Return to clinic as necessary until CHF is compensated.
- Once compensated, routine follow-up is every 1 to 3 months.
- Refer client to physician if CHF is refractory to intervention.

REFERENCES

Deedwania, P., & Carbajal, E. (1995). Congestive heart failure. In M. Crawford (Ed.), *Current diagnosis and treatment of cardiology* (pp. 140-162). Norwalk, CT: Appleton & Lange.

Hoole, A., Pickard, C., Ouimette, R., Lohr, J., & Greenberg, R. (1995). *Patient care guidelines for nurse practitioners* (4th ed.). Philadelphia: J. B. Lippincott.

Konstam, M., & Dracup, K. (1994). *Heart failure: Evaluation and care of patients with left ventricular systolic dysfunction*, Clinical Practice Guideline No. 11. AHCPR Publication 94. Agency for Health Care Policy and Research, Public Health Service, U.S. Department of Health and Human Services.

Miller, M. (1994). Current trends in the primary care management of chronic congestive heart failure. *Nurse Practitioner: The American Journal of Primary Health Care, 19*(5), 64-70.

Smith, T., Braunwald, E., & Kelly, R. (1992). The management of heart failure. In *Heart disease: A textbook of cardiovascular medicine* (pp. 464-509). Philadelphia: W. B. Saunders.

REVIEW QUESTIONS

1. Which of the following is not a compensatory mechanism of CHF?

    a. Progressive left ventricular dilatation and hypertrophy
    b. Activation of the sympathetic nervous system
    c. Activation of the renin-angiotensin system
    d. Decrease in systemic vascular resistance

2. Which of the following is **not** considered a precipitating risk factor for CHF?

    a. Hypertension
    b. CAD
    c. Severe anemia
    d. Family history

3. A 68-year-old man with known systolic dysfunction seeks treatment with increasing dyspnea and signs of recurrent heart failure. Which of the following medications may be contributing to these symptoms?

    a. Aspirin, 325 mg/day
    b. Digoxin, 0.125 mg/day
    c. Lisinopril, 10 mg/day
    d. Metoprolol, 50 mg bid

4. Which of the following diagnostic tests is indicated for evaluation of left ventricular ejection fraction?

    a. Echocardiogram
    b. ECG
    c. CXR
    d. GXT

5. A 52-year-old woman with known CHF reports dyspnea with minimal exertion (walking from room to room). In what NYHA functional class is she?

    a. Functional class I
    b. Functional class II
    c. Functional class III
    d. Functional class IV

6. All the following are appropriate differential diagnoses for the client seeking treatment for dyspnea **except:**

    a. CHF
    b. Anxiety (panic attacks)
    c. Pulmonary embolus
    d. Pelvic inflammatory disease

7. Which of the following drugs have been proved to decrease mortality and increase survival in persons with CHF?

    a. Diuretics
    b. Digoxin
    c. ACE inhibitors
    d. Nitrates

8. Which of the following is **not** a contraindication to use of an ACE inhibitor?

    a. Hypotension
    b. Serum potassium of ≥5.5 mEq
    c. History of intolerance or reaction to ACE inhibitors
    d. Renal insufficiency

9. A 60-year-old man with a history of CHF and an ejection fraction of 25% comes to the clinic with compensated CHF. His medications include furosemide 80 mg bid, enalapril 5 mg bid, digoxin 0.25 mg/day, and aspirin 325 mg/day. His blood pressure is recorded as 126/70 mm Hg and his pulse is 70 beats/min. What would you do to optimize afterload reduction?

    a. Increase enalapril to 10 mg bid.
    b. Continue his current medication regimen.
    c. Change furosemide to hydrochlorothiazide
    d. Increase digoxin to 0.375 mg/day.

10. Which of the following restrictions is **not** necessary in all clients with CHF related to systolic dysfunction?

    a. Sodium restriction of 2 g/day
    b. Decrease in alcohol consumption
    c. Strict fluid restriction
    d. Reinforcement of medication compliance

ANSWERS AND RATIONALES

1. Answer: d (diagnosis/cardiovascular/NAS)

Rationale: There is an increase in systemic vascular resistance as a result of activation of the sympathetic nervous system and an increase in catecholamines. (Dweedwania & Carbajal, 1995)

2. *Answer:* d (assessment/history/cardiovascular/NAS)

Rationale: Although family history is considered a risk factor for CAD, it is not a precipitating risk factor for CHF. There is an underlying pathophysiologic cause for development of CHF. (Konstam & Dracup, 1994)

3. *Answer:* d (assessment/history/cardiovascular/aging adult)

Rationale: Negative inotropic agents such as beta-blockers, verapamil, diltiazem, and class IA and IC antiarrhythmics can cause a decompensation in CHF. NSAIDs can also contribute to CHF. (Smith, Braunwald, & Kelly, 1992)

4. *Answer:* a (assessment/physical examination/NAS)

Rationale: Echocardiogram or radionuclide ventriculography can be used to measure left ventricular ejection fraction. GXT measures functional capacity but does not provide a definitive measure of left ventricular function unless used with echocardiography or radionuclide ventriculography. (Konstam & Dracup, 1994; Deedwania & Carbajal, 1995)

5. *Answer:* c (diagnosis/cardiovascular/adult)

Rationale: Class I, no limitation in activity; class II, dyspnea with normal to maximal physical activity; class III, dyspnea with minimal activity; class IV, dyspnea at rest. (Smith, Braunwald, & Kelly, 1992)

6. *Answer:* d (diagnosis/cardiovascular/NAS)

Rationale: All the listed diagnoses may feature dyspnea as a presenting symptom. Anxiety disorders usually have an irregular pattern and occur frequently at rest; hyperventilation may be noticed. (Deedwania & Carbajal, 1995)

7. *Answer:* c (plan/management/therapeutic/pharmacologic/cardiovascular/NAS)

Rationale: ACE inhibitors have been shown to reduce mortality and increase functional status in persons with CHF. None of the other drugs listed have been shown to decrease mortality. (Konstam & Dracup, 1994)

8. *Answer:* d (plan/management/therapeutic/pharmacologic/cardiovascular/NAS)

Rationale: ACE inhibitors can be used with caution in clients with elevated creatinine (<3 mEq) but require close monitoring with follow-up seven-item chemistry panel. ACE inhibitors should not be instituted in clients with elevated serum potassium and the presence of hypotension. (Konstam & Dracup, 1994)

9. *Answer:* a (evaluation/cardiovascular/adult)

Rationale: ACE inhibitors optimize afterload reduction. Given the blood pressure of 126/70 mm Hg, this client will tolerate an increase in his enalapril. Reinforce symptoms of side effects, such as signs of orthostasis. Because the client is compensated on his current doses of digoxin and furosemide, these should be continued. (Konstam & Dracup, 1994)

10. *Answer:* c (evaluation/cardiovascular/NAS)

Rationale: Excessive fluid intake should be avoided. However, strict fluid restriction is necessary only in the presence of hyponatremia. (Konstam & Dracup, 1994)

DIZZINESS (SYNCOPE)

OVERVIEW

- *Syncope* is defined as a transient loss of consciousness accompanied by unresponsiveness and loss of postural tone with spontaneous recovery.
- Syncope is most likely to occur in the older adult, increasing with age from 2% in ages 65 to 69 years to 12% in those older than 85 years.
- The pregnant woman is more susceptible to syncopal episodes as a result of a change in her blood flow, particularly when changing position.

ASSESSMENT: SUBJECTIVE/HISTORY

History of Present Illness

- Ask about the circumstances around the syncopal episode; what the client was doing, where he or she was, and a subjective description of the event. For women of childbearing age, ask for date of last menstrual period and about contraceptive use.
- Timing of the syncopal episode is critical. Does it occur after micturition, defecation, coughing, or swallowing? These events may lead to a transient hypotension that results in syncope.
- Another cause of syncope is carotid sinus hypersensitivity. Syncope usually occurs with tight collars or neck turning, such as with shaving. Medications can also provoke carotid sinus hypersensitivity (e.g., digitalis, beta-blockers, alpha-methyldopa, and calcium-channel blockers).

Symptoms

- Chest pain
- Shortness of breath
- Pleuritic chest pain

Past Medical History

- Hypotension
- Cardiovascular or peripheral vascular disease
- Atrial fibrillation
- Ventricular aneurysms
- Aortic stenosis
- Hypoglycemia
- Seizures
- Pulmonary disease
- Carotid artery disease

Medication History

In older adults the medications most likely to cause syncope are phenothiazine, tricyclic antidepressants, and antihypertensive medications.

Family History

- History of cardiovascular disease
- History of CVA

Psychosocial History

- Smoking
- Increased stress

Dietary History

Syncope can be precipitated by swallowing, so the timing in relationship to meals is important. Also, if the client is taking antihypertensive medications with a meal or just before, hypotension can develop, causing a syncopal episode. Poor nutrition can also cause dehydration and hypotension leading to syncope.

ASSESSMENT: OBJECTIVE/ PHYSICAL EXAMINATION

Physical Examination

A complete physical examination is indicated with a chief complaint of syncope. Special attention should be paid to the cardiovascular examination. Orthostatic vital signs should be taken and hydration status should be assessed.

Diagnostic Procedures

LABORATORY TESTS
- CBC
- Electrolytes
- Glucose
- Creatine kinase
- Consider troponin I if possible MI

RADIOLOGIC TESTS
- Obtain echocardiogram if history of heart disease.
- If trauma to head during syncopal episode, consider CT of head.

- Consider carotid artery Doppler study if any indication of central nervous sysem (CNS) problem.

OTHER TESTS

- ECG
- Consider doing 24-hour Holter monitoring.
- Consider tilt table.
- Consider other electrophysiologic testing if all other test results are negative.

DIAGNOSIS

Differential diagnosis includes the following:
- Pulmonary embolus
- MI infarction
- Vasovagal syncope
- Situational syncope
- Drug-induced syncope
- Orthostatic hypotension
- Postprandial hypotension
- Aortic stenosis
- Pulmonary hypertension
- Idiopathic hypertrophic subaortic stenosis
- Carotid sinus syncope
- Subclavian steal
- Coronary artery disease
- Transient ischemic attack
- Seizure
- Psychogenic syncope
- Left atrial myxoma
- Tetralogy of Fallot
- Arrhythmias
- Hypoglycemia
- Pregnancy

THERAPEUTIC PLAN

The therapeutic plan depends on the diagnosis. While working the client up, consider using aspirin 81 mg/day for platelet inhibition.

EVALUATION/FOLLOW-UP

- Clients should be followed up closely until a cause for the syncopal episode is known.
- Clients should be educated to change positions slowly, waiting before actually moving after a position change has been made.

REFERENCES

Hart, G. (1995). Evaluation of syncope. *American Family Physician, 51,* 1941-1948.

Kapoor, W. (1994). Evaluation and management of syncope. *Contemporary Internal Medicine, 6,* 29-39.

McCance, K., & Huether, S. (1994). *Pathophysiology: The biologic basis for disease in adults and children* (2nd ed.). St. Louis: Mosby.

Reuben, D., Yoshikawa, T., & Besdine, R. (Eds.). (1995). *Geriatrics review syllabus.* New York: American Geriatrics Society.

Wilson, J., Braunwald, E., Isselbacher, K., Petersdorf, R., Martin, J., Fauci, A., Root, R. (Eds.). (1991). *Harrison's principles of internal medicine* (12th ed). New York: McGraw-Hill.

Woodley, M., & Whelan, A. (Eds.). (1992). *Manual of medical therapeutics* (27th ed). Boston: Little, Brown.

REVIEW QUESTIONS

1. All the following can lead to a syncopal event **except:**

   a. Micturition
   b. Swallowing
   c. Neck turning with shaving
   d. Sleeping

2. A medication that can cause carotid sinus hypersensitivity is:

   a. Beta-blockers
   b. Aspirin
   c. Acetaminophen
   d. NSAIDs

3. Although a full physical examination is important when assessing a client with syncope, to what part of the examination should special attention be paid?

   a. Pulmonary
   b. GI
   c. Cardiovascular
   d. Ears, nose, and throat

4. Clients receiving antihypertensive medications should be taught which of the following?

   a. Take medications just before meals

   b. Change positions slowly (from lying to standing, waiting a few minutes in sitting position before standing, and standing a few minutes before beginning to walk).

   c. Put the head between the knees before standing up.

   d. Skip medications if feeling light-headed.

5. Clients with a diagnosis of carotid sinus hypersensitivity should be taught which of the following?

   a. Avoid changing positions quickly.

   b. Avoid high-calorie meals.

   c. Avoid tight collars.

   d. Avoid sweets.

6. Clients with syncope should be followed up:

   a. Only as needed

   b. Closely until a diagnosis is made for the syncope

   c. Yearly until a diagnosis is made for the syncope

   d. Every 3 months until a diagnosis is made for the syncope

ANSWERS AND RATIONALES

1. *Answer:* d (diagnosis/cardiovascular/NAS)

   Rationale: Answers *a* and *b* are situational causes of syncope and *c* refers to carotid sinus hypersensitivity; therefore *d* is the correct answer.

2. *Answer:* a (diagnosis/cardiovascular/NAS)

   Rationale: Beta-blockers provoke carotid sinus hypersensitivity by their dilatory effect as well as the slowing of the electrical impulse.

3. *Answer:* c (assessment/physical examination/cardiovascular/NAS)

   Rationale: Although the cause of syncope is often undetermined, the most likely cause is cardiovascular.

4. *Answer:* b (plan/cardiovascular/NAS)

   Rationale: Because of the effect of antihypertensive medications on the vascular tree, if clients are taught to change position slowly, the vascular tree is given a chance to adjust to the change so that the brain continues to be perfused adequately.

5. *Answer:* c (plan/cardiovascular/NAS)

   Rationale: Tight collars may stimulate carotid sinus hypersensitivity by putting pressure on the carotid sinus and partially obstructing flow, particularly if the head is turned.

6. *Answer:* b (evaluation/cardiovascular/NAS)

   Rationale: Clients with syncope should be followed up closely until a diagnosis for the syncope is made. Depending on the diagnosis, treatment can be initiated and the client may not need such close follow-up at that point.

HYPERLIPIDEMIA (HYPERLIPOPROTEINEMIA)

OVERVIEW
Definition

Hyperlipidemia is excessive accumulation of one or more of the lipoproteins in the blood. *Primary hyperlipidemia* is hereditary or spontaneous genetic disorder of metabolism. *Secondary hyperlipidemia* is caused by disease (diabetes mellitus, renal disease, hypothyroid).

Clinical trials have clearly demonstrated a relationship between high cholesterol levels and CAD. Reduction of cholesterol levels reduces the incidence of cardiac events. National Cholesterol Education Project (NCEP) has recommended guidelines for the diagnosis and management of high cholesterol levels (National Cholesterol Education Project [NCEP], 1993).

Incidence

- In the United States, approximately 120 million people have cholesterol ≥200 mg/dl.
- Hypercholesterolemia incidence is 1/500.
- Prevalence increases with age.

- The condition is more common in males than in females.

Pathophysiology

Hyperlipidemia results from excessive production of lipids, defective removal of lipids, or both excessive production and defective removal.

PROTECTIVE FACTORS AGAINST CAD AND INCREASED CHOLESTEROL

- Exercise
- Estrogen
- High-density lipoprotein (HDL) >35 mg/dl

FACTORS INCREASING SUSCEPTIBILITY TO CAD AND INCREASED CHOLESTEROL

- History of CAD, such as MI or angina
- At least two of following:
  —Male gender
  —Family history of CAD (MI, sudden death of parent or sibling younger than 55 years)
  —Cigarette smoking
  —Hypertension
  —Low HDL cholesterol (<35 mg/dl in men, <45 mg/dl in women)
  —Diabetes mellitus
  —History of CVA or peripheral vascular disease
  —Obesity (>30% above desirable weight)
- High intake of saturated fatty acids
- High intake of dietary cholesterol
- High intake of total calories resulting in obesity
- Sedentary lifestyle
- Stress
- Heredity

ASSESSMENT: SUBJECTIVE/HISTORY

Symptoms

No symptoms are pathognomic for hypercholesterolemia; however, 35% to 55% of affected persons may report abdominal pain. These episodes are related to marked elevations of triglyceride levels (>1000 mg/dl). Client may also have nausea, vomiting, borborygmi, and diarrhea.

Past Medical History

Ask about past history of elevated cholesterol, exercise, smoking, and stress.

Medication History

Inquire about oral contraceptives, anabolic steroids, and diuretics.

Family History

Ask about family history of elevated cholesterol.

Dietary History

Inquire about diet. Consider 24-hour diet recall or diet diary. Caffeine may increase cholesterol.

ASSESSMENT: OBJECTIVE/ PHYSICAL EXAMINATION

Physical Examination

A problem-oriented physical examination should be conducted, with particular attention to vital signs, weight (obesity), and general appearance.

SKIN. Xanthomas

EYE. Arcus senilus before 50 years

Diagnostic Procedures

- *Thyroid-stimulating hormone:* Hyperthyroidism can increase cholesterol level.
- *Cholesterol:* <200 mg/dl is desirable, 201 to 239 mg/dl is borderline, and >240 mg/dl is high.
- *HDL:* >35 mg/dl
- *Low-density lipoprotein (LDL):*
  Total cholesterol − HDL − triglycerides = LDL
  —*High LDL:* ≥160 mg/dl
  —*Borderline:* 130 to 159 mg/dl
- *Triglycerides:* <200 mg/dl is desirable, 200 to 400 mg/dl is borderline high, 400 to 1000 mg/dl is high, and >1000 very high. Needs to be fasting specimen.

Children

Screening should be done for children who have a family history of premature CAD (before 55 years) or parental hypercholesterolemia (>240 mg/dl).

DIAGNOSIS

Accurate diagnosis is important. Consider secondary lipoprotein disorders.

THERAPEUTIC PLAN

A therapeutic plan for treatment of hyperlipidemia is shown in Table 3-1.

Table 3-1   Therapeutic Plan for Treatment of Hyperlipidemia

TREATMENT	INITIATION LDL LEVEL	GOAL LDL LEVEL
Dietary Treatment		
Without CAD or <2 risk factors	≥160 mg/dl	<160 mg/dl
>2 risk factors	≥130 mg/dl	<130 mg/dl
Drug Treatment		
Without CAD or <2 risk factors	≥190 mg/dl	<160 mg/dl
Without CAD but >2 risk factors	≥160 mg/dl	<130 mg/dl
With CAD		<100 mg/dl

Modified from National Cholesterol Education Program (1993). Summary of the second report of the National Cholesterol Education Program (NCEP) Expert Panel on Detection, Evaluation, and Treatment of High Blood Cholesterol in Adults (Adult Treatment Panel II). *Journal of the American Medical Association, 269,* 3015.

Table 3-2   Dietary Management of Hyperlipidemia

RECOMMENDED GUIDELINES	STEP ONE	STEP TWO
Total fat	<30% of total calories	<30% of total calories
Saturated fatty acids	<10% of total calories	<7% of total calories
Polyunsaturated fatty acids	≤10% of total calories	≤10% of total calories
Monounsaturated fatty acids	10%-15% of total calories	10%-15% of total calories
Carbohydrates	50%-60% of total calories	50%-60% of total calories
Protein	10%-20% of total calories	10%-20% of total calories
Cholesterol	<300 mg/dl/day	<200 mg/dl/day

Modified from U.S. Preventive Services Task Force (1996). *Guide to clinical preventive services* (2nd ed.). Baltimore: Williams & Wilkins.

Cholesterol Reduction in Older Adults

The benefit of lowering cholesterol in older adults has not been clearly defined. Research shows a decreased mortality among persons with CAD who follow a low-cholesterol diet and take medications.

Cholesterol Reduction in Children

Dietary changes appear to reduce LDL levels in children with familial elevated cholesterol levels. However, long-term benefits of cholesterol reduction in children are unclear. Studies are ongoing to determine long-term benefits and medication safety and efficacy.

Nonpharmacologic Therapy

- Dietary management is first line of defense.
- Step One diet is recommended by the American Heart Association as "prudent" for the U.S. population.
- Step Two diet decreases cholesterol and fat intake further (Table 3-2).

EXERCISE. Regular exercise enhances fatty acid oxidation and glycogen storage, increasing HDL formation, triglyceride clearance, and insulin sensitivity. These changes cause reductions in serum lipid levels. HDL levels rise approximately 20% and LDL levels may decrease as much as 10%.

SMOKING CESSATION. Individuals who smoke tend to have lower HDL and higher VLDL levels. All clients with hyperlipidemias should be counseled to stop smoking.

Pharmacologic Therapy

Pharmaceutical agents should be tried if client does not respond to 3 to 6 months of intensive dietary therapy. If the client has an LDL level >220 mg/dl, drug therapy should be begun after 3 months of diet if no improvement is seen. Dietary therapy should continue during drug therapy.

Four categories of medication are available for reduction of cholesterol levels (Table 3-3).

Table 3-3 Categories of Medication for Reduction of Cholesterol Levels

DRUG CATEGORY	BEST FOR THESE CLIENTS	EFFECT ON LDL	EFFECT ON HDL	EFFECT ON TRIGLYCERIDE	COMMENTS ABOUT DRUG
Nicotinic acid	Use for clients with ↑ LDL and triglycerides	−15% to 20%	+30% to 35%	−25% to 30%	Cutaneous flushing; GI complaints; gradually increase dose; take with aspirin to ↓ flushing
Bile acid sequestrants	Young men and premenopausal women (no other risk factors) with moderate ↑ LDL	−15% to 25%	+5%	+10%	Unpleasant sandy, gritty taste; GI complaints; compliance a problem
Fibric acid derivatives	Clients with diabetes and clients with type 3 elevated lipids, not as useful for secondary prevention	−15%	+15% to 20%	−45% to 50%	Well tolerated; some GI complaints; ↑ in cholelithiasis
3-Hydroxy-3-methylglutaryl coenzyme A "statins"	Good for both familial and nonfamilial ↑ cholesterol	−20% to 45%	+10%	−20%	Well tolerated; ↑ in liver function tests; GI complaints; good compliance

COMBINATION DRUG THERAPY. If response with one drug and diet is inadequate, consider adding a second drug.

OTHER DRUG THERAPY. Estrogen may increase HDL levels and lower LDL levels. Estrogens have been shown to be beneficial to postmenopausal women with preexistent CAD.

Client Education

- For clients 20 to 70 years old, measure cholesterol level every 5 years.
- Discuss healthy diet; encourage use of diet diary, exercise, smoking cessation.

Referral

Referral may be made to cholesterol specialists if blood cholesterol is not responsive to medication. Those with genetic hyperlipidemias should be followed up by specialists.

EVALUATION/FOLLOW-UP

- After drug therapy is started, lipids should be checked in 4 weeks and at 3 months.
- Once target goals of LDL and cholesterol have been achieved, total cholesterol should be measured every 4 months, with a full lipid analysis every year.

REFERENCES

American Heart Association. *Dietary guidelines.* Dallas, TX: Author.

Blackman, M., & Busby-Whitehead, M. (1995). Clinical implications of abnormal lipoprotein metabolism. In L. Barker, J. Burton, & P. Zieve. (Eds.). *Principles of ambulatory medicine* (4th ed., 1075-1101).Baltimore: Williams & Wilkins.

National Cholesterol Education Program. Summary of the second report of the National Cholesterol Education Program (NCEP) Expert Panel on Detection, Evaluation, and Treatment of High Blood Cholesterol in Adults (Adult Treatment Panel II) (1993). *Journal of the American Medical Association, 269,* 3015.

U.S. Preventive Services Task Force (1996). *Guide to clinical preventive services* (2nd ed.). Baltimore: Williams & Wilkins.

REVIEW QUESTIONS

1. Calvin Smith (47 years) had an MI 2 years ago. His cholesterol level is 245 mg/dl, with LDL of 159 mg/dl and HDL of 45 mg/dl. The treatment goal for his LDL cholesterol level should be:

   a. 190 mg/dl
   b. 160 mg/dl
   c. 130 mg/dl
   d. 100 mg/dl

2. Which of the following subjective factors would most influence your choice for treatment for hyperlipidemia?

   a. Obesity
   b. Sedentary lifestyle
   c. Family history of elevated cholesterol
   d. High intake of dietary cholesterol

3. Cardiovascular risk and treatment goals related to hyperlipidemia are determined by what factor?

   a. Total cholesterol
   b. LDL
   c. HDL
   d. VLDL

4. Which of the following physical examination findings would lead you to suspect hyperlipidemia?

   a. Increased liver size
   b. Xanthoma of inner canthus of both eyes
   c. Obesity
   d. Arcus senilus of both eyes

5. Initial treatment prescribed for Sylvia (40 years, cholesterol 297 mg/dl, LDL 189 mg/dl) would be:

   a. Lifestyle changes
   b. Step Two dietary plan by the American Heart Association
   c. Increased oat bran in diet
   d. Use of pharmaceutical agents

6. What is the most appropriate recommendation for screening of cholesterol in children?

   a. Screen all children.
   b. Screen children who have family members with elevated cholesterol levels.
   c. Only obese children should be screened.
   d. Because treatment for elevated cholesterol in children is controversial, no children should be screened.

7. Bev, a 50-year-old woman with a history of elevated cholesterol (340 mg/dl), LDL of 220 mg/dl, and a history of recent angioplasty, has been started on a 3-hydroxy-3-methylglutaryl coenzyme A (statin) drug. What information is crucial before beginning this drug?

   a. CBC
   b. Renal panel
   c. Liver panel
   d. Thyroid-stimulating hormone

8. Bev has been taking the statin drug for 1 month. She reports muscle weakness and has noticed brown discoloration of her urine. What is the appropriate action for the nurse practitioner to take at this time?

   a. Continue her antilipemic, but check her laboratory values.
   b. Stop her antilipemic and encourage increased hydration.
   c. Increase her antilipemic dosage.
   d. Send her to the emergency department.

9. Cheryl has started taking niacin she got at a health food store for her elevated cholesterol level. What is a common side effect seen with this drug?

   a. Flushing
   b. Constipation
   c. Bad taste in mouth
   d. Discoloration of urine

10. What are the current recommendations for routine screening for cholesterol?

   a. Every year
   b. Every 2 years
   c. Every 5 years
   d. Every 10 years

ANSWERS AND RATIONALES

1. *Answer:* d (diagnosis/cardiovascular/NAS)
Rationale: Any client with known CAD should have as a treatment goal reduction of LDL levels to <100 mg/dl. (NCEP, 1993)

2. *Answer:* c (assessment/history/cardiovascular/NAS)
Rationale: Clients who have a family history will be more likely to require pharmacologic treatment to reduce their hyperlipidemia. (NCEP, 1993)

3. *Answer:* b (plan/cardiovascular/NAS)
Rationale: Treatment for and risk of CAD are determined by the client's LDL level. (NCEP, 1993)

4. *Answer:* b (assessment/physical examination/cardiovascular/NAS)
Rationale: Xanthomas are dermatologic indications of elevated cholesterol. They are commonly seen in the inner canthus of the eyelids, as well as behind the knees, skin folds, and scars. (Blackman & Busby-Whitehead, 1995)

5. *Answer:* a (plan/cardiovascular/NAS)
Rationale: Initial treatment for most clients consists of dietary changes and exercise. Only clients with known CAD and elevated cholesterol levels should be started immediately on pharmacologic therapy. (NCEP, 1993)

6. *Answer:* b (diagnosis/cardiovascular/child)
Rationale: Only children who have family members with elevated cholesterol levels should be screened. The long-term benefit of cholesterol reduction in children is unclear; however, for those who have known elevated cholesterol levels, dietary changes can be initiated. (NCEP, 1993)

7. *Answer:* c (plan/cardiovascular/adult)
Rationale: Statins may cause elevated hepatic function tests (in approximately 1% of clients.) A baseline liver function test is essential before starting therapy. (Blackman & Busby-Whitehead, 1995)

8. *Answer:* b (evaluation/cardiovascular/adult)
Rationale: Statins can cause myopathy in approximately 0.1% of clients. The myopathy is reversible if the drug is discontinued and hydration is encouraged. If the drug is not stopped, severe myopathy (rhabdomyolysis) can occur. (NCEP, 1993)

9. *Answer:* a (evaluation/cardiovascular/adult)
Rationale: The most common side effect seen with niacin is flushing. This side effect is usually tolerable if the medication is started slowly and increased slowly. Tolerance to the flushes does develop. (NCEP, 1993)

10. *Answer:* c (diagnosis/cardiovascular/adult)
Rationale: Current preventive health recommendations are to screen for cholesterol levels every 5 years. (U.S. Preventive Services Task Force, 1996)

HYPERTENSION

OVERVIEW
Definition

PRIMARY (ESSENTIAL) HYPERTENSION. An elevation of blood pressure to >140 mm Hg systolic and >89 mm Hg diastolic on the average of two or more readings taken at each of two or more visits

URGENT HYPERTENSION. An elevated diastolic blood pressure (DBP) between 120 and 160 mm Hg without symptoms or acute retinopathy

SEVERE, ACCELERATED, OR MALIGNANT HYPERTENSION. Elevation of DBP to >120 mm Hg with evidence of target-organ damage such as retinal hemorrhages, exudates, or papilledema, left ventricular hypertrophy or dysfunction, and renal or cerebrovascular injury

ISOLATED SYSTOLIC HYPERTENSION (ISH). Persistently elevated systolic blood pressure (SBP) to >160 mm Hg, with DBP of <90 mm Hg

HYPERTENSIVE CRISIS. Severe elevation of DBP to >120 to 130 mm Hg, considered an emergency in the presence of acute or ongoing target-organ damage (rapid or progressive deterioration of central nervous system, myocardial, hematologic, or renal function)

CLASSIFICATION OF HYPERTENSION. The various levels of blood pressure for adults, including four stages of hypertension, are shown in Table 3-4.

Table 3-4   Classification of Blood Pressure for Adults 18 Years and Older*

CATEGORY	SYSTOLIC (mm Hg)	DIASTOLIC (mm Hg)
Normal†	<130	≤85
High normal	130-139	85-89
Hypertension‡		
Stage 1 (Mild)	140-159	90-99
Stage 2 (Moderate)	160-179	100-109
Stage 3 (Severe)	180-209	110-119
Stage 4 (Very severe)	≥210	≥120

From Joint National Committee on Detection, Evaluation and Treatment of High Blood Pressure (1993). *The fifth report of the Joint National Committee on Detection, Evaluation and Treatment of High Blood Pressure.* Bethesda, MD: National Institutes of Health, U.S. Department of Health and Human Services.

*Not taking antihypertensive drugs and not acutely ill. When systolic and diastolic pressures fall into different categories, the higher category should be selected to classify the individual's blood pressure status. For instance, 160/92 mm Hg should be classified as stage 2, and 180/120 mm Hg should be classified as stage 4. *ISH* is defined as SBP ≥140 mm Hg and DPB <90 mm Hg and staged appropriately (e.g., 170/85 mm Hg is defined as stage 2 ISH).

†Optimal blood pressure with respect to cardiovascular risk is SBP <120 mm Hg and DPB <80 mm Hg. However, unusually low readings should be evaluated for clinical significance.

‡Based on the average of two or more readings taken at each of two or more visits after an initial screening.

NOTE: In addition to classifying stages of hypertension based on average blood pressure levels, the clinician should specify presence or absence of target-organ disease and additional risk factors. For example, a client with diabetes and a blood pressure of 142/94 mm Hg plus left ventricular hypertrophy should be classified as "stage 1 hypertension with target-organ disease (left ventricular hypertrophy) and with another major risk factor (diabetes)." This specificity is important for risk classification and management.

Incidence

Approximately 50 million Americans have elevated blood pressure that requires monitoring or drug therapy. The prevalence increases with age and is greater for blacks than for whites. The condition occurs more frequently in the less educated, lower socioeconomic populations. *Children:* There is a higher incidence in children who exhibit other risk factors for cardiovascular disease or have hypertensive parents.

RISK FACTORS. Clients with hypertension are at risk for development of CAD, peripheral vascular disease, stroke, renal disease, and retinopathy. Other risk factors that compound the risk for development of hypertension include hyperlipidemia, cigarette smoking, diabetes mellitus, sedentary lifestyle, and obesity.

Hypertension in Children and Adolescents

Children and adolescents with a persistently elevated blood pressure (higher than 95th percentile for children of the same age and sex) are at risk for development of the same complications as in adults. Secondary hypertension is more common in children than in adults. Secondary hypertension is seen most in infancy and late childhood (Table 3-5).

Pathophysiology

Hypertension results from an increase in the total peripheral resistance caused by arteriolar constriction. This may be due to a primary problem with blood pressure regulation in which there is no identifiable cause. In some cases the arteriolar constriction may be due to some secondary underlying disorder. Secondary causes for hypertension include the following:

- Polycystic kidneys
- Renovascular disease
- Aortic coarctation
- Cushing's syndrome
- Pheochromocytoma
- Oral contraceptives
- Chronic alcohol abuse

The central and autonomic nervous systems regulate blood pressure through the stimulation of alpha and beta receptors on the arterioles and venules. The kidneys also provide a humoral response to maintain blood pressure in the presence of decreased blood flow to the kidneys, which results in the release of renin and its subsequent vasoconstrictors, angiotension and aldosterone. Pathologic disruption in any of these systems can lead to hypertension.

Table 3-5   Classification of Hypertension in the Young by Age Group*

	HIGH NORMAL, 90-94TH PERCENTILE (mm Hg)	SIGNIFICANT HYPERTENSION, 95-99TH PERCENTILE (mm Hg)	SEVERE HYPERTENSION, >99TH PERCENTILE (mm Hg)
Newborns			
7 days		SBP 96-105	SBP ≥106
8-30 days		SBP 104-109	SBP ≥110
Infants	SBP 104-111	SBP 112-117	SBP ≥118
(≤2 years)	DBP 70-73	DBP 74-81	DBP ≥82
Children	SBP 108-115	SBP 116-123	SBP ≥124
(3-5 years)	DBP 70-75	DBP 76-83	DBP ≥84
Children	SBP 114-121	SBP 122-129	SBP ≥130
(6-9 years)	DBP 74-77	DBP 78-85	DBP ≥86
Children	SBP 122-125	SBP 126-133	SBP ≥134
(10-12 years)	DBP 78-81	DBP 82-89	DBP ≥90
Children	SBP 130-135	SBP 136-143	SBP ≥144
(13-15 years)	DBP 80-85	DBP 86-91	DBP ≥92
Adolescents	SBP 136-141	SBP 142-149	SBP ≥150
(16-18 years)	DBP 84-91	DBP 92-97	DBP ≥98

From Joint National Committee on Detection, Evaluation and Treatment of High Blood Pressure (1993). *The fifth report of the Joint National Committee on Detection, Evaluation and Treatment of High Blood Pressure.* Bethesda, MD: National Institutes of Health, U.S. Department of Health and Human Services.
*Note that adult classifications differ.

ASSESSMENT: SUBJECTIVE/HISTORY
Symptoms
Symptoms may include the following:
- Blurred vision
- Chest pain
- Claudication
- Dizziness
- Dyspnea
- Fatigue
- Flushing
- Headaches
- Hematuria
- Muscle cramps
- Palpitations
- Tingling or cold extremities
- Weakness, usually as a result of end-organ damage or the underlying primary disorder

Clients with early primary hypertension are usually free of symptoms.

Past Medical History
Clients may report a history of the following:
- Cardiovascular disease (angina, MI, heart failure)
- Cerebrovascular disease (transient ischemic attack [TIA], CVA, or seizures)
- Renal disease (renal artery stenosis, pheochromocytoma, polycystic kidney disease, Cushing's syndrome)
- Diabetes mellitus, dyslipidemia, gout, or toxemia of pregnancy

Medication History
History should include all recent and current prescribed and OTC medications. Contraceptives, steroids, NSAIDS, nasal decongestants, cold remedies, appetite suppressants, sodium bicarbonate products (antacids), licorice, tricyclic antidepressants, monoamine oxidase inhibitors, cyclosporine, and erythropoietin can increase blood pressure or interfere with blood pressure therapy.

Family History
Ask about anyone in the family with a history of the following:
- Premature CAD
- Peripheral vascular disease
- Diabetes mellitus
- Hypertension
- Stroke, TIA, or seizures
- Renal disease
- Dyslipidemia

Psychosocial History

- Smoking and alcohol use
- Diet (especially sodium, cholesterol, and fat intake)
- Employment and family status
- Educational level
- Leisure activities
- Stress

ASSESSMENT: OBJECTIVE/ PHYSICAL EXAMINATION

Physical Examination

BLOOD PRESSURE EVALUATION

- Two or more blood pressure readings at least 2 minutes apart in supine or seated positions and after standing for 2 minutes
- The client should not have drunk coffee or smoked cigarettes within 30 minutes of the evaluation.
- Check blood pressure in both arms on at least one occasion to verify that results are equivalent.
- The appropriate cuff size should have the bladder encircle at least 80% of the arm above the antecubital space.

HEIGHT AND WEIGHT. Record measurements.

HEAD. Funduscopic examination for arteriolar narrowing, nicking, hemorrhages, exudates, papilledema

NECK. Examination for carotid bruits, distended veins, or thyromegaly

HEART. Examination for increased rate, size, precordial heave, clicks, murmurs, arrhythmias, and S_3 or S_4

ABDOMEN. Examination for bruits, enlarged kidneys, masses, or abnormal aortic pulsations

EXTREMITIES. Examination for decreased or absent peripheral arterial pulsations, bruits, or edema

NEUROLOGIC ASSESSMENT. Screening neurologic examination

Diagnostic Procedures

Laboratory testing may be used to assess cardiovascular risk factors as well as evaluating end organ function or secondary cause of hypertension. Tests may include the following:

- Urinalysis
- Multiphasic panel (potassium, calcium, creatinine, uric acid, cholesterol, triglycerides, magnesium)
- ECG
- Blood glucose
- Thyroid-stimulating hormone

DIAGNOSIS

Differential diagnosis should focus on distinguishing true primary hypertension from pseudohypertension caused by faulty blood pressure reading and from secondary hypertension. Secondary hypertension may be caused by the following:

- Polycystic kidneys
- Aortic coarctation
- Pheochromocytoma
- Renovascular disease (renal artery stenosis)
- Cushing's syndrome
- Oral contraceptives and chronic alcohol abuse

Suspect underlying pathology for secondary hypertension in the following cases:

- Drug therapy is ineffective in the compliant client.
- Elevated blood pressure occurs in individuals younger than 25 or older than 60 years in the absence of family history.
- Associated symptoms occur (edema, abnormal pulses or heart sounds, hirsutism, stria, palpitations, perspiration, and dizziness).

THERAPEUTIC PLAN

High Normal

- SBP 130 to 139, DBP 85 to 89 mm Hg
- Lifestyle modification
- Recheck blood pressure in 1 year

Stages 1 and 2

MILD. SBP 140 to 159, DBP 90 to 99 mm Hg

MODERATE

- SBP 160 to 179, DBP 100 to 109 mm Hg
- Lifestyle modification
- Confirm within 2 months.
- Initiate drug therapy within 3 to 6 months
- In the absence of target-organ disease, longer observation is acceptable if SBP is <150 mm Hg and DBP is <95 mm Hg.
- Monotherapy is preferred.
- Follow up within 1 to 2 months (if without target-organ disease).

Stage 3

- Severe
- SBP 180 to 209, DBP 110 to 119 mm Hg
- Lifestyle modification
- Initiate drug therapy within 1 week.
- It may be necessary to use two or three agents.
- Follow up within 1 to 2 weeks.

Stage 4

- Very severe
- SBP >210, DBP >120 mm Hg
- Lifestyle modification
- Initiate drug therapy on contact.
- It is often necessary to start with two agents.
- Follow up in 1 week.
- If target-organ disease is present, consider hospitalization with immediate drug therapy.
- Hospitalization is almost always required for DBP >130 mm Hg.

The scheduling of follow-up should be modified by reliable information about past blood pressure measurements, other cardiovascular risk factors, or target-organ damage.

Nonpharmacologic Therapy

- Lose weight if overweight.
- Limit alcohol intake to <1 ounce ethanol/day (24 ounces beer, 8 ounces wine, or 2 ounces 100-proof whiskey)
- Perform regular aerobic exercise.
- Reduce sodium intake to <2.3 g sodium or <6 g salt.
- Maintain adequate dietary intake of potassium, calcium, and magnesium.
- Stop smoking and decrease dietary saturated fat and cholesterol.
- Reducing fat intake will decrease caloric intake for weight control.

Pharmacologic Therapy (Table 3-6)

- Diuretics and beta-blockers are preferred because they have shown a reduction in cardiovascular morbidity and mortality in controlled clinical trials.
- Calcium-channel antagonists, ACE inhibitors, alpha$_1$-receptor blockers and alpha-beta–blockers are also effective in reducing blood

Table 3-6   Differential Antihypertensive Therapy in Specific Clinical Situations

	ADVANTAGEOUS	DISADVANTAGEOUS
CHF	ACE inhibitor, diuretic, hydralazine	Beta-blocker, reserpine, calcium-channel antagonist, ACE inhibition
Angina	Beta-blocker, calcium-channel antagonist	Hydralazine, minoxidil
Elderly	Diuretic, alpha-agonist, calcium-channel antagonist, ACE inhibitor	
Black	Diuretic, calcium-channel antagonist	Beta-blocker as initial therapy
Young	Beta-blocker, alpha-agonist, ACE inhibitor	Diuretic
Diabetes	Alpha-agonist, ACE inhibitor, calcium-channel antagonist	Beta-blocker, diuretic
Asthma, COPD	Calcium-channel antagonist	Beta-blocker, ACE inhibitor
Pregnancy	Alpha-agonist, hydralazine	Diuretic, beta-blocker
Depression	ACE inhibitor, hydralazine, calcium-channel antagonist	Methyldopa, reserpine, beta-blocker
Renal insufficiency	Alpha-agonist, calcium-channel antagonist, minoxidil, hydralazine, loop diuretic	Thiazide diuretic
Tachycardia	Beta-blocker, alpha-agonist, reserpine, verapamil, diltiazem	Nifedipine, hydralazine, minoxidil
Hyperlipidemia	Alpha-blocker, ACE inhibitor, calcium-channel antagonist	Diuretic, beta-blocker
Gout/hyperuricemia	Alpha-agonist, alpha-blocker, calcium-channel antagonist, ACE inhibitor*	Diuretic, beta-blocker, ACE inhibitor*

From Dipiro, J., Talbert, R., Hayes, P., Yee, G., Matzke, G., & Posey, L. M. (1996). *Pharmacotherapy: A pathophysiologic approach* (2nd ed.). Norwalk, CT: Appleton & Lange.
*ACE inhibitors may increase urinary clearance of uric acid, reducing hyperuricemia but increasing the risk of uric acid deposition in the urine or kidneys.

pressure, although no long-term studies have been done on mortality and morbidity.

- If initial therapeutic response is inadequate, consider increasing the initial drug dose to maximal levels, substituting another drug, or adding a second or third agent from another class.

Special Considerations

DEMOGRAPHICS. Blacks respond better to diuretics and calcium channel antagonists than to beta-blockers or ACE inhibitors. Older adults respond to all classes. No differences in treatment response have been found between genders.

QUALITY OF LIFE. Undesirable side effects of drug therapy may worsen quality of life and play a role in noncompliance.

ECONOMIC CONSTRAINTS. Drug therapy, routine laboratory tests, follow-up office visits, and time off from work should be considered in selecting therapy.

CONCOMITANT DISEASE. Choose medications that may help treat coexisting disease.

Treatment in Children

- The underlying cause, severity, and potential complications should determine intensity and type of therapy required.
- Lifestyle modifications can be used as initial therapy.
- Drug therapy should be reserved for clients with blood pressure higher than the 99th percentile or those who do not respond to lifestyle modifications.
- Children with insulin-dependent diabetes mellitus and primary renal disease should be treated with drug therapy to slow disease progression.
- Agents used in adults are also effective in young persons.

EVALUATION/FOLLOW-UP

Once the client's blood pressure has stabilized, follow-up should be at 3- to 6-month intervals. Normotensive clients should be evaluated every 1 to 2 years. Annual evaluations should be performed for those clients with hereditary or medical risks.

REFERENCES

Calhoun, D., & Opraril, S. (1990). Treatment of hypertensive crisis. *The New England Journal of Medicine, 323*(17), 1177-1182.

Dipiro, J., Talbert, R., Hayes, P., Yee, G., Matzke, G., & Posey, L. M. (1996). *Pharmacotherapy: A pathophysiologic approach* (2nd ed.). Norwalk, CT: Appleton & Lange.

Hurst, J. W. (1988). Hypertension. In *Atlas of the heart*. Philadelphia: J. B. Lippincott.

Joint National Committee on Detection, Evaluation and Treatment of High Blood Pressure (1993). *The fifth report of the Joint National Committee on Detection, Evaluation and Treatment of High Blood Pressure*. Bethesda, MD: National Institutes of Health, U. S. Department of Health and Human Services.

Moser, M. (1995). Isolated systolic hypertension in the elderly. *Internal Medicine, July*, 33-49.

Task Force on Blood Pressure Control in Children (1987). Report of the Second Task Force on Blood Pressure Control in children. *Pediatrics, 79*, 1-25.

Uphold, C., & Graham, M. (1994). *Clinical guidelines in family practice*. Gainesville, FL: Barmarrae Books.

U. S. Public Health Service, U. S. Department of Health and Human Services. Put prevention into practice. (1997). *Nurse Practitioner, 9* (1), 27-31.

REVIEW QUESTIONS

1. Which of the following diagnostic tests would **not** be appropriate for a hypertension workup?

   a. ECG
   b. CBC
   c. Sedimentation rate
   d. Urinalysis

2. The differential diagnosis for true primary hypertension includes:

   a. Pseudohypertension
   b. Secondary hypertension
   c. Both *a* and *b*
   d. None of the above

3. Lifestyle modifications for controlling blood pressure should include all the following **except:**

   a. Weight reduction
   b. Regular aerobic exercise
   c. Increased sodium intake
   d. Smoking cessation

4. Which of the following does **not** suggest a secondary cause for hypertension?

 a. Drug therapy is ineffective in the compliant client.
 b. No associated symptoms are found.
 c. Elevated blood pressure occurs in client younger than 25 or older than 60 years.
 d. Family history is positive for stroke and hypertension.

5. Which of the following medications should **not** interfere with blood pressure therapy?

 a. Oral contraceptives
 b. Antibiotics
 c. Nasal decongestants
 d. NSAIDs

6. Once their blood pressure has stabilized, hypertensive clients should be evaluated every:

 a. 1 to 2 weeks
 b. 2 to 3 weeks
 c. 2 to 3 months
 d. 3 to 6 months

7. Which of the following is **not** a secondary cause of hypertension?

 a. Renovascular disease
 b. Polycystic kidneys
 c. Cushing's syndrome
 d. Stress

8. Which physical finding is **not** characteristic of hypertensive end-organ disease?

 a. Funduscopically visible hemorrhages
 b. Carotid bruits
 c. Cardiac hypertrophy cushing's syndrome
 d. Pulmonary rhonchi

9. Which of the following statements is true?

 a. Drug therapy should be used as initial therapy for all children with diagnoses of hypertension.
 b. Concomitant disease should have no impact on the drug therapy selected.
 c. Blacks respond better to beta-blockers and ACE inhibitors.
 d. If a therapeutic response is inadequate, you may increase the dose or change to another agent.

ANSWERS AND RATIONALES

1. *Answer:* c (assessment/physical examination/cardiovascular/NAS)
 Rationale: ECG, CBC, and urinalysis are appropriate diagnostic tests used to assess for cardiovascular and renal function; they may exhibit end-organ damage as a result of hypertension. (Dipiro et al., 1996)

2. *Answer:* c (diagnosis/cardiovascular/NAS)
 Rationale: Hypertension may be caused by faulty blood pressure readings as seen in pseudohypertension or due to secondary underlying pathology. (Joint National Committee on Detection, Evaluation and Treatment of High Blood Pressure, 1993)

3. *Answer:* c (plan/cardiovascular/NAS)
 Rationale: Sodium intake should be decreased because it produces fluid retention and increased intravascular volume, which raises blood pressure. Weight reduction, exercise, and smoking cessation have all been shown to lower blood pressure. (Dipiro et al., 1996; Joint National Committee, 1993)

4. *Answer:* b (diagnosis/cardiovascular/NAS)
 Rationale: Secondary hypertension usually is seen with other associated symptoms. (Joint National Committee, 1993)

5. *Answer:* b (assessment/history/cardiovascular/NAS)
 Rationale: Antibiotics do not have any vasoconstrictive properties with respect to the neural and humoral mechanisms that control blood pressure. Oral contraceptives, decongestants, and NSAIDs have been documented to interfere with these mechanisms. (Dipiro et al., 1996)

6. *Answer:* d (evaluation/cardiovascular/NAS)
 Rationale: Hypertensive clients, once their condition has been stabilized, should be evaluated at 3- to 6-month intervals. (Joint National Committee, 1993)

7. *Answer:* d (diagnosis/cardiovascular/NAS)
 Rationale: Renovascular disease, polycystic kidneys, and Cushing's syndrome are all possible secondary causes of hypertension. (Joint National Committee, 1993)

8. *Answer:* d (assessment/physical examination)

Rationale: Funduscopically visible hemorrhages, carotid bruits, and cardiac hypertrophy are indications of end-organ damage. Pulmonary rhonchi are not associated with hypertension. (Joint National Committee, 1993)

9. *Answer:* d (plan)

Rationale: Lifestyle modifications should be initial therapy for all children. Only children with blood pressures higher than the 99th percentile or who do not respond to lifestyle modifications should be considered for drug therapy. Concomitant disease, quality of life, and economic constraints should be considered in selecting drug therapy. Blacks respond better to diuretics and calcium channel antagonists. (Joint National Committee, 1993)

MYOCARDIAL INFARCTION

OVERVIEW
Definition

Myocardial infarction results when there is a lack of oxygen to the myocardium for a prolonged period that leads to necrosis of heart muscle.

Incidence

- Approximately 900,000 people in the United States have MIs annually.
- Approximately 225,000 die; most deaths are secondary to arrhythmia.
- Mortality is greatest within the first 2 hours of onset of symptoms.
- Women on the average are 10 years older than men; however, by 75 years coronary disease in women exceeds that in men.

Pathophysiology

The coronary arteries acquire atherosclerotic changes with superimposed thrombus. These plaques cause a narrowing of the lumen of the arteries, and the development of thrombus further narrows the vessel. This may eventually lead to occlusion of the artery, causing ischemia to a particular area. If this ischemia is prolonged, infarction of muscle occurs.

MI is rare during pregnancy. However, greatest mortality occurs with MI late in pregnancy.

RISK FACTORS
- Cigarette use
- Hyperlipidemia/hypercholesterolemia
- Hypertension
- Family history of premature CAD
- Obesity
- Diabetes mellitus
- Postmenopausal without estrogen replacement therapy
- Sedentary lifestyle

ASSESSMENT: SUBJECTIVE/HISTORY
Symptoms

- Assess pain characteristics (usually occurs at rest, longer duration than angina, usually unrelieved by rest or nitroglycerin).
- Pain can be described as a retrosternal ache, heaviness, or tightness, with radiation to jaw, neck, or left arm, or through to the back. Associated shortness of breath, nausea and vomiting, or diaphoresis.
- May have acute onset of dyspnea, congestive heart failure, or confusion in the absence of chest discomfort as presenting symptoms. This can be seen in persons with diabetes and in older adults.
- Atypical presentations may occur:
  —CHF
  —Atypical location of pain (left arm or jaw pain only)
  —Mental status changes secondary to decrease in cardiac output resulting in decreased cerebral perfusion as a result of associated cerebral arteriosclerosis (older adults may have confusion)
  —Syncope
  —Indigestion-like presentation

Past Medical History

Assess presence of risk factors for CAD
- Family history of premature CAD
  —Age 65 years in women
  —Age 45 years in men
- Previous history of arteriosclerotic heart disease, diabetes, hypertension
- Recent surgical procedure that may have resulted in a large blood loss.

Medication History

- Previous and current medications
- Medication allergies

Psychosocial History

Assess client for recent use of recreational drugs. Cocaine can cause coronary spasm.

ASSESSMENT: OBJECTIVE/ PHYSICAL EXAMINATION

Physical Examination

- General appearance: Anxiousness, restlessness; Levine's sign (clenched fist against chest), diaphoresis, pallor
- Vital signs: Heart rate may vary from bradycardia to tachycardia. Premature ventricular contractions are common. Blood pressure may vary from hypotensive to hypertensive. A fever may develop within 24 to 48 hours after onset of MI as a result of tissue necrosis. Respiratory rate may be tachypneic.
- Neck: Elevated jugular venous pressure (volume overload)
- Chest: Presence of rales, left ventricular dysfunction
- Cardiac Status: S_4 gallop is frequently present. This indicates decreased left ventricular compliance. S_3 gallop indicates left ventricular dysfunction. Murmurs are commonly audible.
  —New systolic murmurs are important (e.g., mitral regurgitation and VSD).
  —Pericardial friction rubs: These most commonly occur during the second or third day postinfarction.

Diagnostic Procedures

- ECG: ST-T changes, ST-segment elevation with or without T-wave inversions; Q-wave development; Q-wave absence in non–Q-wave MI, nontransmural

- Laboratory studies
  —Cardiac enzymes: Creatine kinase–MB current standard elevate in first 6 to 8 hours, peak within 24 hours, and are resolved within 72 hours.
  —Troponin I and troponin T are markers for acute MI; increased serum levels occur early after muscle damage. Troponin I is present for as long as 7 days postinfarction; troponin T may be present for 10 to 14 days.
  —Lactic dehydrogenase (LDH): LDH elevation is detectable 12 hours after chest pain and peaks within 24 to 49 hours.
- Echocardiography: Assess left ventricular wall motion abnormalities, valvular structures.
- Other laboratory studies: CBC, electrolytes, prothrombin time, partial thromboplastin time
- CXR: pulmonary venous congestion

DIAGNOSIS

MI has occurred if two of the following criteria are present:
- Prolonged ischemic-type chest discomfort
- ECG changes consistent with ischemia
- Elevated cardiac enzymes

Differential diagnosis includes the following:
- Pericarditis: Usually there are some pleuritic components to pain.
- Pulmonary embolus: $\dot{V}/\dot{Q}$ scan; inferior ST-segment elevation
- Aortic dissection: ST-segment elevation or depression; nonspecific ST-T changes; chest CT, MRI, or transesophageal echocardiography
- Gallbladder disease
- Costochondritis
- Pancreatitis

THERAPEUTIC PLAN

Refer to physician if suspected MI; acute intervention decreases mortality.
1. Hospitalize immediately.
2. Pharmacologic intervention
   - Thrombolytics at the discretion of the physician and if no contraindications
   - Aspirin if no contraindication or allergy

- Nitrates: SL nitroglycerin provides vasodilation; avoid long-acting nitrates in early course of MI.
- Analgesics: IV morphine sulfate
- Beta-blockers decrease myocardial oxygen demand and reduce morbidity and mortality during an evolving infarction. Secondary prevention occurs with long-term use.
- Heparin IV
- ACE inhibitors within first 24 hours if blood pressure stable and thrombolytic therapy completed
- Calcium-channel blockers: no evidence of reduction in mortality after acute MI with use
3. Oxygen in initial course
4. Continuous ECG monitoring
5. Bed rest for 24 hours and as condition warrants

Complications
- Cardiogenic shock
- Cardiac arrest
- Arrhythmias
- CHF
- Postinfarction angina
- Pericarditis
- Dressler's syndrome

Client Education
- Importance of medication compliance: side effects, mechanism of action, benefits
- Lifestyle and risk factor modification
- Smoking cessation
- Low-fat and low-cholesterol diet: Consult with a dietitian if necessary, especially with associated medical conditions (renal failure, diabetes mellitus).
- Activity limitations
- Disease process and long-term implications and treatment

EVALUATION/FOLLOW-UP
- GXT to assess functional capacity, assess efficacy of current treatment plan, and perform risk stratification.
- Consider cardiac rehabilitation program if appropriate.
- Follow up with health care provider 1 to 2 weeks after discharge and then as indicated.
- Evaluation of lipid profile should be performed as appropriate.

REFERENCES

Arnstein, P., Buselli, E., & Rankin, S. (1996). Women and heart attacks: Prevention, diagnosis, and care. *Nurse Practitioner: The American Journal of Primary Health Care, 21*(5), 57-69.

Douglas, P. (1993). *Cardiovascular health and disease in women.* Philadelphia: W. B. Saunders.

Pasternak, R., Braunwald, E., & Sobel, B. (1992). Acute myocardial infarction. In *Heart disease: A textbook of cardiovascular medicine* (pp. 1200-1291). Philadelphia: W. B. Saunders.

Ryan, T. J., Anderson J. L., Antman, E. M., Braniff, B. A., Brooks, N. H., Califf, R. M., Hillis, L. D., Hiratzka, L. F., Rapaport, E., Riegel, B. J., Russell, R. O., Smith, E. E., III, & Weaver, W. D. (1996). ACC/AHA guidelines for the management of patients with acute myocardial infarction: A report of the American College of Cardiology/American Heart Association Task Force on Practice Guidelines (Committee on Management of Acute Myocardial Infarction). *Journal of the American College of Cardiology, 28*(5), 1328-1428.

REVIEW QUESTIONS

1. Which of the following is **not** a risk factor for coronary artery disease?

a. Family history of premature CAD
b. Cigarette use
c. Hyperlipidemia
d. Postmenopausal with estrogen replacement therapy

2. An 80-year-old man with a known history of a previous MI and CAD follows up on a regular basis. What listed symptoms could represent angina?

a. Dyspnea
b. Confusion
c. Indigestion
d. All of the above

3. Which of the following laboratory tests is most useful in the diagnosis of an acute MI?

  a. Liver profile
  b. Chemistry panel 20
  c. CBC
  d. Creatine kinase MB

4. A new systolic murmur is detected in a client 2 days after MI. What is the best method to evaluate the significance of the murmur?

  a. ECG
  b. CXR
  c. Echocardiogram
  d. Stress testing

5. A 48-year-old woman reports 2 hours of retrosternal chest pain. Her ECG reveals 2.5 mm ST-segment elevation in leads II, III, and aVF. What type of MI is present?

  a. Acute anterior MI
  b. Acute inferior MI
  c. Acute lateral MI
  d. Acute anterolateral MI

6. Which of the following criteria is **not** associated with an acute MI?

  a. Prolonged ischemic-type chest discomfort
  b. Elevated cardiac enzymes
  c. Chest discomfort with activity and relieved with rest
  d. ECG changes consistent with ischemia

7. Which of the following is **not** given during initial presentation of an acute MI?

  a. ACE inhibitors
  b. Oxygen
  c. Aspirin
  d. Heparin

8. Which of the following classification of drugs has been shown to reduce mortality when used long-term in MI survivors?

  a. Calcium-channel blockers
  b. Beta-blockers
  c. Nitrates
  d. Antioxidants (vitamin E)

9. A 42-year-old man 6 weeks after MI with subsequent coronary bypass grafting comes in for follow-up. He has been walking 30 minutes a day, has maintained a low-fat and low-cholesterol diet, and has quit smoking. A lipid profile is performed. According to NCEP guidelines, what is his goal LDL?

  a. <190 mg/dl
  b. <160 mg/dl
  c. <130 mg/dl
  d. <100 mg/dl

10. A 54-year-old woman comes in for follow-up with reports of chest discomfort with increased exertion (walking 1 mile) that is relieved with rest. She had a coronary angiogram approximately 3 years ago. At that time she had a 50% blockage in her right coronary artery. Which of the following is best used to evaluate progression of the blockage?

  a. ECG
  b. Echocardiogram
  c. GXT without imaging
  d. GXT with nuclear imaging

ANSWERS AND RATIONALES

1. *Answer:* d (assessment/history/cardiovascular/NAS)

  Rationale: Several studies have shown that the use of estrogen replacement therapy reduces the risk of coronary disease. (Arnstein, Buselli, & Rankin, 1996)

2. *Answer:* d (assessment/history/cardiovascular/aging adult)

  Rationale: All the above may be complaints representative of angina. In the older adult, confusion and mental status changes may be characteristic of angina or MI. Indigestion may be an atypical presentation. (Pasternak, Braunwald, & Sobel, 1992)

3. *Answer:* d (assessment/physical examination/cardiovascular/NAS)

  Rationale: Creatine kinase MB remains the current standard for diagnosing an acute MI. Troponin I and troponin T can also be markers for acute MI. (Ryan et al., 1996)

4. *Answer:* c (assessment/physical examination/ cardiovascular/NAS)

Rationale: Development of a new systolic murmur may indicate papillary muscle rupture, resulting in mitral regurgitation, or septal rupture, resulting in a VSD. An echocardiogram is the best diagnostic test to evaluate the severity of a valvular abnormality or VSD. (Pasternak, Braunwald, & Sobel, 1992)

5. *Answer:* b (diagnosis/cardiovascular/adult)

Rationale: ST-segment elevations in leads II, III, and aVF represent inferior ischemia. ST-segment elevations in leads V_1 through V_4 represent anterior ischemia. ST-segment elevations in leads I, aVL, and V_6 represent lateral ischemia. ST-segment elevations in leads I, aVL, and precordial leads represent anterolateral ischemia. (Pasternak, Braunwald, & Sobel, 1992)

6. *Answer:* c (diagnosis/cardiovascular/NAS)

Rationale: Two of the three criteria listed above as *a, b,* and *d* should be present to make a definitive diagnosis of acute myocardial infarction. (Ryan et al., 1996)

7. *Answer:* a (plan/management/therapeutics/cardiovascular/NAS)

Rationale: ACE inhibitors can be started within the first 24 hours of an acute MI. However, administration should be held until after thrombolytics are completed and blood pressure is stable. Oxygen, aspirin, and heparin should be started at time of initial presentation. (Ryan et al., 1996)

8. *Answer:* b (plan/management/therapeutics/cardiovascular/NAS)

Rationale: Chronic beta-blocker use reduces mortality by decreasing incidence of sudden cardiac death. Beta-blockers should be used if no contraindications are present. Calcium-channel blockers have not been shown to reduce mortality after MI. Use of calcium-channel blockers should be reserved if angina or blood pressure is inadequately controlled in clients with intolerance to beta-blockers. No convincing evidence is available to support use of antioxidants to reduce mortality. (Ryan et al., 1996)

9. *Answer:* d (evaluation/cardiovascular/adult)

Rationale: According to NCEP guidelines, a goal LDL of <100 mg/dl is established in clients with known CAD.

10. *Answer:* d (evaluation /cardiovascular/adult)

Rationale: An ECG may not reveal changes in absence of pain. Routine echocardiography can detect wall-motion abnormalities consistent with previous MI. Conventional GXT has decreased sensitivity and specificity when compared with GXT with imaging. Baseline abnormalities on ECG decrease the sensitivity of routine GXT. GXT with associated nuclear or echocardiographic imaging increases sensitivity and specificity of the test, as well as assisting in determining extent of ischemia in clients with known coronary disease. (Ryan et al., 1996)

THROMBOPHLEBITIS

Superficial and Deep Venous Thrombophlebitis

OVERVIEW
Definition

Superficial thrombophlebitis (SVT) is the presence of thrombus and inflammation of the superficial veins. *Deep vein thrombosis* is the presence of thrombus and inflammation in the deep venous system.

Incidence

- Occurs more commonly in women.
- All races are affected equally.

- Incidence increases with advancing age.
- Although thrombophlebitis does occur in children, incidence is low.

Pathophysiology

PROTECTIVE FACTORS. Body's natural fibrinolytic system prevents thrombus formation.

FACTORS INCREASING SUSCEPTIBILITY. Stasis of blood flow, endothelial injury, hypercoagulability

CONDITIONS ASSOCIATED WITH INCREASED RISK
- Trauma

- Old age
- Varicosities
- Previous thrombophlebitis
- Immobility
- Cancer
- CHF
- MI
- Abdominal condition
- Pelvic and lower extremity surgery
- Obesity
- Pregnancy
- Oral contraceptives and hormone replacement therapy

COMMON SITES
- Superficial thrombophlebitis: The greater or lesser saphenous veins or their tributaries are most often involved
- Deep vein thrombophlebitis: The calf veins are most frequently affected, but the popliteal, femoral, and ileofemorals are also common.

ASSESSMENT: SUBJECTIVE/HISTORY
Symptoms

SUPERFICIAL THROMBOPHLEBITIS. Sudden onset of pain localized to the site of the thrombus, a tender palpable cord, erythema and warmth without generalized edema. Low-grade fever may be present.

DEEP VEIN THROMBOPHLEBITIS. The physical signs for diagnosing DVT are unreliable. Calf pain, tenderness, unilateral swelling, low-grade fever, warmth, erythema, engorged, prominent superficial veins, and pain during dorsiflexion (Homan's sign) may occur but are nonspecific.

Past Medical History

Ask about conditions that predispose toward immobility, such as recent trauma, surgery, sedentary lifestyle, MI, or stroke. Inquire concerning previous SVT or DVT, pregnancy, recent childbirth, or coagulopathies.

Medication History

- Recent use of oral contraceptives
- Hormone replacement therapy
- Aspirin or NSAIDs

Family History

Ask about a family history of blood clotting disorders, varicose veins, or DVTs.

Psychosocial History

Ask client about tobacco use.

ASSESSMENT: OBJECTIVE/ PHYSICAL EXAMINATION
Physical Examination

A problem-oriented physical examination should be conducted with particular attention to vital signs, including temperature.

- Examine for thigh or calf tenderness on palpation, warmth, erythema, swelling, and palpable cord.
- Palpate femoral, popliteal, posterior tibial, and pedal pulses.
- Feel for enlarged, tender inguinal lymph nodes.

Test of Homan's sign is considered unreliable by some sources. Classic signs will only be found in 25% of cases of DVT.

- Pulmonary embolism may be the first clinical indication of thrombosis.

Diagnostic Procedures

SUPERFICIAL THROMBOPHLEBITIS. SVT is readily diagnosed on physical examination.

DEEP VEIN THROMBOPHLEBITIS. Refer for venous Doppler studies to measure blood flow and detect venous obstruction with good sensitivity and specificity. Venography is considered one of the most accurate means for diagnosis of DVT.

DIAGNOSIS

Differential diagnosis includes the following:

SUPERFICIAL THROMBOPHLEBITIS
- Ruptured calf muscle
- Cellulitis
- Severe muscle cramp
- Trauma

DEEP VEIN THROMBOPHLEBITIS
- Ruptured calf muscle
- Baker's cyst
- Trauma
- Cellulitis
- Lymphedema

THERAPEUTIC PLAN

SUPERFICIAL THROMBOPHLEBITIS
- Aspirin or other NSAIDs
- Discontinue oral contraceptives or hormone replacement therapy.
- Elevation of the extremity, local heat, compression with elastic stockings, and smoking cessation

DEEP VEIN THROMBOPHLEBITIS. DVT requires referral and hospitalization for initiation of antithrombotic therapy.

Client Education

- Proper use of compression stockings
- Avoid leg crossing at knees and prolonged inactivity, including sitting and standing.
- Need for a balance of exercise and rest
- Effects of oral contraceptives and hormone replacement therapy on blood clotting
- Hazards of smoking
- Do not massage calf to reduce pain.

Referral

SUPERFICIAL THROMBOPHLEBITIS. Phlebitis of a varicose vein is generally an indication for surgical removal.

DEEP VEIN THROMBOPHLEBITIS. DVT requires a referral and hospitalization.

PREGNANT WOMEN. Pregnant women should be followed up by obstetrician/gynecologist as well.

EVALUATION/FOLLOW-UP

SUPERFICIAL THROMBOPHLEBITIS. Follow-up for symptom assessment and directed physical examination. Migrating SVT may be a marker for a carcinoma and requires investigation.

DEEP VEIN THROMBOPHLEBITIS. Client should be managed in consultation with a physician.

REFERENCES

Creager, M. A., & Dzau, V. J. (1994). Vascular diseases of the extremities. In K. J. Isselbacher, E. Braunwald, J. Wilson, J. Martin, A. Fauci, & D. L. Kasper (Eds.). *Harrison's principles of internal medicine* (13th ed.). New York: McGraw-Hill.

Eftychiou, V. (1996). Clinical diagnosis and management of the patient with deep venous thromboembolism and acute pulmonary embolism. *The Nurse Practitioner, March,* 50-69.

Feied, C., & Stephen, J. (1995). Venous thrombosis: Lifting the clouds of misunderstanding. *Postgraduate Medicine, 97* (1), 36-47.

Spittell, J. A., & Spittell, P. C. (1996). Diseases of peripheral arteries and veins. In J. S. Alpert (Ed.). *Cardiology for the primary care physician.* Philadelphia: Current Medicine.

Uphold, C., & Graham, M. (1994). *Clinical guidelines in family practice.* Gainesville, FL: Barmarrae Books.

REVIEW QUESTIONS

1. Risk factors for the development of DVT include:

a. Abdominal, pelvic, and lower extremity surgery
b. Middle-class Asian female
c. Jogging more than 3 miles a day
d. Pernicious anemia

2. Twenty-nine-year-old Betty Harris works as an operating room nurse. She seeks treatment with sudden onset of left calf pain, a tender, palpable cord, erythema, and warmth to palpation. She is afebrile. Her most likely diagnosis is:

a. Ruptured Achilles tendon
b. Baker's cyst
c. Ruptured calf muscle
d. SVT

3. Diagnostic studies useful in confirming the diagnoses of SVT include:

a. Prothrombin time
b. CBC with differential
c. Doppler studies
d. Physical findings usually confirm the diagnosis.

4. Which of the following statements regarding the treatment of DVT is true?

a. A low-dose antibiotic should be used.
b. Only clients with symptoms should be treated.
c. Coumadin should be started immediately.
d. Begin aspirin therapy.

5. Clients with DVT:

a. Do not require hospitalization
b. Must have their varicose veins stripped
c. Should be managed in consultation with a physician
d. Can continue their hormone replacement therapy

6. What one factor reported by Ms. Harris is most helpful to you in making your diagnosis?

    a. "I am in an exercise class."
    b. "I do not smoke."
    c. "I am 4 weeks postpartum."
    d. "I stand a lot at work."

7. The primary emphasis in the treatment of DVT is:

    a. Early ambulation
    b. Prevention of pulmonary emboli
    c. Hypercoagulability
    d. Prevention of secondary infections

8. DVT:

    a. Can easily be diagnosed by physical findings
    b. Causes hypocoagulability
    c. May not be clinically apparent
    d. Is unusual in people older than 85 years

9. Client education for Ms. Howard, a 30-year-old postpartum woman with SVT, includes the:

    a. Side effects of antithrombotic medication
    b. Avoidance of prolonged limb dependency
    c. Need for complete bed rest
    d. Need for vena cava umbrella

ANSWERS AND RATIONALES

1. *Answer:* a (assessment/history/cardiovascular/NAS)

Rationale: Abdominal, pelvic, and lower extremity surgery are conditions associated with an increased risk for development of thrombophlebitis. Pernicious anemia, jogging, and Asian ethnicity are not risk factors. (Eftychiou, 1996)

2. *Answer:* d (diagnosis/cardiovascular/adult)

Rationale: Tender, palpable cord, erythema and warmth to palpation are more indicative of SVT. Ruptured Achilles tendon, Baker's cyst, and ruptured calf muscle would not feature the classic symptoms listed. (Uphold & Graham, 1994)

3. *Answer:* d (assessment/physical examination/cardiovascular/NAS)

Rationale: The physical signs of SVT are extremely reliable in diagnosing the disease. Pro-thrombin time and CBC with differential are nonspecific tests. Doppler studies are used to diagnose DVT. (Feied & Stephen, 1995)

4. *Answer:* c (plan/management/therapeutics/cardiovascular/NAS)

Rationale: Client requires hospitalization and the initiation of anticoagulation therapy. Antibiotics are not used in the treatment of thrombophlebitis, and all clients with DVT are treated because the primary goal of treatment is prevention of pulmonary embolism. (Eftychiou, 1996)

5. *Answer:* c (evaluation/cardiovascular/NAS)

Rationale: Clients with DVT are managed in consultation with a physician to regulate their antithrombotic medications. (Uphold & Graham, 1994)

6. *Answer:* c (assessment/history/cardiovascular/adult)

Rationale: Women are more susceptible to development of thrombophlebitis within the first 6 postpartum weeks. Standing (depending on length of time) may or may not be a risk factor. Exercise helps prevent clot formation, and not smoking is also a positive finding. (Eftychiou, 1996)

7. *Answer:* b (plan/management/therapeutics/cardiovascular/NAS)

Rationale: The primary emphasis for treatment of DVT is prevention of pulmonary embolism. (Feied & Stephen, 1995)

8. *Answer:* c (diagnosis/cardiovascular/NAS)

Rationale: The physical signs for diagnosing DVT may not be apparent. Hypocoagulability may cause bleeding, not clotting. (Uphold & Graham, 1994)

9. *Answer:* b (plan/management/client education/cardiovascular/NAS)

Rationale: Prolonged limb dependency is a risk factor for development of thrombophlebitis. Antithrombotic medication is not prescribed for SVT, nor is complete bed rest. (Creager & Dzau, 1994)

TRANSIENT ISCHEMIC ATTACKS

OVERVIEW

Definition

Defined as cerebral ischemia that is transient or reversible in nature, a *transient ischemic attack* is characterized by an acute focal neurologic deficit. It usually lasts less than 20 minutes but may last as long as 24 hours. Signs of cerebral ischemia lasting more than 24 hours and less than 7 days are defined as a *reversible ischemic neurologic deficit (RIND)*.

Incidence

The incidence of cerebral ischemia has declined for clients younger than 70 years, probably as a result of aggressive hypertension and cardiovascular management. TIAs precede 50% to 75% of strokes caused by carotid artery thrombosis. Among all stroke types, however, TIAs precede only about 10%. Approximately one third of clients who have a TIA will have a cerebral infarction within 5 years.

Pathophysiology

Atherosclerosis and inflammatory disease processes damage arterial walls, leading to the development of cerebral thromboses. TIAs represent thrombotic particles causing an intermittent blockage of circulation. There is increased risk of vascular damage with prolonged hypertension, degeneration of the endothelial wall of vessels, and the adherence of platelets and fibrin.

ASSESSMENT: SUBJECTIVE/HISTORY

Most Common Symptoms

Sudden onset of the following:
- Paralysis or paresis of one extremity or extremities on one side of the body
- Numbness
- Tingling
- Clumsiness of an extremity or both extremities on one side of the body
- Aphasia
- Visual disturbances
- Facial paralysis or drooping

Associated Symptoms
- Headache
- Drooling

Past Medical History
- Hypertension
- Diabetes
- Hyperlipidemia
- Cardiovascular or peripheral vascular disease
- Gout
- Atrial fibrillation
- Ventricular aneurysms
- Heart valve replacement

Medication History

Inquire about the possible use of oral contraceptives.

Family History
- History of cardiovascular disease
- History of CVA

Psychosocial History
- Smoking
- Increased stress levels

Dietary History

Ask about increases or excessive intake of salt, carbohydrates, and fats.

ASSESSMENT: OBJECTIVE/ PHYSICAL EXAMINATION

Physical Examination
- General appearance: Confusion, facial drooping
- Vital signs: Hydration status, orthostatic changes
- Eyes: Check reactivity of pupils (remember in the older adult they may not have a brisk response), check for visual field deficit.
- Throat: Check ability to swallow.
- Neck: Check whether neck is supple, listen to carotid arteries for bruits, check for diminished or absent carotid pulsations.
- Cardiovascular status: Listen for irregular rhythms, murmurs, artificial heart valves.
  —Check extremities for possible signs of DVT.

- Neurologic status: Cranial nerve deficits, especially facial paresis or paralysis, possible abnormalities of the gag reflex, tongue, extraocular movements
  —Deep tendon reflexes may be normal or increased in upper extremities.
  —Level of consciousness, memory, speech, walking, balance, sensory perception, motor ability (hand grips, lifting leg off the table and holding against pressure)

Diagnostic Procedures

These clients need to be referred to a physician, or at least consultation with a physician should occur. Other diagnostic tests should include ECG, CT of the head (which should have normal results), and lumbar puncture if suspect septic embolism from bacterial endocarditis.

LABORATORY TESTS. CBC, biochemical survey 19

RADIOLOGIC TESTS. Another radiologic test that may be considered would be carotid artery duplex Doppler study to determine the patency of the carotid arteries. If there is significant stenosis of the carotid arteries (>70%), arteriography should be performed.

DIAGNOSIS

Differential diagnosis includes the following:
- TIA
- RIND
- Stroke
  UNDERLYING CAUSES
  - Atrial fibrillation
  - Infective endocarditis
  - Meningitis
  - Recent anteroseptal MI
  - Valvular heart disease or heart valve replacement
  - Carotid stenosis
  - Polycythemia
  - Blood dyscrasias (especially those resulting in hypercoagulable states)
  - Connective tissue diseases
  - Hypertension
  - Chemical imbalances, particularly glucose and sodium

THERAPEUTIC PLAN

The therapeutic plan depends on whether an underlying condition was determined. Treatment of the underlying condition is imperative.

Pharmacologic Treatment

- Inhibit platelet aggregation
- Aspirin 81 mg daily; enteric coated best in the older adult
- Ticlopidine 250 mg bid

Surgical Treatment

If carotid artery stenosis is significant, carotid endarterectomy may be indicated.

EVALUATION/FOLLOW-UP

Clients with TIAs should be followed up closely, depending on the underlying mechanism of the TIA. If unidentified, frequency of check-ups will vary from clinic to clinic. However, clients should be evaluated every 4 to 6 months, and immediately should symptoms recur.

REFERENCES

McCance, K., & Huether, S. (1994). *Pathophysiology: The biologic basis for disease in adults and children* (2nd ed.). St. Louis: Mosby.

Reuben, D., Yoshikawa, T., & Besdine, R. (Eds.). (1995). *Geriatrics review syllabus.* New York: American Geriatrics Society.

Wilson, J., Braunwald, E., Isselbacher, K., Petersdorf, R., Martin, J., Fauci, A., & Root, R. (Eds.). (1991). *Harrison's principles of internal medicine* (12th ed.). New York: McGraw-Hill.

Woodley, M., & Whelan, A. (Eds.). (1992). *Manual of medical therapeutics* (27th ed.). Boston: Little, Brown.

REVIEW QUESTIONS

1. TIAs represent:
   a. Total, permanent occlusion of circulation to a small area of the brain
   b. Hemorrhage of a small vessel in the brain
   c. Intermittent occlusion of circulation in the brain
   d. Permanent occlusion of circulation to a large area of the brain

2. Diseases associated with TIAs include all the following **except:**

    a. Atrial fibrillation
    b. Hyperlipidemia
    c. Cardiovascular or peripheral vascular disease
    d. Arthritis

3. If a client has a possible TIA, which of the following objective findings may be related to the TIA?

    a. Heberden's nodes
    b. Carotid bruit
    c. Tenderness in both wrists
    d. Increased grip in both hands

4. Polycythemia can result in a TIA because:

    a. The blood is too thin, resulting in decreased perfusion.
    b. The blood is too thick, resulting in clotting.
    c. The tissue is resistant to insulin.
    d. The platelets are inhibited.

5. Ticlopidine may be used for inhibition of platelets in clients with TIA instead of aspirin because of:

    a. Allergy to aspirin
    b. Allergy to acetaminophen
    c. Allergy to eggs
    d. Allergy to tetanus

6. The treatment for significant carotid stenosis (>70%) is:

    a. Heart catheterization
    b. Cardiac arterial bypass surgery
    c. Carotid endarterectomy
    d. Vagotomy

7. Until a cause is determined for the TIA, the client should be followed up:

    a. Closely
    b. Every 6 months
    c. Yearly
    d. Only as symptoms occur

ANSWERS AND RATIONALES

1. *Answer:* c (diagnosis/cardiovascular/NAS)
   Rationale: By definition, the occlusion is intermittent. (Wilson et al., 1991)

2. *Answer:* d (assessment/history/cardiovascular/NAS)
   Rationale: The other diseases are associated with the potential for emboli formation and a resultant TIA. (Wilson et al., 1991)

3. *Answer:* b (assessment/physical examination/cardiovascular/NAS)
   Rationale: Carotid bruits indicate turbulence of blood flow in the carotid artery that may be stenosis or ulceration in the carotid from which emboli can come. (McCance & Huether, 1994)

4. *Answer:* b (assessment/history/cardiovascular/NAS)
   Rationale: Polycythemia is an increase in the number of RBCs that makes the blood have a higher viscosity and may result in abnormal clotting. (McCance & Huether, 1994)

5. *Answer:* a (plan/cardiovascular/NAS)
   Rationale: If the client is allergic to aspirin, the platelets can still be inhibited with ticlopidine. (Reuben, Yoshikawa, & Besdine, 1995)

6. *Answer:* c (plan/cardiovascular/NAS)
   Rationale: Carotid endarterectomy cleans up the carotid artery such that if there are tiny emboli being sent to the brain from the carotid, resulting in TIA, this will be stopped and the possibility of stroke will be decreased. (McCance & Huether, 1994)

7. *Answer:* a (evaluation/cardiovascular/NAS)
   Rationale: The client needs to be followed up closely to determine the cause and prevent stroke. (Wilson et al., 1991)

4

Gastrointestinal System

ABDOMINAL PAIN

OVERVIEW
Incidence

Abdominal pain accounts for 5% of all emergency department visits and is the most frequently described reason for ambulatory visits within general adult and family practice settings.

Pathophysiology

Common pathogenic mechanisms underlying acute (surgical) abdominal pain include *perforation* (hollow viscus), *obstruction* (intestinal, sigmoid volvulus), *ischemia* (mesenteric infarction), *inflammation* (diverticulitis with perforation, peritonitis), and hemorrhage (abdominal aneurysm, ulcers, ectopic pregnancy).

Nonemergency causes may include hepatitis, cholecystitis, gastritis, nephrolithiasis, pneumonia, hernia, pyelonephritis, endometriosis, and colon carcinoma.

ASSESSMENT: SUBJECTIVE/HISTORY
History of Present Illness

When the chief complaint is abdominal pain, the client should be asked about the location at onset and at present; radiation; aggravating factors (movement, coughing, respiration); mitigating factors (position, lying still, vomiting, antacids, food); mode of onset with progression (better, same, worse); abruptness of onset; duration; and the character (intermittent, steady, colicky), severity, and previous similar episodes of the pain.

WOMEN. Regardless of age, inquire about vaginal bleeding (including last normal menses). Ask women of childbearing age about sexual history, obstetric history, ectopic risk factors (pelvic inflammatory disease (PID), intrauterine contraceptive device (IUD), previous ectopic pregnancy, history of tubal surgery), and infertility treatment.

MEN. Ask men about urologic history, including sexual history.

CHILDREN. Question child, parent, or both about general indicators of illness: activity level, appetite, food intake, history of recent infection, current infections, and presence of fever.

Symptoms

Anorexia, nausea and vomiting, and diarrhea generally are nonspecific symptoms, but they are significant in the presence of abdominal pain. In an acute surgical abdomen, pain generally precedes vomiting; the opposite is true in medical conditions. Clients with an acute developing abdomen usually have no desire for food. Diarrhea is usually associated with medical etiologies.

Clients with an acute abdomen often have a paralytic ileus, so it is important to determine whether the common and often subjective report of constipation is really obstipation (absence of both stool and flatus). True obstipation is strongly suggestive of a mechanical bowel obstruction, especially when accompanied by progressively increasing abdominal distention or repeated vomiting.

Past Medical History

Ask about the following:
- Previous abdominal surgery
- Cardiovascular disease

- Analgesic use (acute or chronic)
- Alcohol use
- Other substance abuse (tobacco or recreational drugs)
- Weight change
- Past illness
- Risk factors such as recent travel (travel history may direct the examiner to the possibility of gastroenteritis or dysentery), environmental exposure, or immunologic suppression
- Medications
- Allergies
- Family history (family history of appendicitis increases risk)
- Previous surgery, especially abdominal or gynecologic operations, is a common predisposing factor in bowel obstruction caused by adhesions.
- Social history indicating domestic violence

In female clients, a menstrual and obstetric history is pertinent to rule out ectopic pregnancy, mittelschmerz, and endometriosis.

Medication History

- Anticoagulant therapy has been implicated in the development of abdominal hematomas.
- Oral contraceptives have been associated with hepatic adenomas and with mesenteric infarction.
- Corticosteroids may mask the symptoms of advanced peritonitis.
- Nonsteroidal antiinflammatory drugs (NSAIDs) can lead to peptic ulcer disease.

Review of Systems

A complete review of systems should be done (as allowed by the client's condition). Special attention should be given to cardiac, pulmonary, gynecologic and genitourinary systems, because abdominal pain may originate from these systems (e.g., angina, basal pneumonia, PID, pyelonephritis).

ASSESSMENT: OBJECTIVE/ PHYSICAL EXAMINATION

Physical Examination

Perform a complete history and physical examination when possible. Important areas to stress include the following:

- Vital signs
- General observation
- Cardiopulmonary system
- Abdominal, rectal, and pelvic examinations

Special maneuvers to be performed during the physical examination are shown in Table 4-1.

PEDIATRIC ABDOMINAL EXAMINATION

- As much as possible, examine young child while he or she is seated with the parent.
- Place the child's hand over your hand for palpation.
- Normal abdomen is rounded and scaphoid in the school-aged and younger child.
- Attempts to ellicit psoas and obturator signs in the young child are seldom helpful.
- Gentle percussion should be used instead of the usual test for rebound tenderness.
- Liver and spleen should be palpated in all children, as should the kidney in the neonate.
- The inguinal canal should be examined for hernias.

Diagnostic Procedures

About 65% of acute surgical abdomen cases can be diagnosed by history and physical examina-

Table 4-1 Special Maneuvers for Physical Examination

SIGN	ORGAN	PHYSICAL FINDINGS
Murphy's sign	Gallbladder	Temporary inspiratory arrest with palpation of right subcostal margin
Iliopsoas	Peritoneal irritation	Psoas muscle pain with active hip flexion or passive extension
Obturator	Peritoneal irritation	Pain with internal/external rotation of flexed thigh
Punch tenderness	Liver, splenic, or adjacent structure	Tenderness with firm palpation to lower costal (anterior) margin
Costovertebral angle	Kidney	Tenderness over posterior costal margin

Modified from Burkhardt, C. (1992). Guidelines for the rapid assessment of abdominal pain indicative of acute surgical abdomen. *Nurse Practitioner, 17*(6), 43-46.

tion alone. However, supplemental examinations are necessary for diagnosis or exclusion of non-surgical abdominal pain. Laboratory tests that should be ordered for all clients with severe abdominal pain include the following:

Table 4-2 Most Common Causes of Acute Abdominal Pain

AGE (YR)	COMMON	LESS COMMON
0-1	Intussusception	Appendicitis
	Incarcerated hernias	Testicular torsion
	Gastroenteritis	
	Hernia	
2-5	Appendicitis	Intussusception
	Constipation	UTI
	Gastroenteritis	Testicular torsion
	Pneumonia	
6-11	Appendicitis	Intussusception
	Pneumonia	Testicular torsion
	Constipation	Incarcerated inguinal hernia
	Gastroenteritis	
	UTI	
12-21	Appendicitis	UTI
	Testicular torsion	Pneumonia
	Pelvic inflammatory disease	Constipation
	Mittelschmerz	
	Pregnancy	
	Ectopic pregnancy	

From Finelli, L. (1991). Evaluation of the child with acute abdominal pain. *Journal of Pediatric Health Care,* 5(5), 251-256.

- CBC with differential
- Urinalysis
- Stool sample for occult blood
- Renal and liver function test (alanine aminotransferase (ALT), aspartate aminotransferase (AST), and alkaline phosphatase) amylase
- Serum pregnancy test in women, if the possibility of pregnancy exists (a necessity for women of childbearing age)
- Chest x-ray (CXR) to rule out conditions that may mimic an acute abdomen, such as basal pneumonia or pleural effusion
- Flat and upright films of abdomen to detect the presence of free air (perforated viscus), necessary before operation

DIAGNOSIS

Conditions to be considered in differential diagnosis of abdominal pain are shown in the accompanying box. The most common causes of acute abdominal pain are presented by age group in Table 4-2.

THERAPEUTIC PLAN

- Clients with minimal symptoms may be managed initially with clear liquids and analgesics (after surgical consultation).

DIFFERENTIAL DIAGNOSIS WITH ABDOMINAL PAIN

A. Significant vomiting or diarrhea
  1. Bowel obstruction
  2. **Gastroenteritis**
  3. Gastroparesis
  4. **Pregnancy**
  5. Volvulus
B. Hematemesis or melena
  1. Aortic enteric fistula
  2. **Diverticular disease**
  3. **Malignancy**
  4. Polyps
  5. **Ulcers**
  6. Varices
C. Syncope
  1. Aortic aneurysm
  2. **Ectopic pregnancy**
  3. Gastroenteritis
  4. **Gastrointestinal bleed**
  5. **Myocardial Infarction**
D. Dysuria, urgency, frequency, or hematuria
  1. **Pyelonephritis**
  2. Renal colic
E. Constipation
  1. Bowel ischemia
  2. **Bowel obstruction**
  3. Diverticular disease
  4. **Volvulus**
F. Rectal pain
  1. Ovarian cyst
  2. **Prostatis**

Modified from American College of Emergency Physicians. (1994). Clinical policy for the initial approach to patients with a chief complaint of nontraumatic abdominal pain. *Annals of Emergency Medicine, 23*(4), 906-922.
NOTE: The most common diagnoses are shown in **bold** type.

- Therapy for moderate to severe pain and vomiting includes IV fluids, nasogastric suction, and correction of electrolyte imbalance. Antibiotics should be considered if the client has fever. Histamine (H_2) blockers may be indicated for the relief of gastritis and colicky pain.
- Advise client to avoid spicy or gas-producing foods.
- Physician or surgeon referral when appropriate

EVALUATION/FOLLOW-UP

Advise adult client to return immediately in the following cases:

- Pain gets worse or is now only in one area.
- Bloody emesis or stool
- Dizziness or syncope
- Abdomen becomes swollen
- Elevated temperature (>102° F orally)
- Difficulty passing urine
- Shortness of breath

Advise parent of pediatric client to return immediately in the following cases:

- Pain increases or is only in one specific area.
- Child begins to vomit blood or blood is present in stool.
- The child is walking bent over or holding the abdomen, or refuses to walk.
- Pain is in the testicle or scrotum.
- Child's abdomen becomes swollen or quite tender to the touch.
- Child has difficulty urinating.
- Child is short of breath.

Follow up abdominal pain in 1 week, sooner if the client has fever or prostrating pain. If no problems in 1 week, follow up in 1 month and then 6 months.

REFERENCES

American College of Emergency Physicians (1994). Clinical policy for the initial approach to patients with a chief complaint of nontraumatic acute abdominal pain. *Annals of Emergency Medicine, 23*(4), 906-922.

Burkhardt, C. (1992). Guidelines for the rapid assessment of abdominal pain indicative of acute surgical abdomen. *Nurse Practitioner, 17*(6) 43-46.

Finelli, L. (1991). Evaluation of the child with acute abdominal pain. *Journal of Pediatric Health Care, 5*(5), 251-256.

Mead, M. (1996). Detecting appendicitis. *Practice Nurse, 11*(7), 486-487.

A one-antibiotic regimen for ruptured appendix. (1992). *Emergency Medicine, 24*(2), 742.

Rothrock, S. (1996). When appendicitis isn't "classic." *Emergency Medicine, 28*(3), 108-124.

REVIEW QUESTIONS

1. For which female client should a serum pregnancy test be ordered to evaluate abdominal pain?

   a. 8-year-old
   b. 75-year-old
   c. 50-year-old
   d. 30-year-old

2. Common differential diagnosis in vomiting and diarrhea includes all the following **except:**

   a. Bowel obstruction
   b. Gastroenteritis
   c. Pregnancy
   d. Malignancy

3. Which indicators of illness should **not** be included in the history of a child with abdominal pain?

   a. Activity level
   b. Appetite
   c. Recent infections
   d. History of sexual abuse

4. True obstipation is strongly suggestive of a mechanical bowel obstruction, especially when accompanied by:

   a. Pain after vomiting
   b. Diarrhea
   c. Increasing abdominal distention and repeated vomiting
   d. Nausea

5. If the client's presenting symptom is vague abdominal pain, with no abdominal tenderness or systemic symptoms, what should the nurse practitioner do?

   a. Consult with surgeon right away.
   b. Reassess the client in 3 to 4 hours.
   c. Order needed laboratory tests.
   d. Send client home.

ANSWERS AND RATIONALES

1. Answer: d (assessment/physical examination/gastrointestinal/childbearing female)

Rationale: Any female of childbearing years should have a serum pregnancy test to rule out pregnancy (American College of Emergency Physicians, 1994).

2. Answer: d (diagnosis/gastrointestinal/NAS)

Rationale: Diagnoses in *a* through *c* need to be considered when the client has vomiting or diarrhea. Bleeding is associated with malignancy. (American College of Emergency Physicians, 1994)

3. Answer: d (assessment/history/gastrointestinal/child)

Rationale: Symptoms in *a* through *c* provide information related to how seriously ill the child is. (Finelli, 1991)

4. Answer: c (diagnosis/gastrointestinal/NAS)

Rationale: True obstipation is strongly suggestive of a mechanical bowel obstruction. (Burkhardt, 1992)

5. Answer: b (plan/management/therapeutic/gastrointestinal/NAS)

Rationale: If there are no systemic symptoms with no abdominal pain on examination, the client can be reevaluated to determine progression of the illness. (Mead, 1996)

APPENDICITIS

OVERVIEW
Definition

Appendicitis is an inflammation of the appendix caused by bacterial infection.

Incidence

* In the United States, appendicitis develops in approximately 1 in 15 persons.
* The incidence rises after 3 years, until it peaks during the late teen years. Sixty-nine percent of cases occur before 30 years.
* It is the most common surgical condition, with the greatest incidence in preadolescence, adolescence, and early adult age groups.
* Males are more often affected than females, by a ratio of 1.5:1.
* As many as two thirds of cases occur between October and May.
* Persons with a family history of appendicitis are at increased risk.

Pathophysiology

Appendicitis arises from obstruction of the appendiceal lumen, usually by a fecalith but also by foreign bodies such as seeds, barium, bones, wood, metal fragments, or plastic. Conditions that can induce obstruction include Crohn's disease, respiratory infections, measles, mononucleosis, amebiasis and bacterial gastroenteritis.

Obstruction prevents emptying of the intraluminal fluid into the cecum. The fluid accumulates and distends the appendix. The increased luminal pressure inhibits lymphatic and venous drainage. Luminal bacteria multiply and then invade the appendiceal wall.

RISK FACTORS (ABDOMINAL PAIN)
* Dietary factors (fatty diet)
* Medications (erythromycin, theophylline, amoxicillin with clauvulanate)
* Sexual activity
* Consumption of contaminated food
* Dysfunctional coping methods
* Stressful situations

PROTECTIVE FACTORS. Dietary fiber lessens the risk of appendiceal lumen obstruction by decreasing the viscosity of feces, reducing bowel transit time and subsequently diminishing the likelihood of fecalith formation.

COMMON PATHOGENS
* *Escherichia coli*
* *Bacteroides* species
* *Enterococcus* species
* *Pseudomonas* species

ASSESSMENT: SUBJECTIVE/HISTORY

The most common symptoms are as follows:
* Abdominal tenderness is not always dull at first and may be intense and persistent later on. Migration of pain from umbilical area

to right lower quadrant occurs in only 50% to 65% of clients.

- After age 2 years, clinical symptoms of appendicitis become more typical. Right-sided abdominal pain is at first vague and progresses to become more intense and persistent.
- In a child, right lower quadrant tenderness should never be considered insignificant, no matter how mild it is.
- Older adults have few or no prodromal symptoms.
- Nausea is common but not universal.
- Emesis almost always follows pain onset, except in a few children. Children may be systemically ill with vomiting rather than with abdominal pain and tenderness.
- Anorexia is common, but 10% to 40% have no loss of appetite.

ASSESSMENT: OBJECTIVE/ PHYSICAL EXAMINATION
Physical Examination

Examination should be problem oriented, with particular attention to the following:

- Vital signs: Low-grade fever
- Heart and lungs
- Abdomen: Bowel sounds, guarding, distention, tenderness, masses, inability to jump, walk, or cough without pain
- Rectal: Especially note tenderness on the right.
- Pelvic examination is indicated for females who are sexually active.

NOTE: In *pregnancy*, the appendix is pushed higher, with pain and tenderness outside the classic position. In *very young children*, the abdomen is commonly distended and they look toxic. These children are usually lethargic with irritability and vomiting. In *acute appendicitis* the child is likely to exhibit guarding and to lie on his or her left side with the legs drawn up to reduce tension on the rectus muscle. Suspect appendicitis in anyone with nonspecific complaints who is taking *oral steroids*.

Diagnostic Procedures

RADIOGRAPHY. Plain abdominal films are of little value except for those clients, usually children, with a calcified fecalith in the right lower quadrant.

ULTRASONOGRAPHY. Ultrasonography is 80% to 90% sensitive and 90% to 100% specific for appendicitis. It can be used safely during pregnancy.

LABORATORY TESTS

- There is no specific test for the diagnosis of appendicitis.
- The WBC count is usually normal for the first 24 hours of symptoms.
- Leukocytosis (>15,000 cells/mm^3) may be seen.
- Urinalysis is used to exclude genitourinary conditions in clients of all ages.

DIAGNOSIS

Differential diagnosis includes the following:

- Crohn's disease (any age group)
- Mesenteric adenitis (most common differential diagnosis in children)
- Pain in the abdomen after an upper respiratory tract infection (URI)
- Diverticulitis (in older adult)
- Gastroenteritis
- Henoch-Schönlein purpura
- Psychogenic abdominal pain
- Pneumonia

In young women appendicitis is most often confused with PID, mittelschmerz, dysmenorrhea, tubal pregnancy, ovarian torsions, ruptured follicles with bleeding, and ruptured cysts.

Appendicitis is the most common atraumatic abdominal surgical emergency in pregnancy. Whenever a pregnant woman reports right-sided abdominal pain, obtain a surgical consultation, especially in the second or third trimester.

Think of appendicitis in every child, regardless of age, who has GI or other abdominal complaints.

THERAPEUTIC PLAN
Referral

- Seek early consultation with a surgeon for a child with a gastrointestinal (GI) or abdominal complaint if the child appears toxic.
- Obtain an obstetric consultation for a pregnant woman with right-sided abdominal pain, especially in the second or third trimester.
- Whenever appendicitis is suspected, a prompt surgical consultation is critical.

Preoperative Care

- Before an emergency appendectomy, start IV fluid replacement.
- Do not give the client anything by mouth; rectal metronidazole may be given 3 hours before surgery to prevent infection.
- Give broad-spectrum antibiotics immediately if the client appears septic.
  - —In children use single-dose cefoxitin.
  - —Accepted therapies for perforation or abscess formation include an aminoglycoside (gentamicin; always obtain a baseline creatinine before starting this drug) with one or more of the following: ampicillin, clindamycin, metronidazole, and cefoxitin.
  - —An alternative to gentamicin is ticarcillin with clavulanate or cefotaxime with clindamycin.

EVALUATION/FOLLOW-UP

- Routine postoperative visits at 2 and 6 weeks
- The postoperative follow-up is normally limited to checking the wound and providing a work release.
- The most common complication is wound infection, which may require antibiotics, dressings, or packings.

REFERENCES

Finelli, L (1991). Evaluation of the child with acute abdominal pain. *Journal of Pediatric Health Care, 5*(5), 251-256.

Fox, J. (1997). *Primary health care of children.* St. Louis: Mosby.

Griffith, H., & Dambro, M. (1997). *The 5-minute clinical consult* (4th ed.). Philadelphia: Lea & Febiger.

Mead, M. (1996). Detecting appendicitis. *Practice Nurse, 11*(7), 486-487.

A one-antibiotic regimen for ruptured appendix. (1992). *Emergency Medicine, 24*(2), 742.

Rothrock, S. (1996). When appendicitis isn't "classic." *Emergency Medicine, 28*(3), 108-124.

1. The pain of appendicitis:
   a. Always starts at the umbilical area and migrates to the right lower quadrant
   b. Is not always dull at first, changing to an intense and persistent pain later
   c. Has a specific sign of right lower quadrant tenderness
   d. Is dull and radiates to the costovertebral angle

2. Which of the following is **not** a common physical finding in appendicitis?
   a. The appendix is pushed lower, with pain and tenderness outside quadrant.
   b. Young child with distended abdomen
   c. Right-sided rectal tenderness
   d. Inability to jump up and down as a result of abdominal pain

3. In young women appendicitis is most often confused with all the following **except:**
   a. PID
   b. Mittelschmerz
   c. Ovarian torsion
   d. Normal pregnancy

4. Melissa is an 11-year-old girl with abdominal pain. She has had one episode of nausea and vomiting. Her examination is unremarkable. What is the best approach for you to take at this time?
   a. Send her immediately to a surgeon for surgery.
   b. Keep her in your office for the next 2 to 3 hours for close observation.
   c. Tell her that it is gastroenteritis.
   d. Advise watchful waiting; describe symptoms for which the family should be alert.

5. Which of the following signs and symptoms might indicate that Melissa's condition is worsening and warrants a referral?
   a. Able to jump up and down without pain
   b. Low-grade fever, localized mass on digital rectal examination
   c. Able to eat pizza with nausea and vomiting
   d. Costovertebral angle tenderness and low-grade fever

ANSWERS AND RATIONALES

1. *Answer:* b (assessment/history/gastrointestinal/NAS)

Rationale: The pain of appendicitis may not always start with a dull quality, increasing in intensity and persistence. It may start as an intense pain. (Rothrock, 1996)

2. *Answer:* a (assessment/physical examination/gastrointestinal/NAS)

Rationale: In a pregnant woman, the appendix may be pushed out of the classic position. Right-sided rectal tenderness, inability to jump up and down, and a distended abdomen are typical with appendicitis.

3. *Answer:* d (diagnosis/gastrointestinal/adult)

Rationale: Gynecologic conditions frequently mimic the signs and symptoms of appendicitis. (Mead, 1996; Rothrock, 1996)

4. *Answer:* d (plan/gastrointestinal/adolescent)

Rationale: Most of the diagnosis of appendicitis is based on the history and clinical examination. At this point Melissa does not have any of the typical symptoms of appendicitis, so watchful waiting is an appropriate plan. (Fox, 1997)

5. *Answer:* b (evaluation/gastrointestinal/adolescent)

Rationale: A low-grade fever, a localized rectal mass, and right-sided abdominal tenderness are hallmarks of appendicitis that warrant an immediate referral to a physician. (Fox, 1997)

CHOLECYSTITIS/CHOLELITHIASIS (GALLBLADDER DISEASE)

OVERVIEW
Definition
Cholecystitis is an inflammation of gallbladder caused by cystic duct irritation or obstruction.

Cholelithiasis is stone formation with or without obstruction. Gallbladder disease may be asymptomatic or may be accompanied by recurrent bouts of abdominal discomfort. With asymptomatic disease the probability of biliary pain developing is <20% at 20 years.

Incidence
- It is more common in women than men and more common in overweight women older than 40 years; at 65 years the two sexes are affected equally. It also occurs in young, thin to normal-weight women.
- Persons with diabetes are more likely to acquire gallstones.
- Cholesterol stones occur more frequently in women with advancing age and are present in half of all Americans older than 70 years.
- The most common cause of acute abdomen in older clients.
- Acute cholecystitis is fatal in nearly 10% of elderly clients.
- Highest in industrial countries and in certain native North Americans especially females.

Pathophysiology
Gallbladder disease is caused by cystic duct irritation or obstruction, usually from stone or inflammation. Bile becomes supersaturated with cholesterol. A tiny nucleus of cholesterol crystals can form and ultimately grow into a macroscopic stone.

PROTECTIVE FACTORS
- Low-calorie diet in a normal-weight individual without family history of gallbladder disease
- Young age

RISK FACTORS
- Diabetes
- Thiazides
- Estrogen replacement therapy
- Young age

COMMON PATHOGENS. Pigmented stones are associated with infection and tend to be black or brown. Bacteria have been found in some cases.

ASSESSMENT: SUBJECTIVE/HISTORY

CHOLECYSTITIS. Sudden pain that builds over time is localized to the right upper quadrant, with radiation to the right or left scapula and lasting 2 to 4 hours. Nausea and vomiting are associated. Right-sided pain worsens with deep inspiration associated with acute cholecystitis. Fever, itching, or jaundiced skin may be present.

CHOLELITHIASIS. Symptoms are the same as in cholecystitis, but the condition may be asymptomatic.

OLDER ADULTS. Abdominal pain, fever, and altered mental status are common. Symptoms may be vague.

Symptoms

- Nausea and vomiting
- Possible jaundice
- Itching skin
- Low-grade fever sometimes present
- Bloating, indigestion, and upper abdominal fullness

Past Medical History

- Diabetes
- Frequent starvation diets or recent high-calorie meal
- Previous episodes of gallbladder problems or right upper abdominal pain

Medication History

Estrogens, progesterone, and thiazides should be discontinued or decreased in dosage to avoid stone formation. Calcium supplements have also been implicated.

Family History

Sometimes positive family history is present.

Psychosocial History

Social intake of alcohol may decrease incidence of gallstones.

Dietary History

Ask about frequent dieting or starvation diets and/or high caloric intake.

ASSESSMENT: OBJECTIVE/ PHYSICAL EXAMINATION

Physical Examination

- Jaundice may or may not be present.
- Low-grade fever
- Lungs clear
- Slight tachycardia may be present.
- Colicky right upper quadrant tenderness with guarding or rigidity
- Respiratory pause with deep inspiration and palpation (Murphy's sign)
- Vomiting
  OLDER ADULTS
  - Most have typical signs and symptoms.
  - Some may have vague abdominal pain, no previous episodes.
  - Elevated WBCs
  - Fever
  - Altered mental status
  - More prone to ascending cholangitis, disseminated intravascular coagulation, subphrenic and liver abscess, small-bowel obstruction

Diagnostic Procedures

- Total bilirubin
- Alkaline phosphatase (elevation indicates cholangitis)
- Transaminases (AST and ALT), gamma-glutamyl transpeptidase; elevated levels indicate obstruction of biliary tree.
- Prothrombin and partial thromboplastin times
- Serum amylase
- Abdominal ultrasonography and/or radionuclide scan (confirms diagnosis)
- Hepato–iminodiacetic acid scan confirms diagnosis
- ECG in clients older than 50 years
- Urinalysis
- Slightly elevated WBC count (12,000 to 15,000 cells/mm^3; if higher, may be complication)
  OLDER ADULTS
  - ECG
  - Upright chest
  - Radiography of kidneys and upper bladder sometimes detects air in the wall of the gallbladder or emphysematous cholecystitis.

DIAGNOSIS

Differential diagnosis includes the following:
- Biliary disease
- Peptic ulcer disease
- Bowel obstruction
- Pancreatitis
- Appendicitis
- Diverticular disease
- Mesenteric ischemia
- Cardiovascular
- Urogenital
- Pneumonia
- Pulmonary emboli
- Pneumothorax
- Congestive heart failure with hepatic congestion
- Herpes zoster
- Diabetic ketoacidosis
- Porphyria
- Hypercalcemia
- Gastroesophageal reflux with or without hiatal hernia

THERAPEUTIC PLAN
Pharmacologic Treatment

NSAIDs such as indomethicin have been shown to relieve pain and prevent stones and to prevent recurrence in some cases. For medical management of cholesterol stones with the use of ursodiol (Actigall), recurrence is a factor. NSAIDs have been shown to decrease recurrence. Criteria for treatment of gallstones with ursodiol include a functioning gallbladder, stones <15 mm in diameter, stones that float on oral cholecystogram or are lucent, clients who are poor candidates for surgery, clients with mild symptoms, single stone, or multiple stones in a client receiving long-term NSAID therapy.

Cholecystitis

Demonstrating the presence of gallstones is sufficient indication for surgical treatment. Refer client for definitive treatment.

Cholelithiasis

Refer clients with symptoms for evaluation for surgery. Treatment of choice is laparoscopic cholecystectomy. Use of medical therapies must be prescribed by a specialist; these are usually reserved for cases of high surgical risk or in which surgery is contraindicated.

Client Education

- Asymptomatic gallstones do not grow rapidly and rarely dissolve or pass spontaneously; surgery is not generally performed.
- Gradual weight reduction through caloric restriction
- Avoid fasting or starvation diets; restricting fat and cholesterol is of little benefit.
- Notify health care providers of previous presence of gallstones.
- Client should know signs and symptoms of acute disease and when to seek emergency help.

Referral

Refer clients with symptoms.

EVALUATION/FOLLOW-UP
Cholecystitis

Refer client for treatment. If surgery not performed, ask about symptoms at each visit.

Cholelithiasis

If surgery is performed, ask about symptoms during visits because of the possibility of new stone formation in duct.

REFERENCES

Barnes, W. (1995). Cholecystitis. *Australian Journal of Emergency Care, 2*(1), 18-22.

Birnbaumer, D. (1993). Abdominal emergencies in later life. *Emergency Medicine, 25*(5), 75-98.

Nahrwold, D. (1993). Update: Diagnostic dilemmas, therapeutic options. *Consultant, 33*(8), 27-29.

Rhodes, V., & Madison, J. (1991). Gallbladder disease: Confirming the diagnosis. *Academy of Physician Assistants, 4*(6), 457-469.

Shaw, B. (1996). Primary care of women. *Journal of Nurse-Midwifery, 42*(2), 155-167.

Shaw, M. (1993). Current management of symptomatic gallstones. *Postgraduate Medicine, 93*(1), 183-187.

Van Ness, M., & Chobanian, S. (1994). Gallstones and acute and chronic cholecystitis. In *Manual of clinical problems in gastroenterology* (2nd ed., pp. 242-253). Boston: Little, Brown.

REVIEW QUESTIONS

1. Asymptomatic cholelithiasis in clients without other complicating factors is best treated by:

   a. Surgical intervention
   b. Actigall therapy
   c. NSAIDs
   d. Observation

2. In the older adult symptoms of gallbladder disease may be:

   a. More pronounced
   b. Generalized over abdomen
   c. Accompanied by chest pain
   d. Vague

3. Typical symptoms of cholelithiasis may:

   a. Include pain down left arm
   b. Be absent
   c. Include low hemoglobin
   d. Be more frequent in poor countries

4. The most useful test result in diagnosing gallbladder disease is:

   a. Oral cholecystography
   b. Cholescintigraphy
   c. Ultrasonography
   d. CT

5. A complication of cholecystitis caused by stone formation and indicated by an elevated serum amylase would be:

   a. Cardiac disease
   b. Pancreatitis
   c. Liver disease
   d. Bowel perforation

6. A 73-year-old man comes in with reports of abdominal pain, altered mental status, and a low-grade fever. You suspect biliary disease because of which of the following?

   a. Biliary colic leads differential diagnoses in this age group.
   b. Biliary colic is the second most common cause of abdominal pain in this age group.
   c. Incidence of gallstones increases with age.
   d. All are correct.

7. A 70-year-old client with serious heart disease has been found to have gallstones on abdominal ultrasonography. The ultrasonography was performed because of occasional abdominal pain. Only one stone, measuring less than 15 mm, is present. Your plan is to:

   a. Start oral Actigall therapy
   b. Send for lithotripsy
   c. Schedule surgery
   d. Refer to GI specialist

8. The plan for a client without symptoms with documented gallstones is to:

   a. Refer for surgery
   b. Monitor for symptoms
   c. Start oral dissolution therapy
   d. Order further laboratory tests

9. Clients with asymptomatic gallstones should be instructed to:

   a. Lose weight as quickly as possible
   b. Restrict fat and cholesterol to prevent stone formation
   c. Eat a high-calorie diet
   d. Notify health care providers of presence of stones

10. Education of clients with gallbladder disease must include which of the following?

   a. Preparation for surgery
   b. Signs and symptoms of attacks
   c. Stones may pass spontaneously.
   d. Weight must remain stable.

ANSWERS AND RATIONALES

1. *Answer:* d (plan/gastrointestinal/NAS)
   Rationale: Observation is appropriate for symptom-free clients with gallstones. Medical therapy is recommended for poor surgical risks only. (Van Ness & Chobanian, 1994)

2. *Answer:* d (assessment/history/gastrointestinal/aging adult)
   Rationale: In the older adult symptoms may be vague. The pain should not include chest pain, and some older adults will report only of indigestion in epigastrium. Symptoms may be less severe and the cause of abdominal pain may be difficult to locate. (Birnbaumer, 1993)

3. *Answer:* b (assessment/history/gastrointestinal/NAS)

Rationale: Symptoms of gallstones may be absent. Stones may be found incidentally during imaging studies for other causes. Low hemoglobin is not associated with gallstones. Poor countries have lower incidence of gallstones. Left arm pain is not considered a symptom of gallstones. (Birnbaumer, 1993; Shaw, 1996)

4. *Answer:* c (diagnosis/gastrointestinal/NAS)

Rationale: Ultrasonography is the most useful test because it is least invasive and more cost-effective, as well as capable of being performed in a short time. Oral cholecystography is the second choice. Cholescintigraphy does not reveal the presence or absence of calculi. CT scan may be useful in difficult cases, but it is not the first choice. (Van Ness & Chobanian, 1994)

5. *Answer:* b (diagnosis/gastrointestinal/NAS)

Rationale: Elevated serum amylase is indicative of pancreatitis or obstruction of the bile duct. Serum amylase has no role in cardiac disease or bowel perforation. Liver disease is indicated by elevated liver enzymes. (Rhodes & Madison, 1991)

6. *Answer:* d (diagnosis/gastrointestinal/aging adult)

Rationale: All are correct, according to clinical studies and statistical information of morbidity in the older adult. (Birnbaumer, 1993)

7. *Answer:* d (plan/gastrointestinal/aging adult)

Rationale: Referral for evaluation regarding oral dissolution therapy is appropriate. The client is a poor surgical risk because of severe cardiac disease. The gallstones meet the criteria for oral therapy. (Shaw, 1993)

8. *Answer:* b (plan/gastrointestinal/NAS)

Rationale: Monitoring the symptom-free client with incidental gallstones is an appropriate plan. Answers *a, c,* and *d* are actions best left to a consultant if treatment is an option. (Rhodes & Madison, 1991)

9. *Answer:* d (evaluation/gastrointestinal/NAS)

Rationale: Notifying health care providers is important because this enables the provider to provide necessary education as well as assisting the provider in identifying signs and symptoms. Losing weight rapidly and eating a high-calorie diet are inappropriate. Clients may lose weight gradually by eating a low-calorie diet. Low fat and cholesterol diets, although healthful for most people, have not been proved to prevent gallstone formation. (Rhodes & Madison, 1991; Shaw, 1996)

10. *Answer:* b (plan/evaluation/gastrointestinal/NAS)

Rationale: Clients should be taught the signs and symptoms of gallbladder disease and acute episodes. Clients in whom symptoms develop may be candidates for cholecystectomy. Answers *c* and *d* are incorrect information. Surgical preparation is not indicated and is better done by surgeon as a client becomes a candidate for surgery. (Shaw, 1996)

CONSTIPATION/DIARRHEA

Constipation

OVERVIEW
Definition

Constipation is defined as a decrease in the frequency, size, or liquid content of stool. The term refers more to the consistency of stool than to the frequency of stools. Constipated stools are small, hard, and dry.

Incidence

- Constipation is common among children, adolescents, and older adults
- It accounts for 2.5 million health care visits annually and 4% of all pediatric visits.

Pathophysiology

Distention of the bowel wall from stool passing into the rectum stimulates mass peristalsis, producing the defecation reflex. The urge to defecate can be voluntarily controlled through tightening of the external sphincter. When this occurs, stool remains in the rectum and produces relaxation and cessation of the defecation reflex. Liquid content is continually reabsorbed, producing hard, dry stool that is difficult and painful to pass.

Most constipation is functional, with no organic cause. Contributing factors are low fiber in the diet, sedentary lifestyle, low fluid intake, and voluntarily ignoring the urge to defecate because of lack of privacy or painful anal fissures or hemorrhoids.

Causes include the following:

- Organic causes include Hirschsprung's disease, strictures, anal-rectal stenosis, and volvulus.
- Neuromuscular defects include spinal cord lesions.
- Metabolic causes include hypokalemia, dehydration, and hypothyroidism.
- Adverse drug effects may be seen from narcotics, psychoactive drugs, and antidepressants.
- Eating disorders, such as anorexia nervosa, may contribute.

ASSESSMENT: SUBJECTIVE/HISTORY

- Decrease in the number of stools from normal stooling patterns
  —Breast-fed babies may stool after every feeding.
  —Bottle-fed babies stool less often, neonates stool more often than 4 per day.
  —Four-month-olds produce 2 stools per day.
  —Four-year-olds through adults generally produce 1 stool per day. Stool size increases with age.
- Hard, dry, small stools
- Straining required to push stool out (normal during neonatal period)
- Pain with defecation
- *Children:* Nausea, vomiting, excessive urination, blood in stools, soiling of underclothes, behavioral problems
- *Adults:* Abdominal pain, blood in stools, weight loss, depression, diarrhea

History should include client's definition of constipation, usual bowel pattern including recent changes, dietary recall, activity level, and current or recent use of medications, including laxatives.

ASSESSMENT: OBJECTIVE/ PHYSICAL EXAMINATION
Abdominal Examination

- Abdomen is distended with a palpable mass in the midline or lower left quadrant.
- Auscultate bowel and percuss for dullness over fecal mass.

Rectal Examination

Check for fissures, hemorrhoids, irritation, fecal impaction, and sphincter tone. NOTE: Clients with functional constipation usually have normal sphincter tone and large rectal vaults.

Diagnostic Tests

An x-ray examination of the abdomen is sometimes helpful to estimate the amount of stool retained. In adults, three separate stools should be obtained for occult blood testing.

DIAGNOSIS

Diagnosis of functional constipation is made by detailed history and physical examination. Differential diagnosis includes the following:

- Toilet-training resistance
- Normal straining on infancy-soft stools
- Hirschsprung's disease–constipation from birth, rectal ampulla empty
- Encopresis
- Partial bowel obstruction
- Irritable bowel syndrome (IBS)
- Rectal fissures or hemorrhoids
- Hypothyroidism

THERAPEUTIC PLAN
Infant

- At 0 to 4 months, discontinue solids, increase water and fruit juice in the diet.
- At 4 to 12 months, introduce fruits and nonstarchy vegetables into diet. Encourage an occasional juice or water bottle. Avoid rice cereal. It may be necessary to use Maltsupex, 1 to 2 teaspoons tid.

Child

- 1 to 12 years
  —If significant constipation is seen on initial examination, give one or more pediatric Fleet enemas to evacuate the bowel.

—Retrain bowels; have the child sit on the toilet for 20 minutes after meals. Educate child and parents on gastrocolic reflex.

—Encourage dietary changes, an increase of fiber, fluids, vegetables, and fruit.

- Toddlers: If child is not completely potty-trained, put the child back in diapers and remove all pressure related to toileting.
- Use stool softeners only if other measures fail.

—Docusate sodium (Colace), 5 mg/kg/day

—Maltsupex: Age 1 to 5 years, 1 teaspoon bid, may increase to 2 tablespoons bid; age 5 to 15 years, 2 teaspoons bid, may increase to 2 tablespoons bid

—Reduce daily dose once stools are soft.

—Continue for 2 to 3 months until regular bowel habits are established.

Adult

- Increase fluid intake to 1.5 to 2 L daily.
- Increase fiber in the diet, add fresh fruits and vegetables, bran cereals, whole-grain breads.
- Increase daily exercise.
- Retrain bowel habits; client should sit on the toilet for 15 minutes after meals. Client should not ignore the urge to defecate.
- Instruct the client to avoid chronic laxative use.
- Use pharmacologic measures if general measures fail.

—Stool softeners: Docusate sodium (Colace), 50 to 300 mg/day; docusate calcium (Doxidan), 240 mg/day; short-term use only

—Bulk-forming agents: Polycarbophil (Fibercon), methylcellulose (Citrucel), or psyllium (Effersylium); beginning with 1 tablespoon daily and increasing as needed to 3 tablespoons daily; must be accompanied by plenty of fluids; may be used long term

EVALUATION/FOLLOW-UP

Schedule follow-up visits every 2 weeks until normal bowel function resumes. Refer the following clients to gastroenterologist:

- Any child who has a poor response to therapy or who exhibits emotional problems
- Adults older than 50 years with constipation representing a change from their usual pattern
- Any client who has Hemoccult-positive stools

Diarrhea

OVERVIEW
Definition

Diarrhea is defined as an increase in the frequency and fluid content of stools.

Incidence

- Diarrhea accounts for approximately 20% of all pediatric office visits in the United States.
- It affects approximately 10% of all infants younger than 1 year in the United States.
- Incidence varies with age, causative organism, geographic location, season, and host susceptibility.

Pathophysiology

CONTRIBUTING FACTORS
- Poor hand washing
- Improper food handling
- Recent antibiotics
- Immunocompromised host
- Poor sanitation
- Recent travel

ACUTE DIARRHEA. Viral or bacterial toxins stimulate the active transport of electrolytes into the small intestines. The mucosal lining of the intestines becomes irritated resulting in secretion of excess amounts of fluid and electrolytes from the cells.

LACTOSE INTOLERANCE. Inflammation of the intestinal mucosal cells decreases the ability to absorb nutrients, electrolytes, and water.

OVERFEEDING AND SOME MEDICATIONS. With overfeeding or medications such as antibiotics, laxatives, and antacids, excess fluid in the gut produces increased motility and rapid emptying.

CAUSES OF CHRONIC DIARRHEA
- Malabsorption
- AIDS
- Hyperthyroidism
- Fecal impaction
- Functional bowel disease
- Congenital (short-gut syndrome, gastroschisis, etc.)

ASSESSMENT: SUBJECTIVE/HISTORY

- Possible elevated temperature
- Anorexia

- Lethargy
- Sudden or gradual increase in number and liquidity of stools
- Crampy abdominal pain
  In addition, ask about the following:
  - Onset
  - Description of stools
  - Frequency of stools
  - Usual pattern of elimination
  - Associated symptoms, such as vomiting or localized abdominal pain
  - Current or recent drugs
  - Exposure to others with diarrhea
  - Detailed dietary history, including introduction of new foods
  - Recent travel
  - Psychologic upsets
  - Treatments tried
  - Urinary output

ASSESSMENT: OBJECTIVE/ PHYSICAL EXAMINATION
Physical Examination

- Weight
- State of hydration:
  —Mucous membranes
  —Skin turgor
  —Urinary output
  —Fontanel
  —Tears
  —Heart rate
  —Level of consciousness
- Temperature elevation may be related to dehydration or infection.
- Abdominal examination:
  —Distention
  —Hyperactive bowel sounds
  —Diffuse tenderness
  —Increased tympany to percussion
  —Splenomegaly (bacterial)
- Look for other infections that can produce diarrhea and vomiting:
  —Streptococcal pharyngitis
  —Pneumonia
  —Otitis media

Diagnostic Procedures

- Diagnosis can usually be made by careful history alone.

- With duration less than 48 hours, no tests are usually needed.
- If dehydration is present, especially in small children, check serum electrolytes.
- Wet preparation for WBCs
- Stool for ova and parasites
- Stool culture for enteric pathogens

DIAGNOSIS

Summary information for diagnosis of acute diarrhea is included in Table 4-3.

Acute Diarrhea

Differential diagnosis includes the following:
- Diarrhea induced by food or drug sensitivities
- Starvation diarrhea
- Parenteral infections: urinary tract infection (UTI), URI
- Sepsis in neonates

Chronic Diarrhea

Differential diagnosis includes the following:
- Malabsorption (cystic fibrosis, lactose deficiency, celiac disease)
- Reye's syndrome
- AIDs
- Inflammatory bowel disease
- Food allergies
- Metabolic disease
- Pseudomembranous colitis

THERAPEUTIC PLAN
Infants and Children

Diarrhea is usually self-limiting and requires no aggressive therapy. The family nurse practitioner's treatment plan should be based on careful assessment of the degree of dehydration. Treat as follows;

DIARRHEA WITHOUT DEHYDRATION
- Continue breast milk, formula, or age-appropriate diet.
- Push oral fluids at a rate of 150 ml/kg/day.
- Follow each stool with 10 ml/kg electrolyte solution (Pedialyte or Infalyte).

MILD DEHYDRATION
- Oral rehydration therapy (ORT) with a solution containing 75 to 90 mEq/L sodium.

Table 4-3 Diagnosis of Acute Diarrhea

AGENT	AGE	SOURCE	SYMPTOMS	STOOL CHARACTERISTICS	TREATMENT
Viral					
Rotavirus Norwalk, adenovirus, enterovirus	Any	Food, person-to-person contact	Nausea, vomiting, low-grade fever may precede diarrhea, URI	Large and liquid, variable odor; negative for blood and leukocytes	Varies with age; see text
Bacterial					
Campylobacter jejuni	Any Most common bacterial diarrhea in ages 1–5 yr	Fecal-oral, food and water, person-to-person contact	Vomiting, fever	Profuse bloody and watery, with mucus in streaks; positive for blood and leukocytes	Erythromycin: children, 40 mg/kg q 6 hr × 5–7 days; adults, 250 mg q 6 hr × 5–7 days
Salmonella	Any	Fecal-oral, animal or human source, food	Vomiting, fever, abdominal pain	Loose, slimy, and green, with "rotten egg" odor; positive for leukocytes and blood	Ampicillin (used rarely): children, 200 mg/kg q 4 hr × 14 days; adults, 500 mg qid × 14 days
Shigella	Any; peaks at 2–10 yr	Fecal-oral, rarely food	Vomiting, fever, abdominal pain	Watery, yellow-green, mucoid, and bloody; no change in odor; positive for blood and leukocytes	Trimethoprim-sulfamethoxazole (Bactrim): children, 8 mg/kg trimethoprim and 40 mg sulfamethoxazole bid × 5 days; adults, 160 mg trimethoprim & 800 mg sulfamethoxazole bid × 5 days
Escherichia coli (leading cause of traveler's diarrhea)	Any; peaks at <1 yr	Fecal oral, food and water	Low-grade fever, abdominal cramps, gradual onset of diarrhea	Green, slimy, and foul-smelling; positive for leukocytes	Same as *Shigella*
Parasitic					
Giardia lamblia	Any; peaks at 4 yr	Waterborne, seen in day care centers and communities with inadequate water treatment	Nausea, vomiting, anorexia, abdominal distention and cramping	Pale, bulky, and greasy, with foul odor; negative for blood and leukocytes; 30% to 60% are positive for casts	Metronidazole (Flagyl): children, 100 mg tid × 7 days

World Health Organization rehydration salts. Give 40 to 50 ml/kg over 4 hours.

—Reassess hydration status every 2 to 4 hours.

—When dehydration is corrected, move to maintenance therapy.

- Maintenance therapy; resume breast milk, formula, or age-appropriate diet.

—Push oral fluids at a rate of 150 ml/kg/day.

—Follow each stool with a solution containing 40 to 60 mEq/L sodium (Pedialyte or Infalyte) at 10 ml/kg and follow each emesis with 2 ml/kg.

MODERATE DEHYDRATION

- ORT at 100 ml/kg over 4 hours
- Reassess hydration status every 2 to 4 hours.
- When dehydration is corrected, move to maintenance therapy.

SEVERE DEHYDRATION. Consult physician and refer for hospitalization and IV rehydration.

Pharmacologic Therapy

Usually it is not indicated, and at times it may prolong the course. Pharmacotherapy may be used in severe cases to shorten course, prevent complications, or decrease excretion of the causative agent (see Table 4-3).

Oral Rehydration Therapy

- Give children younger than 2 years ½ cup ORT solution every hour.
- Give children older than 2 years ½ to 1 cup ORT solution every hour.
- If vomiting occurs, give 1 teaspoon ORT solution every 2 to 3 minutes until vomiting stops, and then continue ORT as above.
- Have parent notify the family nurse practitioner if diarrhea is not improved in 24 hours, there is an increase in the frequency or amount of vomiting or diarrhea, or if blood appears in either the stool or the emesis.
- Avoid using antidiarrheal agents, including OTC preparations.

Adults

- For acute episodes discontinue solids for 12 hours.
- Reintroduce food as soon as possible and advance as tolerated.

- Pharmacologic therapy is usually not indicated. It may be used in severe cases to shorten course, prevent complications, or decrease excretion of the causative agent.
- Give kaolin-pectin (Kaopectate) 60 ml PO every 3 to 4 hours. Use is not to exceed 2 days.
- Give loperamide (Imodium) 4 mg PO initially then 2 mg after each loose stool, to a maximum dose of 16 mg/24 hr. Use is not to exceed 2 days.
- See Table 4-3 for treatment of bacterial infections.

Client Education

Teach parents signs and symptoms of dehydration:

- Dry mouth
- No tears
- Less moisture in diaper
- Lethargy
- Weight loss
- Irritability
- Sunken fontanel

EVALUATION/FOLLOW-UP

- Infants and small children
  —Conduct telephone follow-up in 12 hours and then daily until diarrhea has subsided. Infants need daily weight checks.
  —Instruct caregiver to call if fluids are refused or continually vomited.
- Adults: Return to clinic in 3 days if diarrhea has not resolved.
- Consult and/or refer in the following cases:
  —Infants younger than 3 months
  —Severe dehydration
  —Diarrhea persisting longer than 3 days in children and longer than 2 weeks in adults
  —Bloody diarrhea or emesis

REFERENCES

Arvin, A. M., Behrman, R. E., Kliegman, R. M., & Nelson, W. E. (Eds.). (1996). *Nelson textbook of pediatrics* (15th ed.). Philadelphia: W. B. Saunders.

Boynton, R. W., Dunn, E. S., & Stephens, G. R., (Eds.). (1994). *Manual of ambulatory pediatrics* (3rd ed.). Philadelphia: J. B. Lippincott.

Dershewitz, R. A. (Ed.). (1993). *Ambulatory pediatric care* (2nd ed.). Philadelphia: J. B. Lippincott.

Goepp, J. G., & Santosham, M. (1993). Oral rehydration therapy. In M. D. Oski & J. A. McMillan (Eds.), *Principles and practice of pediatrics updates.* Philadelphia: J. B. Lippincott.

Groothuis, J. R., Hay, W. W., Hayward, A. R., & Levin, M. J. (Eds.). (1995). *Current pediatric diagnosis and treatment* (12th. ed.). Norwalk, CT: Appleton & Lange.

McCargar, L. J., Hotson, B. L., & Nozza, A. (1995). Fibre and nutrient intakes of chronic care elderly patients. *Journal of Nutrition for the Elderly, 15*(1), 13-31.

Rosenthal, M. (1997). Diarrhea organisms are becoming media stars. *Infectious diseases in children, 10*(1), 10-11.

Straughn, A., & English, B. (1996). Oral rehydration therapy: a neglected treatment for pediatric diarrhea. *Maternal Child Nursing, 6*(5), 144-147.

Uphold, C. R., & Graham, M. V. (1994). *Clinical guidelines in family practice.* Gainesville, FL: Barmarrae Books.

REVIEW QUESTIONS

1. A 3-year-old comes to the clinic with a 24-hour history of vomiting, diarrhea, fever (103° F), and severe abdominal tenderness. What should the family nurse practitioner do?

 a. Reassure the mother that this is gastroenteritis and it should be self-limiting.
 b. Conduct a complete dietary history and physical examination before making a diagnosis.
 c. Take a complete dietary history, looking especially for other family members who might have eaten the same contaminated foods.
 d. Send a stool culture for ova and parasites and for enteric pathogens.

2. While taking a history on a 30-year-old woman, the nurse practitioner learns that the client has a bowel movement every third day. What should the family nurse practitioner do?

 a. Prescribe a bulk-forming agent such as polycarbophil (Fibercon).
 b. Instruct the client to take a laxative if she fails to have a bowel movement by bedtime.
 c. Take a detailed dietary history, looking especially for high-fiber foods.
 d. Ask the client whether this represents a change from her usual pattern before assessing further.

3. The family nurse practitioner would need to consult the physician for which of the following cases?

 a. An 8-month-old infant with a 24-hour history of diarrhea and mild dehydration
 b. An 8-year-old with a familial tendency toward constipation who reports having a bowel movement once a week
 c. A 55-year-old woman who reports a bowel history of stools QOD
 d. A 60-year-old man who reports constipation after having previously been regular

4. During the physical examination of an elderly client with a history of chronic constipation, the family nurse practitioner would expect to find all the following **except:**

 a. Occult blood in the stool
 b. Hemorrhoids or rectal irritation
 c. Hard, impacted stool in the rectal vault
 d. Mild abdominal tenderness, with a fecal mass palpable in the left lower quadrant

5. The family nurse practitioner has prescribed ORT for a 14-month-old with mild dehydration. The mother asks what she should do if the child vomits the solution. What instructions should the family nurse practitioner give?

 a. Hold the ORT solution until the child stops vomiting.
 b. Continue to give the ORT solution in small, frequent amounts (1 teaspoon every 1 to 2 minutes).
 c. Hold the ORT solution for 2 to 3 hours until the child's stomach has settled and then resume feeding.
 d. Continue to give the ORT solution as ordered.

6. Four hours after beginning ORT on an infant with moderate dehydration, the family nurse practitioner phones to check the child's progress. The mother reports that he has vomited all the ORT solution and is continuing to have liquid stools. The family nurse practitioner should do which of the following?

 a. Ask the mother to continue ORT in the clinic under a controlled situation.
 b. Ask the mother to observe the child for 1 hour and then attempt to restart ORT.
 c. Change the ORT solution to juice or gelatin water.
 d. Consult the physician about the need for parenteral fluid therapy and refer to the ED.

ANSWERS AND RATIONALES

1. Answer: b (assessment/history/gastrointestinal/child)

Rationale: Significant abdominal tenderness suggests a more serious problem than gastroenteritis. A thorough history and physical examination should always be conducted before making any diagnosis.

2. Answer: d (assessment/history/gastrointestinal/adult)

Rationale: Bowel habits are unique to individuals. A daily bowel movement may not be normal for everyone. The family nurse practitioner should first determine whether the pattern is a problem for this individual before attempting to treat. A dietary history and perhaps a bulk-forming agent would be appropriate if it is determined that constipation exists. Regular laxative use should always be discouraged. (Boynton, Dunn, & Stephens, 1994)

3. Answer: d (plan/gastrointestinal/NAS)

Rationale: A physician should be consulted for any adult older than 50 years with constipation that represents a change from his or her usual pattern. Both the 8-month-old and the 8-year-old could be managed by the family nurse practitioner. The 55-year-old is continuing in an established pattern that would be considered normal. (Uphold & Graham, 1994)

4. Answer: a (assessment/physical examination/gastrointestinal/aging adult)

Rationale: Older clients with chronic constipation often have fecal impaction. Rectal irritation and hemorrhoids frequently accompany constipation as a result of straining to pass large, hard stools. The presence of occult blood in any client's stool is an indication of a more serious problem and warrants a consultation. (Uphold & Graham, 1994)

5. Answer: b (plan/gastrointestinal/child)

Rationale: Giving the ORT in very small quantities will limit gastric distention while at the same time helping to correct dehydration and acidosis. Vomiting is generally triggered by gastric distention and acidosis. Both choices *a* and *d* would fail to give the child fluid and would contribute to increasing dehydration. Choice *c* would require large quantities of solution, which would lead to gastric distention and more vomiting. (Goepp & Santosham, 1993)

6. Answer: d (evaluation/gastrointestinal/infant)

Rationale: Children who continue with a negative fluid balance 4 hours into ORT should receive IV fluids (Goepp & Santosham, 1993). High-osmolar fluids, such as gelatin water and fruit juices, tend to draw water into the intestines and actually increase the number of stools. (Straughn & English, 1996)

DIVERTICULAR DISEASE

OVERVIEW
Definition

Diverticula are abnormal herniations of mucosa through the muscle layer of the colon wall. Asymptomatic diverticular disease is referred to as *diverticulosis.* Often diverticulosis is diagnosed serendipitously when searching for other diagnoses. *Diverticulitis* represents inflammation caused by infection.

Incidence

Diverticular disease affects men and women equally. Although there is no known genetic pattern, it is present in 20% of the adult population older than 40 years, increasing progressively with age. It is estimated that 70% of those older than 70 years have diverticular disease. Diverticulitis occurs in about half of those individuals with diverticulosis. Thirty-three percent of those treated for diverticulitis will likely have subsequent episodes. Two or three occurrences during 1 to 2 years is an indication to consider surgical removal of that portion of the bowel.

Pathophysiology

Diverticula most commonly occur in the sigmoid colon, where the colon is narrowest and the pressure is highest. However, diverticula can occur anywhere in the GI tract. The saclike outpouchings occur at a weak point in the colon, often where arteries penetrate the tunica musculars. Thickening, hypertrophy, and contraction of the muscles in the colon wall increase intraluminal pressure and the degree of the herniation. Trapped undigested food and bacteria in the diverticular sacs can result in an infection.

COMPLICATIONS OF DIVERTICULITIS
- Abscess formation (abscess may rupture)
- Peritonitis
- Obstruction
- Bleeding
- Fistula development into bladder, gut, or vagina

RISK FACTORS
- Age older than 40 years
- Low-residue diets reduce fecal bulk, reducing the diameter of the colon.
- Previous episodes of diverticulitis

ASSESSMENT: SUBJECTIVE/HISTORY
Diverticulosis

- Symptoms may be vague or absent; fewer than 25% of individuals with diverticulosis have symptoms.
- Intermittent lower left quadrant abdominal pain, worse after eating; some relief after bowel movement or flatulence
- Constipation alternating with diarrhea

Diverticulitis

Symptoms will vary; any of the following symptoms may be present:
- Pain is localized to the left lower quadrant and is usually sudden in onset.
- Fever and chills
- Poor appetite
- Nausea and vomiting
- Constipation or diarrhea
- Guarding, rebound tenderness
- Gas and flatulence
- Rectal bleeding

ASSESSMENT: OBJECTIVE/ PHYSICAL EXAMINATION
Physical Examination

A problem-oriented physical examination should include vital signs, height, and weight. Age and level of acuity may require a more comprehensive examination than an assessment of the abdomen and rectum.

DIVERTICULOSIS
- Abdomen may be distended and tympanic.
- Flatulence
- Rectal examination may reveal a palpable mass in left lower quadrant, firm and tender.
- Melena if diverticular bleed
- Brisk rectal bleeding

DIVERTICULITIS
- Rigid abdomen, or distended and tympanic
- Tender, firm, fixed palpable mass in left iliac fossa
- Bowel sounds depressed, or increased if obstruction
- Rectum may be tender on examination; there may be a mass in the cul de sac.
- Melena if diverticular bleed
- Brisk rectal bleeding
- Leukocytosis

Diagnostic Procedures

- CBC with differential (WBCs elevated with immature polymorphs in diverticulitis)
- Hemoglobin low if bleeding
- Sedimentation rate elevated in diverticulosis
- Imaging
  —Abdominal flat-plate supine and upright radiographs (useful in peritonitis and perforation)
  —Barium enema is used to diagnose diverticulosis. It is controversial for diagnosing diverticulitis in the acute phase because it may cause rupture of the diverticula. Diagnostic accuracy of the barium enema in distinguishing between diverticular disease and cancer has been questioned.
  —Colonoscopy and flexible sigmoidoscopy are helpful in differentiating diverticulosis, ulcerative colitis, and cancer.
  —CT scan, although expensive, is an excellent alternative diagnostic procedure to the barium enema.

DIAGNOSIS

Differential diagnosis includes the following:
- IBS
- Lactose intolerance
- Appendicitis
- Gastroenteritis
- Fecal impaction

- Ulcerative colitis, Crohn's disease
- Carcinoma
- Ectopic pregnancy
- UTI

THERAPEUTIC PLAN
Diverticulosis

PHARMACOLOGIC TREATMENT
- Manage pain with antispasmodic dicyclomine [Bentyl], 10 to 20 mg bid to qid with meals. Anticholinergics need to be used with caution (they may reduce the painful spasm but they increase the risk of constipation).
- Manage constipation and diarrhea similarly to irritable bowel syndrome.
  —Loperamide (Imodium), 2 mg after each diarrheal stool, or diphenoxylate, (Lomotil), 2.5 to 5 mg after each diarrheal stool
  —Psyllium products, Metamucil 1 tablespoon bid or tid for constipation or Fiberall 1 to 2 wafers bid or tid with 8 ounces water
  —Antiflatulents, simethicone (Flatulex), 80 mg after meals and at bedtime

Diverticulitis

Only treat mild, nontoxic individuals in primary care (temperature <101° F, WBCs 13,000 to 15,000 cells/mm^3).
PHARMACOLOGIC TREATMENT
- Metronidazole (Flagyl), 250 to 500 every 8 hours for 7 days, and amoxicillin, 500 mg combination every 8 hours, or Ciprofloxacin, 500 mg bid (to cover enterococcal and gram-negative aerobes)
- A client should respond within 3 days.
- Use mild analgesics (nonopiates) for pain.

Client Education

- Diet: In acute diverticulitis, reduce diet to clear liquids, graduating to soft foods as symptoms improve. Progress to high fiber when normal bowel function returns.
- Maintain adequate fluid intake (2000 ml/day).
- Good sources of fiber include bran, raw carrots, and fruit. Bran can cause bloating or flatulence, which resolves with continued use.
- Avoid foods with seeds or those that are indigestible, such as nuts, popcorn, corn, cucumbers, tomatoes, strawberries, or caraway seeds on buns. These can block the neck of the diverticulum.
- Avoid laxatives, enemas, and opiates because they can lead to chronic constipation.
- Signs and symptoms of complications: Severe abdominal pain, vomiting, temperature >101° F, hard or firm abdomen, no bowel movements, frank rectal bleeding
- Stress management: Discuss ways to reduce stress; consider relaxation techniques. Participate in support groups if helpful to manage symptoms.
- Activity: There are no activity restrictions for diverticulosis. Restrict activity in diverticulitis, with bed rest during the acute phase. Develop and maintain a regular exercise program (walking exercise increases peristalsis and decreases constipation).

EVALUATION/FOLLOW-UP
Diverticulosis

Follow-up in 1 to 2 weeks, then every 3 months to 1 year, then annually as needed. Barium enema may be repeated every 3 to 5 years (if maximal or no symptoms), followed by a colonoscopy if needed.

Diverticulitis

- Do telephone follow-up at 24 to 72 hours; if there is no progress or symptoms are worse, client should return to clinic for further evaluation.
- Follow-up in 10 days to 2 weeks if recovery has progressed as expected.
- Follow-up at 1- to 3-month intervals, expanding to annual check-ups based on symptoms.

Referral

- Refer very ill older clients with history of diverticulosis (older clients may not look toxic yet have an acute abdomen with no pain and no fever).
- Toxic clients with diverticulitis (septicemia, peritonitis)
- Failure to resolve in 48 to 72 hours
- Brisk rectal bleeding
- If client's condition is worsening, consider hospitalization immediately if temperature is >101° F, there is a marked change in abdomi-

nal pain and continuous increase in WBCs and peritoneal signs develop.
- Two or more episodes of diverticulitis during a 1- to 2-year period may be an indication for surgery.

Consultation

If there is no change in symptoms regardless of management regimen

REFERENCES

Goroll, A., May, L., & Mulley, A. (Eds.). (1995). *Primary care medicine: Office evaluation and management of the adult patient*. Philadelphia: J. B. Lippincott.
Hurst, J. W. (1996). *Medicine for the practicing physician*. Norwalk, CT: Appleton & Lange.
Isselbacher, K., Braunwald, E., Wilson, J., Martin, J., Fauci, A., & Kasper, D. (1994). *Harrison's principles of internal medicine* (13th ed.). New York: McGraw Hill.
Lonergan, E. (Ed.). (1996). *Geriatrics: A clinical manual*. Norwalk, CT: Appleton & Lange.
Rakel, R. (Ed.). (1995). *Textbook of family practice* (5th ed.). Philadelphia: W. B. Saunders.

REVIEW QUESTIONS

1. Which of the following is most indicative of diverticulosis?

  a. Generalized abdominal pain, better after eating
  b. Lower right quadrant abdominal pain, worse after eating
  c. Intermittent epigastric pain
  d. Intermittent lower left quadrant abdominal pain, worse after eating

2. B.B., a 58-year-old man reports to the clinic with a temperature of 100° F, bloating, and cramping abdominal pain throughout his entire abdomen for the past 2 days. He notes mild constipation and increasing nausea. He has a 5-year history of diverticulosis. He reports no surgeries. He ate popcorn 3 days ago. His WBCs are 15,000 cells/mm³. On physical examination, you note generalized abdominal tenderness, no rebound tenderness, no rectal point tenderness, and a negative guaiac test result. On the basis of this history, what is the most likely diagnosis?

  a. Diverticulitis
  b. Gastroesophageal reflux disease (GERD)
  c. IBS
  d. Appendicitis

3. Bruce is a 58-year-old man reporting a fever, bloating, cramping, and abdominal pain throughout his entire abdomen for 2 days. He notes mild constipation. He has a 5-year history of diverticulosis. He ate popcorn 2 days ago. His WBCs are 15,000 cells/mm³. On his examination you note generalized abdominal tenderness, no rebound tenderness, no rectal point tenderness, and a negative guaiac test result. What would be the best treatment for Bruce?

  a. Lifestyle changes and H_2 blockers
  b. Anticholinergic agents
  c. Hydrocodone bitartrate (Vicodin) for pain
  d. Antibiotics

4. Steve is a 52-year-old client you are treating with antibiotics for diverticulitis. How would you follow up once he leaves your office?

  a. After his discharge from the hospital
  b. In 1 to 2 weeks
  c. With a telephone call in 24 hours to reevaluate
  d. As needed

5. Which of the following is most indicative of diverticulitis?

  a. Nausea and vomiting, distended abdomen
  b. Epigastric pain radiating upward
  c. Pain improving with eating
  d. Pain improving with bowel movement

6. Which of the following findings are most common in persons with diverticulitis?

  a. Elevated WBCs, fever, left lower quadrant abdominal pain
  b. Elevated WBCs, fever, right lower quadrant abdominal pain
  c. Rectal bleeding
  d. Constipation

ANSWERS AND RATIONALES

1. *Answer:* d (assessment/history/gastrointestinal/NAS)

Rationale: Increased bulk and motility after eating result in pressure irritation of the diverticula, most commonly found in the sigmoid colon located on the left lower side of the abdomen. Right-sided pain is rarely worse after eating and is most frequently associated with appendicitis; intermittent epigastric pain is more likely gastric or cardiac in nature. (Goroll, May, & Mulley, 1995; Hurst, 1996; Rakel, 1995)

2. *Answer:* a (diagnosis/gastrointestinal/adult)

Rationale: The elevated temperature, elevated WBCs, abdominal tenderness, and history of diverticulosis are strongly indicative of a diagnosis of diverticulitis. However, appendicitis also needs to be a consideration because the client has had no surgeries. Although you would expect right-sided pain, presenting symptoms of disease processes are not always predictable. The client's history and physical findings do not support a diagnosis of GERD or IBS. (Goroll, May, & Mulley, 1995; Hurst, 1996; Rakel, 1995)

3. *Answer:* d (management/therapeutics/pharmacologic/gastrointestinal/adult)

Rationale: Antibiotics are an appropriate treatment for a person with diverticulitis. The client notes mild constipation, so you would avoid constipating medications, such as anticholinergic medications or Vicodin. Lifestyle changes may be relevant after this acute phase, but they and H$_2$ blockers are more appropriate therapy for a diagnosis of GERD or peptic ulcer disease. (Goroll, May, & Mulley, 1995; Hurst, 1996; Rakel, 1995)

4. *Answer:* c (evaluation/gastrointestinal/adult)

Rationale: This client is at risk for rapid progression of illness. Remember, diverticulitis can cause abscess formation, obstruction, hemorrhage, and peritonitis. Antibiotic therapy should result in improvement within 24 to 72 hours. A rise in temperature, severity of pain, or rigidity in the abdomen may be signs of pending complications. It is important to know this within 24 hours, especially with an older individual. (Goroll, May, & Mulley, 1995; Hurst, 1996; Rakel, 1995)

5. *Answer:* a (assessment/history/gastrointestinal/ NAS)

Rationale: The inflammatory process in the bowel often results in an alteration in motility, leading to abdominal distention, nausea, and vomiting. These symptoms may also be accompanied by abdominal pain. Epigastric pain radiating upward is often referred to as *heartburn,* common in GERD. Pain that improves with eating is associated with a duodenal ulcer. Pain improvement with bowel movements is noted among individuals with IBS. Such improvement may also occur with diverticulosis. (Goroll, May, & Mulley, 1995; Hurst, 1996; Rakel, 1995)

6. *Answer:* a (assessment/physical examination/gastrointestinal/NAS)

Rationale: Elevated WBCs and fever are signs of an infection and inflammation. The left-sided abdominal pain is common in diverticulitis (the sigmoid colon seems to be somewhat more vulnerable to the development of diverticula). Right-sided lower quadrant pain is more common in appendicitis. Rectal bleeding and constipation may be present regardless of any inflammatory process. (Goroll, May, & Mulley, 1995; Hurst, 1996; Rakel, 1995)

GASTROESOPHAGEAL REFLUX DISEASE

OVERVIEW
Definition

Gastroesophageal reflux disease (GERD) is characterized by an abnormal reflux of gastroduodenal contents into the esophagus, which may result in esophageal inflammation. It is a chronic disease; without therapy, individuals are prone to have relapses.

Incidence

- The incidence is increasing in the United States, where more than 60% of the adult population have had "heartburn."

- From 70% to 80% of women who are pregnant report the symptom of heartburn.
- More than 20% of affected adults have had symptoms for longer than 10 years.
- Approximately 10% of affected adults experience symptoms daily.
- Children may also be affected, usually in the first year of life.
- Males and females are affected equally.
- GERD causes complications in less than 2% of the general population.
- Without long-term therapy, 50% to 80% of persons with GERD have a relapse within 6 to 12 months of healing of the acute disease.

- An increasing number of individuals are observed to have GERD-induced asthma.

Pathophysiology

GERD is caused by a reflux of gastric contents into the esophagus, which may be due to an abnormal antireflux barrier, defective esophageal clearance, increased gastric secretions, and delayed gastric emptying. The pathophysiology of the asthma-GERD connection is less clear. It is suggested that the esophageal broncheal reflux triggers bronchospasm, which promotes acid reflux, leading to further bronchospasms.

RISK FACTORS. Inappropriate relaxation of lower esophageal sphincter may be idiopathic. This relaxation may be transient rather than low basal tone. Lower esophageal sphincter relaxation may also be due to food or drugs, which may affect motility, gastric secretions, and sensory response.

- Foods that influence symptoms
  —Chocolate
  —Citrus fruit
  —Caffeine
  —Alcohol
  —High-fat diets
- Medications that reduce lower esophageal sphincter pressure
  —Anticholinergics
  —Progesterone
  —Calcium channel blockers (nifedipine and verapamil)
  —Calcium
  —Theophylline
  —Diazepam
  —Meperidine
  —Transdermal nicotine
- There may be decreased pressure of the lower esophageal sphincter during pregnancy as a result of progestational hormones.
- Sphincter competence and peristaltic clearing of acid may be impaired in individuals with hiatal hernia.
- Smoking lowers sphincure pressure.

Complications

- Reflux esophagitis results in inflammation in the esophageal wall, increasing capillary permeability, edema, tissue fragility, and erosion.
- Fibrosis may result.

- Chronic GERD may be associated with strictures, hemorrhage, and increased risk of adenocarcinoma. There is no genetic predisposition.
- Age increases the risk of malignancy.
- Asthma

ASSESSMENT: SUBJECTIVE/HISTORY
History of Current Illness

- Burning substernal pain radiates upward, often called "heartburn," usually within 30 to 60 minutes of eating.
- Note frequency, onset, progression, and duration of pain.
- Pain is aggravated by large meals, lying down, or bending over.
- Pain is relieved by antacids or nonprescription doses of H_2-receptor antagonists.
- Dysphagia, cough, weight loss, or blood loss may suggest other problems.
- Does the client smoke, chew tobacco, or use alcohol?
- Regurgitation of fluid or food particles may occur.
- Reflux may trigger angina-like chest pain.
- Hoarseness, sore throat, and feeling of lump in throat may be symptoms of GERD.
- Wheezing, nocturnal coughing, and shortness of breath may suggest an asthmatic component.

Past Medical History

- Chronic diseases
- Similar episodes
- History of asthma

Medication History

Note whether any prescribed, OTC, or herbal remedies are taken.

ASSESSMENT: OBJECTIVE/ PHYSICAL EXAMINATION
Physical Examination

A problem-oriented physical examination is necessary, with attention to vital signs, height and weight, and general appearance.

- Lungs: Evaluate for adventitious sounds.
- Abdomen: Check for bowel sounds, distention, obesity, masses, pain.

- Rectal: Assess for masses, tenderness, occult blood.
- A comprehensive examination should be scheduled to evaluate other problems.

Diagnostic Procedures

- Usually no laboratory studies are required.
- Do CBC with differential to rule out anemias and infections.
- Do chemistry profile (to evaluate for other chronic problems, such as diabetes and liver problems).
- Procedures include endoscopy if dysphagia, weight loss, blood loss, or treatment failure.
- Follow cardiac guidelines if it is suspected that symptoms are cardiac in origin.
- Evaluate respiratory symptoms according to guidelines.
- Perform a guaiac evaluation of stool for occult blood.

DIAGNOSIS

Differential diagnosis includes the following:
- Cardiac chest pain
- Peptic ulcer disease
- Esophageal infection (*Candida*, herpes, HIV, cytomegalovirus)
- Esophagitis from pill taking (doxycycline, ascorbic acid, quinidine, etc.)
- Esophageal carcinoma
- Asthma may coexist with GERD.

THERAPEUTIC PLAN

Management of GERD involves a stepped approach to care. The client needs to be an active member of the management team. NOTE: The medications listed below are expensive.

Phase I

- Dietary changes
- Lifestyle modifications (if necessary lose weight, stop smoking, and reduce alcohol consumption; eat small, frequent meals and take no food 2 to 3 hours before bed)
- Antacids (after meals and at bedtime)
- Nonprescription H_2
- Raise head of bed 4 inches (do not use pillows because this may worsen problem).

Pharmacologic Treatment

- *Phase II:* Add an H_2-receptor antagonist orally:
  —Cimetidine (Tagamet), 400 mg bid
  —Ranitidine (Zantac), 150 mg bid
  —Famotidine (Pepcid), 20 bid
  —Nizatidine (Axid), 150 bid
- Alternatives to H_2-receptor antagonists:
  —Cisapride (Propulsid), alone or in combination with an H_2-receptor antagonist
  —Sucralfate (Carafate), may be used but is controversial. Studies in the United States have not supported higher effectiveness than Propulsid or H_2-receptor antagonists.
- If second-phase therapy fails, proton-pump inhibitors (PPIs) may be used:
  —Omeprazole (Prilosec), 20 mg/day
  —Lansoprazole (Prevacid), 30 mg
  —Short-term therapy, 8 to 12 weeks
  —Long-term therapy, longer than 12 weeks to lifetime
- Be alert to the manufacturer's profile regarding dosing, side effects, possible drug interactions, and precautions for use.

For example:

1. H_2-receptor antagonist dosage may need to be lower if client has renal disease.

2. Cimetidine interacts with many drugs, such as theophylline, warfarin, and phenytoin.

3. Theophylline and beta$_2$-agonists used in treatment of asthma may decrease lower esophageal sphincter pressure.

- Antacids can be used on an as-needed basis. Remember that magnesium-based antacids may cause diarrhea; aluminum-based antacids may cause constipation.
- If possible, avoid drugs that may injure the esophageal mucosa (doxycycline, quinidine, NSAIDs).
- Long-term maintenance therapy with an H_2-receptor antagonist and lifestyle modifications are essential to prevent exacerbation of GERD. Maintenance therapy is usually half the therapeutic dose taken at bedtime. Both Prilosec and Prevacid may be indicated in long-term treatment, but there have been negative long-term effects associated with the use of these drugs (cell hyperplasia, atrophic gastritis).

Pregnant Clients

Heartburn among pregnant women is worse in the first and second trimesters. Treatment is self-managed: frequent small meals, avoidance of meals 2 to 3 hours before lying down, and elevating the head of bed for sleeping.

Pediatric Clients

Gastroesophageal reflux is common in the first year of life. Symptoms include vomiting, weight loss, and failure to thrive. The symptoms, which may include apnea and bradycardia secondary to vagal response, generally resolve by 18 months. Antacids and liquid H_2-receptor antagonists (Zantac syrup) are used to manage symptoms. Placing the infant upright in a car seat 2 to 3 hours after feeding and thickening the feedings with rice cereal may be helpful to minimize symptoms. Surgical treatment may be indicated if there is apnea, persistent vomiting, or difficulty in breathing or swallowing.

Geriatric Clients

Older adults may be at an increased risk for complications.

Client Education

- Stop smoking.
- Elevate head of bed.
- Lose weight if >130% of ideal body weight.
- Avoid lying down immediately after meals.
- Eat smaller meals, low-fat diet.
- Avoid foods that cause symptoms.
- Avoid alcohol and coffee.
- Avoid stooping, bending, and tight clothes.
- Avoid drugs that decrease lower esophageal sphincter pressure.
- Exercise daily.
- Refer client to local support groups if available.

Referral

- Dysphagia, weight loss, blood loss, myocardial infarction
- Recurrence after full course of therapy with two different medications
- Clients receiving protein pump inhibitors
- Pregnant women whose symptoms persist despite lifestyle modifications
- Failure to thrive in children

- Persistent or worsening symptoms in children (apnea, vomiting, difficulty in swallowing or breathing)

Consultation With Physician

- First treatment failure
- Weight loss and vomiting in children

EVALUATION/FOLLOW-UP

- Initial follow-up in 1 to 2 weeks to assess improvement; recheck in 4 weeks
- At 8 weeks adjust follow-up on the basis of recurring signs and symptoms

REFERENCES

Behrman, R., & Kliegman, R. (1994). *Nelson essentials of pediatrics* (2nd ed.). Philadelphia: W. B. Saunders.

Brady, W. M., & Ogorek, C. P. (1996). Gastroesophageal reflux disease. *Postgraduate Medicine, 100*(5), 76-89.

Clark, C. L., & Horwitz, B. (1996). Complications of gastroesophageal reflux disease. *Postgraduate Medicine, 100*(5), 95-113.

Dumont, J. A., & Richter, J. E. (1997). Gastroesophageal reflux masquerading as asthma. *Internal Medicine, February,* 19-37.

Fennerty, M., Castell, D., Fendrick, A., Halpern, M., Johnson, D., Kahrilas, P., Leiberman, D., Richter, J., & Sampliner, R. (1996). The diagnosis and treatment of gastroesophageal reflux disease in a managed care environment: Suggested disease management guidelines. *Archives of Internal Medicine, 156*(5), 477-484.

Goroll, A., May, L., & Mulley, A. (Eds.). (1995). *Primary care medicine: Office evaluation and management of the adult patient.* Philadelphia: J. B. Lippincott.

Hancock, L., & Selig, P. (1994). Gastrointestinal disease. In E. Youngkin & M. Davis (Eds.), *Women's health: A primary care clinical guide* (pp. 603-605). Norwalk, CT: Appleton & Lange.

Harding, S., Richter, J., Guzzo, M., Schan, C., Alexander, R., & Bradley, L. (1996). Asthma and gastroesophageal reflux: Acid suppressive therapy improves asthma outcome. *American Journal of Medicine, 100*(4), 395-405.

Larsen, R. (1997). Gastroesophageal reflux disease. *Postgraduate Medicine, 101*(2), 181 to 187.

Lonergan, E. (Ed.). (1996). *Geriatrics: A clinical manual.* Norwalk, CT: Appleton & Lange.

Rakel, R. (Ed.). (1995). *Textbook of family practice* (5th ed.). Philadelphia: W. B. Saunders.

Uphold, C., & Graham, M. (1994). *Clinical guidelines in family practice* (2nd ed.). Gainesville, FL: Barmarrae Books.

REVIEW QUESTIONS

1. Which of the following is most indicative of GERD?

   a. Abdominal pain is relieved by bowel movement.
   b. Food intake makes the pain worse.
   c. Pain is relieved by food intake.
   d. Burning, substernal pain is noted 1 hour after eating.

2. Which of the following findings is common in a client with GERD?

   a. Abnormal liver function studies
   b. Normal physical findings
   c. Angina pectoris
   d. Occult blood

Situation: *T.M., a 57-year-old man, seeks treatment for chest pain after eating. This symptom has been intermittent for 3 months. He uses antacids as needed, with relief. He smokes 2 packs/day, drinks 2 beers/night, and is 130% of his ideal body weight. He points to his chest and describes his chest pain as burning, substernal pain that moves upward. He takes no other medications and denies chronic diseases. He was last seen 1½ years ago for a similar episode. He coughed frequently during the office visit. Results of his examination are normal. (Questions 3 through 5)*

3. On the basis of this history, what is the most likely diagnosis for T.M.?

   a. GERD
   b. Inflammatory bowel disease
   c. Angina
   d. Peptic ulcer disease

4. What would be the best treatment for this individual?

   a. H_2-receptor antagonist only
   b. Lifestyle changes and H_2-receptor antagonist
   c. Lifestyle modifications, dietary changes to lose weight, and antacids
   d. Beta-blocker only

5. You would instruct T.M. to return for follow-up:

   a. In 8 weeks
   b. In 1 to 2 weeks
   c. In 3 months
   d. As needed

6. Which of the following percentages best describes the incidence of GERD?

   a. Eighty percent of pregnant women have symptoms.
   b. Eighty percent of adults have symptoms for more than 10 years.
   c. Seventy percent of those older than 70 years have it.
   d. GERD occurs in 20% of the adult population.

Situation: *A 33-year-old client who is 4 months' pregnant reports heartburn. You suspect that she may have a weakened lower esophageal sphincter, which is a risk factor for GERD. (Questions 7 and 8)*

7. You suspect lower esophageal sphincter relaxation is due to which of the following?

   a. Pressure caused by increasing size of pregnancy
   b. Progestational hormones associated with pregnancy
   c. Not related to her pregnancy
   d. Caused by foods she is eating

8. What would you recommend for her to alleviate symptoms?

   a. Omeprazole (Prilosec)
   b. H_2-receptor antagonist
   c. Smoking cessation
   d. Frequent, small meals

Situation: *A 68-year-old man seeks treatment with burning substernal pain that radiates upward and lasts 30 to 60 minutes after meals. His weight is 210 pounds, his height is 5 feet 9 inches, and he takes nifedipine (90 ml) for hypertension. He currently has a transdermal nicotine patch to quit smoking. (Questions 9 and 10)*

9. A major consideration when making your diagnosis is which of the following?

   a. Nifedipine and nicotine patch are drugs that relax the lower esophageal sphincter.
   b. Substernal pain may be cardiac in nature.
   c. The client is overweight.
   d. All the above

10. What basic tests would you order to help confirm your diagnosis for a 68-year-old man who has burning, substernal pain that radiates upward, lasts 30 to 60 minutes after meals, a weight of 210 pounds, and a height of 5 feet 9 inches. He takes nifedipine (90 mg/day) for hypertension, and is using a transdermal nicotine patch to quit smoking.

    a. CXR, treadmill
    b. Chemistry panel, ECG
    c. CBC with differential
    d. Sedimentation rate

ANSWERS AND RATIONALES

1. *Answer:* d (assessment/history/gastrointestinal/NAS)

Rationale: Burning substernal pain 1 hour after eating is a classic definition of GERD's symptom of heartburn. Pain relieved by bowel movements is associated with IBS. Food often makes the pain worse in gastric ulcers, whereas pain may be relieved by food among individuals with duodenal ulcers. (Goroll, May, & Mulley, 1995; Larsen, 1997)

2. *Answer:* b (assessment/physical examination/gastrointestinal/NAS)

Rationale: Often physical findings are normal and diagnostic tests are not required to make a diagnosis of GERD. If there is any question that the history is suggestive of angina, liver problems or anemia, tests would need to be done to rule out these conditions. (Goroll, May, & Mulley, 1995; Larsen, 1997)

3. Answer: a (diagnosis/gastrointestinal/adult)

Rationale: It is most likely GERD because of the nature and duration of the chest pain, especially when it is relieved by antacids. His weight, alcohol, and smoking behavior increase his risk for symptoms of GERD. However, given his age and symptoms, heart disease, gastric ulcer disease and malignancy also need to be ruled out. (Clark & Horwitz, 1996; Goroll, May, & Mulley, 1995; Larsen, 1997)

4. *Answer:* c (plan/gastrointestinal/adult)

Rationale: In a step approach, lifestyle modifications (stop smoking, eat small meals, etc.), dietary changes (to avoid selected foods and reduce types and amounts to lose weight), and antacids or nonprescription H_2-receptor antagonists are the appropriate first step. If this does not work, the second phase is to add

H_2-receptor antagonists in conjunction with lifestyle and dietary modifications. Beta-blockers are commonly used to treat hypertension. (Brady & Ogorek, 1996; Goroll, May, & Mulley, 1995)

5. *Answer:* b (evaluation/gastrointestinal/adult)

Rationale: This is a new client starting a new regimen of care. Follow-up in 1 to 2 weeks allows you to spot any changes in his heartburn and to provide support and reinforcement of the lifestyle changes and dietary modification. If symptoms are *not* better, you may want to add the H_2-receptor antagonist at this time. Follow-up intervals of 8 weeks and 3 months are both too long if the client is not getting better. As-needed follow-up may be interpreted by the client as a message not to come back. When implementing a plan involving lifestyle and dietary changes, "structured" or scheduled support visits may be reinforcing for the client. (Brady & Ogorek, 1996; Goroll, May, & Mulley, 1995; Larsen, 1997)

6. *Answer:* a (incidence/gastrointestinal/NAS)

Rationale: From 70% to 80% of women who are pregnant experience heartburn, one of the symptoms of GERD. Only 20% of adults have symptoms longer than 10 years. Seventy percent of 70-year-old clients have diverticular disease. Both diverticular disease and IBS occur in 20% of the adult population. (Goroll, May, & Mulley, 1995; Hancock & Selig, 1994; Rakel, 1995; Uphold & Graham, 1994)

7. *Answer:* b (risk factors/gastrointestinal/childbearing female/adult)

Rationale: There may be decreased pressure of the lower esophageal sphincter during pregnancy as a result of progestational hormones; pressure caused by increasing uterine size does not usually influence lower esophageal sphincter relaxation. You lack a dietary history to make any conclusions relating the cause to foods. (Goroll, May, & Mulley, 1995; Hancock & Selig, 1994; Rakel, 1995; Uphold & Graham, 1994)

8. *Answer:* d (plan/gastrointestinal/childbearing female/adult)

Rationale: Starting with frequent, small meals may reduce her symptoms. Prilosec is a category C drug for pregnancy. H_2-receptor antagonists are category B drugs for pregnancy and could be prescribed; however, most providers encourage minimal or no prescription drug use during pregnancy. (Goroll, May, & Mulley, 1995; Hancock & Selig, 1994; Rakel, 1995; Uphold & Graham, 1994)

9. ***Answer:*** d (diagnosis/gastrointestinal/adult)

Rationale: All the above need to be considered when making the diagnosis for this client. (Goroll, May, & Mulley, 1995; Hancock & Selig, 1994; Rakel, 1995; Uphold & Graham, 1994)

10. ***Answer:*** b (plan/gastrointestinal/adult)

Rationale: Of all the choices available, the chemistry panel and the ECG will provide the most immediate and useful information to make a diagnosis for this client. They help you assess liver function, electrolytes, and cardiac function. A CXR may be helpful related to cardiomegaly. You would not order a treadmill test without basic ECG data related to the client's cardiac status. The CBC and sedimentation rate may complement your other tests but would not be the first that you would do to confirm a diagnosis. (Goroll, May, & Mulley, 1995; Hancock & Selig, 1994; Rakel, 1995; Uphold & Graham, 1994)

HEPATITIS

OVERVIEW
Definition

Hepatitis is a general term denoting inflammation of the liver. It can be caused by viral or bacterial sources or by chemical damage. Some viral infections (Epstein-Barr, mononucleosis, cytomegalovirus) can systemically inflame the liver; however, those hepatotropic viruses that primarily cause hepatitis will be the focus of this chapter.

Incidence

Incidence depends on exposure to situations predisposing one to the virus.

HEPATITIS A. Hepatitis A (HAV) is found in infected water and food and is common in crowded situations, such as low-income housing, schools, and dormitories. Clinical manifestations of HAV may be silent, especially in children.

HEPATITIS B. Hepatitis B (HBV) is common among individuals exposed to needle punctures or blood products and those who engage in unprotected sexual intercourse. Users of intravenous drugs and homosexual men have the highest incidence. Health care workers who are not vaccinated for HBV have an incidence of 15% to 30%. When a pregnant woman has HBV, a cesarean section is performed to protect the infant. Chronic HBV occurs in more than 90% of neonates infected with HBV at birth. About 10% in other populations are subject to a chronic HBV disease state.

HEPATITIS C. Hepatitis C (HCV) is the leading cause of posttransfusion hepatitis, and individuals receiving repeated blood transfusions therefore have a higher incidence. Hepatitis C is also seen in individuals who are exposed to blood, such as health care workers or those whose habits expose them to trauma resulting in exposure to blood, such as homosexual men. Chronic liver disease is seen in approximately 10% to 40% of individuals with HCV infection.

HEPATITIS D. Hepatitis D only occurs in conjunction with hepatitis B, with the same routes of transmission.

HEPATITIS E. Hepatitis E viral infection is rare in the United States; it is usually a mild disease in clients older than 15 years. Hepatitis E carries a considerable (10% to 20%) mortality rate in pregnant women and does not progress to chronic liver disease.

Pathophysiology

The liver performs numerous metabolic and regulatory functions. It is the largest gland in the body and normally weighs approximately 1.4 kg (3 pounds). The liver processes nearly every nutrient class absorbed from the GI tract. It is able to withstand and repair damage remarkably. Complete regeneration can take place even when 70% of the liver is destroyed. Cirrhosis is due to necrosis of the hepatic cells, leading to fibrosis of hepatic tissue, loss of hepatic architecture, and eventual loss of hepatic function.

The physiologic function of the liver can be divided into six categories:

1. Metabolism of carbohydrates, proteins and lipids, some hormones, and vitamins A, D, and K; conservation of iron salvaged from destruction of RBCs; regulation of temperature; major role in regulating plasma cholesterol

2. Excretion of bile salts and bile pigment, heavy metals, and dyes; conversion of ammonia into urea to be excreted
3. Phagocytic abilities of the Kupffer cells in removing specific pathogens; prevention of intravascular coagulation
4. Detoxification of drugs, endotoxins, alkaloids, steroids, alcohol, etc.
5. Storage of glycogen, vitamins, and iron; packaging fatty acids into forms for storage or transportation
6. Circulatory functions are systemic and portal transfer of blood, regulation of blood volume, and production of lymphatic fluid. Invasion of the liver by hepatotropic viruses yields a range of assorted syndromes, and the pattern or predictability of how host factors come into play is not well understood.

TRANSMISSION
- HAV infection is transmitted through the fecal-oral route. Incubation period is 2 to 6 weeks.
- HBV infection is transmitted through blood and body fluids. Incubation period is 6 weeks to 6 months.
- HCV infection is transmitted through blood and body fluids. Incubation period is 5 to 10 weeks.
- Hepatitis D viral infection is only present as a coinfection with HBV. Concurrent infection results in a more virulent manifestation than if individual had hepatitis B alone.
- Hepatitis E viral infection is transmitted through the fecal-oral route. Incubation period is 2 to 9 weeks.

FACTORS INCREASING SUSCEPTIBILITY. High-risk groups are as follows:

Hepatitis A. Persons at day care centers and institutions (such as those caring for mentally challenged individuals), individuals engaging in foreign travel

Hepatitis B. Users of intravenous drugs who share needles, homosexual men, individuals on hemodialysis, persons with hemophilia, health care personnel (such as nurses, laboratory personnel, surgeons, and personnel performing hemodialysis), and sexually promiscuous persons (the same high-risk groups for hepatitis D).

Hepatitis C. Individuals receiving frequent blood transfusions, male homosexuals and hospital personnel.

ASSESSMENT: SUBJECTIVE/HISTORY

NOTE: The subjective symptoms presented are ambiguous in nature and are related to an alteration in the normal function of the liver.

Symptoms
- *Hepatitis A:* Signs and symptoms appear at the end of prodromal period and include fatigue, weakness, and mild GI disturbances. A striking aversion to cigarettes may occur. Some may have joint pain, fever, hepatomegaly, lymphadenopathy, and jaundice.
- *Hepatitis B:* General malaise, joint swelling, rash pruritus, hepatomegaly, and GI symptoms are seen. Jaundice is seen with more nausea and vomiting.
- *Hepatitis C:* Acute illness with fever, chills, malaise, nausea, and vomiting
- Assess for presence of weight loss, cough, dyspnea, and history of yeast infections, which would be significant to help rule out HIV.
- Assess for history of menorrhagia in females or constipation in both genders; may help rule out hypothyroidism.

Past Medical History

The individual may remember the exposure to the viral agent; but past medical history may also be inconclusive in identifying how and where the individual was exposed.

Psychosocial History
- Significant for sexual practices, recreational use of drugs, or other habits or occupations that place the individual at risk for viral hepatitis infection
- For hepatitis A it is important to determine whether other contacts have demonstrated the same illness. With food contamination, events (such as weddings or other gatherings), school cafeterias, or any other common source should be identified.

ASSESSMENT: OBJECTIVE/ PHYSICAL EXAMINATION
Physical Examination
- A general skin examination should note jaundice, rashes (mononucleosis), dryness (hypothyroidism), or spider angiomas.
- Conduct a head, eyes, ears, nose, and throat ex-

amination to rule out mononucleosis. Oral lesions or lymphadenopathy may indicate HIV infection.

- Abdominal examination is imperative to assess liver size and tenderness, splenomegaly, and presence of ascites.
- A neurologic examination will help rule out thyroid dysfunction.
- Presence of occult blood loss should be evaluated with a stool specimen, optimally obtained by voluntary evacuation because there is a percentage of false-positive results with a digital rectal examination specimen.

Diagnostic Procedures

- Do Monospot test to rule out mononucleosis.
- Perform thyroid screen (thyroid-stimulating hormone, triiodothyronine, thyroxine) to rule out hypothyroidism. Thyroid-stimulating hormone will be elevated and free thyroxine will be low in hypothyroidism.
- Electrolytes, renal panel, and liver function tests are important because of the hepatic involvement. AST is maximally elevated in the acute phase of hepatitis (>1000 IU/L) then tapers off. Remember that AST and ALT levels do not always correlate with the degree of liver damage. Total and direct bilirubin will be elevated with hepatitis. Jaundice is usually detectable, with a total bilirubin level >2 mg/dl. Jaundice does not reflect the severity of the illness.
- Do HIV screen to rule out HIV infection.
- Liver biopsy will determine the extent of the disease but is not usually performed until the disease is believed to be chronic, as defined by clinical history of unresolved symptoms with AST and ALT elevations for 6 months or longer. This test does not provide useful prognostic value in the acute phase of hepatitis. CBC with differential provides information regarding anemia and possible infection. Lymphocytosis with >10% atypical cells is characteristic for Epstein-Barr, and leukopenia is common with HAV.
- CXR can be delayed until the serologic test results are known; however, if the history and physical examination strongly indicate a cytomegaloviral infection, a CXR would be useful. If cytomegaloviral infection is present, the x-ray may demonstrate bilateral, diffuse white infiltrates.

Table 4-4   Laboratory Interpretation of Hepatitis Tests

HBsAG	Anti-HBs	Anti-HBc	IgM	INTERPRETATION
+	−	−	−	Early acute HBV infection
+	−	+	+	Acute HBV infection
+	−	+	−	Chronic HBc carrier
−	−	+	−/+	Early convalescence, HBV
−	+	+	−	Recovery/immunity to HBV
−	+	−	−	Immunity to HBV infection

HBsAg, Hepatitis B surface antigen; *anti-HBs,* antibody to HBsAg; *anti-HBc,* antibody to hepatitis B core antigen; *IgM,* immunoglobulin M.

- Hepatitis screening will determine which viral infection is responsible for the illness and the stage of the infection (Table 4-4).

DIAGNOSIS

Differential diagnosis includes the following:
- Anemia
- Cytomegaloviral infection
- Epstein-Barr virus
- Viral infection
- Hepatitis
- Chronic fatigue syndrome
- Acquired hypothyroidism
- Depression

THERAPEUTIC PLAN

The main therapeutic plan will be to track the liver enzyme levels and closely observe symptoms.

Hepatitis A

HAV infection commonly requires no treatment. If an epidemic of HAV is noted in the community from a common source of food or water contamination, close contacts should be offered passive immunity with serum immunoglobulin (Gamastan, Gammar), 0.02 ml/kg IM. This vaccine is safe and inexpensive. Usually, casual contacts such as coworkers do not need to be vaccinated. Individuals expecting to be exposed to HAV (travelers, institutional workers, day care employees, military personnel, etc.) should receive an inactivated HAV vaccine (Havrix). Clients aged 2 to 18 years receive two IM injections of 360 enzyme-linked immunosorbent assay (ELISA) units (0.5 ml) given 1 month apart. Adults receive one dose of 1440 ELISA units. Both populations should receive a booster injection at 6 months.

Hepatitis B

HBV treatment consists of observation of liver enzymes and hepatitis markers to identify individuals who may benefit from interferon therapy. Interferon is used to eradicate viral replication and end chronic hepatitis infection. Common side effects of interferon are flulike symptoms, especially at initiation of treatment, which tend to decrease with continued therapy. The flulike symptoms can be minimized by keeping the client well hydrated and administering the dose at bedtime. Acetaminophen 30 minutes before the interferon dose may also help.

Immunoprophylaxis for HBV can be achieved by both passive (high-titered antibody to hepatitis B surface antigen [anti-HBs] immunoglobulin [HBIG]) and active immunization (HBV vaccine; Recombivax HB, Engerix-B). Prophylaxis before exposure consists of three deltoid IM injections of HBV vaccine at 0, 1, and 6 months. Dosage depends on the formulation of the vaccine. Immunocompromised individuals should receive a higher dose.

Prophylaxis for unvaccinated individuals exposed to HBV should be with both HBIG and HBV vaccine. Adult dosage of HBIG is 0.06 ml/kg IM, followed by a complete course of HBV vaccine. Another dose of HBIG can be repeated 1 month later. This is the same protocol used for infants born to hepatitis B surface antigen (HBsAg)–seropositive mothers or for sexual contacts of persons seropositive for HBsAg.

When the previously vaccinated individual is exposed to HBsAg-positive blood or body fluids, serum anti-HBs titers should be obtained. If the antibody level is less than 10 mIU/ml, the individual should be treated the same as an unvaccinated person.

Hepatitis C

HCV exposure prophylaxis of serum immunoglobulin is used but has no proven effec-

tiveness. One regimen is two IM injections of 0.06 ml/kg within the first 2 weeks of exposure.

Client Education

RELATED TO HEPATITIS A
- Transmitted through fecal-oral route
- Usually a 6-week course of illness with a high recovery rate
- No carrier state; no chronic state
- Immunoglobulin (Ig)M–anti-HAV assay is diagnostic for HAV infection. It is usually detectable at the time of clinical presentation and persists for several months.
- Detectable serum IgG–anti-HAV confirms HAV immunity.
- Preventive measures include handwashing. Pooled human immune serum globulin (0.02 mg/kg IM) is effective only when administered within 2 weeks of the exposure.
- Fulminant hepatitis A is infrequent; however, when it does occur, it has a 50% mortality rate.

RELATED TO HEPATITIS B
- Detectable in blood, breast milk, saliva, tears, nasal secretions, menstrual fluid, urine, semen, and blood-sucking insects that have bitten infected individuals
- Appears in blood as a virion called the *Dane particle*
- HBV may occasionally exist in a quiescent nonhepatotoxic state (chronic carrier state)
- Hepatitis B e antigen (HBeAg) is present when the liver is making large quantities of hepatitis B core antigen (HBcAg) during viral replication. When HBeAg is present for longer than 3 to 4 months, a chronic HBV state is likely. HBeAg is used to manage the client in the chronic state and signifies ongoing viral replication and liver damage. Antibody to HBeAg is associated with resolution of the infection.
- Chronic HBV exists when transaminases remain elevated for 6 months or longer. It may be transient and spontaneously resolve. Occasionally it progresses to an active ongoing hepatocellular necrosis (chronic active hepatitis) and eventually cirrhosis, with a dramatically increased risk for hepatocellular carcinoma (hepatoma).
- HBV is responsible for almost 80% of the primary cases of hepatoma worldwide.

- Icteric phase lasts 2 to 6 weeks; peaks in 14 days with a variable period of disappearance.
- Prompt administration of HBIG and HBV vaccine to neonates is highly effective in prevention of vertical transmission of HBV. This protocol is also recommended for accidental needle sticks or splashes.

Related to Hepatitis C

- Seroconversion may not occur for as long as 6 months.
- Half of the individuals who acquire posttransfusion HCV will have chronic hepatitis develop, with potential for cirrhosis.

Related to Hepatitis D (Delta)

- Hepatitis D virus only causes infection in coinfection with HBV.
- It is clinically important because it is associated with a higher rate of fulminant hepatitis and a high fatality rate. There is also a substantially higher risk for development of chronic hepatitis B liver disease.
- Hepatitis D viral superinfection usually correlates to a more severe and rapid progression of HBV infection.
- Serum anti–hepatitis D virus proteins are diagnostic for hepatitis D virus infection.

Related to Impact on Family

- The family impact of any infectious disease is worrisome at the least, and people are guilt ridden if the disease is inadvertently passed on to their loved ones. Support is needed throughout the course of the workup, diagnosis, and treatment.
- Safe sexual practices should be reviewed because hepatitis B, C, and D are sexually transmitted. Condom use should be encouraged.
- Resources include the American Liver Foundation Hepatitis/Liver Disease Hotline for printed material and reference to the nearest support group (1-800-223-0179). The local health department is a good resource as well.
- Fatigue is a common symptom of hepatitis, and the client should be educated about appropriate behavioral management. Assist the client in assessing the home and work situations to identify where energy can be conserved. Give permission to ask for assistance and to take the needed rest breaks.

Referral

If the liver function test results remain elevated or progressively elevate, the client should be referred to a gastroenterologist for a possible liver biopsy to assess the extent of hepatic damage.

EVALUATION/FOLLOW-UP

Follow-up should be on a monthly basis to assess disease progression. If the client has an increase in severity of symptoms, the follow-up will be more frequent. Blood work should be done every 2 months, more frequently if the symptoms worsen.

REFERENCES

Groer, M., & Shekleton, M. (1979). Disorders of digestions, absorption, excretion, and metabolism. In M. Groer & M. Shekleton (Eds), *Basic pathophysiology: A conceptual approach*. St. Louis: Mosby, 344-376.

Norris, J. (1992). Infection. In E. McMahon, M. Ambrose, & D. Deutsch (Eds), *Diseases* (pp. 209-211). Philadelphia: Springhouse.

Norris, J. (1993). Gastrointestinal disorders. In J. Norris, et al. (Eds), *Diseases*. Springhouse, PA: Springhouse.

Shulman, S. (1992). Viral hepatitis. In S. Shulman, J. Phair, & H. Sommers (Eds.), *The biologic and clinical basis of infectious diseases.* (pp. 312-326). Philadelphia: W. B. Saunders.

Uphold, C., & Graham, M. (1994). *Clinical guidelines in family practice* (2nd ed.). Gainesville, FL: Barmarrae Books.

Zeldis, J. B., & Friedman, L. S. (1997). Acute and chronic viral hepatitis. In R. E. Rakel (Ed.), *Conn's current therapy* (pp. 488-495). Philadelphia: W. B. Saunders.

REVIEW QUESTIONS

Situation: *Rose is a 36-year-old female who has had a history of tiring easily for 2 months. She is able to work all day as a secretary but needs to rest as soon as she gets home. She has no energy left for family activities and her libido is low.*

1. Which of the following findings rules out chronic fatigue syndrome?

  a. The fact that Rose is female
  b. Her age
  c. Unknown etiology with 2-month duration
  d. Fatigue resolution with bed rest

2. Which of the following diagnostic tests will best assist you in narrowing your diagnosis for Rose?

    a. Liver enzymes, liver biopsy, HIV
    b. HIV, liver enzymes, CXR
    c. CBC, CXR, liver enzymes
    d. Liver enzymes, HIV, Monospot

3. With the history, you have narrowed the diagnosis down to one of the hepatitis infections. Rose's laboratory results are as follows: hemoglobin 15.6, hematocrit 43.1, WBCs 7.4 cells/mm^3, AST 60 IU/L, ALT 121 IU/L, alkaline phosphatase within normal limits, total bilirubin 2 mg/dl, anti-HBs negative, HBsAg positive, and HBcAg positive. Your diagnosis is:

    a. Acute hepatitis B infection, resolving
    b. Acute hepatitis C infection
    c. Chronic hepatitis B infection
    d. Acute hepatitis A infection

4. Elmer has a diagnosis of hepatitis C. His level of function has not changed in the past 6 months. Although he has been able to carry out activities of daily living, his AST and ALT levels have remained elevated. Your next best interaction would be which of the following?

    a. Monitor Elmer for 6 more months; monitor his disease progress for 2 more months.
    b. Initiate interferon therapy and prophylactically medicate him before therapy.
    c. Refer Elmer to a gastroenterologist for a liver biopsy.
    d. Advise Elmer that the disease continues to destroy hepatic cells and that there is nothing else to be done.

5. Mary is a nurse who just stuck herself with an HBV contaminated needle. She has received her full course of HBV vaccine but does not know her titers. Mary washes the puncture with copious amounts of soap and water. She asks you what else needs to be done. What is your response?

    a. Mary needs to have a booster of HBV vaccine.
    b. Mary needs to have a titer level drawn, and if it is <10 mIU/ml, she should receive a regimen of HBIG and HBV vaccine.
    c. Mary should receive a dose of HBIG.
    d. Mary should receive no further treatment because she received the full course of HBV vaccine.

6. As a nurse practitioner, your role in caring for Rose, a 36-year-old woman (described in question 1), would include all the following **except:**

    a. Referral to a gastroenterologist as soon as possible for a liver biopsy
    b. Education related to the disease process and possible treatment options
    c. Following Rose's progress on a periodic basis to determine disease progression
    d. Assistance in identifying resources and offering support in notifying spouse

7. All the following are true about hepatitis A viral infection **except:**

    a. Found in infected food, it often runs its course without diagnosis.
    b. It has a chronic carrier state.
    c. It is common in crowded situations.
    d. IgM antibody (anti-HAV) denotes active infection.

8. Which of the following statements about hepatitis B viral infections is **false?**

    a. It is considered a sexually transmitted disease.
    b. At-risk groups are homosexual men, health care workers, and IV drug users sharing needles.
    c. It is associated with hepatitis D viral infection.
    d. It is treated with interferon on diagnosis.

9. Hepatitis infections associated with chronic carrier states are:

    a. HAV and HBV
    b. HBV only
    c. HBV and HCV
    d. HCV only

ANSWERS AND RATIONALES

1. *Answer:* d (assessment/history/gastrointestinal/NAS)

    Rationale: One of the defining characteristics of chronic fatigue syndrome is fatigue unresolved with rest. (Norris, 1992)

2. *Answer:* d (diagnosis/gastrointestinal/NAS)

    Rationale: Liver biopsy is inappropriate as a workup test. CXR will not be useful in narrowing down a diagnosis, and the only answer that has useful tests is *d.* (Groer & Shekleton, 1979; Shulman, 1992)

3. *Answer:* a (diagnosis/gastrointestinal/NAS)

Rationale: On the basis of HBsAg and HBcAg, the diagnosis has to be narrowed to HBV infection. Anti-HBs would have to be present for it to be a chronic infection, so this is therefore an acute hepatitis B infection. (Groer & Shekleton, 1979; Shulman, 1992)

4. *Answer:* c (evaluation/gastrointestinal/NAS)

Rationale: Six-month duration is the definition of chronic hepatitis infection. Elmer should be evaluated by a gastroenterologist who can conduct a liver biopsy. Initiating interferon therapy is premature, and there is no foundation to tell him that the disease is continuing to destroy liver cells. (Groer & Shekleton, 1979; Shulman, 1992)

5. *Answer:* b (plan/gastrointestinal/adult)

Rationale: If titer is low, the person is treated as though he or she has not received vaccine. (Groer & Shekleton, 1979; Shulman, 1992)

6. *Answer:* a (plan/gastrointestinal/adult)

Rationale: Liver biopsy is not appropriate in the acute stage. Education and assistance in identifying resources and offering support is always a correct approach, as is periodic assessment to determine progression. (Groer & Shekleton, 1979; Norris, 1992; Shulman, 1992)

7. *Answer:* b (diagnosis/gastrointestinal/NAS)

Rationale: HAV is never a chronic infection. IgM denotes active (it has *me*) whereas IgG (it's *gone*) denotes recovery and immunity stages. (Groer & Shekleton, 1979; Shulman, 1992)

8. *Answer:* d (diagnosis/gastrointestinal/NAS)

Rationale: Treatment is observation for as long as you can, and interferon treatment is not entered readily. All the other choices are true concerning HBV. (Groer & Shekleton, 1979; Shulman, 1992)

9. *Answer:* c (plan/gastrointestinal/NAS)

Rationale: Hepatitis A never has a chronic carrier state, whereas HBV and HCV do. (Groer & Shekleton, 1979; Shulman, 1992)

IRRITABLE BOWEL SYNDROME

OVERVIEW
Definition

IBS is a functional disturbance of intestinal mobility characterized by both diarrhea and constipation, (constipation is predominant), bloating, and abdominal and rectal pain. There is a high correlation between emotional factors and signs and symptoms. IBS sometimes is referred to as *mucous colitis, spastic bowel,* or *spastic colitis.* Care should be taken to differentiate IBS from diverticular disease. IBS often becomes chronic, with varying symptoms.

Incidence

Estimated incidence between 15% and 20% of the adult population. IBS is uncommon in children and teenagers. The syndrome is predominant in ages 20 to 35 years. In the United States, females are twice as likely as males to have IBS, whereas men are more frequently afflicted in other parts of the world. Because of the concern for organic disease, IBS accounts for 50% of the referrals to gastroenterologists. Comprehensive care emphasizing client-provider relationships is critical to the management of this syndrome.

Pathophysiology

It is believed that IBS is a functional disturbance in motor activity and visceral perception of the bowel. Triggers include psychologic factors and luminal irritants. Motor activity abnormalities (decreased or excessive contractility) account for the diarrhea and constipation. Excessive sensitivity of the viscera may explain the abdominal and rectal pain caused by pressure of stool or bloating.

FACTORS INCREASING SYMPTOMS. Individuals with persistent symptoms have been found to have a greater prevalence of situational stress, which is thought to modify the underlying pathophysiology and influence the severity of symptoms. Intraluminal factors that cause bloating and diarrhea include lactose (in dairy products), fructose (in citrus fruits), and sorbitol (often found in "sugar-free" candies and gum). There is no detectable pathology.

RISK FACTORS
- Other family members with IBS or other GI disorders
- History of sexual abuse in child
- Sexual or domestic abuse in women

ASSESSMENT: SUBJECTIVE/HISTORY
History of Present Illness
- Continuous or recurrent symptoms for at least 3 months
- Abdominal pain and cramps, often relieved by bowel movement
- Diarrhea or constipation, or alternating between both (note frequency and consistency of stool)
- Abdominal pain may be in left lower quadrant.
- Diet (note whether milk products, citrus fruit, and sugar-free products with sorbitol make symptoms worse)
- No change in appetite
- Mucus in stool; no blood in stool
- Bloating and distention, often flatulence, especially after meals
- Stressful life events exacerbate symptoms.
- Client may be depressed (loss of appetite, lack of energy, poor concentration, insomnia, etc.).
- Determine whether there has been weight loss (should not occur with IBS).
- No temperature elevations
- Urinary frequency
- Note travel, camping history (or any possibility of drinking contaminated water)

Past Medical History
- Client may "physician hop" because of unrelieved symptoms or lack of "cure."
- Note any previous episodes with similar clinical course.
- Any chronic disease, any food or drug allergies
- Family history of IBS or other GI problems
- Ask about sexual or domestic abuse (past or current). Sensitive information may not be revealed until client feels trust for provider.

Psychosocial History
- Stress level and how it is managed
- Past or current counseling

Medication History
Note all medications currently being taken (prescription, OTC, vitamins, or herbal therapies), including use of laxatives or enemas.

ASSESSMENT: OBJECTIVE/ PHYSICAL EXAMINATION
Physical Examination
- A problem-oriented physical examination should include vital signs, height, and weight.
- *Abdomen:* Assess for bowel sounds, distention, pain, organomegaly.
- *Rectal:* Assess for tenderness, masses, stool for occult blood.
- Schedule a comprehensive examination to rule out other pathologies.

Diagnostic Procedures
- CBC with differential and sedimentation rate (to rule out anemia, infection, and inflammatory causes)
- Chemistry panel (to identify any other pathology, such as diabetes, abnormal liver function). Elevated magnesium may indicate diuretic or laxative abuse.
- Stool (guaiac, usually six times), maybe ova and parasites (usually three times) or culture (to rule out bowel symptoms caused by other pathologies, malignancy, bacterial infections, or parasites)
- *Procedures:* If indicated, obtain abdominal x-ray (flat-plate and upright). If symptoms are severe (excessive bloating pain, rule out obstruction), procedures include barium enema, abdominal ultrasonography or flexible sigmoidoscopy, and possible colonoscopy (to rule out diverticular disease, inflammatory bowel disease, or malignancy).

DIAGNOSIS
Consider IBS if abdominal pain is recurrent or continuous for 2 to 3 months, pain is relieved with defecation, and bowel changes such as diarrhea or constipation are seen. The diagnosis is made by careful history and the absence of clinical findings. Caution is in order not to overutilize medical services (see previous diagnostic procedures).

Differential diagnosis includes the following:
- Inflammatory bowel disease (ulcerative colitis, Crohn's disease)
- Lactose intolerance
- Diverticulosis
- Chronic appendicitis
- Malignancy
- Diabetes (may be seen as diarrhea)
- Obstruction
- Parasites (giardiasis)
- Psychologic pathology

THERAPEUTIC PLAN
Pharmacologic Treatment
- Bulk-producing agents such as psyllium (Metamucil) bid or tid, 1 tablespoon (helps with constipation and diarrhea)
- Loperamide (Imodium) 2 mg PO or dephenoxylate (Lomotil) 2.5 to 5.0 mg after each unformed stool
- Antispasmodics and anticholinergics such as dicyclomine (Bentyl, Levsin), 10 to 20 mg bid to qid with meals, for postprandial cramping
- Lactaid, 1 to 3 caplets with meals, for lactose intolerance
- Relieve bloating and flatulence with simethicone (Mylicon), 80 mg, with meals and at bedtime.
- Consider anticholinergic agent amitriptyline (Elavil) 50 to 100 mg at bedtime for depressed clients with diarrhea. Use fluoxetine (Prozac) 20 mg/day, for depressed clients with constipation.

Client Education
GENERAL INTERVENTIONS
- Heat to abdomen may help (contraindicated if suspected inflammation such as appendicitis or diverticulitis).
- Biofeedback may help.
- Stress reduction
- Avoid straining with bowel movements and respond promptly to urges to defecate.
- Teach the need for patience and tolerance to work out what will work best for the client. Validate client's symptoms.

Diet
- Increase fiber intake.
- Avoid intraluminal factors (lactose, fructose, and sorbitol) in foods (milk products, citrus fruits and juices, and sugar-free candies and gums) if they increase symptoms.
- Avoid large meals and spicy and fatty foods.
- Increase fluid intake (water) to 2000 ml/day.
- A food diary may be needed.

Exercise
Encourage 20 to 45 minutes of walking at least four or five times a week.

Referral
- For uncontrolled IBS, refer to primary care physician or gastroenterologist.
- For psychopathology (anxiety, depression, posttraumatic stress disorder) refer for counseling and stress relief.
- Nutrition counseling
- Self-help and support groups

Consultation
- Newly diagnosed
- Worsening IBS

EVALUATION/FOLLOW-UP
- Initial follow-up is done in 1 to 2 weeks to assess improvement.
- Every 1 to 3 months, adjust follow-up on the basis of recurring signs and symptoms.
- Consider more frequent visits or develop support group to establish client-provider relationship.

REFERENCES
Bonis, P., & Norton, R. (1996). The challenge of irritable bowel syndrome. *American Family Physician, 53*(3), 1229-1239.
Cerda, J., Drossman, D., & Scherl, E. (1996). Effective, compassionate management of IBS. *Patient Care, 30*(1), 131-142.
Dalton, C. B., & Drossman, D. A. (1997). Diagnosis and treatment of irritable bowel syndrome. *American Family Physician, 55*(3), 875-880.
Goroll, A., May, L., & Mulley, A. (Eds.). (1995). *Primary care medicine: Office evaluation and management of the adult patient.* Philadelphia: J. B. Lippincott.

Hancock, L., & Selig, P. (1994). Irritable bowel disease. In E. Youngkin & M. Davis (Eds.), *Women's health: A primary care clinical guide* (pp. 609-611). Norwalk, CT: Appleton & Lange.

Hurst, J. W. (1996). *Medicine for the practicing physician.* Norwalk, CT: Appleton & Lange.

Isselbacher, K., Braunwald, E., Wilson, J., Martin, J., Fauci, A., & Kasper, D. (1994). *Harrison's principles of internal medicine* (13th ed.). New York: McGraw Hill.

Johnson, T. R., & Apgar, B. (1995). Irritable bowel syndrome. *The Female Patient, 20,* 48-58.

Lonergan, E. (Ed.). (1996). *Geriatrics: A clinical manual.* Norwalk, CT: Appleton & Lange.

Rakel, R. (Ed.). (1995). *Textbook of family practice* (5th ed.). Philadelphia: W. B. Saunders.

Uphold, C., & Graham, M. (1994). *Clinical guidelines in family practice* (2nd ed.). Gainesville, FL: Barmarrae Books.

REVIEW QUESTIONS

1. Which of the following symptoms are most indicative of IBS?

   a. Fever, nausea, and diarrhea for 10 days

   b. Right lower quadrant abdominal pain with fever

   c. Left lower quadrant abdominal pain with bloody diarrheal stools

   d. Intermittent abdominal pain with diarrhea for 3 months

2. Which of the following findings would most likely be observed in a client with IBS?

   a. No detectable pathology, generalized abdominal pain

   b. Elevated sedimentation rate

   c. Splenomegaly

   d. Positive guaiac test result

Situation: *M.J. is a 28-year-old woman with a history of rape 6 months ago. She seeks treatment with vague symptoms of abdominal pain and bloating after meals for the past 3 months. Her abdominal pain is relieved by a bowel movement. She denies diarrhea or constipation. (Questions 3 through 5)*

3. Which of the following diagnoses is most appropriate for this woman?

   a. Posttraumatic stress disorder

   b. Probable IBS

   c. Probable peptic ulcer

   d. Early stages of ulcerative colitis

4. The client states that the symptom that is causing her the most problems is bloating. Which of the following pharmaceutic agents is likely to be most therapeutic?

   a. Bentyl

   b. Imodium

   c. Simethicone

   d. Prozac

5. M.J.'s symptoms of abdominal pain are getting worse despite treatment with simethicone for the past 6 weeks. Constipation is an occasional problem. Which of the following is the most appropriate plan of action for you to take?

   a. Consult with primary care physician.

   b. Refer to gastroenterologist after colonoscopy.

   c. Refer to counseling.

   d. Reassure client and have her return in 6 weeks.

6. What would you do for an individual with "cramping" after meals associated with IBS?

   a. Elavil, 50 mg at bedtime

   b. Bentyl, 10 mg qid with meals

   c. Simethicone, 80 mg with meals and at bedtime

   d. Metamucil, bid

7. For clients with IBS, it is important to teach which of the following?

   a. Respond to urges to defecate immediately.

   b. Avoid exercises such as walking.

   c. Eat large meals to create bulk.

   d. Avoid alcohol.

8. Which of the following tests used during a workup for IBS is most expensive?

   a. Stool hematocrit

   b. Echocardiogram

   c. Colonoscopy

   d. Flat-plate and upright abdominal x-ray

9. What past medical history is most relevant to ask someone with suspected IBS?

   a. Tuberculosis exposure

   b. Immunization

   c. Surgeries

   d. Previous episodes

ANSWERS AND RATIONALES

1. *Answer:* d (assessment/history/gastrointestinal/NAS)

Rationale: Fever, bloody stools, nausea, right lower quadrant pain, and diarrhea for short durations are more like an inflammatory or infectious condition, such as appendicitis. Criteria for diagnosis of IBS include continuous or recurrent abdominal pain and a change in bowel habits (diarrhea, constipation, or both) for a 2- to 3-month period. (Dalton & Drossman, 1997; Goroll, May, & Mulley, 1995; Hurst, 1996; Rakel, 1995; Uphold & Graham, 1994)

2. *Answer:* a (assessment/physical examination/gastrointestinal/NAS)

Rationale: IBS features symptoms of abdominal pain and altered bowel habits with no detectable pathology. Elevated sedimentation rates, splenomegaly, and a positive guaiac result are indicative of infection or inflammatory disorders or of a malignancy, which requires further follow-up. (Cerda, Drossman, & Scherl, 1996; Dalton & Drossman, 1997; Goroll, May, & Mulley, 1995; Hurst, 1996)

3. *Answer:* b (diagnosis/gastrointestinal/adult)

Rationale: This individual fits the profile of persons vulnerable to IBS: female, age 28 years, and previous experience with sexual violence. Her symptoms are typical of IBS, more so than of any other listed diagnoses. Additional information would be required to rule out the other diagnoses listed. (Dalton & Drossman, 1997; Goroll, May, & Mulley, 1995; Hurst, 1996; Rakel, 1995; Uphold & Graham, 1994)

4. *Answer:* c (plan/management/therapeutics/pharmacology/gastrointestinal/NAS)

Rationale: Simethicone is an antiflatulent, which will help with symptoms of bloating. Bentyl is an antispasmodic, Imodium is a constipating agent, and Prozac is given for individuals with depression who have constipation. (Cerda, Drossman, & Scherl, 1996; Goroll, May, & Mulley, 1995; Hurst, 1996; Uphold & Graham, 1994)

5. *Answer:* a (evaluation/gastrointestinal/NAS)

Rationale: M.J.'s circumstances are getting worse, so a consultation with a primary care physician would be in order. Colonoscopy is expensive, and given the symptoms and history it would not be justified at this time. Counseling may be a relevant referral, but the client's priority is management of symptoms. Reassuring the client and returning in 6 weeks or sending her to counseling while she still has pain is not appropriate at this time.

6. *Answer:* b (plan/management/therapeutics/pharmacology/gastrointestinal/NAS)

Rationale: Bentyl is an antispasmodic and anticholinergic agent suitable for relief of postprandial cramping. Elavil is an anticholinergic agent used at night for depressed clients with diarrhea. Simethicone is an antiflatulent agent, and Metamucil is a bulk-producing agent. (Goroll, May, & Mulley, 1995; Hurst, 1996; Uphold & Graham, 1994)

7. *Answer:* a (plan/management/client education/gastrointestinal/NAS)

Rationale: It is important to promote bowel habits that will minimize problems associated with constipation and to promote normal bowel function, so responding promptly to urges to defecate is important. Exercise (such as walking) should be encouraged for general health, and it is not contraindicated. Alcohol (if tolerated) is not contraindicated in moderation. Small meals rather than large meals are encouraged. (Goroll, May, & Mulley, 1995; Hurst, 1996; Uphold & Graham, 1994)

8. *Answer:* c (plan/management/diagnostics/gastrointestinal/NAS)

Rationale: Colonoscopy is most expensive. It may be used to rule out diverticular disease, inflammatory bowel disease, or malignancy. Stool Hemoccult is the least expensive. An x-ray is moderately expensive. Echocardiograms are expensive and are not part of an IBS workup. (Goroll, May, & Mulley, 1995; Hurst, 1996; Uphold & Graham, 1994)

9. *Answer:* d (assessment/history/gastrointestinal/NAS)

Rationale: Clients may "doctor hop" because of lack of cure. Previous episodes with similar clinical courses are an important piece of information with respect to a diagnosis of IBS. Tuberculosis exposure, surgeries, and immunization are important to know for any client, regardless of the diagnosis. (Goroll, May, & Mulley, 1995; Hurst, 1996; Uphold & Graham, 1994)

PEPTIC ULCER DISEASE

OVERVIEW
Definition

Pepti ulcer disease is defined as an ulcer, a sore, or a lesion that forms in the lining of the stomach or duodenum where acid and pepsin are present.

DUODENAL ULCERS. These affect the proximal part of the small intestine. They follow a chronic course characterized by remissions and exacerbations.

GASTRIC ULCERS. These affect the stomach mucosa. They are most common in middle-aged and elderly men, especially among the poor and undernourished, and in chronic users of aspirin, alcohol, or NSAIDs.

Incidence

Approximately 20 million Americans have at least one ulcer develop during their lifetimes. Ulcers are rare in teenagers and even more uncommon in children. Duodenal ulcers usually occur for the first time between the ages of 30 and 50 years, and they occur more frequently in men than in women. Of all ulcers, approximately 80% are duodenal and 20% are gastric. Approximately 5% of all gastric ulcers are malignant. Each year ulcers affect about 4 million people. More than 40,000 people anually undergo surgery because of persistent symptoms or problems from ulcers; about 6000 people die of ulcer-related complications.

Pathophysiology

PROTECTIVE FACTORS. The stomach's natural defenses include:
- *Mucous production:* Lubricant-like coating shields stomach tissues.
- *Bicarbonate production:* Bicarbonate neutralizes and breaks down digestive fluids.
- *Good blood supply:* This increases cell renewal and repair.

FACTORS INCREASING SUSCEPTIBILITY
- Bacterial virulence
- Physiologic stress: Surgical procedures, severe trauma, burns, shock
- Medications: Corticosteroids, NSAIDs
- Gender and age: Male age 30 to 50 years, female age older than 60 years
- Familial predisposition

- Physiologic incompetences: Bile reflux from incompetent pyloric sphincter, delayed or abnormal gastric emptying

COMMON PATHOGENS. The common etiologic source is *Helicobacter pylori.*

ASSESSMENT: SUBJECTIVE/HISTORY
Most Common Symptoms

DUODENAL ULCERS. Intermittent epigastric pain (gnawing or burning, heartburn) often occurs between meals and in the early hours of the morning and may awaken the client at night. Nausea, vomiting, loss of appetite; fatigue and weakness; tarry stools; dyspepsia

GASTRIC ULCERS. Pain is often aggravated or triggered by food; weight loss. Older adults may be free of symptoms until disease has advanced (GI bleeding, pancreatitis).

Associated Symptoms
- Chest pain
- Diarrhea

Past Medical History
- Obtain a clear statement of the chief complaint.
- Ask about the manifestation of pain, noting the location, intensity, whether the pain radiates and is relieved or aggravated by food, and measures taken to alleviate pain, including OTC medications.
- Explore GI symptoms of nausea, vomiting, changes in bowel habits, dysphagia, weight loss or gain, change in appetite, heartburn, and acid taste in mouth.
- Past history of ulcer disease, previous upper GI or endoscopies done
- Ask about other symptoms, such as history of testicular atrophy, gynecomastia, and alopecia (may be indicative of hepatic cirrhosis).
- Blood type: Type O has been associated with the adherence of *H. pylori.*
- Allergies
- Older adults: Ask about excessive belching, bloating, flatulence, nausea and vomiting, diarrhea, rectal bleeding, number of bowel movements per day, and dietary history.

Medication History

Inquire about NSAIDs and other medications.

Family History

Ask about family history of polyps, GI cancers, alcohol consumption, smoking, and psychologic disorders.

Psychosocial History

- Habits: Alcohol, smoking, tobacco juice, swallowing tobacco juice
- Older adults: Consider losses and role changes in the past year. May need to ask about death of loved ones, retirement, changes in living situations.

Dietary History

- Ask about the consumption of caffeine and foods that increase or relieve the symptoms
- Ask about patterns of consumption and elimination.
- Older adults: Ask the client to record diet for 3 days; this will give a more accurate pattern.

ASSESSMENT: OBJECTIVE/ PHYSICAL EXAMINATION

Physical Examination

A problem-oriented physical examination should be conducted with particular attention to the following:

- Vital signs, weight, general appearance, hydration status (including turgor and orthostatic changes)
- Cardiovascular: Rule out cardiac insufficiency.
- Abdomen: Do complete examination; especially note areas of tenderness, bruits, hums, or rubs. Note size of organs, costovertebral angle tenderness.
- Genital and rectal: Examine external genitalia for atrophy, perform digital rectal examination.

Diagnostic Procedures

- *H. pylori:* All clients with a new ulcer should be tested for *H. pylori* if they are in a high-risk category. *H. Pylori* test is for antibodies, so titer will remain positive for life.
- Upper GI series: This will detect 90% of peptic ulcers.

- CBC: Check for anemia.
- Hemoccult
- Albumin and renal: Tests are useful if signs of nutritional deficit is present.
- Endoscopy is becoming the test of choice because it is more sensitive; ulcers can be diagnosed photographically and tissue can be taken for biopsy at the time of the procedure.
- Indicate whether clinical symptoms persist despite negative results of barium studies. Rule out malignancy of gastric ulcers; locate bleeding site in those with diagnosed or suspected blood loss.

DIAGNOSIS

Differential diagnosis includes the following:
- Gastric cancer
- Angina
- Depression with somatic complaints
- Cholecystitis
- Pancreatitis
- GERD

THERAPEUTIC PLAN

The goal is to relieve the pain, aid healing, prevent recurrence, and prevent complications.

Nonpharmacologic Treatment

- Smoking cessation
- Discontinue the use of NSAIDs.
- Discontinue or decrease the consumption of alcohol and caffeine.
- Stress management

Pharmacologic Treatment

Treatment is based on the presence of *H. pylori*.

H. PYLORI NEGATIVE
- Antacids reduce total acid load for less than 1 hour; administer 1 hour after meals.
- Coating agents
- H_2-receptor antagonists

H. PYLORI POSITIVE. Most effective therapy is 2-week triple therapy with metronidazole (Flagyl), tetracycline, or amoxicillin and bismuth subsalicylate (Pepto-Bismol); may consider adding an acid-suppressing drug such as omeprazole (Prilosec). Multiple combinations of therapy are now available.

NSAID-INDUCED ULCERS. Misoprostol (Cytotec).

NEW FOOD AND DRUG ADMINISTRATION–APPROVED DRUGS

- Tritect (ranitidine-bismuth-citrate combination), to be coprescribed with clarithromycin
- Helidac (combines bismuth subsalicylate, metronidazole, and tetracycline hydrochloride), designed to eradicate *H. pylori* and can be coprescribed with an H_2-receptor antagonist to heal existing ulcers

Client Education

- Disease process, expected outcomes, and possible complications
- There is no specific diet; avoid irritating foods.
- Decrease caffeine intake.
- Use stress reduction techniques.
- Stop smoking.
- Medications, especially NSAIDs

Referral

- Failure to respond to treatment
- Significant weight loss
- Symptoms of peritonitis (abdominal rigidity, rebound tenderness, fever)
- Suspected gastric ulcers

EVALUATION/FOLLOW-UP

Follow up within 2 to 4 weeks of initial visit and every 6 to 8 weeks thereafter until condition is stable.

REFERENCES

Cornell, S. (1997). New treatments for peptic ulcer disease. *Advance for Nurse Practitioners, 5*(3), 57-59.

Cryer, B., & Feldman, M. (1995). Treatment and prevention of NSAID-induced ulcers. *Federal Practitioner, December,* 22-37.

Goroll, A. H., et al. (1995) *Primary care medicine* (3rd ed., pp. 309-443). Philadelphia: J. B. Lippincott.

Hogstel, M. O., & Keen-Payne, R. (1993). *Practical guide to health assessment: Through the lifespan.* Philadelphia: F. A. Davis.

Johnson, D. A. (1996). New dimensions in *Helicobacter pylori* infection. *Emergency Medicine, 28*(2), 74-85.

Loeb, S. (1993). *Diseases: Causes and complications—Assessments, findings, nursing diagnoses, and interventions.* Springhouse, PA: Springhouse.

Millonig, V. (1994). *Adult nurse practitioner certification review guide* (2nd ed.). Potomac, MD: Health Leadersh Association.

National Institutes of Health (1995). *Stomach and duodenal ulcers* (NIH publication no. 95-38). Bethesda, MD: National Digestive Diseases Information Clearinghouse.

Salerno, M. (1994). Gastrointestinal disorders. In V. L. Millonig (Ed.), *Adult nurse practitioner certification review guide* (pp. 240-250). Potomac, MD: Health Leadership Associates.

Van Schaik, T. (Ed). (1993). *Gastroenterology nursing: A core curriculum.* St. Louis: Mosby.

REVIEW QUESTIONS

1. Mr. T., a 55-year-old white man, seeks treatment with a sharp left upper quadrant abdominal pain associated with nausea and vomiting. The pain seems to come on as a sharp spasm or cramping discomfort, which turns into a burning sensation that goes to the chest. The pain sometimes awakens him at night. He reports that he has taken Mylanta for 7 years for indigestion. Which of the following would most likely be the cause of Mr. T.'s pain?

  a. Diverticulitis
  b. Pancreatitis
  c. Peptic ulcer disease
  d. Coronary artery insufficiency

2. Your next step would be which of the following?

  a. Give sublingual nitroglycerin to relieve the associated chest pain.
  b. Change his antacid.
  c. Obtain additional medical history data.
  d. Check his vital signs.

3. The fact that Mr. T.'s pain is not associated with activity and awakens him at night makes it less likely that his problem is:

  a. Coronary artery insufficiency
  b. Peptic ulcer disease
  c. Pancreatitis
  d. Diverticulitis

4. The most commonly used test that detects 90% of peptic ulcers is:

  a. Flat plate radiograph of abdomen
  b. Upper GI series
  c. Stool Hemoccult
  d. Bernstein acid perfusion

5. All the following are reasons for endoscopy **except:**

   a. Clinical symptoms persist despite negative barium studies.
   b. Rule out malignancy.
   c. Locate site in those with diagnosed or suspected blood loss.
   d. History of NSAID use.

6. About 80% of all peptic ulcers occur in the:

   a. Stomach
   b. Duodenum
   c. Ileum
   d. Jejunum

7. Predisposing factors for duodenal ulcers include all the following **except:**

   a. Genetic factors
   b. Bacterial virulence
   c. Constipation
   d. Medications (NSAIDs, corticosteroids)

8. For optimal effect, antacids should be given:

   a. 1 hour before meals
   b. 1 hour after meals
   c. Immediately after meals
   d. Immediately before meals

9. The most effective therapy for a client who is *H. pylori* positive is:

   a. 2 weeks with metronidazole (Flagyl), tetracycline, and bismuth subsalicylate (Pepto-Bismol), with omeprazole (Prilosec)
   b. 4 weeks with Mylanta, ranitidine (Zantac), and dicyclomine hydrochloride (Antispas)
   c. Discontinue the use of NSAIDs, start misoprostol (Cytotec), and teach stress reduction.
   d. Place on bland diet (no caffeine, no alcohol), discontinue NSAIDs, follow up in 4 weeks.

10. Mr. T. returns to your office for a follow-up. He has lost 15 pounds, and has had an increase in nausea, vomiting, and pain. You should:

   a. Change his medications.
   b. Refer him to a gastroenterologist.
   c. Assure him that the symptoms always get worse before they get better.
   d. Tell him that if he does not stop smoking, there is nothing anyone can do to help him get better.

ANSWERS AND RATIONALES

1. *Answer:* c (diagnosis/gastrointestinal/adult)
   Rationale: Manifestations of peptic ulcer disease include intermittent epigastric pain. Pain begins 1 to 3 hours after eating, frequently awakening the person at night. Pain is relieved by food, antacids, dyspepsia. (Millonig, 1994)

2. *Answer:* c (assessment:subjective/history/gastrointestinal/adult)
   Rationale: More information is needed about Mr. T.'s symptoms and history before an informed decision can be made for treatment. (Van Schaik, 1993)

3. *Answer:* a (diagnosis/gastrointestinal/adult)
   Rationale: Pain associated with coronary artery insufficiency is usually precipitated by physical activity, persists no more than a few minutes, and subsides with rest. (Loeb, 1993)

4. *Answer:* b (diagnosis/gastrointestinal/adult)
   Rationale: An upper GI series will detect 90% of peptic ulcers. It may show anatomic deformity created by ulcer crater and delayed gastric emptying if partial obstruction is present. The upper GI series is also less expensive than endoscopy. (Millonig, 1994)

5. *Answer:* d (diagnosis/gastrointestinal/NAS)
   Rationale: History of NSAID use is no reason for an endoscopy. Endoscopy allows visualization of the ulcer site and determination of healing stage. It also allows biopsies to be performed to rule out gastric cancers or malignant gastric ulcers. (Millonig, 1994)

6. *Answer:* b (diagnosis/gastrointestinal/NAS)
   Rationale: Duodenal ulcers are about four times more common than gastric ulcers. They occur most often between 40 and 60 years of age and are three times more common in men than women. (Van Schaik, 1993)

7. *Answer:* c (assessment: subjective/history/gastrointestinal/NAS)
   Rationale: Predisposing factors for duodenal ulcers include bacterial virulence, physiologic stress (surgical procedures, trauma, burns, etc.), medications (NSAIDs), male gender, and familial predisposition. (Johnson, 1996; Loeb, 1993; National Institutes of Health [NIH], 1995)

8. *Answer:* b (plan/gastrointestinal/NAS)

Rationale: Antacids are given to reduce the total acid load in the GI tract and to elevate the gastric pH to reduce pepsin activity. Duration of activity is less than 1 hour. To be most effective, they must be given 1 hour after meals. (Van Schaik, 1993)

9. *Answer:* a (plan/gastrointestinal/NAS)

Rationale: The most effective therapy, according to an NIH panel, is 2-week triple therapy. This regimen eradicates the bacteria and reduces the risk of ulcer recurrence. (National Institutes of Health, 1995)

10. *Answer:* b (evaluation/gastrointestinal/adult)

Rationale: A referral should be made for persons who fail to respond to treatment in 2 to 4 weeks and have significant weight loss, symptoms of peritonitis, or suspected gastric ulcers. (Millonig, 1994)

5

Genitourinary System

Enuresis

OVERVIEW
Definition

Involuntary voiding after the age when control should have been established (usually 5 years old) is called *enuresis*. It may be nocturnal (85%) or diurnal (15%). Enuresis is subdivided into two categories. In *primary enuresis* bladder control has never been established. In *secondary enuresis* there is loss of bladder control in a child who has been consistently dry for at least 6 months.

Incidence

- More common in boys than girls
- Familial tendency
- More common in large families and in the lower socioeconomic groups
- Approximate incidence by age group
  —10% to 15% of 6-year-olds
  —5% of 10-year-olds
  —3% of 12-year-olds
  —1% of 15-year-olds

Pathophysiology

PRIMARY ENURESIS
- Urinary control is a function of the CNS.
- Delayed maturation of that portion of the CNS that permits bladder control results in the child not sensing bladder fullness and therefore not awakening to void.
- Contributing factors include the following:
  —Immature bladder with small capacity

  —Arousal from non–rapid eye movement sleep
  —Psychologic or emotional problems (new sibling, divorce, etc.)
  —Neurologic deficit (neurogenic bladder, spinal cord lesion)
  —Urologic abnormalities (urinary tract infection [UTI], vesicoureteral reflex, bifurcated bladder, tumors)
  —Diabetes mellitus/diabetes insipidus

SECONDARY ENURESIS
- Psychologic problems
- Urinary tract infections: The presence of bacteria is irritating to the bladder mucosa, producing frequency, urgency, and dysuria.
- Sexual abuse
- Diabetes mellitus/diabetes insipidus

ASSESSMENT: SUBJECTIVE/HISTORY

- Primary enuresis: Involuntary voiding one or more times a day, at least once a week without ever having achieved full bladder control
- Secondary enuresis: Involuntary voiding one or more times a day, at least once a week after having achieved bladder control for at least 6 months

History of Present Illness

- Onset, frequency, time frame (At what time of night does the bed-wetting usually occur? Is it consistent?)
- Fluid intake related to bedtime
- Method used by parents to correct the problem

167

- Attitude of parents and the child regarding the enuresis
- Depending on the child, the family nurse practitioner might choose to conduct a portion of the interview with the parents and child separated.

Symptoms

- Frequency, urgency, pain, or burning on urination
- Nocturnal seizures (bitten tongue or sore muscles on awakening)

Past Medical History

- UTI
- Congenital anomalies
- Toilet training methods (Were parents demanding or punitive?)

Family History

- Enuresis, especially in father
- Diabetes

Psychosocial History

- Births
- Deaths
- Divorce
- Moves
- School problems

ASSESSMENT: OBJECTIVE/ PHYSICAL EXAMINATION

Physical Examination

- Perform complete physical and neurologic examinations; findings from these examinations are usually within normal limits.
- Focus on constant dribbling, external anomalies of the genitalia, rectal sphincter tone, café au lait spots, abdominal masses, spinal bony defects, hairy tufts, and masses and gait.
- Assess for chronic urinary tract disease; suspect disease if the client's height and weight are below the 5th percentile and/or the client's average blood pressure is above the 95th percentile for age and sex.

Diagnostic Procedures

- Urinalysis and clean voided culture are recommended. More invasive procedures (cystoscopy, ultrasound) are not indicated unless

an abnormality is discovered on physical examination, or the problem persists past age 6 years and all other diagnostic procedure results are negative.

DIAGNOSIS

The differential diagnosis includes the following:

- Normal developmental enuresis
- Toilet training resistance
- Altered parenting
- UTI or anatomic abnormalities
- Diabetes mellitus, diabetes insipidus
- Seizure disorder, excessive fluid
- Intake and CNS deficit

NOTE: In the majority of cases, no organic pathologic condition can be found.

THERAPEUTIC PLAN

- Involve the child in the treatment plan.
- Decision to treat or not to treat must be made jointly by the child and the parents.
- Treat only children who are 8 years old or older and who have a bladder capacity of 200 ml or greater (determined by measuring output after having the child wait to as long as possible).
- Investigate and treat the cause of secondary enuresis.

Nonpharmacologic Treatment

- Bladder stretching exercises: Increase fluid and have child hold off voiding as long as possible.
- Positive reinforcement for dryness: Use a gold-star chart.
- Education: Support and reassure the child; avoid punishing or embarrassing the child.
- "Enuresis alarm": The alarm is worn at night and is triggered by moisture. A success rate up to 80% has been reported. The typical course is 4 months. The alarm must be worn until 21 consecutive nights of dryness are achieved. There is roughly a 25% relapse rate.

Pharmacologic Treatment

- Imipramine (Tofranil): The initial dose is 15 to 25 mg PO hs, which may be increased to a maximum dose of 50 mg for children younger than 12 years and 75 mg for children older than 12 years.

—Prescribe a 6- to 8-week treatment, then taper the dose during a 4- to 6-week period.

—Drug tolerance is common.

—Watch for cardiac side effects (dysrhythmia, postural hypotension, anemia) and anticholinergic effects (dry mouth).

—Overdose may be fatal; warn parents to keep medicine out of child's reach.

- Desmopressin acetate (DDAVP; antidiuretic hormone): Use 20 to 40 mg intranasally with children age 6 years and older.

—Treatment is expensive.

—Effectiveness is controversial.

—There is a high relapse rate.

Client Education

REFERRAL

- Refer for any anatomic abnormalities.
- Once a UTI has been ruled out, children with chronic enuresis should have a thorough urologic workup simultaneously with behavioral therapy.

EVALUATION/FOLLOW-UP

Primary Enuresis

- Contact by telephone in 2 weeks to check progress.
- Schedule a return visit in 1 month.
- Continue follow-up at 2- to 4-week intervals. Phone calls and office visits may alternate.

Secondary Enuresis

- Draft an individualized counseling contract.
- Schedule initial follow-up in 10 to 14 days.
- If medication is prescribed, the client should be seen monthly.
- If a UTI is diagnosed, follow up after antibiotics are completed.

Encopresis

OVERVIEW
Definition

Encopresis is repeated fecal soiling in the absence of organic defect or illness in children older than 4 years. The condition is usually secondary to constipation or incomplete defecation.

Incidence

- Two percent to three precent of preschool and elementary school-age children
- Greater incidence in boys than girls

Pathophysiology

Encopresis frequently results from voluntary withholding of stool, which creates a functional megacolon. The defecation reflex occurs when the walls of the rectum become distended with stool, stimulating mass peristalsis. When stool is retained via voluntary constriction of the external sphincter, the rectum relaxes, decreasing peristalsis and the urge to defecate. The megacolon requires progressively larger stools to stimulate defecation. As the rectal vault becomes enlarged, control of the external sphincter is lost, and liquid stool involuntarily seeps past the fecal bolus.

ASSESSMENT: SUBJECTIVE/HISTORY

- "Dribbling" stool; staining of underpants
- Abdominal pain and distention
- Anorexia
- Enuresis

Determine the usual pattern of elimination and description of stools including frequency, dietary history, use of laxatives, any treatments tried and effectiveness, availability of bathrooms including degree of privacy, and any psychosocial factors.

ASSESSMENT: OBJECTIVE/ PHYSICAL EXAMINATION
Physical Examination

- Abdominal: Usually normal; may reveal soft, nontender mass in midline or left lower quadrant
- Rectal: May reveal anal fissures, decreased tone, or hard formed stool in rectal vault

Diagnostic Procedures

Obtain an abdominal x-ray examination to rule out obstruction and look for fecal mass.

DIAGNOSIS

The differential diagnosis includes the following:

- Hirschsprung's disease
- Neuromuscular defect

- Spinal cord lesion
- Cerebral palsy
- Anal stricture/fissure
- Lead poisoning
- Irritable bowel syndrome
- Chronic diarrhea
- Crohn's disease
- Ulcerative colitis

THERAPEUTIC PLAN

- Education
  —Remove blame by explaining that the soiling is involuntary.
- Initial treatment
  —Relieve constipation and/or impaction.
  —Prescribe hypertonic phosphate enemas 3 ml/kg bid until return is free of solid stool.
  —Prescribe mineral oil 1 to 2 ml/kg bid until incontinence develops; reduce dose until child has two to three loose stools daily.
- Bowel retraining
  —Taper laxatives as tolerated.
  —Prescribe stool softeners (docusate sodium [Colace] 5 mg/kg/day).
  —Have child sit on the toilet immediately after meals for 15 to 20 minutes at the same time every day.
  —Increase the child's intake of fiber, fruits, vegetables, and fluids.

EVALUATION/FOLLOW-UP

- Follow up by telephone prn and in 1 week.
- Recheck every month until rectal vault is normal size.
- Taper stool softeners once regular elimination pattern is established.

REFERENCES

Arvin, A. M., Behrman, R. E., Kliegman, R. M., & Nelson, W. E. (Eds.). (1996). *Nelson textbook of pediatrics* (15th ed.). Philadelphia: W. B. Saunders.

Boynton, R. W., Dunn, E. S., & Stephens, G. R. (Eds.). (1994). *Manual of ambulatory pediatrics* (3rd ed.). Philadelphia: J. B. Lippincott.

Chaney, C. A. (1995). A collaborative protocol for encopresis management in school-aged children. *Journal of School Health, 65*(9), 360-364.

Dershewitz, R. A. (Ed.) (1993). *Ambulatory pediatric care* (2nd ed.). Philadelphia: J. B. Lippincott.

Groothuis, J. R., Hay, W. W., Hayward, A. R., & Levin, M. J. (Eds.). (1995). *Current pediatric diagnosis and treatment* (12th ed.). Norwalk, CT: Appleton & Lange.

Loening-Baucke, V. (1996a). Balloon defecation as a predictor of outcome in children with functional constipation and encopresis. *The Journal of Pediatrics, 128*(3), 336-340.

Loening-Baucke, V. (1996b). Encopresis and soiling. *Pediatric Clinics of North America, 43*(1), 279-299.

Sprague, J. M., Lamb, W., & Homer, D. (1993). Encopresis: A study of treatment alternatives and historical and behavioral characteristics. *Nurse Practitioner, 18*(10), 52-63.

REVIEW QUESTIONS

1. Seven-year-old Robert is brought to the clinic for his annual physical examination. When the family nurse practitioner asks how things are going, Robert's mother flashes him an angry look and says "everything would be fine if I could just get him to stop pooping in his pants every afternoon." To evaluate this situation the family nurse practitioner would need to:

   a. Ask about other behavioral problems.
   b. Ask for a complete description of Robert's stooling patterns.
   c. Ask about psychosocial upsets such as divorce or the birth of a sibling.
   d. Assist the mother in planning a program of behavior modification.

2. Robert's mother goes on to explain that one of the most frustrating components of his soiling is that "he tries to hide his underwear, and when I find it, he acts like he just doesn't care." Which of the following statements about encopresis would help the family nurse practitioner explain this behavior?

   a. Children with encopresis frequently have major psychosocial problems.
   b. Boys with encopresis generally do not consider it a problem.
   c. Since Robert only soils in the afternoon, he is probably just trying to get his mother's attention.
   d. Hiding soiled clothing and acting indifferent are common coping strategies used by children with encopresis.

3. All the following would help the family nurse practitioner rule out an organic cause for secondary enuresis **except:**

    a. Urine specific gravity 1.011
    b. No evidence of glycosuria and acetonuria from urinalysis
    c. Presence of protein and leukocytes in the urine
    d. No evidence of bacteria in the urine

4. Before a diagnosis of encopresis is made, the family nurse practitioner should consider all the following **except:**

    a. Hirschsprung's disease
    b. Lead poisoning
    c. Chronic diarrhea
    d. Iron deficiency anemia

5. The therapeutic plan of care for a 5-year-old diagnosed with enuresis who has a negative physical examination would include all the following **except:**

    a. Reassure the parents and wait for maturation.
    b. Refer for a renal ultrasound and a voiding cystogram.
    c. Suggest the use of exercises to increase bladder capacity.
    d. Suggest the use of a behavior modification program such as "gold stars" for dryness.

6. Sam, a 12-year-old who has been undergoing treatment for encopresis, returns to the clinic for his 1-month follow-up. He is currently taking 2 teaspoons of mineral oil bid and is having regular soft-to-loose stools. The family nurse practitioner should:

    a. Praise Sam for his success and continue current treatment.
    b. Increase the amount of mineral oil until stools are liquid.
    c. Discontinue all pharmacologic intervention and continue dietary therapy.
    d. Discontinue the mineral oil, begin docusate sodium (Colace) 10 mg/kg/day, and continue a high-fiber diet.

ANSWERS AND RATIONALES

1. *Answer:* b (assessment/history/genitourinary/child)

    Rationale: Soiling in the afternoon is suggestive of encopresis. Knowledge of stooling patterns will either support or rule out this diagnosis. The soiling involved with encopresis is involuntary and not a reflection of a behavioral problem or a psychosocial upset. It would be inappropriate to develop a plan prior to conducting a complete assessment. (Boynton, Dunn, & Stephens, 1994)

2. *Answer:* d (assessment/history/genitourinary/child)

    Rationale: Children who experience soiling are usually ashamed and embarrassed. Hiding soiled clothing and pretending indifference are frequently used coping strategies. (Chaney, 1995)

3. *Answer:* c (plan/genitourinary/child)

    Rationale: A urine specific gravity >1.006 rules out diabetes insipidus, absence of glycosuria and acetonuria rules out diabetes mellitus, and absence of bacteriuria rules out a UTI. The presence of protein and leukocytes in the urine might be indicative of glomerulonephritis or nephrotic syndrome. (Boynton, Dunn, & Stephens, 1994)

4. *Answer:* d (diagnosis/genitourinary/child)

    Rationale: Hirschsprung's disease is characterized by chronic constipation sometimes accompanied by liquid seepage. Lead poisoning also frequently produces constipation, abdominal pain, and anorexia. Soiling may occur with any case of diarrhea. Iron deficiency anemia may be characterized by anorexia but usually does not produce soiling, constipation, or abdominal pain. (Arvin, Behrman, Kliegman, & Nelson, 1996)

5. *Answer:* b (plan/genitourinary/child)

    Rationale: The majority of cases of primary enuresis have no organic cause. Extensive or invasive laboratory or radiologic examination should be avoided in the absence of physical findings. An estimated 10% to 15% of all 6-year-olds continue to be incontinent at night. At age 5 years this is probably a normal variant; if the parents desire treatment, the least invasive methods should be tried first. (Arvin, Behrman, Kliegman, & Nelson, 1996)

6. *Answer:* d (evaluation/genitourinary/child)

Rationale: Mineral oil therapy should be continued at 3 to 4 teaspoons bid until liquid stools develop. The dose should then be reduced to 1 to 2 ml/kg until soft stools occur bid. The client can then be treated with dietary therapy and stool softeners until regular bowel habits are well established. Mineral oil therapy is unpleasant, and clients usually will not comply for extended periods. Moving the client toward nonpharmacologic therapy should always be the goal. (Boynton, Dunn, & Stephens, 1994)

PROSTATE DISEASE

Acute and Chronic Bacterial Prostatitis, Benign Prostatic Hyperplasia, Prostate Cancer

OVERVIEW
Definition

Acute bacterial prostatitis is an infection usually caused by gram-negative rods, especially *Escherichia coli* and *Pseudomonas* species, and less commonly by gram positive organisms, such as *Enterococcus.* The signs and symptoms include fever, irritative voiding symptoms (frequency, nocturia, urgency), perineal or suprapubic pain, exquisitely tender prostate on physical examination, and positive results from culture.

Chronic bacterial prostatitis is an infectious process that may evolve from acute bacterial prostatitis, but not always. Gram-negative rods are the most common etiologic agent, and only one gram-negative rod, *Enterococcus,* is associated with chronic infection.

Benign prostatic hyperplasia (BPH) is defined as urinary outflow obstruction with decreased force/caliber of urinary stream, nocturia, sensation of incomplete emptying, hesitancy, frequency, urgency, and high postvoid residual.

Malignant neoplasm of the prostate gland is called *prostate cancer.*

Incidence

Bacterial prostatitis is the most important cause of urinary tract infections in men. Both acute and chronic bacterial prostatitis can occur in men of any age but are not seen in children.

BPH affects one in every four men by age 80 in the United States. Symptomatology is reported in nearly half the men 50 to 64 years old in the general population.

Prostate cancer has overtaken lung and colon cancers to be the most common cancer in males, comprising 21% of all newly discovered cancers in males. The lifetime probability that a man will have prostate cancer is between 6% to 9%, but the probability of death as a result of prostate cancer is approximately 2%.

Pathophysiology

Bacterial prostatitis is most likely caused by ascending urethral infection, reflux of infected urine, extension of rectal infection, or hematogenous spread. The most common pathogen is *E. coli;* others may be *Klebsiella* or *Pseudonomas* organisms.

The causes of BPH are not fully understood. The disorder is associated with two factors: male sex and increasing age. The cause of age-related hyperplasia is unknown, although is thought to be related to androgenic changes at the cellular level. The earliest changes of BPH occur in the periurethral glands, with nodular hyperplasia. As these nodules grow and coalesce during a period of years, true prostatic tissue is compressed outward. As the gland enlarges, urethral resistance to urine flow increases and muscular hypertrophy of the bladder ensues.

Prostate cancer incidence increases with age, and blacks have a threefold higher incidence than whites; however, there is no clear cut etiologic relationship to environment, socioeconomic status, fertility, or endogenous androgen level. Regional differences do exist and may reflect unknown environmental factors or variation in detection methods.

PROTECTIVE FACTORS
- Acute and chronic bacterial prostatitis: Young age
- BPH: Young age
- Prostate cancer: White, young age

FACTORS INCREASING SUSCEPTIBILITY
- Acute and chronic bacterial prostatitis: Advancing age, prior history of prostatitis
- BPH: Advancing age
- Prostate cancer: Black, advancing age

ASSESSMENT: SUBJECTIVE/HISTORY
Acute Bacterial Prostatitis

- Fever
- Urgency
- Nocturia
- Frequency
- Perineal or suprapubic pain
- Acute onset
- Lower back pain
- Fatigue
- Occasional hematuria or penile tip pain
- Pain with bowel movements
  Older adults may be asymptomatic, and fever may not be as pronounced.

Chronic Bacterial Prostatitis

- Fever
- Urgency
- Nocturia
- Frequency
- Perineal or suprapubic discomfort that is often dull and poorly localized
- Hematospermia or painful ejaculation
  Older adults may be asymptomatic.

Benign Prostatic Hyperplasia

- Decreased force and caliber of urinary stream
- Nocturia
- Feeling of incomplete emptying
- Hesitancy
- Dribbling
  In older adults, symptoms may be more pronounced.

Prostate Cancer

- Hesitancy
- Frequency
- Nocturia
- Decreased force and caliber of stream
- Urge incontinence

Approximately 20% of individuals with prostate cancer have symptoms of metastastic cancer, such as spinal/bone pain and gross hematuria.

In older adults, symptoms are more likely to be present.

Past Medical History

- Previous episode(s) of prostatitis
- Family history for prostatic disease(s)
- Medication history
- Delayed sexual drive
- Early cessation of sexuality
- Smoking

Medication History

Inquire about use of decongestants, antidepressants, or antihypertensives.

Family History

Ask about prostate/urinary diseases.

Psychosocial History

Ask about multiple sexual partners and multiple STDs (especially in considering prostate cancer).

Dietary History

Ask about the amount of fat in the diet.

ASSESSMENT: OBJECTIVE/ PHYSICAL EXAMINATION
Physical Examination

A problem-oriented approach should be conducted, paying particular attention to vital signs, weight, general appearance, and hydration. Given the wide variety of signs and symptoms in clients with BPH, a complete physical examination may be necessary.
- Abdominal: Check for distended bladder and abdominal pain.
- Musculoskeletal: Check for pain in back with range of motion or palpation.
- Genital/rectal: Perform an examination of the external genitalia. Assess for prostate tenderness, enlargement, or nodules.

Diagnostic Procedures

- Acute and chronic bacterial prostatitis: Obtain a CBC or urinalysis. Expressed prostatic secretions are usually obtained by a urologist.

- BPH: A postvoid urine residual of >100 ml suggests BPH or other obstruction, urinalysis. The American Urological Association Index is an important aspect of the initial examination.
- Prostate cancer: Always obtain a prostate specific antigen prior to rectal examination or 1 week later. Obtain a prostate biopsy, renal functions, acid phosphatase, postvoid urine residual to check for obstruction.

DIAGNOSIS

The differential diagnosis includes the following:
- Chronic nonbacterial prostatitis
- Prostatodynia
- STD
- Urethral stricture
- Acquired or congenital bladder neck contracture
- Chronic urethritis

THERAPEUTIC PLAN
Pharmacologic Treatment

Antibiotic treatment for acute bacterial prostatitis includes quinolones or trimethoprim-sulfamethoxazole (TMP-SMX) for at least 2 weeks and perhaps for 30 days. Chronic bacterial prostatitis is treated with the same medications but for at least 12 weeks. Other medications for both acute and chronic bacterial prostatitis include trimethoprim or erythromycin for the specified periods of time.

Pharmacologic treatment for BPH includes consideration of antiandrogrens (finasteride) and alpha-adrenergic antagonists (prazosin, doxazosin, terazosin) given at bedtime to minimize side effects. Titrating the medications up to the desired/effective dose may be accomplished during a 3- to 4-week period. Before the dose is increased, blood pressure and the presence of orthostatic changes should be monitored.

Nonpharmacologic Treatment

Nonpharmacologic treatment for BPH can include herbal therapy, saw palmetto at 80 mg bid for 8 weeks, vitamin B_6 500 to 1000 mg/qd, or zinc 50 to 100 mg/qd. If zinc is taken for more than 1 month, copper at 1 to 2 mg/day should be added as zinc depletes the body's stores of copper.

A nurse practitioner should immediately refer cases of suspected prostate cancer to a urologist.

Client Education

- A seated position may enhance voiding with obstruction.
- Increased water intake is important.
- Reduction of fat and caffeine in diet is essential.
- Taking sitz baths may be beneficial.
- Compliance with medication regimen is essential.
- Bacterial prostatitis has a chronic/relapsing nature.
- Isolated bacterial prostatitis does not cause impotency or infertility.
- Adding lycopenes (tomatoes, sauces containing tomatoes) to the diet is recommended.

Referral

Refer men with BPH, suspected prostate cancer, or chronic/relapsing cases of bacterial prostatitis to a urologist.

EVALUATION/FOLLOW-UP

Indications for urologic investigation include treatment failures with appropriate medications, chronic/relapsing cases of bacterial prostatitis, BPH, or suspected prostate cancer.

REFERENCES

Fugh-Berman, A. (1996, January). A better way to shrink an enlarged prostate. *Health Confidential*, p. 10.

Gorroll, A. H., May, L. A., & Mulley, A. G. (1995). *Primary care medicine: Office evaluation and management of the adult patient* (3rd ed.). Philadelphia: J. B. Lippincott.

Hollander, J. B., & Diokno, A. C. (1995). Prostatism. *Urologic Clinics of North America, 23*(1), 75-86.

Hostetler, R. M., Mandel, I. G., & Marshburn, J. (1996). Prostate cancer screening. *Medical Clinics of North America, 80*(1), 83-99.

Liebman, B. (1996, March). Clues to prostate cancer. *Nutrition Action Healthletter*, pp. 12-13.

Peters, S. (1997, April). For men only: An overview of three top health concerns. *Advance for Nurse Practitioners*, pp. 53-57.

Tierney, L. M., McPhee, S. J., & Papadakis, M. A. (1996). *Current medical diagnosis and treatment* (35th ed.). Norwalk, CT: Appleton & Lange.

Uphold, C., & Graham, M. (1994). *Clinical guidelines in family practice.* Gainesville, FL: Barmarrae Books.

U.S. Department of Health and Human Services (1994). *Benign prostatic hypertrophy: Diagnosis and treatment* (AHCPR Publication No. 94-0583). Rockville, MD: U.S. Department of Health and Human Services.

Zippe, C. D. (1996). Benign prostatic hyperplasia: An approach for the internist. *Cleveland Clinic Journal of Medicine, 63*(4), pp. 226-236.

REVIEW QUESTIONS

1. Which symptom is most indicative of acute bacterial prostatitis?

　　a. Poorly localized pain
　　b. Hesitancy
　　c. Acute onset of symptomatology
　　d. Urge incontinence

2. An exquisitely tender prostate is most likely to be associated with:

　　a. Acute bacterial prostatitis
　　b. BPH
　　c. Prostate cancer
　　d. Chronic bacterial prostatitis

3. A 70-year-old man has nocturia, frequency, and dribbling. Which of the following diagnoses would you **not** consider as a possible diagnosis?

　　a. Prostate cancer
　　b. Acute bacterial prostatitis
　　c. BPH
　　d. UTI

4. Alpha-adrenergic antagonists, used in the treatment of BPH, may be titrated to the desired dose during a period of:

　　a. 5 to 6 weeks
　　b. 1 to 2 weeks
　　c. 1 to 2 months
　　d. 3 to 4 weeks

5. A man who has shown no response to treatment for his fourth episode of chronic bacterial prostatitis in the last 5 months should:

　　a. Receive a prescription for medication effective against gram-positive organisms
　　b. Be referred to a urologist
　　c. Be counseled about his adherence to prescribed treatment
　　d. Be asked to return to the clinic in 1 week

ANSWERS AND RATIONALES

1. *Answer:* c (assessment/history/genitourinary/adult male)

Rationale: Perineal/suprapubic pain that is poorly localized is more indicative of chronic bacterial prostatitis, whereas urge incontinence and hestitancy may be associated with BPH or prostate cancer. (Gorroll, May, & Mulley, 1995; Tierney, McPhee, & Papadakis, 1996)

2. *Answer:* a (assessment/physical examination/genitourinary/adult male)

Rationale: With chronic bacterial prostatitis the prostate gland may or may not be tender but not exquisitely tender. With BPH there is enlargement of the gland, and with prostate cancer nodules are most likely palpated. (Gorroll, May, & Mulley, 1995; Tierney, McPhee, & Papadakis, 1996; Uphold & Graham, 1994)

3. *Answer:* b (assessment/history/genitourinary/adult male)

Rationale: Prostate cancer and BPH are both more common in older men; dribbling is not often seen in acute bacterial prostatitis but may be seen with urinary tract infection. (Gorroll, May, & Mulley, 1995; Hostetler, Mandel, & Marshburn, 1996)

4. *Answer:* d (plan/genitourinary/adult male)

Rationale: Because of the orthostatic side effects and the older age of the men being treated, the medications should be started at a low dose and titrated upward to reach the desirable dose. (Hollander & Diokno, 1995)

5. *Answer:* b (evaluation/genitourinary/adult male)

Rationale: Nurse practitioners should refer clients with chronic/relapsing episodes of bacterial prostatitis to a urologist.

URINARY TRACT INFECTION

Cystitis/Pyelonephritis

OVERVIEW

Definition

Cystitis is the presence of bacteria in urine, causing a change in urinary patterns. It is considered a lower UTI.

Pyelonephritis is an infection of the renal pelvis or parenchyma. It is considered an upper UTI.

Two infections that occur within 6 months or three infections within 1 year constitute a *recurrent UTI.*

Incidence

- UTI is the second most common infection.
- Twenty percent of women complain of UTI symptoms every year; occurrence of UTI becomes more common with increasing age.
- Newborn boys have UTIs more frequently than girls, but after the newborn period most UTIs occur in girls.
- Twenty percent of UTIs are recurrent.
- UTIs cost $1 billion per year.

Pathophysiology

PROTECTIVE FACTORS
- Urinary acidity and osmolality
- Antimicrobial properties of the mucosa
- "Flushing" effect of urination
- Cervical immunoglobulins

FACTORS INCREASING SUSCEPTIBILITY
- Bacterial virulence
- Behavioral factors: Poor hygiene, wiping back to front
- Abnormal urinary flow: Stones, BPH, vesicoureteral reflux (structural abnormalities)
- Other host factors: Decreased immunity, pregnancy, alcoholism, indwelling catheter, increased sexual activity, urinary instrumentation, bubble baths (girls only)

COMMON PATHOGENS
- *E. coli* (70% to 85% of cystitis; 90% of pyelonephritis)
- *Staphylococcus saprophyticus* (10% to 20%)
- *Enterococcus* species

ASSESSMENT: SUBJECTIVE/HISTORY

Most Common Symptoms

CYSTITIS
- Adults: Typical symptoms include dysuria, urinary frequency, urinary urgency, hematuria, urine odor, suprapubic discomfort, pressure, acute onset.
- Infants: Irritability, failure to thrive, systemic illness (fever), vomiting/diarrhea, abdominal pain and distention, decreased urination, change in urination pattern (enuresis), foul odor (UTI is the most common cause of fever of undetermined origin in infants. The younger the infant, the more likely sepsis and structural abnormalities will be found.)
- Toddlers: Abdominal discomfort, fever, altered voiding patterns, malodorous urine
- Preschool: Voiding discomfort, enuresis
- School-age/teens: Typical signs and symptoms
- Older adults: May be asymptomatic, fever uncommon

PYELONEPHRITIS
- Adults/school-age children and older: Fever, malaise, prostration, nausea, more gradual onset, toxic appearance
- Children <6 years old: Nonspecific symptoms similar to cystitis
- Older adults: Generalized symptoms common; in 50% of women older than 65 possibly no fever until later in the course

Associated Symptoms

- Back or flank pain
- Nausea/vomiting
- Incontinence in children (previously toilet trained) or older adults
- Fever
- Decreased force of urine stream
- Nocturia
- Diarrhea
- Constipation
- Vaginal discharge
- Urethral discharge
- Perianal itching

Past Medical History

- Kidney stones, UTIs, kidney, bladder or prostate disease
- Diabetes, hypertension, multiple sclerosis
- Last menstrual period, use of barrier birth control methods, birth control methods
- Allergies, date of last sexual contact, new sexual partner within last 6 months
- Pregnant female: Recent group A beta-streptococcus (GABS) infection

Medication History

Inquire about recent use of antibiotics or any other medications.

Family History

Ask about family history of kidney problems.

Psychosocial History

In children, consider possible sexual abuse. Do not ask the child about possible sexual abuse until a comfortable nurse-client relationship is established.

Dietary History

- Increased ingestion of caffeine or carbonated drinks
- Abnormal water intake

ASSESSMENT: OBJECTIVE/ PHYSICAL EXAMINATION

Physical Examination

A problem-oriented physical examination should be conducted with particular attention to vital signs and weight, general appearance, and general hydration status, including orthostatic changes.

- Abdominal: Perform a full abdominal examination and check for costovertebral angle (CVA) tenderness (common in pyelonephritis).
- Genital: In females, perform a complete pelvic examination if abdominal or laboratory results do not provide data for a diagnosis of UTI. In males, perform a complete examination of external genitalia and assess for prostate tenderness or enlargement.
- Children: Assess for dehydration and activity level. Physical examination results may be essentially within normal limits.

Diagnostic Procedures

The choice of procedure is based on the documented presence of pyuria/bacteriuria in a clean catch urine sample. Children may require catherization to obtain a specimen.

- Urine dipstick
  —Presence of leukocyte esterase
  —Presence of nitrites
- Microscopic urinalysis
  — >2 to 5 leukocytes/field
  — >2 to 5 RBCs/field
  — >1+bacterial organisms

A urinanalysis with >0 to 5 epithelial cells should be considered contaminated and should be redone.

The following are indications for urine culture:

- Symptoms without pyuria or bacteriuria
- Complicated UTIs (see the following list)
- Suspected pyelonephritis
- Females who failed prior treatment

The following is a standard definition of positive results from urine culture:

- 10^5 colony-forming units (CFU)/ml
- CFU of 10^2 is considered a positive result if all of the following are present:
  —Male
  —Symptomatic client
  —Presence of pyuria

NOTE: Fifteen percent to twenty percent of symptomatic women have negative culture results.

- Wet mount of vaginal secretions/penile discharge
  —Only needed if STD is suspected. Wet mount will reveal trichomoniasis. Send culture for chlamydia and gonorrhea screening.
  —Consider doing wet mount and vaginal cultures if female has had new sexual partner in last 3 months.
- Obtain CBC with differential, electrolytes, BUN and creatinine.
  —Only needed if the client is severely ill or systemic illness or pyelonephritis is suspected.

DIAGNOSIS

The differential diagnosis includes the following:

- Nephrolithiasis
- Pyelonephritis

- Trauma
- Prostatitis
- Diabetes
- STD
- Acute urethral syndrome
- Tumor
- Pelvic inflammatory disease
- Vulvovaginitis
- Cervicitis
- Epididymitis
- BPH
- Renal tuberculosis
- Poststreptococcal glomerular nephritis
- Children: Sexual abuse, constipation, appendicitis
- Older adults: Menopause

THERAPEUTIC PLAN
Pharmacologic Treatment
Antibiotic treatment for UTI is based on how involved or complicated the condition is:

SIMPLE **UTI**
- Three days' duration
- Choice of antibiotics, first considerations
  —TMP-SMX, second-generation cephalosporins, nitrofurantoin
  —Fluoroquinolones for resistant pathogens
- Consider use of phenazopyridine (Pyridium) as urinary tract analgesic

COMPLICATED **UTI**
- Symptoms >6 days' duration
- Male clients, children, and pregnant women
- Nosocomial infections
- Postinstrumentation infection
- Abnormal urinary flow
- Compromised host

The following describes antibiotic treatment for complicated UTIs:
- Diabetic clients, pregnant women: 7 to 10 days
- Children: 10 days
- Pyelonephritis: 10 to 14 days
- Frequent postvoid urine residual: Treat symptoms only
- Permanent Foley catheter: Treat symptoms only

PYELONEPHRITIS. Clients who are healthy and at low risk for complications with no nausea or vomiting can be treated on an outpatient basis.

Clients who are more ill, children, and pregnant women (increased chance of premature labor) at risk for complications must be treated with IV antibiotics with broad activity against gram-negative bacteria. Possible drug choices include TMP-SMX (Bactrim) or an aminoglycoside. Referral to a urologist is required.

Client Education
- Use of correct postvoiding wiping technique
- Use of barrier methods of birth control
- Use of tampons, deodorants, douches
- Need to void before and after intercourse
- Local trauma: Certain sexual positions, horseback riding, etc.
- Adequate fluid intake: Increased when symptoms are noted, but avoiding overhydration
- Self-administered treatment at first symptoms of UTI
- Need for good perineal hygiene
- Effect of estrogen depletion on vaginal tissues
- Use of phenazopyridine (Pyridium): Red discoloration of urine and all body fluids that may stain contact lenses and clothes

Children
- Teach children to avoid a full bladder. Children in toilet training require a regular schedule.
- Teach children not to delay urination. Advise children to avoid taking bubble baths and sitting in soapy bath water.
- Stress the implications of a UTI. Ensure that parents understand that most infection causing renal scarring occurs in infancy and childhood. The consequences of UTI in children is not the same as the "annoyance" experienced by adults.

Referral
- Children: Hospitalize children with symptomatic pyelonephritis or sepsis.
- Men: Refer men with a UTI to a urologist.
- Pregnant females: Refer pregnant females to an OB/GYN/urologist. Pregnant females may need maintenance antibiotics during pregnancy.

EVALUATION/FOLLOW-UP

The following are indications for urologic investigation (intravenous pyelogram or ultrasound with KUB):

- All male clients
- Children <8 years (ultrasound less invasive)
- Clients with renal colic
- Clients with gross or persistent hematuria
- Persistent UTI
- Recurrent UTI/relapses
- Voiding cystourethrogram (VCUG)
- Clients with evidence of renal scarring

Cystitis

Simple UTIs do not require follow-up unless symptoms persist.

CHILDREN

- Obtain a second culture in 2 to 3 days after treatment begun to check for sterile urine.
- Schedule routine follow-up cultures in 1 month, every 3 months for 1 year, then yearly for 2 to 3 years.

PREGNANT FEMALES

- Schedule once-a-month urine cultures during pregnancy after initial UTI is treated.
- Because of a higher incidence of asymptomatic bacteriuria, schedule once-a-month screenings for pregnant females with sickle cell trait.

COMPLICATED UTIS

- For all UTIs confirmed by urine culture, reassess by urinalysis in 2 weeks after treatment.
- For complicated UTIs, schedule a follow-up urine culture after treatment.

MEN OLDER THAN 50. Follow-up after 4 to 6 weeks is recommended.

Pyelonephritis

- Monitor urinary output.
- Follow up for evaluation of symptom assessment and directed physical examination in 24 to 48 hours.
- Schedule a test of cure 1 to 4 weeks after completion of antibiotic therapy.
- Special diagnostic studies are needed in men and children after an episode of pyelonephritis. Referral to a urologist is warranted.

REFERENCES

Forland, M. (1993). UTI—How its management has changed. *Postgraduate Medicine, 93*(5), 71-86.

French, M. (1995, November). UTI in elderly. *Advance for Nurse Practitioners*, pp. 25, 26, 28, 52.

Johnson, J. (1992, February 29). Recognizing and treating acute pyelonephritis. *Emergency Medicine*, pp. 25-33.

Mulholland, S. (1995, April). UTI in women. *Consultant*, pp. 534-540.

Nygaard, I., & Johnson, M. (1996). UTI in elderly women. *American Family Practice, 53*(1), 175-182.

Pollen, J. (1995, July-August). Short-term course for uncomplicated UTI. *Contemporary Nurse Practitioner*, pp. 21-30.

Uphold, C., & Graham, M. (1994). *Clinical guidelines in family practice.* Gainesville, FL: Barmarrae Books.

REVIEW QUESTIONS

1. Which of the following physical findings would **not** usually be found in a client with cystitis?

a. CVA tenderness
b. Urethral discharge
c. Mild abdominal pain
d. Suprapubic tenderness

2. You suspect 23-year-old Marcy has pyelonephritis. Which of the following symptoms would you expect?

a. Spasmodic flank pain and hematuria
b. Urethral discharge and dysuria
c. Flank pain, CVA tenderness, and nausea/vomiting
d. Urinary urgency, frequency, and suprapubic pain

3. A 38-year-old man complains of flank pain, fever, and nausea and vomiting. Which of the following diagnoses is **not** appropriate for this client?

a. Cystitis
b. Acute bacterial prostatitis
c. Gastroenteritis
d. Pyelonephritis

4. Treatment for a pregnant female with cystitis would include:

a. Tetracycline
b. Amoxicillin
c. Ciprofloxacin
d. TMP-SMX (Bactrim)

5. Which of the following actions indicates that Tracy, a 19-year-old woman with frequent UTIs, understands the teaching given regarding her care?

   a. Tracy stops taking her antibiotic as soon as her symptoms are gone.
   b. Tracy drinks 10 quarts of water a day during the treatment.
   c. Since her roommate has similar symptoms, Tracy gives some of her pills to her roommate.
   d. Tracy returns to the office in 2 weeks for a urine culture.

ANSWERS AND RATIONALES

1. *Answer:* a (assessment/physical examination/genitourinary/NAS)

Rationale: CVA tenderness is most indicative of pyelonephritis. Urethral discharge, mild abdominal pain, and suprapubic tenderness may be found during the examination of a client with cystitis. (Uphold & Graham, 1994; Forland, 1993)

2. *Answer:* c (assessment/history/genitourinary/NAS)

Rationale: Spasmodic flank pain and hematuria may be seen with a kidney stone. Urethral discharge and dysuria are more common with an STD. Urinary urgency, frequency, and suprapubic pain are most commonly seen with cystitis. (Mulholland, 1995)

3. *Answer:* c (diagnosis/genitourinary/adult)

Rationale: Cystitis, acute bacterial prostatitis, and pyelonephritis must be considered in a male with flank pain, fever, and nausea and vomiting. Although gastroenteritis is a possibility in a 38-year-old client, the other diagnoses must be considered first. (Uphold & Graham, 1994; Johnson, 1992)

4. *Answer:* b (plan/genitourinary/childbearing female)

Rationale: TMP-SMX (Bactrim) and ciprofloxacin are category C drugs during pregnancy. Tetracycline is not appropriate for generic treatment of UTIs, as well as not being recommended for pregnant females or for children because of teeth staining. (Mulholland, 1995)

5. *Answer:* d (evaluation/genitourinary/adult)

Rationale: The client should complete the whole course of antibiotic therapy for a UTI. Although having an adequate fluid intake is recommended, 10 quarts is too much since the urinary antibiotics depend on the concentration of drug in the bladder to achieve their maximum effect. Women with frequent UTIs are considered as having a complicated UTI and should return for a follow-up urine culture. (Mulholland, 1995; Pollen, 1995)

6

Reproductive System

AMENORRHEA

OVERVIEW
Definition

Amenorrhea is the absence of menstrual periods. It is classified as either primary or secondary. *Primary amenorrhea* is defined as no bleeding by age 16 years, regardless of the presence of normal growth and development, with the appearance of secondary sex characteristics. *Secondary amenorrhea* occurs in a woman who has previously been menstruating and misses at least three menstrual cycles.

The most common cause of amenorrhea is pregnancy. Aside from pregnancy, common causes of amenorrhea include pituitary disease, uterine disease, and ovarian failure. Secondary amenorrhea may also be caused by stress, alterations in nutritional status, eating disorders, medications, strenuous exercise, thyroid disease, altered adrenal function, or polycystic ovary disease.

ASSESSMENT: SUBJECTIVE/HISTORY
History of Present Illness

A careful menstrual, sexual, and pregnancy history should include the following:
- Past and current methods of contraception
- Recent medications (including illicit drugs)
- Any signs and symptoms of menopause
- Any chronic or acute illnesses
- Sources of emotional stress
- Present weight and weight 1 year ago
- Amount of daily exercise

Symptoms

Clients should be questioned regarding breast discharge, hirsutism, male pattern baldness, deepening of voice, and signs and symptoms of hypothyroidism. Also to be noted are severe fluctuations in weight and excessive exercising (e.g., long-distance running, gymnastics).

Past Medical History

Any history of hypothyroidism, galactorrhea, pituitary disease, fibroids, or endometriosis should be assessed.

Medication History

Drugs that may cause amenorrhea include the following:
- Contraceptives (oral contraceptives, medroxyprogesterone acetate [Depo-Provera], levonorgestrel [Norplant])
- Antipsychotics
- Digitalis
- Calcium-channel blockers
- Tricyclic antidepressants
- Marijuana
- Methyldopa

ASSESSMENT: OBJECTIVE/ PHYSICAL EXAMINATION
Physical Examination

Examination should focus on the neck (thyroid), breasts (assessing for discharge), and complete pelvic examination, looking at mucosa, hymen, size of uterus, and adnexa. Baseline vital signs, including weight, should be obtained.

Diagnostic Procedures

1. The first-line test for any report of amenorrhea should be a pregnancy test.
2. If the client is not pregnant, then thyroid-stimulating hormone (TSH) and prolactin levels should be drawn, along with administration of a progesterone challenge (10 mg medroxyprogesterone [Provera] for 5 days). If bleeding occurs 3 to 5 days after completing Provera and both TSH and prolactin levels are normal, the amenorrhea is due to anovulation. This means that hypothalamus-pituitary-ovarian axis is intact.
3. If no bleeding occurs, a combination oral contraceptive pill is then initiated (or estrogen, 1.25 mg days 1 through 21, with medroxyprogesterone, 5 to 10 mg on days 16 through 21). Withdrawal bleeding excludes anatomic causes.
4. Refer client to a physician if no withdrawal bleeding occurs.
5. Clients with prolonged amenorrhea and signs of estrogen or androgen excess should be referred for endometrial biopsy before initiating withdrawal bleeding.

DIAGNOSIS

Irregular menses are not uncommon early in menarche. Differential diagnosis includes the following:

- Pregnancy
- Pituitary tumor
- Menopause
- Excessive dieting
- Excessive exercise
- Use of hormonal contraceptive methods
- Changes in lifestyle (e.g., stress)
- Thyroid disease (usually hypothyroidism)
- Polycystic ovary
- Eating disorders
- Premature ovarian failure or ovarian dysfunction

THERAPEUTIC PLAN

Evaluate lifestyle (stress, nutritional status). If contraception is desired, the use of a combination birth control pill is suitable. If the client desires to become pregnant, referral to a fertility specialist is warranted. If amenorrhea is due to hypothyroidism or pituitary disease, treatment of that disease is indicated.

EVALUATION/FOLLOW-UP

Perform evaluation as indicated by diagnostics. Women with chronic anovulation with adequate estrogen are at increased risk for endometrial cancer from the unopposed estrogen.

REFERENCES

Dunnihoo, D. R. (1992). Amenorrhea. In *Fundamentals of gynecology and obstetrics* (2nd ed.). Philadelphia: J. B. Lippincott.

Hawkins, J. W., Roberto-Nichols, D. M., & Stanley-Haney, J. L. (Eds.) (1995). *Protocols for nurse practitioners in gynecologic settings* (5th ed.). New York: Tiresias Press.

Johnson, C. (1996). Amenorrhea. In C. A. Johnson, B. E. Johnson, J. L. Murray, & B. S. Apgar (Eds.), *Women's health care handbook.* St. Louis: Mosby.

McMillan, A. (1995). Gynecologic problems in the family planning consultation. In N. Loudon, A. Glaiser, & A. Gebbie (Eds.), *Handbook of family planning and reproductive health* (3rd ed.). New York: Churchill Livingstone.

Speroff, L. (1993). Amenorrhea. In R. H. Glass (Ed.), *Office gynecology* (4th ed.). Baltimore: William & Wilkins.

Uphold, C.R., & Graham, M. V. (Eds.). (1994). *Clinical guidelines in family practice.* Gainesville, FL: Barmarrae Books.

REVIEW QUESTIONS

1. A 45-year-old woman (secundigravida, secundipara) comes to the office reporting amenorrhea for the past 3 months. Before this her menses had been becoming irregular, occurring anywhere between 21 and 36 days apart. She reports fatigue and constipation along with "mood swings." First-line testing includes:

a. TSH and prolactin levels
b. Follicle-stimulating hormone (FSH) and luteinizing hormone (LH) levels
c. Complete blood cell count (CBC) with differential
d. Human chorionic gonadotropin (hCG) level

2. Why is breast discharge a significant finding in women with amenorrhea?

   a. Hyperprolactinemia occurs in one third of women with amenorrhea.
   b. It is a way of determining pregnancy.
   c. It determines pituitary disease.
   d. It indicates probable breast cancer.

3. A 23-year-old woman with previously normal menses who reports amenorrhea with an increase in acne, increased muscle mass, decreased breast size, deepening of voice, and temporal balding should:

   a. Respond to the progesterone challenge and have withdrawal bleeding
   b. Have elevated prolactin levels, indicating galactorrhea
   c. Have elevated FSH levels, indicating ovarian failure
   d. Be evaluated by a physician before initiation of withdrawal bleeding

4. A 39-year-old woman with amenorrhea who has an elevated TSH should:

   a. Be sent for a thyroid scan
   b. Be started on a thyroid replacement regimen
   c. Begin propylthiouracil (PTU) to decrease the amount of circulating thyroid hormone
   d. Be sent to have a CT scan to evaluate for a pituitary-secreting tumor

5. A 13-year-old girl started menstruating 11 months ago. Physical examination shows that she is Tanner stage III. She reports that she has a regular period for a couple of months, followed by a month or two without menstruating. She is currently menstruating. What does the nurse practitioner do?

   a. Suggests checking FSH level to evaluate ovarian function.
   b. Suggest keeping a menstrual calendar to evaluate cycles.
   c. Obtain urine for a pregnacy test.
   d. Check TSH and prolactin levels.

6. Amenorrhea is the most common side effect of which medication?

   a. Levothyroxine (Synthroid)
   b. Beta-blockers
   c. Levonorgestrel (Norplant)
   d. Medroxyprogesterone (Depo-Provera)

7. Women with a diagnosis of chronic anovulation should be regulated with hormones for which of the following reasons?

   a. They are at higher risk for endometrial and breast cancer.
   b. They will have an increasingly difficult time becoming pregnant if they are not "primed" with estrogen on a regular basis.
   c. They are at higher risk for osteoporosis and heart disease.
   d. They have an increased risk for development of endometriosis and fibroid tumors.

ANSWERS AND RATIONALES

1. *Answer:* d (diagnosis/reproductive/adult)
   Rationale: The most common cause of amenorrhea in women of childbearing years is pregnancy. Women in the perimenopausal period may incorrectly believe that they are unable to become pregnant and become lax in their use of birth control. Further testing should take place only after pregnancy is ruled out. (Dunnihoo, 1992)

2. *Answer:* a (assessment/history/reproductive/adult)
   Rationale: Although breast discharge may occur late in pregnancy and may also signify a possible pituitary disease, it most often indicates an elevated prolactin level, which occurs in one third of women with amenorrhea. Breast discharge by itself does not indicate probable breast cancer. (Dunnihoo, 1992)

3. *Answer:* d (plan/reproductive/adult)
   Rationale: These symptoms, signs of androgen excess that may indicate polycystic ovarian disease, should be evaluated by a physician before initiation of hormone therapy. Because these symptoms are a change in her normal status, a more serious condition must be ruled out. (Dunnihoo, 1992)

4. *Answer:* b (plan/reproductive/adult)
   Rationale: Hypothyroidism is a fairly common cause of amenorrhea and with treatment should result in regular menstrual cycles. PTU is the treatment for hyperthyroidism. A thyroid scan is not necessary if the client responds to replacement therapy, and neither is a CT scan. (Glass, 1992)

5. *Answer:* b (plan/reproductive/adolescent)

Rationale: Irregular menstrual cycles are common for the first year or two as a result of irregular ovulatory cycles. It is not necessary to do further testing as long as she continues to menstruate at least once every 6 months. (Dunnihoo, 1992)

6. *Answer:* d (evaluation/reproductive/NAS)

Rationale: One of the side effects of medroxyprogesterone (Depo-Provera) is irregular menstrual cycles, often including amenorrhea. Levonorgestrel (Norplant) may cause breakthrough bleeding. Neither levothyroxine (Synthroid) nor beta-blockers are known to cause amenorrhea. (Hawkins, Roberto-Nichols, & Stanley-Haney, 1995)

7. *Answer:* a (plan/reproductive/NAS)

Rationale: Although anovulatory women may have a difficult time becoming pregnant, "priming" them with low-dose estrogen will not increase their fertility. Withdrawal bleeding indicates sufficient estrogen to prevent osteoporosis and heart disease, which may occur from a decrease in estrogen production. They are also at no greater risk for development of endometriosis and uterine fibroids. However, unopposed estrogen may predispose these women toward endometrial cancer, and hormonal regulation is therefore necessary.

BREAST LUMPS

OVERVIEW
Definition

A *breast lump* is a three-dimensional, dominant, palpable lump or area of thickening distinct from the surrounding breast tissue and generally asymmetric in comparison with the other breast.

Incidence

Four of five masses are benign; but malignancy must always be ruled out. According to the American Cancer Society (ACS), a woman has a 1:8 lifetime risk for breast cancer and a 1:28 lifetime risk for dying of breast cancer.

Pathophysiology

The most common benign breast masses, fibrocystic disease and fibroadenoma, represent a normal glandular response to fluctuating levels of estrogen.

FIBROCYSTIC DISEASE
- Not really pathologic, fibrocystic disease is rather a change in breast tissue associated with fluid-filled cysts within glandular structure.
- Such a change is experienced by 50% of all women.
- Breast lumps are cyclic in nature. Areas of thickness, nodularity, or cystic masses may be palpable and tender 7 to 14 days before menses.
- The condition ceases at menopause unless the client receives estrogen replacement therapy.
- Masses are multiple, round or lobular, soft and rubbery to thick, well circumscribed, and mobile, with no nipple retraction. Client can have tender, palpable axillary nodes. Fine, granular tissue or gross lumpiness can be palpated. Masses are most often found in upper outer quadrant. Local edema or overall enlargement may be present, with symmetrical findings in both breasts.
- Common ages for benign breast masses are 30 to 55 years.

FIBROADENOMA
- This is the most common benign breast tumor.
- It is an abnormal growth of fibrous and ductal tissue under hormonal influence.
- Not cyclic, with 10% to 20% recurrence rate
- Surgery provides definitive diagnosis and cure.
- Fibroadenoma is not associated with increased risk of breast cancer.
- Mass is single, nontender, soft or firm, freely moveable, and round or lobular in shape, with clear margins.
- Common ages are 20 to 40 years; the condition is rare after menopause.

- Excessively large fibroadenoma *(cystosarcoma phyllodes)* grows rapidly and may stretch the skin to the point of ulceration. It is a benign condition.

INTRADUCTAL PAPILLOMA
- Small, wartlike growth in lining of mammary duct, usually near nipple
- Most common cause of nipple discharge, usually bloody or serous and spontaneous
- Palpable mass occurs in approximately half of cases.
- Condition occurs commonly in women 45 to 55 years and increases after menopause.

FAT NECROSIS
- Onset of mass, usually palpated superficially, in direct response to trauma in half of cases
- It resolves slowly.
- No increase in cancer risk
- Findings: Ecchymosis possible, painless mass, nipple retraction common
- It is common in overweight women with large breasts or after breast surgery.
- It occurs at any age.

DUCT ECTASIA
- Result of dilation of subareolar ducts, with fibrosis and inflammation behind nipple.
- Areola may be reddened.
- No increase in cancer risk
- It causes burning pain exacerbated by cold, itching nipple, and nipple discharge (thin watery in young women and thick, sticky, pasty in older women); nipple retraction is possible.
- It is common in women 45 to 55 years old.
- Treated with antibiotics

BREAST CANCER
- Breast cancer is the second leading cause of cancer death in women (first is lung cancer).
- Malignant cells invade breast tissue, with malignant potential for spread.
- Findings suggestive of malignancy are as follows: Mass, often single, irregular, or stellate; fixed, not clearly distinct from surrounding tissue; firm to rock hard; unilateral; nipple retraction common; bloody discharge common; prominent vascular pattern on affected breast; peau d'orange (thick skin resembling orange peel) because of blocked lymphatic drainage.
- There may or may not be pain.

- Common ages are 30 to 80; prevalence significantly increases after menopause.
- Breast cancer is more than 100 times more common in women than men.

PAGET'S DISEASE. This type of breast cancer affects the epidermis of the nipple or areola. Its presenting symptoms include an eczema-like rash with excoriation and scaling.

PROTECTIVE FACTORS. Breast-feeding, early first pregnancy, and oral contraceptive use provide some protection against certain breast masses and breast cancer.

FACTORS INCREASING SUSCEPTIBILITY. Eighty-five percent of women who get breast cancer have one of the following risk factors:
- Age older than 50 years
- Personal history of breast cancer
- Family history, first-degree relatives with breast cancer
- History of fibrocystic disease with epithelial hyperplasia
- Early menarche (younger than 12 years) and late menopause (older than 55 years)
- Nulliparity
- Age greater than 30 years at first pregnancy
- Exposure to ionizing radiation
- Prolonged hormone replacement with unopposed estrogen
- Excessive alcohol use
- Exposure to toxic substances
- Smoking
- Increased fat in diet
- Obesity
- Diethylstilbestrol (DES) exposure
- Ashkenazi Jewish heritage (increased probability of inherited breast cancer gene)

ASSESSMENT: SUBJECTIVE/HISTORY

Most breast masses are discovered by the client herself. The following subjective data should be elicited from the client with a breast mass:
- Location and description of mass
- When discovered
- What changes, if any, in mass since discovery
- Relationship to menstrual cycle
- Any changes in skin over area of mass
- Any trauma to breast
- Change in breast
- Previous mass (if yes, elicit details)

- Last menstrual period (LMP)
- Menstrual and obstetric history, age at menarche
- Last breast self-examination (BSE), last clinical examination, last mammogram or breast ultrasound
- Evidence of risk factors for breast cancer
- Hormone replacement therapy

Symptoms

- Pain or tenderness: If present, describe when, where, how much on a 0- to 10-point scale, what makes it better, and what exacerbates it?
- Nipple discharge: If present, describe duration, color, and characteristics of fluid and whether it occurs spontaneously or is elicited.
- Palpable, tender axillary lymph nodes

Past Medical History

- Previous breast mass: Provide details about diagnosis and treatment.
- Previous breast, ovary, colorectal or other cancer
- Trauma to breast

Medication History

Ask about use of the following medications:

- Oral contraceptives
- Medications associated with nipple discharge:
  —Tricyclic antidepressants
  —Diuretics
  —Phenothiazines
  —Steroids
  —Phenytoin
  —Digitalis
  —Reserpine
  —Methyldopa
- Medications with significant levels of methylxanthines, which exacerbate fibrocystic disease, are thought to increase mastalgia:
  —Aspirin plus caffeine (Anacin)
  —Aspirin, caffeine, and cinnamedrine (Midol)
  —Caffeine plus ergotamine tartrate (Cafergot)
  —Aspirin (Empirin)
  —Butalbital (Fiorinal)
  —Chlorpheneramine maleate plus phenylephrine hydrochloride, with or without aspirin (Dristan)
  —Theophylline
  —Aspirin plus oxycodone hydrochloride (Percodan)
  —Cimetidine, associated with gynecomastia

Family History

Ask about family history of breast, ovarian, and colorectal cancer; such history is especially significant in first-degree maternal relatives or men. Ask about other cancers.

Psychosocial History

Ask about OTC, prescription, and leisure drug use. Ask about smoking, caffeine use, and alcohol use. Determine client's feelings of uncertainty and anxiety and responses of her partner and family to the news of her finding the breast lump. The nurse practitioner must appreciate that few findings are as alarming to a woman and her partner than a breast mass, because the potential for malignancy always exists. Many fear the consequences of a cancer diagnosis and the possibility of pain, debilitating illness, disfiguring surgery, and death.

Dietary History

Ask about methylxanthines (coffee, tea, cola, chocolate) in diet since restricting these, although not research-proven, seem to help relieve some cyclic breast pain. For the same reason, ask about caffeine use, vegetables, especially those with carotene, and dietary sodium use. Ask about the amounts of beef and fat in diet; excesses are believed to increase susceptibility to cancer.

ASSESSMENT: OBJECTIVE/ PHYSICAL EXAMINATION

Physical Examination

A problem-oriented physical examination should be conducted with particular attention to the following:

- General appearance and examination of the breasts
- Axilla
- Supraclavicular and infraclavicular lymph nodes

CLIENT SITTING ON EXAMINATION TABLE WITH ARMS AT SIDES. Observe uncovered breasts for symmetry, contour, change in vascular pattern.

Note discoloration or peau d'orange skin, retraction of nipple, crusting of areola and nipple, and local edema. Repeat observation with arms over head and with arms pressing against hips.

CLIENT SUPINE. Inspect breasts and skin. Begin palpation on opposite side from identified mass. Palpate entire breast, including tail of Spence, for masses. Palpate for axillary, supraclavicular, and infraclavicular lymphadenopathy. Massage entire breast toward nipple to attempt to elicit nipple discharge. If client has breast implants, check for location, extent of healing, symmetry, and presence of bulging.

CLIENT WITH PENDULOUS BREASTS. Examine with client sitting up and leaning forward. Support breast with inferior hand and use other hand to palpate. Note the following:

- Locate, with distance of mass from nipple in centimeters
- Size
- Shape: Oval, spherical, lobular, indistinct, stellate, irregular
- Consistency: Soft, firm, rubbery, hard
- Mobility: Freely movable vs fixed on chest wall
- Solitary vs multiple
- Nipple retraction
- Dimpling
- Discharge
- Tenderness

MEN. Men may have breast masses, too. Examination is the same as in women.

PREPUBERTAL MALE. Breast enlargement is normal in the prepubertal male, usually with bilateral enlargement. Recheck in 6 months. If the client is embarrassed or distressed, refer him to a surgeon.

Diagnostic Procedures

MAMMOGRAM. Mammography is used in women older than 35 years to locate suspect lesions. Can localize masses <1 cm, which is the smallest clinically detectable mass, increasing the survival potential and decreasing the necessity for extensive surgery. Mammography cannot distinguish benign from malignant disease; 10% of normal results occur with actual presence of breast cancer. Radiation dose approximates that received during a day in the sun. Indications are as follows:

- Ages 35 to 40 years: Baseline
- Ages 40 to 49 years: Every 2 years
- Ages 50 years and older: Every year
- With first-degree relative with premenopausal breast cancer, schedule first mammogram 5 to 10 years before the age of the relative at diagnosis.
- Men with breast mass (any age)

BREAST ULTRASONOGRAPHY

- Is more effective for women younger than 35 years who have denser breast tissue.
- Differentiates cystic from solid masses.
- Exposes the client to less radiation.

FINE-NEEDLE ASPIRATION (FNA). Aspiration of fluid from cystic mass with sterile technique, with or without local anesthesia, followed by cytologic analysis by a pathologist. (NOTE: Papanicolaou smear of breast fluid yields inconclusive results).

GENETIC STUDIES. BRAC-1 (long arm of chromosome 17) and BRAC-2 (chromosome 13) are transmitted by autosomal dominant inheritance pattern. There is an increased risk of breast cancer in those who inherit an abnormal gene.

DIAGNOSIS

Differential diagnosis includes the following:

- Fibrocystic breast disease
- Mammary duct ectasia
- Fat necrosis
- Carcinoma
- Intraductal papilloma
- Paget's disease
- Mastitis
- Normal premenstrual breast tissue
- Costal cartilage disorder (Tietze's syndrome)
- Fibroadenoma

THERAPEUTIC PLAN
Pharmacologic Treatment

- Oral contraceptives daily or medroxyprogesterone acetate (Provera) days 15 to 25 of cycle may be used for cyclic pain.
- For fibrocystic disease: Vitamin E daily, evening primrose oil, vitamin B_6 (pyridoxine)
- As a last resort in cases of severe mastalgia, these drugs may be used (consultation with physician is advised): danazol (Danocrine), only drug approved by Food and Drug Administration for fibrocystic disease), tamoxifen, and bromocriptine (Parlodel). All have

significant side effects. A pregnancy test is advised because of teratogenicity.

Client Education

- Monthly BSE with ACS standards, reinforcing at each follow-up visit as necessary
- With fibrocystic disease:
  —Restriction of caffeine, alcohol, and methylxanthines may lessen pain.
  —Decrease alcohol use to <3 drinks/week.
  —Increase vegetables, especially those with carotene.
  —Decrease sodium 10 days before menses.
  —Do not smoke.
  —Decrease weight if obese.
  —Wear support bra, day and night.
  —Avoid trauma.
  —Take mild analgesics.
  —Use warm compresses.
  —Low-fat, high-fiber diet may offer protective effect against cancer.
- Advise client regarding ways to alter lifestyle to decrease risk of breast cancer.

Referral

- Mass suspect for cancer
- Cystic mass persisting after aspiration or 1 week past next menses
- Palpable lymph nodes
- Solid mass

EVALUATION/FOLLOW-UP

Ideal time for clinical breast examination is 7 to 9 days after menses. If office examination is performed during premenstrual phase and a mass is found, advise return in 2 to 3 weeks for re-check.

For soft, mobile mass or thickness with suspicion of fibrocystic changes in low-risk clients, consider reexamination week after next menses terminates. Refer if mass persists on reexamination.

Plan for follow-up of cystic mass:

- Do FNA; if cyst resolves, observation for 6 weeks. If it recurs, refer to surgeon.
- Do FNA; if cyst persists, obtain fluid for cytologic testing and refer to surgeon.

Treatment for breast cancer usually involves surgery, with or without breast reconstruction. Systemic treatment—adjuvant therapy with radiation, chemotherapy, hormonal therapy, or immune system stimulants—generally follows.

Survivors of breast cancer should continue monthly BSE and have a yearly mammogram and clinical examination with evaluation for a new breast cancer or metastasis. Special attention is paid to the increased risk of bowel, endometrial, and ovarian cancer in this population.

REFERENCES

Bowman, M. A., Braly, P. S., Johnson, S., & Mikuta, J. J. (1996). Who are you screening for cancer and when? *Patient Care, 30,* 54-87.

Carlson, K. J., Eisenstat, S. A., Frigoletto, F. D., & Schiff, I. (1995). *Primary care of women.* St. Louis: Mosby.

Conry, C. (1994). *Evaluation of a breast complaint: Is it cancer? American Family Physician, 49*(2), 445-452.

Donegan, W. L. (1992). Evaluation of a palpable breast mass. *New England Journal of Medicine, 327*(13), 937-941.

Fiorica, J. V., Schorr, S. J., & Sickles, E. A. (1997). Benign breast disorders—First rule out cancer. *Patient Care, 31,* 140-154.

Fogel, C. I., & Woods, N. F. (1995). *Women's health care: A comprehensive handbook.* Thousand Oaks, CA: Sage.

Lichtman, R., & Papera, S. (1990). *Gynecology well-woman care.* Norwalk, CT: Appleton & Lange.

Ma, J. C., & Easter, D. W. (1995). Current guidelines for breast cancer screening. *Contemporary Nurse Practitioner, 1,* (5), 10-17.

Marchant, D. J. (1994). Contemporary management of breast disease II: Breast cancer. Risk factors. *Obstetrics and Gynecology Clinics of North America, 21*(4), 561-586.

Reifsnider, E. (1990). Educating women about benign breast disease. *AAOHN Journal, 38*(2), 121-125.

Star, W. L., Lommel, L. L., & Shannon, M. T. (1995). *Women's primary health care—Protocols for practice.* Washington, DC: American Nurses Publishing.

Treinen, A. D. (1997). Breast cancer screening—Making sense of controversies. *Advance for Nurse Practitioners, 5*(5), 17-23.

Uphold, C., & Graham, M. V. (1994). *Clinical guidelines in family practice.* Gainesville, FL: Barmarrae Books.

White, G. L., Griffeth, C. J., Nenstiel, R. O., & Dyers, D. L. (1996). Breast cancer: Reducing mortality through early detection. *Clinician's Review, 6,* (10), 77-106.

Youngkin, E. Q., & Davis, M. S. (1994). *Women's health: A primary care clinical guide.* Norwalk, CT: Appleton & Lange.

REVIEW QUESTIONS

1. Which factor in a woman's history would be considered positive protection against breast cancer?

    a. She has breast-fed four children.
    b. She experienced menarche at age 10 years.
    c. She drank alcohol excessively for years but quit recently.
    d. Her mother and grandmother had early menopause.

2. Which objective finding is **not** usually associated with breast cancer?

    a. Rubbery, well-circumscribed, tender lesion
    b. Eczema-like scaling on one aerola and nipple
    c. Peau d'orange dimpling of skin over breast
    d. Unilateral deviated and retracted nipple

3. The examination of a 27-year-old woman reveals the following: irregular, unilateral, stony-hard mass, poorly defined, with spontaneous bloody discharge from a retracted nipple. What diagnosis is most appropriate?

    a. Fibroadenoma
    b. Paget's disease
    c. Breast cancer
    d. Intraductal papilloma

4. For which client should ultrasonography be ordered to evaluate a breast mass?

    a. 27-year-old Gail
    b. 39-year-old Merry
    c. 51-year-old Anna
    d. 68-year-old Thelma

5. Twenty-year-old Ms. Stelly comes in for an annual examination. Her next menstrual period is due to start in 3 days. The family nurse practitioner notes multiple cystic areas bilaterally, and the client's breasts are extremely tender. What follow-up will be most appropriate?

    a. Client should return for re-check 7 to 10 days after her period ends.
    b. No follow-up is necessary because she is problem free.
    c. Ultrasonography of breasts should be performed within 24 hours.
    d. Client should return for recheck in 1 month.

6. A breast biopsy is considered mandatory with which of the following findings?

    a. Straw-colored fluid aspirated with FNP
    b. Nonpalpable lesion found on mammogram
    c. Ecchymotic area on the breast of a woman injured in a fall
    d. Production of milky discharge after sexual stimulation of the breasts

7. Ms. Strauss, age 26 years, is a new client who comes in for a preemployment physical examination. History reveals that her mother had breast cancer diagnosed at age 38 years. In addition to a clinical examination and monthly BSE, this client should be advised to have a baseline mammogram:

    a. At 28 to 33 years of age
    b. At 40 to 45 years of age
    c. Within the next 6 months
    d. Anytime before her 50th birthday

ANSWERS AND RATIONALES

1. *Answer:* a (assessment/history/reproductive/NAS)
    Rationale: Breast-feeding appears to impart a protective effect against breast cancer. (Marchant, 1994)

2. *Answer:* a (assessment/physical examination/reproductive/NAS)
    Rationale: Peau d'orange and nipple retraction are common features of breast cancer; the cancer of Paget's disease reveals nipple and areola scaling, erythema, and erosion similar to eczema. (Star, Lommell, & Shannon, 1995)

3. *Answer:* c (diagnosis/reproductive/adult)
    Rationale: Cancerous masses are usually unilateral, hard, and rough-edged. Nipple retraction and bloody discharge are common manifestations. (Fiorica, Schorr, & Sickles, 1997)

4. *Answer:* a (plan/management/diagnostics/reproductive/NAS)
    Rationale: Ultrasonography is more effective for evaluating the dense breasts of the woman younger than 35 years. (Fiorica et al., 1997)

5. *Answer:* a (evaluation/reproductive/adult)
    Rationale: Clinical breast examination is best performed a week or so after the onset of menses, when the breast is least congested. (Fiorica et al., 1997)

6. *Answer:* b (plan/management/diagnostics/reproductive/NAS)

Rationale: Mammography identifies masses <1 cm earlier than when they are clinically palpable. (Fiorica et al., 1997)

7. *Answer:* a (evaluation/reproductive/adult)

Rationale: If a first-degree relative had breast cancer develop before menopause, start screening the client when she is 5 to 10 years younger than that relative was at diagnosis. (Bowman, Braly, Johnson, & Mikuta, 1996)

CHLAMYDIA

OVERVIEW
Definition

- Chlamydia is a sexually transmitted disease (STD) caused by *Chlamydia trachomatis.*
- Chlamydial infection is one of the most common STDs in the United States today.
- It is often asymptomatic in both men and women.
- Routine screening of young adult women is currently recommended, particularly those not using barrier methods of birth control or those who have new or multiple partners.
- Transmission to the infant occurs in 70% of untreated women with chlamydial infection during pregnancy.
- It is frequently found in conjunction with gonorrhea.

Pathophysiology

Chlamydia infects the genital tract of women at the transition zone of the endocervix. It is an obligate intracellular organism.

RISK FACTORS INCREASING SUSCEPTIBILITY
- Sexual promiscuity, multiple sexual partners
- No use of barrier contraceptives
- Lower socioeconomic status
- Inversely related to age

ASSESSMENT: SUBJECTIVE/HISTORY
History of Present Illness

Obtain information regarding the following:
- Sexual practices
- Use of barrier methods of protection
- Changes in partners or in number of partners
- Any previous infections and treatments
- Last contact with partner(s)

Symptoms

In women the disease is often asymptomatic. If left untreated, however, the affected woman reports abdominal pain, vaginal pain, dysuria, and postcoital bleeding. Men may also be free of symptoms; however, more often they report a thick, cloudy penile discharge with dysuria.

ASSESSMENT: OBJECTIVE/ PHYSICAL EXAMINATION
Physical Examination

MEN. Examination should include examination of the penis, including "milking" of the shaft to assess for presence of a discharge, and examination of the testes.

WOMEN. Examination should focus on the abdomen (checking for guarding and rebound tenderness), genitalia (looking for excoriation, lesions, and ulcerations), and pelvic examination (assessing the cervix for friability). Look for any mucopurulent discharge. The bimanual examination may demonstrate motion tenderness, adnexal tenderness, or uterine fullness.

Diagnostic Procedures

Wet preparation may show increased WBCs and decreased normal vaginal flora. There are multiple laboratory tests available; sensitivities and specificities may vary. Cultures should also be done to check for gonorrhea at the same time. Consider testing for syphilis and HIV if history indicates.

DIAGNOSIS

Differential diagnosis includes gonorrhea, appendicitis, and cystitis.

Men

- Urethritis
- Epididymitis
- Proctitis

Women

- Cervicitis
- Urethral symptoms
- Bartholinitis
- Endometritis
- Pelvic inflammatory disease (PID)

Infants

- Conjunctivitis
- Pneumonitis

THERAPEUTIC PLAN

Doxycycline 100 mg PO bid for 7 days or azithromycin 1 g PO in a single dose. Azithromycin's safety and efficacy has not been established for persons 15 years old or younger. (NOTE: This will change in the Centers for Disease Control and Prevention [CDC] 1998 treatment guidelines for sexually transmitted diseases.) Ofloxacin, erythromycin, and sulfisoxazole are also available for treatment.

Pregnant or Lactating Clients

Erythromycin or amoxicillin is recommended; however, a test of cure 1 month after completion of therapy is necessary. (NOTE: The 1998 CDC guidelines will include azithromycin 1 g PO in a single dose for pregnant women and will not require a test of cure.)

Neonates

Erythromycin with follow-up to determine resolution.

Public Health

Partners must be treated to prevent reinfection, including any partner within the past 60 days, regardless of symptoms. Also, in most states *Chlamydia* is a reportable disease.

Complications

Complications in women include PID, pelvic abscess, infertility, and abnormal Papanicolaou smear secondary to cervicitis; those in men include epididymitis and Reiter's syndrome; those in neonates include conjunctivitis and pneumonia.

Client Education

- Use of barrier protection to decrease STD transmission.
- A possible sequela of untreated chlamydial infection is infertility.
- Perform tests for other STDs.

EVALUATION/FOLLOW-UP

Clients do not need to be retested for *Chlamydia* after completing treatment with doxycycline or azithromycin unless symptoms persist or reinfection is suspected.

REFERENCES

Centers for Disease Control and Prevention (1993). Sexually transmitted diseases treatment guidelines. *MMWR, Morbidity Mortality Weekly Report, 42* (RR-14), 50-55.

Dunnihoo, D. R. (1992). *Fundamentals of gynecology and obstetrics* (2nd ed.). Philadelphia: J. B. Lippincott.

Griffith, H., & Dambro, M. (1997). *The five-minute clinical consult* (4th ed.). Philadelphia: Lea & Febiger.

Hawkins, J. W., Roberto-Nichols, D. M., & Stanley-Haney, J. L. (1995). In *Protocols for nurse practitioners in gynecologic settings* (5th ed.). New York: Tiresias Press.

Johnson, C. A., Johnson, B. E., Murray, J. L., & Apgar, B. S. (1996). *Women's health care handbook.* St. Louis: Mosby.

Landers, D., & Sweet, R. (1993). Sexually transmitted infection. In R. H. Glass (Ed.), *Office gynecology* (4th ed.). Baltimore: Williams & Wilkins.

McMillan, A. (1995). Sexually transmittable diseases. In N. Loudon, A. Glaiser, & A. Gebbie (Eds.), *Handbook of family planning and reproductive health* (3rd ed.). New York: Churchill Livingstone.

Uphold, C. R., & Graham, M. V. (1994). *Clinical guidelines in family practice.* Gainesville, FL: Barmarrae Books.

REVIEW QUESTIONS

1. Reevaluating for a "test of cure" is not necessary with which medication?

   a. Amoxicillin
   b. Azithromycin
   c. Erythromycin
   d. Ofloxacin

2. A 13-year-old boy comes to the office with a report of pain with urination. On examination, the nurse practitioner sees a thick, milky discharge from the meatus. Treatment of choice for *Chlamydia* for this client includes:

   a. Azithromycin
   b. Doxycycline
   c. Erythromycin
   d. Ofloxacin

3. *Chlamydia* may cause what abnormal result in which test?

   a. Urinalysis
   b. Veneral Disease Research Laboratory Test (VDRL)
   c. Rapid plasma reagin test (RPR)
   d. Papanicolaou smear

4. Women who are treated for *Chlamydia* with doxycycline should receive which of the following cautions?

   a. They need to be recultured before they can be considered free of infection.
   b. Take medication before being considered free of infection.
   c. Use a backup method of birth control if using oral contraceptives.
   d. Use condoms if having sexual intercourse before partner is treated.

5. Clients treated with doxycycline should be cautioned that which of the following side effects may occur?

   a. Medication may cause gastrointestinal (GI) upset if taken with meals.
   b. Medication may cause a reaction in clients with allergies to sulfa.
   c. Medication may cause urine to change color.
   d. Medication may cause photosensitivity.

ANSWERS AND RATIONALES

1. *Answer:* b (evaluation/reproductive/NAS)
Rationale: Retesting may be considered after treatment with erythromycin and ofloxacin. Also, erythromycin and amoxicillin are used in pregnant women, and both require a test of cure in pregnancy. Azithromycin does not require a test of cure unless symptoms persist or reinfection is suspected. (CDC, 1993)

2. *Answer:* b (plan/reproductive/adolescent)
Rationale: Treatments of choice for *Chlamydia* include both azithromycin and doxycycline; however, the safety and efficacy of azithromycin have not been established for persons younger than 15 years. Erythromycin and ofloxacin are alternative methods of treatment. (CDC, 1993)

3. *Answer:* d (assessment/physical examination/reproductive/NAS)
Rationale: VDRL and RPR are tests for syphilis, and results of a urinalysis should be normal. A Papanicolaou smear may be abnormal, showing either inflammation or cellular changes related to cervicitis.

4. *Answer:* c (plan/reproductive/NAS)
Rationale: Persons treated with doxycycline do not require a test of cure. Clients should also be counseled not to have sexual intercourse until both parties have completed therapy. Although GI upset may occur with doxycycline, it is more important to instruct a woman using oral contraceptives to use a "backup" form of birth control, because many antibiotics decrease the efficacy of birth control pills. (Hawkins, Roberto-Nichols, & Stanley-Haney, 1995)

5. *Answer:* d (plan/reproductive/NAS)
Rationale: Doxycycline should be taken with meals to prevent GI upset. There is no connection between doxycycline and sulfa medications, and it has not been shown to discolor the urine. It may, however, increase photosensitivity, and the client should be warned appropriately. (Hawkins, et al., 1995)

DYSFUNCTIONAL UTERINE BLEEDING

OVERVIEW
Definition

Dysfunctional uterine bleeding (DUB) is abnormal uterine bleeding without readily identifiable cause. Diagnosis is by exclusion because of numerous etiologies.

ADENOMYOSIS. This is growth of endometrial tissue within and under the myometrium.

LEIOMYOMAS. These are benign, slow-growing tumors made up of smooth muscle that develop in the uterus during reproductive years.

METORRHAGIA. This is irregular bleeding or bleeding between periods.

MENORRHAGIA. This is heavy or prolonged bleeding.

POLYMENORRHEA. This is menstruation less than 22 days.

CONTACT BLEEDING. Postcoital bleeding is called *contact bleeding*.

DYSMENORRHEA. Painful menstruation is known as *dysmenorrhea*.

Pathophysiology

Sometimes a cause cannot be identified. Usually DUB is caused by anovulation (without LH surge or with insufficient progesterone, endometrial lining begins to shed), as with menarche or menopause. Other causes are obesity, hyperthyroidism, hypothyroidism, coagulation disorder, polycystic ovaries, trauma, leiomyoma, STD, malignancy, contraception, trauma, spontaneous abortion, endometritis, medications, or hypothalamic, pituitary, or ovarian dysfunction.

ASSESSMENT: SUBJECTIVE/HISTORY
Menorrhagia

Client may have single occurrence of heavy bleeding or recurrent prolonged, heavy bleeding. Client may or may not report pelvic pain.

Metorrhagia

Client may have spotting, hemorrhage, or bleeding between menses, with oral contraceptives and levonorgestrel (Norplant) (most often at midcycle), with medroxyprogesterone acetate, and perimenopause.

Leiomyoma

- Pelvic heaviness
- Low abdominal pressure
- Constipation
- Urinary incontinence
- Dysmenorrhea
- Spotting throughout cycle

Adenomyosis

- Dysmenorrhea
- Menorrhagia
- Premenstrual spotting

Past Medical History

Ask about the following:
- Menstrual history (menarche, cycle length and duration)
- Birth control method
- History of liver disease
- Diabetes
- Hypertension
- Obesity
- Thyroid disorder
- Blood dyscrasia or coagulation abnormality
- Dysmenorrhea
- Date of last sexual contact
- Number of sexual partners
- Vaginal discharge
- Pelvic pain or bleeding after intercourse
- Date of last Papanicolaou smear
- Past Papanicoloau smear results

Ask client to describe the abnormal bleeding pattern. If she has been saturating one pad per hour for 7 days, blood loss is significant.

Medication History

- Major tranquilizers
- Anticoagulants
- Oral contraceptives
- Steroids
- Chemotherapy
- Medroxyprogesterone (Depo-Provera)
- Levonorgestrel (Norplant)

Family History

Ask about family history of leiomyoma. Ask about age of client's mother at menopause.

Dietary History

Ask about dietary history, particularly if client is obese.

Psychosocial History

Ask about history of psychiatric illness. Ask about smoking (smoking decreases the chance of leiomyoma).

ASSESSMENT: OBJECTIVE/ PHYSICAL EXAMINATION

Every physical examination for DUB should include a thorough pelvic examination with careful Papanicolaou smear.

Bimanual Examination

Bimanual examination may suggest adenomyosis (globular, boggy enlargement of uterus), pregnancy (even, smooth enlargement), or leiomyoma (smooth, spherical, firm masses). Note amount of bleeding coming through cervical os and presence of polyps. Perform cervical culture or microscopic examination if indicated. If using intrauterine contraceptive device (IUD), visualize strings. Palpate thyroid.

Diagnostic Procedures

Perform endometrial biopsy (especially if client is perimenopausal or menopausal) to rule out endometrial carcinoma or hyperplasia. Ultrasonography is useful for identifying leiomyomas, polyps, or adnexal masses; it is not useful with adenomyosis. Laboratory tests depend on age, history, and physical examination and include urine hCG if suspected pregnancy, thyroid function studies if indicated and hemoglobin and hematocrit if excessive bleeding. Determine FSH levels if suspected menopause (>30 mIU/ml suggests menopause). If client uses oral contraceptives, draw FSH level on fifth day of placebo pills. Perform coagulation studies on any woman younger than 35 years with excessive bleeding and hemoglobin <10 g/dl.

DIAGNOSIS

Differential diagnoses includes the following:
- Pregnancy
- Uterine or cervical polyps
- Leiomyomas
- Carcinoma
- STD
- Adenomyosis
- Anovulation
- Endocrine disorders
- Thyroid disorder

THERAPEUTIC PLAN

Treatment depends on specific cause.

Pharmacologic Treatment

- If bleeding is severe, obtain gynecologic consultation with hospitalization for IV conjugated estrogens or dilatation and curettage.
- Oral therapy includes iron therapy and dietary adjustment if anemia is identified. Thyroid replacement may be indicated.
- Give hormonal therapy if there are no contraindications. If endometrial biopsy is not required, initial therapy includes medroxyprogesterone acetate, 10 mg PO daily for 10 days (each month days 19 through 28 of menstrual cycle).
- Nonsteroidal antiinflammatory drugs (NSAIDs) decrease endometrial blood through an antiprostaglandin effect.
- Monophasic oral contraceptives promote atrophy of endometrial lining and provide lacking progestin. If client is having heavy bleeding and is not pregnant, give oral contraceptives twice daily for 1 week, then once daily for next 2 weeks, or give conjugated estrogens at 1.25 mg bid for 1 week, then once daily with medroxyprogesterone at 10 mg/day for 2 weeks. If unsuccessful, obtain gynecologic consultation.
- If biopsy reveals proliferative endometrium, give medroxyprogesterone at 10 mg/day for 10 days each month for 3 months, with a repeated biopsy at 3 months.
- Long-term therapy (especially if birth control is desired) includes monophasic oral contraceptives or medroxyprogesterone acetate at 150 mg IM every 3 months. Monthly luteal phase medroxyprogesterone (10 mg daily for 10 days) may be used if birth control is not desired. Antibiotics are indicated for STDs or endometritis.

Client Education

- Stress importance of safe sex practices.
- Explain side effects of medications, treatment plan, treatment options, and signs and symptoms to report.
- Stress importance of scheduled Papanicolaou smears and gynecologic examination.
- Discuss fertility concerns or client concerns surrounding menopause.
- If client chooses myomectomy for leiomyoma, risk of recurrence is unknown. Polyps often return after removal. Hysterectomy is often successful for carcinoma.

Referral

Refer client if abnormal bleeding resumes after being controlled (suspect malignancy), if ectopic pregnancy is suspected, if bleeding occurs 6 or more months after menopause (suspect malignancy), or if bleeding is severe or uncontrolled. Refer client if leiomyoma is larger than 12-week size or is rapidly increasing in size, if significant anemia is present, or if adenomyosis is suspected.

EVALUATION/FOLLOW-UP

- Repeat Papanicolaou smears per protocol for abnormal Papanicolaou smear.
- Schedule return visit 3 months after hormonal treatment.
- Perform test of cure for STDs 2 weeks after completion of therapy.

Special Considerations

- Leiomyomas may mask malignant uterine tumors (leiomyosarcoma).
- Any bleeding 6 months or longer after menopause suggests malignancy.
- Postcoital bleeding may indicate *either* STD or malignancy.
- Leiomyomas usually resolve with menopause.

REFERENCES

Brown, J. S., & Crombleholme, W. R. (1993). *Handbook of gynecology and obstetrics.* Norwalk, CT: Appleton & Lange.

DeCherney, A., & Pernoll, M. L. (Eds.). (1994). *Current obstetrics and gynecology: Diagnosis and treatment.* Norwalk, CT: Appleton & Lange.

Fogel, C. I., & Woods, N. F. (1995). *Women's health care.* Thousand Oaks, CA: Sage.

Lemke, D. P., Pattison, J., Marshall, L. A., & Cowley, D. S. (1995). *Primary care of women.* Norwalk, CA: Appleton & Lange.

Strickland, K. (1996). Primary care management of leiomyoma-induced abnormal bleeding. *Journal of the American Academy of Nurse Practitioners, 8*(11), 541-545.

REVIEW QUESTIONS

1. A 55-year-old woman reports vaginal bleeding. She is distressed because she has not had a period for the past 12 months and says, "I didn't anticipate this period." What condition would you suspect given this situation?

   a. Perimenopause
   b. Leiomyoma
   c. Anovulation
   d. Malignancy

2. Which of the following laboratory studies should be done on any woman with excessive vaginal bleeding?

   a. Urine hCG
   b. FSH
   c. Hematocrit and hemoglobin
   d. TSH

3. Which of the following statements is true regarding education of a 42-year-old woman with diagnosed leiomyoma?

   a. Myomectomy ensures that leiomyomas will never return.
   b. Leiomyomas usually resolve with menopause.
   c. Hysterectomy is the only choice of treatment.
   d. Leiomyomas become larger with the withdrawal of estrogen.

4. After a pregnancy test, which of the following laboratory tests would you order for an anemic 16-year-old with heavy vaginal bleeding?

   a. FSH and LH
   b. Thyroid studies
   c. Estrogen levels
   d. Prothrombin time, partial thromboplastin time and platelets

5. Which of the following must be included in the physical examination of a 38-year-old woman who reports contact bleeding?

    a. Uterine biopsy

    b. Papanicolaou smear

    c. Palpation of thyroid

    d. IUD string visualization

6. Which of the following symptoms is common with leiomyoma?

    a. Midcycle spotting

    b. Pelvic pain

    c. Pelvic heaviness

    d. Premenstrual syndrome

7. A 51-year-old client returns 2 months after treatment with a report of return of heavy bleeding. Which of the following should be the next step in her therapy?

    a. Begin progesterone at 10 mg PO daily for 10 days.

    b. Reinstitute therapy as previously ordered.

    c. Refer client for further evaluation.

    d. Schedule client for leiomyoma excision.

8. Which of the following questions should be included in the history taking of a 36-year-old woman with reports of dysmenorrhea, vaginal spotting, and constipation?

    a. Does she drink alcohol?

    b. Does she smoke?

    c. Does she use oral contraceptives for birth control?

    d. How many times has she been pregnant?

9. Differential diagnosis for a woman with a uterine contour distorted by several spherical, firm masses includes which of the following?

    a. PID vs ectopic pregnancy

    b. Leiomyoma vs polycystic ovaries

    c. Adenomyosis vs leiomyoma

    d. Leiomyoma vs leiosarcoma

10. Which of the following is the treatment of choice when uterine biopsy reveals proliferative endometrium?

    a. Progesterone at 10 mg daily for 10 days

    b. Oral contraceptives for 21 days

    c. Conjugated estrogens at 3.75 mg for 21 days

    d. Medroxyprogesterone (Depo-Provera) at 150 mg IM monthly for 3 months

ANSWERS & RATIONALES

1. **Answer:** d (diagnosis/reproductive/adult)
Rationale: With any bleeding 6 months or more after menopause, suspect malignancy. (Fogel & Woods, 1995)

2. **Answer:** c (diagnosis/reproductive/NAS)
Rationale: With excessive bleeding in any woman, an evaluation for anemia is necessary. (Lemke, Pattison, Marshall, & Cowley, 1995)

3. **Answer:** b (plan/reproductive/adult)
Rationale: Leiomyomas regress after menopause as a result of estrogen decrease. (Strickland, 1996)

4. **Answer:** d (plan/reproductive/adolescent)
Rationale: Coagulation studies are indicated for a woman younger than 35 years with heavy bleeding and a hemoglobin <10 g/dl. (Brown & Crombleholme, 1993)

5. **Answer:** b (assessment/physical examination/reproductive/adult)
Rationale: Contact bleeding must be considered a sign of cervical cancer until proved otherwise. (DeCherney & Pernoll, 1994)

6. **Answer:** c (assessment/reproductive/NAS)
Rationale: Leiomyomas are rarely painful, but pelvic heaviness is a common complaint. (DeCherney & Pernoll, 1994)

7. **Answer:** c (evaluation/reproductive/adolescent)
Rationale: Recurrent abnormal bleeding warrants further investigation. (Brown & Crombleholme, 1993)

8. **Answer:** b (assessment/history/reproductive/childbearing female)
Rationale: Smoking decreases the risk for leiomyomas, probably by decreasing estrogen levels. (Strickland, 1996)

9. **Answer:** d (diagnosis/reproductive/childbearing female)
Rationale: The most serious consequence of leiomyoma is that it may mask malignant uterine tumors. (Strickland, 1996)

10. **Answer:** a (evaluation/reproductive/NAS)
Rationale: Proliferative endometrium diagnosed by biopsy can be treated with progesterone to promote atrophy of endometrial lining. (Lemke et al., 1995)

DYSMENORRHEA: PRIMARY AND SECONDARY

OVERVIEW
Definition

Primary dysmenorrhea is defined as painful menstruation, occurring with ovulatory menstrual cycles and in the absence of pelvic pathology. *Secondary dysmenorrhea* is defined as painful menses caused by pelvic pathology (endometriosis is the most common cause).

Incidence

PRIMARY DYSMENORRHEA
- Primary dysmenorrhea is the most common medical problem in young women and the most common gynecologic problem.
- It is estimated that 50% of all menstruating women have dysmenorrhea, with 10% having symptoms severe enough to interfere with school, work, or other activities.
- Onset is usually at least 6 to 12 months after menarche, or when ovulatory cycles begin.
- Incidence increases and peaks in the late teens and early 20s, then gradually declines with age.
- Incidence is increased in women who are obese, smoke, are sexually inactive, are nulliparous, or delay childbearing.

SECONDARY DYSMENORRHEA
- Incidence is unknown.
- Onset is usually after age 25 to 30 years.
- Incidence gradually increases with age.

Pathophysiology

PRIMARY DYSMENORRHEA
- It is due to increased levels of prostaglandins during the luteal phase of the menstrual cycle, causing increased myometrial muscle tone, uterine contractions, and vasopression of uterine vessels, which results in ischemic pain and associated symptoms (see below).
- Prostaglandin synthesis varies from woman to woman, as does degree of pain, but pain can be severe.
- Severity of pain is related to amount of prostaglandin produced.
- Tendency to synthesize prostaglandin tends to be hereditary, so daughters of mothers

with primary dysmenorrhea are more likely than others to have primary dysmenorrhea.
- Women with anovulatory cycles do not have luteal increases in prostaglandins and thus do not have primary dysmenorrhea.

SECONDARY DYSMENORRHEA. Secondary dysmenorrhea is associated with pelvic pathology; this is frequently endometriosis but can be many other causes, including but not limited to the following:
- Extrauterine
  —Congenital malformation
  —Endometriosis
  —Ovarian diseases, ectopic pregnancy
  —PID
  —Adhesive disease as a result of surgery or infection
- Intrauterine
  —Endometriosis
  —Adenomyosis
  —Leiomyomas
  —Polyps
  —Malignant tumors
  —Pregnancy or pregnancy complication
  —Congenital malformation
  —IUD
- Cervical
  —Congenital malformation
  —Polyps
  —Stenosis
- In rare cases of dysmenorrhea, no cause is determined.

ASSESSMENT: SUBJECTIVE/HISTORY

Obtain detailed menstrual and gynecologic history, including menarche, frequency and duration of menses, pain associated with the onset of menses, associated symptoms, sexual and obstetric histories (treatment of STDs, Papanicolaou smear history, contraceptive method, symptoms associated with sexual intercourse).

Symptoms

Description of the most common symptoms follows:

PRIMARY DYSMENORRHEA
- Pain is crampy; spasmodic lower abdominal and pelvic pain are characteristic.
- Pain may radiate to the upper thighs, groin, or lower back.
- Symptoms usually begin several hours before or at the onset of menses and last 24 to 72 hours, at which time they begin to abate.
- Pain may be moderate to severe, with some women having more severe pain than with labor.

Associated Symptoms. Associated symptoms may include nausea, vomiting, diarrhea, constipation, headache, fatigue, weakness, diaphoresis, flushing, anxiety, tension, depression, bloating with weight gain, and breast tenderness. Severe cases may have dizziness and fainting.

SECONDARY DYSMENORRHEA
- Symptoms are more variable, depending on cause.
- Pain may occur at any time during the menstrual cycle and tends to increase with age.
- A detailed menstrual and gynecologic history can often differentiate primary from secondary dysmenorrhea.
- Additional diagnostic tests and usually referral are necessary to diagnose secondary dysmenorrhea.

Associated Symptoms. Associated symptoms of secondary dysmenorrhea depend on the cause.

Past Medical History

Obtain a detailed menstrual and gynecologic history; also ask about hospitalizations, surgery and procedures, liver or renal disease, other chronic medical conditions, and allergies.

Medication History

Ask about any current prescription drugs, all OTC medications, contraceptive agents, and allergies. Query previous use of analgesics.

Family History

Look for positive family history for dysmenorrhea or other gynecologic problems.

Psychosocial History

Assess support systems, coping skills, and previous mechanisms for coping with pain.

Dietary History

Assess for diet high in refined sugar and salt, and for excessive caffeine. Obtain a complete nutritional history for the obese client.

ASSESSMENT: OBJECTIVE/ PHYSICAL EXAMINATION

Physical Examination

A problem-oriented physical examination should be conducted with particular attention to the following:
- General appearance
- Vital signs
- Weight
- Abdomen: Assess for masses, tenderness, other abnormality.
- Pelvic: Speculum visualization of cervix and bimanual examination to assess for cervical motion tenderness, adnexal tenderness and abnormality, uterine tenderness, and uterine enlargement or irregularity

PRIMARY DYSMENORRHEA. Physical examination is normal, although client may have some uterine and cervical tenderness if examined during symptoms. If evaluating for the first time, rule out pregnancy and pelvic infection.

SECONDARY DYSMENORRHEA. Pelvic pathology may or may not be found on examination; additional tests are necessary to confirm diagnosis.

Diagnostic Procedures

- Primary dysmenorrhea:
  —Papanicolaou smear
  —Pregnancy test
  —Vaginal wet mount
  —Cultures (cervical)
- Secondary dysmenorrhea: Tests are based on physical findings and symptoms and may include the following:
  —CBC, erythrocyte sedimentation rate (ESR) to rule out infection or inflammation
  —RPR to rule out syphilis
  —Cervical culture to rule out gonorrhea and *Chlamydia*
  —Vaginal wet mount to rule out bacterial vaginosis, trichomoniasis, and candidiasis
  —Papanicolaou smear to rule out cervical cancer
  —Pregnancy test

- Refer to consultant for additional tests such as the following:
  —Vaginal and pelvic ultrasonography
  —Laparoscopic examination
  —Hysteroscopy
  —Hysterosalpingogram

DIAGNOSIS

Differential diagnosis includes the following:
- Endometriosis
- PID
- Pregnancy complications
- Uterine, ovarian, cervical congenital malformation or other pathology
- Appendicitis
- Intestinal disease
- Renal or biliary colic

THERAPEUTIC PLAN
Primary Dysmenorrhea

PHARMACOLOGIC TREATMENT
1. Prostaglandin synthetase inhibitors (NSAIDs) are effective in 75% to 90% of cases; try various agents for 6 months before considering treatment a failure.
   - Three FDA-approved NSAIDs for primary dysmenorrhea:
     —Ibuprofen (Motrin, Advil, other analogs)
     —Indomethacin (Indocin)
     —Naproxen sodium (Anaprox)
   - Mefenamic acid (Ponstel), aspirin, and other NSAIDs are effective.
   - Treat 2 to 3 days when symptoms are present; best relief is obtained with treatment before onset of pain; may treat 1 to 2 days before onset of menses if (1) menses are regular, (2) client is not pregnant, and (3) client has no side effects or contraindications to medications.
   - Assess for sensitivity before administration.
   - Should take with food or milk to lessen GI side effects.
   - Contraindications: Hypersensitivity, peptic ulcer disease, renal or hepatic disorder, asthma, anticoagulant therapy, bleeding disorder

- Side effects: Nausea, abdominal pain, indigestion, constipation, diarrhea, fluid retention, rash, tinnitus, GI bleeding; renal, hepatic, or central nervous system toxicity
2. Oral contraceptives
   - Combined estrogen-progesterone pill is drug of choice if client also desires contraception and has no contraindications.
   - Effective pain relief is obtained in 90% cases.
3. Antiemetics are used if nausea and vomiting are major symptoms.
4. Surgery is used rarely, in severe cases; presacral neurectomy, laser uterosacral nerve ablation (LUNA), hysterectomy.
5. Vitamin E is recommended by some because of its mild prostaglandin inhibitory properties.
6. Vitamin B_6 is recommended by some for pain relief.
7. Calcium-channel blockers show promising effects in experimental use but are not yet approved for primary dysmenorrhea.

NONPHARMACOLOGIC TREATMENT
1. Local heat, gentle abdominal massage, pelvic tilt, and stretching to increase uterine blood flow and decrease muscle spasm
2. Transcutaneous electrical nerve stimulation to stimulate release of endorphins
3. Regular aerobic exercise, 3 to 4 times/week for 20 to 30 minutes to suppress prostaglandin release, to increase endorphin release, to promote fitness and weight loss, and to improve overall sense of well-being
4. Stress reduction, relaxation techniques
5. Diet: Decreased salt, caffeine, alcohol, refined sugar; increased complex carbohydrates, foods that cause diuresis; moderated amount of protein; weight loss if obese
6. Stop smoking.
7. Sexual activity: Sexual arousal and orgasm cause arteriolar vasodilatation in uterus, decreasing ischemic pain.
8. Pregnancy: Pregnancy reduces number of adrenergic nerves with only partial regeneration after delivery, resulting in decreased pain perception.

Secondary Dysmenorrhea

Treatment of secondary dysmenorrhea depends on the cause.

Client Education

PRIMARY DYSMENORRHEA

- Educate client about menstrual cycle and changes that occur.
- Inform client of nonpharmacologic measures.
- Teach about purpose, dosage, expected results, and potential effects of medications.
- Teach warning signs associated with oral contraceptive use.
- Keep record of menses, symptoms, effects of medications.
- Encourage follow-up with health care provider.

SECONDARY DYSMENORRHEA. Educational needs are determined by cause and treatment.

Referral

- Refer to consultant if secondary dysmenorrhea suspected.
- Refer client with primary dysmenorrhea to consultant for further evaluation if condition fails to improve on aforementioned treatment.

EVALUATION/FOLLOW-UP

PRIMARY DYSMENORRHEA. After initial evaluation, client should return at 2 months and at 4 months to evaluate therapy then annually for Papanicolaou smear and pelvic examination. Client should return to clinic with new or worsening symptoms.

SECONDARY DYSMENORRHEA. Follow up with consultant as instructed or with health care provider when diagnosis and treatment are established.

REFERENCES

Baker, S. (1994). Menstruation and related problems and concerns. In E. Youngkin & M. Davis, *Women's health care: A primary care clinical guide* (pp. 86-90). Norwalk, CT: Appleton & Lange.

Beck, W., Jr. (1993). *The national medical series for independent study: Obstetrics and gynecology* (3rd ed.). Philadelphia: Harwal.

Coupey, S. (1994). Menstrual disorders in adolescents. *Emergency Medicine, 26*(4), 21-36.

Gerbie, M. (1994). Complications of menstruation: Abnormal uterine bleeding. In A. DeCherney & M. Pernoll (Eds.), *Current obstetric and gynecologic diagnosis and treatment* (8th ed., pp. 664-665). Norwalk, CT: Appleton & Lange.

Havans, C., Sullivan, N., & Tilton, P. (Eds.). (1992). *Manual of outpatient gynecology* (2nd ed.). Boston: Little, Brown.

Hawkins, J., Roberto-Nichols, D., & Stanley-Haney, J. (1995). *Protocols for nurse practitioners in gynecologic settings* (5th ed.). New York: Tiresias Press.

Klotz, M. (1995). Dysmenorrhea, endometriosis, pelvic pain. In D. Lemcke, L. Marshall, J. Pattison, & D. Cowley. (Eds.), *Primary care of women* (pp. 420-422). Norwalk, CT: Appleton & Lange.

Murphy, J. (1995). Dysmenorrhea. In W. Star, L. Lommel, & M. Shannon. (Eds.), *Women's primary health care: Protocols for practice* (pp. 12/30-12/35). Washington, DC: American Nurses Publishing.

Stoll, S. (1991). Dysmenorrhea. In H. Frederickson & L. Wilkins-Haug, *Ob/gyn secrets* (pp. 12-18). St. Louis: Mosby.

Uphold, C., & Graham, M. (1994). *Clinical guidelines in family practice* (2nd ed.). Gainesville, FL: Barmarrae Books.

Webb, T. (1996). Common menstrual disorders. *Advance for Nurse Practitioners, 4*(1), 21-23.

REVIEW QUESTIONS

1. The cause of pain in primary dysmenorrhea is due to:

   a. Uterine muscle dysfunction
   b. Shedding of uterine lining
   c. Prostaglandin release and synthesis
   d. Endometriosis

2. Of the following, all are suggestive of secondary dysmenorrhea **except:**

   a. Spasmodic abdominal cramps and low back pain on days 1 through 3 of menses
   b. Pain intermittently throughout menstrual cycle
   c. Onset of menstrual pain at 38 years, increasing in severity
   d. Menstrual pain with anovulatory cycles

3. Diagnostic tests that may be used to evaluate for secondary dysmenorrhea include all the following **except:**

a. Laparoscopy
b. Sonography
c. Electrolytes
d. RPR

4. Symptoms associated with primary dysmenorrhea include all the following **except:**

a. Syncope
b. Seizures
c. Sweating
d. Spasmodic abdominal pain

5. Mary, 28 years old, seeks treatment. She has intermittent lower abdominal pain, dyspareunia, postcoital bleeding, and foul-smelling vaginal discharge. Of the following, the **least** likely diagnosis is:

a. Primary dysmenorrhea
b. Secondary dysmenorrhea
c. Endometriosis
d. PID

6. Mrs. Brown, 24 years old, has irregular, anovulatory menstrual cycles associated with intermittent abdominal pain. On the basis of this information, the most likely assessment to make is:

a. Primary dysmenorrhea
b. Endometriosis
c. Secondary dysmenorrhea
d. Uterine leiomyoma

7. Which of the following statements is true regarding the treatment of primary dysmenorrhea?

a. Oral contraceptives are the drug of choice when birth control is desired.
b. Mild narcotics are frequently necessary for the pain.
c. NSAIDs are completely safe and have no contraindications
d. Medication is not necessary because the pain and symptoms are psychologic.

8. All the following are routinely used as treatment measures for the associated symptoms of primary dysmenorrhea **except:**

a. Exercise
b. Hysterectomy
c. Local heat
d. Decreased-sodium diet

9. Jane, 29 years old, has just had primary dysmenorrhea diagnosed and has started on a regimen of NSAIDs. She should be evaluated:

a. As needed
b. Annually
c. In 2 months, then in 4 months
d. Weekly for 2 months

10. Betty, 35 years old, was referred to a consultant and secondary dysmenorrhea was diagnosed. Her treatment and follow-up will:

a. Be determined by the cause of the secondary dysmenorrhea
b. Include a Papanicolaou smear every 6 months
c. Consist of low-dose narcotics
d. Include annual endometrial biopsy

Answers and Rationales

1. *Answer:* c (assessment/history/reproductive/NAS)
Rationale: Prostaglandin release and synthesis occur during the luteal phase of the menstrual cycle. Prostaglandins stimulate uterine contractions, which results in menstrual cramps. (Beck, 1993)

2. *Answer:* a (assessment/history/reproductive/NAS)
Rationale: Secondary dysmenorrhea is associated with pelvic pathology and can occur at any time during the menstrual cycle. Although it can occur at any age, it typically occurs in the third and fourth decades and increases in intensity. (Baker, 1994)

3. *Answer:* c (diagnosis/reproductive/NAS)
Rationale: Many diagnostic tests may be used in the evaluation for secondary dysmenorrhea. Tests may include but are not limited to sonography, laparoscopy, hysteroscopy, hysterosalpingography, CBC, RPR, pregnancy tests, and cervical culture. Electrolytes serve no purpose in the diagnostic evaluation of secondary dysmenorrhea. (Murphy, 1995)

4. *Answer:* b (assessment/physical examination/reproductive/NAS)
Rationale: Symptoms associated with primary dysmenorrhea include but are not limited to nausea, vomiting, diarrhea, constipation, spasmodic abdominal cramping, lower back pain, pain in the groin or upper thighs, and diaphoresis. Fainting, weakness, fatigue, and nervousness have also been

identified. Seizures have not been identified as an associated symptom of primary dysmenorrhea.

5. *Answer:* a (diagnosis/reproductive/adult)

Rationale: Primary dysmenorrhea is characterized by pain associated with ovulatory cycles, with the pain occurring just before or with the onset of menses and lasting for 2 to 3 days. Pain between menstrual periods, dyspareunia, postcoital bleeding, and foul-smelling vaginal discharge are not associated with primary dysmenorrhea. (Webb, 1996)

6. *Answer:* c (diagnosis/reproductive/adult)

Rationale: Primary dysmenorrhea is associated with ovulatory cycles, with pain occurring just before or with the onset of menses. On the basis of the information provided, this client has secondary dysmenorrhea. Further diagnostic tests would be necessary to establish the diagnosis of endometriosis or uterine leiomyoma. (Beck, 1993)

7. *Answer:* a (plan/reproductive/NAS)

Rationale: A combined estrogen and progesterone oral contraceptive is the drug treatment of choice for primary dysmenorrhea when birth control is also desired and there are no contraindications to taking oral contraceptives. Narcotics are rarely indicated. Although NSAIDs are relatively safe, there are potential side effects and contraindications to their use (such as hypersensitivity, renal or liver disease, asthma, and peptic ulcer disease). (Baker, 1994)

8. *Answer:* b (plan/reproductive/NAS)

Rationale: As many as 90% of all primary dysmenorrhea cases are successfully treated with pharmacologic and nonpharmacologic approaches. Hysterectomy would be indicated extremely rarely as a treatment for primary dysmenorrhea. (Gerbie, 1994)

9. *Answer:* c (evaluation/reproductive/adult)

Rationale: Evaluation of treatment should be at 2 months and then at 4 months to evaluate effectiveness and to assess for any problems. Other choices listed are inappropriate. (Uphold & Graham 1994)

10. *Answer:* a (evaluation/reproductive/adult)

Rationale: There are many potential causes of secondary dysmenorrhea, and further diagnostic testing is required to establish the diagnosis. Specific treatment and follow-up are determined by the cause of secondary dysmenorrhea. (Hawkins, Roberto-Nichols, Stanley-Haney, 1995)

GONORRHEA

OVERVIEW
Definition

Gonorrhea is an STD caused by the organism *Neisseria gonorrhoeae.*

Incidence

Gonorrhea occurs in 1400/100,000 population, or approximately 1 million new cases a year. Often there are no (or few) symptoms in the early stages (25% in men, 80% in women).

Pathophysiology

Gonorrhea is caused by gram-negative diplococcus with an incubation period of 2 to 7 days.

FACTORS INCREASING RISK
- Sexual exposure to infected individuals
- No use of barrier protection
- Multiple sexual partners
- Infants born through infected birth canal
- Sexual abuse of child
- Autoinnoculation
- Presence of IUD

ASSESSMENT: SUBJECTIVE/HISTORY
History

History includes the following:
- Previous vaginal, urethral, and prostatic infections and treatments
- Any chronic illnesses
- Sexual history (including specific practices)
- Type of contraceptive used
- Most recent contact
- Any changes in menstrual flow
- HIV risk or exposure
- Any medications being taken

WOMEN. Women should be asked whether there is any dysuria, leukorrhea, labial pain or swelling, or abdominal pain. In later disease stages, female clients may report fever, purulent vaginal discharge, abnormal menses, joint pain or swelling, and tenderness in the pelvic region.

MEN. Men may report dysuria and a whitish discharge from the penis. Later, this discharge may become yellow-green and the male client may report testicular pain.

ASSESSMENT: OBJECTIVE/ PHYSICAL EXAMINATION

Physical Examination

FEMALE CLIENTS. The abdomen should be assessed for guarding, tenderness, and rebound pain. The pelvic examination should include inspection of the glands (Skene's and Bartholin's) and of the urethra. There may be a mucopurulent discharge from the cervix. The bimanual examination may demonstrate motion tenderness and generalized pelvic tenderness. The throat should also be assessed for tonsillar exudate, edema, and erythema.

MALE CLIENTS. The penis should be assessed for discharge, the testicles should be assessed for tenderness or swelling, and a rectal examination should be done to evaluate the prostate.

Diagnostic Procedures

- Wet preparations may show increased WBCs and decreased normal vaginal flora.
- There are multiple laboratory tests available; sensitivities and specificities may vary. Gram stain or DNA probes are used to identify the causative organism.
- Cultures of the throat, urethra, and anus should also be considered, depending on sexual practices.
- Testing for *Chlamydia* should be done at the same time.
- HIV testing should also be offered.

DIAGNOSIS

Differential diagnosis includes the following:
- *Chlamydia*
- Appendicitis
- Ectopic pregnancy
- PID

THERAPEUTIC PLAN

- Ceftriaxone, 125 mg IM in a single dose (causes pain at injection site)
- Cefixime, 400 mg PO in a single dose
- Ciprofloxacin, 400 mg PO in a single dose
- Ofloxacin, 400 mg PO in a single dose
- A treatment regimen for treating *Chlamydia*, azithromycin (Azithromax) or doxycycline, is added to one of the above.
- If pharyngeal infection is a concern, the client should be treated with either ceftriaxone or ciprofloxacin.

Pregnant Women

Pregnant women should be treated with either ceftriaxone or spectinomycin, 2 g IM in a single dose, or cefixime, 400 mg PO in a single dose. They should not be treated with either quinolones or tetracyclines.

Newborns

For the prophylactic management of ophthalmia neonatorum, these medications may be administered: 1% silver nitrate, 0.5% erythromycin ophthalmic ointment, and 3.1% tetracycline ophthalmic ointment.

Client Education

Emphasize the importance of barrier contraceptive methods to prevent recurrence. Discuss the signs and symptoms of the complications, and encourage the client to seek care quickly if he or she exhibits any of the symptoms.

EVALUATION/FOLLOW-UP

- Clients should be instructed to refer partners for treatment and to avoid sexual contact until all parties have been treated.
- All sexual contacts within the past 60 days should be referred for treatment, regardless of symptoms.
- Clients who are treated with any of these regimens do not need to return for a test of cure unless symptoms persist, recur or are exacerbated.
- Serologic testing for syphilis is recommended within 30 days.

Complications

WOMEN. PID, pelvic or Bartholin's gland abscess, infertility, and disseminated gonococcal infection

PREGNANT WOMEN. Spontaneous abortion, premature rupture of membranes, preterm delivery, and chorioamnionitis

MALES. Proctitis, infertility related to epididymitis, proctitis or seminal vesiculitis, ureteral stricture, and disseminated gonococcal infection

NEONATES. Ophthalmia neonatorum, sepsis, arthritis, meningitis, and scalp abscess

MALES AND FEMALES. Meningitis, endocarditis, and gonococcal conjunctivitis

REFERENCES

Centers for Disease Control and Prevention (1993). Sexually transmitted diseases treatment guidelines. *MMWR Morbidity Mortality Weekly Report, 42* (RR-14), 50-55.

Dunnihoo, D. R. (1992). *Fundamentals of gynecology and obstetrics* (2nd ed.). Philadelphia: J. B. Lippincott.

Hawkins, J. W., Roberto-Nichols, D. M., & Stanley-Haney, J. L. (1995). *Protocols for nurse practitioners in gynecologic settings* (5th ed.). New York: Tiresias Press.

Johnson, C. (1996). Gonorrhea. In C. A. Johnson, B. E. Johnson, J. L. Murray, & B. S. Apgar (Eds.), *Women's health care handbook.* St. Louis: Mosby.

Landers, D., & Sweet, R. (1993). Sexually transmitted infection. In R. H. Glass (Ed.), *Office gynecology* (4th ed.). Baltimore: Williams & Wilkins.

McMillan, A. (1995). Sexually transmittable diseases. In N. Loudon, A. Glaiser, & A. Gebbie (Eds.), *Handbook of family planning and reproductive health* (3rd ed.). New York: Churchill Livingstone.

Uphold, C. R. & Graham, M. V. (1994). *Clinical guidelines in family practice.* Gainesville, FL: Barmarrae Books.

REVIEW QUESTIONS

1. A common side effect of ceftriaxone is:
   a. Stevens-Johnson syndrome
   b. Pain at injection site
   c. GI upset
   d. Nausea

2. Clients with pharyngeal gonorrhea should be treated with which of the following antimicrobials?
   a. Doxycycline
   b. Erythromycin
   c. Azithromycin
   d. Ciprofloxacin

3. Prophylactic management of ophthalmia neonatorum includes which of the following medications?
   a. Bacitracin ophthalmic ointment
   b. Silver nitrate aqueous solution
   c. Sulfacetamide sodium (Sodium Sulamyd)
   d. Prednisolone acetate and sulfacetamide sodium (Blephamide) ophthalmic solution

4. Which of the following symptoms is **least** indicative of gonorrhea?
   a. Odorous, musty vaginal discharge
   b. Dysuria
   c. Abdominal pain
   d. Asymptomatic presentation

5. What objective measure is most suited for diagnosis of gonorrhea?
   a. Vital signs
   b. Menstrual symptom checklist
   c. CBC, clotting profile
   d. Vaginal Gram stain

ANSWERS AND RATIONALES

1. *Answer:* b (plan/reproductive/NAS)
   Rationale: Stevens-Johnson syndrome is a rare disease, not often seen with ceftriaxone. GI upset is common, so the medication is given IM. Although nausea is a side effect of most drugs, it is not at all common with ceftriaxone. However, ceftriaxone is a painful injection, and whenever possible it should be mixed with lidocaine (Xylocaine) before injection. (Hawkins, Roberto-Nichols, & Stanley-Haney, 1995)

2. *Answer:* d (plan/reproductive/NAS)
   Rationale: Erythromycin is not indicated in the treatment of gonorrhea. Both doxycycline and azithromycin are the treatments for chlamydial infections. Ciprofloxacin and ceftriaxone are indicated for pharyngeal infections. (CDC, 1993)

3. *Answer:* b (plan/reproductive/infant)
   Rationale: Silver nitrate, erythromycin ophthalmic ointment, and tetracycline ophthalmic ointment are all used for prophylactic management of ophthalmia neonatorum. (CDC, 1993)

4. *Answer:* a (assessment/history/reproductive/NAS)

Rationale: Dysuria, abdominal pain, and lack of symptoms are typical presentations of gonorrhea. The musty, odorous vaginal discharge is a hallmark of bacterial vaginosis. (Uphold & Graham, 1994)

5. *Answer:* d (assessment/physical examination/reproductive/NAS)

Rationale: Gram stain is the usual diagnostic method for diagnosing gonorrhea. (CDC, 1993)

HERPES*

Herpes Zoster and Herpes Simplex

Herpes Zoster

OVERVIEW
Definition

Herpes zoster, or shingles, is an acute dermatomal infection associated with reactivation of varicella-zoster virus (VZV) that has been dormant in a dorsal root ganglion. It is characterized by unilateral pain and a vesicular or bullous eruption limited to dermatomes innervated by a corresponding sensory ganglion.

Incidence

More than 66% of those affected are older than 50 years; only 5% of cases occur in children <15 years of age. Herpes zoster occurs in 10% to 20% of the population at some time, equally in males and females.

RISK FACTORS
- The most common risk factor is diminishing immunity with advancing age, with most cases occurring in those older than 55.
- Malignancy
- Immunosuppression
- Radiotherapy
- HIV-infected individuals have an eightfold increased incidence of zoster.

TRANSMISSION. Zoster is about one third as contagious as varicella, and susceptible contacts can contract varicella by the airborne route.

CLASSIFICATION. Herpes zoster manifests in three distinct clinical phases: prodromal, active, and chronic stages.

ASSESSMENT: SUBJECTIVE/HISTORY
History of Present Illness

- Ask about when and how the eruption began and about appearance and distribution of the lesions.
- Ask whether there was preeruption pain, itching, or burning in the affected dermatome several days before the eruption.
- Ask about immunosuppressed status.

PRODROMAL STAGE
- Headache, malaise, and fever occur in 5% of affected persons.
- Tenderness, neuritic pain, or paresthesia (itching, tingling, or burning) in the involved dermatome precedes cutaneous eruption by 3 to 5 days but can have a range of 1 to 14 days.
- Pain is described as stabbing, pricking, boring, penetrating, or shooting.
- Allodynia, which is a heightened sensitivity to mild stimuli, may also be reported.

ACTIVE VESICULATION
- Headache, malaise, and fever
- Lasts 3 to 5 days
- Neuritic pain
- Pain in the involved skin
- Crust formation occurs from days to 2 to 3 weeks.

CHRONIC POSTHERPETIC NEURALGIA
- Depression is common.
- Burning pain can persist for weeks, months, or even years after the cutaneous involvement has resolved.

---

*NOTE: This discussion of herpes infections includes both genital and integumentary conditions.

ASSESSMENT: OBJECTIVE/ PHYSICAL EXAMINATION

Physical Examination

- Examine skin for characteristic lesions and distribution.
- Determine whether there is ophthalmic involvement.

Skin Lesions

TYPE. Progress from papules (24 hours) to vesicles and bullae (48 hours) to pustules (96 hours) to crusts (7 to 10 days). New lesions continue to appear for as long as 1 week. Necrotic and gangrenous lesions may also occur.

COLOR. Lesions have erythematous, edematous base, with superimposed clear or hemorrhagic vesicles.

SHAPE. The vesicle or bulla is oval or round and may be umbilicated.

ARRANGEMENT. Herpetiform clusters of lesions are characteristic.

DISTRIBUTION. Distribution is unilateral and dermatomal. Two or more contiguous dermatomes may be involved. Noncontiguous dermatomal zoster is rare. Hematogenous dissemination to other skin sites occurs in 10% of healthy individuals.

SITES OF PREDILECTION. Site is thoracic in 50%, trigeminal in 10% to 20%, and lumbosacral and cervical in 10% to 20%. In HIV-infected persons, lesions may be multidermatomal or recurrent.

MUCOUS MEMBRANES. Vesicles and erosions occur in mouth, vagina, and bladder, depending on dermatome involved.

Lymphadenopathy

Regional nodes draining the area are often enlarged and tender.

Sensory or Motor Nerve Changes

Changes are detectable by neurologic examination. Sensory defects and motor paralysis may occur.

Eye

In ophthalmic zoster, nasociliary branch involvement of the trigeminal nerve occurs in about one third of cases and is heralded by vesicles on the side and tip of the nose. Complications include uveitis, keratitis, conjunctivitis, retinitis, optic neuritis, glaucoma, proptosis, cicatricial lid retraction, and extraocular muscle palsies.

Diagnostic Procedures

In addition to tests specific for herpes zoster and to rule out other conditions, consider HIV testing.

ELECTROCARDIOGRAM. Rule out ischemic heart disease in prodromal stage.

IMAGING. In prodromal stage, rule out organic, pleural, pulmonary, or abdominal disease.

TZANCK SMEAR. Smear of vesicle base or fluid shows giant or multinucleated epidermal cells.

VARICELLA-ZOSTER VIRUS ANTIGEN DETECTION. Direct fluorescent antibody detects VZV antigen in smear of vesicle base or fluid. The test is specific and very sensitive.

VIRAL CULTURE. Perform viral culture for isolation of VZV.

DIAGNOSIS

Differential diagnosis is different for the prodromal and the dermatomal eruption phases.

PRODROMAL PHASE
- Migraine
- Cardiac or pleural disease
- Acute abdomen
- Vertebral disease

DERMATOMAL ERUPTION
- Varicella
- Herpes simplex virus (HSV)
- Cellulitis
- Poison oak or poison ivy
- Contact dermatitis
- Erysipelas
- Bullous impetigo
- Necrotizing fasciitis

THERAPEUTIC PLAN

- Suppression of pain, inflammation, and infection is goal of therapy.
- Use NSAIDs for pain and fever.
- Wet compresses with Burrow's solution or cool tap water can be applied for as long as 30 minutes several times a day.
- Isolate client from neonates, pregnant women, people who have not had chickenpox, and immunosuppressed persons because the active lesions are potentially infectious, although such infection is rare.
- Refer all clients with eye or facial involvement or dissemination beyond two dermatomes to an ophthalmologist or an infectious disease specialist.

- Antiviral therapy is indicated for acute herpes zoster in immunosuppressed persons, older adults, and debilitated clients.
  —Acyclovir, 800 mg 5 times per day for 5 to 7 days if client seeks treatment within first 72 hours of neuralgic symptoms
  —After all vesicles have resolved, topical capsaicin cream may be used qid for 21 days for postherpetic neuralgia.
  —Use of antiviral therapy is not warranted in the young, immunocompetent population.

EVALUATION/FOLLOW-UP

- Follow up in 7 days, or in 2 to 3 days for clients who are immunosuppressed, old, or debilitated.
- Monitor renal function in people taking acyclovir.

Herpes Simplex

OVERVIEW
Definition

Herpes simplex refers to cutaneous infections with HSV; HSV-1 is usually associated with oral infections and HSV-2 with genital infections. Nongenital HSV infection, whether primary or recurrent, is characterized by grouped vesicles arising on an erythematous base on keratinized skin or mucous membrane.

Incidence

Herpes simplex occurs most commonly in young adults (genitalis) and in children (gingivostomatitis). Incubation period is 2 to 20 days.

Physiology

TRANSMISSION. Usually skin to skin, skin to mucosa, or mucosa to skin contact. Increased HSV-1 transmission is associated with crowded living conditions.

RISK FACTORS. Risk factors for herpes include the following:
- Skin or mucosal irritation (ulraviolet radiation)
- Altered hormonal milieu (menstruation)
- Fever
- The common cold
- Altered immune states

- Site of infection
- Neonates
- Occupational exposure
- Previous HSV
- Immunocompromising factors: HIV infection, malignancy, transplantation, chemotherapy, systemic corticosteroids, irradiation, immunosuppressive drugs

ASSESSMENT: SUBJECTIVE/HISTORY
History of Present Illness

- Ask about location, onset, duration, and appearance of lesions.
- Ask whether pain, burning, or paraesthesia was present before eruption.
- Ask about associated symptoms of fever, myalgia, or malaise.
- Ask about previous occurrence.
- Ask about exposure to infected persons.

Symptoms

Many persons have no symptoms or have only minor symptoms with primary herpes. If present, symptoms may include regional lymphadenopathy, intense itching, pain, fever, headache, malaise, and myalgia peaking within 3 to 4 days of onset. Gingivostomatitis (sore throat, fever, and vesicles on pharynx and oral mucosa) is the most common symptom in children. Recurrent herpes may have prodrome of tingling, itching, or burning.

ASSESSMENT: OBJECTIVE/ PHYSICAL EXAMINATION
Physical Examination

- Examine lesions for characteristic location, distribution, and appearance.
- Check for cervical lymphadenopathy.

Skin Findings

Erythema is often noted initially, followed by grouped, often umbilicated vesicles, which may evolve into pustules. These may become eroded and may enlarge into ulcers. They may heal in 2 to 4 weeks. Vesicles on the end of fingers are characteristic of herpetic whitlow.

General Findings

- Fever is often present
- Gingivostomatitis
- Regional lymphadenopathy

Diagnostic Tests

- Tzanck smear
- Viral culture

DIAGNOSIS

Differential diagnosis includes the following:
- Erythema multiforme
- Pemphigus

THERAPEUTIC PLAN

- Treatment is primarily supportive.
- Lidocaine 2% for lesions of the mouth/lip, directly to lesion or as a rinse
- For oral lesions, apply hydrocortisone acetate (Orabase Hca)
- Diphenhydramine (Benadryl) may also be used as a rinse
- For lip lesion, apply ice, Blistex, and sunscreen
- Acetaminophen (Tylenol) for pain
- Acyclovir has been approved to treat herpes in immunosuppressed persons; consult physician.

EVALUATION/FOLLOW-UP

No follow-up is indicated for herpes simplex infection.

REFERENCES

Barker, L. R., Burton, J. R., & Zieve, P. D. (Eds.). (1995). *Principles of ambulatory medicine.* (4th ed.). Baltimore: Williams & Wilkins.

Decherney, A. H., & Pernoll, M. L. (Eds.). (1994). *Current obstetrics and gynecology: Diagnosis and treatment* (8th ed.). Norwalk, CT: Appleton & Lange.

Fitzpatrick, T. B., Johnson, R. A., Wolff, K., Polano, M. K., & Suurmond, D. (1997). *Color atlas and synopsis of clinical dermatology.* (3rd ed.). New York: McGraw-Hill.

Homes, K. K., Mardh, P., Sparling, P. F., Weisner, P. J., Cates, W., Jr., Lemon, S. M., & Stamm, W. E. (1990). *Sexually transmitted diseases* (2nd ed.). New York: McGraw-Hill.

Uphold, C. R., & Graham, M. V. (1994). *Clinical guidelines in family practice* (2nd ed.). Gainesville, FL: Barmarrae Books.

Youngkin, E., Davis, M. (1994). *Women's health: A primary care clinical guide.* Norwalk, CT: Appleton & Lange.

REVIEW QUESTIONS

1. The skin lesions most suggestive of herpes is:
   a. Thick, crusted plaques, varying in size
   b. Erythematous papular rash
   c. Topical, grayish white burrows of varying lengths
   d. Erythematous, vesicular rash

2. A cardinal symptom of herpes simplex and zoster is:
   a. Burning sensation on trunk
   b. Nocturnal itching
   c. Generalized itching
   d. Painful vesicles

3. Which of the following is **not** included in a list of differential diagnoses when herpes is suspected?
   a. Drug eruption
   b. Hand-foot-mouth disease
   c. Pediculosis
   d. Erythema multiforme

4. Which of the following is the treatment of choice for herpes zoster?
   a. Acyclovir, 800 mg 5 times a day
   b. Prednisone, 40 mg/day
   c. Burow's solution q 4 hours
   d. Vicodin, 1 tablet q 4 hours for pain

5. Mr. Smith, a 66-year-old man with lung cancer, reports persistent pain on the face where he had herpes zoster 4 weeks ago. These symptoms sound like what complication of herpes zoster?
   a. Chronic pain syndrome
   b. Postherpetic neuralgia
   c. Chronic cutaneous herpes
   d. Drug-seeking behavior

6. Appropriate diagnostic tests for a client in whom you suspect genital herpes is:
   a. CBC
   b. Viral culture
   c. Tzanck smear
   d. VZV antigen detection

ANSWERS AND RATIONALES

1. Answer: d (assessment/physical examination/reproductive/NAS)

Rationale: The diagnosis of herpes is suggested by finding an erythematous, vesicular rash. (Fitzpatrick, Johnson, Wolff, Polano & Suurmond, 1997, pp. 792-816)

2. Answer: d (assessment/history/reproductive/NAS)

Rationale: A cardinal symptom of herpes infections is painful lesions. (Fitzpatrick et al., 1997, p. 792)

3. Answer: c (diagnosis/reproductive/NAS)

Rationale: Pediculosis does not have erythematous, vesicular lesions. (Fitzpatrick et al., 1997, p. 836)

4. Answer: a (plan/reproductive/NAS)

Rationale: Although the other medications help with symptoms of herpes zoster, acyclovir is a viral inhibitory agent that hastens healing and decreases viral shedding. (Fitzpatrick et al., 1997, p. 818)

5. Answer: b (evaluation/reproductive/aging adult)

Rationale: Postherpetic neuralgia occurs in approximately 40% of clients older than 60 years. The incidence is even higher when the zoster is ophthalmic. (Fitzpatrick et al., 1997, p. 816)

6. Answer: c (assessment/physical examination/reproductive/NAS)

Rationale: The most cost-effective diagnostic test for herpes is the Tzanck smear. Other tests take longer and are more expensive because they are very sensitive and specific. (Fitzpatrick et al., 1997, p. 816)

INFERTILITY

OVERVIEW
Definition

Infertility is the inability to achieve fertilization and pregnancy after 1 year of unprotected intercourse. Sterility is the inability to reproduce.

Incidence

- Incidence of infertility is at least 14%, one of every seven couples.
- From 1% to 2% of couples are involuntarily sterile.

Physiology

RISK FACTORS
- Increasing age of woman (age at least 35 years, with a sharp decrease in fertility at 40 years)
- Previous contraceptive use (IUD)
- Increased number of sexual partners, leading to greater possibility of STDs

ETIOLOGY. Female factors include pelvic cause in 25% of cases, ovulatory cause in 20% of cases, and cervical factor in 10% of cases.
- Male infertility accounts for 35% of infertility in couples.

ASSESSMENT: SUBJECTIVE/HISTORY
General Current History

- Previous obstetric history
- Length of time attempting conception
- Frequency of intercourse
- Use of lubricants (which can be spermicidal)
- Anorgasmia
- Impotence
- Dyspareunia

Medical History for Female Factor Infertility*

- In utero DES exposure
- History of sexual development and pubertal development, including onset of menses
- Menstrual cycle characteristics (length, duration, molimina), LMP
- Contraceptive history, including use of IUD
- Previous pregnancies and outcome, including history of ectopic pregnancy or septic abortion
- Previous surgeries especially pelvic surgery including ruptured appendix and adnexal or ovarian mass or cyst

---

*Modified from DeCherney & Pernoll, 1994.

- Previous infection, including STDs, PID
- Leiomyomas
- Endometriosis
- Obesity or eating disorders
- History of cervicitis, abnormal Papanicolaou smear, abnormal cone biopsy sample, cautery, obstetric trauma
- Thyroid disease
- Hirsutism, galactorrhea, hot flushes, severe psychologic stress
- General health (diet, weight stability, medications, exercise, alcohol consumption)
- Use of nicotine, alcohol, and illegal substances, such as marijuana and other street drugs

Medical History for Male Factor Infertility*

- In utero DES exposure
- Congenital abnormalities, including hypospadias
- Previous paternity
- Frequency of intercourse
- Exposure to toxins
- Previous surgery, including testicular, prostate, or hernia repair surgery
- Retrograde ejaculation
- Previous infections and treatments, including STDs and postpubertal mumps
- Drugs and medications, including genital radiation, chemotherapy, and anabolic steroids
- Excessive exposure to heat (hot tubs, saunas), toxic chemicals, and pesticides
- General health (diet, medications, exercise, review of systems)
- Use of nicotine, alcohol, or illegal substances, such as marijuana and other street drugs

ASSESSMENT: OBJECTIVE/PHYSICAL EXAMINATION

Physical Examination

- Height, weight, and vital signs
- A complete physical examination should be performed, including notation of the overall body habitus and appropriate hair distribution for both males and females.
- The thyroid gland should be palpated for evidence of enlargement or nodules.

- Breast development in women and the presence of gynecomastia in men should be noted.
- Abdominal and genital inspection for scars from previous reproductive surgery
- Male: Testicular descent, size, consistency; examination of the epididymis and vas deferens; check for penile lesions
- Female: Pelvic examination for assesing the clitoris, labia, Skene's and Bartholin's glands, vulva, perineum, and uterine mobility and contour

Diagnostic Procedures

- Papanicolaou smear
- Cultures of vaginal fluid, penile discharge
- Ovulation testing by way of basal body temperature (temperature will increase at time of ovulation), progesterone level (>15 ng/ml indicates ovulation), and endometrial biopsy
- Postcoital test to examine sperm–cervical mucus interaction (sample 2 to 8 hours after intercourse)
- Hysterosalpingogram to assess tubal patency
- Laparoscopy to determine whether endometriosis is a factor
- Presence of sperm antibodies in serum, sperm, and cervical mucus
- Sperm penetration assay to assess ability to initiate fertilization
- Semen analysis (semen collected after 2 to 3 days of abstinence and examined within 1 hour of ejaculation)

DIAGNOSIS

Differential diagnosis includes the following:

- Primary or secondary hypothalamic or pituitary failure
- Obstructive disorders of the reproductive system
- STDs
- Urinary tract infection (UTI)
- Endometriosis

THERAPEUTIC PLAN

- Develop an infertility testing plan according to the couple's financial situation, motivation to become parents, and risks of the testing.
- Provide contact for an infertility support group.

---

*Modified from DeCherney & Pernoll, 1994.

- Refer to a reproductive endocrinologist for reproductive technology such as in vitro fertilization and embryo, gamete, and zygote transfer.
- Provide information on artificial insemination if appropriate.
- Provide information about adoption.

EVALUATION/FOLLOW-UP

Most infertility evaluations occur during the course of 12 to 18 months.

REFERENCES

DeCherney, A. H., & Pernoll, M. L. (1994). Infertility. In *Current obstetrics and gynecology: Diagnosis and treatment* (8th ed., pp. 996-1006). Norwalk, CT: Appleton & Lange.

Gray, M. (1992). *Genitourinary disorders* (pp. 275-298). St. Louis: Mosby.

Hawkins, J. W., Roberto-Nichols, D. M., & Stanley-Haney, J. L. (1993). *Protocols for nurse practitioners in gynecologic settings* (4th ed., pp. 67-69). New York: Tiresias Press.

Infertility. (1989). *ACOG Technical Bulletin, 125,* 1-6.

Loriaux, T. C. (1991). Male infertility: A challenge for primary health care providers. *The Nurse Practitioner, 16*(3) 38-45.

Male infertility. (1990). *ACOG Technical Bulletin, 142,* 2.

Medical induction of ovulation. (1998). *ACOG Technical Bulletin, 120,* 1-2.

New reproductive technologies. (1990). *ACOG Technical Bulletin, 140,* 1-4.

Wilson, B. (1991). The effects of drugs on male sexual function and fertility. *The Nurse Practitioner, 16*(9), 12-22.

REVIEW QUESTIONS

1. Which of the following symptoms is more indicative of a male infertility factor?

    a. DES exposure
    b. Pituitary insufficiency
    c. Thyroid disease
    d. Mumps orchitis

2. Which of the following physical findings on a pelvic examination might be significant in terms of an infertility evaluation?

    a. A retroflexed uterus
    b. An enlarged, irregular uterine contour

    c. A mobile uterus
    d. Bacterial vaginosis

3. Infertility is defined as which of the following?

    a. The inability to conceive with multiple sexual partners
    b. The inability to conceive for 9 months of unprotected intercourse if partners are younger than 30 years
    c. The inability to conceive after 1 full year of unprotected intercourse
    d. The lack of desire for pregnancy

4. The definition of sterility is which of the following?

    a. Unexplained infertility
    b. The inability to reproduce
    c. A decrease in the ability to conceive
    d. Infertility greater than 1 year

5. A referral to a reproductive endocrinologist for infertility would be appropriate for which of the following?

    a. To advise on assisted reproduction technologies
    b. To advise on basic infertility workup
    c. To advise on an adoption plan
    d. To advise on the treatment of PID

6. Sperm antibodies can be found in all the following **except:**

    a. Serum
    b. Semen
    c. Tissue
    d. Cervical mucus

ANSWERS AND RATIONALES

1. *Answer:* d (assessment/history/reproductive/adult male)

    Rationale: DES exposure, pituitary insufficiency, and thyroid disease are both male and female factors. Mumps orchitis, however, is specific to male infertility. (DeCherney & Pernoll, 1994)

2. *Answer:* b (assessment/physical examination/reproductive/childbearing female)

    Rationale: A retroflexed uterus and or mobile uterus are both normal findings. Bacterial vaginosis is a common, easily treated infection that is not typically significant in terms of an infertility evaluation. An enlarged, irregular uterine contour may be indicative of uterine fibroids and warrants further evaluation. (ACOG Technical Bulletin, 1991)

3. *Answer:* c (diagnosis/reproductive/childbearing female)

Rationale: Infertility is defined as the inability to conceive after 1 full year of unprotected intercourse.

4. *Answer:* b (diagnosis/reproductive/childbearing female)

Rationale: Sterility is the inability to reproduce, whereas infertility implies a decrease in the ability to conceive in a certain time frame, with the potential for conception remaining a possibility. (Gray, 1992)

5. *Answer:* a (plan/reproductive/childbearing female)

Rationale: The primary care provider would be responsible for the basic workup, treatment of infections, including PID, and advising the couple on options such as adoption. A reproductive endocrinologist would be an appropriate referral if a couple's infertility was unexplained or if the couple could benefit from advanced assisted reproduction technologies.

6. *Answer:* c (plan/reproductive/adult male)

Rationale: Sperm antibodies can be found in serum, semen, and cervical mucus and may impair the sperm's ability to penetrate an egg. Tissue is not identified as a location of sperm antibodies.

OVARIAN CYSTS

OVERVIEW
Definition

Most *ovarian cysts,* fluid-filled sacs on the ovary, are functional in nature—normal and usually transient with a diameter ≤8 cm.

Incidence

Most women have functional ovarian cysts that never cause problems; nor do they come to medical attention unless found on coincident pelvic examination. Ovarian cysts represent one of most common causes of adnexal mass and tenderness in women of childbearing age. Ovarian cysts generally do not occur before puberty or after menopause.

Pathophysiology

There are two types of functional ovarian cysts: *follicle* and *corpus luteum cysts.*

Follicle Cysts. *Follicle cysts,* physiologic structures resulting from faulty resorption of fluid from incompletely developed ovarian follicles, are the most common ovarian cysts. Their size ranges from microscopic to 8 cm. They are usually asymptomatic, disappearing spontaneously within 60 days. Follicle cysts may be associated with an abnormally long or short intermenstrual interval, thus causing irregular periods.

Corpus Luteum Cysts. A less common, transient structure resulting from failure of the corpus luteum to degenerate after ovulation is referred to as a *corpus luteum cyst* if >3 cm. This cyst causes local pain and tenderness on examination.

Multiple Inactive Ovarian Cysts. Associated with polycystic ovary or Stein-Leventhal syndrome, *multiple inactive ovarian cysts* are caused by androgen excess and anovulation. This pathology affects 15- to 30-year-olds and causes infertility. In addition to bilateral polycystic ovaries, the affected woman has small breasts, large clitoris, obesity, secondary amenorrhea, enlarged muscle mass, acne, and oily skin. Fifty percent have hirsutism, with male pattern distribution.

NOTE: With an adnexal mass, the practitioner must always suspect cancer until proved otherwise.

Ovarian Cancer. *Ovarian cancer,* potentially lethal malignancy of ovarian tissue, is asymptomatic in early stages. Its cause is unknown. In many cases, malignancy has spread before symptoms occur. Vague GI symptoms (anorexia, early satiety, dyspepsia, bloating, and increased belching) are sometimes seen 6 months or less before disease is discovered. Mass is irregular and adheres to surrounding tissue; firm nodules are frequently noted in the cul de sac or along the uterosacral ligaments. It is most common among women of childbearing age.

PROTECTIVE FACTORS. Use of oral contraceptives and pregnancy protect against ovarian cysts by suppressing ovarian activity, including ovulation. Factors decreasing the risk of ovarian cancer include the following:

- Oral contraceptive use
- Multiparity
- Breast-feeding
- Early first pregnancy

FACTORS INCREASING SUSCEPTIBILITY TO OVARIAN CYSTS. Susceptibility is increased in women of childbearing age.

FACTORS INCREASING RISK OF OVARIAN CANCER

- Anovulation
- Nulliparity
- Infertility
- Irradiation of pelvis
- Endometriosis
- Late childbearing
- Family history of breast or ovarian cancer (especially first-degree relatives)
- Personal history of breast, colorectal, or endometrial cancer
- Menopause before 45 years
- Menarche after 14 years
- Talc on perineum
- Increased fat in diet

ASSESSMENT: SUBJECTIVE/HISTORY
Functional Ovarian Cysts

Presenting symptoms may include vague, local pressure, heaviness, and aching in affected side. Follicle cysts occur in the first half of the menstrual cycle. Corpus luteum cysts occur in the last half of the menstrual cycle.

Ask about the following:

- Menstrual history: LMP, age at menarche or menopause.
- Pregnancy history
- Type and extent of pain.
- Sexual history: Use of contraception, exposure to STD.
- High-risk behaviors that might lead to PID, confusing the diagnosis
- Any other physical problems
- Dyspareunia
- Radiation exposure
- Use of talc on perineum

Polycystic Ovary Syndrome

Ask about menstrual and sexual histories and about attempts to become pregnant.

Suspicion of Torsion or Rupture of Functional Cyst

Ask about the following:

- LMP: Usually occurs 14 to 60 days after last period.
- General aching followed by sudden severe abdominal pain.
- Weakness, syncope, and dizziness that may occur with sudden blood loss
- Activity that preceded sudden pain (client often will report exercise, trauma, or sexual intercourse immediately preceding)

Ovarian Cancer

Ask about the following:

- Increasing abdominal girth
- Vague GI complaints (dyspepsia, anorexia, early satiety, increased bloating and belching)
- Weight loss

Medication History

- Note use of oral contraception
- Ask about use of analgesia for discomfort
- Ask about use of medications for indigestion, nausea, and constipation.

Family History

Ask about first-degree relatives who have had cancer.

Psychosocial History

- Ask about smoking, alcohol use, and other drug use.
- Inquire about sexually risky behavior, including multiple sexual partners.
- Ask how pelvic aching affects lifestyle, including sexual relationship.

Dietary History

Determine whether high-fat diet places client at risk for ovarian cancer.

ASSESSMENT: OBJECTIVE/ PHYSICAL EXAMINATION

Physical Examination

- Perform a problem-centered physical examination, with special attention to general appearance, vital signs, and abdominal, and pelvic examinations.
- Weight and height
- Note abdominal girth, presence of ascites, and fluid wave.
- Check bowel sounds and palpate for general tenderness.
- Check for hirsutism and note hair distribution pattern (male vs female)
- Perform pelvic examination gently to avoid inadvertent rupture of ovarian cyst.
- Note size, contour, and position of uterus.
- Note cervical motion tenderness and presence of cervical or vaginal discharge.
- Assess adnexa for tenderness and presence of mass or enlarged ovary.
- Perform rectovaginal examination to confirm size of adnexal mass and to locate in relation to uterus (usually lateral).
- Note nodularity posterior cul de sac and along uterosacral ligaments.
- If client has a history of sudden, severe abdominal pain, note position on examination table. With ruptured cyst, client will usually lie quietly, with knees drawn up toward abdomen.
- Assess for acute abdomen, looking for pain, rigidity, rebound, and other peritoneal signs.

Diagnostic Procedures

PELVIC OR TRANSVAGINAL ULTRASONOGRAPHY. This test differentiates between cyst and solid mass and aids in determining which should be followed up and which referred.

BLOOD WORK. CBC should be done, with special attention to WBC and existence of shift to left. Urine or serum HCG should be determined to rule out intrauterine or ectopic pregnancy when client has acute abdomen or possible ruptured ovarian cyst. Physician may also perform culdocentesis to check for presence of hemorrhagic bleeding.

CALCIUM 125 RADIOIMMUNOASSAY

- Tumor-sensitive antigen for clients at high risk for ovarian cancer

- This test cannot be used as screening test for ovarian cancer because not all cancers increase level
- Low sensitivity and specificity in early stages
- Levels are also elevated in other conditions, including PID, leiomyoma, and endometriosis.

FSH, LH, URINARY 17 KETOSTEROIDS. Check level of these in clients with polycystic ovaries.

DIAGNOSIS

Rule out the following:
- Functional ovarian cyst
- Solid ovarian mass
- Ovarian cancer

When client has findings suggestive of ruptured cyst, rule out the following:
- Ectopic pregnancy
- Appendicitis
- Diverticulitis
- Tuboovarian abscess
- PID

THERAPEUTIC PLAN

- Functional cyst: consider reevaluating in 2 to 3 weeks, just before ovulation.
- Cyst <8 cm in premenopausal patient: Treat conservatively and wait to resolve (4 to 8 weeks); repeat pelvic examination every 3 to 4 weeks. Repeat ultrasonography as needed to confirm size.

Pharmacologic Treatment

Use of oral contraception may aid resolution in 80% of functional cysts

Client Education

- Discuss possible cause and course of functional cysts.
- Teach what to expect if torsion or hemorrhage occurs; reassure client that these are rare complications but prepare her to respond by notifying caregiver or going directly to emergency department.
- Advise about lifestyle changes that decrease risk of ovarian cancer.

Referral

- For cysts >8 cm or persisting for two cycles, refer client to surgeon for evaluation and treatment. Large cysts are more subject to torsion and hemorrhage.
- If lesion is suspected not to be a functional cyst, refer client.
- In postmenopausal client, if cyst is <5 cm and client does not have other risk factors, observe. Recheck at 6 weeks, 3 months, and 6 months. Refer client if there is any increase in size of mass.
- Refer any child who is prepubertal and has an adnexal mass.
- Refer any postmenopausal older woman who has an enlarged ovary.
- In the event of symptoms of rupture or torsion, refer for emergency care.
- Clients with polycystic ovary syndrome should be referred for initial diagnosis and early management; however, depending on the setting, they may be comanaged by the primary care provider.

EVALUATION/FOLLOW-UP

Most functional cysts resolve in 8 weeks, either spontaneously or with the aid of oral contraception. Clients taking oral contraceptives should be followed up for untoward effects. Women with a history of functional ovarian cysts should continue to have annual clinical examinations. Cysts sometime recur.

If an adnexal mass occurs during pregnancy, ectopic pregnancy must be ruled out. A fetal sac of intrauterine pregnancy should be seen on pelvic ultrasonography with an hCG level of 6500 IU and on transvaginal ultrasonography with an HCG level of 2000 IU. Physician management is warranted.

Clients with polycystic ovaries should have an annual examination to reevaluate the appropriateness of oral contraception and to determine the desire for childbearing, which would require ovulation induction. Because of their anovulatory status without treatment, these clients need to be followed up carefully for endometrial cancer related to prolonged unopposed endogenous estrogen.

Follow-up for ovarian cancer depends on the client's situation. It is usually done by physician and oncology team. Because of its insidious nature, most ovarian cancer has spread before diagnosis. Despite aggressive treatment, 5-year survival is only 0% to 30%.

REFERENCES

Barber, H. K., Creasman, W. T., & Knapp, R. C. (1993). A rational approach to ovarian masses. *Patient Care, 27,* 50-67, 74.

Benson, R. C., & Pernoll, M. L. (1994). *Handbook of obstetrics and gynecology.* New York: McGraw-Hill.

Bowman, M. A., Braly, P. S., Johnson, S., & Mikuta, J. J. (1996). Who are you screening for cancer and when? *Patient Care, 30,* 54-87.

Carlson, K. J., Eisenstat, S. A., Frigoletto, F. D., & Schiff, I. (1995). *Primary care of women.* St. Louis: Mosby.

Lemke, D. P., Pattison, J., Marshall, L. A., & Cowley, D. S. (1995). *Primary care of women.* Norwalk, CT: Appleton & Lange.

Lichtman, R., & Papera, S. (1990). *Gynecology well-woman care.* Norwalk, CT: Appleton & Lange.

Mann, W. J. (1994). Diagnosis and management of epithelial cancer of the ovary. *American Family Physician, 49*(3), 613-618.

Star, W. L., Lommel, L. L., & Shannon, M. T. (1995). *Women's primary care: Protocols for practice.* Washington, DC: American Nurses Publishing.

Youngkin, E. O., & Davis, M. S. (1994). *Women's health: A primary care clinical guide.* Norwalk, CT: Appleton & Lange.

REVIEW QUESTIONS

1. Which of the following clinical manifestations is associated with a diagnosis of polycystic ovary syndrome?

a. Infertility
b. Excessive menstrual flow
c. Reports of dry, flaking skin
d. Unexplained weight loss

2. In Miss Logan, a 26-year-old with a history suggestive of ruptured ovarian cyst, which objective finding best supports that diagnosis?

a. She is thrashing about on the examination table.
b. She is lying quietly on the examination table, with her legs drawn up toward her abdomen.
c. She has excessive dark, bloody vaginal drainage.
d. She has dry, hot skin and a high fever.

3. Which of the following are appropriate differential diagnoses when an ovarian cyst ruptures?

  a. Ruptured ectopic pregnancy
  b. Appendicitis
  c. Tuboovarian abscess from salpingitis
  d. All the above

4. An enlarged left ovary is found on a prepubescent girl. What is the most appropriate action?

  a. Advise the girl and her mother that menses should be starting soon.
  b. Start low-dose oral contraceptives for 3 months.
  c. Refer the client to a surgeon immediately.
  d. Document the presence of a cyst and plan to follow up in 2 weeks.

5. Ms. Slade, a 30-year-old woman, has a family history of ovarian cancer. In consultation with the physician, the nurse practitioner orders oral contraceptives as a protective factor for Ms. Slade. What follow-up is appropriate in these circumstances?

  a. Annual examination and ultrasonography
  b. Monthly calcium 125 radioimmunoassay
  c. Biannual endometrial biopsy
  d. Papanicolaou smear every 3 months

6. Which symptom group below would make the practitioner suspect ovarian cancer in a 45-year-old woman?

  a. Anorexia, early satiety, and dyspepsia
  b. Pelvic pain, vaginal bleeding, and dyspareunia
  c. Weight gain, pedal edema, and hirsutism
  d. Diarrhea, breast enlargement, and abdominal tenderness

7. Which of the following statements concerning calcium 125 in relation to ovarian cancer is **false**?

  a. Calcium 125 is the ideal screening test for ovarian cancer because of its specificity.
  b. Not all ovarian cancers increase the calcium 125 level.
  c. Other disorders, such as leiomyoma, cause an elevated calcium 125 level.
  d. Calcium 125 lacks sensitivity as a screening test for ovarian cancer.

8. Gertrude Ewing, who is 49 years old and postmenopausal, comes in for an annual physical. She reports dyspepsia, anorexia, and bloating. Pelvic examination reveals a fixed left adnexal mass (>8 cm) and firm irregular nodules in the cul de sac. The most likely diagnosis is:

  a. Ovarian cancer
  b. Diverticulitis
  c. Uterine fibroid
  d. Appendiceal abscess

9. Which of the following findings **fails** to justify immediate referral to a surgeon?

  a. Cystic mass, 2 cm, slightly tender, in a 20-year-old
  b. Cystic mass, 10 cm, persisting 12 weeks, in a 25-year-old
  c. Solid mass at any age
  d. Any adnexal mass in a 68-year-old

ANSWERS AND RATIONALES

1. *Answer:* a (assessment/history/reproductive/NAS)
  Rationale: Infertility, acne, oily skin, weight gain, and amenorrhea are classic features of polycystic ovary syndrome. (Carlson, Eisenstat, Frigoletto, & Schiff, 1995)

2. *Answer:* b (assessment/physical examination/reproductive/adult)
  Rationale: Peritoneal irritation caused by ruptured ovarian cyst causes clients to attempt to minimize pain by lying quietly, with the knees drawn up toward the chest. (Barber, Creasman, & Knapp, 1993)

3. *Answer:* d (diagnosis/reproductive/NAS)
  Rationale: Ruptured ovarian cysts mimic appendicitis, ruptured ectopic pregnancy, and salpingitis. (Lichtman & Papera, 1990)

4. *Answer:* c (plan/management/consult/referral/reproductive/adolescent)
  Rationale: An adnexal mass in a premenstrual girl needs immediate referral. (Barber et al., 1993)

5. *Answer:* a (evaluation/reproductive/adult)
  Rationale: With a family history, annual clinical examination and ultrasonography is recommended. (Carlson et al., 1995)

6. ***Answer:*** a (assessment/history/reproductive/adult)

Rationale: Common signs of ovarian cancer include a 6- to 12-month history of increased belching, bloating, acid indigestion, early satiety, and anorexia. (Barber et al., 1993)

7. ***Answer:*** a (assessment/physical examination/reproductive/NAS)

Rationale: Calcium 125 cannot be used as a screening test for ovarian cancer because it lacks sensitivity and specificity. (Barber, et al., 1993)

8. ***Answer:*** a (diagnosis/reproductive/adult)

Rationale: Digestive symptoms for 6 to 12 months and increasing abdominal girth are signs of ovarian cancer. (Barber et al., 1993)

9. ***Answer:*** a (evaluation/reproductive/NAS)

Rationale: A small cystic mass in a young woman is not a referrable problem. (Star, Lommel, & Shannon, 1995)

PELVIC INFLAMMATORY DISEASE

OVERVIEW
Definition

Pelvic inflammatory disease (PID) is an infection of many or all of the pelvic structures (cervix, uterus, ovaries, fallopian tubes, and peritoneum). It is generally considered to be sexually transmitted. PID may be acute, chronic, or atypical.

Incidence

Approximately one in seven females of childbearing age in the United States has been treated for PID.

Pathophysiology

PROTECTIVE FACTORS
- Condom use
- Monogamous relationship
- Age older than 25 years
- Oral contraceptive use

FACTORS INCREASING SUSCEPTIBILITY
- Age younger than 25 years
- Cigarette, alcohol, and illicit drug use
- Previous history of PID
- History of STDs
- Multiple or new sex partners
- Nulliparity
- Pelvic instrumentation
- Use of IUD
- Douching or menses within 1 week of symptoms

COMMON PATHOGENS
- *C. trachomatis*
- *N. gonorrhoeae*
- Anaerobes, such as *Bacteroides* or *Peptostreptococcus*
- Usually more than one pathogen is present.
- Bacterial vaginosis and trichmoniasis may also be present.

ASSESSMENT: SUBJECTIVE/HISTORY
Past Medical History

- Previously diagnosed STD or PID
- History of IUD use, therapeutic abortion, or dilation and curettage (D&C)
- Date of LMP
- Unprotected intercourse

Medication History

Inquire about recent or current antibiotic use.

Psychosocial/Sexual History

- Age
- Cigarette, alcohol, or illicit drug use
- Number of sexual partners
- Recent new partner
- Use of contraception and type used

Symptoms

- Lower abdominal pain, fever, nausea, and vomiting in acute PID
- Dysuria, postcoital bleeding
- Atypical or chronic PID features vague symptoms, such as abnormal vaginal bleeding and dyspareunia.

- *C. trachomatis* infection may feature very few symptoms and is often the cause of atypical PID.

ASSESSMENT: OBJECTIVE/ PHYSICAL EXAMINATION

Physical Examination

- Lower abdominal tenderness, bilateral adnexal tenderness, and cervical motion tenderness (Chandelier sign)
- Guarded gait, with client taking small steps while holding her lower abdomen.
- Oral temperature >100.4° F (>38° C)
- Mucopurulent discharge
- Cervical friability

Diagnostic Procedures

LABORATORY TESTS
- Wet preparation to assess for WBCs, *Trichmonas,* and yeast
- Do cervical cultures for *N. gonorrhoeae.** Do *not* wait for culture results before treating acute PID.
- Cervical culture or nonculture test (DNA probe) for *C. trachomatis.**
- Do pregnancy test; results will influence treatment plan.
- CBC with differential; WBC will be elevated >10,000 cells/mm^3 unless client is immunocompromised.
- Urinalysis
- ESR may be elevated above 15 to 20 mm/hr (not commonly performed).
- C-reactive protein level may be elevated (not commonly performed).
- Serologic tests for syphilis and HIV.* Results will influence treatment plan.

DIAGNOSTIC TESTS
- PID is diagnosed on the basis of the clinical examination. It is confirmed by wet preparation and cultures.
- Laparoscopy is considered for clients not responding to treatment or to rule out another diagnosis.
- Ultrasonography may rule out other causes of symptoms (e.g., tuboovarian abscess, ectopic pregnancy, appendicitis).
- Endometrial biopsy sample will show histopathologic evidence of endometritis.

Combined with transvaginal ultrasonograpy, biopsy may be an alternative to laparoscopy when the diagnosis is in question. If pregnancy is suspected, endometrial biopsy is contraindicated.

DIAGNOSIS

Differential diagnosis includes the following:
- Ectopic pregnancy
- Appendicitis
- Ovarian torsion
- Ovarian cyst
- Tuboovarian abscess
- Endometriosis
- Pyelonephritis
- UTI
- Vaginitis
- Uterine fibroids
- Threatened abortion
- Diverticulitis

THERAPEUTIC PLAN

Because of the serious complications of untreated PID, most references suggest treatment even when the diagnosis is only probable, not positive.

Outpatient Care

REGIMEN A. Cephalexin (Rocephin), 250 mg IM, plus azithromycin (Zithromax), 1 g PO, once in the office (both are approved for pregnancy), followed by metronidazole (Flagyl), 500 mg PO bid for 7 days if client is not pregnant. Instruct client to avoid alcohol.

REGIMEN B. Cefoxitin sodium (Mefoxin) 2 g IM, plus probenecid (Benemid) 1 g PO in a single dose, concurrently; *or* ceftriaxone (Rocephin) 250 mg IM, or other parenteral third-generation cephalosporin plus doxycycline,* 100 mg PO bid, for 14 days.

REGIMEN C. Ofloxacin (Floxin),† 400 mg bid, for 14 days, plus clindamycin (Cleocin), 450 mg PO qid, for 14 days‡; *or* metronidazole (Flagyl), 500 mg PO bid, for 14 days.

---

*Positive results on any of these tests must be reported to the Health Department.

*Use during pregnancy is controversial. Routine use during pregnancy is not recommended.

†Not for use in clients younger than 18 years or during pregnancy.

‡Compliance may not be good with any medication that must be taken four times a day.

Inpatient Care

REGIMEN A. Cefoxitin (Mefoxin), 2 g IV q 6 hours, or cefotetan (Cefotan), 2 g IV q 12 hours, *plus* doxycycline, 100 mg PO or IV q 12 hours. Continue this regimen for at least 48 hours after clinical improvement. Continue doxycycline, 100 mg PO bid, for 14 days.

REGIMEN B. Clindamycin phosphate (Cleocin phosphate), 900 mg IV q 8 hours, *plus* gentamicin (Garamycin), in a loading dose of 2 mg/kg IV or IM, followed by a maintenance dose of 1.5 mg/kg q 8 hours. Continue this regimen for at least 48 hours after clinical improvement. Continue doxycycline, 100 mg PO bid, *or* clindamycin hydrochloride (Cleocin hydrochloride), 450 mg PO qid, for 14 days+.

Addendum and Notes

Erythromycin, 500 mg PO qid, for 14 days, may be used during pregnancy and for clients intolerant or allergic to doxycycline.

Referral

Hospitalization is warranted in the following cases: acute surgical abdomen (appendicitis or ectopic pregnancy), possible pelvic abscess, pregnancy, suspected sepsis or other serious illness, temperature >102.2° F (>39° C), client unable to tolerate oral medications, failure to respond to outpatient medications, arrangement of follow-up in 72 hours not possible, young adolescent, or any client whose compliance is unreliable.

Client Education

- Abstain from sexual intercourse until treatment is completed and symptoms have resolved.
- Partner should be tested and treated for any STD.
- Use condoms and spermicide consistently.
- Abstain from sexual intercourse if symptoms recur.
- Complete all medication, even when feeling better.
- Return for follow-up as instructed.

EVALUATION/FOLLOW-UP

Client should return for follow-up 72 hours after initiation of medication, sooner if symptoms worsen. If there is no clinical improvement at 72 hours, hospitalization is required for IV treatment. Further studies are also warranted at this time to assess for other possible diagnoses. *C. trachomatis* will continue to be excreted after treatment. Repeated cultures must wait 3 to 6 weeks for accuracy.

Complications

Fitz-Hugh–Curtis syndrome occurs in 5% to 30% of cases of pelvic infection. It is caused by inflammation of the capsule surrounding the liver. Affected clients have right upper quadrant pain that is intense enough to obscure the symptoms of pelvic pain.

Infertility as a result of tubal scarring occurs in 10% to 30% of clients after the first episode of PID, depending on the severity of the infection. Infertility rates continue to rise with each subsequent episode of PID, reaching 50% to 75% after three or more cases. Ectopic pregnancy rates also increase as a result of scarred fallopian tubes. Chronic pelvic pain, etiology unknown, may be a complication.

REFERENCES

Apuzzio, J., & Hoegsberg, B. (1992). PID: Hard to find, essential to treat. *Patient Care, 26*(6), 30-40.

Bowie, W., Hammarschlag, M., & Martin, D. (1994). STDs in '94: The new CDC guidelines. *Patient Care, 28*(7), 29-53.

Centers for Disease Control and Prevention. *CDC prevention guidelines* [On-line]. (1997). Available http://wonder.cdc.gov.

Deutsch, N. (1995). PID while pregnant. *Canadian Nurse, Aug.,* 23.

Howes, D., Marrazzo, J., & Scott, C. (1993). Recognizing pelvic inflammatory disease. *Patient Care, 27*(6), 186-204.

Jossens, M., & Sweet, R. (1993). Pelvic inflammatory disease: Risk factors and microbial etiologies. *JOGNN, 22*(2), 169-176.

Kottman, L. (1995). Pelvic inflammatory disease: Clinical overview. *JOGNN, 24*(8), 759-766.

Newkirk, G. (1996). Pelvic inflammatory disease: A contemporary approach. *American Family Physician, 53*(4), 1127-1139.

The challenges of diagnosing PID…Pelvic inflammatory disease. (1994). *Emergency Medicine, 26*(8), 56, 59-60.

REVIEW QUESTIONS

1. What are the minimum diagnostic criteria for PID?

   a. Right upper quadrant pain, fever, and vomiting
   b. Cervical motion tenderness, left adnexal pain, and vaginal discharge
   c. Lower abdominal pain, cervical motion tenderness, and bilateral adnexal pain
   d. Abnormal vaginal bleeding, dyspareunia, and elevated WBCs

2. Which of the following physical findings is suggestive PID?

   a. Vaginal discharge mucopurulent
   b. Right lower quadrant pain
   c. Cervical friability
   d. Cervical motion tenderness

3. Which of the following regimens would be appropriate for 21-year-old client who is having her first episode of PID, is afebrile, and is in her first trimester of pregnancy?

   a. Ofloxacin, 400 mg bid, for 14 days, plus metronidazole, 500 mg bid, for 14 days
   b. Cefoxitin, 2 g IV q 6 hours, plus doxycycline, 100 mg bid, for 14 days
   c. Ceftriaxone, 250 mg IM, and doxycycline, 100 mg, bid for 14 days
   d. Clindamycin, 900 mg IV q 8 hours, with gentamicin loading dose, 2 mg/kg IV, and maintenance dose, 1.5 mg/kg q 8 hours.

4. Your client has been treated for 4 days with IV cefoxitin and IV doxycycline for PID with culture positive for *N. gonorrhoeae.* When should she initially return for follow-up after her discharge from the hospital?

   a. In 4 to 6 weeks for repeated culture
   b. Only if symptoms recur
   c. In 72 hours
   d. In 7 to 10 days after completion of medication

5. In atypical PID, the most probable causative organism is:

   a. *C. trachomatis*
   b. *N. gonorrhoeae*
   c. *Bacteroides*
   d. *Peptostreptococcus*

6. Your client has been taking ofloxacin, 400 mg, and metronidazole, 500, mg both PO bid, for 14 days. At her initial 72-hour follow-up appointment, she has minimal resolution of her symptoms. All the following are appropriate courses to follow **except:**

   a. Hospitalize client.
   b. Order abdominal ultrasonography.
   c. Start cefotetan, 2 g, and doxycycline, 100 mg, IV every 12 hours.
   d. Recheck on outpatient basis in 24 hours.

ANSWERS AND RATIONALES

1. *Answer:* c (assessment/physical examination/reproductive/childbearing female)

   Rationale: Right upper quadrant pain is a symptom of complications from PID. Unilateral pain is more indicative of appendicitis or ectopic pregnancy. Abnormal uterine bleeding, dyspareunia, and elevated WBCs are associated with PID but are not minimum diagnostic criteria. (Newkirk, 1996)

2. *Answer:* d (assessment/physical examination/reproductive/childbearing female)

   Rationale: The pain of PID originates from the cervix. The pain should be with motion of cervix. Pregnancy may accompany PID but is not diagnostic. (Howes, Marrazzo, & Scott, 1993)

3. *Answer:* d (plan/management/therapeutic/pharmacologic/reproductive/childbearing female)

   Rationale: Hospitalization is warranted for the pregnant client. *D* is the regimen used for hospitalized patients. *A,* in addition to being an outpatient regimen, also contains ofloxacin, which is not for use during pregnancy. *C* includes doxycycline, which is best avoided during pregnancy. (Kottman, 1995)

4. *Answer:* d (evaluation/reproductive/childbearing female)

   Rationale: A 4- to 6-week follow-up is in addition to the 7- to 10-day follow-up. The 72-hour time is from initiation of therapy. The client should not be discharged from the hospital without clinical improvement. (Kottman, 1995)

5. *Answer:* a (pathophysiology/reproductive/child-bearing female)

Rationale: C. trachomatis is an often asymptomatic STD, including cases of PID. Choices *b, c,* and *d* are also causes of PID, but these are less likely to be asymptomatic. ("The Challenges of Diagnosing PID," 1994)

6. *Answer:* d (plan/management/therapeutic/pharmacological/childbearing female)

Rationale: This client has not improved after 72 hours of treatment. She warrants hospitalization and IV antibiotics. Further diagnostic tests are indicated to determine if she is simply not responding to oral medications or there is another possible diagnosis. (CDC, 1997)

PREMENSTRUAL SYNDROME

OVERVIEW

Definition

Premenstrual syndrome (PMS) is a cluster of unpleasant, often distressing, physical, psychologic, and behavioral symptoms (>100 have been identified) that occur in the second half (premenstrual or luteal phase) of the menstrual cycle and disappear dramatically within 1 to 2 days after onset of menses.

Incidence

As many as 90% of all menstruating women have some recurring premenstrual symptoms. For 20% to 40%, symptoms are severe enough to require medical intervention; 5% suffer debilitating symptoms. Peak incidence is during the 20s and 30s; PMS rarely occurs in teenagers.

Pathophysiology

The exact cause has not been established, but there are numerous theories of cause:

- Hormonal imbalance
- Low blood glucose
- Excess prolactin
- Excess prostaglandin
- Vitamin deficiency
- Endorphin malfunction
- Fluid retention
- Food allergy

PROTECTIVE FACTORS

- Regular exercise
- Current use of oral contraceptives
- Menopause

FACTORS INCREASING SUSCEPTIBILITY

- Being of reproductive age
- Increased parity
- Stressful lifestyle

ASSESSMENT: SUBJECTIVE/HISTORY

- Symptoms are best assessed through a daily symptom diary, calendar, or checklist. Retrospective recall is less accurate.
- Assess current health status.
- Conduct obstetric history.
- Note current and past contraceptive use and any relationship to symptoms.
- Conduct detailed menstrual history: Menarche; LMP; history of dysmenorrhea; when PMS symptoms first noted; and usual frequency, duration, and flow.
- Ask about typical day and stress level. Determine how this varies throughout cycle.
- Self-diagnosis is common. If this is the case, ask what made the client draw the conclusion that she has PMS.
- Let the client identify which symptoms she finds most distressing and which she considers a priority for intervention.

Past Medical History

- History of chronic illness, noting particular effects of PMS on chronic illness
- Ask specifically about lupus, fibrocystic disease, thyroid disease, chronic fatigue syndrome, and mood or anxiety disorders, which may mimic PMS.
- History of psychiatric illness
- History of surgery
- Drug or other allergies

Medication History

Ask about current use of prescription or OTC medications, including those for menstrual-related symptoms.

Family History

- Ask about first degree relatives with PMS.
- Ask about family history of psychiatric illness.

Psychosocial History

- Ask how symptoms affect work or school, leisure, and relationships.
- Ask about use of alcohol, tobacco, or street drugs.
- Determine how significant others have responded to diagnosis, if applicable. (Remember that PMS diagnosis is controversial and sometimes discounted by others, including health care professionals. For some, diagnosis is stigmatizing. For those reasons, syndrome should be validated and treated seriously by the nurse practitioner.)

Dietary History

- Ask about food cravings.
- Use dietary recall to determine fat, refined sugar, and sodium intakes.

ASSESSMENT: OBJECTIVE/ PHYSICAL EXAMINATION

Physical Examination

Problem-oriented physical examination should be performed, with attention to symptom-related clusters, vital signs, weight and presence of edema, skin, heart, thyroid, breasts, abdomen, and pelvis.

Diagnostic Procedures

There is no single test diagnostic for PMS because no physiologic or biochemical factors are consistently altered. Laboratory tests may be ordered on the basis of individual symptoms or to rule out organic causes.

Diagnosis is made on the basis of evaluation of a menstrual symptom calendar, diary, or checklist that indicates 30% increase in luteal phase symptoms—10 to 14 days before the menses when compared with those during and 10 to 14 days after. To be diagnosed as PMS, symptoms must occur in three consecutive cycles and be serious enough to require medical intervention. The hallmark feature is presence of minimum 7-day symptom-free interval in the first half of the cycle. The client should keep this record for 2 to 3 months to provide enough data for evaluation.

DIAGNOSIS

Rule out the following:
- Endocrine, metabolic, neurologic, and gynecologic disorders
- Underlying chronic illness with exacerbation related to menstrual cycle
- Acute illness with coincidental occurrence during luteal phase
- Psychiatric illness

THERAPEUTIC PLAN

Pharmacologic Treatment

- PMS is treated symptomatically. Oral contraception may help by suppressing ovulation.
- Use of mild diuretics, such as spironolactone, during luteal phase may decrease edema and bloating.
- Bromocriptine during luteal phase may help breast tenderness.
- Synthetic androgens, such as danazol (Danocrine), or gonadotropin-releasing hormone analogs, such as leuprolide (Lupron), may also be used in consultation with a physician, usually as a last resort.
- Several drugs are effective for many women but without fully documented rationale: vitamin B_6, evening primrose oil, progesterone vaginal suppositories, prostaglandin inhibitors (NSAIDs), and multivitamins with magnesium and zinc.
- Psychotropic drugs may be necessary for anxiety or depression.

Client Education

- Teach record-keeping system with menstrual-symptom diary, checklist, or calendar. Being actively involved in management is sometimes therapeutic.
- Provide understandable information about menstrual cycle and its relationship to symptoms.
- Educate client's significant others about illness to enlist their support.
- Role play assessment of needs and dealing with difficult situations.
- Suggest scheduling difficult situations for symptom-free intervals as much as possible.
- Assist with stress reduction and management.

- Discourage client from placing blame for all negative circumstances on PMS, to avoid perceptual victim role.
- Advise regular aerobic exercise.
- Advise frequent small meals—low in calories, fat, and refined sugar; with minimal sodium; and high in complex carbohydrates and water.
- Advise reduction of caffeine and methylxanthines (coffee, tea, chocolate).
- Suggest limiting alcohol intake and eliminating smoking.

Referral

- Refer client to PMS support group, PMS clinic, or subspecialty if available.
- Refer client for psychotherapy if indicated by symptoms.
- Refer client to physician if no response to treatment or with exacerbation of chronic illness.

EVALUATION/FOLLOW-UP

Return to clinic monthly for 3 months, then annually or as needed for evaluation of symptom management. Closely monitor effectiveness of treatment and side effects.

REFERENCES

Carter, J., & Verhoef, M. J. (1994). Efficacy of self-help and alternative treatments of premenstrual syndrome. *Women's Health Institute, 4*(3), 130-136.

Chuong, C. J., Pearsall-Otey, L. R., & Rosenfeld, B. L. (1995). A practical guide to relieving PMS. *Contemporary Nurse Practitioner, 1*(3), 31-37.

DeCherney, A. H., & Pernoll, M. L. (1994). *Current obstetrics and gynecology: Diagnosis and treatment.* (8th ed.). Norwalk, CT: Appleton & Lange.

Endicott, J., Johnson, S. R., & Keye, W. R. (1990). Helping the patient with PMS. *Patient Care, 24*(3), 44-48.

Hawkins, J. W., Roberto-Nichols, E. M., & Stanley-Haney, J. L. (1994). *Protocols for nurse practitioners in gynecologic settings.* New York: Tiresias Press.

Hsia, L. S., & Long, M. H. (1990). Premenstrual syndrome—Current concepts in diagnosis and management. *Journal of Nurse Midwifery, 35*(6), 351-353.

Lemke, D. P., Pattison, J., Marshall, L. A., & Cowley, D. S. (1995). *Primary Care of Women.* Norwalk, CT: Appleton & Lange.

Lindow, K. B. (1991). Premenstrual syndrome: Family impact and nursing implications. *Journal of Obstetric, Gynecologic, and Neonatal Nursing, 20*(2), 135-138.

Mastrangelo, R. (1994). Taming the beast known as PMS. *Advance for Nurse Practitioners, 2*(10), pp. 11-14.

Star, W. L., Lommel, L. L., & Shannon, M. T. (1995). *Women's primary health care: Protocols for practice.* Washington, DC: American Nurses Publishing.

Taylor, D. L. (1994). Evaluating therapeutic change in symptom severity at the level of individual women experiencing severe PMS. *Image: Journal of Nursing Scholarship, 26*(1), 25-33.

Youngkin, E. Q., & Davis, M. S. (1994). *Women's health: A primary care clinical guide.* Norwalk, CT: Appleton & Lange.

REVIEW QUESTIONS

1. Which of the following psychologic symptoms is **least** indicative of a diagnosis of PMS?

    a. Irritability

    b. Anxiety

    c. Aggression

    d. Manic affect

2. Before a diagnosis of PMS may be made, the practitioner must determine when in the menstrual cycle symptoms occur. In which case is a diagnosis of PMS most justified?

    a. Symptoms consistently occur on day 14 of a 28-day cycle.

    b. Symptoms consistently occur in the first 5 days after menstrual flow ceases.

    c. Symptoms occur throughout the entire menstrual cycle every other month.

    d. Symptoms occur during the premenstrual phase of the cycle.

3. Which of the following suggestions is **least** appropriate for the 25-year-old client with PMS?

    a. Eat frequent, small meals with limited refined sugars, fats, and sodium; limit alcohol intake.

    b. Schedule difficult activities for symptom-free days if possible.

    c. Remind any significant other that conflicts and confrontations in the relationship may be blamed on her diagnosis.

    d. Schedule regular aerobic exercise weekly.

4. Which of the following factors most justifies more frequent follow-up of the client with PMS?

   a. She has become engaged to marry her college boyfriend.
   b. She recently changed to a part-time management position so that she can enroll in graduate school.
   c. She has bought a puppy.
   d. She joined a gym to make exercise easier to schedule.

5. Which objective measure is most suited to diagnosing PMS?

   a. Vital signs
   b. CBC and clotting profile
   c. Chemistry panel 20
   d. Menstrual symptom checklist

6. Ann Kovick is a 25-year-old who comes in for an annual examination. She mentions recent onset of symptoms suggestive of PMS. Which factor in Ann's history increases her risk for PMS?

   a. Her job is as a flight attendant.
   b. Both her sisters have significant premenstrual symptoms.
   c. She jogs and swims regularly at a health club.
   d. She uses oral contraceptives for birth control.

7. Which symptom documented in Ann's menstrual diary is most diagnostic of PMS?

   a. Severe menstrual cramps and backache
   b. Premenstrual frothy, slightly malodorous vaginal discharge
   c. Leg cramps more noticeable immediately after menses
   d. Irritability and tearfulness in the 4 days before her period

8. The practitioner spends time counseling Ann about symptom management. Which comment that Ann might make would indicate her need for additional instruction?

   a. "I will start eating less fried and salty foods."
   b. "I can expect these symptoms to get progressively worse until I go through menopause."
   c. "Attending a support group with other women who experience PMS may help me to deal better with the problem."

   d. "Limiting my coffee, tea, cola, and chocolate intake may help alleviate some of the breast tenderness."

9. To determine whether the therapeutic plan has been effective, when should Ann's next visit be scheduled?

   a. 14 days before her next menstrual period
   b. 7 to 10 days after her next menstrual period
   c. The day her menstrual flow begins
   d. At any time convenient to Ann, regardless of the cycle

ANSWERS AND RATIONALES

1. *Answer:* d (assessment/history/reproductive/NAS)
   Rationale: Irritability, anxiety, and aggression are common features of PMS. Depressed, not manic, affect is common. (Hsia & Long, 1990)

2. *Answer:* d (diagnosis/reproductive/NAS)
   Rationale: A hallmark of the PMS diagnosis is occurrence of the symptoms during the luteal or premenstrual phase of the menstrual cycle. (Hsia & Long, 1990)

3. *Answer:* c (plan/reproductive/adult)
   Rationale: Blaming everything negative on the diagnosis of PMS causes the client to become a perpetual victim. (Endicott, Johnson, & Keye, 1990)

4. *Answer:* b (evaluation/reproductive/NAS)
   Rationale: A stressful lifestyle that includes balancing career, family, and other commitments predisposes toward PMS. (Hsia & Long, 1990)

5. *Answer:* d (assessment/physical examination/reproductive/NAS)
   Rationale: A menstrual symptom checklist, diary, or calendar is the most effective measure for assessing PMS symptoms. (Hawkins, Roberto-Nichols, & Stanley-Haney, 1994)

6. *Answer:* b (assessment/history/reproductive/adult)
   Rationale: PMS in a first-degree relative is a factor that increases the probability of the client having PMS. (Hsia & Long, 1990)

7. *Answer:* d (diagnosis/reproductive/adult)
   Rationale: PMS symptoms occur in the luteal or premenstrual phase of the menstrual cycle. (Hawkins et al., 1994)

8. *Answer:* b (plan/reproductive/adult)

Rationale: Symptoms of PMS are most common in the 20s and 30s but do not necessarily progress. With appropriate intervention, most can be managed effectively. (Endicott et al., 1990)

9. *Answer:* b (evaluation/reproductive/adult)

Rationale: To determine whether symptom management has been effective, the follow-up visit should be scheduled for 7 to 10 days after menstruation. (Endicott et al., 1990)

VAGINITIS

OVERVIEW
Definition

Vaginitis is infection of the vagina, either inflammatory or noninflammatory.

Incidence

Approximately 40% of vaginal infections are caused by bacterial vaginosis. It is not considered an STD, yet it is uncommon in virginal females. Trichimoniasis occurs in approximately 10% of vaginal infections. Candidiasis is the cause of approximately 50% of all vaginal infections.

Pathophysiology

The most common causes of vaginal infections include bacterial vaginosis *(Gardnerella vaginalis)*, *Candida albicans (Monilia)*, and trichomoniasis. Bacterial vaginosis is caused by a change in the natural ecology of the vagina, whereas *Candida* infections occur when the natural flora of the vagina proliferates. Trichomoniasis is caused by a protozoan flagellate. All three are considered sexually associated, but *not* sexually transmitted.

RISK FACTORS FOR *CANDIDA* AND BACTERIAL VAGINOSIS. Risk factors include use of vaginal douches and deodorant sprays, recent changes in contraceptives, use of tampons and diaphragms, use of spermicides, latex allergy, medications, chronic illness, and personal hygiene habits. Pregnancy also appears to be a contributing factor.

RISK FACTORS FOR TRICHOMONIASIS. Risk factors include poor hygiene, lack of concurrent treatment of partner, and changes in sexual partner.

ASSESSMENT: SUBJECTIVE/HISTORY
Bacterial Vaginosis

Women with bacterial vaginosis may report increased vaginal discharge, vaginal burning after intercourse, and a strong, usually "fishy" odor.

There are generally no associated symptoms of inflammation (hence the term *vaginosis* instead of *vaginitis,* which indicates inflammation).

Candidiasis

Women with candidiasis frequently report itching (often severe), burning with urination, and dyspareunia or burning during or after intercourse. Discharge is thick, white, and curdlike.

Trichomoniasis

Frequently presenting symptoms of trichomoniasis are foul-smelling vaginal discharge, external itching and burning, dyspareunia, and postcoital bleeding. Partners may have similar symptoms.

History

- Previous infections and treatments
- Vaginal discharge (color and odor)
- Sexual activity
- LMP
- Last intercourse
- Method of birth control
- Other medications (antibiotics, steroids, or estrogens with *Candida*)
- History of chronic illness (especially seizure disorders, diabetes, and HIV)
- Relationship of symptoms to sexual contact
- It is also important to evaluate the possibility of pregnancy because it will affect treatment.

ASSESSMENT: OBJECTIVE/ PHYSICAL EXAMINATION
Physical Examination

A problem-oriented physical examination should be conducted, with particular attention to abdominal examination and pelvic examination. Objective signs that may also be seen are listed in Table 6-1.

Table 6-1   Objective Signs of Vaginitis

	CANDIDIASIS	BACTERIAL VAGINOSIS	TRICHOMONIASIS
External genitalia	Excoriated, erythema, edema, ulcerations, lesions	Normal	Excoriated, erythema, edema, ulcerations, lesions
Vaginal mucosa	Erythema; irritated, white patches along walls	Normal	May notice red papules
Cervix	Normal	Normal	Strawberry-like appearance
Discharge	Thick, odorless, white, curdlike	Adherent, homogenous, grayish in color, with a fishy, musty odor	Greenish, yellow, malodorous, and frothy
Wet preparation	Hyphae, pseudohyphae	Clue cells, positive whiff	Highly motile, oval cells

DIAGNOSIS

NOTE: Frequently, two or more of the types of vaginitis will coexist.

Differential diagnosis includes the following:

CANDIDIASIS
- Herpes
- Chemical vaginitis
- Contact dermatitis
- Candidias related to diabetes
- Other, less frequently seen *Candida* infections
- Trichomoniasis
- Bacterial vaginosis
- *Chlamydia*
- Gonococcal infections
- Atrophic vaginitis

BACTERIAL VAGINOSIS
- Trichomoniasis
- Presence of a foreign body

TRICHOMONIASIS
- Candidiasis
- Bacterial vaginosis
- UTI
- Gonorrhea
- *Chlamydia*

THERAPEUTIC PLAN

Candidiasis

Clotrimazole, miconazole (Monistat), butoconazole (Femstat), terconazole (Terazol), and fluconazole (Diflucan). Terazol will treat most atypical species in candidiasis. Women in whom candidiasis develops after antibiotic treatment may consider the use of either vitamin C, 500 mg bid to qid, or oral acidophilus tablets, 40 MU to 1 GU (1 tablet).

Bacterial Vaginosis

Use metranidazole cream (Flagyl), clindamycin (Cleocin) vaginal cream, or metronidazole gel (MetroGel, treatment of choice). In the past, Cleocin vaginal cream was the treatment of choice during pregnancy. New studies, however, indicate that MetroGel is safe to use during pregnancy and carries a lower instance of preterm labor and other complications.

Trichomoniasis

Use Flagyl. If client is pregnant, she may use clotrimazole vaginal suppositories or amoxicillin. MetroGel is *not* indicated for treatment of trichomoniasis. Partner must also be treated.

Client Education

Instruct client that there should be no intercourse until symptoms subside and treatment is complete. Douching is to be avoided. Instruct client on hygiene measures.

EVALUATION/FOLLOW-UP

There is no "test of cure"; however, if client has chronic infections, consider evaluating for underlying disease process, incomplete treatment course, or concomitant infections.

REFERENCES

Centers for Disease Control and Prevention (1993). Sexually transmitted diseases treatment guidelines. *MMWR Morbidity Mortality Weekly Report, 42* (RR-14), 67-75.

Dunnihoo, D. R. (1992). Vaginal disease. In *Fundamentals of gynecology and obstetrics* (2nd ed.). Philadelphia: J. B. Lippincott.

Glass, R. H. (1993). Sexually transmitted infection. In *Office gynecology* (4th ed.). Baltimore: Williams & Wilkins.

Hawkins, J. W., Roberto-Nichols, D. M., & Stanley-Haney, J. L. (1995). Vaginal discharge, vaginitis, and sexually transmitted diseases. *Protocols for nurse practitioners in gynecologic settings* (5th ed.). New York: Tiresias Press.

Johnson, C. A., Johnson, B. E., Murray, J. L., & Apgar, B. S. (1996a). Gynecological infections. In C. A. Johnson et al. (Eds.), *Women's health care handbook.* St. Louis: Mosby.

Johnson, C. A., Johnson, B. E., Murray, J. L. & Apgar, B. S. (1996b). Sexually transmitted diseases. In C. A. Johnson et al. (Eds.), *Women's health care handbook.* St. Louis: Mosby.

Loudon, N., Glaiser, A., & Gebbie, A. (1995). Sexually transmittable diseases. In *Handbook of family planning and reproductive health* (3rd ed.). New York: Churchill Livingstone.

Uphold, C. R., & Graham, M. V. (1994). Sexually transmitted disease. In *Clinical guidelines in family practice.* Gainesville, FL: Barmarrae Books.

REVIEW QUESTIONS

1. Complaints of dyspareunia, postcoital bleeding, itching, and a foul-smelling discharge suggest which condition?

   a. Bacterial vaginosis
   b. UTI
   c. Candidiasis
   d. Trichomoniasis

2. On examination, the nurse practitioner notices a bright red cervix and a thin, frothy, green discharge. There are highly motile, oval cells located on wet preparation. The practitioner suspects which condition?

   a. Bacterial vaginosis
   b. *Chlamydia*
   c. Trichomoniasis
   d. Gonorrhea

3. Hyphae and pseudohyphae are visible with potassium hydroxide on wet preparation with which condition?

   a. Bacterial vaginosis
   b. Trichomoniasis
   c. Candidiasis
   d. UTI

4. A 24-year-old woman reports dysuria with external burning. Her urine dip result is negative. She reports douching weekly. Her pelvic examination is unremarkable, except for edematous mucosa and vulva. Before checking a wet preparation and solely on the basis of her history and symptoms, the nurse practitioner would suspect which condition?

   a. A sterile cystitis
   b. Bacterial vaginosis
   c. Candidiasis
   d. Subclinical herpes

5. The treatment of choice for women in their first trimester of pregnancy who have bacterial vaginosis is what?

   a. Metronidazole cream (Flagyl)
   b. MetroGel vaginal gel
   c. Clindamycin
   d. Cleocin vaginal cream

6. Clients with a diagnosis of trichomoniasis who are allergic to Flagyl may be treated with what antibiotic?

   a. Clindamycin
   b. Amoxicillin
   c. Erythromycin
   d. All other treatment choices are not as effective as metronidazole (Flagyl).

7. Women who are predisposed toward *Candida* infections while or after taking antibiotics may consider using what supplements when antibiotics are necessary?

   a. Vitamin E
   b. Vitamin C
   c. Calcium
   d. B-complex vitamins

ANSWERS AND RATIONALES

1. *Answer:* d (diagnosis/reproductive/NAS)

Rationale: Bacterial vaginosis does not cause inflammation, so it would not cause dyspareunia, postcoital bleeding, or itching. UTI will cause neither vaginal discharge nor postcoital bleeding. Candidiasis does not have a foul-smelling discharge. A trichomoniasis vaginitis will cause these symptoms. (Johnson, Johnson, Murray, & Apgar, 1996b)

2. *Answer:* c (diagnosis/reproductive/NAS)

Rationale: On a wet preparation, the practitioner will see increased WBCs and decreased normal flora with both *Chlamydia* and gonorrhea infections. Bacterial vaginosis will produce clue cells. Trichomoniasis has highly motile oval cells, as well as a strawberry-red cervix with frothy, thin, green discharge. (Johnson et al., 1996b)

3. *Answer:* c (diagnosis/reproductive/NAS)

Rationale: Bacterial vaginosis produces clue cells on wet preparation, whereas trichomoniasis produces highly motile oval cells. UTI does not produce either hyphae or pseudohyphae, which are present with candidiasis. (Hawkins, Roberto-Nichols, & Stanley-Haney, 1995)

4. *Answer:* c (diagnosis/reproductive/adult)

Rationale: A sterile cystitis will produce a sensation of internal burning, and subclinical herpes produces a fairly localized area of pain. Both bacterial vaginosis and candidiasis are caused by a change in the vaginal environment, often from frequent douching, but bacterial vaginosis does not cause inflammation. Therefore, on the basis of history and gross examination, the practitioner will suspect candidiasis. (Glass, 1993)

5. *Answer:* b (plan/reproductive/childbearing female)

Rationale: Metronidazole is contraindicated in the first trimester of pregnancy. Clindamycin and Cleocin both care category B and may be used. The treatment of choice is MetroGel. (CDC, 1993)

6. *Answer:* d (plan/reproductive/NAS)

Rationale: Currently there is no other approved treatment for trichomoniasis in the United States (CDC, 1993)

7. *Answer:* b (plan/reproductive/adult)

Rationale: Although each of these vitamin and mineral supplements has additional value to women, vitamin C, 500 mg bid to qid, will increase the acidity of vaginal mucosa. (Hawkins et al., 1995)

Musculoskeletal System

ARTHRITIS

Osteoarthritis and Rheumatoid Arthritis

OVERVIEW

Definition

Osteoarthritis (OA) is a degenerative disease of the cartilage of joints with reactive formation of new bone at auricular margins.

Primary OA is the most common form of OA and is of unknown origin. It affects most commonly the distal interphalangeal (DIP) joints and less commonly the proximal interphalangeal (PIP) joints, the metatarsophalangeal (MTP) and carpometacarpal joints of the hip, the knee, the MTP joint of the big toe, and the cervical and lumbar spine.

Secondary OA may occur in any joint as a result of articular injury (fracture, overuse of joint, or metabolic disease) resulting from either intraarticular (including rheumatoid arthritis) or extraarticular causes.

Rheumatoid arthritis (RA) is an immunologically mediated chronic inflammatory disease of unknown origin that primarily affects joints but may have generalized manifestations.

Juvenile rheumatoid arthritis (JRA) has three major presentations: (1) acute febrile form with salmon macular rash, arthritis, splenomegaly, leukocytosis, and polyserositis; (2) polyarticular (five or more joints involved) pattern that resembles adult disease, with chronic pain and swelling of many joints; and (3) pauciarticular (fewer than five joints) disease characterized by chronic arthritis of a few joints, often the large weight-bearing joints, in asymmetric distribution. Up to 30% of children (1 to 16 years old) with this form of disease develop iridocyclitis, which can cause blindness if untreated.

Incidence

OA is the most common form of arthritis and affects approximately 20 million Americans. Ninety percent of people have radiographic evidence of OA by age 40 in weight-bearing joints.

RA affects approximately 7 million Americans (females more than males, based on diagnostic criteria). The incidence increases with age and peaks in the fourth decade. The onset of JRA is between 2 and 4 years of age; the rate of JRA in girls is almost twice that of boys.

Pathophysiology

PROTECTIVE FACTORS
- Normal weight
- Male gender

FACTORS INCREASING SUSCEPTIBILITY
- Obesity
- Positive family history
- Posttraumatic injury
- Fracture/immobilization
- Increasing age
- Female gender
- History of gout, hemochromatoses, psoriasis, avascular necrosis, congenital dysplastic hip
- Intraarticular steroid overusage
- Metabolic abnormalities (Wilson's disease, acromegaly)

229

ASSESSMENT: SUBJECTIVE/HISTORY
Most Common Symptoms

OSTEOARTHRITIS

- Insidious onset
- Morning stiffness of less than 30 minutes
- Pain on movement
- Limitation of movement

RHEUMATOID ARTHRITIS

- Prodromal systemic symptoms (malaise, fever, weight loss)
- Morning stiffness lasting 30 to 60 minutes

JUVENILE RHEUMATOID ARTHRITIS

- Nonmigratory arthropathy (one or more joints)
- Tends to involve larger joints or PIP joints
- Lasts more than 3 months with systemic manifestations of fever, rash, nodules, leukocytosis
- Onset related to age of child with systemic involvement
- More likely in younger children

Associated Symptoms

OSTEOARTHRITIS

- Crepitus
- Pain relieved by rest
- Joint instability
- Edema and joint effusion minimal (or absent)
- Minor erythema or warmth of joint may be present
- Nocturnal pain after vigorous exercise
- Joint deformity
  - —Bony enlargement
  - —Heberden's nodes
  - —Flexion contracture/valgus/varus deformity of the knee
  - —Quadricep atrophy

RHEUMATOID ARTHRITIS

- Articular inflammation with swelling, pain, erythema, and warmth
- Progression of joint involvement centripetal and symmetric
- Tenosynovitis
- Rheumatoid nodules
- Systemic manifestations
  - —Vision loss
  - —Conjunctivitis
  - —Pain associated with pleural effusion
  - —Carpal tunnel syndrome (CTS)
  - —Cutaneous lesions
  - —Rashes
  - —Neuropathies
  - —Vasculitis

JUVENILE RHEUMATOID ARTHRITIS

- Characteristic salmon maculopapular rash in 25% to 50% of affected children
- May be intermittent, associated with fever spikes and increased splenomegaly
- May precede joint symptoms by 3 years

Past Medical History

- Steroid articular injections
- Occupational/leisure activity and/or injuries
- History of metabolic, endocrine, autoimmune, or other musculoskeletal disease (postural or developmental defects, joint instability, past meniscectomy)
- May affect ADLs
  Children: Past medical history may be unremarkable.

Medication History

Ask about use of antiinflammatory or analgesic agents (results, any other prescribed or OTC medications).

Family History

- OA
- RA
- Musculoskeletal disease
- Endocrine disease
- Autoimmune disease
- Metabolic disease

Psychosocial History

- Adults/older adults: Inquire how OA or RA affects their ADLs or instrumental activities of daily living (IADLs) (e.g., shopping, check writing)
- Children: Consider how RA may affect their daily life and school performance.

Dietary History

Obtain overall nutritional assessment with emphasis on weight reduction, if necessary.

ASSESSMENT: OBJECTIVE/ PHYSICAL EXAMINATION
Physical Examination

- Conduct a problem-oriented physical examination, keeping in mind potential systemic manifestations of RA (dermatologic, pleurisy, splenomegaly, ocular manifestations, etc.) that might necessitate a complete physical examination.

- Pay attention to vital signs, weight, blood pressure, and pulse.
- Note general appearance, gait, and activity level.

Musculoskeletal Examination

- Inspect affected joints for deformities, nodes, numbers of affected joints, symmetry of affected joints, and erythema.
- Observe affected joints in active/passive ROM.
- Palpate affected joints for warmth, tenderness, crepitus, and edema.
- Assess muscle strength.
- Assess joint stability.

Diagnostic Procedures

OSTEOARTHRITIS. There are no definitive tests for OA; however, radiographic findings of the affected joint may reveal narrowing of joint space, soft tissue swelling, and marginal osteophytes. Other tests (ESR, CBC, electrolytes) are often not needed unless ordered to support OA as a diagnosis of exclusion.

RHEUMATOID ARTHRITIS. No test can exclude or prove this diagnosis. ESR provides useful but nonspecific information in confirming inflammatory disease. An ESR >60 mm/hr indicates severe inflammation. The ESR is useful in following the client's response to treatment but is not useful when inflammatory disease is in remission.

Rheumatoid factor is not pathognomonic of RA but is present in 70% to 80% of persons meeting the criteria for RA. A significant titer is a finding of 1:80 or greater, although the result may be negative in early disease.

The WBC count from CBC is normal or slightly elevated and may reveal normocytic, hypochromic anemia. The platelet count is often elevated.

JUVENILE RHEUMATOID ARTHRITIS
Rheumatoid factor results by latex fixation are positive in about 15% of cases. Antinuclear antibodies (ANAs) may be present in pauciarticular disease. ESR results may be normal in the presence of active disease.

DIAGNOSIS
Osteoarthritis

Because articular inflammation is absent or minimal and systemic manifestations are absent, OA

is seldom confused. However, diagnosis is not always straightforward. In those instances, the following conditions may be included in the differential diagnosis of OA:

- Rheumatoid arthritis
- Gout
- Pseudogout
- Psoriatic arthritis
- Septic arthritis
- Malignancy
- Osteoporosis
- Tendinitis (bursitis)

Rheumatoid Arthritis

- Osteoarthritis
- Polymyalgia rheumatica
- Systemic lupus erythematosus (SLE)
- Sjögren's syndrome
- Vasculitis
- Gout
- Pseudogout
- Scleroderma
- Septic arthritis
- Psoriatic arthritis
- Lyme disease
- Malignancy
- Polymyositis

Juvenile Rheumatoid Arthritis

- Rheumatic fever
- Osgood-Schlatter disease
- Fracture
- Slipped capital femoral epiphysis
- Schönlein-Henoch purpura
- Infections
- SLE
- Lyme disease
- Neoplasms (leukemia, lymphoma, neuroblastoma)
- Syndromes of psychoorganic origin

THERAPEUTIC PLAN

The objectives of therapy are to restore function, relieve pain, and maintain joint motion.

Pharmacologic Treatment

OSTEOARTHRITIS
Because there is no major inflammation with OA and because OA is a chronic disease, pure analgesics that are inexpensive and safe such as acetaminophen (<4 g/day) and aspirin (1.2 to 2.4 g/day) should be considered. Enteric-coated as-

pirin to reduce gastrointestinal tract bleeding is recommended. NSAIDs may also be used.

RHEUMATOID ARTHRITIS

NSAIDs are the first choice in the treatment of RA. Aspirin is effective, inexpensive, and usually the first NSAID employed. Dosages of 3.6 to 4.8 g/day are usually necessary to achieve therapeutic serum levels of 15 to 20 mg/dl. Enteric-coated aspirin or misoprostol with regular aspirin or NSAIDs is recommended to reduce the chance of gastrointestinal tract bleeding.

Second-line drugs are employed if NSAIDs prove ineffective or the client shows evidence of progression of the disease (physician consultation recommended):

- Gold salts injectable or PO
- Antimalarials
- Sulfasalazine 1 g/day initially and increase after 1 to 2 weeks to 2 g/dl
- Hydroxychloroquine 200 mg qd or bid

Third-line drugs are employed for those clients who do not respond to second-line drugs:

- Corticosteroids
- Prednisone 5 mg/day
- Intraarticular injections of corticosteroids (no more than every 3 months)
- Penicillamine
- Cytotoxic drugs (usually prescribed by rheumatologist): Azathioprine (Imuran) 1 to 2.5 mg/kg/day; methotrexate 7.5 mg/wk to start

Older Adults. As with other pharmacologic treatment, it may be necessary to start with lower dosages and titrate upward until symptoms are controlled.

JUVENILE RHEUMATOID ARTHRITIS.

Consider a consultation with a pediatric rheumatologist at diagnosis. NSAIDs have replaced salicylates in liquid form; the decreased dosage frequency and diminished side effects of NSAIDs enhance compliance. Treatment includes naproxen 7.5 mg/kg bid; ibuprofen 10 mg/kg qid; tolmetin sodium 10 mg/kg tid. Aspirin 75 to 100 mg/kg in 3 divided doses is equally effective. (Do not use aspirin if the client was exposed to chickenpox or Asian flu.) For those children who fail to respond to NSAIDs, methotrexate is a second-line medication (5 to 10 mg/m^2/wk). Injectable gold salts are an alternative. Children with ophthalmic involvement should be referred to an ophthalmologist.

Client Education

- Weight loss
- Exercise to maintain ROM and increase strength
- Rest during day
- Selective rest of affected joints to prevent contracture (example: splinting at night)
- Heat and cold to relieve muscle spasm and provide pain relief
- Physical therapy
- Proper posture
- Assistive devices: Canes, walkers, crutches
- Surgery

Referral

For children and adults who do not respond to therapy or have severe disease, treatment is a team approach and should include referrals for nutritional counseling, physical and/or occupational therapy, and surgery when necessary.

EVALUATION/FOLLOW-UP

Follow-up depends on the severity of the disease. If medications are to be advanced weekly, laboratory evaluations should be performed. Clients should be seen on a weekly basis until symptoms are controlled. At the evaluation/follow-up visits, reinforce client education measures and assess for psychosocial adaption/coping to the disease.

Children

Disease activity progressively diminishes with age and in 95% of cases ceases by puberty. In a few cases, disease persists into adulthood. Problems after puberty relate to joint damage, but JRA in adolescence may precede adult disease.

REFERENCES

Barker, L. R., Burton, J. R., & Zieve, P. D. (1995). *Principles of ambulatory medicine* (4th ed.). Baltimore: Williams & Wilkins.

Burns, C. E., Barber, V., Brady, M. A., & Dunn, A. M. (1996). *Primary pediatric care: A handbook for nurse practitioners.* Philadelphia: W. B. Saunders.

Gorroll, A. H., May, L. A., & Mulley, A. G. (1995). *Primary care medicine.* Philadelphia: J. B. Lippincott.

Hery, W. W., Groothius, J. R., Hayward, A. R., & Leven, M. J. (1997). *Current pediatric diagnosis and treatment.* Norwalk, CT: Appleton & Lange.

Hooker, R. S. (1996, January). Osteoarthritis of the hip and knee: Managing a common joint disease. *Clinicians Review,* pp. 54-67.

Hurst, J. W. (1996). *Medicine for the practicing physician.* Norwalk, CT: Appleton & Lange.

Tierney, L. M., McPhee, S. J., & Papadakis, M. A. (1996). *Current medical diagnosis and treatment.* Norwalk, CT: Appleton & Lange.

Uphold, C., & Graham, M. (1994). *Clinical guidelines in family practice.* Gainesville, FL: Barmarrae Books.

REVIEW QUESTIONS

1. JRA is characterized by all the following **except:**

   a. Polyarticular
   b. Acute febrile form
   c. As a result of articular injury
   d. Pauciarticular

2. Morning stiffness in RA lasts:

   a. 30 to 60 minutes or longer
   b. Less than 30 minutes
   c. Throughout the day
   d. Indefinite period of time

3. The typical client with RA is:

   a. Male
   b. 40 years or older
   c. Overweight
   d. Older than 65 years of age

4. The anemia often associated with RA is:

   a. Microcytic, hypochromic
   b. Macrocytic, normochromic
   c. Normocytic, hypochromic
   d. Microcytic, normochromic

5. The differential diagnosis of RA includes all the following **except:**

   a. Gout
   b. Osteoarthritis
   c. Tendinitis
   d. Polymyalgia rheumatica

6. Aspirin, to reach therapeutic serum levels in adults, usually requires:

   a. Enteric coating
   b. 1.6 to 2.4 g/day
   c. >5 g/day
   d. 3.6 to 4.8 g/day

7. After treatment with sulfasalazine is initiated, the client should be seen in:

   a. 1 month
   b. 1 to 2 weeks
   c. 1 to 2 days
   d. 3 to 5 days

ANSWERS AND RATIONALES

1. **Answer:** c (assessment/physical examination/musculoskeletal/NAS)

   Rationale: JRA has three major presentations: (1) acute febrile form with salmon maculopapular rash, arthritis, splenomegaly, leukocytosis, and polyserositis; (2) polyarticular (five or more joints) pattern with swelling and chronic pain; (3) pauciarticular (fewer than five joints) disease with chronic arthritis of a few joints, often weight-bearing joints, in an asymmetric distribution. (Burns, Barber, Brady, & Dunn, 1996; Hery, Groothius, Hayward, & Leven, 1997)

2. **Answer:** a (assessment/history/musculoskeletal/NAS)

   Rationale: RA typically has a history of morning stiffness lasting 30 to 60 minutes or even longer, whereas OA morning stiffness lasts 15 to 30 minutes. (Gorroll, May, & Mulley, 1995)

3. **Answer:** b (assessment/history/musculoskeletal/NAS)

   Rationale: The typical client with RA is female with the incidence peaking in the fourth decade of life. (Gorroll et al., 1995)

4. **Answer:** c (plan/musculoskeletal/NAS)

   Rationale: Clients with RA often exhibit anemia that is referred to as "anemia of chronic disease." This anemia is a normocytic, hypochromic anemia with reduced RBC mass.

5. **Answer:** c (diagnosis/musculoskeletal/NAS)

   Rationale: Because of joint involvement and/or inflammatory characteristics, OA, gout, and polymyalgia should be considered in the diagnosis of RA. (Uphold & Graham, 1994)

6. *Answer:* d (plan/musculoskeletal/adult)

Rationale: The usual dosage of aspirin needed to reach therapeutic levels is 3.6 to 4.8 g/day. Enteric coating has no relevance to therapeutic levels, 1.6 to 2.4 g/day is too low a dosage, and >5 g/day is too high a dosage. (Gorroll et al., 1995)

7. *Answer:* b (evaluation/musculoskeletal/NAS)

Rationale: The usual time frame for follow-up after initiation of treatment with sulfasalazine is 1 to 2 weeks to consider adjusting the dosage upward. This time frame allows for adequate blood levels and a trial for symptomatic relief. (Gorroll et al., 1995)

CARPAL TUNNEL SYNDROME

OVERVIEW
Definition

Carpal tunnel syndrome (CTS) is compression of the median nerve at the wrist with associated symptoms of tingling, numbness, or pain of the affected fingers and wrist. CTS is associated with occupations/hobbies with frequent repetitive motion of the wrist.

Incidence

- CTS is a common wrist-hand disorder.
- CTS occurs 3 to 5 times more in women than in men.
- The highest frequency is in the age group of 30 to 60.
- Hormones and fluid retention may have a role in women.
- Incidence is increasing in industry with repetitive forceful flexion/extension, vibration, or awkward positioning of wrist without sufficient rest.
- Pregnancy: There is an increased incidence of CTS in pregnancy, typically third trimester. Most cases resolve after childbirth.
- Childhood: CTS is not typically found in children.
- Statistics: The National Institute for Occupational Safety and Health (1989) estimates there are 20 million workers at risk for CTS; 23,000 new cases are reported every year; 100,000 CTS release surgeries are performed annually. Treatment is expensive, including surgery costing $25,000 to $30,000.

Pathophysiology

The median nerve is easily compressed as it runs through the carpal tunnel of the wrist. The tunnel is made of carpal bones on the dorsal side and the transverse carpal ligament (flexor retinaculum) on the ventral (volar) side. The median nerve lies in this 2- to 3-cm tunnel along with the nine flexor tendons of the fingers. Any swelling, trauma, or systemic metabolic process can affect the tunnel and cause compression on the median nerve with accompanying symptoms. Frequent wrist flexion/extension causes increased friction of tendons against the carpal bones or ligaments with inflammation and swelling. The median nerve supplies sensory fibers to the thumb, second and third fingers, and radial side of the fourth finger. Pressure on the nerve produces symptoms of tingling, numbness, pain. CTS resulting from repetitive factors can take weeks to years to develop with intermittent symptoms.

RISK FACTORS

Causes of CTS are complex and multicausal; not everyone with exposure develops CTS. There are three categories of causes:

- Occupational/hobbies: The major types are computer keyboard typists, checkout clerks, meatcutters, seamstress, hairdressers, those who use vibrating tools, musicians, mail-handlers/sorters, domestics, cooks, bowlers, knitters, and gardeners.
- Trauma: Fractures, dislocations, a blow to wrist, and structural defects are common.
- Metabolic/pregnancy: An increased incidence of CTS is associated with diabetes, RA, gout, hypothyroidism, birth control pill use, degenerative joint disease, and congenital defects of wrist. CTS is frequently seen in pregnancy.

ASSESSMENT: SUBJECTIVE/HISTORY
History of Present Illness

- Do symptoms wake up the client at night?
- What aggravates the symptoms?
- What impact do symptoms have on life activities?

- Problem with sensation, weakness, fine motor tasks?
- Discomfort while driving a car?
- Length of symptoms, intermittent or continuous?
- Are symptoms getting worse?

Symptoms

- Numbness, tingling, and pain to thumb and second, third, and fourth fingers of affected hand
- Most often wakes the person at night
- Onset insidious
- Symptoms sometimes intermittent for months

Associated Symptoms

- Wrist, forearm, and shoulder pain
- Chronic/late stages: Thenar wasting (muscle pad of thumb), weakness of hand with decreased grip strength, and decreased sensitivity of fingers

Past Medical History

OCCUPATIONAL/HOBBIES

- Past job/work history and extensive current job description?
- Repetitive forceful work, vibration, small tools, keyboard?
- Length of rest periods and breaks?
- Postures and motions?
- Does discomfort decrease when away from work/vacations?
- Type of hobbies? How often?
- Type of discomfort?

TRAUMA AND METABOLIC/PREGNANCY

- Diabetes (most commonly associated risk factor)
- Thyroid disease
- Any similar past problems during prior pregnancies
- Arthritis
- Use of oral contraceptives
- Medications/hormones
- Cancer
- Trauma

Family History

There is some indication of familial association with familial thickening of transverse carpal ligament.

ASSESSMENT: OBJECTIVE/ PHYSICAL EXAMINATION

Physical Examination

- Skin: Dry skin of affected area
- Musculoskeletal: Palpate affected area, grip strength, active and passive ROM
- Cardiovascular: Pulses
- Neurologic: Two-point discrimination
- Specific maneuvers
  —Tinel's sign: Tap at the volar surface of wrist. A positive result is reproduced symptoms or tingling into the median nerve distribution (50% accuracy).
  —Phalen's maneuver: This maneuver has the greatest sensitivity. Flex wrists maximally and hold 60 seconds. A positive result is reproduced symptoms.
  —Carpal compression: Compress the median nerve with thumbs for 30 seconds. A positive result is reproduced symptoms.

Diagnostic Procedures

The following examinations may be considered. Diagnosis can be made based on history and physical examination with further studies used as confirmatory.

- Quantitative grip and pinch studies: Loss of strength
- Laboratory work: Indicated by history of or suspected metabolic disorder; CBC, thyroid, glucose, renal, uric acid, ESR, rheumatoid factor
- Nerve conduction tests: EMG/nerve conduction studies to show abnormality in time/velocity of nerve conduction and aids to verify clinical diagnosis
- Radiographic: Used to assess trauma, fracture, tumor, structural defect; MRI and CT for detailed studies

DIAGNOSIS

The differential diagnosis includes the following:

- Cervical radiculopathy (pressure on the nerve root as it exits the cervical spine)
- Thoracic outlet syndrome (pressure of vascular or neurogenic compression at neck/ shoulder)
- de Quervain's disease (tenosynovitis of the thumb)
- Primal median nerve compression (median nerve compression higher in the arm)
- Guyon's canal (ulnar nerve compression)

THERAPEUTIC PLAN

Noninvasive Treatment

Conservative treatment is 50% to 75% effective if started early, without thenar wasting, severe pain, or weakness.

- Limit activities/work that stress wrist. May need specific work restrictions.
- Apply cock-up splint to affected wrist with wrist in slight extension. Wear at night to prevent hyperflexion in sleep. Use during the day, if activity is restricted.
- Apply cold to wrist to decrease inflammation.
- Take NSAIDs with food daily 4 to 8 weeks (example: ibuprofen 600 mg tid for 6 to 8 weeks).
- May consider physical therapy in conjunction with above, bioconductive therapy, and interference currents.
- Treat concurrent conditions (diabetes mellitus, thyroid disorders).
- Pregnancy: Avoid repetitive activities, splinting most effective, cold to wrist. Educate that CTS usually abates after delivery.

Invasive Treatment

- Refer to an orthopedic hand specialist for invasive treatments after noninvasive measures fail.
- Steroid injection into the carpal tunnel may provide temporary relief, but there is an associated risk of infection, damage to nerve, and scarring.
- Surgical intervention is required to treat continued pain, thenar wasting, and progressive weakness.
  - Surgery is highly successful with 90% to 95% improvement of symptoms (if not chronic disease).
  - The transverse carpal ligament is incised; this opens the tunnel and releases the pressure.
  - There are two procedures: An open procedure with ability to visualize and explore the tunnel and an endoscopic procedure, which has less visualization but faster recovery.
  - Postoperative care consists of splinting for 1 week or more, continued job restriction, and sutures out in 10 to 14 days.

Client Education

- Prevention is the key. Modification of environment for proper joint alignment at worksite is essential. Advise the client to seek ergonomic assessment from company of work tasks and tools. This strategy is important especially in high-risk jobs. Conditioning exercises for hands and wrists with mild stretching and strengthening may help prevent CTS in nonsymptomatic clients.
- CTS takes a long time to heal following the treatment regimen. It may be months. If activities not modified, symptoms will return.
- Wear a splint at night. Avoid use of splint during the work day. Wear the spint if there is no interference with activities.
- Pregnancy cases usually resolve. If symptoms continue after delivery and the client is not nursing, consider initiation of NSAIDs and referral.

Referral

If no improvement occurs after 1 to 2 months of conservative treatment, refer to orthopedic hand specialist for surgical evaluation.

EVALUATION/FOLLOW-UP

- Schedule initial follow-up in 2 to 4 weeks for noninvasive treatment. Assess for decrease in symptoms, grip and pinch strength, and thenar wasting (deterioration sign).
- Expect a decrease in symptoms 2 weeks after complaint noninvasive treatment and avoidance of cause. If CTS is work related, specific restrictions of job may be required (example: no typing more than 20 minutes every 2 hours). Work closely with occupational health nurse at worksite if needed.
- If caught early, symptoms usually resolve following surgical intervention. If the client returns to the same activity postoperatively without modification and correct joint positioning, symptoms may recur.

REFERENCES

Dorwart, B. D. (1984). Carpal tunnel syndrome: A review. *Seminars In Arthritis and Rheumatism, 14*(2), 134-139.

Magee, D. J. (1987). *Orthopedic physical assessment.* Philadelphia: W. B. Saunders.

Miller, B. K. (1993). Carpal tunnel syndrome: A frequently misdiagnosed common hand problem. *Nurse Practitioner, 18*(12), 52-56.

National Institute of Occupational Safety and Health (1989, March). *Carpal tunnel syndrome selected references* (DHHS Publication No. 1992-648-179/60023). Cincinnati: U.S. Department of Health and Human Services.

Putz-Anderson, V. (1988). *Carpal tunnel disorder: A manual for musculoskeletal diseases of the upper limbs.* Pennsylvania: Taylor & Francis.

Siebenaler, M. J., & McGovern, P. (1992). Carpal tunnel syndrome. *American Association of Occupational Health Nursing, 40*(2), 62-71.

Tomal, D. R. (1992, December). Reduce carpal tunnel syndrome through safety training. *American Society of Safety Engineers*, pp. 27-29.

Williams, K. (1992). Doing business with carpal tunnel syndrome. *Work, 2*(4), 2-7.

Wright, P. E. (1992). Carpal tunnel and ulnar tunnel syndromes and stenosing tenosynovitis. In A. H. Crenshaw (Ed.), *Campbell's operative orthopaedics* (pp. 3435-3450). St. Louis: Mosby.

REVIEW QUESTIONS

1. Which is **not** a common risk factor for CTS?

   a. Repetitive, forceful flexion, and/or extension wrist

   b. Metabolic disease such as diabetes and thyroid disorders

   c. Trauma to wrist

   d. Parkinsonism

2. Which best describes Phalen's maneuver?

   a. Perform ROM test for wrist.

   b. Tap on median nerve.

   c. Flex wrist maximally for 60 seconds and evaluate for symptoms.

   d. Compress median nerve with thumbs.

3. Which is **not** a diagnostic test used to assess for CTS?

   a. Grip and pinch test

   b. Phalen's maneuver, Tinel's sign

   c. Two-point discrimination

   d. Abduction of the shoulder

4. Preventive teaching is effective if clients recall all the following **except:**

   a. Keep joints in neutral positions at work.

   b. Increased speed and force of movements helps decrease symptoms.

   c. Rest breaks for recovery time are helpful to prevent CTS.

   d. Preventive mild conditioning exercises may be helpful for asymptomatic people in high-risk jobs.

5. Bridgett, an occupational health nurse practitioner, has responsibility for worksite management of CTS at the diamond processing plant where she works. Which of the following is the first strategy she must employ in implementing this program?

   a. Splints for high-risk workers

   b. Easy access to ice machines for ice therapy

   c. Preventive teaching

   d. Prophylactic NSAIDs for workers at risk

6. Which of these occupations/hobbies are at least risk for CTS?

   a. Checkout clerks, seamstress, typists

   b. Swimmers, opera singers, salesman

   c. Bowlers, knitters, musicians

   d. Meatcutters, jackhammer users, hairdressers

ANSWERS AND RATIONALES

1. *Answer:* d (assessment/history/musculoskeletal/NAS)

   Rationale: Parkinsonism is not a risk factor for CTS. Prior trauma, metabolic disorders, and forceful repetitive motions are risk factors. (Siebenaler & McGovern, 1992)

2. *Answer:* c (assessment/physical examination/musculoskeletal/NAS)

   Rationale: The Phalen's maneuver is to maximally flex wrists for 60 seconds. (Magee, 1987)

3. *Answer:* d (assessment/physical examination/musculoskeletal/NAS)

   Rationale: Phalen's maneuver, Tinel's sign, grip and pinch test, and two-point discrimination are diagnostic maneuvers for CTS. Abduction of the shoulder is not a typical diagnostic maneuver for CTS. (Siebenaler & McGovern, 1992)

4. *Answer:* b (evaluation/musculoskeletal/NAS)

Rationale: Neutral positions, conditioning, and rest/recovery time for joints may help prevent CTS. Forceful repetitive movements increase risk for CTS. (Tomal, 1992)

5. *Answer:* c (plan/management/client education/musculoskeletal/NAS)

Rationale: Prevention of CTS is the key, especially in large at-risk populations. Prevention is accomplished through plantwide programs and teaching, which includes neutral joint positioning, rotation of jobs, rest periods, and knowledge of high-risk movements. (Williams, 1992)

6. *Answer:* b (assessment/history/musculoskeletal/NAS)

Rationale: Occupations/hobbies with repetitive forceful motions are risks for CTS. It is not a known problem in swimmers. (National Institute of Occupational Safety and Health, 1989)

CONGENITAL DISLOCATION OF THE HIP/DEVELOPMENTAL DYSPLASIA OF THE HIP

OVERVIEW
Definition

Developmental dysplasia of the hip (DDH) is displacement of the femoral head with respect to normal orientation with the acetabulum. *Dislocation* refers to hips that completely move out of the socket. *Subluxation* describes hips that have movement within the joint. The movement feels like "popping out" or "click."

Incidence

- One to two for every 1000 births
- Girls more than boys
- Unilateral dislocation twice as frequent as bilateral
- Unknown genetic link; association of first-born females with positive family history of affected first-degree relatives

Pathophysiology

In utero, the acetabulum starts as a flat surface, which later cups around the head of the femur. This is completed during the first months of extrauterine life. DDH is the failure of formation of this normal cup around the head of the femur.

FACTORS INCREASING SUSCEPTIBILITY. Congenital dislocation can be divided into two types: idiopathic and teratogenic.

Idiopathic
- More frequent and often related to family history; can range from subluxed to dislocated but reducible or dislocated and irreducible
- Abnormal intrauterine positioning
- Relaxing effect of hormones acting on soft tissue during pregnancy
- History of breech presentation, exhibits generalized increased ligamentous laxity

Teratogenic
- More severe form of the disorder
- Associated congenital anomalies common in infants; significant association with clubfoot deformities and neuromuscular conditions

COMMON PATHOGENS. There are no known infectious etiologic factors.

ASSESSMENT: SUBJECTIVE/HISTORY
Symptoms

INFANT (DDH)
- Legs held in adduction and external rotation
- Asymmetry of skinfolds of thighs and buttocks; not true of bilateral dislocation
- Limited abduction
- Irritability on leg motion

CHILDREN
- Gait disturbance
- Inability to crawl
- Hip or medial knee pain
- Low activity level

Past Medical History

INFANT
- Birth order
- Family history
- Abnormal intrauterine positions
- Infant with congenital deformities
- Muscle disorder
- Progress of ambulation

CHILDREN
- Abnormal gait
- Uneven length of legs
- Difficult diapering

Psychosocial History

This information is noncontributory.

Dietary History

This information is noncontributory.

ASSESSMENT: OBJECTIVE/ PHYSICAL EXAMINATION

Physical Examination

INFANTS
- Conduct a problem-oriented examination with particular attention to height and general appearance.
- Skin: Assess for asymmetry of skinfolds of thighs and buttocks.
- Lower extremities: Do a complete examination of the legs and hips. Perform the Barlow's test and Ortolani's sign.
  - Ortolani's sign: Place the infant in the supine position with the pelvis on a flat surface, abduct and externally rotate the hip with middle finger of the examiner over the greater trochanter. A palpable "clunk" confirms reduction of the dislocated hips.
  - Barlow's test: Place the infant in the supine position with pelvis flat. Adduct and internally rotate the hips. A palpable "clunk" confirms the hip dislocation.

CHILDREN
- Assess gait status for limping, swayback, toe walking, lurch gait, or delay of ambulation.
- Skin: Assess for excessive thigh or buttocks folds.
- Galeazzi's sign: Place the child in the supine position with the knees fully adducted and held together. If one femur shorter than the other, the result is positive.

Diagnostic Procedures

Based on documented positive hip click or clunk, the following radiographic studies should be performed:
- Ultrasound: Confirms real-time dislocation of the femoral head in an immature, unossified anatomy
- X-ray examination: After 4 months of age
  - Frog-legged view
  - Upright anteroposterior view; hips internally rotated
- Hip arthrography: Injection of radiopaque dye into hip joint; may require sedation
- CT/MRI

DIAGNOSIS

The differential diagnosis includes the following:
- Spina bifida
- Arthrogryposis
- Lumbosacral agenesis
- Neonatal Marfan syndrome
- Fetal hydantoin syndrome
- Larsen's syndrome
- Septic hip
- Proximal femoral epiphyseal separation
- Coxa vara

THERAPEUTIC PLAN

- Always refer to a pediatric orthopedic surgeon for evaluation.
- Therapy depends on the age of the child at the time of diagnosis and the age of the abnormality on clinical examination.
  - Age 0 to 6 months: A Pavlik harness permits a relaxed motion of the hip while maintaining a flexed and abducted position for natural development of joint space, until the capsule tightens at approximately 6 weeks.
  - Age 6 months to 2 years: Consider a possible Pavlik harness, closed reduction vs open reduction, spica cast, or preliminary traction
- The prognosis is excellent if treated early. Failure to diagnose early can result in more extensive management and less favorable outcome.

- Complications if untreated include no stable reduction, avascular necrosis of the femoral head, and decreased ROM.

Client Education

- Despite traditional use of double and triple diapering, there is no clinical evidence to support the benefit of these treatments. These therapies are not recommended since the adductor muscles of the thigh usually overpower saturated diapers and abduction is not maintained.
- Pavlik harnesses should stay in place during all sleep and wake hours with the exception of bathing.
- Harness straps should be adjusted by a medical professional only.
- Parents may apply skin moisturizer in areas of strap erosions.
- Without therapy DDH will result in permanent degenerative changes of the hip that will eventually lead to arthritis.

EVALUATION/FOLLOW-UP

- Even though spontaneous reduction of the hip may occur in 6 weeks, it is recommended that the Pavlik harness be continued for several months until the hips are stable.
- Spica cast should be changed every 6 weeks to allow for the child's growth. The cast should not be used for more than 6 months.

REFERENCES

Behrman, R., & Vaughan, V. (1997). *Nelson textbook of pediatrics* (14th ed.). Philadelphia: W. B. Saunders.

Swartz, M. W. (1997). *The 5-minute pediatric consult.* Baltimore: Williams & Wilkins.

Zitelli, B., & Davis, H. (1994). *Atlas of pediatric physical diagnosis* (2nd ed.). London: Mosby-Wolfe.

REVIEW QUESTIONS

1. Abnormal development of all the following structures can cause congenital dislocation of the hip **except:**

a. Femoral metaphysis
b. Acetabulum
c. Surrounding capsule
d. Soft tissues

2. Signs associated with DDH in an infant would include all the following **except:**

a. Asymmetric or extra skinfolds of the thigh
b. Legs adducted and externally rotated
c. Hip clunk
d. Full or unlimited abduction

3. A maneuver used to detect DDH is named for:

a. Phalen
b. Ortolani
c. Pavlik
d. Galeazzi

4. All the following diagnostic procedures can be useful in diagnosing DDH **except:**

a. Radiographics
b. Ultrasound
c. Arthrography
d. Rheumatoid factor with ANA

5. A 4-year-old girl visiting from Mexico has a 2-year history of a progressively increasing limp. She is diagnosed with DDH. Her prognosis for correction will likely be:

a. Excellent
b. Complicated management and less favorable outcome
c. Unknown
d. No correction possible

6. DDH affects:

a. Girls more often than boys
b. Boys more often than girls
c. Both boys and girls equally
d. Boys later in life than girls

7. Physical examination of infant's hip is **least** helpful when an infant is:

a. Sleeping
b. Feeding
c. Crying
d. Quietly awake

8. For a hip that is dislocatable and relocatable, a reliable form of fixation such as a Pavlik harness is used. The Pavlik harness:

a. Should be removed only for each diaper change
b. Should be removed only for bathing
c. Should be removed as desired
d. Should never be removed

9. At his first well-child visit, a 14-day-old infant is noted to have a positive result from a Barlow's test but negative results from Galeazzi's sign and Ortolani tests. Appropriate management would include:

a. Reassuring the mother that this may be a variant of normal and reexamining the hip at 2 months of age

b. Obtaining anteroposterior and frog-legged views of the pelvis to confirm the diagnosis

c. Obtaining a hip ultrasound to confirm the diagnosis

d. Immediately placing the child in a Pavlik harness

ANSWERS AND RATIONALES

1. *Answer:* a (assessment/physical examination/musculoskeletal/child)

Rationale: Abnormal development results from the acetabulum, femoral head, surrounding capsule, and soft tissue. (Behrman & Vaughan, 1997)

2. *Answer:* d (assessment/physical examination/musculoskeletal/infant)

Rationale: In the neonate each thigh should abduct to almost 90 degrees; abduction less than 60 to 70 degrees indicates abnormality. (Behrman & Vaughan, 1997)

3. *Answer:* b (assessment/physical examination/musculoskeletal/infant)

Rationale: Ortolani's sign and Barlow's test are used to determine hip stability; Galeazzi's sign determines shortness of the femur. Pavlik is the type of harness used in the treatment of DDH. (Behrman & Vaughan, 1997)

4. *Answer:* d (plan/management/diagnostics/infant)

Rationale: No laboratory tests are helpful in diagnosing DDH.

5. *Answer:* b (evaluation/musculoskeletal/child)

Rationale: Evaluation if diagnosed early, prognosis is uniformly excellent. (Zitelli & Davis, 1994)

6. *Answer:* a (diagnosis/musculoskeletal/child)

Rationale: Girls are more commonly affected than boys. (Behrman & Vaughan, 1997)

7. *Answer:* c (assessment/physical examination/infant)

Rationale: A crying infant's hip is nearly impossible to examine accurately. (Swartz, 1997)

8. *Answer:* b (plan/management/therapy/nonpharmacologic/musculoskeletal/infant)

Rationale: The harness should not be removed with each diaper change. (Behrman & Vaughan, 1997)

9. *Answer:* c (plan/management/diagnostics/musculoskeletal/infant)

Rationale: By 14 days of age normal ligamentous laxity should be resolved; however, the diagnosis of DDH should still be confirmed before instituting prolonged therapy because Pavlik harness placement can cause necrosis of the femoral head. The femoral head is not calcified, and its relationship to the acetabulum cannot be seen on x-ray examination. However, these same structures are easily visualized on ultrasound, and the motion of the femoral head over the acetabulum can be confirmed. This has the added advantage of not subjecting the infant to unnecessary radiation. Delay of diagnosis and treatment by 2 months may provide a less favorable outcome.

FIBROMYALGIA

OVERVIEW
Definition

The American College of Rheumatology's definition of *fibromyalgia* includes both a 3-month history of widespread pain and pain in 11 of 18 tender points using a digital palpation force of 4 kg.

Incidence

- 2% of general population
- 5% to 10% of clients in internal medicine practices
- 4% to 20% of clients in rheumatology practices
- Women: 73% to 90% of affected clients

- Average age: 40 to 60, with the peak incidence at age 45 to 55

Pathophysiology

Although there is no clearly documented pathophysiology, there are some abnormalities that may account for the pain, poor sleep, and fatigue observed in fibromyalgia:

- Sleep abnormality: Restorative delta-wave stage IV (non-REM) sleep is disrupted by nonrestorative alpha-wave sleep.
- Psychologic abnormality: Emotional stressors may alter CNS serotonin, which is a chemical mediator of deep sleep and pain perception.
- Activity abnormality: Pain and fatigue often result in decreased activity, which increases depression and sleep difficulties, which result in more pain and fatigue.

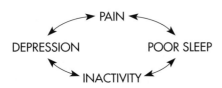

ASSESSMENT: SUBJECTIVE/HISTORY
Symptoms

- Pain: Most common areas are axial skeleton (especially cervical and low back), shoulder, and pelvic girdles.
  —Two thirds report pain to palpation all over not just at the tender points.
  —Pain may be due to a decreased pain threshold.
- Sleep abnormality: Ninety percent wake up tired and unrefreshed, but may not be aware of a sleeping problem per se.
- Fatigue: 55% to 100%
- Morning stiffness: 76% to 91%
- Depression: 26%
- Subjective sensation of swollen joints
- Headache (migraine, tension)
- Symptoms similar to Raynaud's disease (pallor, cyanosis, and paresthesias)
- Irritable bowel or bladder symptoms or both
- Paresthesias
- Anxiety

- Functional disability: The client is unable to perform work or other tasks because of pain/fatigue.
  AGGRAVATING FACTORS
  - Cold, humid weather
  - Physical/mental fatigue
  - Extremes of physical activity (too much/little)
  - Stress
  RELIEVING FACTORS
  - Warm, dry weather
  - Hot showers, baths
  - Moderate activity

Past Medical History

- Major depression: Seventy-one percent have a current or past history of depression.
- Rheumatologic disorders: Fibromyalgia frequently complicates existing rheumatic disorders.
- Hypothyroidism: If not well controlled, hypothyroidism may mimic fibromyalgia.
- Chronic fatigue syndrome: Both conditions have similar symptoms, except fibromyalgia causes more pain.

Medication History

Ask about previous relief from steroids or NSAIDs (do not usually help with fibromyalgia).

Family History

Ask about rheumatic or autoimmune disorders.

Psychosocial History

- Functional impairment: Clients often are unable to perform normal household and work-related tasks.
- History of depression
- History of a traumatic event preceding the current symptoms

ASSESSMENT: OBJECTIVE/PHYSICAL EXAMINATION
Physical Examination

Physical examination includes manual palpation of tender points employing a rolling motion with either the thumb or first two fingers (using 4 kg of pressure). According to the American College of Rheumatology 1990 Criteria for the Classification of Fibromyalgia (Multicenter Criteria Committee, 1990), pain must be elicited in 11 of 18 tender points to diagnose fibromyalgia:

- Occiput: Bilateral, at the suboccipital muscle insertions
- Low cervical: Bilateral, at the anterior aspects of the intertransverse spaces at C5-C7
- Trapezius: Bilateral, at the midpoint of the upper border
- Supraspinatus: Bilateral, at origins, above the scapula spine near the medial border
- Second rib: Bilateral, at the second costrochondral junctions, just lateral to the junctions on the upper surfaces
- Lateral epicondyle: Bilateral, 2 cm distal to the epicondyles
- Gluteal: Bilateral, in the upper outer quadrants of the buttocks in the anterior fold of muscle
- Greater trochanter: Bilateral, posterior to the trochanteric prominence
- Knee: Bilateral, at the medial fat pad proximal to the joint line

Tender points must be differentiated from trigger points. Pressure on trigger points causes radiating pain, which is associated with myofascial syndromes but not with fibromyalgia.

Physical examination results are otherwise negative. There should be no visible swelling or objective weakness unless it is caused by other concomitant illnesses. (This is despite subjective complaints of swelling and weakness.)

Diagnostic Procedures

Fibromyalgia is a diagnosis of exclusion. All test results should be negative in the absence of concomitant disease:

- Initial workup includes CBC, ESR, chemistries, and TSH.
- If other causes are suspected, perform creatine phosphokinase (CPK), serum protein electrophoresis, ANA, and rheumatoid factor.
- Radiographs are appropriate if pain is more localized.

DIAGNOSIS

The differential diagnosis includes the following:

- RA
- Metabolic myopathies
- Endocrine disorders (thyroid, parathyroid)
- Adrenal disorders (most commonly hypothyroidism)
- Polymyositis
- Polymyalgia rheumatica
- OA
- Metastatic cancer
- Myofascial pain syndrome
- Ankylosing spondylitis
- Depression/anxiety
- Disk herniation
- Connective tissue disease
- Chronic fatigue syndrome

THERAPEUTIC PLAN
Pharmacologic Treatment

- Tricyclics help induce stage IV sleep and provide nonspecific analgesia for chronic pain:
  —Cyclobenzaprine (Flexeril) 10 to 30 mg
  —Amitriptyline (Elavil) 10 to 50 mg
- If there is no relief of the sleep disorder, use the following with caution:
  —Chlorpromazine (Thorazine) 100 mg
  —Alprazolam (Xanax) 0.25 to 0.50 mg
- NSAIDs and corticosteroids are not helpful.
- Prescribe fluoxetine 20 to 40 mg, especially if there is a depressive component.

Nonpharmacologic Treatment

- Reassurance
  —Give a name to the symptoms. The clients have probably often been told, "It's all in your head."
  —Relate symptoms to modifiable factors (stress, sleep, exercise) to give clients a sense of control over their body and symptoms.
  —Reassure clients that fibromyalgia is not a progressive, crippling disease.
- Exercise: Aerobic exercise for at least 30 minutes 3 times per week is essential to overall management.
- Refer to support groups, biofeedback programs, relaxation therapy, and hypnotherapy as appropriate.
- Contact the Arthritis Foundation and Fibromyalgia Network for client education booklets.
- Emphasize that goals are to reduce, not eliminate, pain and sleep disorders.

EVALUATION/FOLLOW-UP

- Since there are no diagnostic tests for fibromyalgia, evaluation must be based on the client's subjective feeling of decreased pain, fatigue, and stiffness. The examiner should also be able to either elicit fewer tender points or less tenderness at these points.
- Follow monthly at first until some improvement in symptoms is noticed. Then decrease the frequency of visits as symptoms warrant.
- It is essential to emphasize the importance of ongoing aerobic exercise because it is the treatment modality that gives the most consistent positive results.
- Approach must be very emotionally supportive with the philosophy of collaborating with the client to individually tailor his or her treatment regimen. No one treatment regimen works for all clients with fibromyalgia.
- Consult with a physician about additional testing if there is any reason to suspect other disorders.

REFERENCES

Bennett, R. M., Gatter, R. A., Campbell, S. M., Andrews, R. P., Clark, S. R., & Scarola, J. A. (1988). A comparison of cyclobenzaprine and placebo in the management of fibrositis. *Arthritis and Rheumatism, 31,* 1535-1542.

Cunningham, M. D. (1996). Becoming familiar with fibromyalgia. *Orthopedic Nursing, 15*(2), 33-36.

Geel, S. E. (1994). The fibromyalgia syndrome: Musculoskeletal pathophysiology. *Seminars in Arthritis and Rheumatism, 23,* 347-353.

Harmon, C. E. (1996). Fibromyalgia: Treatments worth trying. *Internal Medicine, 17*(1), 64-75.

Hench, P. K. (1989). Evaluation and differential diagnosis of fibromyalgia. *Rheumatic Disease Clinics of North America, 15*(1), 19-28.

Johnson, S. P. (1997). Fluoxetine and amitriptyline in the treatment of fibromyalgia. *Journal of Family Practice, 44*(2), 128-130.

Kennedy, M., & Felson, D. T. (1996). A prospective long-term study of fibromyalgia syndrome. *Arthritis and Rheumatism, 39,* 682-685.

Martin, L., Nutting, A., MacIntosh, B. R., Edworthy, S. M., Butterwick, D., & Cook, J. (1996). An exercise program in the treatment of fibromyalgia. *Journal of Rheumatology, 23,* 1050-1053.

Multicenter Criteria Committee (1990). The American College of Rheumatology 1990 Criteria for the Classification of Fibromyalgia. *Arthritis and Rheumatism, 33,* 160-172.

Unger, J. (1996). Fibromyalgia. *Journal of the American Academy of Nursing Practitioners, 8*(1), 27-29.

White, K. P., & Harth, M. (1996). An analytical review of 24 controlled clinical trials for fibromyalgia syndrome (FMS). *Pain, 64,* 211-219.

Wilke, W. S. (1995). Treatment of "resistant fibromyalgia." *Rheumatic Disease Clinics of North America, 21,* 247-257.

Wolfe, F. (1989). Fibromyalgia: The clinical syndrome. *Rheumatic Disease Clinics of North America, 15*(1), 1-16.

REVIEW QUESTIONS

1. The most critical objective data to diagnose fibromyalgia are:

a. Negative ESR, TSH, ANA
b. Negative ANA, rheumatoid factor, CPK
c. Tenderness at 11 or more of the 18 tender points on one side of the body
d. Tenderness at 11 or more of the 18 tender points on both sides of the body

2. Which of the following constellations of symptoms are most common in fibromyalgia?

a. Paresthesias, headache, anxiety
b. Pain, sleep abnormality, fatigue
c. Functional disability, depression, stiffness
d. Irritable bowel symptoms, anxiety, depression

3. Fibromyalgia may be distinguished from chronic fatigue syndrome by:

a. More severe fatigue because of disruptions of delta-wave sleep
b. Higher levels of depression
c. More severe and widespread pain
d. Functional disability

4. The main difference between trigger points and tender points is:

a. The amount of pressure needed to elicit them is different.
b. Trigger points are usually found in myofascial syndromes but not in fibromyalgia.
c. Tender points are usually found in myofascial syndromes but not in fibromyalgia.
d. Tender points cause radiating pain, whereas trigger points do not.

5. The most effective medication for fibromyalgia is:

  a. Naproxen (Naprosyn) 500 mg PO bid
  b. Fluoxetine (Prozac) 40 mg PO qd
  c. Amitriptyline (Elavil) 50 mg PO qhs
  d. Alprazolam (Xanax) 0.5 mg PO qhs

ANSWERS AND RATIONALES

1. *Answer:* d (assessment/physical examination/musculoskeletal/NAS)

  Rationale: Many other diseases listed in the differential diagnosis list may have negative results from blood work. However, the distinguishing characteristic of fibromyalgia is the presence of these tender points. They are bilateral in 9 locations, and 11 of them must be painful to palpation to diagnose fibromyalgia. (Multicenter Criteria Committee, 1990)

2. *Answer:* b (assessment/history/musculoskeletal/NAS)

  Rationale: Although all the symptoms may occur in fibromyalgia, pain, sleep abnormality, fatigue, morning stiffness, and depression are the most common. (Wolfe, 1989)

3. *Answer:* c (assessment/history/musculoskeletal/NAS)

  Rationale: All the symptoms may occur in both chronic fatigue syndrome and fibromyalgia. However, the primary symptom in fibromyalgia is pain, whereas fatigue is the dominating symptom in chronic fatigue syndrome. (Hench, 1989)

4. *Answer:* b (assessment/physical examination/musculoskeletal/NAS)

  Rationale: Trigger points are areas that when palpated cause radiating pain. Their presence is indicative of myofascial disorders rather than fibromyalgia. In fibromyalgia only tender points should be present. (Hench, 1989)

5. *Answer:* c (plan/musculoskeletal/NAS)

  Rationale: Naprosyn is not helpful with fibromyalgia. The other medications have limited usage, but cyclobenzaprine (Flexeril) and amitriptyline (Elavil) are still the mainstays of pharmacologic treatment. (Wilke, 1995)

GOUT

OVERVIEW
Definition

Gout is an inflammatory arthritis, caused by deposition of monosodium urate (MSU) crystals in joints, resulting from an inborn error of purine metabolism and uric acid excretion.

Prevalence

An estimated 2.2 million Americans have gout. Prevalence is 0.5% to 0.7% for men and 0.1% for women. Gout is rare before puberty in boys and before menopause in women. It is the most common cause of inflammatory arthritis in men older than 40.

Incidence

- Risk of gout increases as serum uric acid level rises; 0.1% with serum uric acid <7 mg/dl to 4.5% with levels at or >9 mg/dl.
- Age, obesity, and alcohol intake are factors in gout but to a lesser extent than uric acid levels.
- Incidence of gout is 3 times greater for hypertensive men taking diuretics (hyperuricemic effect) when compared to normotensive men.
- Other associated disorders are hyperlipidemia and diabetes.

Pathophysiology

PRIMARY GOUT. Primary gout is caused by either decreased excretion or increased production of uric acid. Hereditary underexcretion is the most common cause of gout. After many asymptomatic years of chronic hyperuricemia (30 years mean), acute gout will develop in 25% of these individuals. Women are protected until menopause by estrogen since it promotes uric acid excretion.

SECONDARY GOUT. Secondary gout is caused by acquired conditions causing overproduction or underexcretion of uric acid:

- Overproduction: Polycythemia vera, leukemia, multiple myeloma, psoriasis, hemolytic anemia, disseminated carcinoma

- Underexcretion: Chronic renal insufficiency, lead poisoning, acidosis, drug ingestion (nicotinic acid, levodopa, pyrazinamide, ethambutol, cyclosporine, diuretics, low-dose salicylates)

Any sudden change in uric acid levels can bring on symptoms of gouty arthritis. Factors causing a rise in uric acid levels include the use of diuretics, alcohol, and low-dose aspirin. Lowering of uric acid is attributed to sudden cessation of alcohol use, high-dose salicylates, or initiation of allopurinol or uricosuric drugs. Acute illness or surgery may alter uric acid levels and bring on an attack.

Though not related to uric acid levels, minor trauma can trigger symptoms. Gout may infrequently co-exist with a joint infection.

Untreated chronic gout can lead to tophaceous destruction of bone and cartilage or gouty nephropathy.

ASSESSMENT: SUBJECTIVE/HISTORY
Symptoms

Classic symptoms are significant pain and erythema (usually of the great toe), followed by desquamation of the overlying skin. Onset of symptoms is rapid, increasing during a period of a few hours and lasting a few days to weeks, with complete recovery.

The MTP joint, instep, or ankle is often the target of a first attack. MSU crystals are soluble at body temperature. With the temperature of the great toe being lower, the crystals are predisposed to precipitate into the joint, thereby causing symptoms. Low-grade fever and leukocytosis may or may not be present.

Women often have more than one joint involved, with 70% having polyarticular instead of monoarticular symptoms of gout (hands most common). Chronic gout or interval gout may affect multiple joints of upper and lower extremities and can be confused with RA or OA.

Past Medical History

Note history of previous attacks including location, duration, type of treatment, and response to therapy. History of chronic conditions (listed previously under Secondary Gout) may be helpful. Inquire about joint trauma, recent illness, or surgery.

Medication History

Ask about history of diuretic, aspirin, and alcohol use.

Family History

Twelve percent of individuals with gout have a positive family history of the condition.

ASSESSMENT: OBJECTIVE/ PHYSICAL EXAMINATION
Physical Examination

- Assess weight and vital signs with attention to temperature and blood pressure.
- Evaluate affected joints for redness, increased warmth, tenderness, effusion, and ROM.
- Check for nonpainful tophi on Achilles tendon, extensor surfaces of the forearms, or helix of the ear. Tophi may ulcerate, leaving a white urate deposit on the surface.
- Look for joint deformity, particularly of the hands and feet, and joint stiffness characteristic of chronic gout.

Diagnostic Procedures

Consult with or refer to a physician for joint aspiration; this is the gold standard and only definite means to confirm the diagnosis. Presence of needle-shaped MSU crystals in the phagocytes or free in the tophi is diagnostic. These crystals are visible under a polarized microscope. If symptoms are classic, clinical judgment should guide the decision whether to defer this step and treat empirically with antiinflammatory medications.

Serum uric acid levels are limited in diagnostic value since 20% to 30% of persons with acute gout have normal values.

When uric acid is elevated in young men or premenopausal women, order a 24-hour urine collection for uric acid to look for a secondary cause. A 24-hour urine collection is also helpful to determine risk for kidney stone formation.

X-ray examinations have limited diagnostic value in initial attacks of gout, but they may assist in excluding other disorders. In advanced chronic gout, x-ray examinations have a characteristic punched-out appearance with asymmetric bony erosions and sclerotic joint margins.

If there is concern about a joint infection alone or co-existing with gout, order a CBC with differential plus a Gram stain and culture of synovial fluid. A WBC count of synovial fluid exceeding 50,000 to 100,000 cells/mm indicates a likelihood of septic joint. The serum CBC with differential and ESR may be elevated in a severe attack. X-ray examinations are usually ordered but may not reveal any abnormality.

DIAGNOSIS

The primary differential diagnosis includes pseudogout and septic joint infection.

Pseudogout is only slightly more common in men and causes both acute and chronic arthritis, generally affecting the knee. Synovial fluid aspiration shows calcium pyrophosphate dihydrate crystals. X-ray examinations of the knees, wrists, and symphysis pubis demonstrate characteristic findings of chondrocalcinosis.

Reiter's syndrome, ankylosing spondylitis, psoriatic arthritis, sarcoidosis, and gonococcal arthritis are other diseases that may be characterized by acute monoarthritis. Also consider acute rheumatic fever, cellulitis, tendinitis, bursitis, and thrombophlebitis.

Gout of the great toe is frequently referred to as podagra (George & Mandell, 1996).

THERAPEUTIC PLAN
Pharmacologic Treatment

ACUTE GOUT

- NSAIDs are symptom relieving and considered the first line of therapy. Naproxen (Naprosyn) and indomethacin (Indocin) have been the most studied, but any in this class can be used. Naproxen (Naprosyn) 500 mg tid or indomethacin (Indocin) 25 to 50 mg tid to qid for 1 week, tapering during a period of 3 to 5 days, is very effective. These agents should be used cautiously, if at all, in older adults with congestive heart failure or renal insufficiency. Use the low-dose range for other older adults and use a drug other than indomethacin (Indocin) because of side effects. NSAIDs should be avoided in clients with a history of peptic ulcer disease, gastrointestinal tract bleeding, cirrhosis, or anticoagulant therapy. Do not recommend salicylates since they affect uric acid excretion.
- Colchicine helps speed resolution of acute gout symptoms at a dose of 0.6 mg/hr until symptoms are relieved, up to a maximum of 4 to 8 mg. Decrease doses in individuals with renal insufficiency. Gastrointestinal tract side effects of nausea, vomiting, and diarrhea are common and may necessitate discontinuation of the drug before relief is achieved.
- Corticosteroids are an alternative to NSAIDs and colchicine. There is no advantage of parenteral vs oral medication in terms of effectiveness. A typical short course is prednisone 30 to 50 mg/day, tapered during a period of a week.

Intraarticular joint injections are given to relieve symptoms without the side effects of parenteral or oral therapy. Joint aspiration before injection of corticosteroid should be done to rule out infection. Physician consultation or referral is recommended.

PREVENTION OF RECURRENT ATTACKS

One attack of gout does not necessarily require lifelong treatment with medication, but recurrent attacks justify treatment. Options include the following:

- Colchicine 0.5 to 1.8 mg/day help reduce recurrence; if renal insufficiency is present, give 0.6 mg every other day.
- Serum uric acid–lowering drugs can aggravate an acute attack and should not be started for 2 to 3 weeks. The client should take an antiinflammatory agent in the interim. The goal for serum uric acid–lowering drugs is <6 mg/dl.

The xanthine oxidase inhibitor allopurinol decreases the production of uric acid. The usual dose is 300 mg/day but should be adjusted for renal function. Adverse reactions include rash, fever, hepatitis, eosinophilia, vasculitis, and renal insufficiency.

Probenecid and sulfinpyrazone (uricosuric agents) work by blocking uric acid reabsorption in the proximal tubules of the kidney. The agents are fairly well tolerated but require ample fluid intake and multiple doses per day. They are contraindicated in clients with a history of renal lithiasis. Clients must have a glomerular filtration rate higher than 30 to 50 ml/min.

ASYMPTOMATIC HYPERURICEMIA. Treatment is generally not required for clients with uric acid levels less than 10 mg/dl, but follow regularly and consider secondary causes.

Client Education

- Avoid alcohol binges, fasting, or low-calorie diets since these can trigger can attack. The diet is unrestricted otherwise, although generous fluid intake is important if the client is at risk for kidney stones. A low-purine diet has only modest impact on reducing uric acid levels.
- Discuss the pros and cons of treatment options, including the side effects of the drugs.
- Avoid salicylates and diuretics.

Referral

Refer to orthopedic surgeon or rheumatologist if there is concern about septic joint, the diagnosis is in question, or the client is unresponsive to therapy.

EVALUATION/FOLLOW-UP

- Recheck within 48 hours if not responding to treatment for acute attack. Return in 4 to 8 weeks to discuss further treatment or evaluation.
- Arrange annual examination for follow-up of chronic gout.

REFERENCES

George, T. M., & Mandell, B. F. (1996, May-June). Individualizing the treatment of gout. *Cleveland Clinic Journal of Medicine, 63*(3), 150 to 155.

Goroll, A. H., May, L. A., & Mulley, A. G. (1995). *Primary care medicine* (3rd. ed.). Philadelphia: J. B. Lippincott.

Hershfield, M. S. (1996). Gout and uric acid metabolism. In J. C. Bennett & F. Plum (Eds.), *Cecil textbook of medicine* (20th ed.). Philadelphia: W. B. Saunders.

Holland, N. W., & Agudelo, C. A. (1997). Hyperuricemia and gout. In R. Rakel (Ed.), *Conn's current therapy.* Philadelphia: W. B. Saunders.

Joseph, J., & McGrath, H. (1995, April). Gout or 'pseudogout': How to differentiate crystal-induced arthropathies. *Geriatrics, 50*(4), 33-39.

Michet, C. J., et al. (1995, December). Common rheumatologic diseases in elderly patients. *Mayo Clinic Proceedings, 70*,1205-1213.

Towheed, T. E., & Hochberg, M. C. (1996, November 15). Acute monoarthritis: A practical approach to assessment and treatment. *American Family Physician, 54*(7), 2239-2243.

Uphold, C. R., & Graham, M. V. (1994). *Clinical guidelines in family practice.* Gainesville, FL: Barmarrae Books.

REVIEW QUESTIONS

1. Which one of the following statements about gout is true?

    a. Gout is caused by joint deposition of pyrophosphate dihydrate crystals.

    b. Gout is more prevalent in men than in women.

    c. Gout is primarily a result of a poor diet high in purines.

    d. Most cases of gout are the result of secondary conditions.

2. Which of the following scenarios is most indicative of gout?

    a. 35-year-old woman with swollen painful fingers

    b. 30-year-old man with MTP joint pain, iritis, and penile discharge

    c. 55-year-old alcoholic man with recurrent instep pain and redness

    d. 75-year-old hypertensive man with hip pain and limp

3. Which of the following best describes the pathophysiology of gout?

    a. Gout is most commonly a result of increased uric acid production.

    b. The onset of gout is caused by a gradual change in uric acid levels.

    c. Secondary gout is a hereditary chronic disorder.

    d. The lower temperature of the toe causes precipitation of uric acid crystals.

4. Which one of the following statements is **not** true?

    a. Symptoms of gout evolve during a period of several days.

    b. Surgery may bring on an attack of acute gout.

    c. Gout can be confused with cellulitis.

    d. As gout resolves, skin over the joint desquamates.

5. Which statement is **not** correct regarding the treatment of gout?

　　a. Any NSAID can be given to relieve symptoms.
　　b. With renal insufficiency, corticosteroids are an alternative treatment.
　　c. Colchicine provides good relief and is well tolerated.
　　d. Intraarticular injections should be preceded by joint aspiration.

6. The following statements about long-term treatment of recurrent gout are true with which **exception?**

　　a. Serum uric acid–lowering agents should be started immediately after an attack.
　　b. Allopurinol can cause a sensitivity reaction with rash and fever.
　　c. Uricosuric drugs require intake of large quantities of fluid.
　　d. Colchicine can be given to reduce recurrence of gout symptoms.

7. Which of the following client education teaching points about gout is **incorrect?**

　　a. Binge drinking of alcohol can bring on an attack.
　　b. Only high doses of aspirin can bring on symptoms of gout.
　　c. Medication for acute gout should reduce pain within 48 hours.
　　d. A low-purine diet has limited impact on uric acid levels.

ANSWERS AND RATIONALES

1. *Answer:* b (assessment/history/musculoskeletal/adult)

　　Rationale: Gout is primarily a disease of adult men. MSU crystals are found in gout; pyrophosphate dihydrate crystals are found in pseudogout. Dietary sources are responsible for only 10% of blood purines, which has limited impact on gout. (Goroll, May, & Mulley, 1995) Gout is primarily due to an inborn error of metabolism and less often to secondary diseases. (Holland & Agudelo, 1997)

2. *Answer:* c (assessment/history/musculoskeletal/adult)

　　Rationale: Gout is more common after the fifth decade and is associated with alcohol use, and the instep is a common site of inflammation. The hip is a rare location for gout. (Goroll et al., 1995) Symptoms in women are rare before menopause; findings described suggest RA. The 30-year-old man's triad points to Reiter's syndrome. (Towheed & Hochberg, 1996)

3. *Answer:* d (diagnosis/pathophysiology/musculoskeletal/adult)

　　Rationale: Uric acid is soluble in serum at body temperature, but at lower temperatures uric acid precipitates into a joint. Only 10% of gout is due to overproduction of uric acid. Onset of gout symptoms is due to a rapid change in uric acid levels. Secondary gout is due to an acquired disease and is not hereditary. (Hershfield, 1996)

4. *Answer:* a (assessment/pathophysiology/musculoskeletal/adult)

　　Rationale: Gout evolves rapidly, usually during a period of hours or a day. (Towheed & Hochberg, 1996)

5. *Answer:* c (plan/management/therapeutics/pharmacological/adult)

　　Rationale: Colchicine does provide good relief for gout symptoms but often must be discontinued because of gastrointestinal tract side effects. (Michet, 1995)

6. *Answer:* a (plan/management/therapeutics/pharmacologic/adult)

　　Rationale: Serum uric acid–lowering agents should be delayed until at least 1 month after an acute attack for gout. During this time, antiinflammatory medication is started to prevent recurrence when the serum uric acid–lowering agents are initiated. (Uphold & Graham, 1994)

7. *Answer:* b (plan/management/client education/adult)

　　Rationale: Both high and low doses of aspirin can trigger symptoms of acute gout. (Joseph & McGrath, 1995)

LOWER BACK PAIN

Lumbosacral Strain and Herniated Nucleus Pulposa

OVERVIEW

Definition

Lumbosacral strain (LBS) is a stretching or tearing of muscles, tendons, ligaments, or fascia of the lumbosacral area secondary to trauma or mechanical injury. Symptoms of less than 3 months' duration constitute *acute lower back pain.*

Herniated nucleus pulposa (HNP) is a rupture of an intervertebral disk with herniation of the nucleus pulposa into the spinal canal. *Sciatica* refers to pain and paresthesias extending down the leg in a dermatomal pattern; the most common cause is HNP at L4-5 and L5-S1.

Incidence

- Lower back problems affect virtually everyone at some point in their life; 50% of working adults are affected every year, and 15% to 20% seek health care.
- For persons younger than 45, lower back problems are the most common cause of disability.
- Lower back pain is more common between 20 to 40 years of age and costs approximately $30 billion per year in direct and indirect costs.
- Only about 10% of clients with lower back pain experience HNP.
- Children: Sprains of the ligaments/muscles of the back are unusual in children unless they occur as a result of trauma, infection, inflammation, or malignancies.

Pathophysiology

The cause of LBS is unclear; herniation occurs with tears in annulus fibroses, which allows contents of pulposa to protrude.

PROTECTIVE FACTORS
- Proper body mechanics
- Appropriate weight maintenance
- Conditioned state

FACTORS INCREASING SUSCEPTIBILITY
- Overweight
- Mechanical disorders (i.e., scoliosis, kyphosis)
- Nonmechanical disorders (i.e., ankylosing spondylitis, prostate cancer, pelvic and renal disease)
- Occupational strain
- Leg length differences
- Poor posture
- Poor body mechanics with lifting

ASSESSMENT: SUBJECTIVE/HISTORY

The client's history is the initial diagnostic approach.

Symptoms

LUMBOSACRAL STRAIN
- Pain that was minimal at time of or immediately after activity, but increases, with stiffness, later as soft tissue swells.
- Pain that is located primarily in the back but may radiate to the buttock(s) or thigh(s).
- Pain increased with movement and relieved with rest.
- Older adults: Symptoms are less severe.

HERNIATED NUCLEUS PULPOSA
- Radicular pain (shooting, electric) below the knee
- Deep tendon reflexes (DTRs) absent or diminished along nerve root distribution
- Possible paresthesia or numbness along sensory distribution of nerve root
- Older adults: Nucleus pulposa more fibrotic making the incidence and/or symptoms much less

History of Present Illness

- LBS and HNP
- Pain (new or recurrent problem)
- Character, distribution of pain
- Mechanism of injury
- Treatment to date and response
- Concurrent health problems
- Previous treatment(s) response
- Level of compliance with other treatment method(s)

Associated Symptoms

- Weakness, hypoesthesia, weight loss, fever, malaise
- Sleep disturbance
- Presence of genitourinary tract symptoms (i.e., dysuria, vaginal discharge, prostatism symptoms)
- Precipitating factor(s)
- Night sweats
- Occupational/leisure activities

Past Medical History

- Back pain, compliance, outcome
- Use of alcohol, tobacco products
- Last normal menstrual period
- Weight loss, systemic disease, malignancy
- Affective disorder(s)

Medication History

- Recent use of acetaminophen, NSAIDs or other OTC preparations and their effectiveness
- Other current medications

Family History

- Back problems
- Treatment
- Outcome(s)
- Malignancies

Psychosocial History

- Stresses in workplace/job satisfaction
- Financial resources
- Support systems
- Prior pain
- Internal/external locus of control

Dietary History

- Overall nutrition pattern
- Emphasis on weight reduction (if needed) and a balanced diet

ASSESSMENT: OBJECTIVE/ PHYSICAL EXAMINATION

Physical Examination

The physical examination should be conducted with attention to vital signs, weight, general appearance, and systems other than musculoskeletal to rule out mechanical, systemic, or psychosocial causes for back pain. The examination should be conducted in a systematic head-to-toe fashion, incorporating standing, sitting, and lying positions of the client for the examination.

GAIT

- Assess client's ability to walk to the examination room, remove shoes, and get up on the examination table.
- Note flexion or other difficulties during performance of these functions.

STANDING

- If possible, begin with observation of gait.
- The client should be undressed with back exposed.
- Note posture in bare feet.
- The client will be unable to walk on heels (L4-5) and toes (S1-2) if there is nerve root irritation.
- Back: Examine the spinal column from the front, back, and side. Note any scoliosis and abnormalities of expected S-curvature.
- Lumbar lordosis may be seen in acute LBS.
- Note the level of the shoulder tips, scapular ranges, iliac crests, and gluteal folds. Popliteal creases should be equal. In LBS, unequal levels may be present.
- Perform spinal ROM (flexion, extension, lateral bending, and rotation). Severe guarding may support a diagnosis of fracture, spinal infection, or tumor.
- Palpate paravertebral muscles for spasm and/or tenderness, which may be seen in acute LBS.

SITTING

- Lungs: Check for signs of pleural effusion or consolidation.
- Heart: Note rate, rhythm, and any signs of recent cardiac event (rub, effusion).
- Extremities/neurologic: Check DTRs of knees (L4) and Achilles (S1).
- Check for Babinski's sign. Observe for bilaterally equal responses. If responses are unequal, consider nerve root irritation. Test strength, vibratory, and proprioceptive sensation bilaterally. They should be equal. Weakness in dorsiflexion of ankle or great toe (L4-5) suggests nerve root dysfunction.
- Perform light touch sensation of medial (L4), dorsal (L5), and lateral (S1) aspects of foot.
- Perform sitting straight-leg raise (SLR). The client should be able to extend the knee

without radiation of pain below the knee. SLR is also one way to check for malingering behavior as results should equal those of SLR performed in lying position.

- Check for ankle and toe (L5) dorsiflexion strength bilaterally. They should be equal.

SUPINE

- Abdomen: Check for tenderness of peptic ulcer disease and/or bruits/enlargement of dissecting aortic aneurysm.
- Extremities: Flexion, abduction, external rotation (FABER or Patrick's test) of the hips may demonstrate decreased ROM, which may indicate a hip or sacroiliac joint problem.
- Neurologic
  —Standard SLR: Normally the hip can be flexed to 80 degrees without pain, except in the thigh. A positive test result is one that elicits (shooting, sharp, electric) pain that radiates below the knee or the affected side at 30 degrees of flexion or less.
  —Crossed SLR (SLR of unaffected leg): A positive test result causes radicular pain to be reproduced in the affected side.
  —Perform sensory assessment of the buttocks and perineum to rule out saddle anesthesia of cauda equina syndrome (compression of nerves at L4-5 level, which requires emergency surgical decompression).

INDICATORS FOR PELVIC EXAMINATION

- The client reports abdominal pain, dyspareunia, or vaginal discharge.
- The rest of the examination results are unequivocal.
- Perform a complete pelvic examination (without Pap smear) to check for discharge, lesions, cervical motion tenderness, and tubal enlargement.

INDICATORS FOR RECTAL EXAMINATION

- Men older than 50
- Rest of examination results equivocal

SPECIALIZED EXAMINATION TECHNIQUES FOR MALINGERING BEHAVIOR. "Pain behaviors" of distress such as amplified grimacing, distorted gait or posture, or rubbing of painful body parts may cloud the picture. Interpreting inconsistencies of pain behaviors as malingering may not be useful. They could be viewed as a plea for help. The goal is to facilitate recovery and avoid the development of chronic lower back disability.

- Waddell signs: The following lists a standardized group of nonorganic physical signs:
  —Tenderness: Nonanatomic or superficial tenderness on palpation
  —Simulation: Simulate movement without actually performing it to see if client responds
  —Axial loading: Pressure to the top of the head should not produce pain.
  —Distraction: Examine SLR while the client is in the sitting and supine positions and compare the results.
  —Regionalization: Inappropriate location of pain from normal neuroanatomy during palpation
  —Overreaction: Disproportionate verbalization, facial expression, or tremor on movement or palpation
- Other tests
  —Magnuson's test: Mark areas that were tender when palpated; return to the marked areas later in the examination to see if pain can be reproduced. With malingering behavior, those marked areas are not likely to reproduce pain.
  —Hoover's sign: The examiner puts his or her hands under both the client's heels. (The client can be standing, sitting, or lying.) The examiner asks the client to raise the affected leg. If the pain is real, the heel on the other leg will push into the examiner's hands.

Diagnostic Procedures

X-ray examinations or laboratory testing are generally not necessary at the initial visit unless there is a history of trauma or suspicion of systemic or structural changes.

DIAGNOSIS

The differential diagnosis includes the following:

- LBS
- HNP
- Pelvic inflammatory disease
- Prostate tumor/infection
- Aortic aneurysm
- Abdominal tumor
- Uterine fibroids
- Vertebral fracture
- Possible cauda equina syndrome

- Malingering behavior
- Renal colic
- Bladder infection
- Malignancy
- Spinal cord disease
- Pyelonephritis
- Osteoporosis
- OA
- Spinal stenosis
- Bursitis

The preceding list is not all inclusive but should remind the nurse practitioner to consider the following as possible causes of lower back pain:

- Discogenic causes
- Malignancies
- Vascular lesions
- Infections
- Intraabdominal or pelvic causes
- Neurologic complications
- Congenital abnormalities
- Trauma
- Metabolic bone diseases
- Children: Pain resulting from sprains of ligaments and muscles unusual; consideration of inflammation, infections, tremors, and trauma as possible causes

THERAPEUTIC PLAN
Pharmacologic Treatment

Nonprescription drugs such as acetaminophen, aspirin, or ibuprofen provide relief for most persons. If these analgesics are not effective, other NSAIDs, such as nabumetone (Relafon) and tolmetin sodium (Tolectin), that have a rapid onset of action are appropriate.

Muscle relaxants do not appear to be more effective than NSAIDs and should be reserved for those whom NSAIDs do not help or those in whom NSAIDs are contraindicated. If muscle relaxants are used, they should be limited to a course of 1 to 2 weeks; they should be avoided in older adults who are at risk for falling.

Opiates are not necessary in the management of acute LBS; if they are used for more severe pain, they should be taken for a short period of time only. Poor client tolerance, drowsiness, clouded judgment, decreased reaction time, and the potential for misuse (dependence) may occur.

Client Education

EXPECTED OUTCOMES

- When to return to work: A goal is to return to light work in 4 to 7 days and to normal duty within 1 to 2 weeks.
- Continuation of daily activities is preferred.
- Aerobic conditioning exercises (walking, swimming, stationary biking, light jogging) may be recommended to avoid debilitation. If the client was sedentary before this event, walking is preferred; if the client was more active, light jogging is permitted.
- Exercise may increase pain, but most clients work through pain unless it is intolerable
- Back braces/belts, transcutaneous electric nerve stimulation (TENS) units, shoe lifts (unless leg length discrepancy), biofeedback, and traction have *not* been shown to be beneficial.
- Adjunct therapies, such as ultrasound and massage, may be used for 3 weeks or less.
- Chiropractic manipulation, if used in the first month, has been found to be safe and effective.
- Bed rest is reserved for those clients with rare severe leg pain and should not exceed 2 to 4 days. The emphasis for other clients is on maintaining physical activity.
- If the client must stand, the client can rest one foot on a low stool to relieve pressure on the back. Every 5 to 15 minutes, the client should switch the foot resting on the stool.
- Sleeping may be facilitated by lying on either side with the knees flexed; if the client sleeps on the back, place pillows under the knees and a small pillow under the lower back.
- Men should lift no more than 20 pounds if pain is severe and no more than 60 pounds if pain is mild; women should lift no more than 20 pounds if pain is severe and no more than 35 pounds if pain is mild.
- Local application of ice may help initially in decreasing edema and/or pain; after 2 to 3 days either ice or heat may be applied.
- Discuss ergonomic issues involved in work, home, or leisure activities and how to remedy any problems identified.
- Explore available community resources (exercise programs, swimming pools, physical therapists, walking trails).

- One of the most important aspects of client education involves prevention. Stress education regarding proper body mechanics in lifting, weight loss (if needed), and overall muscular conditioning.
- The client should not sit longer than 20 minutes if back pain is severe. Even if back pain is not present, the client should sit no longer than 50 minutes without getting up and walking around 5 to 10 minutes.

Referral

Refer clients in whom HNP, fractures, malignancies, aortic aneurysms, cauda equina syndrome, spinal cord disease, or renal colic is suspected.

EVALUATION/FOLLOW-UP

- Most episodes of acute LBS will resolve spontaneously within 4 weeks if not, referral to an orthopedist or neurosurgeon for more advanced testing is indicated.
- Consider scheduling a return visit in 2 weeks with instructions to call/return if the client has questions or there is no improvement.
- If recovery does not go as expected, perform the following:
  —Briefly assess the family, support systems, difficulty getting/taking medications, and transportation/financial resources.
  —Attempt to build a trusting relationship, emphasizing self-care and minimizing the chance of chronic pain.

REFERENCES

Barker, L. R., Burton, J. R., & Zieve, P. D. (1995). *Principles of ambulatory medicine.* Baltimore: Williams & Wilkins.

Bigos, B. S., Bowyer, R. O., Braen, G., Brown, K. C., Deyo, R. A., Haldeman, S., Hart, J. L., Johnson, E. W., Keller, R. B., Kido, D. K., Liang, M. H., & Nelson, R. M. (1994, December). Acute low back problems in adults. In *Clinical practical guideline, quick reference guide, number 14* (AHCPR Publication No. 95-0643). Rockville, MD: U.S. Department of Health and Human Services, Public Health Service, Agency for Health Care Policy and Research.

Deen, H. G. (1996). Concise review for primary care physicians. *Mayo Clinic Proceedings, 71,* 283-287.

Gillette, R. D. (1996a). A practical approach to the patient with back pain. *American Family Physician, 53,* 670-676.

Gillette, R. D. (1996b). Behavioral factors in the management of back pain. *American Family Physician, 53,* 1313-1318.

Gorroll, A. H., May, L. A., Mulley, A. G. (1995). *Primary care management.* Washington, DC: American Psychological Association.

Tierney, L. M., McPhee, S. J., & Papadakis, M. A. (Eds.). (1996). *Current medical diagnosis and treatment.* Norwalk, CT: Appleton & Lange.

Uphold, C. R., & Graham, M. V. (1994). *Clinical guidelines in family practice.* Gainesville, FL: Barmarrae Books.

Weinstock, M. B., & Neides, D. M. (1996). *The resident's guide to ambulatory care.* Columbus, OH: Anadem Publishing.

REVIEW QUESTIONS

1. Which of the following symptoms are more indicative of acute LBS?

    a. Paresthesia, numbness
    b. Pain that increases over time as soft tissue swelling occurs
    c. Radicular pain
    d. Severe pain at onset

2. A client with a chief complaint of lower back pain who was unable to walk on heels and/or toes would be suspected of having:

    a. Nerve root irritation
    b. Acute LBS
    c. Spinal column stenosis
    d. Structural abnormality

3. The SLR and crossed SLR tests are used to help diagnose:

    a. Acute LBS
    b. Pelvic inflammatory disease
    c. HNP
    d. Prostate infection

4. In which of the following conditions, in a client with a herniated lumbar disk, is emergency surgical treatment required?

    a. Cauda equina syndrome
    b. Sciatica
    c. Diabetic peripheral neuropathy
    d. L5 radiculopathy

5. Which of the following statements of the use of medications in the treatment of acute LBS is **not** true?

    a. Muscle relaxants should be limited to 2 weeks.

    b. Opiates are not generally indicated.

    c. Muscle relaxants are as effective as NSAIDs.

    d. NSAIDs, with rapid onset of action, are preferred.

6. A complaint of lower back pain often interferes with sleep. The client may experience pain when sleeping on the back. The nurse practitioner should suggest:

    a. The client could switch to sleeping on the side that is most comfortable.

    b. The client could sleep propped up with two to three pillows.

    c. Pillows under the head make pain increase.

    d. Pillows under the knees and lower back may help.

7. Most episodes of acute LBS will spontaneously resolve in:

    a. 6 to 8 weeks

    b. 2 weeks

    c. 4 weeks

    d. More than 8 weeks

ANSWERS AND RATIONALES

1. *Answer:* b (assessment/history/musculoskeletal/NAS)

    Rationale: Pain that increases with movement, is relieved with rest, and increases over time as soft tissue swelling occurs is more indicative of LBS. (Tierney, McPhee, & Papadakis, 1996; Uphold & Graham, 1994)

2. *Answer:* a (assessment/physical examination/musculoskeletal/NAS)

    Rationale: Heel walking (L5) and toe walking (S1) cannot be accomplished if there is nerve root irritation. (Bigos et al., 1994)

3. *Answer:* c (assessment/physical examination/musculoskeletal/NAS)

    Rationale: The SLR is considered sensitive for HNP, and the crossed SLR is more specific for HNP. (Barker, Burton, & Zieve, 1995; Uphold & Graham, 1994)

4. *Answer:* a (plan/musculoskeletal/NAS)

    Rationale: Cauda equina syndrome is considered a surgical emergency diagnosis. (Barker et al., 1995; Tierney et al., 1996; Uphold & Graham, 1994)

5. *Answer:* c (plan/musculoskeletal/NAS)

    Rationale: NSAIDs appear to be more effective than muscle relaxants. (Bigos et al., 1994)

6. *Answer:* d (plan/musculoskeletal/NAS)

    Rationale: Pillows under knees and lower back reduce the strain of muscles and consequently reduce pain, making sleeping on the back better tolerated. (Bigos et al., 1994)

7. *Answer:* c (evaluation/musculoskeletal/NAS)

    Rationale: With a diagnosis of acute LBS, recovery should occur within 4 weeks; if recovery does not occur, additional assessment, examination, and diagnostic testing should be performed. (Deen, 1996)

MUSCULOSKELETAL INJURIES

Common Sprains and Fractures

OVERVIEW
Definitions

An injury to one of the ligamentous structures of the body is termed a *sprain*. A *strain* is trauma to a muscle or musculoskeletal unit of the body from an excessive forcible stretch. Loss in continuity in the substance of the bone is called a *fracture*.

Pathophysiology

FRACTURE. Fractures are classified as either open or closed. Open fractures are exposed to the external environment and are highly prone to serious infection. Description of a fracture includes the anatomic location and degree of displacement, rotation, translation, or shortening. Fractures into the joint are called intraarticular fractures. Fracture patterns are described as transverse, oblique, spiral, comminuted, or greenstick. The Salter-Harris classification is commonly used to describe growth plate fractures in children.

SPRAIN. Ligaments, which connect bones together, can sustain injuries. Ligamentous injuries are classified as first degree, second degree, or third degree, depending on the extent of injury. A completely torn ligament is classified as a third-degree sprain, whereas a mildly stretched ligament is classified as a first-degree sprain.

Common Injuries/Fractures

- Elbow: *Nursemaid's elbow* (radial head subluxation) is a dislocation of the radial head in which the head becomes caught beneath the annular ligament. *Tennis elbow* (lateral epicondylitis) is a tendinitis at origins of the wrist extensors that originate at the lateral epicondyle of the humerus.
- Wrist: *Colles' fracture* is a fracture of the distal radius and is the most common type of adult wrist fracture. *Scaphoid fractures* are common carpal bone fractures because of the scaphoid bone's anatomic location where it spans both rows of carpal bones.
- Hand: *Gamekeeper's thumb/skier's thumb* (ulnar collateral ligament injury of the metacarpophalangeal [MCP] joint) is caused by a forced hyperabduction of the thumb. *Boxer's fracture* is a fifth metacarpal fracture.
- Fingers: *Mallet finger* is a flexion deformity of the distal interphalangeal joint of the finger. *Distal phalanx fractures* are fractures of the distal tip of the fingers.
- Knee: *Meniscus injuries* usually result from a tear in either the lateral or medial meniscus secondary to some type of sport involvement. *Ligament injuries* involving the anterior cruciate (ACL), posterior cruciate (PCL), medial collateral (MCL), and lateral collateral (LCL) ligaments commonly occur during athletic activities.
- Ankle: *Ankle sprains* are most commonly caused by inversion of the ankle, resulting in injury to one or more of the lateral ankle ligaments (anterior talofibular ligament, calcaneofibular ligament, and posterior talofibular ligament). Eversion ankle injuries commonly injure the deltoid ligament of the medial an-

kle. *Ankle fractures* involve either the medial malleolus, the lateral malleolus, or both.
- Foot: *Jones fracture* (fracture of the fifth metatarsal) frequently occurs with ankle sprains.
- Toes: *Toe fractures* occur from direct trauma.

ASSESSMENT: SUBJECTIVE/HISTORY
History of Present Illness
- Exact mechanism of injury
- Timing of injury
- Description/location of pain
- Radiation
- Quality
- Timing
- Severity
- Aggravation/relief
- Previous treatment

Symptoms
- Swelling
- Deformity
- Masses
- Paralysis
- Gait changes

Past Medical History
- Previous injuries
- Surgery
- Exercise
- Allergies

Medication History
Ask about recent or present use of pain medications, NSAIDs, and other medications.

Family History
Inquire about orthopedic problems.

Psychosocial History
- Occupational job description
- Smoking
- Alcohol intake
- Conditioning

History of Common Injuries/Fractures
- Elbow: *Nursemaid's elbow* commonly occurs in children 1 to 3 years of age as they are being pulled up by an extended arm. *Tennis elbow* results after repetitive wrist and elbow activity in persons with limited conditioning.

- Wrist: *Colles' fracture* is associated with a fall on an outstretched hand. *Scaphoid fractures* are usually seen in young adults who have sustained a fall on an outstretched hand.
- Hand: *Gamekeeper's thumb/skier's thumb* includes a history of forced hyperabduction of the thumb such as when skiers fall while holding onto ski poles. *Boxer's fracture* is associated with a forceful punch with a closed fist.
- Fingers: *Mallet finger* is usually caused by a jamming injury of the finger or a forced flexion of the distal phalanx. *Distal phalanx fractures* are frequently associated with crush injuries.
- Knee: *Meniscus injuries* occur in all age groups and are frequently associated with athletic activity in which a hyperextension, hyperflexion, or rotational injury occurs. *Collateral ligament injuries* occur as a result of varus or valgus stress to the knee. *ACL injuries* occur with twisting motion, a quick stop, or a hyperextension. ACL injuries are also associated with an audible pop. *PCL injuries* are associated with a direct blow to the anterior portion of the tibia.
- Ankle: *Ankle sprains* usually result from an inversion injury in which the lateral ligaments of the ankle are damaged. *Ankle fractures* may occur as a result of inversion or eversion injuries.
- Foot: *Jones fracture* usually occurs as a result of an inversion injury of the foot and frequently accompanies an ankle sprain.
- Toes: *Toe fractures* usually occur from direct trauma such as stubbing or secondary to an object striking the toe.

ASSESSMENT: OBJECTIVE/ PHYSICAL EXAMINATION

Physical Examination

A problem-oriented physical examination should be conducted with particular attention to vital signs, general assessment, musculoskeletal area of complaint, adjacent musculoskeletal areas, and neurovascular status distal to the injury.

VITAL SIGNS. These should be relatively normal with common, non–life-threatening injuries.

GENERAL ASSESSMENT. This should note the client's response to pain, gait, and how the client holds the injured extremity.

MUSCULOSKELETAL ASSESSMENT. This examination should include observation for swelling and effusion, palpation of adjacent and actual areas of injury, evaluation of ROM, and special physical testing to diagnose specific conditions.

NEUROVASCULAR ASSESSMENT. This should be performed distal to the injury. Check pulses, sensation, and capillary refill.

Specific Physical Findings of Common Injuries/Fractures

- Elbow: *Nursemaid's elbow* is characterized by a child holding the affected arm limply in adduction and pain elicited with palpation of the radial head and resistance to ROM. *Tennis elbow* is characterized by pain over the lateral epicondyle aggravated with resisted finger and wrist extension.
- Wrist: *Colles' fracture* is characterized by the classic "dinner fork" appearance, with considerable pain and resistance to ROM with palpation. Concomitant median nerve injury commonly occurs with Colles' fracture; numbness and tingling of the thumb, index and long fingers, and radial half of the ring fingers should be noted. *Scaphoid fractures* are characterized by wrist pain localized to the snuffbox area with palpation.
- Hand: *Gamekeeper's thumb/skier's thumb* is characterized by a painful ulnar aspect of the MCP joint of the thumb, with a possible abnormal opening of the MCP joint with stress. *Boxer's fractures* demonstrate swelling along the dorsum of the hand with pain elicited on palpation of the fifth metatarsal. Commonly a malrotation of the involved digit also exists.
- Fingers: *Mallet finger* is a flexion deformity of the distal phalanx and inability to actively extend the distal interphalangeal joint. *Distal phalanx fractures* are often associated with crush injuries and therefore are associated with lacerations, contusions, and subungual hematoma.
- Knee: *Meniscus injuries* are characterized by mild swelling, joint line tenderness, and positive results from a McMurray's test. *MCL injuries* are associated with joint line pain, mild swelling, +/− joint effusion, pain, and/or laxity with valgus stress. *LCL injuries* include joint line pain, +/− swelling or effusion, and pain and/or laxity with varus stress. *ACL injuries* frequently include a joint effusion with a positive anterior drawer sign or positive Lachman's

sign. *PCL injuries* are associated with minimal swelling but positive posterior drawer sign or a positive sag sign of Godfrey.

- Ankle: *Ankle sprains* include mild-to-severe swelling over the area involved with mild-to-severe pain over the lateral ligaments and lateral malleolus. Inversion ankle sprains are often difficult to differentiate from distal fibular avulsion fractures since both have similar physical findings. Include palpation of the distal tibia, fibula, all ankle ligaments, and the fifth metatarsal base. Joint laxity reveals a positive anterior drawer sign and indicates a significant ligamentous injury.
- Foot: *Jones fracture* is associated with a painful, swollen lateral foot with pain elicited on palpation of the fifth metatarsal.
- Toes: *Toe fractures* are swollen, contused, and painful with palpation.

Diagnostic Procedures

Consider x-ray examinations with significant pain, swelling, effusion, or contusion.

Radiographic Findings of Common Injuries/Fractures

- Elbow: *Nursemaid's elbow* and *tennis elbow* show no specific x-ray findings.
- Wrist: *Colles' fractures* reveal a fractured distal radius with a dorsally angulated distal fragment. *Scaphoid fractures* typically do not show up on initial x-ray examination but may be evident on follow-up x-ray examination 7 to 10 days after injury.
- Hand: *Gamekeeper's thumb/skier's thumb* usually demonstrate normal findings on film, but occasionally an avulsion fracture of the ulnar aspect of the distal thumb metacarpal exists. *Boxer's fractures* reveal a fracture of the fifth metatarsal, which frequently is medially angulated.
- Fingers: *Finger fractures* may reveal crush injuries to the distal phalanx; transverse or spiral fractures of the phalanges may be present. Intraarticular fractures must be referred to an orthopedic surgeon.
- Knee: Soft tissue injuries *(ACL, MCL, PCL, LCL, and meniscus injuries)* usually reveal normal findings on films with the exception of a visible joint effusion or soft tissue swelling.

Occasionally a ligament rupture reveals a small avulsion fracture.

- Ankle: *Ankle sprains* usually reveal normal findings on film with soft tissue swelling but can include avulsion fractures of the distal fibula or tibia. *Ankle fractures* may reveal malleolar fractures of the tibia or fibula or bimalleolar fracture of both the tibia and fibula. Trimalleolar fractures reveal a bimalleolar fracture and a fracture of the posterior tibial malleolus.
- Foot: *Jones fractures* reveal a fracture to the fifth metatarsal.
- Toes: *Toe fractures* are usually very obvious on x-ray film.

DIAGNOSIS

The differential diagnosis includes the following:
- Sprain
- Strain
- Fracture
- Tendinitis
- OA
- RA
- Cellulitis
- Gout
- Gonococcal arthritis
- Tumors
- Degenerative changes
- Congenital disorders
- Overuse syndromes
- Infections
- Bursitis
- Plantar fascitis

THERAPEUTIC PLAN
RICE

- **Rest** any injured part of the musculoskeletal system. Rest time varies according to the seriousness of the injury.
- **Ice** all musculoskeletal injuries in an attempt to control swelling. Continue ice application as long as swelling exists. Ice can be applied for 15 minutes at a time.
- **Compression** controls edema and provides comfort and/or support. Compression can be accomplished with Ace wraps, neoprene braces, custom-made splints, and commercially made splints.

- Elevate all injured extremities. Upper extremities should be elevated with a sling.

Joint Protection/Immobilization

- The injured joint should be protected with application of a splint.
- Splinting allows for postinjury swelling.
- Never apply a circumferential cast to an acutely injured extremity.
- Use crutches for lower extremity injuries.
- Many splints are commercially made, and easy-to-apply custom-made splinting material includes plaster and fiberglass.
- Immobilization also assists in pain control.

Splints for Particular Injuries

- Volar cock-up: Wrist sprains, Colles' fractures
- Sugar tong upper extremity: Colles' fracture, forearm fractures
- Posterior splint upper extremity: Radial head fractures, fractures about the elbow and forearm
- Thumb spica: Gamekeeper's thumb, scaphoid fractures
- Ulnar gutter: Boxer's fractures
- Metal finger splint: Finger sprains
- Stax splint: Mallet finger
- Knee immobilizer: Knee injuries
- Bimalleolar splint: Ankle sprains
- Posterior splint lower extremity: Ankle sprains, Jones fracture, foot fractures, fractures of the lateral or medial malleolus
- Posterior splint with stirrups: Severe ankle sprains, malleolus fractures, foot fractures

Pharmacologic Treatment

Antiinflammatory drugs and muscle relaxants are the drugs of choice for musculoskeletal injury.

- NSAIDs are indicated for musculoskeletal injury. NSAIDs inhibit prostaglandin synthesis, which decreases pain. Common NSAIDs include ibuprofen (Motrin), naproxen (Naprosyn), etodolac (Lodine), and diclofenac (Voltaren). Do not prescribe NSAIDs to clients with peptic ulcer disease, allergy to NSAIDs/aspirin, renal dysfunction, or pregnancy
- Myorelaxants are indicated for pain related to muscle spasm. Common muscle relaxants include cyclobenzaprine (Flexeril) and chlorzoxazone (Parafon Forte). Muscle re-

laxants should be prescribed for short periods of time (3 to 5 days).
- OTC analgesics such as acetaminophen are for less severe pain and for clients who are unable to take NSAIDs.
- Narcotic analgesics are indicated only for fractures with severe pain and should be given for only several days.

Client Education

- RICE: Emphasize the importance of rest, ice application, use of splints/Ace wraps, and elevation. These measures tend to decrease swelling and help to control pain.
- Pathophysiology: Explain injury pathophysiology with expected outcomes.
- Cast/splint care: Give detailed information concerning splint care including bathing instructions, removal/application if indicated, and observation for signs of neurovascular compromise.
- Medications: Include potential medication side effects and instructions for administration. Advise the client to take NSAIDs with food to avoid abdominal discomfort. Muscle relaxants/narcotic analgesics may cause drowsiness; advise the client not to operate machinery or work above ground level.

Referral

- Immediate referral to an orthopedic surgeon for long bone fractures, displaced fractures, intraarticular fractures, all fractures with neurovascular compromise, and knee injuries with significant effusion and/or instability
- Three- to five-day referral to an orthopedic surgeon for simple nondisplaced fractures, and grade II to III ankle sprains of the ankle and knee after appropriate splinting and client education
- Referral to an orthopedic surgeon for all minor injuries that do not respond to conservative management

EVALUATION/FOLLOW-UP

- Recheck all minor injuries/sprains in 1 week. For those that do not show improvement, consider a referral to an orthopedic surgeon.

- Begin rehabilitation for minor injuries/sprains as soon as possible to prevent contractures and loss of conditioning.
- Continue prescribing NSAIDs with food.

REFERENCES

Alonso, J. (1996). Ankle fractures. In V. Masear (Ed.), *Primary care orthopedics* (pp. 122-127). Philadelphia: W. B. Saunders.

Anderson, B. (1995). *Office orthopedics for primary care.* Philadelphia: W. B. Saunders.

Balano, K. (1996). Anti-inflammatory drugs and my-orelaxants. Pharmacology and clinical use in musculoskeletal disease. *Primary Care, 23*(2), 329-334.

Connolly, J. (1996, August). Acute ankle sprains: Getting and keeping patients back up on their feet. *Consultant,* 1631-1639.

DiChristina, D. (1996). Fractures and ligamentous injuries of the ankle. In V. Masear (Ed.), *Primary care orthopedics* (pp. 117-122). Philadelphia: W. B. Saunders.

Dvorkin, M. (1993). *Office orthopedics.* Norwalk, CT: Appleton & Lange.

Garth, W. (1996). Knee injuries in sports. In V. Masear (Ed.), *Primary care orthopedics* (pp. 88-101). Philadelphia: W. B. Saunders.

Lillegard, W. A. (1996, March). Common upper extremity injuries. *Archives of Family Medicine, 5,* 159-168.

Martin, J. (1996). Initial assessment and management of common fractures. *Primary Care, 23*(2), 405-409.

McRae, R. (1989). *Practical fracture treatment* (2nd ed.). Edinburgh: Churchill Livingstone.

Meislin, R. (1996). Managing collateral ligament tears of the knee. *The Physician and Sports Medicine, 24*(3), 67-80.

Savage, P. L. (1996). Casting and splinting techniques. In V. Maeser (Ed.), *Primary care orthopedics* (pp. 337-346). Philadelphia: W. B. Saunders.

Swenson, E. J. (1995, June). Diagnosing and managing meniscal injuries in athletes. *The Journal of Musculoskeletal Medicine,* 35-45.

Thordarson, D. B. (1996). Detecting and treating common foot and ankle fractures. *The Physician and Sportsmedicine, 24*(9), 29-38.

Torburn, L. (1996). Principles of rehabilitation. *Primary Care, 23*(2), 335-343.

REVIEW QUESTIONS

1. ACL knee injuries usually show which one of the following x-ray findings?

   a. No radiographic findings
   b. Soft tissue swelling or effusion
   c. Tibial plateau fractures
   d. Distal fibula avulsion fractures

2. Which one of the following knee injuries is associated with a "pop" that is either felt or heard?

   a. PCL injuries
   b. ACL injuries
   c. MCL injuries
   d. LCL injuries

3. Which one of the following fractures is characterized by the classic "dinner fork" appearance?

   a. Jones fractures of the foot
   b. Mallet finger deformity
   c. Boxer's fracture of the hand
   d. Colles' fracture of the wrist

4. Ankle injuries are most commonly associated with which one of the following?

   a. Inversion injuries in which the lateral ligaments are damaged
   b. Eversion injuries in which the deltoid ligament is injured
   c. Fractures of the first metatarsal
   d. Proximal fibula fractures

5. Radiographic findings consistent with a Colles' fracture include which one of the following?

   a. A fractured distal radius with a dorsally angulated fragment
   b. A fractured distal radius with a volar displaced fragment
   c. An avulsion fracture of the lateral fibula
   d. A fractured midshaft radius

6. Nursemaid's elbow is associated with which one of the following mechanisms of action?

   a. Repetitive wrist motion
   b. Pulling up of a young child by an extended arm
   c. Repetitive forearm motion as seen with golf and tennis
   d. A fall on an outstretched hand in young children

7. Which one of the following is the most common type of adult wrist fracture?

    a. Boxer's fracture
    b. Scaphoid fracture
    c. Colles' fracture
    d. Mallet finger

8. Which one of the following best describes the mechanism of action for NSAIDs?

    a. NSAIDs inhibit H_2 receptors in the gastric mucosa.
    b. NSAIDs alter pain receptors in the brain by altering serotonin release.
    c. NSAIDs inhibit prostaglandin synthesis, thereby decreasing pain.
    d. NSAIDs relax skeletal muscle by decreasing stimulation along the axons.

9. Which one of the following describes appropriate follow-up time for minor injuries or sprains?

    a. Recheck all injuries in 24 hours.
    b. No follow-up is needed for minor injuries.
    c. Recheck minor sprains and injuries in 1 week.
    d. Recheck common injuries in 4 to 6 weeks.

ANSWERS AND RATIONALES

1. *Answer:* b (assessment/physical examination/ musculoskeletal/NAS)

    Rationale: Radiographs are routinely obtained with suspected ACL tears. Routine findings usually include only soft tissue swelling or effusion. Occasionally an avulsion fracture is visible. (Garth, 1996)

2. *Answer:* b (assessment/history/musculoskeletal/NAS)

    Rationale: The client with an ACL injury may give a history of a shifting sensation of the knee with a pop being felt or heard. (Garth, 1996)

3. *Answer:* d (assessment/physical examination/ musculoskeletal/NAS)

    Rationale: When viewed from the side, the wrist with a displaced Colles' fracture resembles a dinner fork, with the tines resembling the fingers. (McRae, 1989)

4. *Answer:* a (assessment/history/musculoskeletal/NAS)

    Rationale: Lateral ankle ligaments are weaker than medial ankle ligaments and are injured with common inversion of the ankle. (DiChristina, 1996)

5. *Answer:* a (assessment/physical examination/ musculoskeletal/NAS)

    Rationale: In a Colles' fracture the distal radius is fractured. The fragment is dorsally angulated with shortening at the fracture site. (Dvorkin, 1993)

6. *Answer:* b (assessment/history/musculoskeletal/ child)

    Rationale: Nursemaid's elbow typically is characterized by a history of a jerk on the upper extremity of a young child who has an extended elbow. (Lillegard, 1996)

7. *Answer:* c (assessment/history/musculoskeletal/ adult)

    Rationale: Colles' fracture is the most common adult wrist fracture and is associated with a fall on an outstretched hand. (Dvorkin, 1993)

8. *Answer:* c (plan/management/therapy/pharmacologic/NAS)

    Rationale: NSAIDs decrease prostaglandin synthesis via inhibition of cyclooxygenase. Prostaglandins are associated with the development of pain after trauma. (Balano, 1996)

9. *Answer:* c (evaluation/musculoskeletal/NAS)

    Rationale: Most athletes with grade I ankle sprains are able to return to full activity in 1 to 2 weeks. (DiChristina, 1996) Therefore follow-up is indicated at about 1 week after injury.

OSTEOPOROSIS

OVERVIEW

Definition

Osteoporosis is a systemic skeletal disease characterized by low bone mass and microarchitectural deterioration of bone tissue, leading to enhanced bone fragility and consequent increase in fracture risk.

Incidence

- Osteoporosis is the major cause of bone fracture in postmenopausal women.
- Forty percent of women age 50 and older will experience an osteoporotic fracture in their lifetime.
- Incidence increases with age. In women, at age 50, risk of hip fracture doubles every 10 years.
- As men live longer, there is an age-correlated increase in osteoporotic fracture.
- Before the seventh decade, osteoporosis in men is often due to a secondary cause such as hypogonadism and gastrectomy.

Pathophysiology

- Normally osteoclasts remove damaged bone from microfractures that are caused by everyday stresses; osteoclasts then attract osteoblasts that replace bone matrix.
- Bone is lost if osteoclasts create a cavity of excessive depth or if osteoblasts incompletely fill a cavity.
- Two main types of bone: Dense cortical bone forms the outer layer. Spongy, trabecular bone forms the inner supporting structures. Turnover is most rapid in trabecular bone. Sites with a high proportion of trabecular bone such as the spine, pelvis, distal radius, and primal femur are generally the first to show osteoporotic changes.
- Menopause-related bone loss (type I) is associated with high bone turnover and osteoclastic overactivity. The greatest loss occurs in vertebral bodies and long bones (vertebral and Colles' fracture).
- Age-related bone loss (type II) is due to impaired bone formation and osteoclastic underactivity. Greatest bone loss is in cancellous and cortical bone (hip fracture).

  RISK FACTORS
  - Increasing age
  - Caucasian or Asian race
  - Family history
  - Small stature
  - Smoking
  - Physical inactivity
  - Female gender
  - Early menopause
  - Low body weight
  - Low calcium intake
  - Excessive alcohol intake
  - High caffeine intake

  SECONDARY CAUSES. Table 7-1 lists the causes of secondary osteoporosis.

Table 7-1   Secondary Causes of Osteoporosis

Endocrinopathies
Hypercortisolism
Hyperthyroidism
Hyperparathyroidism
Hypogonadism
Hyperprolactinemia

Drugs
Corticosteroids
Levothyroxine
Heparin
Barbiturates
Phenytoin
Methroxate
Alcohol
Aluminum-containing antacids
Tobacco
Isoniazid

Other Conditions
Immobilization
Diabetes mellitus
Chronic renal failure
Hepatic disease
Scurvy
Malabsorption
Chronic obstructive lung disease
Rheumatoid arthritis
Osteomalacia
Systemic mastocytosis
Osteogenesis imperfecta
Sarcoidosis

Modified from Abrams, W., Beers, M., & Berkow, R. (1995). *The Merck manual of geriatrics* (2nd ed., p. 901). Whitehouse Station, NJ: Merck.

PROTECTIVE FACTORS
- Black race, obesity, early menarche
- Estrogen replacement therapy immediately after menopause (retards menopause-related acceleration of bone loss)

ASSESSMENT: SUBJECTIVE/HISTORY
History of Present Illness
- Often asymptomatic
- Negative self-image with clothes not fitting right
- With vertebral fractures, acute pain with a sudden onset, localized to specific vertebrae with local tenderness and radiating bilaterally; pain that subsides within 2 to 6 weeks
- Constipation secondary to painful bowel irritation and compression
- Possible modest-to-moderate scoliosis or kyphosis, especially if fracture occurs at T2-T11
- Chronic pain in the paraspinal muscles that localizes to the lumbar area even when a fracture occurs in the thoracic area
- Hip fractures associated with falls that are painful, with distortion of the leg and an inability to bear weight on the leg
- Kyphosis
- Protuberant abdomen
- Abdominal discomfort
- Back pain

Past Medical History
- Fractures
- Scoliosis
- Loss of 1.5 cm or more of height (based on maximum self-reported height)
- Age of menarche
- Late menarche
- Athletic amenorrhea
- Amenorrhea secondary to anorexia nervosa
- Hyperprolactinemia
- Gonadotropin-releasing hormone agonist therapy
- Premature or surgical menopause
- Irregular menses
- Oligomenorrhea
- Malignancies such as multiple myeloma
- Endocrinopathies such as hypogonadism if male (see Table 7-1)
- Seizures (treatment with phenytoin)

Medication History
- Current and past medications (see Table 7-1)
- Estrogen replacement therapy

Family History
- Osteoporosis
- Maternal hip fracture (most strongly associated with osteoporosis)

Psychosocial History
- Ask about current and lifetime physical activity patterns (include types of exercise and recreational sports).
- Calculate pack-years of cigarette smoking.
- Evaluate for alcohol use more than two drinks per day.

Dietary History
- Review over the lifetime anything affecting nutrition
  —Bulimia
  —Anorexia
  —Gastrectomy
  —Intestinal bypass
  —Malabsorption syndrome
  —Chronic renal failure
  —Diet high in protein, caffeine, sodium, and phosphate and/or low in calcium
- Use of dairy products: A good guide to evaluating calcium intake (Table 7-2)

ASSESSMENT: OBJECTIVE/ PHYSICAL EXAMINATION
Physical Examination
- Generally a complete history and physical examination is indicated to rule out other pathology.
- Observe for visible deformity of the spine (e.g., dorsal kyphosis).
- Record height and compare with self-reported maximum height.

Diagnostic Procedures
LABORATORY PROCEDURES
- Obtain laboratory data to rule out other pathology and to identify secondary causes of osteoporosis.
- CBC, ESR, serum calcium, phosphorus, alkaline phosphatase, creatinine levels, liver

Table 7-2   Foods High in Calcium

FOOD	CALCIUM CONTENT
Yogurt, plain, nonfat (1 cup)	450 mg
Milkshake, chocolate (10 fluid ounce)	320 mg
Sardines, canned, with bones (3 ounce)	320 mg
Milk, skin or lowfat (1 cup)	300 mg
Cheese, Swiss (1 ounce)	270 mg
Cheese, cheddar (1 ounce)	200 mg
Salmon, canned with bone (3 ounce)	200 mg
Tofu, without calcium sulfate (½ cup)	150 mg
Turnip greens, cooked (½ cup)	100 mg
Frozen yogurt, vanilla (½ cup)	90 mg
Ice cream or ice milk (½ cup)	90 mg
Broccoli, cooked (½ cup)	90 mg
Cottage cheese, 2% lowfat (½ cup)	80 mg

Data from Tresolini, C. P., Grid, D. T., & Lee, L. S. (1996). *Work with patients to prevent, treat, and manage osteoporosis.* San Francisco: San Francisco National Fund for Medical Education.

function tests, thyroid function tests, urine calcium, and glucose are normal in uncomplicated osteoporosis.
- Abnormalities suggest secondary pathology.
- Deoxypyridinoline and N-telopeptides are biochemical markers of bone resorption. In a client unable to obtain dual-energy x-ray absorptiometry (DEXA), a high level of urinary deoxypyridinoline or N-telopeptide suggests active bone turnover and high future fracture risk.

RADIOGRAPHIC PROCEDURES
- Measurement of bone mass confirms the existence of osteoporosis. Low bone mass increases the risk of fracture.
- Dual-energy x-ray absorptiometry (DEXA) is the preferred method because of DEXA's 10-minute scan time, precision, and low radiation exposure. The spine and hip are commonly scanned. DEXA is a good technique for assessing future fracture risk.
- Dual-energy photon absorptiometry (DPA) is the next preferred method; however, the scan time is longer than with DEXA.
- Single-energy photon absorptiometry (SPA) is limited to peripheral sites.
- Quantitative computed tomography (QCT) has a higher cost and radiation exposure.

BONE DENSITY TESTING. The National Osteoporosis Foundation Clinical Guidelines recommend determining bone mass measurements for the following:
- Estrogen-deficient women
- A vertebral abnormality that is seen on radiography
- Initiation of glucocorticosteroid therapy
- Presence of primary hyperparathyroidism

Interpretation of Bone Density Testing
- Normal bone density is not more than 1 SD below the young adult mean (T score above -1)
- Osteopenia is a low bone mass that lies between 1 and 2.5 SD below the young adult mean (T score between -1 and -2.5)
- Osteoporosis is a bone density that is more than 2.5 SD below the young adult mean (T score less than -2.5) or the presence of fragility fractures irrespective of the bone density.

EXPECTED FINDINGS. The following lists expected findings in osteoporotic women:
- Decreased radiodensity
- Changes in vertebral body shape
- Generalized osteopenia
- Fractures (particularly vertebral compression fractures)

DIAGNOSIS

For information on differential diagnosis, refer to Table 7-1.

Children

- Physical activity and dietary calcium influence the bone mass of the developing skeleton; these may each contribute up to 40% of the total variance in bone density.
- Weight-bearing recreational activities such as basketball, soccer, and tennis are associated with a modest increase in bone mass at the radius and hip and to a lesser extent in the spine.
- Participation in non–weight-bearing activities such as bicycling and swimming is associated with either no change or a reduction in bone mass.

Adolescents

Early behavioral factors such as diet, smoking, alcohol use, and exercise are major determinants of peak bone mass in later life and therefore osteoporosis.

THERAPEUTIC PLAN

- The objective is to increase bone mineral density and decrease the risk of osteoporotic fractures.
- Consult with a physician regarding suspected fractures in the presence of secondary causes and/or complicated cases.
- The plan depends on client problems (e.g., care of patient with fracture, physical therapy for soft tissue trauma).

Prevention

- Prevention begins in childhood and continues through life.
- The nurse practitioner should consider teaching the following to every client of any age as appropriate.
  EXERCISE
  - Assist the client to develop a plan that allows for gradual buildup of muscle strength and endurance.
  - Advise the client to avoid excessive exercise (marathon running).
  - Encourage regular, diverse, weight-bearing exercise 2 to 3 times weekly
  - Treadmill, climbing a Stairmaster, tennis, using a Nordic-track apparatus, and low-impact aerobics are desirable.
  CALCIUM INTAKE
  - See Table 7-2 for dietary sources (preferred).
  - See Table 7-3 for optimal requirements.
  - Average calcium intake in diet at age 40 to 65 is 450 to 650 mg per day.
  - Calcium is needed on a consistent basis.
  - Only elemental calcium is absorbed. Elemental calcium by type of calcium is as follows:

Calcium carbonate	40%
Calcium phosphate	39%
Calcium citrate	24%
Calcium lactate	13%
Calcium gluconate	9%

  - Taking calcium supplements between meals increases bioavailability.
  - Calcium carbonate absorption is impaired in persons who have an absence of gastric acid; these persons should take calcium carbonate with food.

Table 7-3 Optimal Calcium Requirement Recommended by the National Institutes of Health Consensus Panel

AGE GROUP	OPTIMAL DAILY INTAKE OF CALCIUM (mg)
Infant	
Birth-6 mo	400
6 mo-1 yr	600
Children	
1-5 yr	800
6-10 yr	800-1200
Adolescents/Young Adults	
11-24 yr	1200-1500
Men	
25-65 yr	1000
Older than 65 yr	1500
Women	
25-50 yr	1000
Older than 50 (post- menopausal)	
Taking estrogens	1000
Not taking estrogens	1500
Older than 65 yr	1500
Pregnant and nursing	1200-1500

Data from NIH Consensus Conference (1994). Optimal calcium intake. *Journal of the American Medical Association, 272*, 1943.

- Calcium citrate does not require gastric acid for absorption and can be used in older adults who have reduced gastric acid.
- Advise the client to take 500 mg calcium hs. Take 500 mg bid if a larger dose is required
- Advise the client to add a multivitamin with 400 mg vitamin D qd to ensure adequate absorption.
- There is a risk of ectopic calcium deposition if too much vitamin D is ingested.
  ESTROGEN REPLACEMENT THERAPY (ERT)
  - Counsel postmenopausal women regarding estrogen replacement therapy; never too late but immediate replacement preferable
  - Benefits: Prevents bone loss and osteoporotic fractures; protects from coronary artery disease; elevates HDL levels; relieves menopausal/genitourinary symptoms

- Risks and side effects: Intermittent bleeding, breast tenderness, abdominal fullness, weight gain
- More serious side effects: Hypertension, thrombosis, migraine headaches, endometrial hyperplasia; relationship to breast cancer undetermined
- Progesterone: Used in conjunction with estrogen if uterus present to avoid endometrial cancer; omitted after hysterectomy
- No difference in increase in bone mass with type or method of estrogen
- Regular breast examinations, mammograms, pelvic and Papanicolaou smears
- Tamoxifen: Increases bone mass but not used for primary treatment

Fall Prevention (Older Adults)

- Flat, rubber-soled shoes
- Cane or walker as needed
- Proper lifting techniques
- Assess number and types of medications
- Check visual acuity
- Home safety modifications
- Hand grips, safety mats, removing clutter, lighting

Screening

- Bone density testing: Use with clients who have several osteoporotic risk factors and as a baseline measurement before pharmacologic treatment.
- National Osteoporosis Foundation Clinical Guidelines: Bone mass measurements should be obtained in estrogen-deficit women as part of the consideration for the use of hormone replacement or the need for other treatment modalities.
  —For women whose bone mass is 1 SD below the mean peak bone mass, hormone replacement or some other form of treatment should be recommended.
  —Women with bone mass 1 SD above the mean require no intervention.
  —Women with bone mass within 1 SD of the mean should be followed with measurements taken at 1- to 5-year intervals, depending on the initial value.

Pharmacologic Treatment

ESTROGEN REPLACEMENT THERAPY. This treatment may be used if not contraindicated.

BIPHOSPHONATE: ALENDRONATE (FOSAMAX)

- Biphosphonate decreases bone resorption and prevents bone loss.
- Biphosphonate binds to hydroxyapatite and specifically inhibits the activity of osteoclasts; inhibits osteoclastic resorption
- Prescribe 10 mg/day to be taken 30 minutes before breakfast with full glass of water.
- Instruct the client to wait at least 30 minutes in an upright position before eating or drinking anything else.
- Instruct the client to take with calcium and vitamin D supplement to increase bone mass
- Persons living in northern climates in winter may need to increase their vitamin D during this time.
- Side effects: Nausea and abdominal pain are common side effects.

INTRANASAL CALCITONIN

- Suppresses osteoclast activity and subsequently bone resorption
- Analgesic effect on osteoporotic fracture pain
- 200 IU/day; 1 puff in one nostril, alternating nostrils each day
- Adequate calcium and vitamin D concurrently
- Reserved for clients with severe osteoporotic fractures and skeletal pain

CALCIUM SUPPLEMENTS

- Prescribe calcium carbonate, citrate, or phosphate usually 1000 to 1500 mg/day divided into two separate doses to be taken between or after meals or at bedtime.
- Tums and several other brands of antacids contain calcium carbonate in varying strengths (read label). Os-Cal is a chewable tablet but generally more expensive than Tums.
- Avoid calcium tablets made from bone meal or dolomite because they contain lead, mercury, or arsenic.

EVALUATION/FOLLOW-UP

- Prevention: Maintenance of adequate bone mass through life without fractures
- Screening: High-risk clients identified and therapy instituted
- Pharmacologic therapy: Resolution of client problems, decrease in advancement of osteo-

porosis, and/or prevention of complications such as excess disability

REFERENCES

Abrams, W., & Berkow, R. (1995). *The Merck manual of geriatrics*. Whitehouse Station, NJ: Merck.

Barrett-Connor, C., Chang, J., & Edelstein, S. (1994). Coffee-associated osteoporosis offset by daily milk consumption. *Journal of the American Medical Association, 271*, 280-283.

Birge, S. J. (1993). Osteoporosis and hip fracture. In T.E. Kaiser (Ed.), *Clinics in geriatric medicine: Care of the older woman* (Vol. 9, pp. 69-86). Philadelphia: W. B. Saunders.

Janis, L. W. (1996). Prevention of osteoporosis. In R. Rubin, C. Voss, D. Derkesen, A. Gateley, & R. Quenzer (Eds.), *Medicine: A primary care approach* (pp. 55-57). Philadelphia: W. B. Saunders.

Kanis, J., Melton, L., Christiansen, C., Johnston, C., & Khaltaev, N. (1994). The diagnosis of osteoporosis. *Journal of Bone Mineral Research, 8*, 1137-1141.

Kessenich, C. R. (1996). Update on pharmacologic therapies for osteoporosis. *Nurse Practitioner, 21*(8), 19-24.

Kupecz, D. (1996). Alendronate for the treatment of osteoporosis. *Nurse Practitioner, 21*(1), 86-89.

Lindsay, R. (1992). *National Osteoporosis Foundation: Osteoporosis: A guide to diagnosis, prevention, and treatment*. New York: Raven Press.

Lufkin, E., & Zilkoski, M. (1996). Diagnosis and management of osteoporosis. *American Family Physician Monograph, 1*, 3-17.

Moussa, J., Elias, Y., & Libanati, C. (1997). Osteoporosis: Prevention and treatment in the primary care setting. *Primary Care Reports, 3*(1), 1-8.

New drugs for osteoporosis (1996). *The Medical Letter, 38*(965), 1-3.

NIH Consensus Conference (1994). Optimal calcium intake. *Journal of the American Medical Association, 272*(24), 1942-1947.

Notelovitz, M. (1994). Osteoporosis in post-menopausal women: Pathophysiology, prevention, and management. *Clinical Geriatrics, 2*, 1-13.

Riggs, A. (1992). The prevention and treatment of osteoporosis. *The New England Journal of Medicine, 327*, 620-627.

Uphold, C., & Graham, M. (1994). *Clinical guidelines in family practice*. Gainesville, FL: Barmarrae Books.

REVIEW QUESTIONS

Situation: *Mrs. Jones, a 57-year-old obese white woman, has a thoracic vertebral fracture. The DEXA reveals generalized osteopenia. Past medical history: Anorexia nervosa between the ages of 14 and 20 years; smoked cigarettes and drank coffee all her life; gastrectomy for peptic ulcer disease, age 40; hysterectomy, age 40; seizure disorder since age 20. Medications: Phenytoin (Dilantin).*

1. Which of the following is **not** a risk factor for osteoporosis?

    a. Gastrectomy

    b. Smoking

    c. Anorexia nervosa

    d. Obesity

2. Which of the following would be expected on Mrs. Jones' physical examination?

    a. Dorsal kyphosis

    b. Scoliosis

    c. Lordosis

    d. No loss of height

3. Given Mrs. Jones' history, she would be classifed as:

    a. Primary, type I osteoporosis

    b. Primary, type II osteoporosis

    c. Secondary osteoporosis

    d. Both primary and secondary osteoporosis

4. Assume that results from breast, pelvic, and Pap smears are normal. Considering Mrs. Jones' age and condition, which of the following should be done?

    a. Discuss starting estrogen replacement therapy immediately.

    b. Delay estrogen replacement therapy for 1 year.

    c. Do not recommend estrogen replacement therapy.

    d. Prescribe only calcium citrate.

5. Mrs. Jones returns 3 weeks later for evaluation. If therapy is successful, all the following should happen **except:**

    a. Acute pain to subside

    b. Absence of pain

    c. Increased mobility

    d. Dorsal kyphosis

ANSWERS AND RATIONALES

1. *Answer:* d (assessment/history/musculoskeletal/aging adult woman)

Rationale: Obesity is a protective factor for osteoporosis.

2. *Answer:* a (assessment/physical examination/musculoskeletal/aging adult woman)

Rationale: Dorsal kyphosis is a likely finding with vertebral fracture at the thoracic level. One would not expect this pathology to cause scoliosis or lordosis. With vertebral fractures there is usually some loss of height.

3. *Answer:* d (diagnosis/musculoskeletal/aging adult woman)

Rationale: It is likely that both types of osteoporosis exist. Mrs. Jones' age, the absence of estrogen replacement therapy combined with premature surgical hysterectomy predisposes her to osteoporosis, which would be accentuated by smoking and caffeine and alcohol intake. Her history of gastrectomy and phenytoin (Dilantin) use predisposes her to secondary osteoporosis.

4. *Answer:* a (plan/musculoskeletal/aging adult woman)

Rationale: It is never too late to benefit from estrogen replacement therapy, and there is no benefit in delaying treatment.

5. *Answer:* b (evaluation/musculoskeletal/aging adult woman)

Rationale: Acute pain should have subsided. Absence of pain and resolution of the dorsal kyphosis are unrealistic therapeutic goals at 3 weeks after the fracture. The kyphosis may not disappear, and it may take several more weeks for the pain to subside.

SCOLIOSIS

OVERVIEW
Definition

A lateral S- or C-shaped curvature of the thoracic and/or lumbar spine is called *scoliosis*.

Incidence

- Scoliosis is most prevalent during prepubertal growth spurt (10 years to adolescence).
- Scoliosis will progress through the growth spurt.
- A greater number of females than males are affected; in cases with curves greater than 20 degrees, girls outnumber boys 5 to 1.
- Two percent of U. S. children have curves greater than 10 degrees.

Types

- Idiopathic: Curve greater than 10 degrees in a well child during active growing years
- Structural: True deformity of the vertebrae rather than a structural problem
- Functional: Lateral curvature without structural change in vertebrae

Etiology

The cause is unknown. It is familial, with 75% of cases idiopathic.

ASSESSMENT: SUBJECTIVE/HISTORY
Past Medical History

- Spinal column abnormalities
- Neuromuscular disease
- Relatives with scoliosis
- Poor posture
- Asymmetry of shoulder height and/or hip height
- Parent noticing a curve in the spine or asymmetry of the back.

    Scoliosis is usually painless; however, if a child with scoliosis has back pain, the child must have a complete neurologic assessment for neuromuscular or intraspinal disorders. A child with a left thoracic curve has an increased incidence of intraspinal disease (i.e., tumor).

ASSESSMENT: OBJECTIVE/PHYSICAL EXAMINATION

Physical Examination

Scoliosis screening examination may reveal any of the following:

- Asymmetry in shoulder height
- Asymmetry in scapula height or prominence
- Asymmetry of hip height
- Evidence of a rib hump
- Lateral curvature of the spine
- Unequal waist angles

Physical examination should also include the following:

- Assessment of leg length symmetry
- Assessment of skin for hairy patches, nevi, café au lait spots, lipomas, or dimples in sacral area
- Neurologic examination
- Cardiac assessment for Marfan syndrome
- Tanner staging

Diagnostic Procedures

Radiographic studies: Spinal x-ray examination

DIAGNOSIS

The differential diagnosis includes the following:

- Functional scoliosis corrects with forward bending (Adam's position); no permanent disability occurs.
- Consider a systemic problem such as cerebral palsy or multiple sclerosis.

THERAPEUTIC PLAN

Nonpharmacologic Treatment

- Curves 20 to 25 degrees or less require regular observation every 4 to 6 months.
- Curves 25 to 40 degrees require referral for possible Milwaukee brace.
- Curves 40 degrees or more require referral for possible surgical management with Harrington rod.

Client Education

- The child may require psychosocial counseling and support because of use of braces, casting, and surgery.
- The child may have concerns about clothing and participation in sports.

Referral

- Refer when there are indications that the curve is progressing (a change in 5 degrees) or when finding a curve that is 15 degrees or greater in a growing child.
- Refer anyone with any degree of scoliosis accompanied by back pain to an orthopedist or neurosurgeon.

EVALUATION/FOLLOW-UP

- Evaluate psychologic adjustment to treatment.
- Evaluate degree of adherence to prescribed treatment.
- Recheck every 6 months in a growing child.

REFERENCES

Burns, C., Barber, N., Brady, M., & Dunn, A. (1996). *Pediatric primary care: A handbook for nurse practitioners.* Philadelphia: W. B. Saunders.

Dershewitz, R. (1993). Ambulatory pediatric care (2nd ed.). Philadelphia: J. B. Lippincott.

Nelson, W. (1996) *Textbook of pediatrics.* Philadelphia: W. B. Saunders.

REVIEW QUESTIONS

1. A parent of a 7-year-old girl, Mary, is concerned that her daughter does not stand straight. She is worried that Mary may have scoliosis because she herself has it and had to wear a brace when she was younger. Which of the following should be done?

a. Reassure her that it is not familial.
b. Inform her that Mary is too young to worry about scoliosis yet.
c. Proceed with a scoliosis screening test.
d. Encourage Mary to have better posture.

2. Which of the following is true about scoliosis?

a. More males than females are affected.
b. It is most prevalent during the prepubertal growth spurt.
c. A specific cause should be identified and alleviated.
d. The majority of children with scoliosis will have a significant scoliosis deformity.

3. The most common cause of scoliosis is:

   a. Poor posture
   b. Familial
   c. Idiopathic
   d. Carrying heavy books on one shoulder over an extended period of time.

4. A scoliosis screening should include:

   a. Observation of the anterior chest for asymmetry
   b. ROM of spine
   c. Heel-to-toe walking
   d. Symmetry of shoulders, scapula, hips, and back

5. Milwaukee braces are required for those children with spinal curves of:

   a. 10 to 20 degrees
   b. 20 to 25 degrees
   c. 25 to 40 degrees
   d. More than 40 degrees

ANSWERS AND RATIONALES

1. *Answer:* c (assessment/physical examination/ musculoskeletal/child)

   Rationale: Because (1) poor posture can be an indication of scoliosis, (2) Mary is at the prepubertal age when scoliosis tends to reveal itself, and (3) scoliosis can be familial, a full scoliosis screening is warranted. (Burns, Barber, Brady, & Dunn, 1996)

2. *Answer:* b (assessment/history/musculoskeletal/ child)

   Rationale: Scoliosis is most prevalent during the prepubertal growth spurt. (Nelson, 1996; Dershewitz, 1993)

3. *Answer:* c (assessment/diagnosis/musculoskeletal/child)

   Rationale: For 75% of the cases of scoliosis the cause is idiopathic. (Nelson, 1996)

4. *Answer:* d (assessment/physical examination/ musculoskeletal/child)

   Rationale: A scoliosis screening should include checking the symmetry of the shoulders, scapula, hips, and back. (Burns et al., 1996)

5. *Answer:* c (plan/management/nonpharmacologic/child)

   Rationale: For children with spinal curves 25 to 40 degrees, a Milwaukee brace is the typical treatment. (Nelson, 1996)

8

Neurologic System

ALZHEIMER'S DISEASE (DEMENTIA, DELIRIUM)

OVERVIEW
Definition

Nonreversible dementia is an acquired syndrome of progressive decline that erodes intellectual abilities. It causes cognitive and functional deterioration and leads to impairment of social and occupational functioning. Symptoms are often treatable. Alzheimer's disease and vascular disease account for most cases (see also section on diagnosis).

Reversible dementia is a cognitive disorder that can be treated effectively to restore normal or nearly normal intellectual function. Depression, alcohol, and drug toxicity are the most common reversible causes. Normal pressure hydrocephalus, neoplasms, metabolic disorders, trauma, and infection are less common causes.

Delirium is a syndrome of marked global disturbances in cognition that develops over a short period of time (hours to days) and exhibits fluctuations in the degree of cognitive impairment. (Table 8-1 presents the diagnostic criteria related to delirium.)

Many healthy older adults experience *age-associated memory impairment* or changes. It is neither progressive nor disabling and is often associated with the slowing of reflexes, fatigue, grief, depression, stress, vision and/or hearing problems, illness, medication, lack of stimulation, isolation, alcohol, and/or nutritional problems.

Alzheimer's disease (AD) is a progressive deterioration of the brain leading to death. It is marked by changes in behavior and personality and by an irreversible decline in intellectual abilities. Prob-

lems with memory are the hallmark of Alzheimer's disease (Table 8-2).

- Prognosis from diagnosis to death
  —Varies from 1 to 20 years; average 8 to 10 years
  —No predictors for length or severity
- Impact of the disease
  —Most common type of nonreversible dementia
  —2 to 4 million Americans affected
  —Fourth leading cause of death among adults
  —Responsible for over 100,000 deaths per year
  —Costs society almost $100 billion per year

Pathophysiology

- AD is not a normal part of aging.
- AD destroys neurons in the hippocampus; as these cells degenerate, short-term memory falters.
- AD attacks the cerebral cortex, especially cells responsible for language and reasoning.
- Pneumonia is often the cause of death.
- Two abnormal structures found in the brain seem to be related to cell destruction:
  —Amyloid (neuritic) plaques
  —Neurofibrillary tangles
  AMYLOID (NEURITIC) PLAQUES
- It is not known if amyloid plaques cause AD or result from it.
- Amyloid plaques are found in areas of the brain related to memory.

Table 8-1   Diagnostic Criteria for Delirium

A. Disturbance of consciousness (i.e., reduced clarity of awareness of the environment with reduced ability to focus, sustain, or shift awareness).

B. A change in cognition (such as memory deficit, disorientation, language disturbance) or the development of a perceptual disturbance that is not better accounted for by a preexisting, established, or evolving dementia.

C. The disturbance develops over a short period of time (usually hours to days) and tends to fluctuate during the course of the day.

D. There is evidence from the history, physical examination, or laboratory findings that the disturbance is caused by the direct physiologic consequences of a general medical condition.

Modified from American Psychiatric Association (1994). *Diagnostic and statistical manual of mental disorders* (4th ed.). Washington, DC: Author.

Table 8-2   Diagnostic Criteria for Dementia of Alzheimer's Type

A. The development of multiple cognitive deficits manifested by both:
   1. Memory impairment (impaired ability to learn new information or to recall previously learned information)
   2. One (or more) of the following cognitive disturbances
      a. Aphasia (language disturbance)
      b. Apraxia (impaired ability to carry out motor activities despite intact motor function)
      c. Agnosia (failure to recognize or identify objects despite intact sensory function)
      d. Disturbance in executive functioning (i.e., planning, organizing, sequencing, abstracting)

B. The cognitive deficits in Criteria A1 and A2 each cause significant impairment in social or occupational functioning and represent a significant decline from a previous level of functioning.

C. The course is characterized by gradual onset and continuing cognitive decline.

D. The cognitive deficits in Criteria A1 and A2 are not due to any of the following:
   1. Other central nervous system conditions that cause progressive deficits in memory and cognition (e.g., cerebrovascular disease, Parkinson's disease, Huntington's disease, subdural hematoma, normal-pressure hydrocephalus, brain tumor)
   2. Systemic conditions that are known to cause dementia (e.g., hypothyroidism, vitamin B_{12} or folic acid deficiency, niacin deficiency, hypercalcemia, neurosyphilis, HIV infection)
   3. The deficits do not occur exclusively during the course of a delirium
   4. The disturbance is not better accounted for by another Axis I disorder (e.g., Major Depressive Disorder, Schizophrenia)

Data from American Psychiatric Association (1994). *Diagnostic and statistical manual for mental disorders* (4th ed.). Washington, DC: Author.

- Amyloid plaques consist of beta-amyloid mixed with dendritic debris from surrounding cells.
- Beta-amyloid is a protein fragment clipped from a larger protein (amyloid precursor protein) during metabolism.
- Beta-amyloid is believed to initiate or is an early finding in a slow multistep process that ultimately leads to brain cell malfunction.
- Beta-amyloid may be toxic to neurons, disrupt potassium channels, reduce choline levels, and/or cause a combination of these effects.

NEUROFIBRILLARY TANGLES
- In healthy neurons, microtubules are formed like train tracks (long parallel rails with crosspieces) that guide nutrients from the bodies of the cells down the ends of the axons. In AD, these structures collapse.
- Tau (a protein) normally forms the crosspieces of the microtubules. In AD, it twists into paired helical filaments (two threads wound around each other). These paired helical filaments are the major components of neurofibrillary tangles.

RISK FACTORS
- Family history of dementia
- Presence of Down syndrome
- Aging
- Gender

Family History of Dementia
- Genetic factors may be involved in more than half the cases of AD.
- By age 90, about half the first-degree relatives of clients with dementia develop dementia.
- Risk is highest if a sibling had AD and increases with the number of first-degree relatives who have AD.
- Three gene alterations are most common in clients with AD:
  —Everyone has apolipoprotein E (ApoE), which helps transport cholesterol in the blood. The gene for ApoE has three possible alleles: $ApoE_2$, $ApoE_3$, and $ApoE_4$.
  —$ApoE_4$ gene locus on chromosome 19 is linked to the most common form of AD (late-onset). People with $ApoE_4$ have 3 times greater risk for late-onset AD.
  —$ApoE_2$ and $ApoE_3$ seem to carry some protection from AD.
- Four autosomal dominant forms of AD exist:
  —The common form is on chromosome 14.
  —Rare forms are on chromosome 1 and 21.
  —These three forms are associated with early onset and early death.
  —Chromosome 12 has recently been implicated in AD disease.

Down Syndrome
- A gene on chromosome 21 is involved in Down syndrome
- Persons with Down syndrome have an extra version of chromosome 21. By age 40, they develop plaques and tangles like those found in AD.

Aging
- Aging is the most strongly associated risk factor for AD.
- Five to ten percent of the U.S. population age 65 and older are affected by a dementing disorder.
- Incidence of dementing disorder doubles every 5 years after age 65.

Gender. The higher rates among women may be due to greater longevity.

Other Possible Risk Factors (Conflicting or Insufficient Data)
- Severe head injury with loss of consciousness: Reported to double the risk for developing AD later in life

- Low level of education and occupation
  —Persons with either low education or low occupation have twice the risk for developing AD.
  —Persons have 3 times greater risk when low occupation and low education occur together.
  —Higher education and occupation may allow people to cope better with the effects of AD for a longer time.
  —More education may lead to development of a protective reserve of brain cells or synapses.
- Family history of Down syndrome

POSSIBLE PROTECTIVE FACTORS (INSUFFICIENT DATA)
- Postmenopausal women who received estrogen replacement therapy
- Long-term use of antiinflammatory drugs
- Cigarette smoking

ASSESSMENT: SUBJECTIVE/HISTORY

Early detection of AD reduces the likelihood of inappropriate treatment, hazardous situations, and unnecessary stress.

Associated Symptoms

NORMAL AGING
- Minimal normal age-related changes in memory
- Begin in 50s
- Lose some ability to learn large amounts of information and retain them after long delays
- Maintain ability to function with memory cues
- Decline in word retrieval and word list generation after age 70

SYMPTOMS THAT MAY INDICATE DEMENTIA. The 1996 AHCPR Guideline Panel for Early Identification of Alzheimer's Disease and Related Dementia (referred to as 1996 AHCPR Panel in future text) (Costa et al., 1996) noted that the client may have problems with the following:

Learning and Retaining New Information. The client is more repetitive; has trouble remembering recent conversations, events, appointments; frequently misplaces objects.

Handling Complex Tasks. The client has trouble following a complex train of thought or performing tasks that require many steps, such as balancing a checkbook or cooking a meal.

Reasoning Ability. The client is unable to respond with a reasonable plan to problems at work or home, such as knowing what to do if the bathroom is flooded, and shows uncharacteristic disregard for rules of social conduct.

Spatial Ability and Orientation. The client has trouble driving, organizing objects around the house, or finding his or her way around familiar places. Becoming lost in a familiar neighborhood may be one of the first difficulties.

Language. The client has increased difficulty with finding the words to express what he or she wants to say and with following conversations.

Behavior. The client appears more passive and less responsive, is more irritable than usual, is more suspicious than usual, or misinterprets visual or auditory stimuli.

The client may exhibit the following:

- Fail to arrive at the right time for appointments
- Have difficulty discussing current events in an area of interest
- Demonstrate changes in behavior or dress

Agitation, mood disturbances, and psychotic symptoms such as hallucinations may be present.

SYMPTOMS IN LATER STAGES

- Procedural memory declines (e.g., remembering how to cook a favorite meal, brush teeth, comb hair).
- New learning is severely curtailed.
- There is increased impairment of judgment.
- Remote memories are gradually lost.
- Progressive deterioration in the ability to read, write, and pronounce words.
- Progressive problems with driving, following medication directions, cooking, etc.
- Incontinence occurs.
- Psychotic behavior and agitation increase in frequency and severity.

Triggers for Initial Assessment

- Evaluate concerns about cognitive decline or function expressed by the client, family, or others or observations by the health care professional working directly with the client (e.g., reports of impaired ability to function as a result of memory loss).
- Consider initial assessment for persons who live alone, have Down syndrome, or are socially isolated (special risk for harmful consequences of dementia).

Focused History

- Combine information from several sources.
- Include relevant medical, family, psychosocial, and medication history and a detailed description of the chief complaint.
- Obtain history from the client *and* a reliable informant:
  —Memory loss poses a problem.
  —Client with AD may lack insight.
- The informant should be the person familiar with the client (e.g., a family member or close friend). It is preferable to include more than one informant.
- Identify any pertinent signs and symptoms (see discussion of associated symptoms).
- Document a chronology of the problems.
- Include a symptom analysis:
  —Abrupt or gradual onset
  —Stepwise or continuous progression
  —Worsening, fluctuating, or improving duration
- Identify evidence of confusional state or delirium and/or dysphoric mood suggesting depression.

Past Medical History

- Ask about relevant systemic diseases, psychiatric disorders, head trauma, and other neurologic disorders.
- Include history of alcohol, substance abuse, and exposure to environmental toxins; occupation may be relevant.
- Indicate intercurrent, infectious, or metabolic illness, such as pneumonia, urinary tract infection, diabetes, or acute or chronic renal failure.

Medication History

- Drug toxicity is the most common cause of reversible dementia.
- Consider any drug including OTC medications and alcohol.
- Ask specifically about nonprescription drugs.
- Encourage the client to bring *all* pills and medication bottles to the appointment.

Family History

Ask about early-onset AD or other genetic conditions leading to dementia, such as Huntington's disease.

Psychosocial History

- Education, literacy, socioeconomic, ethnic, and cultural background
- Recent life events and social support networks: May affect the risk for dementia and performance on mental status examination

Nurse-Client Relationship

- Preserve a good nurse-client relationship.
- Interview the family and other informants away from the client.
- Examine the client alone and before the informant is interviewed.
- Tell the client that others will be interviewed.
- Be aware of possible questionable motives of family members and friends.

ASSESSMENT: OBJECTIVE/ PHYSICAL EXAMINATION

Physical Examination

- Include a brief neurologic evaluation:
  —Focal neurologic signs suggest a potentially treatable intracranial cause.
  —Primitive reflexes such as rooting, grasp, sucking, and spasticity are seen in late dementia.
- Assess for life-threatening or rapidly progressing causes first (refer to discussion of headache later in this chapter):
  —Mass lesions
  —Vascular lesions
  —Infections
- Pay special attention to those conditions that cause delirium (see Table 8-1).
- Measure blood pressure and pulse with the client in the supine and standing positions.
- Assess vision and hearing.
- Evaluate for any evidence of cardiac failure, poor respiratory function, or problems with mobility or balance.
- Include a complete physical examination at some point.
- Assess for signs of caregiver abuse or neglect.
- Pupillary dilation in response to eyedrops has been demonstrated to be greater (23%) in persons with Alzheimer's disease than in normal subjects (5%), but there has been insufficient research to date to use this as a diagnostic sign.

Functional Assessment

Functional ability is a key indicator of dementia. There are two major types of functional ability:
  1. ADLs: Self-maintenance skills (e.g., dressing, bathing, toileting, grooming, eating, and ambulating)
  2. IADLs: More complex, higher order skills (e.g., managing finances, using a telephone, driving a car, taking medications, planning a meal, shopping, and working in an occupation)

The 1996 AHCPR Panel (Costa et al., 1996) recommended that primary care providers use the Functional Activities Questionnaire to assess functional ability.

Mental Status Assessment

- Conduct a quantitative mental status examination to evaluate mental status and establish a baseline for future reference.
- Include the following cognitive elements in your examination:
  —Immediate memory and short-term recall
  —Abstract thinking and judgment
  —Aphasia (language disturbance)
  —Apraxia (impaired ability to carry out motor activities despite intact motor function [e.g., unable to blow out a match])
  —Agnosia (unable to recognize or identify objects or pictures despite intact sensory function)
  —Executive function (planning, organizing, sequencing, and abstracting)
- Four standardized screening tests are recommended by the AHCPR (Costa et al., 1996):
  —Mini-Mental Status Examination (includes all areas except abstract thinking and judgment)
  —Blessed Information-Memory-Concentration Test
  —Blessed Orientation-Memory-Concentration Test
  —Short Test of Mental Status
- Administer the same test at a future session to evaluate progress.
- Interpret scores in conjunction with other signs and symptoms and with the functional status assessment.
- Screening tests are *not diagnostic* and should *not* be used as stand-alone diagnostic tools.

- Assess visual and auditory defects before testing to eliminate these as a cause of response errors:
  —Correct defects before testing; OR
  —Refer for neuropsychologic evaluation that uses the client's unimpaired faculties and capacities, such as tests that do not depend on the ability to read or hear.
- Educational and cultural influences must be considered in interpretation of the results (e.g., the client's ability to read and comprehend the questions). High levels of education can lead to false-negative results.

Assessment for Delirium

- Delirium is a medical emergency that requires immediate evaluation and treatment (e.g., hypoglycemia)
- Unlike dementia, symptoms are associated with treatable, reversible, and acute conditions.
- Delirium may co-exist with a dementing condition.
- Symptoms (see Table 8-1) include the following:
  —Sudden onset of cognitive impairment
  —Disorientation
  —Disturbances in attention
  —Decline in consciousness
  —Perceptual disturbances (e.g., hallucinations)
- Multiple medical conditions can cause delirium.
- Medications commonly causing delirium include the following:
  —Anticholinergic agents
  —Antipsychotic agents
  —Antidepressants
  —Digoxin
  —H_2-blocking agents
  —Antihypertensive agents
- Quantitative mental status examinations can be used as assessment tools.
- Establish the history of onset and the degree of fluctuations.

Assessment for Depression

- Depression is often mistaken for dementia and may co-exist with dementia.
- Memory difficulty, agitation, disrupted sleep cycle, and personality changes such as apathy may be mistaken for depressive signs of poor concentration, decreased interest, changes in psychomotor activity, sleep disturbances, and fatigue.
- Marked visuospatial or language impairment suggests a dementing process.
- Depressed clients often complain of memory problems, whereas clients with AD often try to conceal memory problems.
- Be aware that the physical condition of older adults may account for some of the symptoms listed in the DSM-IV criteria for depression. The following are examples:
  —Changes in sleep patterns or appetite
  —Fatigue
  —Behavioral slowing or agitation
  —Complaints of diminished ability to think or concentrate
- Depression may be so severe that it produces a true cognitive deficit that is reversible with successful treatment.

Diagnostic Procedures

- There is no one clinical test to establish a diagnosis of AD. A battery of tests must be performed to rule out all other conditions that cause similar symptoms.
- The clinician can only establish a probable or possible diagnosis.
- Brain biopsy is the only definitive way to diagnose AD.
  GUIDELINES FOR PERFORMING LABORATORY TESTS
- Laboratory tests are appropriate when there is suspicion of specific medical conditions.
- The 1996 AHCPR Panel (Costa et al., 1996) did not recommend that laboratory tests be used as a screening procedure solely to identify probable early-stage dementia or as a routine part of an initial assessment for dementia.
- Conduct laboratory tests after the following:
  —It has been established that the client has an impairment consistent with the definitions used in the 1996 AHCPR guidelines (i.e., multiple domains, not lifelong, representing a decline from a previous level);
  —Delirium and depression have been ruled out;
  —Confounding factors such as education level have been considered; AND
  —It is relevant to rule out a medical condition.

- See the 1996 AHCPR guidelines for a list of acceptable guidelines for further evaluation by the American Academy of Neurology, Canadian Consensus Conference on Dementia, National Institutes of Health, and the U.S. Department of Veterans Affairs.
- The 1984 National Institute of Neurological, Communicative Disorders, and Stroke—Alzheimer's Disease and Related Disorders (NINCDS-ADRDA) Work Group under the auspices of Department of Health and Human Services Task Force on Alzheimer's Disease recommended that further clinical evaluation include the following tests:
  —CBC
  —ESR
  —Chemistry panel including glucose, electrolyte, calcium, creatinine, and liver function determination
  —Urinalysis
  —Thyroid-stimulating hormone (TSH) level
  —Vitamin B_{12} level
  —Syphilis serology (RPR, VDRL)
  —HIV if indicated by risk factors
- Other tests that may be indicated by history include the following:
  —ECG
  —Chest roentgenogram
  —Lumbar puncture in selected clients with rapidly progressing symptoms indicating inflammation
  —CT or MRI to exclude mass lesions, assess vascular changes, and determine regional atrophy
  —PET if available to assess regional metabolism
  —EEG to exclude Creutzfeldt-Jakob disease or concomitant epilepsy
  —Serum folate to rule out nutritional deficiency
- Psychiatric evaluation may be indicated especially if there is a significant history of depression or other psychiatric illness.

DIAGNOSIS

The differential diagnosis includes the following:
NONREVERSIBLE DEMENTIA
- Vascular dementia
- AIDS-related dementia
- Diffuse Lewy body disease
- Parkinson's disease
- Pick's disease
- Creutzfeldt-Jakob disease
- Huntington's disease
REVERSIBLE DEMENTIA OR DELIRIUM
- Depression
- Drug and alcohol toxicity
- Normal pressure hydrocephalus
- Metabolic changes
- Hepatic disease
- Hyponatremia
- Calcium disorders
- Vitamin B_{12} deficiency
- Thyroid disease
- Hypoglycemia

Clinical Notes

- Vascular dementias are associated with hypertension and cardiovascular disease. The clinical course is stepwise, and the course is variable.
- Pick's disease is a rare brain condition of unknown cause. Atrophy occurs in a relatively circumscribed area of the brain, usually the frontal and temporal regions. The disease occurs in the age range of 40 to 60 and rarely in old age. Autopsy is the only accurate way to diagnose.
- Creutzfeldt-Jacob disease may be caused by a slow-acting virus. Once expressed, it is progressive and fatal with death usually occurring in 2 years. The disease is found in middle-age women and men. It produces ataxia, muscle spasms, seizures, incontinence, psychotic behavior, and visual symptoms. EEG shows a characteristic pattern.

THERAPEUTIC PLAN
Diagnostic Period

- Give clear, continuous information about the purpose of the various diagnostic procedures ordered.
- Make sure caregivers are aware of restrictions on eating and drinking that may relate to the diagnostic tests.
- Explain medical terminology.
- Continuously assess caregivers' understanding of the diagnosis and expected progression of the disease.

Clinical Decisions

The 1996 AHCPR Panel (Costa et al., 1996) recommended the following:

- If results from both mental and functional status tests are normal and no other concerns have been raised in the clinical assessment, reassure the client and family with a suggestion of reassessment at 6 to 12 months.
- If concerns persist despite normal mental status and functional assessment results, refer for a second opinion or further clinical evaluation.
- Conduct further clinical evaluation if abnormal findings are obtained for both mental status and functional status tests.
- Refer for neuropsychologic, neurologic, or psychiatric evaluation if mixed results or abnormal findings on the functional assessment with normal mental status performance, or vice versa, are obtained.
- Reassure the client and family that referral does not mean loss of contact with the primary care provider.

Client Education

For persons diagnosed with Alzheimer's disease or a related disorder, discuss the following with the client, family, and close friends:

- The progressive nature of the disease
- The client's competence to perform the following:
  —Drive and carry out other routine functions such as cooking that raise issues of safety
  —Maintain adequate nutrition and hygiene
  —Manage finances
  —Supervise or care for grandchildren
- Financial, legal, and medical planning including a durable power of attorney for health care

Provide time for the client and family to absorb the diagnosis before giving community resources. Advise them of community support groups and key organizations such as the following:

- The Alzheimer's Association: (800) 272-3900

In follow-up care, support family members' efforts to provide good care, assist them with problem solving, help them secure appropriate resources, and encourage them to maintain their own personal wellness. Assist family members to maintain support of the caregiver.

During Communication of Diagnosis

- Validate the loss.
- Give the family verbal and tactile permission to grieve.
- Be real; share your feelings of distress and sadness with the family.
- Be willing and available to talk.
- Support and encourage the family to participate in the care of the person with AD.
- Encourage the caregivers to care for their own emotional and physical health.
- Encourage the family to participate in local support groups.
- Teach the family about the progression of the disease.
- Give anticipatory guidance regarding what they may experience during the progression of the disease.
- Encourage a healthy lifestyle.

Dealing With Agitated Behavior

Teach families to do the following:

- Simplify the environment; avoid overstimulation.
- Maintain a consistent routine with the same individuals.
- Avoid too many demands.
- Simplify instructions.
- Avoid questions that require an intact memory.
- Do not argue with the client.

Pharmacologic Treatment

TACRINE HYDROCHLORIDE (COGNEX)

- Centrally active, reversible cholinesterase inhibitor that prevents the degradation of endogenously released acetylcholine
- May be of benefit to some clients in the mild-to-moderate stages of AD; improvement in symptoms in 30%
- Works only when the client has functioning neurons (e.g., early and middle stages)
- Dosage titrated over a period of several weeks beginning with 10 mg qid; maximum 160 mg/day
- Taken with meals to decrease gastrointestinal irritation

The nurse practitioner should do the following:
- Monitor ALT/SGPT every week for the first 16 weeks. Dose is modified according to the manufacturer's directions if elevations >2 times the upper limits of normal occur. There may be abrupt worsening of symptoms on withdrawal of the medication.
- Treat for a minimum of 3 months to assess therapeutic response.

ARICEPT (DONEPEZIL HYDROCHLORIDE)
- May improve cognition and behavioral functioning in clients with mild-to-moderate AD
- Reversible inhibitor of acetylcholinesterase, an enzyme that breaks down the neurotransmitter acetylcholine
- May allow greater concentration of acetylcholine in the brain, thereby improving cholinergic function
- Common side effects leading to discontinuation: Nausea, vomiting, and diarrhea (less than 3% of clients in the clinical trials)
- Initial dose: 5 mg
- Possibly greater benefits from increasing to 10 mg after 4 to 6 weeks
- Once daily administration
- Taken in the evening before retiring, with or without food
- Effect of therapy: Depends on administration at regular intervals

CLIENT EDUCATION ABOUT MEDICATIONS
- Clients and families should be advised that neither medication is a cure for AD.
- There may be an improvement in cognitive symptoms.

EVALUATION/FOLLOW-UP

Long-term goals are as follows:
- The client will maintain the highest possible level of wellness for the longest possible period of time. The client will perform the following:
  —Complete the grieving process
  —Participate in the disposition of financial, legal, and other personal affairs (e.g., wills)
  —Not have excess disability
  —Not have avoidable physical illnesses
  —Receive ongoing, timely physical care
  —Live in a supportive environment

- The client will die with dignity and with physical and emotional comfort.
- The family will provide the highest level of physical and emotional care to the client while maintaining their personal health and well-being. The family will perform the following:
  —Maintain a positive relationship with the client (within the constraints of the situation)
  —Experience satisfaction about their caregiving role
  —Maintain physical and emotional health
  —Successfully complete the grieving process

REFERENCES

Alzheimer's Association (1995). *Advances in Alzheimer Research, 5*, 1A-4A, 1-7.

Alzheimer's Association (1997). *Advances in Alzheimer Research, 7*, 1A-4A.

American Psychiatric Association (1994). *Diagnostic and statistical manual of mental disorders* (4th ed.). Washington, DC: Author.

Buckwalter, K., & Hall, G. (1996). Alzheimer's disease. In A. McBride & J. Austin (Eds.), *Psychiatric mental health nursing: Integrating the behavioral and biological sciences* (pp. 348-392). Philadelphia: W. B. Saunders.

Criggs, N., & Forbes, W. (1997). Assessing neurologic function in older patients. *American Journal of Nursing, 97*, 37-40.

Edwards, A. J. (1992). *Dementia*. New York: Plenum Press.

Farlow, M., Gracon, S., Hershey, L., Lewis, K., Sadowsky, C., & Dolan-Ureno, J. (1992). A controlled trial of tacrine in Alzheimer's disease. *Journal of the American Medical Association, 268*, 2523-2529.

Knapp, M., Knopman, D., Solomon, P., Pendlebury, W., Davis, C., & Gracon, S. (1994). A 30-week randomized controlled trial of high-dose tacrine in patients with Alzheimer's disease. *Journal of the American Medical Association, 271*, 985-991.

Manning, F. C. (1996). Dementia. In R. Rubin, C. Voss, D. Derksen, A. Gateley, & R. Guenzer. (Eds.), *Medicine: A primary care approach* (pp. 376-380). Philadelphia: W. B. Saunders.

McKhann, G., Drachman, M., Folstein, M., Katzman, R., Price, D., & Stadlan, E. (1984). Clinical diagnosis of Alzheimer's disease: Report of the NINCDS-ADRDA Work Group under the auspices of Department of Health and Human Services Task Force on Alzheimer's Disease. *Neurology, 34*, 939-944.

National Institute on Aging, National Institutes of Health. (1995). *Progress report on Alzheimer's disease.* (NIH Publication No. 95-3994). Rockville, MD: Author.

Pfeffer, R., Kurosaki, T., Harrah, C., Chance, J., & Filos, S. (1992). Measurement of functional activities of older adults in the community. *Journal of Gerontology,* 37, 323-329.

Physicians' desk reference. (1997). Montvale, NJ: Medical Economics.

Rabins, P., & Storer, D. (1991). Mental illness in the elderly: Principles and common problems (depression, dementia, delirium, psychosis). In L. R. Barker, J. Burton, & P. Zieve (Eds.), *Principles of ambulatory medicine* (3rd ed., pp. 165-172). Baltimore: Williams & Wilkins.

Rubin, R., Voss, C., Derksen, R., Gateley, A., & Quenzer, R. (1996). *Medicine: A primary care approach.* Philadelphia: W. B. Saunders.

Strub, R., & Black, F. (1993). *The mental status exam in neurology* (3rd ed.). Philadelphia: F. A. Davis.

Uphold, C., & Graham, M. (1994). *Clinical guidelines in family practice.* Gainesville, FL: Barmarrae Books.

U.S. Department of Health and Human Services. (1996). *Early identification of Alzheimer's disease and related dementias* (AHCPR Publication No. 97-0703). Rockville, MD: Author.

U.S. Department of Health and Human Services. (1997). Quick reference guide for clinicians: Early identification of Alzheimer's disease and related dementias. *American Academy of Nurse Practitioners, 9,* 85-87.

Woolliscroft, J. O. (1996). *Handbook of current diagnosis and treatment: A quick guide for the general practitioner.* St. Louis: Mosby.

Yanagihara, T., & Petersen, R. (1991). *Memory disorders: Research and clinical practice.* New York: Marcel Dekker.

REVIEW QUESTIONS

1. The single most important source of information in the diagnosis of dementia is:

    a. Neurologic examination
    b. CT or MRI
    c. Mental status examination
    d. Clinical history

2. Which of the following might indicate that the client is suffering from a multiinfarct dementia rather than AD?

    a. CT shows evidence of old strokes.
    b. Blood glucose is elevated.
    c. Folic acid is depressed.
    d. Alcohol and drug abuse are noted.

3. All the following would support the diagnosis of AD **except** the fact that the client:

    a. Forgets where she put things
    b. Is unable to balance her checkbook
    c. Got lost driving home from the grocery store
    d. Cries almost every day

4. All the following tests are included in the 1984 NINCDS-ADRDA recommended battery of laboratory tests to exclude occult causes of dementia **except:**

    a. CBC
    b. Blood glucose
    c. ESR
    d. Full thyroid profile

5. Results of a client's initial testing demonstrated abnormal mental status, impaired functional ability, and absence of depression. Which of the following is the next step?

    a. Reassure the client and family and have them return in 6 months.
    b. Refer for a second opinion.
    c. Conduct a battery of laboratory and radiologic tests to rule out medical conditions.
    d. Refer for a neuropsychologic evaluation.

6. When administering the Mini-Mental State Examination, what elements in the client's history should be used in interpreting the results of the test?

    a. Family history of AD
    b. Past history of concussion
    c. Estrogen replacement therapy
    d. Teaching occupation

7. Successful therapy with tacrine or donepezil is indicated by:

    a. Cessation of the progressive course of AD
    b. Improvements in memory and functional status for an undetermined period of time
    c. Remission of AD
    d. Functional but no mental improvement

ANSWERS AND RATIONALES

1. Answer: d (assessment/physical examination/neurologic/aging adult)

Rationale: The clinical history demonstrates the symptoms and progression that is characteristic of AD.

2. Answer: a (assessment/plan/neurologic/aging adult)

Rationale: Multiinfarct dementia has a stepwise progression unlike the slow, relentless deterioration of AD. It is associated with a history of hypertension and cardiovascular disease. Lacunae on a CT of the brain support a diagnosis of a dementia related to vascular problems, such as multiinfarct dementia.

3. Answer: d (assessment/history/neurologic/aging adult)

Rationale: Although depression may co-exist with dementia, sadness that leads to daily tears is indicative of a depressed state. The depression must be addressed before the possibility of dementia can be fully addressed.

4. Answer: d (assessment/plan/neurologic/aging adult)

Rationale: A TSH level is recommended as the screening test to include in the test battery for occult causes of dementia.

5. Answer: c (plan/neurologic/aging adult)

Rationale: 1996 AHCPR guidelines recommended that if results from the mental and functional assessment are abnormal, the client is likely to have a dementing illness. The client should be clinically evaluated.

6. Answer: d (assessment/history/neurologic/aging adult)

Rationale: It is important to look for cultural and/or educational biases that might influence results. A high educational level increases the likelihood that a cognitively impaired person will test as unimpaired.

7. Answer: b (evaluation/neurologic/aging adult)

Rationale: Because of more effective utilization of acetylcholine, clients experience improvements in cognition or at least a slowing of the decline. The medications do not alter the progressive course of the disease, and functioning will eventually decline. Clients may function at a higher level for a longer period of time.

BELL'S PALSY

OVERVIEW
Definition

Bell's palsy is an acute idiopathic unilateral paralysis of the facial muscles innervated by the seventh cranial nerve.

Incidence

- Most common of all facial neuropathies; accounts for 60% to 80% of all cases.
- Affects all age groups, with frequency increasing with age.
- Women are more often affected before age 50, with men more affected after 50.
- Encompasses all races.
- Occurs seasonally; is more common in winter.
- Higher risk groups: Pregnancy, diabetes mellitus, hypothyroidism, hypertension, family history of Bell's palsy
- May be an early manifestation of HIV infection.

Pathophysiology

Inflammation of the seventh cranial nerve causes edema, which produces compression and entrapment, resulting in ischemia and degeneration of the nerve. The cause is unknown.

A theory of a viral cause (herpes viruses) most frequently implicated in some studies. Other causal theories include autoimmune processes and inflammatory diseases such as sarcoidosis and Lyme disease.

ASSESSMENT: SUBJECTIVE/HISTORY
Symptoms

- The onset of unilateral facial paralysis is sudden, usually during a period of a few hours, with progression during 1 to 3 days.
- The individual may wake up and notice the problem.
- Associated symptoms include pain in or behind the ear.
- Mild transient tinnitus, slightly decreased hearing on affected side, and low-grade fever are possible at the onset.
- Other reported symptoms are taste disorder, hypersensitivity to sound, and drooling.

Past Medical History

- Current pregnancy
- Diabetes mellitus
- Hypothyroidism
- Hypertension
- Trauma
- Infection
- Risk factors for heart disease or stroke

Family History

Inquire about family members with Bell's palsy.

Psychosocial History

Consider the impact of the facial paralysis on the individual.

ASSESSMENT: OBJECTIVE/ PHYSICAL EXAMINATION
Physical Examination

- General appearance: Note facial asymmetry with loss of voluntary and involuntary movement in both the upper and lower portions of the face. The forehead is smooth, the nasolabial fold is flattened, and the eyelid on the affected side does not close.
- Inspect for Zosteriform lesions behind the ear or in the ear canal; expanding target lesion, erythema chronicum migrans; Lyme disease; and neurofibroma.
- Ear: Look for cholesteatoma (pressure on the facial nerve) and otitis media (invasive infection).
- Nose/jaw: Observe for trauma; palpate jaw for tenderness.
- Neck: Check for lymphadenopathy.

- Lungs: Auscultate for adventitious sounds (sarcoidosis).
- Neurologic: Perform a neurologic examination with assessment of cranial nerves; corneal reflex may be decreased.

Diagnostic Procedures

- No diagnostic procedures are required unless the diagnosis is uncertain.
- In severe cases, an EMG obtained at least 72 hours after the onset of symptoms, and preferably in 7 to 10 days from onset, is indicated if there is no sign of improvement. The EMG helps predict the final prognosis.
- If there is no significant recovery in 6 months, a CT or MRI is indicated to rule out other causes.
- If the onset of symptoms is in summer and the client lives in an endemic area for Lyme disease, consider serology testing.

DIAGNOSIS

The differential diagnosis includes the following:
- Surgery: Past history of middle ear or mastoid surgery
- Neoplasms: Tumors, neurofibroma, cholesteatoma (put pressure on or invade the facial nerve)
- Blunt trauma: Fracture of temporal bone
- Infections of the ear, parotid, mastoid, or facial nerve
- Lyme disease
- Infiltrations from sarcoidosis (can produce facial weakness)
- Guillain-Barré syndrome
- Hemiparesis

THERAPEUTIC PLAN
Pharmacologic Treatment

The following lists treatment options with prednisone (after physician consultation):
- Prednisone 1 mg/kg PO for 5 to 6 days, with tapering dose during a period of 7 to 10 days, best started within 72 hours of onset of symptoms; OR
- Prednisone 60 mg PO for 3 days, then tapering by 10 mg/day; OR
- Prednisone 60 mg PO for 5 days; if improved during this period, taper for 10 more

days. If not improved in the first 5 days, continue 60 mg for another 5 days, then taper for 10 more days.

- For children, prednisone 2 mg/kg for 1 week, then 1 mg/kg for another week.
- A double-blind trial randomized two groups of clients with Bell's palsy. One group took prednisone plus acyclovir 400 mg 5 times a day for 10 days, and the other group took prednisone plus placebo. The prednisone/acyclovir group had better facial recovery than the prednisone/placebo group. (Bauer & Coker, 1996)
- In some cases, Bell's palsy may not be treated aggressively enough, with defective healing in up to 40% of cases. This urges more aggressive treatment with antiinflammatory IV therapy using a combination of three drugs. On the opposite end of the treatment spectrum, some internists and neurologists do not treat with any medication. Surgical decompression of the nerve is sometimes used for recurrent facial palsy. (Stennert & Sittel, 1997)

Physical Therapy

- Electric stimulation can lead to irreversible facial contractures and should be used cautiously if at all.
- Safer alternatives are massage and facial exercises, which may be helpful during the recuperative phase.

Client Education

- Advise the client to use artificial tears twice daily to prevent drying of the cornea; may need to tape eyelid shut at night. Instruct the client to report symptoms of eye pain or visual problems.
- Discuss symptoms that might be expected such as altered taste, hypersensitive hearing, decreased tearing, and saliva production. Defective regeneration of damaged nerves can lead to "crocodile tears" or lacrimation when eating.
- The prognosis is generally considered favorable, but with varying rates of complete recovery ranging from 60% to 90%. Symptoms usually resolve within 3 to 4 weeks.
- Follow up in 3 to 4 days and again in 2 to 4 weeks.

Referral

- Provide an *urgent* referral for any facial palsy associated with an acute otitis media since this indicates an invasive process.
- Neurology referral is indicated for facial palsy where the diagnosis is not clear for Bell's palsy.
- Evaluate and refer for sign of corneal abrasion.

REFERENCES

Bauer, C. A., & Coker, N. J. (1996, June). Update on facial nerve disorders. *Otolaryngologic Clinics of North America, 29*(3), 445-455.

Bonner, J. S., & Bonner, J. J. (1991). *The little black book of neurology* (2nd ed.). St. Louis: Mosby.

Pruitt, A. A. (1995). Management of Bell's palsy. In A. H. Goroll, L. A. May, A. G. Mulley (Eds.), *Primary care medicine* (3rd ed.). Philadelphia: J. B. Lippincott.

Stennert, E., & Sittel, C. (1997). Acute peripheral paralysis. In R. Rakel (Ed.), *Conn's current therapy*. Philadelphia: W. B. Saunders.

Uphold, C. R., & Graham, M. V. (1994). *Clinical guidelines in family practice*. Gainesville, FL: Barmarrae Books.

REVIEW QUESTIONS

1. The incidence of Bell's palsy increases in which season of the year?

- a. Spring
- b. Summer
- c. Fall
- d. Winter

2. Bell's palsy is more common in:

- a. Children
- b. Adolescents
- c. Men older than 50
- d. Women older than 50

3. The facial paralysis of Bell's palsy does **not** cause which one of the following?

- a. Bilateral forehead wrinkles
- b. Incomplete eyelid closure
- c. Drooling
- d. Flattened nasolabial fold

4. If the facial paralysis of Bell's palsy has not improved in 2 weeks, the diagnostic test sometimes used to predict outcome is:

a. CT of the head
b. MRI
c. EMG
d. Lumbar puncture

5. Improvement of the symptoms of Bell's palsy can generally be expected by:

a. 1 week
b. 4 weeks
c. 3 months
d. 6 months

6. The differential diagnosis considered in making the diagnosis of Bell's palsy might include all the following **except:**

a. Lyme disease
b. Trauma
c. Epilepsy
d. Tumor

7. The most frequently prescribed treatment for Bell's palsy is:

a. Corticosteroids
b. Surgical decompression
c. NSAIDs
d. Electric stimulation

ANSWERS AND RATIONALES

1. *Answer:* d (assessment/diagnosis/neurologic/NAS)
Rationale: Bell's palsy is slightly more common in winter. (Pruitt, 1995)

2. *Answer:* c (assessment/diagnosis/neurologic/NAS)
Rationale: Bell's palsy increases in frequency with increasing age, but after the age of 50, men are more often affected. (Pruitt, 1995)

3. *Answer:* a (assessment/physical examination/neurologic/NAS)
Rationale: Bell's palsy affects the upper and lower portions of the face unilaterally, so the forehead is smooth on the affected side. (Pruitt, 1995)

4. *Answer:* c (plan/management/diagnostics/neurologic/NAS)
Rationale: EMG testing of facial muscles after 72 hours can determine the degree of nerve degeneration, which helps predict the outcome. (Pruitt, 1995)

5. *Answer:* b (evaluation/neurologic/NAS)
Rationale: Client education regarding the expected time frame for improvement in the majority is usually 4 weeks, although more severe cases may take 3 to 6 months. (Stennert & Sittel, 1997)

6. *Answer:* b (diagnosis/neurologic/NAS)
Rationale: Lyme disease, trauma, and tumor are considerations in the differential diagnosis of facial palsy. Epilepsy would not cause symptoms of facial nerve paralysis. (Uphold & Graham, 1994)

7. *Answer:* a (plan/management/therapeutics/pharmacologic/neurologic/NAS)
Rationale: Although the treatment of Bell's palsy is controversial, the most common treatment is with prednisone. NSAIDs may be used as adjunctive, but not primary, treatment. Surgical decompression and electric stimulation are not frequently used options. (Pruitt, 1995)

CONFUSION

OVERVIEW
Definition

Confusion is a change in mental status. Two forms of confusion are *delirium* (a reversible alteration) and *dementia* (a progressive mental deterioration). (Refer to discussion of Alzheimer's disease earlier in this chapter for more information.)

Incidence

- Seventy percent of clients with confusion in the form of dementia have AD.
- Ten percent of clients with confusion have a form of vascular dementia.

Pathophysiology

Delirium can be caused by hypoxia, infection, dehydration, acute metabolic disturbance, trauma, CNS pathology, endocrinopathies, myocardial infarction, toxins, and drug withdrawal.

RISK FACTORS. According to Simon, Jewell, & Brokell (1997), the risk factors include age over 80, impaired vision and hearing, dementia, history of previous delirium, multiple medications, and multiple coexistent diseases.

ASSESSMENT: SUBJECTIVE/HISTORY

History of Present Illness

- Mode of onset (abrupt or gradual)
- Progression of symptoms (fluctuating, continuous decline, improving)
- Duration of symptoms
- Perceptual disturbances (hallucinations? If so, what type?)
- Cognitive impairment such as memory loss, concentration, orientation
- Speech changes
- Ability to perform ADLs and IADLs (balance a checkbook, make a telephone call)
- New physiologic symptoms such as incontinence (suggesting urinary tract infection and delirium) or shortness of breath
- New medications

Past Medical History

- Alcohol abuse
- Toxin exposure
- Head injury
- Hypertension

Medication History

- Antiarrhythmics
- Antibiotics
- Anticholinergics
- Antidepressants
- Antiemetics
- Antihypertensives
- Antineoplastics
- Antimania agents
- Cardiotonics
- Steroids, H_2 antagonists
- Immunosuppressives
- Narcotics
- Muscle relaxants

- NSAIDs
- Radiocontrast agents
- Sedatives

Family History

Inquire about dementia in parents, siblings, or children.

Dietary History

Inadequate food and fluid intake may precipitate dehydration and delirium.

ASSESSMENT: OBJECTIVE/ PHYSICAL EXAMINATION

Physical Examination

- General hygiene
- Weight loss
- Complete neurologic examination
- Cardiac and pulmonary examination to rule out pneumonia and dysrhythmia
- Thyroid assessment (hypothyroidism may dull mental state)

Diagnostic Procedures

- Mental status evaluation: Administer a Mini-Mental State Examination; further neurocognitive testing may be beyond the primary care office's capabilities, and appropriate referral should be made.
- Depression inventory: Determine if depression is contributing to the presentation.
- Laboratory tests: Determine if treatable conditions exist (multichem, TSH, CBC, RPR, B_{12}, RBC, folate).
- Genetic testing: Determine presence of AD genetic marker $ApoE_4$ (of limited value at this time).
- CT/MRI: Determine presence of small vessel disease, brain focal abnormalities, evidence of stroke, or hydrocephalus.

DIAGNOSIS

- Major criteria for delirium: Sudden onset, disorientation, disturbance in attention, and perceptual disturbances are common.
- Major criteria for dementia: The defining criterion is the history of a progressive decline in global cognitive function.

THERAPEUTIC PLAN

- Treat the identified cause of delirium (treat infection, modify drug regimen, etc.).
- Consider treatment with donepezil (Aricept) or other acetylesterase uptake inhibitor if client has early dementia of the Alzheimer type.
- Treat depression if applicable.
- Link the family with community resources, such as the Alzheimer Association, for availability of day programs, emotional support, and planning for continued care.
- Determine safety needs of the client such as independent living capabilities and driving.
- Determine the level of caregiver stress and burden. Be alert for suspicion of abuse.

EVALUATION/FOLLOW-UP

Ask the client and family to return to the office on a scheduled, routine basis to monitor changes and provide support and information to caregivers.

REFERENCES

Costa, P. T. Jr., Williams, T. F., Somerfield, M., et al. (1996, November). *Early identification of Alzheimer's disease and related dementias. Clinical practice guideline, Quick reference guide for clinicians, No 19* (AHCPR Publication No. 97-0703). Rockville, MD: U.S. Department of Health and Human Services, Public Health Service, Agency for Health Care Policy and Research.

Geldmacher, D., & Whitehouse, P. J. (1996). Evaluation of dementia. *New England Journal of Medicine, 335*(5), 330-335.

Hebert, L. E., Scherr, P. A., Becket, L. A., et al. (1995). Age specific incidence of Alzheimer's disease in a community population. *Journal of the American Medical Association, 273*, 1354-1359.

Simon, L., Jewell, N., & Brokel, J. (1997). Management of acute delirium in hospitalized elderly: A process improvement process. *Geriatric Nursing, 18*, 150-154.

REVIEW QUESTIONS

1. Which of the following suggests delirium rather than dementia?

- a. Lifelong inability to manage stress
- b. Disorientation beginning on Sunday, with onset of urinary incontinence
- c. Progressive inability to manage finances
- d. Lack of appetite, insomnia

2. Progressive decline in ability to perform ADLs and IADLs:

- a. Are a normal part of the aging process
- b. Are associated with the use of multiple medications
- c. Are signs of a dementing process
- d. Require thorough cardiovascular workup

3. In the physical examination of a client with delirium, the nurse practitioner should focus on:

- a. The neurologic examination
- b. A complete physical examination
- c. The specific client complaint
- d. Discussion with the family regarding nursing home placement

4. During the interview, hints that the client may be demented include all the following **except:**

- a. Vague answers
- b. Looking to the family member for answers
- c. "I don't pay attention to that" answers
- d. Continuing to ask questions of the examiner

5. Laboratory tests commonly ordered for dementia workup include:

- a. Chemistry panel, CBC, aluminum level
- b. CBC, urinalysis, ESR
- c. RPR, alcohol level
- d. TSH, chemistry panel, CBC

ANSWERS AND RATIONALES

1. *Answer:* b (assessment/history/neurologic/NAS)
Rationale: Delirium is abrupt and often associated with other physiologic signs of illness.

2. *Answer:* c (assessment/history/neurologic/NAS)
Rationale: Although people may assume that memory loss and infirmity are an expected part of aging, this is not true. Memory loss, declining function of visual-spatial skills reasoning, and difficulty with expressing oneself are signs of dementia.

3. *Answer:* a (assessment/physical examination/neurologic/NAS)
Rationale: When assessing confusion, a complete examination is warranted because a systemic infection can frequently produce delirium. The neurologic examination deserves greater emphasis.

4. *Answer:* d (assessment/history/neurologic/NAS)

Rationale: All these signs hint at inability to answer questions and lack of memory except *d.*

5. *Answer:* d (assessment/physical examination/neurologic/NAS)

Rationale: The object of any laboratory testing is to eliminate physiologic causes for a decline in global mental status. Serum aluminum and ESR would be of little value. Long-term alcohol use can produce a dementia, but an elevated blood alcohol level at the time of evaluation would not contribute to the diagnosis of dementia.

HEADACHE

OVERVIEW

Definition

Headache is an acute or chronic, diffuse pain in different portions of the head, not confined to any nerve distribution area. It is usually a benign symptom and only occasionally is a manifestation of a serious illness.

Incidence

- Headache is the most common complaint experienced by humans.
- Disabling headaches are experienced annually by at least 40% of the world population and account for a significant proportion of visits to health care providers and about 2.5% of visits to emergency departments.
- Headache affects 30% of children and teens (ages 5 to 17) and 34% of adults (ages 25 to 44).
- Headache is a frequent complaint of older adults; most reports indicate women have headaches more often than men.

Pathophysiology

A headache can be a symptom indicating another disease, rather than representing a disease in itself. Headache can originate from activation of peripheral nociceptors in the presence of a normally functioning nervous system or as a result of injury or activation of the CNS or peripheral nervous system.

Headaches may arise from dysfunction, displacement, or encroachment on pain-sensitive cranial structures. Headaches can occur as the result of (1) distention, traction, or dilation of intracranial or extracranial arteries; (2) traction or displacement of large intracranial veins or their dural envelope; (3) compression, traction, or inflammation of cranial and spinal nerves; (4) spasm, inflammation, and trauma to cranial and cervical muscles; (5) meningeal irritation and raised intracranial pressure; and (6) disturbance of intracerebral serotonergic projections.

Classification

Headaches are broadly classified into the categories of primary (benign or idiopathic) headache disorders and secondary (organic or malignant) headache disorders.

Primary headaches include common tension-type (muscle-contraction) headaches, migraine headaches, and cluster headaches. These types of headaches comprise 99% of headache complaints.

Secondary headaches are due to some underlying pathophysiology, are responsible for less than 1% of headache complaints, and include such precipitants as cerebrovascular lesions, meningeal irritation, intracranial pressure changes, arteritis, infections, and facial (trigeminal neuralgia), cervical (osteoarthritis), systemic, or traumatic causes.

Precipitating Factors of Primary Headaches

Factors that trigger migraine headaches include stress and mental tension, excess and lack of sleep, irregular eating habits, certain foods, alcohol, certain types of drugs, hormonal changes, hypoglycemia, bright lights, exercise, orgasm, and weather changes.

Factors that trigger tension-type headaches include stressful events or emotional upset and depression.

Factors that trigger cluster headaches may be changes in length of daylight. Alcohol and nitroglycerin may trigger an attack once the cluster has started.

ASSESSMENT: SUBJECTIVE/HISTORY

The following is a description, symptoms, and diagnostic criteria of the most common types of primary and secondary headaches:

Primary Headaches

MIGRAINE HEADACHE

Migraine Without Aura (Common Migraine)

- Usually a moderate-to-severe, throbbing, unilateral headache in the temple region or around the eye in persons with a family history of migraine
- Higher incidence in children and younger adults
- Greater occurrence in women than in men
- Equal occurrence in boys and girls
- Typical onset in the second and third decades, between ages 10 and 25
- Peak prevalence around age 40 in women and age 35 in men

Diagnostic Criteria for Migraine Without Aura. The International Headache Society (IHS) (1988) diagnostic criteria are as follows:

1. Headache attack lasts 4 to 72 hours
2. At least five attacks fulfilling two to four of the following:
   a. Unilateral location
   b. Pulsating quality
   c. Moderate or severe intensity (inhibits OR prohibits ADL)
   d. Aggravation by walking stairs or similar routine physical activity
3. During headache, at least one of the following:
   a. Nausea and/or vomiting
   b. Photophobia and phonophobia
4. No evidence of organic disease OR if organic disorder present, migraine attack not temporally related

Migraine With Aura (Classic Migraine). In addition to the symptoms associated with migraine without aura, migraine with aura is characterized by typical neurologic symptoms preceding the headache: visual scotomata (flashing lights), visual field defects (hemianopsia: blindness in one half of the visual field; quadrantanopsia: diminished visual acuity in one fourth of the visual field), fortification scintillations (zigzag lines or waves), vertigo, and rarely aural or olfactory hallucinations.

Usually the symptoms of an aura cease soon after the headache starts and have no lasting impairment.

Diagnostic Criteria for Migraine With Aura. The IHS (1988) diagnostic criteria for migraine with aura are in addition to the criteria for migraine without aura:

1. At least two attacks fulfilling criterion *2*
2. At least three of the following characteristics:
   a. One or more fully reversible aura symptoms indicating focal cerebral, cortical, and/or brain stem dysfunction:
      (1) Homonymous visual disturbance
      (2) Unilateral paresthesias and/or numbness
      (3) Unilateral weakness
      (4) Aphasia or unclassified speech difficulty
   b. At least one aura symptom that develops gradually during a period of more than 4 minutes OR two or more symptoms that occur in succession
   c. No aura symptoms that last more than 60 minutes; if more than one aura symptom present, accepted duration proportionally increased
   d. Headache before, concurrent with, or following aura in less than 60 minutes
3. No evidence of organic disease, OR if organic disorder present, migraine attack not temporally related

Older Adults. Frequency and severity of migraine diminishes as one ages.

TENSION-TYPE HEADACHE

- A tension-type headache can be episodic or chronic.
- It is usually a bilateral, steady aching pain of mild-to-moderate intensity that lasts from minutes to days.
- The pain gradually builds with time.
- Tension-type headache accounts for 20% to 30% of headaches that occur more than once a month.
- There is female-to-male ratio of 1:1 until puberty, and after puberty there is a ratio of 5:4.
- Current thoughts indicate that tension-type headaches and migraine headaches occur together along a continuum with tension-type headache at one end and migraine at the other end.

Diagnostic Criteria for Episodic Tension-Type Headache. The IHS (1988) diagnostic criteria for episodic tension-type headache are as follows:

1. At least 10 previous headache episodes fulfilling criteria *2* through *4*; number of days with headache <180 per year or <15 per month
2. Headache lasting from 30 minutes to 7 days
3. At least two of the following pain characteristics:
   a. Pressing/tightening (nonpulsating) quality
   b. Mild or moderate intensity (may inhibit but does not prohibit activities)
   c. Bilateral location
   d. No aggravation by walking stairs or similar routine physical activity
4. Both of the following:
   a. No nausea or vomiting (anorexia may occur)
   b. Photophobia and phonophobia absent, or one but not the other present
5. May include one of the following:
   a. Increased tenderness of pericranial muscles demonstrated by manual palpation of pressure algometer
   b. Increased EMG level of pericranial muscles at rest during physiologic tests
6. No evidence of organic disease OR organic condition present, tension-type headache, not temporally related

Diagnostic Criteria for Chronic Tension-Type Headache

1. Average headache frequency 15 days per month (180 days per year) for 6 months fulfilling criteria *2* through *4*
2. At least two of the following pain characteristics:
   a. Pressing/tightening quality
   b. Mild or moderate severity (may inhibit but does not prohibit activities)
   c. Bilateral location
   d. No aggravation by walking stairs or similar physical activity
3. Both of the following:
   a. No vomiting
   b. No more than one of the following: Nausea, photophobia, or phonophobia
4. No evidence of organic disease OR if comorbid, no temporal relation

CLUSTER HEADACHE (MIGRAINOUS NEURALGIA)

- Pain begins unilaterally, usually in or around the eye or anywhere on one side of the head.
- The pain quickly progresses to involve the whole side of the head and is described as a severe and boring mixture of jabs and pressure.
- Radiation of the pain to the teeth on one side may occur.
- The eye on the side of the pain tears and turns red, and sometimes the lid droops.
- Attacks of pain are associated with extracranial vasodilation, increased cerebral blood flow, and internal carotid artery changes.
- Each attack lasts anywhere from 10 minutes to 3 hours.
- Individuals may experience one to three attacks per day with many of the attacks occurring at night, especially about 90 minutes after onset of sleep.
- The cluster period lasts on an average of 2 months and appears to be related to seasonal photoperiod changes (length of daylight), which often occur in the spring or fall with remission periods between clusters.
- Cluster headaches account for less than 1% of headaches.
- Cluster headaches can begin at any age and are more prevalent in men with a male to female ratio of 6-8:1

Diagnostic Criteria for Cluster Headache. The IHS (1988) diagnostic criteria for cluster headache are as follows:

1. At least five attacks fulfilling criteria *2* through *4*
2. Severe unilateral orbital, supraorbital, and/or temporal pain lasting 15 to 180 minutes untreated
3. Headache associated with at least one of the following signs, which must be present on the side of the pain
   a. Conjunctival injection
   b. Lacrimation
   c. Nasal congestion
   d. Rhinorrhea
   e. Forehead and facial sweating
   f. Miosis
   g. Ptosis
   h. Eyelid edema
4. Frequency of attacks from one every other day to eight per day
   a. Episodic cluster headache: At least two periods of headache (cluster periods) lasting (untreated) from 7 days to 1 year, separated by remissions of at least 14 days

b. Chronic cluster headaches: Attacks occurring for more than 1 year without remission or with remission lasting less than 14 days

5. No evidence of organic disease OR if organic disease present, cluster headache not temporally related

Secondary Headaches

Many organic causes can produce secondary headaches of varying types, characteristics, and location. (The most common and potentially lethal causes are discussed here.)

CEREBROVASCULAR LESION. Headache depends on location, type, and extent of vascular lesion.

SUBARACHNOID HEMORRHAGE
- Approximately 98% to 100% associated with headache
- Can occur at any age; average age about 51
- Sudden onset; described as the worst headache of life; referred to as the thunderclap headache
- May have a sentinel headache (the sudden, unusual headache)
- Occasional family history of polycystic kidney disease or coarctation of the aorta
- Nuchal rigidity about 75% of the time
- Neurologic abnormalities common but may be absent
- CT can be falsely negative (15%)
- CSF bloody; ECG results abnormal; may have leukocytosis, albuminuria/glycosuria

INTRAPARENCHYMAL HEMORRHAGE
- >50% of cases associated with headache
- Occurs in 3% to 10% of all strokes
- Hypertension in >50%
- Sudden onset of profound ataxia in cerebellar hemorrhage

ISCHEMIA CEREBROVASCULAR DISEASE
- Headache frequency of 17% to 54%
- Headache generally mild to moderate in intensity

CAROTID ARTERY DISSECTION
- Rare, usually occurs in young adult
- Headache present in >80% of cases
- Ipsilateral Horner's syndrome (ptosis, myosis, anhydrosis) a diagnostic clue
- Infarcts in approximately one third of individuals

HYPERTENSION
- Hypertension usually does not cause pain unless diastolic pressure is >120 mm Hg.

- When headache is present, it is generally mild and occurs on waking but improves on rising.

CERVICAL DISEASE
- Most common cause of headache that begins to occur in middle to late life; wide variety of cervical (neck) disease processes involved
- Pain usually occipital, frequently asymmetric, nonthrobbing aching quality and associated with shoulder and lower back pain
- Course chronic and relapsing

DRUG OVERUSE OR WITHDRAWAL
- Drug overuse or withdrawal may contribute to as many as 20% of chronic headache syndromes.
- Medications that may cause withdrawal and rebound headaches include barbiturates, opioids, ergotamine tartrate compounds, benzodiazepines, and caffeine-containing analgesic preparations.

INFECTIOUS DISEASES
- Headache is common and predominant in bacterial meningitis.
- Severe headache is the most frequent symptom in viral meningitis.
- Headache is common and prominent with fever.
- Severe headache is common with acute sinusitis (a dull, nonpulsating aching headache); the location depends on the sinus involved.

INFLAMMATORY DISEASE
Temporal Arteritis
- Usually seen in women (4 times more than in men) older than 50
- Typically a new kind of headache for the individual
- Focal pain unvarying in location, at the temporal artery (tenderness in this area) and behind the eye
- Possible sudden blindness without warning; visual impairment in one third to one half of individuals
- ESR elevated with a mean of 100 mm/hr
- Malaise, fever, weight loss, and jaw claudication early symptoms; symptoms associated with polymyalgia rheumatica

Granulomatous Angiitis. Headache is a common complaint (in two thirds) in this rare small artery vasculitis of small vessels restricted to the CNS.

NEOPLASTIC DISEASE
- Headache associated with a brain tumor is usually deep, aching, nonthrobbing, often generalized, and intermittent.
- Headache is occasionally associated with vomiting and may be worse with exertion (e.g., coughing or straining) by increasing intracranial pressure.
- Posterior fossa tumors frequently produce headaches.
- Acute hydrocephalus produces severe headache.
- Pseudotumor cerebri produces headache in >80% of individuals with this condition. It is usually insidious and generalized, may be mild but can be described as "worst ever" headache, and is often worse in the morning or after exertion.

NEURALGIA

Postherpetic Neuralgia
- Up to 50% of individuals older than 60 develop postherpetic neuralgia following shingles.
- Pain is described as an intense burning pain punctuated by stabbing exacerbations and may persist for months to years.
- Cranial nerve V division 1 is the most frequently involved cranial nerve.

Trigeminal Neuralgia (Tic Douloureux)
- This severe, disabling, lancinating pain in distribution of cranial nerve V (trigeminal) division 1 or 2 lasts a few seconds to minutes interspersed with a minute or so of relief.
- Pain may recur several times per day and become more frequent.
- Exposure to environmental irritants such as wind and cold may precipitate pain.

Other Neuralgias. These include glossopharyngeal neuralgia, occipital neuralgia, and neck-tongue syndrome (C-neuralgia).

OPHTHALMOLOGIC DISORDERS

Eyestrain (Refractory Errors). When pain is present, it is increased with use of the eyes.

Narrow-Angle Glaucoma
- Episodic pain in and around the eye
- A severe, boring ache centered in the eye (though may be diffused on that side of the head)
- Possible nausea and vomiting
- Can cause blindness if not treated

Optic Neuritis. The pain is in or behind the eye and may be exacerbated by pressure over the eye or by ocular movement.

Tolosa-Hunt Syndrome. Single or recurrent attacks of unilateral retroorbital continuous boring pain are followed by ophthalmoplegia.

OTALGIC PAIN. Headache from ear pain may originate from external canal foreign bodies, external otitis, external or middle ear neoplasia, otitis media, acoustic neuroma, and external/middle ear trauma.

SPINAL PUNCTURE
- Headache occurs in 10% to 30% of individuals who receive a spinal puncture. It usually begins 15 minutes to 4 days after the procedure and lasts 4 to 8 days. The female-to-male ratio is 2:1.
- The pain is described as either frontal or occipital or diffuse, which is a pounding or a dull ache. The pain is present when the individual is in the upright position, and the pain is relieved when the individual is lying flat.

TEMPOROMANDIBULAR JOINT DYSFUNCTION
- Localized facial pain, limitation of jaw motion, muscle tenderness, and temporomandibular joint crepitus
- Pain in front of and behind ear of affected side; may radiate over cheek and face; "full" feeling in ear possible

TOXIC AND METABOLIC CAUSES

Toxic Causes (Carbon Monoxide, Hypercapnia, and Acute Mountain Sickness). A gradual intensification of headache is followed by impaired consciousness.

Chinese Restaurant Syndrome. Chinese restaurant syndrome is caused by the ingestion of monosodium glutamate (MSG) by individuals who are sensitive to it. Symptoms include headache, nausea, light-headedness, and numbness and burning of head, chest, and arms.

Chronic Hemodialysis. Individuals receiving long-term dialysis therapy frequently have headaches.

Endocrine Disorders. Headache occasionally occurs in individuals with endocrine disorders such as hormonal disorders associated with the menstrual cycle and use of birth control pills, diabetes, hyperthyroidism, and adrenal and pituitary abnormalities.

TRAUMA

Hematomas. Conscious individuals with epidural or acute hematomas without exception complain of headache. In subacute or chronic subdural hematoma, headache occurs in up to 60% of individuals. The headache is more severe than with that associated with brain tumor. Suspect a hematoma in individuals with headache who are alcoholic, uncontrolled epileptics, older than 60, or receiving dialysis or anticoagulant therapy or in those who have a history of a fall or blow to the head.

Head Injury. An immediate transient headache follows almost all head injuries. Prevalence of chronic posttraumatic headache varies from 33% to 83%.

ASSESSMENT: SUBJECTIVE/HISTORY
History of Present Illness

Since headaches tend to be subjective, a focused history is the most important diagnostic tool in determining the type of headache.

HEADACHE CHARACTERISTICS. Gather the following information:

- Age at onset
- Duration (range)
  —Without treatment
  —With treatment
- Frequency
- Location (unilateral, bilateral)
  —If unilateral, does it alternate sides?
- Quality of pain (pulsating or constant steady ache)
- Does the pain *prohibit* usual daily activities?
- Is the pain aggravated by mild physical activity (e.g., walking around, climbing stairs)?
- Presence of associated features such as nausea, vomiting, photophobia, or phonophobia
- Presence of an aura
  —If yes, describe the aura
  —Duration of the aura
  —Relation to onset of pain

POTENTIAL PRECIPITATING FACTORS

- Dietary factors (e.g., tyramine and nitrite sensitivity)
- Relationship to menses
- Medications (e.g., oral contraceptives, anticoagulants)

- Psychosocial stressors
- Fear of what headache may represent
- Other factors identified by the client

Past Medical History

- Asthma
- Peptic ulcer
- Anxiety
- Raynaud's disease
- Depression
- Insomnia
- Frequent strenuous activity (e.g., jogging, aerobics)

Medication History

- Drugs tried for symptomatic relief of headache (both OTC and prescription medications; include highest dose reached and reason for discontinuation)
- Prophylactic medications
- Current medications used for the treatment of headache (include dose, length of time the drug has been taken, and effectiveness)
  —Symptomatic
  —Prophylactic
- Medications used for reasons other than headache
- Nonpharmacologic therapies tried (e.g., biofeedback, hot or cold compresses, sleep); note effectiveness

Family History

- Headaches
- Polycystic kidney disease
- Coarctation of the aorta

ASSESSMENT: OBJECTIVE/ PHYSICAL EXAMINATION
Physical Examination

Perform a problem-oriented physical examination that includes all body systems with emphasis on the vital signs, head, neck, ear, eyes, and neurologic aspects of the examination. The physical examination results are usually normal.

Components of the physical examination to be performed are the following:

- Height, weight
- Vital signs: Temperature, blood pressure, pulse, respirations

- Skin
- Head
- Ears
- Eyes
- Face
- Nose
- Mouth
- Neck, including lymph nodes
- Thorax and lungs
- Cardiovascular
- Peripheral vascular
- Breast can be deferred
- Abdomen
- Genitalia and rectal can be deferred
- Musculoskeletal
- Neurologic
  —Cranial nerves I through XII
  —Eyegrounds (fundus of the eye)
  —Reflexes
  —Muscle strengths

Diagnostic Procedures

Most individuals with headache have normal or unrelated diagnostic findings.

LABORATORY STUDIES
- CBC to rule out inflammatory and infectious conditions
  —WBC and differential high in meningitis; WBC left shift if bacterial meningitis
  —Viral syndrome: Moderately elevated WBC and lymphocytosis
- When suspect HIV: WBC and CD_4 count
- Thyroid function test to rule out hyperthyroidism
- Lumbar puncture if suspected meningitis or subarachnoid hemorrhage
- ESR if suspected temporal arteritis (>80% usually supports the diagnosis)
- Glucose tolerance test to detect significant metabolic abnormalities causing headaches
- ABGs to rule out hypoxia and/or hypercapnia

RADIOLOGIC STUDIES
- Radiologic tests only indicated if an individual describes an atypical headache pattern, changes in headache pattern, or recent onset of persistent headaches
- Head CT when suspected intracranial lesions or sinusitis not responsive to antibiotics
- MRI is preferred when suspected posterior fossa lesions or craniospinal lesions

OTHER STUDIES
- Temporal artery biopsy indicated in older adults with a tender temporal artery and an elevated ESR
- EEG indicated for headaches with seizures

DIAGNOSIS

The differential diagnosis includes the different primary and secondary types of headaches and illnesses that are characteristically associated with a headache.

Illnesses or factors associated with headache includes infectious mononucleosis, systemic lupus erythematosus, chronic pulmonary failure with hypercapnia, Hashimoto's disease, glucocorticoid withdrawal, oral contraceptives, ovulation-promoting medications, inflammatory bowel disease, many of the HIV-associated illnesses, and acute blood pressure elevation that occurs in pheochromocytoma and in malignant hypertension.

THERAPEUTIC PLAN

When a secondary headache is diagnosed, the goal is treatment of the organic cause of the headache or cure of the illness associated with the headache, with referral for medical or surgical interventions. A discussion of the therapeutic plan for secondary headache is beyond the scope of this text.

The goal of treatment of primary headaches is pain alleviation, prevention, and the limitation of dysfunction. A discussion of the nonpharmacologic and pharmacologic treatment of primary headaches follows.

Nonpharmacologic Treatment

- Adequate nutrition with regular meals and adequate fluid intake
- Avoidance of trigger foods and situations
- Adequate rest
- Regular exercise
- Proper posture
- Topical heat or cold applications
- Stress-reduction techniques: Work and home stresses should be discussed and reduced if possible.
- Individual and family counseling
- Lifestyle: Lifestyle modifications should be implemented before considering medications.

Pharmacologic Treatment

- Pharmacologic treatment consists of abortive (symptomatic) therapy and prophylactic (preventive) therapy:
  - *Abortive therapy* is used to treat symptoms once they occur or to prevent headaches after warning signs (such as an aura) have appeared.
  - *Prophylactic therapy* should be considered for the individual who has at least one headache per week that interferes with ADLs.
- The choice of therapy is guided by the type of headache, prior and concurrent use of typical medication, the client's preference and needs as to route of delivery, concurrent symptoms or problems, cost, and length of treatment.
- Prescribe the least potent and least addictive analgesic medication that relieves most of the pain. Opioids and barbiturates have a tendency for addiction.
- Caffeine or ergotamine contribute to rebound headaches. *Rebound headaches* result from too frequent dosing with analgesics, particularly those that contain caffeine and ergotamine. The client must be weaned from these medications before proper management can be initiated. Refer to a neurologist for evaluation.
- Older adults are more susceptible to the cardiovascular effects of the prophylaxis headache medications. Older adults are also more likely to be receiving other medications; therefore drug interactions must be anticipated. Thus medication therapy should be initiated at low dosages and titrate increases slowly.

ABORTIVE THERAPY

Migraine Headache

Analgesics/NSAIDs

- Aspirin or acetaminophen 325 mg (2 tablets every 4 to 6 hours)
- Naproxen 250 to 500 mg bid
- Ibuprofen 300 to 800 mg tid

Analgesic Combinations

- Aspirin/butalbital/caffeine (Fiorinal) 1 to 2 tablets/caplets every 4 hours (maximum 6/24 hours)
- Acetaminophen/isometheptene/dichloralphenazone (Midrin) 2 caplets, then 1 caplet every hour (maximum 5/12 hours)

Narcotics/Opioids

- Acetaminophen/codeine (various fixed dosages) 1 to 2 tablets every 4 hours

- Butorphanol nasal spray (very addictive) 1 spray unilateral to headache, can repeat once in 3 to 5 hours

Ergot Alkaloids

- Ergotamine/caffeine (Cafergot, Wigraine) tablets: 2 tablets, then every 30 minutes up to a maximum of 6 tablets per attack
- Ergotamine/caffeine rectal suppositories: 1 at onset, then may repeat once in 1 hour
- Dihydroergotamine mesylate (DHE, 45) for severe pain 1 ml IV/IM at onset, then every hour (maximum 2 ml IV or 3 ml IM per attack)

Serotonin Receptor Agonist

- Sumatriptan (Imitrex) 6 mg/0.5 ml SC, may repeat once (maximum 2 injections/24 hours)
- Sumatriptan (Imitrex) tablets: 25 to 100 mg (maximum 300 mg/24 hours, 200 mg if SC injection used initially)

*Antiemetics**

- Prochlorperazine (Compazine) 5 to 25 mg
- Metoclopramide (Reglan) 5 to 10 mg

Tension-Type Headache

Analgesics/NSAIDs

- Same as for migraine headache

Analgesic Combinations

- Aspirin/butalbital/caffeine (Fiorinal): Same as for migraine headache
- Acetaminophen/isometheptene/dichloralphenazone (Midrin) 1 to 2 tablets every 4 hours (maximum 6/24 hours)

Antidepressants

- Amitriptyline (Elavil) 50 to 100 mg qhs
- Buspirone (Buspar) 15 to 80 mg qd
- Sertraline (Zoloft) 50 to 200 mg qd

Muscle Relaxant

- Cyclobenzaprine (Flexeril) 10 to 40 mg qd

Cluster Headache

Oxygen Therapy

- 100% oxygen at 7 L/min via face mask (first line of treatment)

Ergot Alkaloids

- Ergotamine sublingual or medihaler: Inhaled at the onset of attack, then may be repeated 3 times 5 minutes apart if needed
- Ergotamine/caffeine (Cafergot, Wigraine) 2 tablets, then every 30 minutes (maximum 6 tablets per attack)

---

*Enhances effect of analgesics, especially if nausea is present.

—Dihydroergotamine mesylate 1 ml IV/IM at onset, then every hour (should be reserved for emergency department use; maximum 2 ml IV or 3 ml IM per attack)

Serotonin Receptor Agonist

—Sumatriptan: Same as for migraine headache

Lidocaine

—Viscous lidocaine 4% intranasally on side of headache, 1 inhalation every hour

PROPHYLACTIC THERAPY

Migraine Headache

Beta-Adrenergic Blockers*

—Propranolol (Inderal) 40 to 100 mg qd

—Timolol (Blocadren) 10 to 30 mg bid

—Nadolol (Corgard) 20 to 40 mg qd

—Atenolol (Tenormin) 50 mg qd

Calcium Channel Blockers

—Verapamil (Calan) 40 to 120 mg tid

—Nifedipine (Procardia) 10 to 30 mg tid

Antidepressants

—Amitriptyline (Elavil) 50 to 200 mg qd

—Sertraline (Zoloft) 50 to 200 mg qd

—Buspirone (Buspar) 15 to 80 mg qd

—Imipramine (Tofranil) 75-200 mg qd

Serotonin Inhibitors

—Methysergide (Sansert) 2 to 4 mg bid (maximum 8 mg/day)

—Cyproheptadine (Periactin) 4 to 20 mg qd

Tension-Type Headache

Antidepressants

—Amitriptyline (Elavil) 25 to 200 mg qd

—Nortriptyline (Aventyl, Pamelor) 75 to 150 mg qd

Muscle Relaxant

—Cyclobenzaprine (Flexeril) 10 to 40 mg qd

NSAIDs

—Naproxen (Naprosyn) 250 mg bid

—Ibuprofen (Advil, Motrin, etc.) 200 mg bid

Cluster Headache

Calcium Channel Blocker

—Verapamil (Calan, Isoptin) 120 mg tid

Antidepressant

—Lithium carbonate (Lithium) 300 mg tid

Ergot Alkaloid

—Methysergide (Sansert) 4 to 8 mg qd

Corticosteroid

—Prednisone 40 mg qd in divided doses

---

*First line of preventive treatment.

Client Education

- Instruct the client to recognize triggers and early warning signs of headaches.
- Instruct the client to use protective or preventive factors against headache.
- No preventive measures have been clearly indicated for individuals at risk for migraine and tension-type headaches.
- Migraine headaches are made more severe by lying down and are relieved by standing or sitting.
- The use of the following can reduce the incidence of tension-type headache:
  —Use of glare screen on computer terminals
  —Use of proper ergonomics at work stations to reduce neck strain
  —Use of good ventilation systems at worksites with exposure to chemical fumes
  —Use of stress-reducing behaviors
- No protective factors for cluster headaches have been identified.
- Discuss with the client protective factors for secondary types of headaches as appropriate to the individual case (e.g., wearing of seat belts and safety helmets to prevent head injury).
- Client needs to seek clinician input early when therapies do not work.
- Advise the client to keep a headache diary.
- Inform the client of available resources for managing treatment of headaches.
- Ensure the client understands the benefits, proper use, and side effects of medications and other treatments.
- Provide the client with information on headaches, need for stress reduction, and dangers of drug overuse.

Referral

Any of the following presentations should be referred to a neurologist or a physician:

- "First or worst" headache, particularly with acute onset or abnormal neurologic findings
- Headache (particularly in those older than age 50) with subacute onset that progressively worsens over days or weeks
- Headache related with fever, nausea, and vomiting that cannot be explained by a systemic disorder
- Headache associated with focal neurologic findings

- No obvious identifiable headache etiologic factor

EVALUATION/FOLLOW-UP

Clients with chronic headaches should be monitored regularly (monthly) to evaluate the headache diary, effectiveness of medications, and client's compliance in taking medication and for counseling, education, and support in maintaining the treatment plan.

REFERENCES

Coutin, I. B., & Glass, S. F. (1996). Recognizing uncommon headache syndromes. *American Family Physician, 54*(7), 2247-2252.

Dalessio, D. J. (1994). Diagnosing the severe headache. *Neurology, (Suppl. 3),* 21-30.

Dodick, D. (1997). Headache as a symptom of ominous disease. *Postgraduate Medicine, 101*(5), 46-64.

Headache Classification Committee of the International Headache Society (1988). Classification and diagnostic criteria for headache disorders, cranial neuralgia and facial pain. *Cephalagia,* 8 (Suppl 7), 1-96.

Isselbachler, K. J., Braunwald, E., Wilson, J. D., Martin, J. B., Fauci, A. S., & Kasper, D. L. (1994). *Harrison's principles of internal medicine* (13th ed.). New York: McGraw-Hill.

Kumar, K. L., Mathew, N. T., & Silberstein, S. D. (1995). Migraine: Finding the road to relief. *Patient Care, 29*(14), 90-110.

Pruitt, A. (1995). Neurologic problems: Approach to the patient with headache. In A. H. Gorroll, L. A. May, & A. G. Mulley (Eds.), *Primary care medicine* (3rd ed., pp. 821-829). Philadelphia: J. B. Lippincott.

Weiss, J. (1993). Assessment and management of the client with headaches. *Nurse Practitioner, 18*(4), 44-57.

REVIEW QUESTIONS

1. Which of the following symptoms are suggestive of a secondary type of headache?

a. Moderate pulsating pain on the right side of the head for more than 24 hours, nausea, and phonophobia

b. Around four episodes per day of 30 minutes of severe pain on the left side of the head in and around the eye, nasal congestion, and conjunctival infection

c. Pain in the right temporal area and behind the right eye, fever, and jaw claudication

d. Bilateral, nonpulsating, moderate, steady aching pain for more than 48 hours, no aggravation by performance of routine physical activities

2. Mrs. Smith, a 30-year-old housewife has a severe pulsating pain on the left side of the head, which has been present more than 48 hours with nausea and phonophobia; she has some numbness on the left side of the face. Mrs. Smith reports "having this type of headache since she was 18 years old and usually has one headache per month." Mrs. Smith's physical examination results are normal. Which of the following types of primary headache is Mrs. Smith most likely experiencing?

a. Cluster headache

b. Episodic tension-type headache

c. Chronic tension-type headache

d. Migraine headache

3. Which of the following statements regarding the use of pharmaceuticals for alleviating pain in migraine headaches is **not** correct?

a. NSAIDs have been found to be as effective as the ergotamine-caffeine preparations in relieving migraine headaches.

b. The use of metoclopramide (Reglan) and phenothiazines enhances the effectiveness of analgesics in the treatment of migraine headache.

c. Narcotic analgesics should be used with caution in the treatment of migraine headache.

d. Administration of 7 L of oxygen by face mask should be given as early as possible after the onset of a migraine headache.

4. Mrs. Webb, a 40-year-old woman is being treated for chronic tension-type headaches. She should receive follow-up on a regular basis for all the following **except:**

a. Continuity of care

b. Instructions on various triggers of headaches and how to avoid them

c. Instructions on relaxation and stress-reduction techniques

d. Routine CBC and urinalysis

5. Mr. Douglas, a 32-year-old white man is being treated for headaches. He has been requested to keep a diary of his headaches, sleep patterns, diet, anger, and other possible contributing factors for a month and bring the diary with him on his follow-up visit. The purpose of a diary is to:

   a. Provide information for establishing the specific type of headache
   b. Assist the health care provider to get to know the client personally
   c. Provide a form of therapy for the client
   d. Is not necessary

ANSWERS AND RATIONALES

1. *Answer:* c (assessment/history/neurologic/NAS)
   Rationale: Moderate pulsating pain on right side of the head for more than 24 hours, nausea, and phonophobia are more indicative of a moderate migraine headache without an aura, whereas around four episodes per day of 30 minutes of severe pain on the left side of the head in and around the eye, nasal congestion, and conjunctival injection are more likely to occur with a cluster headache. Bilateral, nonpulsating, moderate, steady pain not aggravated by performance of routine physical activities is identified with a tension-type headache. (Coutin & Glass, 1996; Dalessio, 1994; Dodick, 1997)

2. *Answer:* d (diagnosis/neurologic/NAS)
   Rationale: Cluster, episodic tension-type, and chronic tension-type headaches should be considered as the differential diagnosis for the symptoms

presented. Typically with migraine headache, the individual has a unilateral moderate-to-severe pulsating pain that may last from 4 to 72 hours and be accompanied by nausea, and/or vomiting, phonophobia, or photophobia. (Dalessio, 1994)

3. *Answer:* d (plan/neurologic/NAS)
   Rationale: According to Kumar, Mathew, and Silberstein (1995), NSAIDs have been found to be as effective as the ergotamine-caffeine preparations in relieving migraine headaches, the use of metoclopramide (Reglan) and phenothiazines enhances the effects of analgesics, and narcotic analgesics should be used with caution in treatment of migraine headaches because of possible addiction. Administration of oxygen is the first line of treatment for cluster headaches. (Kumar, Mathew, & Silberstein, 1995; Pruitt, 1995).

4. *Answer:* d (evaluation/neurologic/NAS)
   Rationale: Clients with headaches should be followed regularly to assure continuity of care; provide instructions on participator factors, relaxation and stress reduction techniques, effects and side effects of medications; counseling; and support. (Pruitt, 1995)

5. *Answer:* a (evaluation/neurologic/NAS)
   Rationale: A diary of when the headache starts, duration, events occurring before headache, sleep patterns, stress, anger, environmental irritants exposed to, diet, etc., assist in the establishment of the specific type of headache an individual is experiencing. (Weiss, 1993)

MULTIPLE SCLEROSIS

OVERVIEW
Definition

Multiple sclerosis (MS) is a chronic inflammatory demyelinating disease of the CNS associated with periods of disability (relapsing/flares) alternating with periods of recovery (remission), which often results in progressive neurologic disability. MS may affect all parts of the CNS and produces a multiplicity of symptoms.

There are two phases of disease:

- In the exacerbating-remitting phase the client averages one attack per year.

- After several years, most individuals enter the chronic-progressive phase (50% within 10 years; 60% within 15 years).

Incidence

- 250,000 to 350,000 Americans with increasing incidence both nationally and worldwide
- 30/100,000 prevalence in high-risk areas: Northern Europe, United States, Canada, southern Australia, New Zealand
- Low prevalence around equator

- Most common neurologic disease in individuals younger than 40; average age 30; diagnosed as young as 10 years of age; can occur as late as 60 to 70
- Women: 2 to 3 times the rate of men
- Factors associated with adverse outcome:
  —Older age at onset
  —Male
  —Cerebellar involvement
  —Persisting deficits in brain stem
  —Higher frequency of attacks in first 2 years after onset
  —High levels of disability
  —Short first interattack interval

Pathophysiology

- Cause unknown; autoimmune disease
- Theories of four possible causes
  —Genetics: Presence of genes that code for certain histocompatibility leukocyte antigen (HLA) genes
  —Environmental factors: Documented occurrences of clusters and epidemics required to reinforce this hypothesis; however, no identified environmental factor
  —Immunologic factors: Decreased suppressor T lymphocytes; excess immunoglobulin; high levels of IgG secreted; loss of suppressor cell inducers
  —Viruses: Most widely accepted causal agent; exposure in adolescence that triggers autoimmune response penetrating blood-brain barrier and causing structural lesions in the CNS
- Hormonal factors possibly implicated in the disease; cyclic increase in symptoms associated with menstrual periods, during climacteric and/or pregnancy suggesting hormones may be involved

ASSESSMENT: SUBJECTIVE/HISTORY

- No characteristic clinical pattern; symptoms extremely variable
- Requires careful history with focus on the temporal profile of the neurologic deficit, which usually starts unilaterally or focally and eventually becomes bilateral and progressive

Symptoms

- Most common symptoms
  —Fatigue
  —Limb weakness
  —Paresthesia
  —Aching pain
  —Double vision
  —Monocular impairment of vision
  —Slurred speech
  —Urgency
  —Constipation
  —Imbalance
  —Impotence
  —Depression
  —Temperature lability
- Less common symptoms
  —Facial weakness
  —Hearing loss
  —Trigeminal neuralgia
  —Euphoria
  —Confusion
  —Nystagmus
- Uncommon symptoms
  —Severe apraxia or aphasia
  —Extrapyramidal movement disorders
  —Seizures
  —Perineal pains
  —Hypersomnolence

ASSESSMENT: OBJECTIVE/ PHYSICAL EXAMINATION
Physical Examination

- Most common signs
  —Asymmetric weakness
  —Sensory loss
  —Pale optic disks
  —Nystagmus
  —Positive Babinski sign
  —Spastic gait
  —Ataxia
  —Diminished visual acuity
- Less common signs
  —Hyporeflexia
  —Writhing facial muscles
  —Afferent pupillary defect
  —Deafness
  —Muscle atrophy
  —Significant dementia

- Uncommon signs
  —Aphasia
  —Apraxia

Diagnostic Procedures

- MRI: Gold standard; multiple (two to three) white matter lesions clinically definitive
- CSF: Cell count <40 WBCs; protein <100 mg/dl; oligoclonal immunoglobulin bands (+); IgG index >0.70
- Evoked potential (visual, auditory, somatosensory, motor) studies: Identifies subclinical areas of disease

DIAGNOSIS

MS is difficult to diagnose because many symptoms mimic those of other diseases. Diagnosis is generally made by means of observation of the temporal clinical course in conjunction with a neurologic examination and laboratory tests.

The differential diagnosis includes the following:

- Systemic lupus erythematosus
- Benign myalgic encephalomyelitis/chronic fatigue syndrome
- Lyme disease
- CNS lesions/tumors
- AIDS
- Seizure disorder
- Peripheral neuropathy

THERAPEUTIC PLAN

The goal is to (1) treat acute exacerbations, (2) manage chronic symptoms, and (3) delay progression of disease.

Pharmacologic Treatment

- Acute exacerbations: Adrenocorticotropic hormone (ACTH) and methylprednisolone
- Chronic symptoms
  —Spasticity: Baclofen (Lioresal) drug of choice; diazepam (Valium); dantrolene (Dantrium)
  —Fatigue: Amantadine (Symmetrel); tricyclic antidepressants; selective serotonin
  —Bladder dysfunction: Urgency, frequency—oxybutynin (Ditropan); urinary retention—prazosin (Minipress); nocturia—desmopressin (DDAVP)

  —Ataxia: Carbamazepine (Tegretol); isoniazid; less effective—Clonazapam (Klonopin), valproic acid (Depakene), beta-blockers
  —Pain: NSAIDs; amitriptyline
- Reduce rate of relapse, slow progression: Azathioprine, cyclophosphamide (Cytoxan), cyclosporine, methotrexate, interferon beta-1b (Betaseron)
- Treatment currently under study
  —Most promising: Interferon beta-1a (Avonex)—fewer exacerbations
  —Copolymer 1: Desensitizes myelin sheath
  —Plasma exchange: Met with mixed results

Treatment Recommendations

- Mild relapse of remitting: None
- Moderate-severe relapse of remitting: IV high-dose methylprednisolone infusion (500 mg qd for 5 days)
- Recent accelerated deterioration in chronic progressive disease: Same as above
- Sustained deterioration in severe chronic progressive disease refractory to IV methylprednisolone: Oral low-dose methotrexate

Client Education

- Promote health/maintenance: Physical therapy, exercise, group therapy, individual counseling.
- Inform about safety issues in the home related to leg spasticity, decreased visual acuity, and changes in balance.
- Provide information about illness; treatment is palliative and course is unpredictable.
- Provide current research on multiple sclerosis, medications, and side effects.
- Provide family planning services; pregnancy is not contraindicated; exacerbations are found in postpartum period.
- Encourage to avoid excessive fatigue; maintain well-balanced diet.

Referral

- Multifaceted disease often requires care from neurologists, urologists, physical therapists, home health nurse, and psychologists. Management of acute exacerbations, hospitalizations, and chronic symptoms should be coordinated by a neurologist.

- A positive finding on the neurologic examination requires referral to a neurologist.
- Pregnancy requires referral to an obstetrician.
- Bladder dysfunction requires referral to a urologist.
- Spasticity requires referral to a physical therapist.
- The primary care provider is in an ideal position to care for the client by coordinating services, offering emotional support, and managing episodic illness.
- Additional support can be obtained from the Multiple Sclerosis Society.

EVALUATION/FOLLOW-UP

- Annual laboratory tests: CBC, chemistry profile, urinalysis, screening tests, influenza vaccinations along with thorough examination to assess the client's condition
- Episodic illness: Increased risk of sinusitis; pseudoexacerbations resulting from fever and infection
- Interferon beta-1b may cause depression of WBC and elevation of liver function tests (LFTs). Follow monthly for 3 months, then every 3 months.

REFERENCES

Brod, S. A., Lindsey, J. W., & Wolinsky, J. S. (1996). Multiple sclerosis: Clinical presentation, diagnosis and treatment. *American Family Physician, 54*(4), 1309-1311.

Ford, H. L., & Johnson, M. H. (1995). Telling your patient he/she has multiple sclerosis. *Postgraduate Medical Journal, 71*(838), 449-452.

Kaufman, M. D. (1996). Multiple sclerosis. *Saunders manual of medical practice,* 1058-1060.

Pender, M. P. (1996). Recent advances in the understanding, diagnosis and management of multiple sclerosis. *New Zealand Journal of Medicine, 26,* 157-161.

Poser, C. M. (1994). The epidemiology of multiple sclerosis: A general overview. *Annals of Neurology, 36*(S2), S180-S193.

Swain, S. E. (1996). Multiple sclerosis: Primary health care implications. *Nurse Practitioner, 21*(7), 40-54.

Thompson, A. J. (1996). Multiple sclerosis: Symptomatic treatment. *Journal of Neurology, 243,* 559-565.

van Oosten, B. W., Truyen, L., Barkhof, F., & Polman, C. H. (1995). Multiple sclerosis therapy: A practical guide. *Drugs, 49*(2), 200-212.

REVIEW QUESTIONS

1. A poorer prognosis is associated with the development of MS in which of the following age groups?

a. 10 years old
b. 30 years old
c. 40 years old
d. 60 years old

2. Major presenting symptoms occurring in MS include all the following **except:**

a. Bladder and bowel dysfunction
b. Visual dysfunction
c. Dizziness
d. Fatigue

3. Which of the following symptoms is relatively uncommon but highly indicative of multiple sclerosis?

a. Paresthesia
b. Seizures
c. Constipation
d. Slurred speech

4. All the following signs are associated with MS **except:**

a. Ataxia
b. Decreased visual acuity
c. Increased motor strength
d. Spastic gait

5. Which of the following tests is considered the gold standard in the diagnosis of MS?

a. MRI
b. Cerebrospinal fluid cell count
c. Evoked potential
d. Urine assay

6. One of the most common clinical findings in an individual with MS is which of the following?

a. Aphasia
b. Asymmetric weakness of the legs
c. Apraxia
d. Deafness

7. The single most important feature in diagnosing MS is which of the following?

a. IgG bands in cerebrospinal fluid
b. Temporal profile of neurologic deficit
c. Presence of single lesion on MRI
d. Evoked potential abnormalities

8. In making the diagnosis of MS, which of the following conditions is **not** a differential diagnosis to consider?

    a. Systemic lupus erythematosus
    b. AIDS
    c. Peripheral neuropathy
    d. Diabetes

9. Which of the following is an appropriate treatment for a mild relapse of exacerbating-remitting MS?

    a. Monitor only
    b. Prednisone 60 mg qd
    c. IV methylprednisolone 500 mg qd for 5 days
    d. Low-dose methotrexate

10. Symptomatic treatment of MS is important and frequently includes which of the following medications for spasticity?

    a. Baclofen (Lioresal)
    b. Tricyclic antidepressants
    c. Carbamazepine (Tegretol)
    d. Amantadine (Symmetrel)

11. Which of the following should be included in the client education for an individual with MS?

    a. Maintain a high-protein diet
    b. Avoid moderate exercise
    c. Avoid excessive fatigue
    d. Avoid pregnancy

12. The goals of treatment of MS include all the following **except:**

    a. Treatment of acute attack
    b. Prevention of further deterioration
    c. Symptomatic relief
    d. Cure of disease

13. Ms. Row has been prescribed interferon beta-1b (Betaseron). How frequently should she return to the clinic for follow-up CBC and LFTs?

    a. Every month for the duration of therapy
    b. Every month for 3 months, then every 3 months
    c. Every month for 6 months, then every 6 months
    d. Every 12 months

14. Individuals diagnosed with MS are more prone to which of the following infections?

    a. Cellulitis
    b. Infectious diarrhea
    c. Sinusitis
    d. Bronchitis

15. Which of the following should **not** be included in the annual clinic visit of the client with MS?

    a. CBC
    b. Chemistry profile
    c. Influenza vaccination
    d. ECG

ANSWERS AND RATIONALES

1. *Answer:* d (assessment/history/neurologic/NAS)
    Rationale: Late-onset disease is usually more severe and progresses more quickly. (Swain, 1996)

2. *Answer:* c (assessment/history/neurologic/NAS)
    Rationale: Dizziness is a symptom of benign myalgic encephalomyelitis/chronic fatigue syndrome, which is frequently erroneously called MS on the basis of a single lesion visualized on MRI. (Poser, 1994)

3. *Answer:* b (assessment/history/neurologic/NAS)
    Rationale: Seizures are uncommon and highly indicative of MS, whereas the other choices are all very common symptoms of numerous abnormalities. (Thompson, 1996)

4. *Answer:* c (assessment/physical examination/neurologic/NAS)
    Rationale: Decreased motor strength is associated with MS. (Swain, 1996)

5. *Answer:* a (assessment/physical examination/neurologic/NAS)
    Rationale: MRI imaging shows areas of white matter demyelination within the CNS in 95% of clients with clinically definite MS. (van Oosten, Truyen, Barkhoff, & Polman, 1995)

6. *Answer:* b (assessment/physical examination/neurologic/NAS)
    Rationale: Common findings on examination include decreased motor strength in the legs. (Swain, 1996)

7. *Answer:* b (diagnosis/neurologic/NAS)
    Rationale: The single most important feature in diagnosing inflammatory demyelination of the CNS is the temporal profile of the neurologic deficit. (Pender, 1996; Brod, 1996)

8. **Answer:** d (diagnosis/neurologic/NAS)

Rationale: Because of the variability of MS symptoms, recognizing clinical symptoms is challenging. Important illnesses to include in the differential diagnosis include systemic lupus erythematosus, AIDS, and peripheral neuropathy. (Swain, 1996)

9. **Answer:** a (plan/neurologic/NAS)

Rationale: It is currently considered prudent to not treat mild attacks. There is no evidence that oral corticosteroid therapy has any beneficial effect in multiple sclerosis; in fact, it may increase the risk of relapse of optic neuritis. (Pender, 1996)

10. **Answer:** a (plan/neurologic/NAS)

Rationale: Baclofen is the most widely used antispastic agent. (van Oosten et al., 1996)

11. **Answer:** c (plan/neurologic/NAS)

Rationale: Common advice is to avoid excessive fatigue but otherwise to continue normal activities since there may be a temporary aggravation or induction of symptoms with exertion. Clients are encouraged to maintain a well-balanced diet. There is no contraindication to pregnancy. (Ford & Johnson, 1995)

12. **Answer:** d (plan/neurologic/NAS)

Rationale: An effective curative therapy for multiple sclerosis is not yet available. The main goal of treatment is the alleviation of symptoms of the disease. (van Oosten et al., 1995)

13. **Answer:** b (evaluation/neurologic/NAS)

Rationale: Interferon beta-1b may cause a depression of the WBC and elevation of LFT results. Follow monthly for 3 months and then every 3 months. (Kaufman, 1996)

14. **Answer:** c (evaluation/neurologic/NAS)

Rationale: Clients with MS have an increased incidence of sinusitis but do not have an increased risk for other common infections. (Swain, 1996)

15. **Answer:** d (evaluation/neurologic/NAS)

Rationale: All clients with MS require yearly laboratory tests including CBC, chemistry profile, and influenza vaccinations. (Swain, 1996)

PARKINSON'S DISEASE

OVERVIEW
Definition

Parkinson's disease (PD) is a chronic, progressive neurodegenerative disorder of movement and posture.

Incidence

- Unusual before age 50
- Occurs in 1 in 1000 persons
- Equal frequency among men and women

Etiology

- Unknown
- Current theories: Environmental toxins, genetic predisposition, infectious disease

Classification

- Idiopathic: Most common
- Secondary: Drug induced (neuroleptics, metoclopramide)
- Postencephalitic vascular: After a cerebrovascular accident

Pathophysiology

There is a loss of cells in the substantia nigra of the basal ganglia of the brain that produce dopamine. (Dopamine is a neurotransmitter essential for control of voluntary movement.) There is a resultant increase in acetylcholine pathway activity. Dopamine concentration is decreased by 80% before the symptoms of PD appear.

ASSESSMENT: SUBJECTIVE/HISTORY
Onset

- Gradual
- May be present several years before diagnosis is clear

Cardinal Signs

- Resting tremor: Initial complaint in 70% of clients; usually one sided; "pill-rolling" of forefinger on thumb; accentuated by stress and distraction; disappears in sleep

- Bradykinesia: Slow movements; difficulty initiating movement; "masked face," decreased blink rate, decreased arm swing, shuffling gait
- Rigidity: "Cogwheel" resistance to passive movement; best felt in elbow, wrist, neck
- Postural instability: Flexed at neck, hips, knees, elbows, and fingers; difficulty getting out of a chair, difficulty maintaining balance; festination (tendency to go from walking to running)

Associated Symptoms

- Dysphagia: Usually in later stages; esophageal hypomotility; solids more problematic than liquids
- Dysphonia: Decrease in voice volume
- Seborrhea and excessive perspiration
- Autonomic dysfunction: Constipation, bladder dysfunction, impotence
- Sialorrhea: As a result of diminished initiation of swallowing
- Micrographia: Progressively smaller handwriting
- Postural hypotension
- Visual problems: Impaired upward gaze
- Anxiety
- Depression
- Dementia

Past Medical History

Include onset and progression of symptoms.

Family History

Inquire about tremor (in essential tremor).

Psychosocial History

- Exposure to environmental toxins
- Existing support systems
- Safety of home (e.g., rugs, steps)

Dietary History

Ask about appetite, swallowing problems.

ASSESSMENT: OBJECTIVE/ PHYSICAL EXAMINATION
Physical Examination

- Perform a problem-oriented physical examination with focus on posture, gait, nutritional status, and psychologic adjustment.
- Assess cranial nerves: Check for diminished sense of smell, possible reduced blink reflex, EOMs: impaired upward gaze.

- Test motor and extrapyramidal symptoms: Check for tremor at rest in hands and head, rigidity on passive movement, hand and foot posturing, hyperreactive reflexes, and peripheral neuropathies.

Diagnostic Procedures

There are no specific diagnostic tests for PD. The diagnosis is based on clinical findings. Order a CBC, urinalysis, and chemistry profile as the baseline for general medical assessment. For younger clients with PD symptoms, order LFTs and copper and ceruloplasmin levels after physician consultation. CT or MRI of the head may be necessary if the presentation is atypical.

DIAGNOSIS

The differential diagnosis includes the following:
- Progressive supranuclear palsy: Rapid progression, early falling, early dysarthria and dysphagia, neck extension vs flexion
- Wilson's disease: Autosomal recessive condition; copper accumulation throughout the body; young client

Disease Progression

PD is slowly progressive, but the client's life span is rarely shortened. The majority of clients remain independent and functional. Some progress to incapacitation after many years.

THERAPEUTIC PLAN

- Individualize the plan to the client's specific level of disability.
- General rule: Use the least amount of medication in the lowest dose for the longest time to achieve reasonable control of the symptoms.
- As symptoms progress, use a stepwise approach to medication.
- Drugs can help with symptoms, but they do not halt the progression of PD.
- Institute drug therapy when the condition interferes with ADLs.
- It is best to delay the use of levodopa because of the side effects of prolonged therapy.

Pharmacologic Treatment

- Dopaminergic drugs increase dopamine activity. Dopamine cannot cross the blood-brain barrier in its pure form, so it is given as levodopa, usually with carbidopa (Senemet)

- Anticholinergic drugs (amantadine [Symmetrel]) decrease acetylcholine activity.
- Dopamine agonists (bromocriptine, pergolide, lysuride, apomorphine) increase the level of dopamine.
- Selegiline inhibits the enzyme that breaks down dopamine.

Nonpharmacologic Treatment

PHYSICAL THERAPY. Exercise is important for the client with PD to maintain strength and overall muscle tone so that the client is less disabled by movement problems.

SPEECH THERAPY. Training in control of voice and communication is necessary for the client with PD.

Client Education

- Safety of the client, understanding of the disease process and treatment
- Support groups and literature available for the client with PD and the family
- Dietary teaching regarding use of low-protein diet, since levodopa competes with dietary amino acids for transport across the intestine and blood-brain barrier

EVALUATION/FOLLOW-UP

- There are many treatment problems because of the disease progression and medication side effects.
- Levodopa causes nausea, postural hypotension, and dyskinesia
- Wearing off: Effect of the drug wears off before next dose.
- On-off phenomenon: When the disease is established, the drug response is variable and fluctuates throughout the day. Controlled-release Senemet may reduce response fluctuations.

Research

- Pallidotomy
- Fetal tissue transplantation

REFERENCES

Barker, L. R., Burton, J. R., & Zieve, P. (1995). *Principles of ambulatory medicine* (4th ed., pp. 1220-1228). Baltimore: Williams & Wilkins.

Calne, D. B. (1995). Diagnosis and treatment of Parkinson's disease. *Hospital Practice*, pp. 83-89.

Calne, S. (1994). Examining causes and care of idiopathic parkinsonism. *Nursing Times, 90*(16), 38-40.

Isselbacher, K., Braunwald, E., Wilson, J., Martin, J., Fauci, A., & Kasper, D. (1994). *Harrison's principles of internal medicine* (13th ed., pp. 2275-2278). New York: McGraw-Hill.

Professional Development (1996a). Parkinson's disease. Part I. *Nursing Times, 92*(1), 1-4.

Professional Development (1996b). Parkinson's disease. The role of the nurse. *Nursing Times, 92*(2), 5-8.

Sweeney, P. J. (1995). Parkinson's disease: Managing symptoms and preserving function. *Geriatrics, 50*(9), 24-26, 28-31.

Weekly, N. J. (1995). Parkinsonism, an overview. *Geriatric Nursing, 16*(4), 169-171.

REVIEW QUESTIONS

1. Pharmacotherapy to treat PD is directed toward replacing which substance in the brain?

   a. Serotonin
   b. Epinephrine
   c. Dopamine
   d. Acetylcholine

2. Dyskinesia is a side effect of which drug treatment for PD?

   a. Cogentin
   b. Selegiline
   c. Levodopa
   d. Amantadine

3. Diagnosis of PD is based on:

   a. CT of the head
   b. Clinical findings
   c. Blood levels of dopamine
   d. EEG

4. Two of the most common side effects of drug therapy for PD are:

   a. Hypertension and peripheral edema
   b. Headache and tinnitus
   c. Postural hypotension and nausea
   d. Diplopia and hypertension

5. When a client with PD is receiving regular carbidopa and levodopa, which diet allows optimal absorption of the drug?

    a. High-carbohydrate diet
    b. Low-protein diet
    c. High-protein diet
    d. Low-fat diet

6. Mrs. Miller is a 60-year-old woman who has a hand tremor. What finding would cause you to suspect that this may **not** be a symptom of PD?

    a. Tremor at rest
    b. Her age
    c. Family history of tremors
    d. Unilateral tremor

7. "On-off" reactions are:

    a. Indications that medicine doses must be increased.
    b. Signs of improved mobility
    c. Unpredictable phenomenon with client response to levadopa and carbidopa
    d. Indications that medications must be dosed more frequently

8. Which of the following concerning the controlled release of levodopa and carbidopa is **not** true?

    a. Decreases nausea
    b. Prevents "wearing off" reactions
    c. May reduce dyskinesia problems
    d. Can halt progression of PD

9. It is best to initiate levodopa/carbidopa therapy:

    a. When symptoms interfere with ADLs
    b. When the diagnosis of PD is confirmed
    c. At the onset of bradykinesia
    d. When the tremor is noticeable

Answers and Rationales

1. *Answer:* c (plan/neurologic/NAS)
Rationale: The most powerful drugs currently available for treatment of PD are those that mimic the actions of dopamine, compensating for the client's loss of dopaminergic neurons in the substantia nigra of the brain. (Calne, 1995)

2. *Answer:* c (evaluation/neurologic/NAS)
Rationale: About half of all clients with PD will experience dyskinesias within 5 years of starting treatment with levodopa. (Professional Development, 1996a)

3. *Answer:* b (diagnosis/neurologic/NAS)
Rationale: There are no specific diagnostic tests for PD. Exclusionary tests may be needed to rule out other causes of PD. (Weekly, 1995)

4. *Answer:* c (evaluation/neurologic/NAS)
Rationale: Postural hypotension is both a side effect of levodopa/carbidopa therapy and the disease itself. Levodopa frequently causes nausea. (Calne, 1995)

5. *Answer:* b (plan/neurologic/NAS)
Rationale: Levodopa and carbidopa compete with dietary amino acids for transport across the intestine and blood-brain barrier. (Barker, Burton, & Zieve, 1995)

6. *Answer:* c (assessment/history/neurologic/aging adult)
Rationale: At least 50% of clients with essential tremor have a positive family history of essential tremor. The other choices are factors in PD. (Barker, Burton, & Zieve, 1995)

7. *Answer:* c (evaluation/neurologic/NAS)
Rationale: On-off reactions are due to fluctuations in the client's response to levodopa and carbidopa that develop with continued treatment. On-off reactions are difficult to treat. (Barker, Burton, & Zieve, 1995)

8. *Answer:* d (plan/neurologic/NAS)
Rationale: No therapeutic measures are available to halt the disease process, which consists of neuronal degeneration. (Isselbacher et al., 1994)

9. *Answer:* a (plan/neurologic/NAS)
Rationale: Because of the side effects of prolonged use of levodopa/carbidopa therapy, it is best to delay its use until the disease begins to compromise the client's lifestyle or employment. (Sweeney, 1995)

SEIZURE DISORDERS

OVERVIEW
Definition

Seizure is a paroxysmal, abnormal discharge of neurons of the cerebral cortex that alters neurologic function. *Epilepsy* is a heterogeneous condition characterized by recurrent, unprovoked seizures.

Incidence

- About 2 million people in the United States may have epilepsy. An even larger number seek medical advice for a possible seizure disorder, generating about 5% of visits to physicians and 20% of visits to neurologists.
- Seizures in children are not uncommon, and their incidence in children is much higher than in adults. Four to six percent of all children have seizures, including febrile seizures. The febrile seizure group alone may make up between 2.5% and 4% of that total.
- Epilepsy is especially likely to affect older adults. Common causes of epilepsy in older adults are cerebrovascular disease, neoplasms, metabolic derangements, and head trauma.

Pathophysiology

The final common pathway of many epileptic seizures is a sudden electric depolarization of cortical neurons that is usually seen on the surface EEG as a negative spike. This is frequently followed by a sustained inhibitory hyperpolarization usually seen as a slow wave on the surface EEG.

Etiology

- Neonatal seizures are often related to birth trauma or congenital malformation.
- Seizures in infancy to early childhood (younger than 6 years) are likely due to metabolic disorders, CNS infections, and febrile seizures.
- In children (6 to 10 years) seizures are most often caused by CNS infection, idiopathic epilepsy, and CNS degeneration.
- In childhood to adolescence (10 to 18 years) idiopathic epilepsy, trauma, and alcohol and drug abuse are likely causes.
- Seizures in older adults are often related to trauma, neoplasm, or stroke.

Classification

One of the major developments in epileptology of the last few decades has been the adoption of the International Classification of Epileptic Seizures (ICES). Much of the basis for this classification, as illustrated in the accompanying box, is the recognition that the brain is highly organized, with specific functions represented in discrete anatomic regions.

ASSESSMENT: SUBJECTIVE/HISTORY
Clinical Presentation

PARTIAL SEIZURES (FOCAL SEIZURES)
Simple Partial Seizures
- Simple partial seizures (auras) usually last 20 to 180 seconds and are not associated with impairment of consciousness.
- There are usually no postictal symptoms, but lethargy may occur.

Complex Partial Seizures
- Complex partial seizures are associated with impairment of consciousness but no loss of consciousness.
- Clients typically stare but do not respond to questions or commands.
- The usual duration is 30 to 180 seconds.
- Auras are common.
- Postictal symptoms are common but usually brief (<20 minutes).
- Lethargy and confusion follow the seizure.

Partial Seizures Evolving to Secondarily Generalized Seizures
- Clients may not recall an aura.
- Witnesses may report that the client described an aura or may observe focal movements or automatisms before the convulsion.

GENERALIZED SEIZURES
Absence Seizures (Petit Mal)
- Onset usually 4 to 11 years
- Paroxysmal onset and offset
- Usually brief (<15 seconds) impairment of consciousness
- Precipitated by hyperventilation
- No aura, postictal confusion, or lethargy
- May be frequent (>100/day)

EPILEPTIC SEIZURES: CLASSIFICATION AND CHARACTERISTICS*

Partial Seizures (Focal Seizures)
Simple partial seizures
  With motor signs
  With somatosensory or special sensory
    symptoms
  With autonomic symptoms
  With psychic symptoms
Complex partial seizures
  Simple partial onset followed by impairment of
    consciousness
  With impairment of consciousness at the onset
Partial seizures evolving to secondarily generalized
  seizures
  Simple partial seizures evolving to generalized
    seizures
  Complex partial seizures evolving to generalized
    seizures
  Simple partial seizures evolving to complex par-
    tial seizures evolving to generalized seizures

**Generalized Seizures (Convulsive or
Nonconvulsive)**
Absence seizures
  Typical absence seizures (petit mal)
  Atypical
Myoclonic seizures
Clonic seizures
Tonic seizures
Tonic-clonic seizures (grand mal)
Atonic seizures

Unclassified Epileptic Seizures
All seizures that cannot be classified because of incomplete data or because they defy classification
  into the above categories (for example, neonatal
  seizures with swimming movements).

Status Epilepticus

Data from Leppik, I. E. (1996). *Contemporary diagnosis and management of the patient with epilepsy* (2nd ed.). Newtown, PA: Handbooks in Health Care.
*Proposed by the International Classification of Epileptic Seizures.

Myoclonic Seizures
- Brief, shock-like jerk of muscles or group of
  muscles
- Two types
  —Nonepileptic: Often unilateral
  —Epileptic myoclonus: Usually bilateral,
    symmetric movements

Clonic Seizures
- Bilateral jerking lasts 30 to 180 seconds
- Rate of jerking then slows
- Large jerk with flaccidity follows

Tonic Seizures
- Brief episode with sudden increase in tone
  in trunk or extremities
- Usually <20 seconds

Tonic-Clonic Seizures (Grand Mal)
- May be partial (beginning focally) or primary generalized (bilateral symmetric onset)
- Initial brief tonic phase lasting 2 to 10 seconds with loss of consciousness, extensor
  rigidity, fall, often a cry; superior deviation
  of eyes and pupil dilation
- Secondary clonic phase with bilateral jerking lasting 30 to 180 seconds; rate of jerk-

ing usually slows; often a large jerk followed
  by flaccidity and coma
- May be hypersalivation, tongue biting, and
  urinary incontinence
- Postictal period lasting minutes to hours
  with lethargy, confusion, decreased attention, depression

Atonic Seizures
- Brief episode with sudden decrease in tone
  in trunk or extremities
- Onset usually in childhood
- Duration <15 seconds
- Sudden loss of postural tone from head nod
  to fall with major trauma
- May be accompanied by tonic seizures
- Injury common and these clients often re-
  quire helmets
- Primarily seen in Lennox-Gastaut syndrome

UNCLASSIFIED EPILEPTIC SEIZURES
Lennox-Gastaut Syndrome
- Begins at 1 to 7 years
- Often co-exists with atonic seizures
- Falls common

- Symmetric jerking of proximal arms with twitching of facial muscles (mouth and eyes)

West's Syndrome (Infantile Spasms)
- Begins at 2 months to 1 year
- Sudden flexion of extremities, head, and trunk for limited time
- Untreated, infantile spasms that subside within 1 to 4 years but often are replaced by other forms of seizures; prognosis poor

Febrile Seizures
- Usually occur between 6 months and 5 years and most commonly occur before 13 months
- Brief, generalized, short, and nonfocal
- Client febrile before seizure; no evidence of CNS infection
- Prognosis excellent since fewer than 3% of children with simple febrile seizures will have nonfebrile seizures subsequently

STATUS EPILEPTICUS
- Status epilepticus is a seizure that continues longer than 30 minutes or repeated seizures associated with impaired awareness for more than 30 minutes.
- Those seizures are medical emergencies that can cause brain damage and death.
- Thus, any tonic-clonic seizure lasting longer than 5 to 10 minutes should be treated.

History of Present Illness

- Determine what type of seizure occurred by interviewing the client, family members, and witnesses.
- Obtain a good description of the seizure.
- Determine whether it was focal (involving only the face or one extremity or one side of the body); immediately generalized (involving all extremities); or initially focal and then generalized to involve the extremities.
- Determine how long it occurred.
- Determine whether the client lost consciousness.
- When the client aroused, determine if there was any evidence of an aura.
- Did the client lose control of bowel or bladder?
- Was there a period of postictal lethargy? How long did it occur?
- Was there any associated illness or fever or any sleep deprivation?

- Determine the relationship of seizure to the time of day, meals, fatigue, emotional stress, excitement, menses, discontinuing medication; obtain information about activity before attack and frequency of occurrence.
- Inquire about history of trauma, drug withdrawal (particularly alcohol, barbiturates, or benzodiazepines), and any exposure to toxins.

Past Medical History

- Family history of seizures
- Cardiac arrhythmias, valve disease, stroke, and malignancies
- Diabetes or renal disease
- Birth history and attainment of development in children
- Previous seizures
  —Precipitating factors
  —Similarity with most recent seizure
  —Medication compliance
  —Increased frequency of seizures

Medication History

Ask about current medications.

Family History

Inquire about seizures or neurologic disorders.

Psychosocial History

- Any recent travel
- Occupation
- Alcohol consumption with amount
- Drug abuse with type and amount of drug or drugs
- Type and age of dwelling

Dietary History

Determine the type of foods eaten in the recent past.

ASSESSMENT: OBJECTIVE/ PHYSICAL EXAMINATION
Physical Examination

- Observe for an injury pattern.
- Determine vital signs.
- Do a complete neurologic examination.
- Do a complete cardiovascular examination.
- Observe the skin for any abnormalities (often associated with congenital seizures):

—Café au lait spots: Neurofibromatosis
—Adenoma sebaceum (reddish nodules over the nose, cheeks, and occasionally the chin) or a shagreen patch over the dorsum of the trunk: Tuberous sclerosis
—Hemangioma involving one side of the face or involving one side of the body: Sturge-Weber syndrome

Diagnostic Procedures

- Serum electrolytes, glucose, BUN, creatinine, and urinalysis
- CBC with differential
- Optional lead level if ingestion suspected
- Optional toxicology screen if drug abuse suspected, screening for marijuana, amphetamines, cocaine, barbiturates, and valium
- EEG (although results possibly normal if the client not presently having a seizure)
- Optional CT or MRI
  —Intractable seizures
  —Focal neurologic abnormalities
  —First seizure in an adult
  —Rule out mass

DIAGNOSIS

The differential diagnosis includes the following:
- Syncope
  —Vasovagal attack: Hyperventilation-induced syncope
  —Cardiac disorder: Atrioventricular block, Adams-Stokes attack, sinoatrial block, paroxysmal tachycardia, reflex cardiac arrhythmia, other cardiac causes of decreased cardiac output
  —Hypovolemia
  —Hypotension
  —Cerebrovascular ischemia
  —Micturition syncope
- Nonepileptic seizures of psychogenic origin (pseudoseizures)
- Breath-holding spells
- Paroxysmal REM sleep behavior
- Panic attack

THERAPEUTIC PLAN
Immediate Management

- Maintain clear airway by turning the client on his or her side with the head down; remove vomitus or dentures.

- Do not try to pry tight jaws open to place an object between the teeth.
- Protect the client from injuries.
- Administer oxygen if cyanotic.
- Status epilepticus (seizure longer than 10 minutes duration) necessitates emergency department transport and immediate consultation with physician.

Principles of Treatment

- Consult with a physician for all first-time seizures.
- The decision to treat a first-time seizure is difficult and should be based on the interpretation of the subtle clinical, historical, and/or laboratory findings.
- The final decision about treatment must be made individually for each client and should take into account the potential psychologic, vocational, and physical consequences of further seizures.
- Leppik (1996) outlines steps to follow when considering treatment of the first seizure. A provoked seizure is one in which the factors that precipitated the episode can be identified and remedied, such as physical injury and drug overdose.
- In febrile seizures the initial treatment is lowering the temperature with acetaminophen, ibuprofen, or cool baths. (Generally, febrile seizures do not require anticonvulsant therapy; however, frequent recurrent febrile seizures may require prophylactic treatment with oral phenobarbital.)

Pharmacologic Treatment

Use of the correct antiepileptic drug (AED) for the type of seizure:
- Simple and complex, partial: Carbamazepine, phenytoin, phenobarbital
- Absence: Ethosuximide, valproic acid
- Tonic-clonic: Phenytoin, valproic acid, carbamazepine
- Myoclonic and atonic: Clonazepam
- Special considerations: Felbamate for treatment of Lennox-Gastaut syndrome; gabapentin for use as add-on therapy in refractory simple and complex partial seizures; lamotrigine for treatment of partial seizures and possibly also tonic-clonic, absence, and atonic seizures; vigabatrin for childhood forms of epilepsy

Special Considerations

REPRODUCTIVE HEALTH AND PREGNANCY

- Fertility rates may be lower in women with localization-related epilepsy.
- Family planning may be affected by the high failure rate of oral contraceptives and AEDs.
- Changes in hormones during the menstrual cycle may influence the frequency of seizures.
- Pregnant women with epilepsy may have more frequent seizures, pregnancy complications, and adverse fetal outcomes.
- The probability of teratogenesis in fetuses of epileptic women treated with AEDs is higher than the probability of teratogenesis in fetuses of untreated epileptic women.

OLDER ADULT POPULATION

- Common causes of epilepsy in older adults are cerebrovascular disease, neoplasms, metabolic derangements, and head trauma.
- A slower metabolic rate often requires a decrease in dosage of AEDs.
- The possibility of drug interactions is increased mainly because many older adults take numerous medications.
- The cost of AEDs may be of great concern to older adults living with a fixed income.
- Failing memory can make compliance difficult, especially when the drug requires multiple daily doses.

Client Education

- Ensure the client, parent, or caregiver understands the goals and time frame of treatment. Provide information and support about seizures.
- Teach families what to do in the emergency management of seizures. To avoid unnecessary medical intervention and to ensure that observers respond appropriately to seizures, the client may want to wear an identification bracelet that notes the condition and phone number of the contact person.
- Counseling in children is especially important, emphasizing the significance of seizures, that they can live a normal life within some limits, and that they must learn to cope with some of the attitudes of the public regarding seizures.
- Areas of psychosocial difficulty should be identified early in the course of treatment so that disabilities related to epilepsy can be mini-

mized by making use of the necessary social, educational, vocational, and psychologic support services.
- Review the applicable state law concerning driving a motor vehicle.
- If the client has good control of seizures, only minimum restrictions such as swimming with a buddy or wearing a helmet with some sports are required.
- Stress the importance of drug compliance and instruct the client about the actions and side effects of medications.
  —AEDs reduce effectiveness of oral contraceptives.
  —AEDs are teratogenic.
  —AEDs and other drugs may display numerous interactions.
- Instruct the client to avoid the following factors since they tend to precipitate seizures in some clients:
  —Sleep deprivation
  —Fever
  —Strobe lights
  —Psychologic stress
  —Excessive alcohol
- A client who is not well-controlled should not have a pertussis vaccine because of increased risk of seizures

Referral

- Consult with a specialist for treatment of clients with West's syndrome and Lennox-Gastaut syndrome.
- Consult with a physician on all first-time seizures.
- The nurse practitioner may actively participate in the AED selection process in choosing the AED, monitoring its administration, and assessing the client's response, including side effects.
- Consult with a physician with clients that have complicating factors such as persistent seizures, change in seizure pattern, and serious infection.
- Consult with a physician regarding clients that may require hospitalization such as children with a complex febrile seizure.
- Consultation with a neurologist is recommended before pregnancy in those women contemplating pregnancy to ascertain that AED is indicated and to consider alteration of

the current regimen to one that would have a lower risk to the fetus.

EVALUATION/FOLLOW-UP

• Follow-up is indicated according to the chosen AED for blood work related to hematopoietic and liver function and serum drug concentrations.

• Always ascertain any untoward side effects that the client may be experiencing.

• Reinforce education as described previously.

REFERENCES

Devinsky, O., & Sloviter, R. (1993). *Perspective on epilepsy: Clinical and structural perspectives* [Film]. Spectral Resources, Inc.

Henneman, P. L., DeRoos, F., & Lewis, R. J. (1994). Determining the need for admission in patients with new-onset seizures. *Annals Of Emergency Medicine, 12*(6), 1108-1113.

Kaplan, P. W., & Fisher, R. S. (1995). Seizure disorders. In L. R. Barker, J. R. Burton, & P. D. Zieve (Eds.), *Principles of Ambulatory Medicine* (4th ed., pp. 1178-1197). Baltimore: Williams & Wilkins.

Leppik, I. E. (1996). *Contemporary diagnosis and management of the patient with epilepsy* (2nd ed.). Newtown, PA: Handbooks in Health Care.

Messenheimer, J. A. (1996). [CD-ROM]. Little, Brown.

Mikati, M., & Browne, T. R. (1993). Seizures and epilepsy. In R. A. Dershewitz (Ed.), *Ambulatory pediatric care* (2nd ed.) (pp. 580-587). Philadelphia: J. B. Lippincott.

Morrell, M. J. (1994). XII epilepsy. In D. C. Dale (Ed.), *Scientific American medicine* (pp. 1-19). New York: Scientific American.

Percy, A. K., & Percy, P. D. (1986). Acute management of seizures in children. *Nurse Practitioner, 11*(2), 15-28.

Scheuer, M. L., & Pedley, T. A. (1990). The evaluation and treatment of seizures. *The New England Journal of Medicine, 323*(21), 1468-1473.

Uphold, C., & Graham, M. (1994). *Clinical guidelines in family practice*. Gainesville, FL: Barmarrae Books.

REVIEW QUESTIONS

1. M.J. comes to the emergency department today with his 74-year-old wife stating that he thinks his wife has had a seizure. What presenting symptoms would lead you to believe that a tonic-clonic seizure may have taken place?

    a. Headache, fever, and general malaise

    b. Eyes rolled back in head while laying rigid, then jerking for 30 seconds

    c. Fall on the floor

    d. Unable to speak after waking this morning

2. What is the most important test in classifying and diagnosing epilepsy?

    a. Brain scan

    b. ECG

    c. EEG

    d. CBC

3. What differential diagnosis would be included with a 3-week-old baby girl that turns very red in the face then passes out after crying?

    a. Panic attack

    b. Nonepileptic seizures of psychogenic origin

    c. Breath-holding spells

    d. Partial seizure evolving to secondarily generalized seizure

4. Once it has been determined that a seizure has taken place, it is then important to determine whether the seizure was provoked to determine treatment. Which of the following options would **not** indicate a provoked seizure?

    a. One that occurs without cause

    b. One that occurs with sustained head injury after a motor vehicle crash

    c. One that occurs with a high fever

    d. One associated with acute alcohol withdrawal

5. P.S., a 31-year-old woman, has been treated many years with several AEDs for her seizures and comes to see you because she wants to get pregnant. What would be an appropriate decision to make in her case?

    a. Take her off all AEDs right away to prevent any harm to the fetus should pregnancy occur.

    b. Refer her to a neurologist.

    c. Inform her that pregnancy will cause a decrease in seizures.

    d. Inform her that the fertility rate in women with localization-related epilepsy is the same as that of women without epilepsy.

6. When would a CT be ordered for a client with seizures?

    a. 85-year-old woman who has slowly been getting forgetful

    b. 28-year-old with first-time seizure

    c. 6-month-old infant with first-time seizure and fever (104.2° F [40.1° C])

    d. 22-year-old that has not had a seizure in more than 3 years

7. A woman of childbearing years that requires AED therapy must be educated in all **except** which of the following?

    a. AEDs in women of childbearing age often require an increase in dosage.

    b. AEDs and other drugs may cause numerous interactions.

    c. AEDs are teratogenic.

    d. AEDs reduce effectiveness of oral contraceptives.

ANSWERS AND RATIONALES

1. *Answer:* b (assessment/history/neurologic/aging adult)

Rationale: Tonic-clonic (grand mal) seizures have an initial brief tonic phase with extensor rigidity and superior deviation of the eyes and a secondary clonic phase with bilateral jerking lasting 30 to 180 seconds. Often a large jerk is followed by flaccidity and coma. There may be hypersalivation, tongue biting, and incontinence. The postictal period lasts minutes to hours with lethargy and confusion. (Devinsky & Sloviter, 1993)

2. *Answer:* c (diagnosis/neurologic/NAS)

Rationale: The EEG is the single most important diagnostic test in the diagnosis and classification of seizures, although it is not uncommon for a standard 30-minute recording to show no definite interictal activity in the presence of diagnosed epilepsy. (Scheuer & Pedley, 1990)

3. *Answer:* c (diagnosis/neurologic/infant)

Rationale: Often infants cry so hard while holding their breath that they pass out temporarily. (Mikati & Browne, 1993). The other choices of panic attack and pseudoseizures are not indicated in an infant. The last choice of partial seizure evolving to secondarily generalized seizure is not indicated either because there may be focal movement or automatisms seen before the convulsion that were not seen in this infant.

4. *Answer:* b (plan/neurologic/NAS)

Rationale: A provoked seizure is one in which the factors that precipitated the episode can be identified and remedied such as those mentioned other than the first choice. An unprovoked seizure is one without an outside influence. (Uphold & Graham, 1994)

5. *Answer:* b (evaluation/neurologic/adult)

Rationale: Consultation with a neurologist is recommended before pregnancy in those women contemplating pregnancy to ascertain that an AED is indicated and to consider alteration of the current regimen to one that would have a lower risk to the fetus (Messenheimer, 1996). The other choices are inappropriate.

6. *Answer:* b (diagnosis/neurologic/NAS)

Rationale: CT is warranted in a first-time seizure in an adult. Other cases where the CT is warranted include intractable seizures and focal neurologic abnormalities. (Uphold & Graham, 1994)

7. *Answer:* a (plan/neurologic/adult)

Rationale: There is no evidence to support that women of childbearing age should have an increase in dosage of AEDs. However, the woman of childbearing age should be counseled in the other factors mentioned. (Messenheimer, 1996)

9

Endocrine System

ADDISON'S DISEASE

OVERVIEW
Definition

Addison's disease is a condition caused by an insufficient amount of adrenocorticotropic hormone (ACTH) resulting from a primary or secondary dysfunction of the adrenal cortex.

Incidence

- Found in 4 per 100,000 of the population.
- Can occur among all age groups.
- Appears most commonly between the ages of 30 and 50 years.

Pathophysiology

The destruction of the adrenal cortex leads to a deficiency in glucocorticoids (e.g., cortisol) and mineralocorticoids (e.g., aldosterone). In Addison's disease, 90% of the adrenal cortex must be destroyed before the disease manifests itself. The lack of cortisol causes a decreased gluconeogenesis and liver glycogen and an increased insulin sensitivity with resulting hypoglycemia. The decrease in aldosterone results in hyponatremia and hyperkalemia. Eighty percent of the cases of Addison's disease in adults are due to autoimmune or idiopathic adrenalitis. The remaining 20% is due to tuberculosis. Other sources that contribute to the development are fungal infections, metastases to the adrenal glands, adrenal hemorrhage, surgical procedure of bilateral adrenalectomy, cytomegalovirus infection, AIDS, and medications such as ketoconazole, aminoglutethimide, metyrapone, trilostane, mitotane, suramin, RU 486, etomidate, rifampin, and phenytoin. In adults,

adrenal hemorrhage can occur as a result of anticoagulant therapy and spontaneous coagulopathy.

CHILDREN. In children, hereditary enzyme defects with congenital adrenal hyperplasia and loss of adrenal function are due to autoimmune destruction of the adrenal glands. Adrenal hemorrhage in children is usually due to meningococcal and pseudomonas septicemia.

ASSESSMENT: SUBJECTIVE/HISTORY
Most Common Symptoms

- Adults most commonly complain of weakness, fatigue, and weight loss. Other possibilities include anorexia, nausea, vomiting, abdominal discomfort, diarrhea, dizziness, and salt craving.
- Children may experience fatigue, weakness, failure to gain weight or loss of weight, salt craving, and vomiting.

Associated Symptoms

- Hyperpigmentation of the skin and mucous membranes may give clients the appearance of having a deep suntan.
- Pain may occur in the abdomen, back, or flank areas.
- Mental changes such as depression, apathy, and confusion often occur.

Past Medical History

- Hypoglycemia
- Hypotension
- Amenorrhea
- Recent surgery or trauma

313

Medication History

Ask about recent use of ketoconazole, aminoglutethimide, metyrapone, trilostane, mitotane, suramin, RU 486, etomidate, rifampin, or phenytoin.

Family History

Inquire about autoimmune disorders.

Psychosocial History

- Depression
- Apathy
- Confusion
- Decreased libido

Dietary History

- Salt cravings
- Weight loss

ASSESSMENT: OBJECTIVE/PHYSICAL EXAMINATION

Physical Examination

A complete physical examination should be performed with particular attention to the following:
- Vital signs (orthostatic hypotension)
- Weight (loss of weight)
- Cardiovascular (tachycardia)
- Musculoskeletal (muscle wasting, weakness)
- Skin (hyperpigmentation of buccal mucosa, pressure areas: knuckles, elbows, creases of hands, areolae, and new scars)
- Hair distribution (women: loss of axillary or pubic hair)

Diagnostic Procedures

The best screening tool for Addison's disease is the ACTH stimulation test:
1. Draw baseline serum cortisol, ACTH, and aldosterone levels.
2. Inject synthetic ACTH (Cortrosyn 0.25 mg) intravenously.
3. Measure cortisol levels at 30 and 60 minutes after injection.

INTERPRETATION. A typical response to ACTH stimulation is a minimum 10 μg/dl rise in cortisol levels above baseline and a maximum 18 μg/dl rise in cortisol levels at 60 minutes. An individual with primary adrenal insufficiency exhibits no response to ACTH stimulation. With secondary adrenal insufficiency, the response may be normal or blunted to the ACTH stimulation.

CHEMISTRY PROFILE. Chemistry results may reveal hyponatremia, hypoglycemia, or hyperkalemia.

DIAGNOSIS

The differential diagnosis includes the following:
- Depression
- Anorexia nervosa
- Myasthenia gravis
- Tuberculosis
- Salt-losing nephritis

THERAPEUTIC PLAN

Pharmacologic Treatment

In primary adrenal insufficiency, cortisol and mineralocorticoids must be replaced. Cortisol is replaced with hydrocortisone 20 to 30 mg daily. Mineralocorticoids are replaced with fludrocortisone 0.05 to 2 mg daily. In secondary adrenal insufficiency, cortisol only is replaced.

Client Education

- Signs and symptoms of adrenal insufficiency
- Self-injection of hydrocortisone for occasions when unable to take oral medications
- Emergency kit of hydrocortisone
- Medic-Alert bracelet or necklace
- Family included in education
- Lifelong need for replacement therapy
- Diet with liberal sodium intake (3000 mg/day)

Referral

Refer to a physician or endocrinologist for evaluation and treatment.

EVALUATION/FOLLOW-UP

Monitor electrolytes every 3 to 4 months during the first year of therapy.

REFERENCES

Barker, L. R., Burton, J. R., & Zieve, P. D. (1995). *Principles of ambulatory medicine.* Baltimore: Williams & Wilkins.

Brosnan, C., & Gowing, N. (1996). Addison's disease. *British Medical Journal, 312,* 1085-1087.

Davis-Martin, S. (1996). Disorders of the adrenal glands. *Journal of the American Academy of Nurse Practitioners, 8,* 323-326.

Gumowski, J., & Loughran, M. (1996). Diseases of the adrenal gland. *Nursing Clinics of North America, 31,* 747-768.

Hay, W., Groothius, J., Hayward, A., Levin, M. (1997). *Current pediatric diagnosis and treatment.* Norwalk, CT: Appleton & Lange.

Loriaux, T. (1996). Endocrine assessment: Red flags for those on the front lines. *Nursing Clinics of North America, 31,* 695-712.

Price, S., & Wilson, L. (1997). *Pathophysiology: Clinical concepts of disease processes.* St. Louis: Mosby.

Rusterholtz, A. (1996). Interpretation of diagnostic laboratory tests in selected endocrine disorders. *Nursing Clinics of North America, 31,* 715-724.

REVIEW QUESTIONS

1. An adult with Addison's disease will most likely complain of:

    a. Nausea, diarrhea, depression
    b. Weakness, fatigue, weight loss
    c. Weakness, abdominal pain, fatigue
    d. Diarrhea, weakness, fatigue

2. The most common causes of Addison's disease in children are:

    a. AIDS/syphilis
    b. Tuberculosis/bronchitis
    c. Adrenal hemorrhage/surgery
    d. Autoimmune process/genetic

3. Systems most commonly affected by Addison's disease include:

    a. Cardiovascular, ophthalmic, musculoskeletal
    b. Musculoskeletal, skin, ophthalmic
    c. Musculoskeletal, cardiovascular, skin
    d. Cardiovascular, skin, neurologic

4. A client with Addison's disease caused by a primary insufficiency (normal cortisol increase of 10 μg/dl from baseline) would typically respond to the ACTH stimulation test with which of the following?

    a. Cortisol levels at baseline 5 μg/dl—30 minutes after injection 10 μg/dl, 60 minutes after injection 15 μg/dl
    b. Cortisol levels at baseline 5 μg/dl—30 minutes after injection 5 μg/dl, 60 minutes after injection 5 μg/dl

    c. Cortisol levels at baseline 5 μg/dl—30 minutes after injection 30 μg/dl, 60 minutes after injection 50 μg/dl
    d. Cortisol levels at baseline 5 μg/dl—30 minutes after injection 10 μg/dl, 60 minutes after injection 30 μg/dl

5. A 27-year-old man reports to the nurse practitioner. He has experienced nausea, weight loss, and fatigue. Which of the following would **not** be included in the differential diagnosis?

    a. Adrenal insufficiency
    b. Irritable bowel syndrome
    c. AIDS
    d. Tuberculosis

6. A 40-year-old woman was seen by the nurse practitioner and referred to an endocrinologist for diagnosis and treatment of Addison's disease. Which of the following would **not** be included in the education plan?

    a. 1-g sodium diet
    b. Self-injection of hydrocortisone
    c. Medic-Alert bracelet
    d. Signs and symptoms of adrenal insufficiency

ANSWERS AND RATIONALES

1. ***Answer:*** b (assessment/history/endocrine/NAS)
    Rationale: In Addison's disease, the most common presenting symptoms are weakness, fatigue, and weight loss. Depression, diarrhea, and abdominal pain may or may not occur. (Barker, Burton, & Zieve, 1995)

2. ***Answer:*** d (assessment/history/endocrine/child)
    Rationale: The leading causes of Addison's disease today are hereditary enzyme defects with congenital adrenal hyperplasia and loss of adrenal function resulting from autoimmune destruction of the glands. (Hay, Groothius, Hayward, & Levin, 1997)

3. ***Answer:*** c (diagnosis/endocrine/NAS)
    Rationale: Postural hypotension, muscle wasting, and hyperpigmentation of the skin are the most common physical findings. (Loriaux, 1996)

4. ***Answer:*** b (assessment/plan/endocrine/NAS)
    Rationale: In Addison's disease, cortisol levels are low and do not rise in response to ACTH. (Price & Wilson, 1997)

5. *Answer:* b (diagnosis/endocrine/NAS)

Rationale: A person with irritable bowel syndrome usually does not have weight loss. (Barker, Burton, & Zieve, 1995)

6. *Answer:* a (plan/endocrine/NAS)

Rationale: Salt intake should not be restricted because of the decreased levels of mineralocorticoid therapy causing sodium loss. (Barker, Burton, & Zieve, 1995)

CUSHING'S SYNDROME

OVERVIEW
Definition

Cushing's syndrome is due to extended glucocorticoid excess (hypercortisolism).

Incidence

- Occurs in 2 to 4 persons per million per year
- More common in women age 20 to 50
- Rare in children

Pathophysiology

Hypercortisolism may be due to the pathology of the pituitary gland or the adrenal cortex. Cushing's disease results from pituitary gland pathology. Cushing's syndrome results from adrenal gland pathology. An iatrogenic cause of Cushing's syndrome is long-term corticotropin or glucocorticoid administration. In children, Cushing's syndrome is usually iatrogenic (related to long-term glucocorticoid administration).

ASSESSMENT: SUBJECTIVE/HISTORY
Most Common Symptoms

- Weight gain
- Muscle weakness
- Fatigue
- Difficulty rising from squatting position
- Classic moonface
- Accumulation of fat on upper back and trunk

Associated Symptoms

- Bruising
- Poor wound healing
- Menstrual irregularities
- Decreased libido and impotence
- Hypertension or hyperglycemia symptoms
- Depression
- Mood swings
- Insomnia
- Anxiety
- Unusual body hair in women
- Accelerated bone loss (osteoporosis)

Past Medical History

- Hypertension
- Diabetes
- Amenorrhea
- Rheumatoid arthritis
- Asthma
- Lymphoma
- Skin disorders

Medication History

Ask about use of glucocorticoids.

Family History

- Autoimmune disorders
- Hypertension
- Diabetes

Psychosocial History

- Depression
- Mood swings
- Confusion
- Suicidal ideation
- Anxiety
- Insomnia

Dietary History

- Weight gain
- Increased appetite
- Nausea

ASSESSMENT: OBJECTIVE/ PHYSICAL EXAMINATION
Physical Examination

A complete physical examination should be performed with particular attention to the following:

- Vital signs (hypertension)
- Weight (weight gain)

- Cardiovascular (edema)
- Musculoskeletal (muscle wasting, weakness, increased subcutaneous fat in the face and upper body: Moonface, buffalo hump, truncal obesity)
- Skin (telangiectasia over the face, atrophy and thinning with bruising, ecchymoses, purplish abdominal striae)
- Hair (thinning, coarse, hirsutism)

Diagnostic Procedures

- The best screening test for Cushing's syndrome is urinary-free cortisol. An elevated level would indicate probable Cushing's syndrome.
- An overnight dexamethasone suppression test is done to further aid in the diagnosis. A dose of 1 mg dexamethasone suppresses ACTH secretion, particularly early in the morning, causing a decreased cortisol production. The test is performed as follows:
  —Dexamethasone 1 mg at 11 PM
  —Plasma cortisol levels at 8 AM
  INTERPRETATION. Cortisol levels are normally suppressed to less than 5 μg/dl. Cortisol levels are only suppressed to 10 μg/dl in Cushing's syndrome.
  CHEMISTRY PROFILE. Obtain an electrolyte profile to identify hypokalemia, hypernatremia, or hyperglycemia.

DIAGNOSIS

The differential diagnosis includes the following:
- Obesity
- Diabetes mellitus
- Hypertension
- Depression

THERAPEUTIC PLAN

- Surgical intervention, depending on the source, may include adrenalectomy or hypophysectomy for tumor removal.
- Mitotane is occasionally used to inhibit adrenal steroid synthesis.

Client Education

- Development of symptoms
- Diagnosis

- Treatment
- Medication
- Emotional support to improve body image and self-esteem
- Symptoms of adrenal insufficiency after treatment

Referral

Consult with a physician or endocrinologist for evaluation and treatment.

EVALUATION/FOLLOW-UP

Schedule follow-up appointments at least every 3 months to monitor blood pressure, electrolytes, and symptoms of adrenal insufficiency.

REFERENCES

Barker, L. R., Burton, J. R., & Zieve, P. D. (1995). *Principles of ambulatory medicine.* Baltimore: Williams & Wilkins.

Davis-Martin, S. (1996). Disorders of the adrenal glands. *Journal of the American Academy of Nurse Practitioners, 8,* 323-326.

Gumowski, J., & Loughran, M. (1996). Diseases of the adrenal gland. *Nursing Clinics of North America, 31,* 747-768.

Hay, W., Groothius, J., Hayward, A., & Levin, M. (1997). *Current pediatric diagnosis and treatment.* Norwalk, CT: Appleton & Lange.

Loriaux, T. (1996). Endocrine assessment: Red flags for those on the front lines. *Nursing Clinics of North America, 31,* 695-712.

Price, S., & Wilson, L. (1997). *Pathophysiology: Clinical concepts of disease processes.* St. Louis: Mosby.

Rusterholtz, A. (1996). Interpretation of diagnostic laboratory tests in selected endocrine disorders. *Nursing Clinics of North America, 31,* 715-724.

REVIEW QUESTIONS

1. Adults or children with Cushing's syndrome typically complain of:
a. Mood swings, weight gain, muscle weakness
b. Menstrual irregularities, mood swings, muscle weakness
c. Weight gain, muscle weakness, fatigue
d. Fatigue, mood swings, weight gain

2. Children usually develop Cushing's syndrome because of:

 a. Pituitary microadenoma
 b. Adrenal tumor
 c. Long-term glucocorticoid administration
 d. Adrenal pathology

3. Ms. Jones is a 45-year-old woman seen by the nurse practitioner. She is concerned about weight gain, fatigue, and edema of her lower extremities. What systems of the physical examination will aid in the diagnosis?

 a. Cardiovascular, musculoskeletal, skin
 b. Respiratory, skin, musculoskeletal
 c. Cardiovascular, skin, ophthalmic
 d. Cardiovascular, musculoskeletal, abdominal

4. A person with Cushing's syndrome would have which of the following chemistry values?

 a. Hyponatremia, hypokalemia, hyperglycemia
 b. Hyponatremia, hyperkalemia, hyperglycemia
 c. Hypernatremia, hypokalemia, hyperglycemia
 d. Hypernatremia, hyperkalemia, hyperglycemia

5. An education plan for a client with Cushing's syndrome includes all the following **except:**

 a. Medication, diagnosis, treatment
 b. Development of symptoms of adrenal insufficiency
 c. Injection of hydrocortisone
 d. Emotional support to improve body image

ANSWERS AND RATIONALES

1. *Answer:* c (assessment/history/endocrine/NAS)
 Rationale: The most common presenting symptoms for Cushing's syndrome are weight gain, muscle weakness, and fatigue. The symptoms are due to the excessive glucocorticoid effect. (Barker, Burton, & Zieve, 1996; Hay, Groothius, Hayward, & Levin, 1997)

2. *Answer:* c (diagnosis/endocrine/child)
 Rationale: Children usually develop Cushing's syndrome after long-term therapy with glucocorticoids causing hypercortisolism. (Hay, Groothius, Hayward, & Levin, 1997)

3. *Answer:* a (assessment/physical examination/endocrine/NAS)
 Rationale: The systems with the most noted change from Cushing's syndrome are cardiovascular, musculoskeletal, and skin. The changes include hypertension, edema, increased subcutaneous fat, muscle weakness, and telangiectasia. (Barker, Burton, & Zieve, 1995)

4. *Answer:* c (assessment/plan/endocrine/NAS)
 Rationale: Because of the elevation of glucocorticoids, sodium and glucose usually increase. Potassium is lost. (Price & Wilson, 1997)

5. *Answer:* c (plan/endocrine/NAS)
 Rationale: Hydrocortisone is used in adrenal insufficiency. If a client develops adrenal insufficiency after treatment, then instruct the client regarding injection of hydrocortisone. (Barker, Burton, & Zieve, 1995)

DIABETES MELLITUS

OVERVIEW
Definition

Diabetes mellitus is a disease in which glucose is not metabolized correctly either because of inadequate insulin levels or poor utilization of insulin.

Incidence

• There are approximately 10 million people with diabetes in the United States.
• Of these, 80% to 90% are non-insulin-dependent diabetes mellitus (NIDDM), and 10% to 20% are insulin-dependent diabetes mellitus (IDDM).

Pathophysiology

• In IDDM, the pancreas ceases to produce insulin. The beta-cells of the pancreas are slowly destroyed. IDDM is an autoimmune disorder with a genetic predisposition. IDDM usually occurs before age 40.
• In NIDDM, there is a defect in the insulin receptors. The pancreas continues to produce in-

sulin, but the body is not able to use the available insulin. NIDDM usually occurs after the age of 40.

ASSESSMENT: SUBJECTIVE/HISTORY
Most Common Symptoms
- In adults with NIDDM, the most common symptoms are polyuria, polydipsia, and polyphagia.
- In children and young adults with IDDM, the most common symptoms are rapid onset of polydipsia, polyuria, weight loss, polyphagia, and fatigue.

Associated Symptoms
- In adults with NIDDM, paresthesia, dysesthesias, blurred vision, vaginal candidiasis, or fungal skin infections may occur.
- In IDDM, in addition to the symptoms just mentioned, abdominal pain, nausea, vomiting, or fruity breath may occur.

Past Medical History
- Hypertension
- Hypoglycemia
- Retinopathy
- Obesity
- Gestational diabetes

Medication History
Recent use of steroids or diuretics may raise blood glucose.

Family History
- Diabetes
- Hyperlipidemia
- Hypertension

Psychosocial History
- Smoking
- Alcohol or drug use
- Exercise

Dietary History
- Weight gain or loss
- 24-hour diet recall
- Polyphagia and polydipsia

ASSESSMENT: OBJECTIVE/ PHYSICAL EXAMINATION
Physical Examination
A complete physical examination should be performed with particular attention to the following:
- Vital signs (hypertension, tachycardia, or tachypnea)
- Weight (gain or loss)
- Ophthalmic (fundoscopic examination: Check for retinopathy)
- Oral (mouth and dental: Attention to teeth and gums)
- Cardiovascular (bruits, pulses, or edema)
- Thyroid (palpable or nonpalpable)
- Abdomen (hepatomegaly, bruits)
- Skin (infections, integrity)
- Feet (integrity, callus, infection, or deformity)
- Neurologic (sensation)

Laboratory Data
DIAGNOSTIC LABORATORY DATA
Plasma Glucose. In adults the diagnosis is based on the following:
- Classic symptoms of diabetes, polyuria, polydipsia, polyphagia, and weight loss and a plasma glucose >200 mg/dl; OR
- Fasting plasma glucose >126 mg/dl on two occasions; OR
- Fasting plasma glucose <126 mg/dl and two oral glucose tolerance tests demonstrate a 2-hour postprandial glucose and one other value >200 mg/dl (of the three values obtained). (Glucose tolerance tests are usually only done with gestational diabetes.)

In children the diagnosis is based on the following:
- Classic symptoms of diabetes, polyuria, polydipsia, polyphagia, and weight loss and a plasma glucose >200 mg/dl; OR
- Fasting plasma glucose >140 mg/dl and two oral glucose tolerance tests demonstrate a 2-hour postprandial glucose and one other value >200 mg/dl (of the three values obtained).

Glycosylated Hemoglobin or Hemoglobin A1C. The glycosylated hemoglobin test or the hemoglobin A1C (Hgb A1C) test can give you the average glucose value for the past 3 months. For the Hgb A1C test, the normal value for a person with diabetes is around 7% to get an average of 150 mg/dl. The glycosylated hemoglobin should be maintained around 8% to get an average glucose of 150 mg/dl. The Hgb A1C test can further validate the diagnosis.

OTHER LABORATORY DATA
- Fasting lipid profile
- Serum creatinine: In adults; in children if proteinuria exists
- Urinalysis: Glucose, ketones, protein, sediment
- Urinary microalbuminuria (overnight specimen): On diagnosis with NIDDM or after 5 years diagnosis IDDM
- Thyroid function tests: When indicated by history and examination
- ECG: In adults

DIAGNOSIS

The differential diagnosis includes the following:
- Cushing's disease
- Transient hyperglycemia
- Acromegaly
- Pheochromocytoma
- Diabetes insipidus

THERAPEUTIC PLAN

Insulin-Dependent Diabetes Mellitus

NUTRITION. Many nutrition plans are available. The easiest for most people is no concentrated sugar with 50% to 60% carbohydrate, 30% fat, and 10% to 20% protein (i.e., food guide pyramid). Three meals per day with optional bedtime snack.

EXERCISE. Recommend 30 to 45 minutes for 3 to 4 days/wk. Check blood glucose before exercise. If blood glucose is <60 mg/dl, eat protein. If blood glucose is >250 mg/dl, avoid exercise (may actually raise blood glucose).

HOME GLUCOSE MONITORING. Recommend 4 times a day (ac and hs) at least 3 to 4 days/week, more if blood glucose is elevated or during illness.

INSULIN. See Tables 9-1 and 9-2.

Non-Insulin-Dependent Diabetes Mellitus

NUTRITION. The guidelines are similar to IDDM, except weight loss is focal. More restriction of calories through fat intake reduction is necessary.

ORAL AGENTS. If blood glucose is <250 mg/dl, the exercise and nutrition guidelines for IDDM are sufficient. If blood glucose is >250 mg/dl, an

Table 9-1 Total Daily Insulin Requirement (Total Dose 0.5 U/kg/day)

REGULAR	LONG/INTERMEDIATE
Onset 1-3 hr	Onset 4-8 hr
⅓ of total daily dose	⅔ of total daily dose

Table 9-2 Number of Injections (Minimum of Two)

INJECTIONS	INSTRUCTIONS
Two injections	Split insulin 50/50 for regular and long-acting insulin prebreakfast and presupper.
Three injections	Divide regular insulin between two doses, prebreakfast and supper; long-acting insulin may be divided between prebreakfast and bedtime.
Three injections	Divide regular insulin between three doses, prebreakfast, prelunch, and presupper; take long-acting insulin at supper.
More than three (only after starting with three)	Divide regular insulin between doses, prebreakfast, prelunch, and presupper; take long-acting insulin at bedtime.

oral agent must be started. The following are the current oral medications used to treat NIDDM:
- Sulfonylureas (second generation)
  —Glimepiride (Amaryl) 1-, 2-, 4-mg tablets; maximum dose 8 mg/day
  —Glyburide (Diabeta) 1.25-, 2.5-, 5-, 10-mg tablets; maximum dose 20 mg/day
  —Glyburide (Glynase) 0.75-, 1.5-, 3-, 6-mg tablets; maximum dose 12 mg/day
  —Glipizide (Glucotrol) 5-, 10-mg tablets; maximum dose 20 mg bid
  —Glipizide (Glucotrol-XL) 5-, 10-mg tablets; maximum dose 20 mg/day
- Biguanides:
  —Metformin (Glucophage) 500-mg tablets; maximum dose 2.5 g tid
- Alpha-glucosidase inhibitors:
  —Acarbose (Precose) 50-, 100-mg tablets; maximum dose 100 mg tid

INSULIN. See section/tables under IDDM.

Client Education

Include the family in the education process. It takes several visits to complete the education plan. Goals should be set based on priority for most needed items. The first visit should include the basics for survival (i.e., medications, signs and symptoms of low blood glucose). At the second visit, assess the knowledge base and determine the next level. Some people may not be able to afford home glucose monitoring. Education is based on each individual:

- Pathophysiology of diabetes
- Home glucose monitoring
- Foot care
- Medication
- Insulin administration (Tables 9-1 and 9-2)
- Nutrition
- Complications of diabetes: Retinopathy, neuropathy, nephropathy, and cardiovascular disorders
- Signs and symptoms of hypoglycemia and hyperglycemia and treatment
- Sick days (i.e., fluids, insulin, medicine, monitoring during illness)
- Exercise plan
- Diabetes identification bracelet

Referral

- Refer for an annual dilated eye examination for NIDDM and after 5 years of diagnosis with IDDM (minimum).
- Consult with a physician for any newly diagnosed client with diabetes.
- Children with diabetes should be referred to a pediatric endocrinologist if possible.

EVALUATION/FOLLOW-UP

- After the initial diagnosis, visits should be every 1 to 2 weeks until blood glucose is closer to 180 to 200 mg/dl. For clients starting insulin, visits may need to be every 1 to 2 days. Phone contact can supplement.
- IDDM: Schedule visits every 3 months to monitor Hgb A1C and assess diabetes control.
- NIDDM: Schedule visits every 6 months if condition is well controlled (Hgb A1C < 7%) and the client does not take insulin. If the condi-

tion is poorly controlled (Hgb A1C > 9%), visits should be every 3 months. For clients treated with insulin, follow the recommendations of IDDM (every 3 months).

REFERENCES

Albright, J. (1993). The process of managing the dietary regimen in the elderly people with diabetes. *Health and Social Care, 2*, 41-52.

American Diabetes Association (1996a). Office guide to diagnosis and classification of diabetes mellitus and other categories of glucose intolerance. *Diabetes Care, 19* (Suppl. 4).

American Diabetes Association (1996b). Nutrition recommendations and principles for people with diabetes mellitus. *Diabetes Care, 19* (Suppl. 16-19).

American Diabetes Association (1996c). Standards of medical care for patients with diabetes mellitus. *Diabetes Care, 19,* (Suppl. 8-15).

Baliga, S.B., & Fonseca, V. A. (1997). Recent advances in the treatment of type II diabetes mellitus. *American Family Physician, 55*(3), 817-824.

Barker, L. R., Burton, J. R., & Zieve, P. D. (1995). *Principles of ambulatory medicine.* Baltimore: Williams & Wilkins.

Bohannon, N.J.V., & Jack, D. B. (1995). Type II diabetes: How to use the new oral medications. *Geriatrics, 51,* 33-37.

Cefalu, W. T. (1996). Treatment of type II diabetes. *Postgraduate Medicine, 99*(3), 109-122.

Hay, W., Groothius, Hayward, & Levin, (1997). *Current pediatric diagnosis and treatment.* Norwalk, CT: Appleton & Lange.

Hiss, R. G. (1996). Barriers to care in non-insulin-dependent diabetes mellitus. *Annals of Internal Medicine, 124,* 146-148.

Jaspan, J. B. (1995). Taking control of diabetes. *Hospital Practice, 30*(10), 55-62.

Singh, I., & Marshall, M. C. (1995). Diabetes mellitus in the elderly. *Endocrinology and Metabolism Clinics of North America, 24*(2), 255-272.

Stolar, M. W. (1995). Clinical management of NIDDM patient. *Diabetes Care, 18*(5), 701-707.

Uphold, C. R., & Graham, M. V. (1994). *Clinical guidelines in family practice.* Gainesville, FL: Barmarrae Books.

Willis, J. (1995). Diabetes dietary management. *Nursing Times, 91*(49), 42-44.

REVIEW QUESTIONS

1. An adult who develops NIDDM is most likely to experience all the following symptoms **except:**

- a. Polyuria
- b. Nausea
- c. Polydipsia
- d. Polyphagia

2. Mr. Jones has polyuria and polydipsia at his first visit to the nurse practitioner. The nurse practitioner suspects NIDDM. Which of the following would **not** be included in the physical examination?

- a. Otoscopic
- b. Ophthalmic
- c. Neurologic
- d. Cardiovascular

3. To assess renal function in a client with IDDM, urinary microalbuminuria should be assessed:

- a. On diagnosis
- b. 2 years after diagnosis
- c. 3 years after diagnosis
- d. 5 years after diagnosis

4. Mr. Bates is a 50-year-old man who visits the nurse practitioner for evaluation. He has been experiencing fatigue, polyuria, polydipsia, and nocturia. Plasma glucose is 240 mg/dl. Which of the following would **not** be included in the differential diagnosis?

- a. Diabetes mellitus
- b. Cushing's syndrome
- c. Diabetes insipidus
- d. Pheochromocytoma

5. The nurse practitioner completed an examination of a 15-year-old, 60-kg male with IDDM. After consulting with the physician, it is agreed to prescribe NPH and regular insulin, 0.5 U/kg/day. Two thirds of the total dose will be NPH, and one third will be regular (R) insulin. The total dose will be divided into two doses, before breakfast and supper. What is the correct dose?

- a. 10 U NPH + 5 U R bid
- b. 15 U NPH + 5 U R AM—10 NPH + 5 R PM
- c. 15 U NPH + 5 U R bid
- d. 10 U R + 5 NPH bid

6. Which of the following is the easiest nutrition plan for a client with diabetes to follow?

- a. Carbohydrate counting
- b. Calorie counting
- c. Food guide pyramid
- d. Counting fat grams

7. Ms. King was seen by her nurse practitioner for follow-up on NIDDM. Her Hgb A1C was 9%. Her current treatment is Glipizide (Glucotrol-XL) 10 mg daily. When should Ms. King's next appointment be scheduled?

- a. 6 months
- b. 3 months
- c. 2 weeks
- d. 1 month

ANSWERS AND RATIONALES

1. *Answer:* b (assessment/history/endocrine/adult)
Rationale: Nausea usual only in IDDM. (Barker, Burton, & Zieve, 1995)

2. *Answer:* a (assessment/physical examination/endocrine/NAS)
Rationale: The ear is not associated with any specific changes in NIDDM. The other systems provide pertinent data. (American Diabetes Association, 1996c)

3. *Answer:* d (evaluation/endocrine/NAS)
Rationale: The American Diabetes Association (ADA) recommends screening for renal disease in IDDM after 5 years of diagnosis. It usually takes 5 to 10 years for complications to develop in IDDM. (American Diabetes Association, 1996c)

4. *Answer:* c (diagnosis/endocrine/NAS)
Rationale: In diabetes insipidus, clients experience polyuria and polydipsia but lack hyperglycemia. (Uphold & Graham, 1994)

5. *Answer:* a (plan/endocrine/NAS)
Rationale: 0.5 U × 60 kg = 30 U/day
2 doses/30 U/day = 15 U/dose
15 × 0.66 = 9.9 = 10 U NPH
15 × 0.33 = 4.95 = 5 U R
10 U NPH + 5 U R bid

6. *Answer:* c (plan/endocrine/NAS)
Rationale: The food pyramid is the easiest tool for people with diabetes to use. (Willis, 1995)

7. *Answer:* b (evaluation/endocrine/NAS)
Rationale: The level of glycemic control is 9% for Ms. King. The medication can be increased to the maximum dose and the visit scheduled in 3 months. (American Diabetes Association, 1996c)

THYROID DISORDERS

Hypothyroidism, Hyperthyroidism, and Thyroid Nodules

OVERVIEW
Definition

Hypothyroidism is the undersecretion of thyroid hormones triiodothyronine (T_3) and thyroxine (T_4). It is termed cretinism when it causes brain damage as a congenital condition, and myxedema when it is a life complication of hypothyroidism in adults.

Hyperthyroidism is the oversecretion of thyroid hormone. *Thyroid nodules* refer to tumors that occur in a thyroid gland that is otherwise normal.

Incidence

Hypothyroidism and hyperthyroidism have a prevalence of 0.5% in the general population, but have a higher prevalence in selected groups. Adults have an incidence of approximately 11% to 15% of hypothyroidism. Postmenopausal women are more at risk for developing hypothyroidism. Approximately one in 500 children is treated for hypothyroidism in the United States. About 2% of the adult population have hyperthyroidism, most often in young women, although it can occur in men and at any age.

Thyroid nodules occur in 2% to 3% of adults, usually 3 to 4 times more often in women than in men.

Pathophysiology

Two thyroid hormones are produced by the body, T_3 and T_4. Production and release of T_4 by the thyroid gland is regulated by the anterior pituitary gland by the means of thyroid-stimulating hormone (TSH). Increases in T_4 or T_3 result in decreased production of TSH, whereas decreases in T_4 or T_3 result in increased TSH production. TSH production is primarily regulated by thyrotropin-releasing hormone (TRH), which is produced by the hypothalamus. These mechanisms produce a negative feedback loop maintaining T_4 and T_3 within therapeutic ranges.

PRIMARY HYPOTHYROIDISM. Primary hypothyroidism is an insufficient quantity of thyroid tissue or loss of functional thyroid tissue because of iatrogenic causes such as thyroidectomy or autoimmune responses (Hashimoto's disease).

SECONDARY HYPOTHYROIDISM. Secondary hypothyroidism is less common; it usually occurs along with other anterior pituitary deficiencies and is most often caused by a pituitary tumor.

HYPERTHYROIDISM. Hyperthyroidism is an increased level of thyroid secretion, usually as a result of an autoimmune disorder in which the body produces thyroid-stimulating antibodies against TSH receptors on the thyroid cells pathologically stimulating the thyroid cells (Graves' disease). Graves' disease is the cause of hyperthyroidism in approximately 90% of cases. Various types of thyroiditis cause the other 10% of hyperthyroidism.

THYROID NODULES. Nodules on the thyroid gland are usually thyroid adenoma, thyroid cyst, or thyroid carcinoma. Of these, only thyroid cancer poses a risk to the client.

CONTRIBUTING FACTORS
- Newborns
- Strong familial history of thyroid disease
- Postpartum period
- History of autoimmune disorders
- Iatrogenic, surgery, x-ray treatments
- Medications
- Thyroid carcinoma: Men, young age, history of neck irradiation, positive family history
- Obesity

ASSESSMENT: SUBJECTIVE/HISTORY
Hypothyroidism

CONGENITAL ABNORMALITIES
- Infrequent crying
- Hypoactivity
- Poor feeding
- Inconsistent bowel habits
- Lethargy
- Temperature instability

ADULT

Early Signs
- Fatigue
- Dry skin
- Weight gain
- Cold intolerance

- Constipation
- Heavy menstrual flow

Later Signs

- Excessively dry skin
- Coarse hair texture
- Alopecia
- Increased weight gain
- Decrease in mental awareness
- Depression
- Pain/swelling in neck

Myxedema

- Thick, dry, scaly skin
- Enlarged tongue
- Muscle weakness
- Joint pain

Hyperthyroidism

- Nervousness: Irritability, decreased concentration, restlessness, tremor
- Weight loss: Despite increased appetite; anorexia in older adults
- Heat intolerance: Sweating
- Skin changes: Silky, hyperpigmentation over joints
- Hair loss: Thinning of scalp in women
- Neck mass
- Eyes: Bulging
- Shortness of breath
- Symptoms of heart failure: Palpitations, angina
- Menstrual irregularities/amenorrhea

Thyroid Nodules

- Neck mass
- Neck discomfort
- Hoarseness
- Dysphagia

Past Medical History

- Allergies
- Last menstrual period and characteristics
- Past neck irradiation

Medication History

Inquire about any iodine-containing medication or antithyroid medication taken during pregnancy.

Family History

Ask about other family members with endocrine disorders.

Dietary History

Inquire about the type of diet the client usually eats.

ASSESSMENT: OBJECTIVE/ PHYSICAL EXAMINATION

Physical Examination

A problem-oriented physical examination should be conducted with particular attention to the following:

- Vital signs, weight, and general appearance
- Hypothyroidism
  —Slow movements, lethargy, and irritability
  —HEENT: Hair texture coarse, inspect neck/thyroid, dull facies
  —Cardiovascular: Dull facies; cardiomegaly, slow heart rate
  —Abdominal: Decreased bowel sounds
  —Neurologic: Deep tendon reflexes (DTRs), persistently opened posterior fontanelle; brisk reaction and prolonged reaction, large anterior fontanelle
  —Skin: Plaques with sharp raised margin, with complaints of pruritus
  —Infant: Sometimes symptomatic as early as 2 weeks, but sometimes asymptomatic for up to 1 month; irreversible mental changes sometimes occurring before symptoms become evident
- Hyperthyroidism
  —Eyes: Forward protrusion of globe, lid lag, stare, limitation in ability to converge
  —Thyroid: Enlargement or asymmetric, enlargement in the young, may not find enlargement in older adults, bruit
  —Cardiovascular: Sinus tachycardia, atrial fibrillation, systolic flow murmurs, cardiac failure
- Thyroid nodules
  —Thyroid: Enlargement, consistency, movement

Diagnostic Procedures

- Hypothyroidism
  —T_4 screen of all newborns in the United States; TSH done if T_4 is low
  —Increased TSH and decreased T_4
  —Additional laboratory data: Lytes, BUN, creatinine, glucose, calcium, lipids
- Hyperthyroidism

—TSH undetectable or below normal

—T$_4$ elevated

• Thyroid nodule

—Radioiodine scan and ultrasound are not able to discriminate between benign and malignant lesions.

—Fine-needle aspiration (FNA) is most reliable and useful method of identifying malignancy.

DIAGNOSIS

The differential diagnosis includes the following:

• Hypothyroidism
  —Ischemic heart disease
  —Depression
  —Nephrotic syndrome
  —Liver disease
• Hyperthyroidism
  —Cancer
  —Cardiac: Congestive heart failure, atrial fibrillation
  —Psychologic problems: Anxiety
  —Tremors: Neurologic problems
  —Fibromyalgia
• Thyroid nodule
  —Benign adenoma
  —Thyroid cancer (papillary, follicular, anaplastic, medullary)

THERAPEUTIC PLAN
Pharmacologic Treatment

• Hypothyroidism
  —Levothyroxine: May be increased depending on symptoms and laboratory results
  —Caution with older adults with heart disease: Lower dose initially
• Hyperthyroidism
  —Medications administered for 12 to 24 months: Lugol's solution, propylthiouracil (PTU: Preferred in pregnant women), and propranolol, methimazale (Tapazole), thiocarbamide antithyroid drugs, radioactive iodine, surgical therapy
  —Major side effect: Agranulocytosis
  —Must treat with levothyroxine after client becomes hypothyroid

Nonpharmacologic Treatment

• Thyroid nodule
  —Refer to physician/surgeon for FNA

Client Education

• Congenital hypothyroidism
  —Educate the family concerning the disease process and importance of early treatment to prevent brain damage and assure normal physical growth.
  —Emphasize the importance of follow-up to obtain a euthyroid level.
• Adult hypothyroidism
  —Educate the family concerning the side effects of medication and the signs and symptoms of hyperthyroidism.
  —Alert families to the genetic component of thyroid disorders.
• Thyroid storm is a complication of hyperthyroidism.
  —It is a medical emergency, with symptoms of fever, sinus tachycardia, nervousness, cardiovascular collapse, and shock

Referral

• Congenital hypothyroidism: Refer to physician and pediatric endocrinologist.
• Adult with myxedema, cardiac disease, hypothyroidism caused by pituitary gland or hypothalamus dysfunction, or hyperthyroidism: Refer to endocrinologist.
• Congenital hyperthyroidism: Refer to pediatric endocrinologist.

EVALUATION/FOLLOW-UP

• Congenital hypothyroidism: Monitor T$_4$ and TSH every 2 to 4 weeks after therapy is begun, then monthly until client is 1 year, then bimonthly until client is 3 years.
• Adult hypothyroidism: Reassess thyroid levels after 4 to 6 weeks after treatment and monitor thyroid levels every 6 to 12 months.

REFERENCES

Barker, L. R., Burton, J. R., & Zieve, P. D. (1995). *Principles of ambulatory medicine.* Baltimore: Williams & Wilkins.

Bishnoi, A., & Sachmechi, I. (1996). Thyroid disease during pregnancy. *American Family Physician, 53*(1), 215-220.

Brody, M., & Reichard, R. (1995). Thyroid screening: How to interpret and apply the results. *Postgraduate Medicine, 98*(2), 54-66.

Costa, A. (1995). Interpreting thyroid tests. *American Family Physician, 52*(8), 2325-2330.

Gregerman, R. (1995). Thyroid disorders. In R. Barker, J. Burton, & P. Zieve (Eds.), *Principles of ambulatory medicine* (pp. 1020-1046). Baltimore: Williams & Wilkins.

Schubert, M., & Kountz, D. (1995). Thyroiditis. *Post-graduate Medicine, 98*(2), 101-112.

Youngkin, E. Q., & Davis, M. S., (1994). (pp. 639-642). *Women's health: A primary care clinical guide.* Norwalk, CT: Appleton & Lange.

REVIEW QUESTIONS

1. Which factor in a woman's history would be considered a positive sign for thyroid nodules?

   a. Menopause
   b. Head/neck irradiation
   c. Young age
   d. Normal body weight

2. Which physical finding is most suggestive of hyperthyroidism?

   a. Dull hair
   b. Flat affect
   c. Weight gain
   d. Anxious speech

3. Which of the following laboratory test results are indicative of hypothyroidism?

   a. Increased TSH and decreased T_4
   b. Normal TSH
   c. Decreased TSH and increased T_4
   d. Normal T_4

4. A thyroid biopsy is considered mandatory with which of the following findings?

   a. Increased TSH and decreased T_4
   b. Thyroid nodule
   c. Thyrotoxicosis
   d. Decreased TSH and increased T_4

5. Ellie is a 34-year-old client being treated with levothyroxine for hypothyroidism. Which of the following would **not** indicate that her medication may need to be adjusted?

   a. Tremor
   b. Fatigue
   c. Increased energy
   d. Chest pain

ANSWERS AND RATIONALES

1. ***Answer:*** b (assessment/history/endocrine/NAS)
   Rationale: Head/neck irradiation is considered a risk factor for developing thyroid malignancies. (Youngkin & Davis, 1994)

2. ***Answer:*** d (assessment/physical examination/endocrine/NAS)
   Rationale: Clients with hyperthyroidism may have anxious and pressured speech. Flat affect, weight gain, and dull hair are more characteristic of hypothyroidism. (Youngkin & Davis, 1994)

3. ***Answer:*** a (diagnosis/endocrine/NAS)
   Rationale: Hypothyroidism is confirmed by a high TSH and a low T_4 level. (Youngkin & Davis, 1994; Costa, 1995; Brody, 1995)

4. ***Answer:*** b (plan/endocrine/NAS)
   Rationale: A thyroid biopsy is necessary for a client with a thyroid nodule. (Gregerman, 1995)

5. ***Answer:*** c (evaluation/endocrine/adult)
   Rationale: A tremor and chest pain may indicate increased levels of thyroid, whereas fatigue may indicate a decreased level of thyroid. Increased energy is the desired response. (Youngkin & Davis, 1994; Schubert & Kountz, 1995)

10

Hematopoietic System

ANEMIA

OVERVIEW

Definition

Anemia is a condition in which the concentration of hemoglobin (Hgb) or the number or volume of RBCs is reduced to a below-normal value. Anemia may be caused by impaired production of RBCs, increased destruction of RBCs, or rapid loss of RBCs.

Incidence

Anemia occurs most frequently in young children, women of reproductive age, and older adults. The most common cause of anemia in the United States is iron deficiency. The prevalence of iron deficiency is currently estimated to be around 3% for children 1 to 5 years old. A low hemoglobin level is present in about 9% of women 15 to 44 years old and is especially common during pregnancy. The prevalence of anemia in persons older than 65 years is 2.3% in males and 5.5% in females. Sickle cell anemia affects >70,000 blacks, with one third between 2 and 16 years old.

Pathophysiology

The physiologic defects caused by the anemia are a decrease in the oxygen-carrying capacity of the blood and a reduction in the oxygen available to the tissues. The signs and symptoms of anemia are a result of failure to oxygenate tissues and the degree of acuity (gradual onset of anemia allows time for compensatory mechanisms to increase oxygenation). Anemias can be classified either by causal (etiologic) mechanisms or by RBC mor-phology. On an etiologic basis, anemia results from the following:

- Acute or chronic hemorrhage
- An increased loss or destruction of RBCs
- Production of abnormal Hgb leads to anemia and tissue damage from vascular blockage by trapped, abnormal RBCs. RBCs assume a crescent shape when oxygen tension is lowered (sickle cell).
- Impaired Hgb and RBC formation (nutritional, bone marrow infiltration, chronic disease)

The morphologic classification of anemia includes the following:

- Normocytic/normochromic (blood loss, hemolytic anemia, chronic disease, bone marrow infiltration)
- Microcytic/hypochromic (iron deficiency, lead, thalassemias)
- Macrocytic/normochromic (vitamin B_{12} or folate deficiency, drugs, bone marrow failure)

RISK FACTORS

Age

- Neonates: Most common causes of anemia include blood loss, isoimmunization, congenital infection, and congenital hemolytic anemia.
- Ages 3 to 6 months: Anemia is usually caused by congenital disorders of Hgb synthesis or Hgb structure. Almost never is nutritional iron deficiency seen in an otherwise healthy term infant. Prematurity pre-

disposes toward early development of iron deficiency.

- Older infants or toddlers: Nutritional iron deficiency may be seen in those who switched to whole cow's milk.

Ethnicity

- Hgb S and Hgb C are more common in blacks.
- Beta-thalassemia is more common in people of Mediterranean background.
- Alpha-thalassemia is more common among blacks and Asians.

Diet. Decreased iron, folate, vitamin B_{12}, or vitamin E in diet increases risk of anemia.

Drugs. Anticonvulsants and chemotherapy increase risk of anemias.

TYPES OF ANEMIA

Microcytic/Hypochromic Anemia

- Iron deficiency anemia is caused by increased physiologic requirements, decreased intake of iron, or chronic blood loss. Lead ingestion leads to increased amninolevulinic acid, which leads to deficient Hgb synthesis.
- Thalassemias are genetically caused, related to deficient synthesis of one or more of the polypeptide chains of Hgb.
  —Thalassemia major: Lack of β-chain synthesis, intramedullary hemolysis
  —Thalassemia minor: Heterozygous state
  —Thalassemia alpha: Deletion of one or more alpha-chain genes

Normocytic/Normochromic Anemia

- Hemolytic anemia is reduced survival of circulating RBCs caused by their destruction in the circulation (intravascular) or within the phagocytic cells of the liver, spleen, or bone marrow (extravascular).
- Intrinsic RBC defects are as follows:
  —Congenital spherocytosis is abnormality of RBC membranes as a result of spectrin deficiency.
  —In glucose-6-phosphate dehydrogenase (G6PD) deficiency, a deficient enzyme concentration does not allow detoxification of oxygen free radicals by the reduced form of nicotinamide adenine dinucleotide, precipitating hemolysis.
  —Hemoglobinopathies include Hgb SS and Hgb C (sickle cell).

- Extrinsic RBC defects are as follows:
  —Immune mediated
  —Hemolytic disease of the neonate (ABO incompatibility)
- Anemia of chronic disease may be caused by the following:
  —Chronic infection
  —Osteomyelitis
  —Tuberculosis
  —Pyelonephritis
  —Chronic inflammatory disorders (rheumatoid arthritis, systemic lupus erythematosus (SLE), inflammatory bowel disease [IBD])

Macrocytic Anemia

- Aplastic anemia/Fanconi's anemia: Causes include idiopathic, hepatitis, chemicals, and pregnancy.
- Vitamin B_{12}/folate deficiency: Causes include inadequate intake, malabsorption, and increased body requirements.

ASSESSMENT: SUBJECTIVE/HISTORY

History of Present Illness and Past Medical History

History of symptoms related to anemia include the following:

- Irritability
- Dyspnea
- Fatigue
- Palpitations
- Headache
- Edema
- Jaundice
- Bleeding
- Pallor
- Infection
- Heart murmur
- Chronic illness
- Drug use
- Bone pain
- Past viral infections

Medication History

Ask about use of anticonvulsants.

Pregnancy History

Ask about anemia with previous pregnancies.

Family and Psychosocial History

- Ethnic origin
- Travel
- History of gallstones or splenectomy in other family members
- Alcohol ingestion

Dietary History

- General diet
- Any recent weight gain or loss
- Anorexia
- Nausea or vomiting
- Decreased intake
- Diarrhea

Environmental History

Ask about environmental exposures at home and in the workplace (lead, chemicals, and heavy metals).

ASSESSMENT: OBJECTIVE/ PHYSICAL EXAMINATION

Physical Examination

Perform a complete physical examination with increased attention to the following:

- Vital signs, weight, height
- In mild anemia (Hgb 10 to 14 g/dl) and even moderate anemia (6 to 10 g/dl), few clinical manifestations may be seen. Most commonly palpitations and dyspnea are the first symptoms seen.
- In severe anemia (Hgb <6 g/dl), the following may be seen:
  —General: Sensitivity to cold, weight loss, lethargy
  —Skin: Jaundice, bleeding, pallor, petechiae, purpura
  —Mouth: glossitis, angular stomatitis
  —Eyes: Eyelid edema, retinal hemorrhage
  —Respiratory: Tachypnea
  —Cardiovascular: Tachycardia, murmur, or gallop; angina; myocardial infarction; congestive heart failure
  —Abdominal: Hepatosplenomegaly or other masses, lymphadenopathy, anorexia
  —Musculoskeletal: Bone pain
  —Neurologic: Headache, vertigo, irritability, depression, impaired thought processes

Diagnostic Procedures

- Complete blood cell count (CBC): Including all indexes, mean cell volume (MCV), mean corpuscular Hgb (MCH), mean corpuscular Hgb concentration (MCHC)
- Hgb
- Hematocrit: Volume of packed RBCs (reflects total mass of RBCs)
- Blood smear: Size (anisocytosis, microcytes, macrocytes), inclusions (basophilic stippling, Howell-Jolly bodies, polychromasia)
- Reticulocyte count: Reflects state of erythroid activity of bone marrow (normal 0.5% to 1.5%).
- Bone marrow: Evaluates number of RBC precursors and maturation; rule out infiltration.
- Direct and indirect bilirubin
- Levels of lactate dyhydrogenase (LDH), aspartate aminotransferase (AST), uric acid, total iron, vitamin B_{12}, vitamin E, folic acid
- Direct and indirect Coombs' test
- Total iron-binding capacity (TIBC)
- Ferritin
- Free erythrocyte protoporphyrin

DIAGNOSIS

The client's Hgb and hematocrit should be compared with a set of standards appropriate for age. The corpuscular MCV and reticulocyte count should be analyzed to suggest a potential cause of the anemia.

Differential diagnosis includes the following:

- Autoimmune pancytopenia
- Marrow infiltration with a solid tumor
- Marrow suppression caused by drug toxins or infections
- Bleeding colitis
- Osteomyelitis
- Pyelonephritis
- Blood loss
- Hemolysis
- Chronic IBD
- Rheumatoid arthritis
- SLE
- Leukemia

Age-specific diagnosis (Table 10-1) includes the following:

NEWBORN

- Blood loss
- Hemolysis

Table 10-1   Age-Specific Diagnosis, Findings, and Treatment Plans for Anemia

AGE	DIAGNOSIS	FINDINGS	PLAN
Infant	Iron deficiency anemia	Serum ferritin <10 mg/ml CBC with RBC indexes decreased; MCV <mm Serum iron <30 mEq/dl Reticulocyte count may be low, normal, or slightly elevated Blood smear showing RBCs to be microcytic, hypochromic	Elemental iron in 3 divided doses
Adult	Iron deficiency anemia	Hgb <14g/dl in men, and <12 g/dl in women; hematocrit <42% in men, <36% in women Low MCV (microcytic) and low MCHC (hypochromic) Low RBC count Increased RBC distribution width Low serum iron (<50 mg/ml) TIBC elevated	Almost always from blood loss—identify and correct source of blood loss; oral iron replacement twice daily
All	Sickle cell anemia	Tests: Hgb electrophoresis, solubility test Peripheral smear: Target cells, poikilocytes, and sickled cells Liver function test results abnormal Decreased erythrocyte sedimentation rate Increased platelets	Prevention of infection by standard immunizations; penicillin prophylaxis starting at 2 to 3 months; treat febrile episodes for sepsis
All	Thalassemia	Hgb electrophoresis: Increased Hbg A (minor) and decreased or absent Hgb A (major) CBC: Microcytosis in minor; hypochromic microcytic in major Peripheral smear: Coarse basophilic stippling in minor; target cells and stippling in major	Major: Transfusions, chelating agents for hemosiderosis, splenectomy may be considered Minor: No therapy, genetic counseling, psychosocial support
Adult	Pernicious anemia	Hgb and hematocrit decreased RBCs decreased Reticulocytes normal or low MCV >100 mm, MCHC within normal limits Serum B12 decreased (0.1 μg/ml) Increased LDH Serum folate and/or RBC level normal or low Serum bilirubin increased	B_{12} (cyanocobalamin) injections
All	Aplastic anemia	Urinalysis: Increased urobilinogen Hypoplastic, fatty bone marrow (pancytopenia) Decreased WBCs, RBCs, platelets	Younger than 45: Bone marrow transplant; older than 45: cyclosporin
Pregnant female	Folic acid deficiency	Hgb and hematocrit decreased MCV increased (megaloblastic anemia) Decreased serum iron TIBC increased Serum folate <165 ng/ml	Folic acid supplementation daily (included in all prenatal vitamins); nutrition assessment and counseling

INFANT
- Iron deficiency anemia
- Gastrointestinal (GI) bleeding
- Thalassemia
- Sickle cell anemia
- Lead exposure
- Spherocytosis

TODDLER AND SCHOOL-AGE CHILD
- Fanconi's anemia
- Aplastic anemia
- Anemia of chronic G6PD deficiency
- Transient erythroblastopenia after illness

ADOLESCENT
- Iron deficiency anemia
- Aplastic anemia
- Autoimmune hemolysis
- Sickle cell anemia

ADULT
- Folic acid deficiency
- Pernicious anemia
- Iron deficiency anemia
- Autoimmune hemolysis
- Aplastic anemia

PREGNANT FEMALE
- Acute blood loss
- Iron deficiency anemia
- Folic acid deficiency

THERAPEUTIC PLAN

- The goal of treatment is to eradicate the anemia and its cause.
- Recommend referral to hematologist for multidisciplinary approach and pain management if needed for sickle cell anemia.

Client Education

IRON DEFICIENCY ANEMIA
- Identify causes of low iron and needed treatment plan.
- Teach family about diet high in iron and about side effects of iron therapy.

SICKLE CELL ANEMIA
- Identify causes of sickle cell crisis and disease process.
- Awareness of precipitating factors:
  —Cold exposure
  —Decreased fluid intake
  —Exercise at high altitude
  —Overexertion, emotional or physical stress
  —Increased blood viscosity

  —Viral or bacterial infections
  —Surgery, blood loss
- Need for routine health care
- Psychosocial support

PERNICIOUS ANEMIA
- Etiology and nature of disease
- Need for lifelong B_{12} replacement
- Review side effects of B_{12} injection.

EVALUATION/FOLLOW-UP

Evaluation of treatment response is discussed in the following sections.

Iron Deficiency Anemia

INFANTS. Reticulocyte count should be increased in 2 to 3 days. Hgb is rechecked in 2 to 3 weeks, at which time indices should have returned to normal. Iron therapy is continued for 2 to 3 months after Hgb levels have returned to normal, to replenish iron stores.

ADULTS. Continue iron 3 months after return of normal Hgb, to replenish iron stores.

Pernicious Anemia

- Follow-up older adults and clients with cardiac conditions in 48 hours (a rapid increase in RBC production can lead to hypovolemia).
- Consider iron supplementation.
- Check initial hematologic response in 4 to 6 weeks, then every 6 months for hematocrit, with stool check for occult blood (incidence of gastric cancer increases with pernicious anemia).

Folic Acid Deficiency

- Repeat Hgb measurement and hematocrit in 2 to 4 weeks (should expect increase of 2 points in Hgb within 1 month).
- Refer if anemia is severe.

REFERENCES

Bates, B. (1995). Physical exam and history taking (6th ed.). Philadelphia: J. B. Lippincott.

Cunningham, F., McDonald, P., Gant, N., Levens, K., Gilstrap, L., Hankins, G., & Clark, S. (1997). Hematological disorders. In *Williams obstetrics* (20th ed., pp. 1173-1189). Norwalk, CT: Appleton & Lange.

Jandl, J. H. (1987). The anemias. In J. H. Jandl (Ed.), *Blood: Textbook of hematology* (pp. 111-113). Boston: Little, Brown.

Kalinyak, K. (1997). Anemias. In R. Arceci (Ed.), *Hematology/oncology/stem cell transplant handbook* (2nd ed., pp. 87-116). Cincinnati: Hematology Oncology Division of Children's Hospital Medical Center.

Lane, P., Nuss, R., & Ambruso, D. (1995). Hematologic disorders. In W. Hay, J. Groothuis, A. Hayward, & M. Levin (Eds.), *Current pediatric diagnosis and treatment* (pp. 819-839). Norwalk, CT: Appleton & Lange.

Miller, D. (1989). Anemias: General considerations. In D. Miller, R. Baehner, & L. Miller (Eds.), *Blood diseases in infancy and childhood* (7th ed., pp. 111-136). St. Louis: Mosby.

Mitus, A., & Rosenthal, D. (1995). History and physical examination of relevance to the hematologist. In R. Handlin, S. Lux, & T. Stossel (Eds.), *Blood: Principles and practice of hematology* (pp. 3-19). Philadelphia: J. B. Lippincott.

REVIEW QUESTIONS

1. The most common presenting symptoms in childhood iron deficiency anemia include:

   a. Fever, pallor, and pain
   b. Pallor, lymphadenopathy, and night sweats
   c. Weight loss, pallor, and fever
   d. Pallor, tachycardia, fatigue, and poor dietary intake

2. Risk factors for development of anemia include all the following **except:**

   a. Family history of anemia
   b. History of pica
   c. Hyperbilirubinemia in the neonatal period
   d. Sibling with a history of hepatitis

3. In which of the following clients would you suspect vitamin B_{12} deficiency?

   a. Male, 36 years old, with 2-week history of pallor, fatigue, and anorexia
   b. Female, 60 years old, with a beefy, red, smooth tongue

   c. Male, 70 years old, with a 2- to 3-month history of fatigue, anorexia, and black, tarry stools
   d. Female, 30 years old, with history of 330 pg/ml serum vitamin B_{12} level

ANSWERS AND RATIONALES

1. ***Answer:*** d (assessment/history/hematopoietic/child)

   Rationale: Pallor, tachycardia, fatigue, and poor dietary intake are symptoms most commonly seen in children during the course of iron deficiency anemia. These symptoms reflect iron deficiency, which is always due to nutritional deficits of iron in young children who consume a diet high in nonfortified cow's milk. (Hay et al., 1995, p. 820)

2. ***Answer:*** d (assessment/history/hematopoietic/NAS)

   Rationale: Risk factors in development of anemia include a positive family history, a known history of pica, and hyperbilirubinemia in the neonatal period. Risk factors do not include a sibling with hepatitis. (Kalinyak, 1997, p. 90)

3. ***Answer:*** b (assessment/physical examination/hematopoietic/adult)

   Rationale: The objective assessment of a 60-year-old-woman with the beefy, red, smooth tongue would point to vitamin B_{12} deficiency. For the 36-year-old man, sudden onset of symptoms would lead one to suspect blood loss; for the 70-year-old, one suspects blood loss through the GI tract. The 30-year-old woman's serum vitamin concentration is elevated, not decreased. (Kalinyak, 1997, p. 97)

LEAD POISONING

OVERVIEW
Definition

Lead poisoning is defined as a blood lead level of ≥10 μg/dl.

Incidence

Lead poisoning is primarily a problem for children younger than 6 years because of the increased absorption (approximately 50%) of lead to which they are exposed. Adults generally absorb 10% of the lead to which they are exposed.

Etiology

Lead poisoning is caused by exposure to lead. Sources and pathways of lead exposure in children include the following:

LEAD-BASED PAINT. This remains the most common high-dose source of lead exposure for children 6 years old and younger. Many homes built before 1950 were painted with paint containing 50% or more lead.

PICA. The repeated ingestion of nonfood substances has been implicated in cases of lead poisoning. This includes not only paint chips but also dust or soil contaminated with lead from paint that flaked or chalked as it aged or was disturbed during home maintenance or renovation. These substances are usually ingested during normal, repetitive, hand-to-mouth activity.

SOIL AND DUST. Lead is deposited from paint, gasoline, and industrial sources in soil and dust, where it can serve as a significant source of lead exposure for children.

DRINKING WATER. The 1986 Safe Drinking Water Act Amendments banned the use of lead in public drinking water distribution systems and limited the lead content of brass used for plumbing to 8%. Lead pipes are still found in residences built before the 1920s. Pipes made of copper and soldered with lead came into general use in the 1950s. In general, lead in drinking water is not the predominant source for lead poisoning in children. Some water coolers and fountains have been found to have lead-soldered or lead-lined tanks. Patterns of intermittent water use from these fountains result in the water standing in the tanks longer than in typical residential situations, which can increase the amount of lead that is leached from the tanks. Several babies have been poisoned when hot tap water, which was then boiled (resulting in concentration of the lead), was used to make baby formula.

PARENTAL OCCUPATIONS AND HOBBIES. "Take-home" exposures may result when workers wear their work clothes home or wash them with the family laundry, or when they bring scrap or waste material home from work. Some industries in which workers are commonly exposed to lead are as follows:

- Secondary smelting and refining of nonferrous metals
- Plumbing fixture fittings and trim
- Motor vehicle parts and accessories (tire weights for balancing)
- Pottery
- Automotive repair shops
- Industrial machinery and equipment
- Batteries
- Glass products

AIRBORNE LEAD. Although lead use in gasoline has been markedly reduced, previous use has resulted in widespread contamination of soil and dust. However, airborne lead exposure is still minimal.

FOOD. The quantity of lead in the U.S. diet has decreased markedly in recent years. Improperly fired ceramic ware, leaded crystal, pewter ware, and lead-soldered cans result in lead leaching into foods. Some food-handling practices can increase the lead content of foods.

OTHER SOURCES. Lead exposure may also come from "traditional" or folk medicines, cosmetics, casting ammunition, fishing weights, toy soldiers, making stained glass, making pottery, refinishing furniture, burning lead-painted wood, and some plastic household blinds.

ASSESSMENT: SUBJECTIVE/HISTORY

Assess the following factors:
- Characteristics of home: Age, location, condition of paint, recent remodeling or restoration, pipes
- Pica behavior
- Use of folk remedies
- Use of imported ceramics

- Parent's occupation
- Others in the home with lead poisoning
- Signs and symptoms: Abdominal pain and cramping, irritability, fatigue, frequent vomiting, constipation, headache, excitability, inability to concentrate, behavioral changes, easily upset, sleep disorder, poor appetite, clumsiness, weakness, loss of recently acquired skills, convulsions
- Risk factors: Young age (<6 months), a sibling with lead poisoning, warm season

ASSESSMENT: OBJECTIVE/ PHYSICAL EXAMINATION

Physical Examination

Signs and symptoms as stated above may be noted during examination. Because symptoms do not usually occur until the child has had a significant lead exposure, the presence of any symptoms should be treated as a medical emergency.

Diagnostic Procedures

- Blood lead level ≥10 μg/dl
- Positive x-ray examination of kidneys and upper bladder (KUB) (presence of paint chips in abdomen)

DIAGNOSIS

Differential diagnosis includes the following:
- Attention deficit disorder
- Learning disabilities
- CNS tumor
- Anemia
- Developmental delay
- Colic
- Metabolic disorders

THERAPEUTIC PLAN

The following guidelines are adopted from the 1991 Centers for Disease Control and Prevention risk classification for children without symptoms:

Class I

- Blood lead <9 μg/dl
- Assess risk factors with every well child visit (at least yearly).

Class IIa

- Blood lead 10 to 14 μg/dl
- Rescreen 6 months.
- Assess risk factors for sources of lead exposure.
- Provide education about diet
  - —Increase high-calcium foods (refer to osteoporosis chapter for a listing of these foods). Lead is absorbed more efficiently in the presence of low calcium.
  - —Increase iron-containing foods (organ meats, red meat, green leafy vegetables, dried fruit).
- Provide education about cleaning (wet mopping with trisodium phosphate solution found in many dishwashing detergents).

Class IIb

- Blood lead 15 to 19 μg/dl
- Rescreen 3 months.
- Assess risk factors for sources of lead.
- Provide education about diet, cleaning, etc.
- Consider environmental investigation with a paint and water lead testing kit, found in most hardware stores, or call health department for professional testing.

Class IIIa

- Blood lead 20 to 24 μg/dl
- Complete medical assessment with KUB and long bone x-ray.
- Identify and eliminate environmental lead.
- Provide education about diet, cleaning, etc.
- Refer to local health department for environmental investigation.
- Rescreen 1 month.

Class IIIb

- Blood lead 25 to 44 μg/dl
- As above, plus start oral chelating treatment. Give succimer, 10 μg/kg or 350 mg/m^2 PO q 8 hours for 5 days. Reduce to 10 mg/kg or 350 mg/m^2 q 12 hours for 2 weeks (Table 10-2). A child receiving succimer should have blood lead, CBC, ferritin level, TIBC, calcium, liver enzymes, AST, blood urea nitrogen, creatinine, and medical evaluation done initially, 1 week after starting the medication, and on completion of the course of treatment (total 19-day treatment).
- The course can be repeated after a 3-week interval if lead level has not significantly dropped.

Table 10-2 Succimer Therapy for Lead Poisoning, Classes IIIb and IV

CHILD'S WEIGHT (lb)	CHILD'S WEIGHT (kg)	DOSAGE (mg)	CAPSULES
18-35	8-15	100	1
36-55	16-23	200	2
56-75	24-34	300	3
76-100	35-44	400	4
>100	>45	500	5

NOTE: Succimer dosages are given every 8 hours for 5 days and then every 12 hours for 2 weeks.

- In young children who cannot swallow capsules, succimer can be administered by separating the capsule and sprinkling the medicated beads on a small amount of soft food or putting them in a spoon and following with fruit drink.
- Identification of the source of lead in the child's environment and abatement of this source are critical to a successful therapy outcome. Chelation therapy is not a substitute for preventing further exposure to lead and should not be used to permit continued exposure to lead.

Class IV

- Blood lead 45 to 69 μg/dl
- Treat as above in classes IIIa and IIIb, however, admit child to the hospital for treatment with ethylenediaminetetraacetic acid (EDTA) in the following cases:
  —Client has symptoms.
  —Client is younger than 3 years and lead level is >60 μg/dl.
  —KUB is positive.

Class V

- Blood lead 70 ≥ μg/dl
- Medical emergency
- Treatment options: Chelation therapy with:
  —EDTA
  —Dimercaprol (BAL) and EDTA
  —Dimercaptosuccinic acid (DMSA)

Client Education

Provide detailed education for parents, including the following key points:
- Most homes built before 1950 contain lead paint.
- Many homes built between 1950 and 1978 contain lead paint.

- Check home for peeling paint, especially around door and window frames.
- Wet mop floors with trisodium phosphate solutions, contained in most dishwashing detergents.
- Most hardware stores sell simple lead testing kits for paint and water.
- *Never* attempt to remove lead paint yourself. Regular vacuuming, sanding, and scraping tend to stir up more lead into the air. Lead *must* be removed by a professional.
- Frequent handwashing is extremely important.
- Increase calcium and iron in the child's diet. Deficiencies increase absorption of lead.

EVALUATION

Lead levels may drop below 20 μg/dl within a few months of chelating treatment. Some children with higher levels of lead may take much longer and need to undergo chelation several times. Lead moves from storage in the bones back into the circulating blood, creating a "rebound" phenomenon. It is important to inform parents of this phenomenon so that they do not become discouraged when lead levels rebound.

REFERENCES

Centers for Disease Control and Prevention (1991). *Preventing lead poisoning in young children: A statement by the Centers for Disease Control.* Atlanta, GA: Author.

Illinois Department of Public Health. (1996). *Guidelines for the detection and management of lead poisoning for physicians and health care providers.* Springfield, IL: Illinois Department of Public Health.

Needham, D. D. (1994). Diagnosis and management of lead poisoned children: The pediatric nurse practitioner in a specialty program. *Journal of Pediatric Health Care, 8*(6), 268-273.

REVIEW QUESTIONS

1. Lead poisoning is primarily a problem for children younger than 6 years for which of the following reasons?

    a. Adults absorb less lead into their systems than do children.
    b. Adults are better handwashers
    c. Children are more prone to pica.
    d. Children do more hand-to-mouth activity.

2. The most common high-dose source of lead exposure for children is:

    a. Drinking water
    b. Pica
    c. Paint
    d. Soil

3. Lead poisoning is diagnosed when the blood lead level is:

    a. ≥ 10 μg/dl
    b. ≥ 15 μg/dl
    c. ≥ 20 μg/dl
    d. ≥ 25 μg/dl

4. Lead in dust can be controlled by wet mopping with:

    a. A chlorine bleach solution
    b. An ammonia-based solution
    c. Trisodium phosphate solution
    d. Hydrogen peroxide solution

5. Homes built before which of the following years should be assessed for lead paint:

    a. 1978
    b. 1980
    c. 1983
    d. 1984

6. If a parent suspects that the home's water distribution system contains lead, it is recommended that the parent:

    a. Use hot water from the faucet to make formula
    b. Use cold water to make formula
    c. Boil hot water form the faucet for 5 minutes to make formula.
    d. Boil hot water from the faucet for 10 minutes to make formula.

7. Lead pipes can still be found in homes built before:

    a. 1920
    b. 1930
    c. 1940
    d. 1950

8. A parental occupation that may cause "take home" lead exposure is:

    a. Pencil manufacturing company
    b. Cigarette manufacturing company
    c. Automotive repair shop
    d. Print shop

9. The most important subjective information to obtain when assessing a child's risk for lead exposure is:

    a. Pica behavior
    b. Use of folk remedies
    c. Age, location, and condition of the home
    d. Use of imported ceramics

10. A child with lead poisoning will often be seen with:

    a. Abdominal pain and cramping
    b. Irritability and fatigue
    c. Convulsions and coma
    d. No symptoms

11. A child with a blood lead level of 14 μg/dl should receive:

    a. KUB and long-bone x-ray examinations
    b. Oral chelating treatment
    c. Removal from the home
    d. Assessment of risk factors and rescreening every 3 months

12. If lead is found in the paint of a child's home, the parents should be encouraged to:

    a. Begin immediate home renovations
    b. Move to another location
    c. Leave it alone so not to stir it up
    d. Have it professionally removed

13. A child with lead poisoning should be encouraged to eat more:

    a. Meat and milk
    b. Green and yellow vegetables
    c. Bread and cereal
    d. Lentils

14. A child with a blood lead level of >70 μg/dl:

    a. Requires chelating treatment only

    b. Requires admission to the hospital if symptoms are present

    c. Should be treated as a medical emergency

    d. Needs frequent follow-up appointments in the office

15. If a child with lead poisoning has symptoms, the treatment should be which of the following?

    a. Treat as a medical emergency.

    b. Assess risk factors and recheck in 1 month.

    c. Educate parents on how to check home for lead.

    d. Encourage calcium- and iron-rich foods.

ANSWERS AND RATIONALES

1. *Answer:* a (assessment/physical examination/hematologic/child)

Rationale: Adults only absorb approximately 10% of the lead to which they are exposed, whereas children absorb as much as 50% of the lead to which they are exposed. (Centers for Disease Control and Prevention, 1991)

2. *Answer:* c (assessment/history/hematologic/child)

Rationale: The most common source of lead for children is lead in paint. (Illinois Department of Public Health, 1996)

3. *Answer:* a (assessment/physical examination/hematologic/NAS)

Rationale: Blood lead levels of ≥10 μg/dl are considered lead poisoning. (Needham, 1994)

4. *Answer:* c (plan/hematologic/NAS)

Rationale: Household dust containing lead can best be cleaned with a trisodium phosphate solution, found in most dishwashing detergents. (Centers for Disease Control and Prevention, 1991)

5. *Answer:* a (assessment/history/hematologic/NAS)

Rationale: Lead-based paint was still used in homes built before 1978. In 1978, a ban was placed on this type of paint. (Centers for Disease Control and Prevention, 1991)

6. *Answer:* b (plan/hematologic/infant)

Rationale: Water sitting in an old water tank can absorb lead from the tank or other parts of the distribution system. Heating or boiling water concentrates the lead. Using cold water from the faucet to make formula is the safest course. (Centers for Disease Control and Prevention, 1991)

7. *Answer:* a (assessment/physical examination/hematologic/NAS)

Rationale: Lead pipes can still be found in homes built before the 1920s. (Centers for Disease Control and Prevention, 1991)

8. *Answer:* c (assessment/physical examination/hematologic/NAS)

Rationale: Parents who work in automotive repair shops can bring home lead on their clothes. (Illinois Department of Public Health, 1996)

9. *Answer:* c (assessment/history/hematologic/child)

Rationale: The age (whether built before 1978), location (near a highway), and condition (any peeling old paint) of the home are the most useful pieces of information to obtain to assess the child's risk for lead poisoning. (Centers for Disease Control and Prevention, 1991)

10. *Answer:* d (assessment/history/hematologic/child)

Rationale: A child with lead poisoning often has no symptoms. By the time a child does show symptoms, the lead level is usually remarkably high and often requires exceptionally aggressive and urgent treatment. (Centers for Disease Control and Prevention, 1991)

11. *Answer:* d (plan/hematologic/child)

Rationale: A child with a blood lead level of 14 μg/dl should be assessed for risk factors and re-screened every 6 months. (Centers for Disease Control and Prevention, 1991)

12. *Answer:* d (plan/hematologic/child)

Rationale: Trying to remove lead paint from your home on your own can be very dangerous. It must be professionally removed. (Centers for Disease Control and Prevention, 1991)

13. *Answer:* a (plan/hematologic/child)

Rationale: Children with lead poisoning should be encouraged to eat more foods with calcium and iron. Any deficiency in these minerals increases the absorption of lead. (Centers for Disease Control and Prevention, 1991)

14. *Answer:* c (plan/hematologic/child)

Rationale: A blood lead level of >70 μg/dl is extremely dangerous and should be treated as a medical emergency. (Needham, 1994)

15. Answer: a (plan/hematologic/child)

Rationale: The presence of any symptoms of lead poisoning should be treated as a medical emergency. (Centers for Disease Control and Prevention, 1991)

LEUKEMIA

OVERVIEW
Definition

Leukemia is a proliferation of immature WBCs, originating in the bone marrow.

Pathophysiology

The overproliferation of immature WBCs in the bone marrow can completely replace the normal bone marrow precursors, leading to a decrease in RBCs, platelets, and granulocytes. Leukemic cells may also proliferate in other reticuloendothelial tissues and in other extramedullary sites, such as the central nervous system, testes, bones, or skin (Lampkin, 1997).

The cause is theorized to be ecogenetic. A genetic transformation of the progenitor (stem) cell occurs in response to environmental agents.

RISK FACTORS
- Genetic predisposition
  —Diamond-Blackfan anemia: Increased risk of acute myelocytic leukemia (AML)
  —Down syndrome (trisomy 21): From 10 to 20 times increased incidence
  —Bloom syndrome and Fanconi's anemia: Increased risk of AML
  AML
  —Ataxia-telangiectasia
  —Identical twins: A 25% increased risk of acute lymphocytic leukemia (ALL)
  —Nontwin siblings: Also increased risk of ALL
  —History of fetal loss
  —Advanced maternal age
- Possible environmental factors
  —Ionizing radiation
  —Chronic chemical exposure: Benzene
  —Previous malignancy treated with alkalating agents
  —Exposure to electromagnetic fields
  —Herbicides and pesticides
  —Maternal use of alcohol, contraceptives, diethylstilbestrol, or cigarettes
- Viral infections
  —Human T-cell leukemia/lymphoma virus (HTLV)–I: Linked to adult T-cell leukemia lymphoma
  —HTLV–II: Linked to hairy cell leukemia
  —HTLV–III: Linked to Kaposi's sarcoma
  —Epstein-Barr virus: Associated with L_3 subtype of ALL
- Immunodeficiency
  —Chronic use of immunosuppressive drugs
  —Wiskott-Aldrich syndrome
  —Congenital hypogammaglobulinemia
  —Ataxia-telangiectasia

TYPES AND INCIDENCE. Incidence of all types of leukemia is approximately 13 cases/100,000 population per year. In general, males are affected more than females and whites more than blacks.

Acute Lymphocytic Leukemia
- Abnormal proliferation of immature lymphocytes in the bone marrow
- Approximately 4 cases/100,000 children every year
- Approximately 3500 new cases each year in United States
- Peak incidence is at 3 to 5 years old.
- Males outnumber females (1.3:1).
- ALL accounts for 75% to 80% of all childhood leukemias.

Acute Myelogenous Leukemia
- Abnormal proliferation of immature myeloid stem cells in the bone marrow
- Ratio of AML to ALL is 1:4.
- Accounts for 15% to 25% of childhood leukemia.
- Approximately 10% of childhood AML occurs in infants younger than 2 years.
- Relatively constant incidence from birth through adolescence

Chronic Lymphocytic Leukemia (CLL)
- A persistent absolute lymphocytosis for at least 3 months
- The most common type of leukemia in the United States
- Males outnumber females (2:1 to 3:1)
- About 75% of CLL cases occur in persons 60 years old or older.

Chronic Myelogenous Leukemia (CML)
- Abnormal proliferation of differentiating myeloid cells in blood and bone marrow
- Juvenile CML
  —Rare in children
  —CML accounts for 1% to 5% of all childhood leukemias
  —If seen in children, it is almost always seen in infants younger than 2 years.
  —Relatively rapid course
  —Cytogenetic marker: Philadelphia chromosome
- Adult CML
  —Median age of onset is 45 years.
  —Natural course of disease: Progresses from chronic, to accelerated, and then to the blast phase.

Leukemia in Pregnancy
- Fewer than 1 case/100,000 pregnancies annually
- Limited studies done.
- Two large studies (Caligiuri & Mayer, 1989) of 72 cases of leukemia from 1975 to 1988 found types and incidences:
  —AML, 61%
  —ALL, 28%
  —CML, 7%

ASSESSMENT: SUBJECTIVE/HISTORY
Symptoms
- In acute leukemias, symptoms are present 1 to 2 weeks before diagnosis.
- In chronic leukemias, symptoms are chronic and less obvious.

ACUTE LYMPHOCYTIC LEUKEMIA AND ACUTE MYELOCYTIC LEUKEMIA. Most common presenting symptoms include pallor, bleeding, fever, and pain. These signs and symptoms are due to bone marrow infiltration and failure.
- Anemia: Anemia is present at diagnosis in most cases. Symptoms include malaise, weakness, dyspnea, irritability, fatigue, anorexia, pallor, and heart murmur.
- Thrombocytopenia: Thrombocytopenia is present in 75% of cases of childhood leukemia. Symptoms include petechiae, easy bruising, epistaxis, menorrhagia, GI and intracranial hemorrhage, and hematuria.
- Neutropenia: Fever at diagnosis is present in 60% of cases of childhood leukemia. Other symptoms include persistent infections and abscesses.
- Central nervous system (CNS) involvement: CNS involvement is present in <10% of cases. Symptoms include headache, vomiting, and visual disturbances.
- Bone pain: Bone pain is present at diagnosis in approximately 23% of cases. Pain is from the overproliferation of leukemia cells within the bone marrow space and possibly from bony destruction by leukemic infiltration.
- GI symptoms: GI symptoms are due to proliferation of leukemic cells in the abdominal viscera, liver, and spleen. Symptoms include anorexia, weight loss, abdominal pain, and hepatosplenomegaly.
- Generalized lymphadenopathy: This is common at diagnosis as a result of infiltration by leukemic cells.
- Genitourinary (GU) symptoms: In males, testicular ALL can be seen with a painless, firm, unilateral, or bilateral enlargement, with or without discoloration.

CHRONIC MYELOCYTIC LEUKEMIA. Most cases of CML are diagnosed during the chronic phase. Symptoms at diagnosis may include splenomegaly, hepatomegaly, fever, night sweats, pallor, weight loss, bone pain, and lymphadenopathy. If hyperleukocytosis is present, complications include focal or diffuse neurologic findings, respiratory distress, metabolic disturbances, and priapism.

JUVENILE CHRONIC MYELOCYTIC LEUKEMIA. This condition usually affects children younger than 2 years. Symptoms include cutaneous lesions (eczema, xanthomata, and café au lait spots), generalized lymphadenopathy, marked splenomegaly, hepatomegaly, and hemorrhagic problems. A facial rash (erythematous, maculopapules, or desquamative) is common and may have been present for months before diagnosis. Respiratory symptoms, including cough, expiratory wheezing, and tachypnea, may also be present.

CHRONIC LYMPHOCYTIC LEUKEMIA. Most cases are diagnosed during the chronic phase. Symptoms at diagnosis include malaise, increased fatigability, generalized lymphadenopathy, and splenomegaly. As the disease progresses, hypogammaglobulinema may develop.

Past Medical History

- Exposure to cytotoxic drugs, benzene, chloramphenicol
- Genetic abnormalities
- Exposure to HTLV-I virus
- Family history of cancer
- Recent history of viral illness
- History of previous illnesses or surgery
- Medications, including home remedies, OTC drugs, vitamin and mineral supplements, and borrowed medicines
- Allergies
- Tobacco, alcohol, or drug use
- Immunizations and screening tests
- Psychosocial history: Home situation and significant others, including family and friends.

ASSESSMENT: PHYSICAL EXAMINATION
Physical Examination

Perform a complete physical examination, with increased attention to the following:

- Vital signs
- Weight
- Signs and symptoms of infection
- General appearance
- Skin: Excessive bruising, petechiae, pallor, rashes, infections, leukemia cutis (leukemic skin infiltration associated mostly with AML)
- Lymphatic system: Check for neck, axilla, supraclavicular, infraclavicular, epitrochlear, and inguinal nodal enlargement.
- HEENT: Fundi, papilledema
- Chest: Murmurs from anemia, wheezing and decreased breath sounds from a possible mediastinal mass
- Abdomen: Hepatosplenomegaly
- Male GU: Check testes for unilateral or bilateral firm, painless enlargement, with or without scrotal discoloration

DIAGNOSTIC TESTS

- CBC with differential
  —WBCs >50,000 cells/mm^3 in 20% of clients with ALL
  —Initial WBC is single most important predictor of prognosis.
  —Low absolute neutrophil count is present.
  —Hgb <10 g/dl
  —Thrombocytopenia (platelets <100,000 cells/mm^3) present at diagnosis in 75%.
  —Blast cells may or may not be seen on differential. Bone marrow may be "packed" before blasts are seen on peripheral smear.
- Bone marrow aspiration shows ≥25% blasts; cytogenetics, immunophenotyping, and special stains are done to differentiate type of leukemia.
- Bone marrow biopsy
- Lumbar puncture to rule out CNS involvement
- Chest x-ray film to check for mediastinal mass
- Serum immunoglobulin levels low at diagnosis in 30% of clients with ALL
- Increased serum uric acid levels can lead to uric acid nephrology and renal failure.
- Elevated liver function test results
- Evaluation of calcium phosphate
- Blood cultures if client is febrile

Prognostic Factors

- Initial WBC count: High risk if WBCs >50,000 cells/mm^3
- Age at diagnosis: Poor prognosis for children younger than 2 or older than 10 years
- Hgb level: Poorer prognosis if low
- Platelet count: Poorer prognosis if low
- Ethnicity: Blacks have poorer prognosis.

- Presence of mediastinal mass, organomegaly, or lymphadenopathy: More tumor burden requires more intense chemotherapy.

DIAGNOSIS

Differential diagnosis includes the following:
- Aplastic anemia
- Marrow infiltration with a solid tumor
- Autoimmune pancytopenia
- Immune thrombocytopenia
- Severe megaloblastic anemia
- Overwhelming infection
- Rheumatoid arthritis
- Marrow suppression related to drugs, toxins, or infections

CHILDREN. Most likely diagnosis is ALL, then AML.

ADULTS. Most likely diagnosis is CML or CLL.

PREGNANT FEMALE. Most likely diagnosis is AML, then ALL; least likely is CML.

THERAPEUTIC PLAN

Refer client if CBC, differential, history, and physical examination lead to suspicions of leukemia. The goal of treatment is to eradicate leukemic blast cells so that normal cells can regrow.

Acute Lymphocytic Leukemia

Treatment consists of combination chemotherapy, often according to specific multicenter protocols. Cranial-spinal radiation is used if there is CNS involvement. Length of the treatment would be 2 years plus a few months for girls and 3 years plus a few months for boys.

Acute Myelocytic Leukemia

Treatment consists of extremely intense combination chemotherapy. Duration of treatment is shorter than for ALL. Cranial-spinal radiation is used if there is CNS involvement. Bone marrow transplantation (BMT) is performed if a complete match is found. Most treatment is done in the hospital.

Chronic Myelocytic Leukemia

JUVENILE TYPE. Generally this disease is resistant to therapy. Median survival is less than 9 months from diagnosis. BMT is the only possible curative treatment.

ADULT TYPE. Goal of treatment is to provide symptomatic relief by lowering the WBC count and reducing liver and spleen size. Hydroxyurea or busulfan, given as single agents, can be used to regulate leukocytosis. BMT is the only possible curative treatment.

Chronic Lymphocytic Leukemia

Stable, symptom-free clients, with or without lymphadenopathy or splenomegaly, do not require treatment. Symptoms (weight loss, malaise, anemia, thrombocytopenia) are treated with alkylating agents (chlorambucil) and prednisone.

Leukemia in Pregnancy

- AML or ALL requires immediate and aggressive treatment with combination chemotherapy.
- If AML or ALL is diagnosed in the first trimester, prognoses for both mother and child are extremely poor.
- If AML or ALL is diagnosed and treated in the second or third trimester, there is a 75% chance of remission and only a 1.5% incidence of congenital anomalies.
- CML has a slow, indolent course.

Supportive Care Guidelines

- Hold all immunizations during treatment. Immunizations may be resumed 6 months to 1 year after treatment.
- Avoid live virus vaccines (measles-mumps-rubella, oral polio)
- Siblings of clients also need to avoid live virus vaccines.
- Varicella-zoster immunoglobulin within 72 to 96 hours of varicella exposure in nonimmune children
- Prophylactic trimethoprim-sulfamethoxazole (Bactrim) to prevent *Pneumocystis carinii*, 5 mg/kg/day 3 days/week.
- Monthly use of IV or aerosolized pentamidine if client is allergic to Bactrim
- Empiric use of broad-spectrum antibiotics for fever and neutropenia
- No IM injections
- No rectal temperatures or suppositories
- No tampons
- Use soft toothbrush or toothettes for oral care.
- If central line access is in place, administer antibiotic prophylaxis before dental work.

- If client is febrile, always check a CBC with differential as soon as possible to rule out fever from neutropenia.

EVALUATION/FOLLOW-UP

- Client should be referred to a hematology/oncology specialist in a timely manner.
- Complications related to delays in referral are to be avoided.
- Client and family should be knowledgeable about diagnosis and treatment plan.
- Client and family should be knowledgeable about expected and toxic side effects of chemotherapy.
- Supportive care guidelines should be clear for family and primary care provider.
- Communication between hematology/oncology specialist and primary care provider should be clear, concise, and current.

REFERENCES

Altman, A. J., Barnard, D. R., Iacuone, J. J., Wiener, E. S., Wolff, J. J., & Ablin, A. R., (1993). The prevention of infection. In A. R. Abline (Ed.), *Supportive care of children with cancer.* Baltimore: Johns Hopkins University Press.

Antonelli, N. M., Dotters, D. J., Katz, V. L., & Kueller, J. A. (1996). Cancer in pregnancy: A review of the literature. *Obstetrical and Gynecological Survey 51*(2), 135-142.

Baer, M. R. (1993). Management of unusual presentations of acute leukemia. In C. D. Bloomfield & G. P. Herzig (Eds.), *Hematology/oncology clinic of North America: Management of acute leukemia.* Philadelphia: W. B. Saunders.

Bates, B. (1995). *Physical exam and history taking* (2nd ed.). Philadelphia: J. B. Lippincott.

Bennetts G. A. (1993). Immunization of patients with malignant disease. In A. R. Ablin (Ed.), *Supportive care of children with cancer.* Baltimore: John Hopkins University Press.

Caligiuri, M. A., & Mayer, R. J. (1989). Pregnancy and leukemia. *Seminars in Oncology 16,* 338-396.

Cohen, D. G. (1993). Leukemia in children and adolescents—Acute lymphocytic leukemia. In G. V. Foley, D. Fochtman, & K. H. Mooney (Eds.), *Nursing care of the child with cancer* (2nd ed.). Philadelphia: W. B. Saunders.

Lampkin, B. (1997). Acute lymphoblastic leukemia. In R. J. Arceci (Ed.), *Hematology/oncology/stem cell transplant handbook* (2nd ed.). Cincinnati: Hematology/Oncology Division, Children's Hospital Medical Center.

Panzarella, C., Aitken, T., Patterson, K., Mosher, R., Moore, R., Moore, K., & Wofford, L. (1993). *Pediatric oncology nursing study guide.* Skokie, IL: Association of Pediatric Oncology Nurses.

Reynoso, E. E., Shepherd, F. A., Messner, H. A., Farquharson, M., Garvey, M., & Baker, M. (1987). Acute leukemia during pregnancy: The Toronto leukemia study group experience with long-term follow-up of children exposed in utero to chemotherapeutic agents. *Journal of Clinical Oncology 5,* 1098-1106.

Salerno, M. (1994). Hematological and oncological disorders. In V. L. Millong (Ed.), *Adult nurse practitioner certification review guide* (2nd ed.). Potomac, MD: Health Leadership Associates.

Sambrano, J. (1997). Chronic myelogenous leukemia. In R. J. Arceci (Ed.), *Hematology/oncology/stem cell transplant handbook* (2nd ed.). Cincinnati, OH: Hematology/Oncology Division, Children's Hospital Medical Center.

Skidmore-Roth, L. (1995). *Mosby's nursing drug reference.* St. Louis: Mosby.

Tierney, J. (1994). Hematological/oncological/immunological disorders. In V. L. Millong (Ed.), *Pediatric nurse practitioner certification review guide* (2nd ed.). Potomac, MD: Health Leadership Associates.

Waterburg, L., & Zieve, P. D. (1995). Selected illnesses affecting lymphocytes: Mononucleosis, chronic lymphocytic leukemia, and the undiagnosed patient with lymphadenopathy. In L. R. Barker, J. R. Burton, & P. D. Zieve (Eds.), *Principles of ambulatory medicine* (4th ed.). Baltimore: Williams & Wilkins.

Wiley, F. M. (1993). Leukemia in children and adolescents: Acute myelogenous leukemia. In G. V. Foley, D. Foctman, & K. H. Mooney (Eds.), *Nursing care of the child with cancer* (2nd ed.). Philadelphia: W. B. Saunders.

REVIEW QUESTIONS

1. The most common presenting symptoms in childhood ALL are:

 a. Lymphadenopathy, fever, and night sweats
 b. Pallor, bleeding, fever, and pain
 c. Headache, vomiting, and visual disturbances
 d. Anorexia, abdominal pain, and weight loss

2. Jenny, a 6-year-old with ALL diagnosed 1 year ago, is away from home visiting her aunt. She had a temperature of 102° F last night. Her aunt knows that Jenny is on a "maintenance" chemotherapy regimen consisting of prednisone, 5 day pulses/month, 6 mercaptopurine pills/day, and methotrexate pills once per week. Jenny also takes trimethoprim-sulfamethoxazole (Bactrim) for *P. carinii* prophylaxis. On physical examination, Jenny has no obvious site of infection and is now afebrile and playing. What should you do for Jenny?

   a. Send her home with instructions to take acetaminophen (Tylenol) q 4 hours as needed.
   b. Give her amoxicillin, 250 mg PO tid for 10 days.
   c. Obtain a CBC with differential to rule out neutropenia.
   d. Tell her to hold chemotherapy until she sees her oncologist.

3. Children with ALL are prescribed either trimethoprim-sulfamethoxazole (Bactrim), 5 mg/kg/day on 3 days/week, or pentamidine, IV or aerosolized once per month as prophylaxis against:

   a. Cytomegalovirus retinitis
   b. *Histoplasmosis* pneumonia
   c. Respiratory syncytial virus
   d. *P. carinii* pneumonia

4. John, a 70-year-old male, whose CLL was diagnosed 3 years ago, has been symptom free until recently. He now has weight loss, malaise, anemia, and thrombocytopenia. His oncologist begins treating John with chlorambucil and prednisone. Parameters for evaluating the efficacy of this treatment include all the following **except:**

   a. John and family are able to state possible side effects of medications.
   b. John's weight stabilizes or increases, and symptoms improve.
   c. John keeps his follow-up appointments with his oncologist.
   d. John seeks information about his disease.

5. Which of the following statements is true?

   a. CML is the most common type of leukemia in the United States.
   b. CLL usually affects males older than 60 years.
   c. The median age of onset for adult CML is younger than 30 years.
   d. The ratio of AML to ALL is 4:1.

6. Risk factors in development of leukemia include all the following **except:**

   a. Chronic use of immunosuppressive drugs
   b. Twin with leukemia
   c. Chronic chemical exposure, especially benzene
   d. Chronic aspirin use

7. What are the most common to the least common types of leukemia that can occur in pregnancy?

   a. CLL (60%), CML (25%), AML (15%)
   b. CML (65%), AML (30%), ALL (5%)
   c. ALL (70%), AML (20%), CML (10%)
   d. AML (61%), ALL (28%), CML (7%)

8. A testicular examination is a part of the initial physical examination for males and is done at least monthly during treatment to rule out leukemic infiltration in the testicles. The most common presentation would be:

   a. Swelling, erythema, and tenderness in one or both testes
   b. Painful, sudden enlargement of one testicle
   c. Bilateral or unilateral firm, painless enlargement of the testicles, with or without discoloration.
   d. Testicular torsion

9. Jimmy, a 3-year-old male, comes to his primary care provider with a 2-week history of fatigue, easy bruising, and paleness. A physical examination reveals multiple bruises on his extremities, petechiae on his face, and extremely pale subconjunctiva and lips. Jimmy has a low-grade fever, with a temperature of 99.9° FPO, but the rest of his physical examination is within normal limits. A CBC with a differential is obtained and sent to a local laboratory. With this amount of information, the differential diagnosis could include all the following **except:**

   a. Immune thrombocytopenia
   b. Iron deficiency anemia
   c. Acute viral exanthem
   d. ALL

10. Tim, a 50-year-old male with a 2-year history of CML, comes to his primary care provider with a 2-week history of worsening sinus symptoms. Tim states that his oncologist considers his CML to be in a chronic phase and that he is supposed to be taking "some pill" every day, but admits that he "is not good at taking it." Tim's lack of understanding of his disease and treatment places him at risk for disease progression and complications. This evaluation leads his primary care provider to do all the following **except:**

 a. Call Tim's oncologist for an update on Tim's condition.
 b. Write another prescription for hydroxyurea.
 c. Make sure Tim has a follow-up appointment with his oncologist.
 d. Treat Tim's sinus infection with an appropriate oral antibiotic.

ANSWERS AND RATIONALES

1. *Answer:* b (assessment/history/hematologic/ child)

Rationale: Pallor, bleeding, fever, and pain are early symptoms in the course of the disease and may be present 1 to 2 weeks before the actual diagnosis. These symptoms reflect bone marrow replacement with leukemic cells, resulting in anemia, thrombocytopenia, neutropenia, and pain from bone marrow "packing" with leukemic replacement. (Cohen, 1993)

2. *Answer:* c (assessment/physical examination/ hematologic/child)

Rationale: It is critical to obtain a CBC with differential to determine Jenny's ability to fight infection. An absolute neutrophil count of <500 cells/mm^3 plus a temperature ≥100.5° F could necessitate a hospital admission, complete with blood cultures and IV antibiotics.

3. *Answer:* d (plan/hematologic/child)

Rationale: *Pneumocystis carinii* is the most common opportunistic infection. Prophylaxis includes maintenance Bactrim.

4. *Answer:* d (evaluation/hematologic/aging adult)

Rationale: Although seeking information about the disease is important, it does not indicate the efficacy of the treatment. Knowing the side effects of the medications, increasing weight, and keeping follow-up appointments all help in evaluating the effectiveness of treatment. (Salerno, 1994)

5. *Answer:* b (diagnosis/hematologic/aging adult)

Rationale: CLL usually affects men older than 60. It is the most common type of leukemia. The median onset for adult CML is 45. The ratio of AML to ALL is 1:4. (Lampkin, 1997)

6. *Answer:* d (assessment/history/hematologic/ NAS)

Rationale: Aspirin may cause adverse hematologic reactions, such as increased prothrombin time, partial thromboplastin time, and bleeding time. It can also cause thrombocytopenia, agranulocytosis, leukopenia, neutropenia, and hemolytic anemia.

7. *Answer:* d (diagnosis/hematologic/adult)

Rationale: The most common to least common types of leukemia in pregnancy are as follows: AML, 61%; ALL, 28%; CML, 7%. (Caligiuri & Mayer, 1989)

8. *Answer:* c (assessment/physical examination/ hematologic/NAS)

Rationale: It is theorized that there is a blood-gonad barrier, similar to the CNS blood-brain barrier. These barriers allow "sanctuaries" for leukemic cells. Additionally, the relatively hypothermic environment of the testicles and decreased concentrations of immunoglobulins in the testicles make the testicles less susceptible to cytotoxic agents.

9. *Answer:* c (diagnosis/hematologic/child)

Rationale: A history of a exanthem can possibly lead to these symptoms of bone marrow suppression, but an acute viral exanthem would not have these presenting symptoms.

10. *Answer:* b (evaluation/hematologic/adult)

Rationale: Tim's oncologist should be updated on Tim's condition, and the oncologist should consistently be the one to write for hydroxyurea.

Immune System

AIDS

OVERVIEW
Definition

AIDS, or *acquired immunodeficiency syndrome,* is a transmissible retroviral disease caused by infection with the human immunodeficiency virus (HIV) and manifested by depression of cell-mediated immunity. The outcome of this process is an increase in opportunistic infections with bacterial, fungal, protozoan, or viral pathogens.

Incidence

One in 250 persons in the United States is infected with HIV. The overall seroprevalence estimate for childbearing women in the United States is 0.15%, which reflects approximately 6000 births per year to infected women. The efficiency of vertical transmission of HIV transmission from mother to infant is approximately 12% to 39%.

AIDS Indicator Conditions*

- HIV-seropositivity with CD4 cell count <200 cells/mm³ or a percentage of CD4 cells <14%
- Candidiasis of bronchi, trachea, or lungs
- Candidiasis of esophagus
- Cervical cancer, invasive
- Coccidioidomycosis, disseminated or extrapulmonary
- Cryptococcocis, extrapulmonary
- Cryptosporidiosis, chronic intestinal (longer than 1 month in duration)
- Cytomegalovirus (CMV) disease (other than liver, spleen, or nodes)

- CMV retinitis (with loss of vision)
- Encephalopathy, HIV-related
- Herpes simplex: Chronic ulcers (1 month duration), bronchitis, pneumonitis, or esophagitis
- Histoplasmosis, disseminated or extrapulmonary
- Isosporiasis, chronic intestinal (longer than 1 month duration)
- Kaposi's sarcoma
- Lymphoma, Burkitt's (or equivalent term)
- Lymphoma, immunoblastic (or equivalent term)
- Lymphoma, primary, of brain
- *Mycobacterium avium* complex or *Mycobacterium kansasii,* disseminated or extrapulmonary
- *Mycobacterium tuberculosis,* any site (pulmonary or extrapulmonary)
- *Mycobacterium,* other species or unidentified species, disseminated or extrapulmonary
- *Pneumocystis carinii* pneumonia (PCP)
- Pneumonia, recurrent
- Progressive multifocal leukoencephalopathy
- *Salmonella* septicemia, recurrent
- Toxoplasmosis of brain
- Wasting syndrome from HIV

Table 11-1 presents the revised classification system used by the Centers for Disease Control and Prevention for individuals with HIV infection and AIDS.

Pathophysiology

The major target for HIV is the CD4 T lymphocyte; macrophages and monocytes may also be

---

*Centers for Disease Control and Prevention, 1992.

Table 11-1 CDC 1993 Revised Classification System for HIV Infection and Expanded AIDS Surveillance Case Definition for Adolescents and Adults

CD4 + T-cell categories (cells/mm³)	CLINICAL CATEGORIES		
	(A), asymptomatic, acute (primary) HIV, or PGL	(B), symptomatic, not (A) or (C) conditions	(C), AIDS indicator conditions
(1) >500	A1	B1	C1
(2) 200-499	A2	B2	C2
<200 AIDS-indicator T cell count	A3	B3	C3

From Centers for Disease Control and Prevention (1992). 1993 Revised classification system for HIV infection and expanded surveillance case definition for AIDS among adolescents and adults. *MMWR: Morbidity and Mortality Weekly Report, 44*(RR-17), 1-19. Shaded areas indicate AIDS.
PGL, Persistent generalized lymphadenopathy.

infected. The virus attaches to the CD4 cell, enters the cytoplasma, and uncoats. By means of the viral enzyme reverse transcriptase, a DNA copy of the viral RNA genome is transcribed and duplicated. This new DNA integrates into the DNA of the host cell. This process generates viral buds that separate from the host cell, thereby initiating viral replication.

HIV is transmitted by sexual exposure, by contamination in intravenous drug use (IDU), through contaminated blood and blood products, and from mother to fetus. Within 2 to 6 weeks after exposure and lasting approximately 1 to 2 weeks, there are symptoms indicative of acute retroviral conversion in approximately 50% to 70% of those exposed. These symptoms, characteristic of infectious mononucleosis or flulike in character, include fever, arthralgias, myalgias, and fatigue. Physical examination may reveal a diffuse, erythematous rash and generalized adenopathy. This clinical presentation coincides with high levels of viral replication, which are measured by HIV RNA and the presence of p24 antigen. CD4 cell counts drop dramatically and CD8 cell counts generally rise in response to the virus. Seroconversion generally takes 6 to 12 weeks after transmission. The levels of HIV RNA are sharply reduced and CD4 counts return to higher levels, but generally not to preinfection levels. This stage is followed by a prolonged stage of asymptomatic clinical latency. During this stage, there is a large viral reservoir actively replicating in the lymphoid tissues. As this clinical latency continues and disease progresses, the framework of the lymph tissue disintegrates, accounting for the rise of viral burden detectable in the plasma. Immunologic damage increases, and opportunistic infections develop unabated. The rate of disease progression is outlined in Figure 11-1.

CLIENTS FOR WHOM HIV TESTING IS RECOMMENDED

- Persons who have sexually transmitted diseases (STDs).
- High-risk categories: These include persons with history of IDU, gay and bisexual men, persons with hemophilia, and regular sexual partners of persons in these categories. Lower risk categories: These include prostitutes and persons who received blood or artificial insemination during the years 1978 through 1985.
- Persons who consider themselves at risk or request testing
- Women at risk who are of childbearing age; risk factors include IDU, prostitution, male sexual partner with history of IDU, bisexual or HIV infection, living in a high-prevalence community, birth in a high-prevalence country, or blood transfusion between 1978 and 1985
- All pregnant women
- Clients with clinical or laboratory findings suggestive of HIV infection
- Clients with active tuberculosis (TB)
- Recipients who receive blood or body fluid exposures

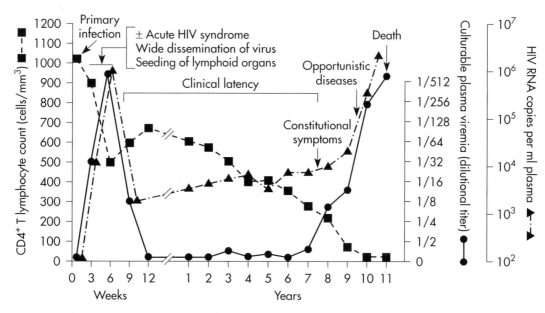

Fig. 11-1   Typical course of HIV infection without therapy. (From Bartlett, J. G., & Finkbeiner, A. [1996]. *The Johns Hopkins Hospital guide to medical care of patients with HIV infection.* Baltimore: Williams & Wilkins.)

- Health care workers who perform exposure-prone invasive procedures
- Hospital admissions for clients 15 to 45 years old in facilities where seroprevalence is ≥1% or the AIDS case rate is ≥1 case/1000 discharges
- Donors of blood, semen, and organs (this is the only category in which testing is mandatory in all states)

ASSESSMENT: SUBJECTIVE/HISTORY
Past Medical History

- Fatigue
- Malaise
- Fevers without cause with oral temperatures ≥100° F
- Night sweats
- Swollen or painful lymph nodes
- Unexplained loss of ≥10% of body weight
- Loss of appetite
- Cough, shortness of breath (SOB), chest tightness, orthopnea, tachypnea, or history of TB or purified protein derivative of tuberculin (PPD) testing
- Oral candidiasis (thrush)
- Changes in central nervous system (CNS) function, including headaches, changes in mental status, stiff neck, seizures, and cognitive, motor, and behavioral changes
- Skin rashes, lesions, bruises
- Herpes zoster (shingles)
- Allergies: Foods, pets, environment
- STDs: Gonorrhea, *Chlamydia*, syphilis, condylomata, hepatitis, herpes simplex
- Sexual preference and safe sex practices
- Female clients: Pregnancy history, Papanicolaou smear history, vaginal infections, contraceptive use
- Children: Gestational history, including drug exposure, labor and delivery history, gestational age at birth, and weight at birth; growth patterns, feeding patterns, developmental milestones, history of illnesses
- Substance abuse
- Smoking
- Assess ongoing high-risk behavioral exposures that may place the client at risk for opportunistic infections or risk of HIV transmission to others.
- Assess the client's perception and knowledge about HIV infection. Has the client ever known anyone infected with HIV? Has the client ever taken care of anyone with HIV infection or AIDS?

Medication History

Medication history should include prescribed and OTC drugs and herbs, vitamins, and other non-traditional therapies.

Family History

- Cardiopulmonary
- Diabetes
- Gastrointestinal
- Cancer
- Depression
- Suicide
- Substance abuse
- Is the client's family aware of the diagnosis? If not, will they be informed?
- Previous family experiences with HIV infection

Psychosocial History

- Signs and symptoms of depression
- Suicidal ideation
- Previous psychologic or psychiatric care
- Support network of family and friends
- Current employment status and medical and dental benefits

ASSESSMENT: OBJECTIVE/ PHYSICAL EXAMINATION

Physical Examination

A summary of physical examination findings and considerations for clients with AIDS is presented in Table 11-2.

Diagnostic Procedures

- HIV serology: Test results are reported as negative, positive, or indeterminate. A positive HIV serologic result requires both a positive enzyme-linked immunosorbent assay (ELISA) and the confirmatory positive Western blot. If the test result is questionable because of the client's history, repeated testing is warranted.
- CD4 count: Results of the CD4 count direct initiation and use of prophylactic antiretrovirals, treatment for opportunistic infections, and diagnostic tests. The test is done initially and repeated every 6 months.
- Complete blood cell count (CBC): Initially then every 3 to 6 months
- HIV RNA: This test is used primarily for disease staging and monitoring of the response to antiretroviral therapies. Frequency of testing should coincide with CD4 screening.

- Venereal Disease Research Laboratory test (VDRL) or rapid plasma reagin test: Initially and yearly, if client is sexually active
- Chemistry panel: Initially and when warranted by disease status or adverse drug reaction
- Hepatitis: The choice of diagnostic test is determined by client history. Hepatitis B immunization status can be determined.
- PPD: This test, done initially and yearly, should be repeated in nonreactors with suspected TB or exposure to TB. Induration ≥5 mm is considered a positive result.
- Chest x-ray film (CXR): When clinically warranted
- Papanicolaou smear: Do initially and repeat every 6 to 12 months according to client's immune status.
- Toxoplasmosis serology: Initially and when client is severely immunocompromised (CD4 ≤100 cells/mm^3)

DIAGNOSIS

Differential diagnosis includes numerous and varied possibilities, depending on client history and physical examination. Most common are the following:

- Persistent generalized lymphadenopathy
- Cytopenias: Anemia, leukopenia, thrombocytopenia
- Pulmonary symptoms suggesting PCP
- Kaposi's sarcoma
- Candidiasis: Vaginal, esophageal, oral
- Constitutional symptoms: Weight loss, night sweats, fatigue, chronic fever or chronic diarrhea for 30 days
- Bacterial infections, primarily pulmonary
- TB
- STDs
- Neurologic syndromes
  —HIV-associated dementia: Difficulty concentrating, memory loss, mental slowing
  —Peripheral syndrome: Pain and paresthesia of the feet

THERAPEUTIC PLAN
Physician Consult

Client returns in 2 weeks to discuss laboratory results. The plan of care is reviewed with the client at that time, allowing client involvement and questions.

Table 11-2   Physical Examination of Clients With AIDS

AREA	FINDINGS	CONSIDER
Mouth	Whitish coating on tongue, gums, roof of mouth	Oral candidiasis
	Fine lines or ridges on sides of tongue	Hairy leukoplakia
	Purple spots or lesions	Kaposi's sarcoma
	Bleeding gums	ITP
	Lesions	Herpes simplex, aphthous ulcers
Eyes	Cotton-wool spots, exudate plus hemorrhage	CMV retinitis
Neck	Swollen, painful lymph nodes	Lymphadenopathy
	Nuchal rigidity	Cryptococcosis
Lungs	Auscultation for extraneous sounds (rales, wheezes, rhonchi)	PCP *Pneumococcus* *M. tuberculosis*
	Cough	Bacterial pneumonia
Abdomen	Abnormal tenderness	ITP
	Enlarged liver/spleen	Hepatitis Cirrhosis Cancers
Genitourinary/rectal	Warts	Venereal warts
	Whitish coating of membranes	Candidal infection
	Ulcers/lesions	Herpes simplex Syphilis
Skin (entire body examination)	Purple lesions	Kaposi's sarcoma
	Vesicular lesions	Herpes simplex or zoster
	Bruising	ITP
	Dry, flaking skin	Seborrheic dermatitis
	Rashes	Drug reactions Syphilis Disseminated disease
	Warts/papules	Molluscum
Neurologic	Memory loss	Cryptococcosis
	Personality changes	Toxoplasmosis
	Decreased cognitive function	CNS lesions
	Decreased or increased reflexes	HIV dementia
	Neuropathies	Progressive multifocal leukoencephalopathy
Gynecologic	Yeast/white discharge	Vaginal candidiasis
	Papular lesions	Condylomata acuminatum

Modified from Bartlett, J. A. (1996). *Care and management of patients with HIV infection.* Durham, NC: Glaxo Wellcome. *ITP,* Immune thrombocytopenia purpura.

Pharmacologic Treatment

- Antiretroviral medication decisions are made in collaboration with a physician. Medication selection according to clinical and laboratory profile of the client is at present highly controversial and subjective, as well as constantly changing with new developments. All recommendations must therefore be periodically reviewed and modified.
- Indications to treat (Bartlett, 1996): CD4 count <500 cells/mm³; it is likely that future strategies will consider initiation of treatment with higher CD4 counts and viral burden of 20,000 to 75,000 copies/dl as a possible independent indicator of treatment.
- Monotherapy is generally not advocated, although some considerations may justify exceptions.
  —Didanosine (DDI)
  —Stavudine (d4T)
- Combination therapy
  —Nucleoside analogs (Zidovudine [AZT] plus lamivudine [3TC])

—Protease inhibitor (Saquinavir, indinavir, or ritonavir) plus nucleoside analog (AZT, ddI, zalcitabine [ddC], d4T, or 3TC)
—Protease inhibitor plus 3TC plus AZT
—AZT plus DDI or ddC
- Pregnant women: AZT is initiated at 14 to 34 weeks' gestation and carried through to delivery
  —Labor: AZT IV infusion
  —Neonate: AZT beginning 8 to 12 hours after birth
- HIV transmission occurs in utero, at delivery, and with breast-feeding. AZT reduces the rate of transmission from 25% in those untreated to 9% in those receiving AZT.

Prevention of Opportunistic Disease

TUBERCULOSIS. HIV and AIDS have substantially increased the prevalence of TB in the United States, as well as of isoniazid (INH)- and rifampin-resistant strains. This represents a significant health threat to those who live and work in crowded facilities and communities. Indications for therapy are as follows:

- PPD ≥5 mm
- Previous positive PPD result without INH prophylaxis
- High-risk exposure

Treatment is as follows:

- INH and pyridoxine (vitamin B_6) for 12 months
- Beware INH-related hepatitis risk. Perform liver function tests at 1 and 3 months after initiating INH.

PNEUMOCYSTIS CARINII PNEUMONIA. PCP is the major AIDS-defining diagnosis and the major identifiable cause of death in persons with AIDS. Indications for therapy are as follows:

- Previous PCP
- CD4 ≤200 cells/mm³
- Thrush

Treatment is as follows:

- Trimethoprim-sulfamethoxazole Bactrim DS
- Adverse reactions reported with trimethoprim-sulfamethoxazole are rash, fever, nausea and vomiting, neutropenia, and hepatitis.

TOXOPLASMOSIS. *Toxoplasma gondii* is a protozoan organism that is ubiquitous in nature. Cats are the primary host and reservoir. Symptoms for clients with immunocompromise include headache, confusion, fever, lethargy, and seizures. In-

dications are: CD4 count <100 cells/mm³ and positive *T. gondii* serologic result. Treatment is trimethoprim-sulfamethoxazole DS.

M. AVIUM COMPLEX. *M. avium* complex refers to a group of atypical mycobacteria, of which *M. avium* and *Mycobacterium intracellulare* are the most important. They are widely isolated from the soil and water and are a threat to those who are immunocompromised. The indication is a CD4 count ≤75 cells/mm³. Treatment is clarithromycin, azithromycin, or rifabutin.

Psychosocial Considerations

- Determine the interest and need for psychologic counseling for the client and those close to him or her. Depression and suicide risk must be assessed by qualified staff.
- Review the natural history of HIV infection and course of disease.
- Assess client's involvement and desired level of participation in health care decisions.
- Notify sexual partners and needle-sharing partners of risk status. Physicians and dentists involved in care should be informed.

Client Education

- Provide resources for education, client services, National Institutes of Health clinical trials, financial aid services, community support groups, and national organizations.
- Review lifestyle behaviors associated with disease prevention: Smoking, alcohol and other substance abuse, exercise, and safe sex practices.
- Household pets are a concern because they may carry microbes that cause diarrhea. If a pet has diarrhea, veterinary care should be sought for the pet. Litter boxes should be cleaned daily and pets should be kept indoors, and not fed raw meat. Wash hands frequently and thoroughly.
- Food preparation: Avoid raw eggs and undercooked poultry, seafood, and meat. Wash produce. Keep utensils used with raw meat washed and keep countertops and cutting boards washed and clean.
- Travel: Avoid contaminated food and water. Review immunization needs for travel.
- Occupational risks: Major occupational settings that pose risks for HIV-infected individuals are health care settings, day care settings, and animal shelters.

EVALUATION/FOLLOW-UP

- Repeat CBC and HIV RNA testing every 6 months when CD4 count is ≥500 cells/mm^3.
- Immunizations
  —Pneumovaxnia vaccine: Initially and consider boosters every 5 to 7 years
  —Influenza: Yearly
  —Tetanus-diphtheria toxoid: Every 10 years
  —HV: Series of 3
- Frequency of subsequent visits will be determined by laboratory data, clinical response, and emotional well-being of the client.

REFERENCES

Bartlett, J. A. (1996). *Care and management of patients with HIV infection.* Durham, NC: Glaxo Wellcome.

Bartlett, J. G., & Finkbeiner, A. (1996). *The Johns Hopkins Hospital guide to medical care of patients with HIV infection.* Baltimore: Williams & Wilkins.

Carpenter, C. C. J., Fischl, M. A., Hammer, S. M., Hirsch, M. S., Jacobsen, D. M., Katzenstein, D. A., Montaner, J. S. G., Richmond, D. D., Saag, M. S., Schooley, R. T., Thompson, M. A., Vella, S., Yeni, P. G., & Volberding, P. A. (1996). Antiretroviral therapy for HIV infection. *Journal of the American Medical Association, 276*(2), 146-154.

Centers for Disease Control and Prevention (1992). 1993 Revised classification system for HIV infection and expanded surveillance case definition for AIDS among adolescents and adults. *MMWR: Morbidity and Mortality Weekly Report, 44* (RR-17), 1-19.

Centers for Disease Control and Prevention (1995). USPHS/IDSA guidelines for the prevention of opportunistic infections in persons infected with human immundeficiency virus: A summary. *MMWR: Morbidity and Mortality Weekly Report, 44*(RR-8), 1-34.

Minkoff, H., DeHovitz, J. A., & Duerr, A. (1995). *HIV infection in women.* New York: Raven Press.

Saag, M. S., Holodniy, M., Kuritzkes, D. R., O'Brien, W. A., Coombs, R., Poscher, M. E., Jacobsen, D. M., Shaw, G. M., Richman, D. D., Volberding, P. A. (1996). HIV viral load markers in clinical practice. *Nature Medicine, 2*(6), 625-629.

REVIEW QUESTIONS

1. All the following clients should be advised to seek HIV testing **except:**

   a. Persons who have any STD
   b. Recipients of blood transfusion since 1990
   c. All pregnant women
   d. Clients with active TB

2. When auscultating the lungs of a client with HIV and suspected PCP, your findings include which of the following?

   a. Crackles and dry rales
   b. Wheezing
   c. Pleural rub
   d. Stridor

3. HIV-infected pregnant women should be counseled for all the following **except:**

   a. HIV transmission occurs in utero, at delivery, and during breast-feeding.
   b. All HIV-infected women must bottle-feed their infants.
   c. AZT significantly reduces HIV transmission.
   d. AZT therapy for the neonate continues for the first year.

4. The workplace can harbor communicable disease exposure. All the following should be of concern for the HIV-infected individual **except:**

   a. Chickenpox and individuals recently vaccinated
   b. TB
   c. *Salmonella*
   d. Esophageal candidiasis

ANSWERS AND RATIONALES

1. *Answer:* b (assessment/history/immunologic/NAS)
   Rationale: Recipients of blood transfusions before 1985 are considered at risk for HIV exposure. (Bartlett, 1996)

2. *Answer:* a (assessment/physical examination/immunologic/NAS)
   Rationale: PCP's presenting symptoms are typically subacute: nonproductive cough, fever, and increasing dyspnea developing during 1 to 4 weeks. This undramatic clinical picture must not be missed by the provider. (Centers for Disease Control and Prevention, 1995)

3. *Answer:* d (plan/immunologic/childbearing female)
   Rationale: Recommendations for the prevention of perinatal HIV transmission to the neonate were

first published by the CDC in 1994. For the pregnant woman, AZT is advised at 14 weeks' gestation and continued through the pregnancy to the time of delivery. The infant receives oral AZT administration every 6 hours for the first 6 weeks, beginning 8 to 12 hours after delivery. The results of ongoing blood tests will determine whether AZT should be continued further. (Minkoff, DeHovitz, & Duerr, 1995)

4. *Answer:* d (plan/immunologic/NAS)

Rationale: Fungal infections are common opportunistic infections seen in clients with immunosuppression; however, they are not transmitted by an airborne route. All others listed can be readily transmitted by indirect contact and therefore must be avoided by the immunosuppressed client. (Bartlett, 1996)

SYSTEMIC LUPUS ERYTHEMATOSUS

OVERVIEW

Definition

Systemic lupus erythematosus (SLE) is a chronic autoimmune disease that causes inflammation of various parts of the body, especially the skin, joints, and kidneys. SLE is highly variable in nature, with periods of exacerbation and remission. Types of SLE are *discoid, systemic,* and *drug-induced.*

- Discoid is limited to skin.
- Systemic is generally more severe than discoid; it affects almost any organ or system of the body.
- Drug-induced is similar to systemic lupus.

Incidence

- 1,400,000 to 2,000,000 cases in 1995
- SLE occurs most frequently in females 15 to 45 years old.
- SLE is 10 to 15 times more frequent in adult females than in adult males.
- Females in late 20s or older comprise 60% of cases.
- Incidence is 3 cases/100,000 children; childhood onset is more severe.
- Increased incidence in black, Native American, and Asian populations.

Pathophysiology

SLE is an autoimmune disorder with environmental and genetic factors.

- Environmental factors: Infection, antibiotics, ultraviolet light, extreme stress, drugs
- Genetic factors: No known gene causes illness; 10% of those affected have close relative with disease and 5% of children born to individuals with SLE have illness develop.
- Hormonal factors: Hormonal factors may be implicated in the disease. Cyclic increases in symptoms associated with menstrual periods or during pregnancy suggest that hormones may be involved.

ASSESSMENT: SUBJECTIVE/HISTORY

No characteristic clinical pattern. May be acute or insidious. Characterized by recurrent seasonal remissions and exacerbations, especially during spring and summer. Requires careful history with focus both on systemic and on single organ symptoms.

Migratory nonerosive polyarthralgia or arthritis has the following characteristics:

- Prolonged morning stiffness in multiple joints
- Less stiffness after using joints
- Spine not involved

Constitutional symptoms include the following:

- Malaise
- Fever
- Anorexia
- Weight loss

Multisystem involvement symptoms are as follows:

- Fatigue
- Rash
- Anemia
- Diffuse adenopathy
- Alopecia
- Oral and nasal ulcers
- Pleuritic chest pain

- Raynaud's phenomenon
- Dry eyes and mouth
- Abdominal pain
- Nausea
- Vomiting
- Diarrhea
- Constipation
- Irregular menstruation or amenorrhea
- Headaches
- Irritability
- Depression
- Renal dysfunction
- Urinary frequency
- Dysuria
- Bladder spasms
- Urinary tract infection (UTI)

Typical presenting picture is a young woman with symmetric polyarthritis or arthralgia, facial rash (butterfly rash), fever, fatigue, and weight loss.

Past Medical History

- Recent viral infection
- Hormonal abnormality
- Ultraviolet radiation
- Seizures
- Visual disturbances

Family History

- SLE
- Autoimmune disorders

Medication History

Drugs that may induce SLE are as follows:
- Hydralazine
- Procainamide
- Penicillin
- INH
- Chlorpromazine
- Phenytoin
- Quinidine

ASSESSMENT: OBJECTIVE/ PHYSICAL EXAMINATION
Physical Examination

- Assess temperature for fever and blood pressure for hypertension.
- Integumentary: Pallor; signs of bleeding, including petechiae and bruising; erythema forming a butterfly pattern on cheeks and nose; lesions and necrosis on fingertips, toes, and elbows; hairline (hair loss)
- Musculoskeletal: Inspect extremities and joints for signs of arthritis, lymphadenopathy, peripheral neuropathy; range of motion (ROM) and joint discomfort.
- Cardiovascular and respiratory: Auscultate lungs and heart to determine presence of pleural or pericardial friction rub.
- Abdomen: Palpate spleen and liver for tenderness, splenomegaly, or hepatomegaly.
- Psychosocial: Determine levels of anxiety, fear, and depression.

Diagnostic Procedures

There is no definitive laboratory test to diagnose SLE. Commonly used tests include the following:
- CBC
- Rheumatoid arthritis (RA) factor
- Erythrocyte sedimentation rate
- VDRL
- Antinuclear antibody (ANA): High titer confirms lupus; low titer confirms autoimmune disease (e.g., RA).
- Anti-DNA or anti–double-stranded DNA: 40% to 75% with SLE
- Anti–*Serratia marcescens* (Sm): 20% to 25% with SLE, for false-positive serologic test for syphilis
- Anti–nuclear ribonucleoprotein: 40% with SLE
- Anti-Ro: 40% with SLE
- Antiphospholipid antibodies: 30% with SLE
- Serum levels of third and fourth components of complement
- Lupus erythematosus cell preparation: This test determines the presence of cells that have ingested swollen, antibody-coated nuclei of other cells. It is used less frequently than ANA, which is more sensitive for SLE.
- Urinalysis: Cellular casts are predictive of early SLE renal disease.

DIAGNOSIS

SLE is difficult to diagnose because many symptoms mimic those of other illnesses. Diagnosis is made by careful review of the entire medical history, current symptoms, and analysis of laboratory tests.

At some point in the disease history, an individual should have four or more of the following 11 criteria for a diagnosis of SLE (American Rheumatism Association):

- Malar rash
- Discoid rash
- Photosensitivity
- Oral and nasal ulcers
- Nonerosive arthritis involving two or more peripheral joints
- Pleuritis or pericarditis
- Persistent proteinuria or casts
- Seizures or psychosis
- Hemolytic anemia, leukopenia, or thrombocytopenia
- ANA
- Anti-DNA antibody, anti-Sm antibody

NOTE: If an individual meets four of the criteria, a positive ANA result confirms the diagnosis and no further testing is necessary. SLE must be considered if *any* of the clinical characteristics is associated with a positive ANA result, but diagnosis is uncertain until more clinical findings develop.

Differential diagnosis includes the following:

- RA
- Psoriatic arthritis
- Reiter's syndrome
- Polyarticular gout
- Pseudogout
- Sarcoidosis
- Lyme disease
- Disseminated gonococcemia
- Rheumatic fever
- Hepatitis B
- Subacute bacterial endocarditis
- Vasculitis
- Scleroderma
- Malignancy
- Ankylosing spondylitis

THERAPEUTIC PLAN

Goals of therapy are: (1) to reduce inflammation, (2) to suppress abnormalities of immune system responsible for tissue inflammation, and (3) to avoid or decrease the severity of flare-ups.

Pharmacologic Treatment

- Nonsteroidal antiinflammatory drugs (NSAIDs): Avoid ibuprofen (Motrin), sulindac (Clinoril),

and tolmetin (Tolectin), which can be associated with aseptic meningitis. NSAIDs are the most common therapy, used to treat arthritis and mild serositis.
- Antimalarials: Chloroquine (Aralen) and hydroxychloroquine (Plaquenil) are used to treat skin and joint manifestations unmanageable with NSAIDs.
- Corticosteroids: Prednisone (Orasone) is reserved for major organ involvement. It is beneficial in the long-term prognosis of SLE nephritis.
- Cytotoxic drugs: Azothioprine (Imuran) and cyclophosphamide (Cytoxan) are used similarly to corticosteroids to reduce inflammation and suppress the immune system.
- Dehydroepiandrosterone: This antiinflammatory agent yields extremely poor results in females; it causes masculinization.

Treatment of common complications includes the following:

- Antihypertensives
- Diuretics
- Anticonvulsants
- Antibiotics

Pediatric recommendations are as follows:

- Long-term hydroxychloroquine is potentially efficacious.
- Methotrexate is promising.
- Aggressive antihypertensive therapy is recommended.
- Do not overtreat with steroids or immunosuppressive agents.
- Cyclophosphamide should be reserved for severe, life-threatening disease (vasculitis, CNS disease, thrombocytopenia).

Client Education

- Encourage regular exercise to maintain full ROM and prevent contractures.
- During exacerbations, rest is indicated.
- Apply heat packs to relieve joint pain and stiffness.
- Use warmth and protect hands from injury in Raynaud's disease.
- Maintain rest and balanced diet.
- Eat cool, bland foods if mouth is sore.
- Avoid infection (meticulous mouth care, handwashing, avoiding crowds and people with known infection).
- Wear protective clothing and sunscreen.

- Avoid precipitating factors: Fatigue, vaccination, allergy shots (immunotherapy), infection, stress, surgery, drugs, exposure to ultraviolet light, food (such as parsley, figs, and celery) and drugs (such as tetracycline) that augment effect of ultraviolet light.
- Watch for signs and symptoms of exacerbation: Increased pain, increased fatigue, fever, abdominal pain, SOB, headache, dizziness, blurred vision, recurring nosebleeds, puffy eyelids, hemoptysis, increasing swelling of feet and legs.

Referral

Consultation or referral to rheumatologist or clinical immunologist should occur in the following cases:

- Severe constitutional symptoms (e.g., disabling fatigue, fever, weight loss)
- Vasculitis, involvement of lungs, heart, kidneys, or central nervous system
- Condition undiagnosed after initial evaluation

Additional support is available from the Lupus Foundation of America and the Arthritis Foundation.

EVALUATION/FOLLOW-UP

Treatment is based on specific needs and symptoms. Ongoing supervision is essential for proper treatment because the course of lupus may vary significantly. Individuals receiving hydroxychloroquine should have an eye examination before starting therapy and every 6 months thereafter.

REFERENCES

Collo, M. C. B., Johnson, J. L., Finch, W. R., & Felicettqa, J. V. (1991). Evaluating arthritic complaints. *Nurse Practitioner, 16*(2), 9-20.

Davis, J. C., Tassiulas, I. O., & Boumpas, D. T. (1996). Lupus nephritis. *Current Opinion in Rheumatology, 8,* 415-423.

Gare, B. A. (1996). Epidemiology of rheumatic disease in children. *Current Opinion in Rheumatology, 8,* 449-454.

Gladman, D. D. (1996). Prognosis and treatment of systemic lupus erythematosus. *Current Opinion in Rheumatology, 8,* 430-437.

Johnson, A. E., Gordon, C., Hobbs, F. D. R., & Bacon, P. A. (1996). Undiagnosed systemic lupus erythematosus in the community. *Lancet, 347,* 367-369.

Khamashta, M. A., & Hughes, G. R. V. (1996). Pregnancy in systemic lupus erythematosus. *Current Opinion in Rheumatology, 8,* 424-429.

Lahita, R. G. (1996). *What is lupus?* Rockville, MD: Lupus Foundation of America.

Sanchez-Guerrero, J., Sands, R. A., & Liang, M. H. (1996). Guidelines for the initial evaluation of the adult patient with acute musculoskeletal symptoms. *Arthritis & Rheumatism, 39*(1), 1-8.

Shmerling, R. H., Fuchs, H. A., Lorish, C. D., Nichols, L. A., Partridge, A. J., Brigham, R. B., & Senecal, J. L. (1996). Learning the signs of lupus flare-ups. *Lupus Foundation of America Newsletter Article Library,* 93-117.

Silverman, E. (1996). What's new in the treatment of pediatric SLE. *Journal of Rheumatology, 23,* 1657-1660.

van Vollenhoven, R. F., Engleman, E. G., & McGuire, J. L. (1995). Dehydroepiandrosterone in systemic lupus erythematosus: Results of a double-blind, placebo-controlled, randomized clinical trial. *Arthritis & Rheumatism, 38*(12), 1826-1831.

West, S. G. (1996). Lupus and the central nervous system. *Current Opinion in Rheumatology, 8,* 408-414.

REVIEW QUESTIONS

1. Use of which of the following drugs increases the risk of SLE?

a. Hydralazine (Apresoline)
b. Nifedipine (Procardia)
c. Verapamil (Calan)
d. Nicardipine (Cardene)

2. Which of the following is one of the most common presenting symptoms in individuals with SLE?

a. Mouth sores
b. Alopecia
c. Fatigue
d. Butterfly-shaped rash across cheeks and nose

3. Which of the following presenting symptoms in a client with acute musculoskeletal complaint might lead a practitioner to suspect SLE?

   a. Asymmetric arthritis, peak period of discomfort after prolonged inactivity, inflamed joint, no constitutional symptoms

   b. Symmetric arthritis, peak period of discomfort after prolonged inactivity, inflamed joint, constitutional symptoms

   c. Symmetric arthritis, peak period of discomfort after prolonged use, no constitutional symptoms

   d. Asymmetric arthritis, peak period of discomfort with use, no constitutional symptoms

4. Which of the following clinical findings would generally **not** be found in an individual with SLE?

   a. Discoid rash

   b. Polyarthralgia

   c. Back pain

   d. Depression

5. Which of the following laboratory tests is most diagnostic of SLE?

   a. Anti-Sm

   b. Anti-Ro

   c. Antiphospholipid antibodies

   d. ANA

6. Which of the following criteria are diagnostic of SLE?

   a. Red, raised patches; oral ulcers; nonerosive arthritis; leukopenia; positive ANA result

   b. Red, raised patches; fever; Raynaud's phenomenon; seizures

   c. Red, raised patches; polyarthralgia; anemia; photosensitivity

   d. Red, raised patches; cellular casts in urine; depression; positive ANA result

7. Systemic lupus erythematosus is difficult to diagnose because many symptoms mimic those of other illnesses. Which of the following should **not** be considered in the differential diagnosis?

   a. AIDS

   b. Rheumatoid arthritis

   c. Fibromyalgia

   d. Psoriatic arthritis

8. The presence of which of the following is the most predictive of the onset of SLE renal disease?

   a. Hematuria

   b. Leukocyturia

   c. Decreasing serum levels of the third component of complement

   d. Cellular casts

9. Mrs. A. has a diagnosis of SLE. You will include which of the following in your initial client education?

   a. Methods of avoiding exposure to sunlight

   b. Application of cosmetics to cover skin lesions

   c. Returning for yearly CXR

   d. Appropriate use of narcotic medications in the management of pain to avoid addiction

10. Which of the following medications frequently used in the treatment of SLE is contraindicated in children **except** in the treatment of severe, life-threatening disease?

   a. Prednisone (Orasone)

   b. Cyclosporine (Sandimmune)

   c. Cyclophosphamide (Cytoxan)

   d. Hydroxychloroquine (Plaquenil)

11. Treatment with hydroxychloroquine (Plaquenil) would be initiated in the presence of which of the following symptoms?

   a. SOB

   b. Fever with temperature >100.5° F

   c. Cellular casts in the urine

   d. Skin rash

12. A client receiving hydroxychloroquine should receive which of the following instructions for follow-up?

    a. Obtain eye examination every 6 months throughout therapy.

    b. Check blood pressure every month throughout therapy.

    c. Return to clinic for CBC every 6 months throughout therapy.

    d. Monitor weight every week throughout therapy.

13. Clients with SLE are advised to avoid flare-ups to extend remission. All the following factors may trigger a flare-up **except:**

    a. Allergy shots

    b. Gammaglobulin

    c. Vaccinations

    d. Ultraviolet light

ANSWERS AND RATIONALES

1. *Answer:* a (assessment/history/immunologic/NAS)

Rationale: Drug-induced lupus may occur after the use of certain prescription drugs, with hydralazine and procainamide being the most common. (Lahita, 1996)

2. *Answer:* c (assessment/history/immunologic/NAS)

Rationale: Eighty-one percent of all individuals are first seen with fatigue, 12% with mouth ulcers, 27% with alopecia, and 42% with butterfly rash. (Lahita, 1996)

3. *Answer:* b (assessment/history/immunologic/NAS)

Rationale: Constitutional symptoms are diagnostically useful clinical features in the initial evaluation of the client with SLE. (Shmerling, et al., 1996)

4. *Answer:* c (assessment/physical examination/immunologic/NAS)

Rationale: Backaches and neck pain are not caused by lupus because the spine is not involved. (Lahita, 1996)

5. *Answer:* d (assessment/physical examination/immunologic/NAS)

Rationale: The best screening test for SLE is ANA. (Lahita, 1996)

6. *Answer:* a (assessment/physical examination/immunologic/NAS)

Rationale: If an individual has signs and symptoms supporting the diagnosis of lupus (e.g., at least four of the American Rheumatism Association criteria), a positive ANA result confirms the diagnosis and no further testing is necessary. If a person has only two or three of the criteria, a positive ANA result supports the diagnosis; however, the diagnosis remains uncertain until more clinical findings develop. (Lahita, 1996)

7. *Answer:* c (diagnosis/immunologic/NAS)

Rationale: Fibromyalgia is a nonarticular disease, consisting of chronic and diffuse muscle aching and stiffness, that mimics arthritis. (Collo et al., 1991)

8. *Answer:* d (diagnosis/immunologic/NAS)

Rationale: Urinalysis is essential in early diagnosis of active renal disease. The appearance of cellular casts is a significantly better predictor than hematuria, leukocyturia, or a decreasing serum level of the third component of complement. (Davis, Tassiulas, & Boumpas, 1996)

9. *Answer:* a (plan/immunologic/NAS)

Rationale: Preventive measures can reduce the risk of flares. Avoidance of sun exposure will generally prevent rashes. (Lahita, 1996)

10. *Answer:* c (plan/immunologic/NAS)

Rationale: Cyclophosphamide does have a role in pediatric SLE, but it should be reserved for severe, life-threatening disease, in which the benefits outweigh the risks. (Silverman, 1996)

11. *Answer:* d (plan/immunologic/NAS)

Rationale: Antimalarials may be useful in some individuals with SLE. They are most often prescribed for skin and joint symptoms. (Gladman, 1996)

12. *Answer:* a (evaluation/immunologic/NAS)
Rationale: Antimalarial drugs may damage the retina of the eye and produce visual disturbances, including blindness. Thorough eye examination before starting treatment and every 6 months throughout therapy is recommended so that therapy can be terminated early if there is any damage to the retina. (Lahita, 1996)

13. *Answer:* b (evaluation/immunologic/NAS)
Rationale: Immunotherapy and exposure to ultraviolet light may cause lupus flare-up. Immunization with vaccines that use live viruses will result in a lupus flare. Gammaglobulin is an example of a vaccine which uses a nonspecific antibody instead of a live virus. (Lahita, 1996)

12

Integumentary System

ACNE VULGARIS

OVERVIEW

Definition

Acne is a chronic follicular eruption at the pilosebaceous unit that begins as a comedone. Papules, pustules, and cysts develop if an inflammatory reaction occurs. Other disorders have been labeled acne, such as neonatal acne and steroid acne. These disorders, better labeled *acneiform*, originate with inflammation, skipping the comedone stage.

Incidence

Acne vulgaris affects nearly 17 million people in the United States. The peak onset is at puberty. Boys are affected more than girls; nearly 100% of boys have acne by the age 16. The prevalence decreases in adulthood; it is 8% among those 25 to 34 years old and 3% among adults 35 to 44 years old. Acne vulgaris usually improves during pregnancy; however, exacerbations may also occur.

Pathophysiology

The exact pathogenesis of acne is still not completely understood. The cause is multifactorial and is most influenced by the following factors:
- Excessive sebum production: The rate of sebum production is determined genetically. The production of sebum is increased by the presence of androgens.
- Comedogenesis: The follicle canal becomes blocked by the sebum, resulting in the formation of comedones. These may be open comedones, or *blackheads*, and closed comedones, or *whiteheads*. Comedogenesis occurs in sebaceous follicles only.

- *Propionibacterium acnes:* The presence of *P. acnes* causes the inflammatory aspects of acne. This bacterium is benign and resides on the skin at all times.

Dietary habits and dirty skin do not contribute to acne.

ASSESSMENT: SUBJECTIVE/HISTORY

Hormonal Influences

Determine the timing of the onset of pubertal changes in relationship to the increase in acne. Females with cystic acne should be assessed for hirsutism and a history of irregular menses to rule out polycystic ovary disease.

Medication History

Oral and injectable steroids, both prescribed and illicit, should be noted. Lithium, isoniazid, and phenytoin are some of the most common drugs that cause drug-induced acne.

Family History

Ask about parental and sibling history of acne.

Home Treatments

Ask about type of soap used, frequency of face washing, OTC treatments tried, and use of cosmetics.

Work History

Is the client working in a fast-food restaurant around hot grease?

Psychosocial History

Is the acne of concern to the client? Does the client's appearance inhibit social interactions?

ASSESSMENT: OBJECTIVE/ PHYSICAL EXAMINATION

Physical Examination

A problem-oriented physical assessment should be conducted, with attention to the skin on the face, chest, neck, and upper back.

- Adolescents: Assess pubertal stage and hirsutism in females with cystic acne.
- Skin: Assess the severity of the lesions. Assess for scarring.
- Determine the grade of the acne.
  —Grade I: Pure comedonal acne
  —Grade II: Mild papular acne
  —Grade II to III: Papulopustular and cystic acne
  —Grade III to IV: Persistent pustulocystic acne
  —Grade V: Pustulocystic nodular acne

Diagnostic Procedures

No diagnostic tests are indicated.

DIAGNOSIS

Differential diagnosis includes the following:

- Acneiform lesions, such as drug-induced acne
- Neonatal acne
- Acne conglobata
- Rosacea

THERAPEUTIC PLAN

Pharmacologic Treatment

Treatment options depend on the severity of the acne lesions. Understanding the pathogenesis is the key to choosing the proper treatment. Treatment may need to be long-term to avoid exacerbations.

TOPICAL TREATMENT

Pure Comedonal Acne. Several formulations of tretinoin (Retin-A) exist, with cream (0.025%, 0.05%, or 0.1%) being the most mild, followed by gel (0.01% or 0.025%) and liquid (0.05%). To avoid overdrying of the skin, the treatment should be initiated on an every-other-day basis.

Mild Papular Acne. Benzoyl peroxide is available only as a 5% or 10% gel by prescription. Begin treatment slowly, with every-other-day application to avoid overdrying of the skin.

Papulopustular Acne. Combination therapy is with tretinoin and benzoyl peroxide, each applied once daily, *or* with tretinoin and a topical antibiotic, especially in inflammatory acne. Topical clindamycin (1%) is available in solution, lotion, and gel formulations.

SYSTEMIC AND COMBINATION TREATMENTS

Grade III or IV Acne. More severe acne may require systemic therapy with oral antibiotics. The first-line choice is most commonly tetracycline, 500 to 1000 mg/day, decreased gradually to a goal of 250 mg/day or every other day. Erythromycin, minocycline, doxycycline, and occasionally trimethoprim-sulfamethoxazole may also be prescribed.

Females With Mild to Moderate Acne. These clients may respond well to topical treatment and the addition of an oral contraceptive pill. Oral contraceptive pills reduce endogenous androgen production and decrease the bioavailability of circulating androgens. Research has demonstrated that combination oral contraceptive pills containing levonorgestrel, gestodene, and desogestrel as the progestin component have decreased acne in women. However, few studies have compared different formulations of pills with each other.

Grade V (Severe Cystic Acne With Scarring). Refer client to dermatology for isotretinoin (Accutane), 1 mg/kg daily for 5 months.

Client Education

- Wash the skin twice daily with a gentle soap.
- Use a moisturizer unless skin is extremely oily.
- All cosmetics should be removed nightly.
- Instruct the client not to pick at lesions.
- Warn the client that improvement will not be noted until 4 to 6 weeks of treatment.
- Sunscreen and sun protection must be used with tretinoin, oral tetracycline, doxycycline, and isotretinoin.
- Tretinoin should be applied with the three-dot method. Dispense a pea-sized amount on the finger, divide it into three smaller dots, and rub it into the affected area.
- Women of childbearing age must be using an effective contraceptive method when taking

isotretinoin and for 1 month after discontinuation.

- Cholesterol and triglyceride levels must be monitored during isotretinoin treatment.
- Clients receiving isotretinoin should be advised to avoid excessive alcohol consumption.

Referral

- Clients in need of isotretinoin treatment
- Females with cystic acne, irregular menses, and hirsutism, for hormonal evaluation
- Clients with significant depressive symptoms as a result of the acne

EVALUATION/FOLLOW-UP

Reevaluate at 4 to 6 weeks and consider combination treatments. Assess for satisfaction with medication and for problems with skin irritation. Note the number and type of lesions present. Consider combination treatment if current treatment is not decreasing the lesions.

REFERENCES

Berson, D. S., & Shalita, A. R. (1995). The treatment of acne: The role of combination therapies. *Journal of the American Academy of Dermatology, 32,* S31-S41.

Hurwitz, S. (1995). Acne treatment for the '90s. *Contemporary Pediatrics, 12*(8), 19-32.

Kaminer, M. S., & Gilchrest, B. A. (1995). The many faces of acne. *Journal of the American Academy of Dermatology, 32,* S6-S14.

Leyden, J. J. (1995). New understandings of the pathogenesis of acne. *Journal of the American Academy of Dermatology, 32,* S15-S25.

Rothman, K. E., & Lucky, A. W. (1993). Acne vulgaris. *Advances in Dermatology, 8,* 347-369.

REVIEW QUESTIONS

1. Acne vulgaris can be differentiated from acneiform causes of acne by the presence of which of the following?

    a. Inflammatory pustules
    b. Comedones
    c. Cystic lesions
    d. Scarring

2. Which of the following is associated with a closed comedone?

    a. A dilated follicular orifice with a black appearance
    b. Most responsibility for the problems seen in clients with acne
    c. A blackhead
    d. A constricted follicular orifice

3. Topical tretinoin (Retin-A) decreases comedone formation through which of the following methods?

    a. Antibacterial properties kill *P. acnes.*
    b. Tretinoin decreases circulating androgens.
    c. Increased cell turnover decreases comedone formation.
    d. Tretinoin decreases inflammatory reactions.

4. Which of the following medication changes would be the most effective for the client with very dry skin and continued inflammatory acne after 6 weeks with topical tretinoin cream?

    a. Discontinue the topical tretinoin and initiate topical antibiotic cream.
    b. Initiate therapy with systemic Isotretinoin.
    c. Change the treatment to topical tretinoin gel.
    d. Continue the topical tretinoin at night with the addition of a topical antibiotic in the morning.

5. Which of the following is the recommended phone triage for an adolescent reporting severe burning sensations after 2 weeks of treatment with tretinoin cream twice daily?

    a. Discontinue treatment immediately and schedule office visit for allergic reaction.
    b. Decrease the use of the medication to once daily.
    c. Encourage the adolescent to apply the medication immediately after washing the face with a mild soap.
    d. Change the prescription to a gel formulation to decrease irritation.

6. Which of the following statements is true?

    a. Benzoyl peroxide is a potent bactericidal agent.
    b. Benzoyl peroxide decreases surface androgen.
    c. Benzoyl peroxide has no keratolytic properties.
    d. Benzoyl peroxide use results in photosensitivity.

7. Which of the following recommendations should be given to a client receiving oral tetracycline treatment for acne?

    a. Sunscreen should be applied for all outdoor activities.

    b. Tetracycline should be taken with food.

    c. Tetracycline can be taken with dairy products to decrease gastrointestinal symptoms.

    d. Topical preparations are no longer necessary after systemic treatment begins.

ANSWERS AND RATIONALES

1. *Answer:* b (physical examination/integumentary/NAS)

    Rationale: True acne vulgaris is characterized by an eruption of the pilosebaceous unit (the sebaceous gland and hair follicles) that begins as a comedone. (Kaminer & Gilchrest, 1995)

2. *Answer:* b (assessment/physical examination/integumentary/NAS)

    Rationale: Closed comedones, or whiteheads, are most responsible for the problems identified with acne. Open comedones, or blackheads, are purely cosmetic and rarely cause additional problems. (Rothman & Lucky, 1993)

3. *Answer:* c (plan/management/therapeutic/pharmacologic/integumentary/NAS)

    Rationale: Tretinoin has no antibacterial properties; it is highly effective in preventing further comedone production. (Hurwitz, 1995)

4. *Answer:* d (evaluation/integumentary/NAS)

    Rationale: Combination therapy with tretinoin and topical antibiotic formulations are highly effective in the treatment of inflammatory acne. (Berson & Shalita, 1995)

5. *Answer:* b (evaluation/integumentary/adolescent)

    Rationale: Topical tretinoin can be highly irritating to the skin, so therapy should begin with daily or every-other-day application. Cream formulations are less irritating than gel formulations. The tretinoin should be applied 20 to 30 minutes after washing with a mild soap to decrease irritation to the skin.

6. *Answer:* a (plan/management/therapeutics/pharmacologic/integumentary/NAS)

    Rationale: Benzoyl peroxide can be used as a single therapy for acne because it has both antibacterial properties and keratolytic properties. Better results can be seen in combination with tretinoin, which has more potent keratolytic properties.

7. *Answer:* a (plan/management/client education/NAS)

    Rationale: Treatment with oral tetracycline, tretinoin, isotretinoin, and doxycycline can result in photosensitivity. Tetracycline must be taken on an empty stomach, and dairy products may decrease absorption. (Rothman & Lucky, 1993)

BURNS

OVERVIEW
Definition

Burns are tissue injuries caused by heat, chemicals, electricity, or irradiation. The depth of the burn is a result of the intensity of the heat and the duration of the exposure. Minor burns are considered those of <10% of the body surface area (BSA) and involving <2% full-thickness injury (Uphold & Graham, 1994).

Incidence

- From 2 to 5 million burns occur each year; 1,000,000 afflicted persons require hospitalization, and 12,000 die.
- Burns are the leading cause of death in children; All ages are affected.
- Male and female prevalences are equal.

Pathophysiology

Burns occur as a result of excessive heat energy transferred to the skin, causing cellular protein coagulation and destruction of enzyme systems (Dershewitz, 1993).

PARTIAL THICKNESS BURN. Partial-thickness burns involve the superficial layers of the epidermis.

- Superficial (first-degree): Erythema is present, skin blanches with pressure, and skin may be tender. Devitalization of superficial layers of epidermis, congestion of intradermal vessels.

- Partial thickness (second-degree): Erythema is present with blisters, skin is extremely tender. There is coagulation of varying depths of epidermis, vesicles are present and skin appendages are intact.

FULL THICKNESS BURN (THIRD-DEGREE). There is destruction of all skin elements, with destruction of subdermal plexus. Third degree: Burned skin is tough and leathery and may be black or white, skin is not tender, and there is necrosis of all skin elements.

FACTORS INCREASING SUSCEPTIBILITY

- Hot-water heaters set too high (>120° F)
- Workplace exposure to chemicals, electricity, or irradiation
- Young children and older adults are more susceptible to burns because of thinner skin.
- Carelessness with cigarettes
- Inadequate or faulty wiring
- Use of alcohol or drugs
- Wearing flammable clothing

CAUSES OF BURNS

- Open flame and hot liquids are the most common causes of burns.
- Burns from caustic chemicals may show little damage for the first few days.
- Electricity may cause significant damage, with little damage seen on the surface.
- Topical medications may cause chemical burns in clients with sensitive skin (e.g., acne medications).
- Excess sun exposure

ASSESSMENT: SUBJECTIVE/HISTORY

- Exposure to cause
- Ask about being in an enclosed location, for possible exposure to smoke.
- Type of burning agent
- Previous treatment
- Use of alcohol or drugs
- Concurrent trauma

Most Common Symptoms

- Pain
- Redness of skin
- Blisters

Associated Symptoms

- Shortness of breath from smoke inhalation
- Palpitations
- Nausea and vomiting
- Chills
- Headache

Past Medical History

Ask about previous skin damage or burns.

Medication History

Determine whether client is taking any regular medications.

Family History

Family history is not applicable.

Dietary History

Ask about time last meal was eaten.

ASSESSMENT: OBJECTIVE/ PHYSICAL EXAMINATION

Physical Examination

A problem-oriented physical examination should be conducted, with particular attention to vital signs, weight, and general appearance.

- Skin: Determine extent of burn with respect to BSA; use "rule of nines."
  —Each upper extremity, 9%
  —Each lower extremity, 18% for adults and 14% for children
  —Anterior trunk, 18%
  —Posterior trunk, 18%
  —Head and neck, 10% for adults and 14% for children
- Perform ENT and chest evaluation to rule out possible smoke inhalation.
- Do cardiovascular check for electrical burns.
- Check for circulation and neurologic status distal to burn.

Diagnostic Procedures

Procedures used are determined by the extent of the burn. Extensive laboratory tests may be necessary for serious burns. Perform ECG with an electrical burn.

DIAGNOSIS

Differential diagnosis includes scalded skin syndrome and abuse.

THERAPEUTIC PLAN

Nonpharmacologic Treatment

- Administer tetanus prophylaxis.
- Remove all rings to avoid tourniquet effect.
- Flush chemical burn copiously with water.
- Do not apply ice to site.

    INITIAL CARE OF FIRST- AND SECOND-DEGREE BURNS. Gently cleanse with a mild detergent (such as Ivory) and water, then débride any broken blisters or dead skin. Blisters that are intact can be left alone. The burned areas should be covered with a thin layer of silver sulfadiazine cream and a fluffy dressing that will absorb drainage.

Pharmacologic Treatment

- Prophylactic antibiotics are not usually needed unless the client has a history of valvular heart disease.
- Pain relief: Aspirin or ibuprofen every 4 hours

Client Education

- Care of burn at home: Cleanse burn of old cream twice daily, dry well, and reapply cream and then dressing. Keep dressings clean and dry.
- Use sunscreens to avoid future burns.
- Identify risk of skin changes in future; monitor skin of area carefully.
- Decrease temperature of hot-water heater to <120° F.
- Store household chemicals in a safe place, away from children.
- Do not smoke in bed.

Referral

All clients with second-degree burns >10% BSA or any third-degree burn should be hospitalized. Clients with any of the following burns should also be hospitalized:

- Any second-degree burns of hands, feet, or perineum
- Electrical burns or lightning strike
- Inhalation burns
- Chemical burns
- Circumferential burns

EVALUATION/FOLLOW-UP

- First-degree burns: Complete resolution in 3 to 6 days without scarring
- Second-degree burns: Epithelialization should occur in 10 to 14 days; deep second-degree burns may require skin grafts.

- Third-degree: Skin grafting is required.
- Follow-up initially in 48 hours and closely thereafter, to make sure that healing is taking place.
- Consider child or elder abuse if burns are seen in a "dripping" pattern or there are cigarette or iron burns.

REFERENCES

Dershewitz, R. A. (1993). *Ambulatory pediatric care* (2nd ed.). Philadelphia: J. B. Lippincott.

Fultz, J., & Messer, M. (1996). Burns. In P. Kidd & P. Sturt (Eds.), *Mosby's emergency nursing reference* (pp. 111-138). St. Louis: Mosby.

Griffith, H., & Dambro, M. (1997). *The 5-minute clinical consult.* Philadelphia: Lea & Febiger.

Latchaw, L. (1993). Burns: The outpatient treatment. In R. Dershewitz (Ed.), *Ambulatory pediatrics* (pp. 535-536). Philadelphia: J. B. Lippincott.

Uphold, C., & Graham, M. (1994). *Clinical guidelines in family practice.* Gainesville, FL: Barmarrae Books.

REVIEW QUESTIONS

1. A client is seen with a tender 10 × 2 cm region on the left lower arm that is red with blisters. The client sustained this injury from boiling water when a pot spilled. The nurse practitioner diagnoses this as a:

   a. Superficial burn
   b. Partial thickness burn
   c. Full thickness burn
   d. First-degree burn

2. When providing anticipatory guidance regarding burns, the nurse practitioner should do which of the following?

   a. Discuss the temperature setting of water heaters with the family of an infant.
   b. Plan a fire escape route for the family.
   c. Demonstrate how to use a fire extinguisher.
   d. Discuss stop, drop, and roll.

3. All the following should be assessed when caring for a client with burns **except:**

   a. Treatment at home
   b. What caused the burn
   c. Family history
   d. Where the burn occurred

4. Which of the following systems should be examined in a client who was burned superficially when putting out a kitchen fire?

  a. HEENT
  b. Chest
  c. Abdomen
  d. Extremities

5. Client education for a client treated for a partial thickness burn should include which of the following?

  a. The future use of sunscreen on the area
  b. The need to return for tetanus immunization within 1 week
  c. Application of ice to decrease pain
  d. Explaining the proper way to débride blisters

6. A person is treated for a partial thickness, second-degree burn. This client should be evaluated in 10 to 14 days for:

  a. Need for skin grafting
  b. Pain control
  c. Swelling
  d. Allergy to the silver sulfadiazine cream

ANSWERS AND RATIONALES

1. *Answer:* b (diagnosis/integumentary/NAS)

  Rationale: A partial thickness (second-degree) burn involves varying levels of epidermis and vesicles. Full thickness burns destroy subdermal layers. A first-degree burn is one type of partial thickness burn, but there are no blisters. (Fultz & Messer, 1996)

2. *Answer:* a (management/plan/client education/integumentary/child)

  Rationale: Although all these actions would be nice, the nurse practitioner does not have the time to perform them all in a visit. The demonstration and discussion of how to extinguish a fire or how to perform in a fire should be left to fire professionals. (Uphold & Graham, 1994)

3. *Answer:* c (assessment/history/integumentary/NAS)

  Rationale: Treatment at home, if incorrect, may have prolonged the burning process. Different agents produce different burning patterns, and severity may not be as readily apparent immediately after the event. A burn received from a fire in an enclosed area may also involve smoke inhalation. Family history is not relevant. (Fultz & Messer, 1996)

4. *Answer:* b (assessment/physical examination/integumentary/NAS)

  Rationale: There is not enough information in the question to determine where on the body the client was burned. However, a kitchen is an enclosed area, and smoke inhalation may have occurred. (Fultz & Messer, 1996)

5. *Answer:* a (management/plan/client education/integumentary/NAS)

  Rationale: A burned area will be more susceptible to injury from thermal energy in the future. Tetanus prophylaxis must be administered within 72 hours. Ice is not used because vasoconstriction may further injure the area. Blisters should remain intact until they break on their own. (Fultz & Messer, 1996)

6. *Answer:* a (evaluation/integumentary/NAS)

  Rationale: Skin grafting may be necessary for second-degree burns. It takes 10 to 14 days for epithelialization to occur and an evaluation regarding grafting to be made. Pain and swelling are worse during the first 48 hours after the burn. Evidence of allergy to the cream occurs quickly after the first application. (Fultz & Messer, 1996)

CELLULITIS

OVERVIEW
Definition

Cellulitis is diffuse, suppurative inflammation involving the subcutaneous tissue. It is usually preceded by a break in skin integrity.

Pathophysiology

Cellulitis is commonly caused by streptococci, *Haemophilus influenzae*, or *Staphylococcus aureus*. In bites, *Pasteurella multocida* is common. *Pseudomonas aeruginosa* may be present in puncture wounds.

Etiology. Cellulitis occurs with trauma to the skin, such as burns, abrasions, bites, and puncture wounds. It may also occur with scratches and insect bites or stings. Tinea pedis may be present, and a portal of entry may be fissures between toes.

ASSESSMENT: SUBJECTIVE/HISTORY
History of Present Illness

When did injury or break in skin occur? What treatment was used at home? The client with cellulitis will report fever, chills, and malaise. There is extreme tenderness at the site.

Past Medical History

- Diabetes
- Peripheral vascular disease (PVD)

ASSESSMENT: OBJECTIVE/ PHYSICAL EXAMINATION
Physical Examination

- Local erythema and warmth
- Lesion not well demarcated or elevated
- Client may have purulent or serous drainage.
- Regional adenopathy
- Superficial blisters may be present.

Diagnostic Procedures

- Wound culture if discharge
- Blood cultures if client appears ill
- Complete blood cell count (CBC) with differential
- X-ray film of site if reason to suspect osteomyelitis (gas present under skin)

DIAGNOSIS

Differential diagnosis includes the following:
- Contact dermatitis
- Erysipelas (a distinct type of cellulitis caused by streptococci, with a sharply demarcated, elevated, advancing edge, usually on the face, abdomen, or legs)
- Hydradenitis suppurativa
- Necrotizing fasciitis
- Candidal infections
- PVD
- Gout

THERAPEUTIC PLAN

Immediately hospitalize any child with facial, orbital, or periorbital involvement.

Pharmacologic Treatment

- Assess tetanus status, administer tetanus-diphtheria toxoid (Td) or tetanus immune globulin (hyper-Tet) as indicated.
- Dicloxacillin, 15 mg/kg/day in 4 divided doses PO for 7 to 10 days
- Amoxicillin-clavulanate, 500 mg PO tid for 7 to 10 days
- If client is intolerant of penicillin, substitute any of the following:
  —Cephalexin, 50 mg/kg/day in 2 divided doses for 7 to 10 days
  —Erythromycin ethylsuccinate, 30 to 40 mg/kg/day in 3 divided doses for 7 to 10 days
  —Azithromycin, 500 mg PO on day 1 then 250 mg PO qd for 4 days
- For cellulitis with puncture wound etiology: Ciprofloxacin, 750 mg bid for 7 days

Client Education

- Fever care instructions
- Wound care instructions
- Return if no improvement within 24 hours
- Stress that hospitalization may be necessary.
- Smoking cessation if appropriate

Referral

- Consult with physician about any client with decreased responsiveness, extremely elevated

WBC count, and diabetes, PVD, or immunocompromise.

- If osteomyelitis is evident on x-ray film or bone scan, refer client to an orthopedic surgeon for surgical débridement to prevent further complications.

EVALUATION/FOLLOW-UP

Recheck in 24 to 48 hours after starting antibiotics if there is no improvement. Recheck at end of antibiotic therapy with improvement.

REFERENCES

Barker, L., Burton, J., & Zieve, P. (1995). *Principles of ambulatory medicine.* Baltimore: Williams & Wilkins.

Bisno, A. (1996). Streptococcal infections of the skin and soft tissue. *New England Journal of Medicine, 334*(4), 240-245.

Callen, I. (1995). *Current practice of dermatology.* Philadelphia: Current Medicine.

Dershewitz, R. A. (1993). *Ambulatory pediatric care* (2nd ed.). Philadelphia: J. B. Lippincott.

Raz, R., & Miron, P. (1996). Oral ciprofloxacin for treatment of infection following nail puncture wounds. *Clinical Infectious Disease, 21*(1), 194-195.

Sanford, J., Gilbert, D., & Sande, M. (1996). *The Sanford guide to antimicrobial therapy.* Dallas: SmithKline Beecham Pharmaceuticals.

REVIEW QUESTIONS

1. Mrs. Jones, a 50-year-old white female, comes to your clinic with a history of warmth, redness, and tenderness of the dorsum of her left foot for 3 days. Which of the following subjective data would be **least** helpful in making a diagnosis?

- a. History of trauma to the affected extremity
- b. History of chronic dependent edema related to venous stasis
- c. Recent initiation of a walking program to promote weight loss
- d. History of fever and chills at home

2. Which of the following past medical problems would influence your decision when treating cellulitis?

- a. Hypertension
- b. Coronary artery disease (CAD)
- c. Obesity
- d. Diabetes

3. Which of the following objective signs are most indicative of cellulitis?

- a. Cool, erythematous, shiny, hairless extremity with diminished pulses
- b. Scattered, erythematous rings with clearing centers
- c. Clearly demarcated, raised, erythematous area of face
- d. Area of poorly differentiated, diffuse redness that is warm and tender to touch

4. Which of the following laboratory tests would be most helpful in diagnosing cellulitis?

- a. Prothrombin time (PT) and INR
- b. CBC count with differential
- c. Culture and sensitivity of nondraining wound
- d. Uric acid

5. Which of the following is **least** likely to be the causal organism in cellulitis?

- a. Staphylococcus
- b. *Escherichia coli*
- c. *P. aeriginosa*
- d. Group A streptococci

6. If your client has no drug allergies, which of the following antibiotics is most appropriate in treating a cat bite wound?

- a. Erythromycin
- b. Penicillin
- c. Dicloxacillin
- d. Ciprofloxacin

ANSWERS AND RATIONALES

1. *Answer:* c (assessment/history/integumentary/NAS)

Rationale: Trauma can be associated with cellulitis if a break in skin integrity has occurred. Decreased circulation to an extremity from any cause contributes to infection once a break in skin integrity occurs. Fever and chills are frequently associated with cellulitis.

2. *Answer:* d (assessment/history/integumentary/NAS)

Rationale: Although obesity, hypertension, and CAD may delay healing, their risks of complications are less than with diabetes, in which both increased blood sugar and decreased circulation may be present. (Bisno, 1996)

3. *Answer:* d (assessment/physical examination/integumentary/NAS)

Rationale: Because cellulitis involves the subcutaneous tissue, it is less demarcated. The infection produces vasodilation and warmth. (Dershewitz, 1993)

4. *Answer:* b (assessment/diagnostics/integumentary/NAS)

Rationale: Of the tests listed, the CBC would be most helpful because the WBC count will be elevated. A nondraining wound should not be cultured.

5. *Answer:* b (pathophysiology/integumentary/NAS)

Rationale: Staphylococci or streptococci are frequently associated with skin infections. *E. coli* is most often associated with internal organs. (Dershewitz, 1993)

6. *Answer:* d (plan/integumentary/NAS)

Rationale: A cat bite produces a puncture wound. This is a more penetrating wound, with greater consequences if not adequately treated. It requires a stronger, broad-spectrum, less frequently used antibiotic for treatment. (Sanford, Gilbert, & Sande, 1996)

DERMATITIS AND MISCELLANEOUS SKIN CONDITIONS

OVERVIEW

Definition

CONTACT DERMATITIS. This is acute or chronic inflammation of the skin caused by external agents or antigens.

LICHEN SIMPLEX (NEURODERMATITIS). *Lichen simplex* is circumscribed area of lichenification resulting from repeated physical trauma (rubbing and scratching).

SEBORRHEIC DERMATITIS. This is a chronic inflammation of areas of the skin where the sebaceous glands are most active (scalp, face, ears, axilla, and pubic areas).

ERYSIPELAS. *Erysipelas* is a superficial bacterial infection of the skin and lymphatics.

ROSACEA. This is a chronic inflammation of the pilosebaceous units of the face associated with increased reactivity of capillaries to heat, leading to flushing.

TINEA VERSICOLOR. *Tinea versicolor* is a saprophytic (yeastlike) organism, a normal inhabitant of the skin, that multiplies excessively, causing a rash.

MOLLUSCUM CONTAGIOSUM. This is a benign epidermal neoplasm caused by a poxvirus.

VITILIGO. *Vitiligo* is depigmented skin, occasionally with a hyperpigmented border.

Incidence

CONTACT DERMATITIS. This condition is less common in elderly and immunocompromised clients, perhaps because of decreased immune function.

LICHEN SIMPLEX. Onset occurs after age 20 years. Higher incidences are seen in Asians and females.

SEBORRHEIC DERMATITIS. This is most common between the ages of 20 and 50 years. It may be seen in infants (cradle cap).

ERYSIPELAS. Erysipelas occurs in immunocompromised clients and those with chronic venous insufficiency.

ROSACEA. Rosacea occurs between the ages of 30 and 50 years. It is more common in females with fair skin.

TINEA VERSICOLOR. Incidence is higher in young adults. The condition is more common in the tropics and in the summer months.

MOLLUSCUM CONTAGIOSUM. Molluscum contagiosum is seen in infants and young children, immunocompromised clients, and sexually active adolescents.

VITILIGO. Incidence is higher in females and in families with an affected member.

Pathophysiology

CONTACT DERMATITIS. This hypersensitivity reaction is caused by sensitized T lymphocytes after contact with an antigen.

SEBORRHEIC DERMATITIS. This is a hypersensitivity reaction to ubiquitous yeast.

ERYSIPELAS. Group A beta-hemolytic streptococci are the most common pathogens.

TINEA VERSICOLOR. Changes in pigmentation are caused by an enzyme produced by the organism that interferes with melanocytes.

MOLLUSCUM CONTAGIOSUM. Poxviruses cause the epidermis to proliferate and form papules.

ASSESSMENT: SUBJECTIVE/HISTORY
Contact Dermatitis

HISTORY OF PRESENT ILLNESS. Rash is seen 10 to 12 hours after exposure. Duration varies from several days to weeks.

PAST MEDICAL HISTORY. Look for history of previous allergen exposure followed by a pruritic rash.

Lichen Simplex

HISTORY OF PRESENT ILLNESS. Lichen simplex is precipitated by an insect bite or minor skin irritation. Scratching the area is pleasurable. Scratching is automatic and reflexive; it is worse during sleep and times of stress.

Seborrheic Dermatitis

HISTORY OF PRESENT ILLNESS. The scalp itches and patient complains of dandruff.

PSYCHOSOCIAL HISTORY. Mother may indicate fear of washing the infant's head or may report "soft spots." Family may have inadequate bathing facilities.

Erysipelas

HISTORY OF PRESENT ILLNESS. Erisypelas has a rapid onset, with fever and chills. Lesion on legs spread.

Rosacea

HISTORY OF PRESENT ILLNESS. Client reports flushing with hot liquid and alcohol consumption.

PAST MEDICAL HISTORY. Look for oily skin and a brunette complexion.

Tinea Versicolor

HISTORY OF PRESENT ILLNESS. Client reports changes in skin color with rash that does not itch. Dark-skinned persons will have loss of pigmentation. Light-skinned persons will have orange-pink, scaly patches.

Molluscum Contagiosum

HISTORY OF PRESENT ILLNESS. Onset is insidious. It begins as a skin-colored, papular lesion.

Vitiligo

HISTORY OF PRESENT ILLNESS. Look for a slowly progressive, irregular area of depigmented skin.

ASSESSMENT: OBJECTIVE/ PHYSICAL EXAMINATION
Contact Dermatitis

PHYSICAL EXAMINATION. Contact dermatitis usually consists of erythematous macules, papules, and vesicles. However, the rash may range from mild redness to large bullae, with a marked amount of oozing. Secondary lesions, crusting, excoriation, and lichenification are common, especially with secondary bacterial infections.

Because all areas of the skin are at risk, the location of the rash helps to provide clues to the offending antigen.

- Generalized: Airborne (paint, ragweed), bath oil or soaps, powders, topical medications
- Scalp: Hair dyes, hair sprays, shampoos, and other hair preparations
- Forehead: Hat bands
- Eyelids: Fingernail polish or polish remover
- Earlobes: Nickel in earrings
- Face: Cosmetics; if linear distribution, think poison ivy.
- Perioral: Lipstick, toothpaste, mouthwash
- Neck: Perfumes
- Hands: Soaps, nickel, lotions, chemicals
- Arms: Wristbands, soaps, poison ivy, chemicals, clothing (new, not yet washed)
- Axilla: Deodorants
- Trunk: Clothing (new, not yet washed), nickel or rubber in clothing (e.g., bra straps, elastic waistbands)
- Anogenital: Menstrual pads, contraceptives (condoms, foam, gels, and creams), powders, poison ivy (camping history without restroom facilities), OTC or prescription salves
- Feet: Powders, shoes, athlete foot medicines

DIAGNOSTIC PROCEDURES. None are necessary. A patch test can be used to confirm a diagnosis.

Lichen Simplex

PHYSICAL EXAMINATION. Look for circumscribed plaque with lichenification (thickened skin with increased markings). There may be areas of scaling and papules. Common areas are the nape of the neck, wrists, arms, and anogenital area.

DIAGNOSTIC PROCEDURES. No diagnostic tests are indicated.

Seborrheic Dermatitis

PHYSICAL EXAMINATION. Characteristic lesion is redness and scaling of skin, frequently on the scalp or behind the ears. On neonates, the scales are yellowish with a "stuck on," dry appearance. If a scale is removed and pressed between tissue paper sheets, an oily residue will be seen. If hygiene is poor, seborrheic dermatitis may become extensive (involving the entire scalp, eyebrows, and eyelashes, and ears and continuing down the neck). Bacterial secondary infections can occur if scratching is severe.

DIAGNOSTIC PROCEDURES. No diagnostic tests are indicated.

Erysipelas

PHYSICAL EXAMINATION. The characteristic lesion, usually located on the lower extremity, is an erythematous, sharply circumscribed plaque with an orange-peel appearance. It is warm to the touch, and local lymphadenopathy is associated.

DIAGNOSTIC PROCEDURES. Tests are not useful in clients who are not systemically ill. Those with marked systemic toxicity should have blood cultures drawn.

Tinea Versicolor

PHYSICAL EXAMINATION. Irregularly shaped, mildly scaly, maculosquamous lesions may appear hypopigmented or have an orange-pink color. The most common distribution pattern is on the chest, back, neck, and arms. Rarely is the rash on the face.

DIAGNOSTIC PROCEDURES. Diagnosis is made through potassium hydroxide (KOH) scraping with direct microscopic examination. The hyphae are short and have a "spaghetti and meatball" appearance, whereas the hyphae of the dermatophytes are long and branching.

Rosacea

PHYSICAL EXAMINATION. This facial eruption (nose and central face) is characterized by pus-tules, papules, and telangiectases. Chronic rosacea can lead to rhinophyma.

DIAGNOSTIC PROCEDURES. No diagnostic tests are necessary.

Molluscum Contagiosum

PHYSICAL EXAMINATION. The lesion is a discrete, pearly white or yellowish, umbilicated, firm papule. The diameter varies from 2 to 5 mm. Many clients have multiple papules. The lesions can occur anywhere, but the most common distribution is on the trunk, face, arms, and genitalia. The center is filled with a cheesy substance.

DIAGNOSTIC PROCEDURES. Most diagnoses are made on the basis of historical and physical findings. Biopsy sampling or microscopic examination of cheesy material (Wright's stain) will show basophilic epidermal cells with inclusions.

Vitiligo

PHYSICAL EXAMINATION. Characteristic appearance is of depigmented areas on the face, dorsum of hands, and the feet.

DIAGNOSTIC PROCEDURES. No diagnostic tests are necessary.

DIAGNOSIS

Differential diagnosis includes the following:
- Contact dermatitis: Rubella, rubeola, acne
- Seborrheic dermatitis: Tinea capitis, psoriasis
- Erysipelas: Cellulitis, thrombophlebitis
- Tinea versicolor: Vitiligo
- Rosacea: Acne, herpes
- Molluscum contagiosum: Acne, miliaria
- Vitiligo: Tinea versicolor, hormonal disease, psoriasis

THERAPEUTIC PLAN
Contact Dermatitis

PHARMACOLOGIC TREATMENT. Use topical corticosteroids (low-potency agents first) and antihistamines for itching. Systemic corticosteroids are not warranted in mild cases and should be reserved for extensive cases, especially if associated with swelling. If oral systemic corticosteroids are used for treatment of poison ivy, the duration of the course of therapy needs to be 10 to 14 days or longer.

NONPHARMACOLOGIC TREATMENT. Cool compresses with astringents (Domeboro) or soaks with oatmeal (Aveeno) are soothing.

Lichen Simplex

PHARMACOLOGIC TREATMENT

- Ice-cold Burrow's solution to lesion every 15 minutes for severe itching
- Moderate-potency fluorinated corticosteroid creams qid
- Antihistamines
- Antibiotics for secondary bacterial infections

Seborrheic Dermatitis

PHARMACOLOGIC TREATMENT

- Selenium sulfide 2½%, tar shampoos, or both daily may remove scaling and alleviate itching.
- Apply triamcinolone (Kenalog) lotion to scalp at night.
- Apply low-potency corticosteroid cream bid to body lesions (do not apply on face or in intertriginous area).
- Ketoconazole 2% cream or clotrimazole (Lotrimin cream) to scalp or body lesions bid may be helpful.

Erysipelas

PHARMACOLOGIC TREATMENT. Oral dicloxacillin, a cephalosporin, or erythromycin is usually effective in the outpatient management of clients who are not systemically ill. Systemically ill clients require hospitalization and more intensive antibiotics. Give tetanus prophylaxis if indicated.

NONPHARMACOLOGIC TREATMENT. Elevate the area and apply warm, moist compresses.

Tinea Versicolor

PHARMACOLOGIC TREATMENT. Management of this disease is usually topical. Topical agents include selenium sulfide shampoo, sodium thiosulfate lotion, ciclopirox, and the imidazoles (see tinea pharmaceutical section for brand names). The ciclopirox and the imidazoles are more effective than the other two older agents. Tretinoin cream (Retin-A) and benzoyl peroxide gel have been reported to be effective. Oral ketoconazole (Nizoral, a single 400 mg dose followed by 200 mg 1 month later and another 200 mg dose a month after the second dose) controls widespread tinea versicolor. It is important to point out that tinea versicolor is not a labeled use for ketoconazole. Oral itraconazole and fluconazole (both are not Food and Drug Administration approved) are also effective against tinea versicolor but require 7 to 10 days of therapy. These two agents are much more costly than ketoconazole. Some dermatologists believe that the organism is harbored in the scalp and that use of selenium shampoo reduces the load of the organism. Selenium shampoo has a repugnant odor.

Rosacea

PHARMACOLOGIC TREATMENT. This condition responds well to oral tetracycline and to topical metronidazole or sulfur-containing preparations. Tretinoin 0.01% to 0.025% creams or gels are used as well.

Molluscum Contagiosum

NONPHARMACOLOGIC TREATMENT. The usual therapy is to leave the lesion alone. The lesions will disappear without therapy within 2 to 3 years. If the client feels that the lesions interfere with self-image, the practitioner may remove the lesion with a curette, electrosurgery, or cryotherapy. These therapies may scar.

Vitiligo

PHARMACOLOGIC TREATMENT

- Staining of skin (Vitadye, Covermark, or walnut juice)
- Corticosteroid cream is effective for early, mild cases

NONPHARMACOLOGIC TREATMENT. Cover depigmented area with cosmetics.

Client Education

CONTACT DERMATITIS. Avoid allergens if possible. Caution clients regarding products with topical diphenhydramine (Benadryl). These products may cause sensitization.

LICHEN SIMPLEX. Explain the scratch cycle and the importance of breaking the cycle. Gloves may be used during sleep.

SEBORRHEIC DERMATITIS. Educate clients that this is a chronic disorder that cannot be cured but can be controlled. It will not cause hair loss, nor is it contagious. Stress that it is more often an oily disorder, rather than one of dry scalp or skin. Good hygiene is essential.

TINEA VERSICOLOR. Expose depigmented area to sunlight gradually. Advise the client that relapses are common.

ROSACEA. Avoid hot fluids and alcohol.

VITILIGO. Avoid sunlight because it accentuates the normal pigmentation and thus makes the depigmented area more noticeable.

Referral

CONTACT DERMATITIS. Refer to dermatologist if no improvement for acute treatment and for patch testing.

MOLLUSCUM CONTAGIOSUM. If lesions are in the genitalia of a small child, consider child sexual abuse.

EVALUATION/FOLLOW-UP

Most skin conditions may last as long as 3 weeks or even longer. Sooner follow-up is indicated for erysipelas. Follow-up can be by telephone or in the office within 24 hours.

REFERENCES

Fenstermacher, K., & Hudson, B. (1997). *Practice guidelines for family nurse practitioners.* Philadelphia: W. B. Saunders.

Boynton, R., Dunn, E., & Stephens, G. (1994). *Manual of ambulatory pediatrics* (3rd ed.). Philadelphia: J. B. Lippincott.

Barker, L. R., Burton, J. R., & Zieve, P. D. (1995). *Principles of ambulatory medicine* (4th ed.). Baltimore: Williams & Wilkins.

REVIEW QUESTIONS

1. Which of the following diagnoses suggests an underlying chronic condition?

  a. Erysipelas
  b. Rosacea
  c. Vitiligo
  d. Molluscum contagiosum

2. A client reports a pruritic rash. Which of the following would help the nurse practitioner differentiate its cause?

  a. Location of the rash
  b. Age of the client
  c. Gender of the client
  d. Skin pigmentation

3. Treatment for tinea versicolor involves:

  a. Steroid ointments
  b. Antihistamines
  c. Ketoconazole (Nizoral)
  d. Tetracycline

4. A child with molluscum contagiosum should:

  a. Remain at home from school until lesions disappear
  b. Cover lesion to prevent transmission
  c. Have the lesions removed
  d. Leave the lesions alone

5. An infant is brought in with a dry, flaky scalp. The nurse practitioner should ask the parent whether he or she:

  a. Has eczema
  b. Fears washing the infant's head
  c. Has been out in the sun
  d. Was exposed to a new detergent

ANSWERS AND RATIONALES

1. *Answer:* a (diagnosis/integumentary/NAS)
  Rationale: The other conditions are not associated with chronic disease. Erysipelas is associated with chronic venous insufficiency and immunocompromise.

2. *Answer:* a (assessment/physical examination/integumentary/NAS)
  Rationale: The conditions with pruritic rashes include contact dermatitis, lichen simplex, and seborrheic dermatitis. Contact dermatitis may appear anywhere on the body. Seborrheic dermatitis is localized to the scalp. Lichen simplex is usually on an extremity and is localized because it occurs after an insect bite or a minor skin irritation.

3. *Answer:* c (management/plan/pharmacologic/integumentary/NAS)
  Rationale: Inflammation is not a problem with this condition, so steroids are not necessary. Itching does not occur, so antihistamines are not needed. This is a fungal infection.

4. *Answer:* d (management/plan/nonpharmacologic/integumentary/NAS)
  Rationale: It is produced by a poxvirus but it is not contagious enough to warrant isolation or covering the lesions. Lesions may last as long as 3 years. Because of the potential for scarring, lesions should not be removed unless self-image is affected.

5. *Answer:* b (assessment/history/integumentary/NAS)

Rationale: These symptoms suggest seborrheic dermatitis. Fear of hurting the baby's "soft spots" prevents thorough washing and may cause the condition. It is not associated with allergies or sun exposure. Contact dermatitis infrequently occurs on the scalp.

ECZEMA AND ATOPIC DERMATITIS

OVERVIEW
Definition

These conditions are both endogenous dermatitis, occurring in three subtypes: infantile (onset 2 months to 3 years), childhood (onset 2 years to adolescent), and adult.

Incidence

- Worse in winter months because of low humidity in schools, homes, and workplaces
- More common in males than females
- Among affected persons, 70% give history of asthma or allergic rhinitis, or a family history of atopy.
- The infantile type may disappear by age 3 to 5 years.

Pathophysiology

Atopic dermatitis is a chronic, pruritic inflammation of the epidermis and the dermis. It is an immunoglobulin (Ig)E–mediated (type I) hypersensitivity reaction that occurs as a result of the release of vasoactive substances from both mast cells and basophils that have been sensitized by the interaction of the antigen with IgE. Primary mediators of the reactions include histamine, chemotactic factors, proteases, and proteoglycans. Secondary mediators are platelet-activating factor, leukotrienes, and prostaglandin.

ASSESSMENT: SUBJECTIVE/HISTORY
History of Present Illness

Client reports dry skin and itching that is worse at night. Rash begins in flexural regions (neck, cheeks, forearms, and knees), and on the face.

Past Medical History

- Allergic rhinitis
- Asthma

Family History

Family history of atopy is significant.

ASSESSMENT: OBJECTIVE/PHYSICAL EXAMINATION
Physical Examination

Very dry skin is present in all persons affected with these conditions.

Infants. Lesions are erythematous papules or vesicles that may weep or crust. The most common areas are the cheeks, forehead, and neck extensor surfaces.

Older Children and Adults. Acute lesions are erythematous papules or vesicles that weep or crust. The chronic lesions are dry and extremely pruritic, which causes secondary excoriation, bacterial infections, and lichenification. Scarring is uncommon, but hypopigmentation or hyperpigmentation of the skin may occur. The neck, anticubital, and popliteal surfaces are common areas of presentation. Less frequent sites include the wrists, hands, eyelids, feet, and face.

DIAGNOSIS

Differential diagnosis includes contact dermatitis, acne, and psoriasis.

THERAPEUTIC PLAN
Pharmacologic Agents

Topical corticosteroids (low-potency agents first) and antihistamines are used for itching; systemic corticosteroids are not warranted in mild cases and should be reserved for extensive cases. Immunotherapy may be used. Appropriate antibiotic therapy is required in secondary infections.

Client Education

Client education is most important. Clients need to understand that atopic dermatitis cannot be cured but can be controlled. Explain that the course of this disorder is unpredictable, either diminishing with age or persisting for life. Breast-feeding of infants may delay onset of atopic dermatitis but will not prevent it. Avoidance of any known allergens is the key to therapy. Because 30% of individuals who have atopic dermatitis have asthma develop, it is essential to encourage clients or caregivers to institute environmental control measures in their homes.

- Avoid excessive bathing and use of soaps.
- Avoid wool and lanolin because these aggravate the condition.
- Keep fingernails short and clean to avoid secondary infections from scratching.

Referral

Refer client to dermatologist if no improvement is seen with steroids.

EVALUATION/FOLLOW-UP

Recheck acute cases within 1 week.

REFERENCES

Barker, L. R., Burton, J. R., & Zieve, P. D. (1995). *Principles of ambulatory medicine* (4th ed.). Baltimore: Williams & Wilkins.

Boynton, R., Dunn, E., & Stephens, G. (1994). *Manual of ambulatory pediatrics* (3rd ed.). Philadelphia: J. B. Lippincott.

Fenstermacher, K., & Hudson, B. (1997). *Practice guidelines for family nurse practitioners*. Philadelphia: W. B. Saunders.

REVIEW QUESTIONS

1. A child has a diagnosis of eczema. Parent education should include which statement?
   - a. It is worse in the summer because of humidity.
   - b. It may disappear by adolescence.
   - c. It is worse in females.
   - d. It is associated with allergies.

2. Characteristics of an eczema rash are:
   - a. Maculopapular without vesicles
   - b. Nonpruritic
   - c. Dry with acute papules or vesicles
   - d. Occurring on the trunk

3. Medications used to treat eczema include all the following **except:**
   - a. Antihistamines
   - b. Acyclovir
   - c. Corticosteroids
   - d. Penicillin

4. When is it appropriate to refer a client with eczema to the dermatologist?
   - a. With the occurrence of secondary infection
   - b. No improvement with steroids
   - c. When the client is allergic to steroids
   - d. When scarring occurs

5. A differential diagnosis for eczema is:
   - a. Scabies
   - b. Contact dermatitis
   - c. Varicella
   - d. Tinea versicolor

ANSWERS AND RATIONALES

1. ***Answer:*** d (management/plan/client education/integumentary/child)
   Rationale: Eczema is worse in the winter because of low humidity. It is more frequently seen in males. Infantile forms may disappear by the age of 5 years.

2. ***Answer:*** c (assessment/physical examination/integumentary/child)
   Rationale: Vesicles may be present. The condition is pruritic and occurs on flexural regions.

3. ***Answer:*** b (management/plan/pharmacologic/integumentary/child)
   Rationale: No viral infections are associated with eczema.

4. ***Answer:*** b (evaluation/integumentary/child)
   Rationale: A client cannot be allergic to steroids. Glucocorticoids are naturally occurring substances in the body and cannot trigger an inflammatory response because they are not recognized as foreign. Scarring would most likely necessitate referral to a

plastic surgeon. It is not common with eczema. Hypopigmentation or hyperpigmentation may occur. A person is referred for alternative treatment (e.g., ultraviolet) when steroids do not improve the condition.

5. *Answer:* b (diagnosis/integumentary/child)

Rationale: Scabies involves burrows and a maculopapular rash. Varicella does not include dry, patchy areas. Tinea versicolor involves only changes in pigmentation.

PITYRIASIS ROSEA

OVERVIEW
Definition

Pityriasis rosea (from the Greek *pityron*, meaning "bran") is an exanthematous, maculopapular, red scaling eruption that occurs largely on the trunk.

Incidence

Pityriasis is mainly a disorder of fair-skinned whites and is uncommon in those with Mediterranean heritage. It is common in ages 10 to 35 years, occurring more in the spring and fall in temperate climates. It accounts for approximately 2% of outpatient dermatologic visits. Male and female prevalences are the same.

Pathophysiology

- Unknown causative organism
- Perhaps a viral or autoimmune disorder
 PROTECTIVE FACTORS. No protective factors are known.
  FACTORS INCREASING SUSCEPTIBILITY
  - Climate
  - Fair complexion

ASSESSMENT: SUBJECTIVE/HISTORY
History of Present Illness

Development of skin lesion, usually on trunk, is followed 1 to 2 weeks later by a generalized secondary eruption. Itching may be reported:
- Absent, 25%
- Mild, 50%
- Severe, 25%

Symptoms

Fever and malaise are rare.

Past Medical History

Past medical history is not contributory.

Medication History

Ask about recent use of corticosteroids.

Family History

Fewer than 5% of those affected give positive family history.

Psychosocial History

Ask about stressful situations.

ASSESSMENT: OBJECTIVE/ PHYSICAL EXAMINATION
Physical Examination

Assess height, weight, and general appearance. Use a problem-oriented approach, with particular attention to the skin:
- General skin lesions: Type, shape, arrangement, distribution
- Hair and nail involvement
- Discrete, erythematous, finely scaling lesions are scattered in a characteristic pattern. The long axes of the lesions follow the lines of cleavage in a "Christmas tree" distribution and are usually confined to the trunk and proximal aspects of arms and legs.
- The condition rarely involves the face. Color is dull pink or tawny.
- A "herald patch" is a 2 to 6 cm patch that precedes the rash by days to weeks. It is an oval, slightly raised patch, bright red, with fine collarette scale at the periphery.

Diagnostic Procedures

- KOH to help rule out tinea corporis
- Rapid plasma reagin to rule out syphilis
- Lyme titer if Lyme disease suspected

DIAGNOSIS

Differential diagnosis includes the following:
- Drug-related eruption
- Secondary syphilis
- Guttate psoriasis
- Lyme disease
- Tinea corporis

THERAPEUTIC PLAN

- Symptomatic treatment
- Colloidal bath
- Topical antipruritics for itching
- Lukewarm oatmeal bath
- Ultraviolet B (UVB) phototherapy or natural sunlight exposure for itching

Client Education

- Reassure client that he or she does not have a "blood disease" and is not contagious.
- Spontaneous remission usually occurs in 6 to 12 weeks.
- Recurrences are uncommon but do happen.

Referral

- Refer client if there is no improvement in expected time frame.
- If rash persists longer than 6 weeks, a skin biopsy is needed to rule out parapsoriasis.

EVALUATION/FOLLOW-UP

Return for reevaluation if lesions last 6 weeks.

REFERENCES

Fitzpatrick, T. B., Johnson, R. A., Polano, M. K., Suurmond, D., & Wolff, K. (1997). *Color atlas and synopsis of clinical dermatology: Common and serious diseases* (3rd ed)., (pp. 104-107). New York: McGraw-Hill.

Habif, T. P. (1996). *Clinical dermatology: A color guide to diagnosis and therapy* (2nd ed, pp. 75-78, 136-154). St. Louis: Mosby.

Millonig, V. L., (1994). *Adult nurse practitioner certification review guide* (2nd ed, pp. 75-79). Potomac, MD: Health Leadership Associates.

Rook, A., Wilkinson, D., & Ebling, F. (1986). *Textbook of dermatology* (pp. 720-735). Oxford: Blackwell Scientific Publications.

Sauer, G. C. (1991). *Manual of skin diseases* (pp. 138-143, 720-723). Philadelphia: J. B. Lippincott.

REVIEW QUESTIONS

1. A 22-year-old female comes in with a slightly pruritic, scaling, red, maculopapular rash on her trunk. The round, dome-shaped lesions are arranged along lines of skin cleavage. She recalls what she thought was a patch of ringworm that appeared before the rash. The probable diagnosis is:

   a. Tinea versicolor
   b. Acne
   c. Seborrheic dermatitis
   d. Pityriasis rosea

2. You examine a scraping from a client's lesions under the microscope with KOH. You would expect to find in pityriasis rosea:

   a. Negative hyphae ("spaghetti and meatballs")
   b. Positive hyphae
   c. Cocci with central black dots
   d. Cocci with central pallor

3. A 12-year-old female comes in with rash on arms and legs for the last 4 days. It does not itch, and fever and chills are not present. She has not used any new products at home. She reports that she first thought it was ringworm but then it spread. Her mother states that she helps at a day care center sometimes after school, and at least one other child has similar symptoms. Which of the following diagnoses would be most appropriate for this scenario?

   a. Tinea versicolor
   b. Lyme disease
   c. Psoriasis
   d. Rosea

4. Your plan of care for the client with rosea would include:

   a. Recommending that she stay home from work until the rash starts to disappear because it is contagious
   b. Selenium sulfide
   c. Coal tar preparations and retinoids
   d. Colloidal baths, calamine lotion, antihistamines, and topical steroids

5. A 16-year-old girl is being treated for rosea. She returns to your office in 3 days, upset that the symptoms have not gone away and that her return appointment is not until 2 weeks.

   a. Inform the client that the 2-week appointment is appropriate to determine progress, but it will take 6 to 12 weeks for the rash to disappear.
   b. Inform her that she should not get so excited; the rash does not look that bad.
   c. Tell her that it is all right that she came back to the office early; lots of people get excited and return early.
   d. Inform her that your schedule is full for the day and she is welcome to change her appointment to an earlier time if there are openings.

ANSWERS AND RATIONALES

1. *Answer:* d (diagnosis/integumentary/adult)
   Rationale: Rosea is usually preceded 2 to 10 days by a larger, single, red, macule, the "herald patch." (Sauer, 1991, p. 159)

2. *Answer:* a (assessment/testing/integumentary/NAS)
   Rationale: For a diagnosis of tinea, microscopic examination of skin scraping with KOH will reveal black clusters of spores and hyphae. You would not expect this in pityriasis rosea. (Habif, 1996)

3. *Answer:* d (diagnosis/integumentary/adolescent)
   Rationale: Rosea is frequently misdiagnosed as ringworm. The single herald patch precedes the general rash by days to a week. (Sauer, 1991)

4. *Answer:* d (plan/integumentary/NAS)
   Rationale: Treatment usually is not necessary; however, the treatments listed in *d* may shorten the duration of the disease. (Sauer, 1991)

5. *Answer:* a (evaluation/integumentary/adolescent)
   Rationale: Teaching clients about the disease process will help them to know what to expect. It takes 6 to 12 weeks for the rash to go away. (Fitzpatrick, Johnson, Polano, Suurmond, & Wolff, 1997)

PSORIASIS

OVERVIEW

Definition

Vulgar psoriasis is a common, plaque-type, genetically determined, chronic disease of the skin. It is characterized by the presence of sharply demarcated, dull-red, scaly plaques, particularly on the extensor prominences and in the scalp. Psoriasis is enormously variable in duration and extent, with common morphologic variants.

   Flexural psoriasis appears in the groin, on the genitalia, in the axilla, at the umbilicus, and in the folds of fat around the abdomen.

Incidence

One of the most common skin disorders, it affects 1% to 2% of the population. It can begin at any age but commonly makes its first appearance in the later 20s and the seventh decade. However, one third of clients are affected before 20 years of age, especially females. Males and females are otherwise affected equally. There is a lower incidence in West Africans, Native Americans, and Asians.

Pathophysiology

Skin lesions are caused by rapid epidermal cell proliferation.

   PROTECTIVE FACTORS. Avoid injury to nonpsoriatic areas.

   FACTORS INCREASING SUSCEPTIBILITY
   • Multifactorial inheritance
   • Minor trauma (Koebner's phenomenon)
   • Certain drugs (systemic corticosteroids, lithium, alcohol, chloroquine)
   • Stress and obesity exacerbate existing psoriasis.
   • Infection (HIV, streptococcal upper respiratory tract infection)
   • Endocrine factors

   ETIOLOGY. The cause of psoriasis remains a mystery. It is clear that there is a genetic component, with an estimated heritability of 90% overall. Certain HLA groupings are also associated with an increased likelihood of the disease.

ASSESSMENT: SUBJECTIVE/HISTORY

Most Common Symptoms

- Skin: Pruritus, pustules, papules, and plaques
- Systemic: Arthritis (resembles rheumatoid arthritis [RA]), fever, acute illness
- Nail involvement: Resembles fungal infection with striping, pitting, fraying, or separation of the distal margin and thickening discoloration and debris under the nail plate.
- Hair growth: Usually unaltered

Associated Symptoms

- Hypothermia
- Hemodynamic changes (shunting of blood to the skin)

Past Medical History

- Medication history
- Other skin disorders
- Trauma (surgeries, minor bumps)
- Infections
- Allergies
- Sexually transmitted disease (STD) and associated risk factors
- Sun overexposure

Medication History

- Corticosteroids
- Lithium
- Alcohol consumption
- Chloroquine
- Beta-blockers
- Interferon-alpha

Family History

Ask about family history of skin disorders.

Psychosocial History

Help client identify stressors.

Dietary History

Obtain dietary history for calorie count, especially in older adults. (Increased metabolic rate and increased calories are needed.)

ASSESSMENT: OBJECTIVE/PHYSICAL EXAMINATION

Physical Examination

A problem-oriented physical examination should be conducted, with particular attention to the following:

- General appearance of client: Uncomfortable, "toxic," or well
- Vital signs
- Skin lesions: Type, shape, arrangement, and distribution of lesions
- Hair and nails
- Mucous membranes

Diagnostic Procedures

- Inconsistent laboratory findings in uncomplicated psoriasis
- Serum HIV test to determine HIV serostatus in at-risk individuals with sudden onset of psoriasis
- Auspitz's sign: Pinpoint areas of bleeding when silvery scales are removed with fingernail
- Throat culture for streptococci: Lesions that are small and red macules that gradually become scaly are usually a result of streptococcal infection.

DIAGNOSIS

Differential diagnosis includes the following:
- Seborrheic dermatitis
- Lichen simplex chronicus
- Candidiasis
- Psoriasiform drug-related eruptions
- Glucagonoma syndrome
- Secondary syphilis

THERAPEUTIC PLAN

Treatment is based on the location of the lesion.
- Elbow, knees, and isolated plaques
  —Apply topical fluorinated corticosteroids in ointment base; cover with plastic wrap and leave on overnight.
  —Apply hydrocolloid dressing; leave on 24 to 48 hours.
  —Topical anthralin preparations: Avoid flexures/eyes
- Scalp
  —Mild: Tar shampoos followed by betamethasone valerate (Betatrex, Valisone)

—Severe: Salicylic acid, 2% to 10% in mineral oil, cover with plastic cap
- Trunk (generalized)
  —Refer client to dermatologist.
  —Topical corticosteroids, anthralin, vitamin D_3
  —UVB phototherapy with emollients
  —Psoralen ultraviolet A-range (PUVA) photochemotherapy
  —Methotrexate given weekly
  —Combination therapy with etretinate (Tegison) or methotrexate and PUVA

Client Education

- Instruct the client to avoid rubbing or scratching the lesions because this trauma stimulates the psoriatic process.
- Medication: Effects and side effects
- Disease process
- Avoid overexposure to the sun.
- Cold may make psoriasis worse.

Referral

- Erythrodermic psoriasis
- Generalized pustular psoriasis
- Subacute psoriasis
- Extensive flexural psoriasis
- Extensive psoriasis vulgaris
- Elderly or incapacitated client
- Psoriasis that interferes with client's functioning
- Psoriatic arthritis or inflammatory disease

EVALUATION/FOLLOW-UP

Initial follow-up is in 2 weeks to assess effectiveness of treatment. Follow-up is at 2-month intervals thereafter.

REFERENCES

Fitzpatrick, T. B., Johnson, R. A., Polano, M. K., Suurmond, D., & Wolff, K. (1997). *Color atlas and synopsis of clinical dermatology: Common and serious diseases* (3rd ed., pp. 42-51). New York: McGraw-Hill.

Marks, R. (1987). *Skin disease in old age* (pp. 49-63). Philadelphia: J. B. Lippincott.

Millonig, V. L. (1994). *Adult nurse practitioner certification review guide* (2nd ed., pp. 75-79). Potomac, MD: Health Leadership Associates.

Parazzini, L. N., Chatenoud, L. P., et al. (1996). Dietary factors and the risk of psoriasis: Results of an Italian case-control study. *British Journal of Dermatology, 134,* 101-106.

Rook, A., Wilkinson, D., & Ebling, F. (1986). *Textbook of dermatology* (Vol. 2, pp. 1460-1478). Oxford, UK: Blackwell Scientific Publications.

REVIEW QUESTIONS

1. A 46-year-old woman comes in with a chief complaint of a 3 cm, red, scaly plaque on her left shin that seems to get better at times. She recalls that her mother had a similar condition. She reports the recent loss of a job at which she had worked for 25 years. She must now work two jobs to make ends meet. She also reports having bumped her leg 1 week before the lesion appeared. You diagnose psoriasis. A discussion of the course and outcome of this disease will include mention of which of the following?

- a. Psoriasis is a chronic disease with no known cure.
- b. The disease has been known to disappear and never return in some people.
- c. Cold weather will make it worse.
- d. All the above are true.

2. The cause of psoriasis remains a mystery. It is clear that there is a genetic component, with an estimated heritability of 90% overall. The other organism associated with psoriasis is:

- a. *S. aureus*
- b. Streptococcus
- c. HIV infection
- d. *Escherichia coli*

3. Which of the following physical findings would usually be found in a client with psoriasis?

- a. Red patches with raised borders on groin and thigh, often in a butterfly pattern
- b. Nails thickened with debris
- c. "Herald patch" of 2 to 6 cm; round, erythematous, scaling plaque resembling ringworm
- d. Auspitz's sign: Pinpoint area of bleeding when silvery scales are removed with the fingernail

4. Psoriatic lesions usually are:

- a. Bilateral, rarely symmetric
- b. Unilateral
- c. Bilateral, usually symmetric
- d. Associated with hair loss with scalp involvement

5. A client with known psoriasis comes in with joint inflammation; your assessment is:

a. RA
b. Osteoarthritis
c. Gout
d. Psoriatic arthritis

6. Laboratory tests ordered include rheumatoid factor levels, erythrocyte sedimentation rate, and uric acid levels. If this is psoriatic arthritis, you would expect the rheumatoid factor to be:

a. Negative
b. <1:40 to 1:160
c. <1:160 to 1:280
d. <1:280 to 1:400

7. For a client with known psoriasis who comes in with joint inflammation, your next step should be which of the following?

a. Start nonsteroidal antiinflammatory drugs to control the pain associated with swollen joints.
b. Refer client to a physician.
c. Recommend physical therapy for moist heat to joints.
d. Do nothing. The symptoms will resolve spontaneously.

8. Treatment for mild psoriasis is likely to start with:

a. Coal tar preparations followed by topical steroids
b. Débridement of necrotic plaques
c. UVB phototherapy
d. Methotrexate given weekly

9. The teaching plan of a client taking anthralin should include all the following **except:**

a. It may cause erythema and burning of the normal skin.
b. It stains clothing, sheets, and bath enamel.
c. It should be used in the flexures and on plaques near the eyes.
d. It will aggravate inflamed psoriasis and may induce pustulation.

10. Which of the following clients with psoriasis would **not** be referred?

a. Older or incapacitated client
b. Client with extensive flexural psoriasis

c. Client in whom psoriasis interferes with function
d. Client with one lesion on elbow

11. Ms. Bernard is a 26-year-old female whom you started on a regimen of coal tar and topical steroids. She should be instructed to return for follow-up:

a. In 2 weeks
b. In 6 months
c. After she completes the medication
d. In the winter, when her symptoms are expected to worsen

12. When Ms. Bernard returns for follow-up, she reports having had a cold since her last visit. She also reports the plaques seem to be spreading. On further examination, you note new lesions—small, round, red macules that have become scaly. Your plan should include which of the following?

a. Change the treatment because this is an allergic reaction to the medicine that she is currently using.
b. Obtain a throat culture for streptococcus.
c. Reassure the client that this is the normal course of her disease.
d. Refer the client to a dermatologist because she has a more severe form of psoriasis.

ANSWERS AND RATIONALES

1. *Answer:* d (plan/integumentary/adult)
Rationale: All are true statements regarding psoriasis. (Fitzpatrick, Johnson, Polano, Suurmond, & Wolff, 1997, p. 42)

2. *Answer:* b (pathophysiology/integumentary/NAS)
Rationale: A history of streptococcal infection ("strep throat") 7 to 10 days before the appearance of the lesions is recognized as a precipitating factor in psoriasis.

3. *Answer:* d (assessment/physical examination/integumentary/NAS)
Rationale: Auspitz's sign is most indicative of psoriasis; the other choices are more indicative of other skin disorders. (Fitzpatrick et al., 1997)

4. *Answer:* a (assessment/physical examination/ integumentary/NAS)

Rationale: The pattern of psoriasis is bilateral, rarely symmetric; hair loss is not a common feature even with severe scalp involvement. (Fitzpatrick et al., 1997)

5. *Answer:* d (diagnosis/integumentary/NAS)

Rationale: Inflammatory changes of the joints are indicative of psoriatic arthritis. (Marks, 1987, pp. 54-58)

6. *Answer:* a (assessment/objective/physical examination/integumentary/NAS)

Rationale: Psoriatic arthritis closely resembles RA and may be equally crippling, but the serum of the affected person contains no rheumatoid factor. (Marks, 1987, pp. 54-58)

7. *Answer:* b (plan/integumentary/adult)

Rationale: Refer clients with extensive disease, psoriatic arthritis, or inflammatory disease to a physician. (Marks, 1987, p. 59)

8. *Answer:* a (plan/integumentary/NAS)

Rationale: Coal tar is effective in psoriasis, although its mode of action is unknown. It is used with topical steroids covered with plastic wrap at night to reverse the inflammatory process. (Fitzpatrick et al., 1997)

9. *Answer:* c (plan/integumentary/NAS)

Rationale: Anthralin should not be used in the flexures because burning is inevitable. It should not be used anywhere near the eyes.

10. *Answer:* d (plan/integumentary/NAS)

Rationale: All the following should be referred: Clients with erythrodermic psoriasis, clients with generalized pustular psoriasis, clients with subacute psoriasis, clients with extensive flexural or vulgar psoriasis, older or incapacitated clients, and clients whose psoriasis interferes with function. (Millonig, 1994)

11. *Answer:* a (evaluation/integumentary/adult)

Rationale: Client should be followed up in 2 weeks to evaluate the effectiveness of the treatment. (Parazzini et al., 1996)

12. *Answer:* b (evaluation/integumentary/NAS)

Rationale: Lesions that are small, round, red macules, which gradually become scaly are usually a result of streptococcus infections. (Fitzpatrick, Johnson, Polano, Suurmond, & Wolff, 1997)

SCABIES

OVERVIEW
Definition

Scabies is an infestation of the skin with an obligate parasite, the human skin itch mite, *Sarcoptes scabiei* var *hominis*.

Incidence

Although most commonly seen in children and young adults, scabies is found in all age, ethnic, and socioeconomic groups, irrespective of standards of cleanliness. A persistently high incidence is found in developing countries and in housing where overcrowding occurs. It is estimated that more than 300 million humans around the world are infested.

Pathophysiology

The male mite stays on the skin surface and impregnates the female. The gravid female mite burrows into the skin, with saliva used to dissolve keratin on the skin surface. Once in the burrow, she remains there for her entire life, approximately 30 days, laying two or three eggs per day. The eggs hatch in 3 to 4 days. The mites reach maturity in about 14 days, migrate to the skin surface, mate, and repeat the cycle. Mites usually require a human host to survive but can live as long as 3 days on inanimate objects. The mites live longer in warmer climates where the humidity is high.

The symptoms occur 4 to 6 weeks after the first infestation and are caused by a hypersensitivity reaction. This response is due to the mite saliva and feces (scybala), which are deposited in the skin. Those who are infested with scabies more than once will have symptoms develop between 24 and 48 hours after the second exposure. The skin reaction is manifested by a rash and burrows.

Burrows are often difficult to distinguish because scratching often destroys them.

In a clinical variant of scabies, Norwegian or crusted scabies, burrows are replaced with granular scales that appear as thick, crusted plaques primarily on the hands and feet, including the palms and soles. This form of scabies is usually seen in immunologically and neurologically impaired older adults, but it is increasing in incidence in immunocompromised hosts, such as persons with HIV infection. Hosts who have this form are highly contagious because they are infested with thousands of mites.

FACTORS INCREASING SUSCEPTIBILITY
- Sexual contact with an infested person
- Close physical contact with an infested person
- Overcrowding
- Sharing linens with or sleeping on a mattress after an infested person

WHO IS MOST SUSCEPTIBLE?
- Children
- Young adults
- Older adults living in nursing homes
- Institutionalized persons of all ages
- Decreased immunity

PROTECTIVE FACTORS. Scabies can be transmitted if, during direct skin-to-skin contact, there is time for the mite to leave its burrow and walk from one body to another. Handwashing will remove scabies mites from the skin before they can burrow. Handwashing and universal precautions are the best protection against scabies infestation for personnel involved in client care.

ASSESSMENT: SUBJECTIVE/HISTORY
Most Common Symptoms

- History of nocturnal itching, particularly on the hands, flexor portion of wrists, elbows, axillary folds, buttocks, breasts, abdomen, and genitals
- Intense itching, more intense at night or with overheating
- Close contacts with the same symptoms
- Persons with a suppressed immune system may not have pruritus.

Associated Symptoms

Ask about history of sleeplessness from intense pruritus.

Family History

Ask about nocturnal itching of other household members.

Psychosocial History

- Multiple sexual partners
- Child enrolled in day care, kindergarten, school, or camp
- Children or adults who are institutionalized
- Older adults in nursing homes
- Other members of the household with same symptoms

ASSESSMENT: OBJECTIVE/ PHYSICAL EXAMINATION
Physical Examination

Strong lighting and a magnifying lens facilitate identification of the burrows. The examiner should always wear gloves when examining persons with skin diseases.

- Primary lesions are burrows, papules, and vesicles.
- Eighty-five percent of infested individuals have burrows on the fingers, interdigital areas, flexor aspects of wrists, lateral palms, nipples of females, and male genitalia.
- Burrows appear as gray to white linear ridges 2 to 14 mm long.
- Erythematous, papular, symmetric rash is found on the trunk, often concentrated in skin folds, including axilla, nipples of women, waistline, buttocks, upper thighs, and external genitalia.
- Rash does not necessarily correspond to where the mite is found.
- Infants and young children have generalized skin eruptions on the scalp, face, knees, palms, and soles. Vesicles and vesiculopustules are common, as well as papules. Burrow lesions are seen on the proximal half of the foot and heel.
- Norwegian or crusted scabies: Thick crusted plaques are seen on the hands and feet, including the palms and soles.

Associated Lesions

- Excoriation from scratching
- Impetigo

Diagnostic Procedures

- Identify burrow. To help identify burrows, go across lesion with a felt-tip marker or gauze soaked with black ink, then wipe dry. Burrows stand out as distinct black lines.
- Place a drop of mineral oil on the burrow. Oil sharpens the appearance of the lesion and makes the specimen adhere to the scalpel blade.
- Obtain specimen and examine it under microscope.
- Scrapings do not always yield mites, so the diagnosis of scabies may often be made on the basis of clinical presentation alone.

DIAGNOSIS

Confirm the presence of the mite, eggs, or mite feces under the microscope. If the presence of any of these substances cannot be identified, confirm the presence of burrows. Rule out atopic dermatitis, allergic and irritant contact dermatitis, pediculoses, insect bites, and secondary syphilis.

THERAPEUTIC PLAN

Pharmacologic Treatment

TREATMENT OF CHOICE. Apply permethrin, 5% cream (Elimite), for its low toxicity and high efficacy.

CONTRAINDICATIONS FOR USE. Infants younger than 2 months, pregnant women, and nursing mothers should not be treated with permethrin.

PROCEDURE FOR APPLICATION. Take a shower or bath before application. With gloves on, apply cream to the entire body from the neck down. Leave on for 8 to 12 hours. One ounce is sufficient for one application.

CHILDREN AND TODDLERS. Apply to head, scalp, and face, as well as to the rest of the body; avoid the eyes, nose, and mouth.

INFANTS, PREGNANT WOMEN, AND NURSING MOTHERS. Sulfur preparations are the treatment of choice.

ALTERNATIVE TREATMENT. Alternative pharmaceutical treatments include lindane 1% lotion (Kwell). The individual should *not* shower or bathe before this treatment. The lotion is to be left on for 8 hours, followed by a second treatment in 7 days. This cream should not be used on clients with neurologic disorders or severe skin disease, infants, or pregnant or nursing women. In geriatric patients and young children, such neurotoxic effects as seizures have occurred. Sulfur preparations are the treatment of choice for infants younger than 2 months and pregnant or nursing women.

CRUSTED OR NORWEGIAN SCABIES. Three treatments are required at 3-day intervals to ensure that all the crusts have been penetrated.

ADDITIONAL TREATMENT. Oral antihistamines and mild topical corticosteroid agents may be needed after treatment to help control the pruritis.

HOME TREATMENT. All laundry should either be washed in hot water with detergent and dried in a hot dryer or be dry cleaned. Bed linen should be washed in hot water daily until the treatment course is finished. Items not washable may be sealed in a plastic bag for 7 to 14 days because the mites cannot survive away from a host for more than 3 days.

Client Education

- Reassure the client that scabies is curable and that it is a common problem in all socioeconomic groups.
- Onset of symptoms occurs 4 to 6 weeks after infestation and coincides with development of the immune response.
- Because of the lag between infestation and symptoms, unrecognized transmission may have occurred.
- All infested family members should be treated simultaneously to avoid reinfestation.
- Symptom-free family members and close contacts should also be treated because of the delay in symptom onset.
- In adults the scabicide should be applied from the neck down to the toes, with special attention to interdigital areas of the fingers and toes, the umbilicus, and skin folds.
- Treatment of infants and young children should include the scalp and face if lesions are present there.
- Relief from itching may not occur from 3 to 6 weeks after treatment. This is because of the skin's hypersensitivity to the debris left in the burrow; itching will continue until the natural turnover of skin.

Referral

Referral to a physician is necessary in the following cases:

- Children younger than 2 years
- Pregnant and lactating women
- Norwegian scabies
- Coexisting dermatologic conditions

EVALUATION/FOLLOW-UP

Clients should be examined 2 weeks after initiation of therapy to assess for irritant dermatitis and treat residual pruritus. A second follow-up examination should be scheduled in 4 weeks to assess for any new lesions. If there are no new lesions at 4 weeks after treatment, the therapy is considered successful. True treatment failures are uncommon and are usually the result of inadequate application of the scabicide or failure to treat all family members and close contacts.

REFERENCES

Belkengren, R., & Sapala, S. (1995). Pediatric management problems. *Pediatric Nursing, 21*(2), 164-165.

Cutter, J. (1996). Scabies: Fighting the mite. *Nurse Prescriber, 2*(8), 44.

Elgart, M. L. (1993). Scabies: Diagnosis and treatment. *Dermatology Nursing, 5*(6), 464-468.

Forsman, K. E. (1995). Pediculosis and scabies: What to look for in patients who are crawling with clues. *Postgraduate Medicine, 98*(6), 94-100.

Goroll, A. H., May, L. A., & Mulley, A. G., Jr. (1995). *Primary care medicine.* Philadelphia: J. B. Lippincott.

Hicks, L. M., & Lewis, D. J. (1995). Management of chronic, resistive scabies: A case study. *Geriatric Nursing, 16*(5), 230-237.

Reeves, J. R. T., & Maibach, H. (1991). *Clinical dermatology illustrated.* Philadelphia: F. A. Davis.

Uphold, C. R., & Graham, M. V. (1994). *Clinical guidelines in family practice.* Gainesville, FL: Barmarrae Books.

REVIEW QUESTIONS

1. After infestation with scabies, symptoms occur:

a. As soon as the infestation occurs
b. Within 1 week of infestation
c. Within 4 to 6 weeks after infestation
d. Within 3 months of infestation

2. The nurse practitioner suspects that Jeff, 18 years old, who has reported to the clinic with a rash on his chest, under his arms, and on his thighs and genital area, may have scabies infestation. Good lighting and which of the following tools are essential in assessing the skin rash?

a. Wood's lamp
b. Spatula for scraping the skin
c. Cotton-tipped swab for retrieving the mite
d. Magnifying glass

3. Which of the following medications is the treatment of choice for scabies?

a. Permethrin 5% cream (Elimite)
b. Lindane 1% (Kwell)
c. Sulfur preparations
d. Nystatin-triamcinolone (Mycolog) cream 1%

4. To ensure successful elimination of scabies from a person and his or her contacts, part of the plan of treatment and evaluation must include treatment of all:

a. Individuals who have shared a bed with the infested individual
b. Individuals living in the same household with the infested individual
c. Sexual contacts of the infested individual
d. Individuals who have had skin-to-skin contact with the infested individual

5. After being treated with a scabicide, a client called the clinic about follow-up care for evaluation of the treatment's effectiveness. Which of the following statements would be the most appropriate?

a. Follow-up care will not be needed because treatment failures are rare.
b. Follow-up care will not be effective in evaluating the treatment because the rash will be present for months.
c. Follow-up appointments will be scheduled for 2 and 4 weeks after treatment to assess for any new lesions.
d. A follow-up appointment will be scheduled for 1 week after treatment to confirm that the rash and burrows have disappeared.

6. Jeff, an 18-year-old, comes to the clinic and reports that he has a rash on his chest, underarms, thighs, and genitalia that itches intensely. Which factor in Jeff's history is most likely associated with scabies infestation?

  a. A sexual contact about 5 weeks ago
  b. Wearing coveralls worn by other workers
  c. Riding in a car with five other people
  d. Camping with no shower for several days

7. After the nurse practitioner examines the erythematous rash on the chest, underarms, thighs, and genitalia of Jeff, an 18-year-old male, she would also examine which of the following areas for the classic lesions found with scabies infestation?

  a. The scalp, hairline and face
  b. Between fingers, flexor portion of wrists, axilla, and penis
  c. Palms of hands and soles of feet
  d. Nape of neck, back, buttocks, and thighs

8. What diagnostic test provides definite evidence of scabies infestation?

  a. Microscopic identification of mites, ova, or feces
  b. Identification of the mite by use of the Wood's lamp
  c. Recovering a scabies parasite from the skin surface
  d. Identification of a burrow

9. When using the recommended pharmaceutical treatment for scabies on a young child, the nurse practitioner knows to apply the preparation to:

  a. The entire body from the neck down, avoiding the palms and soles
  b. The entire body plus the scalp and face
  c. All areas where the rash is seen
  d. All areas with either rash or burrows

10. Older adults in nursing homes are subject to a form of scabies known as Norwegian or crusted scabies. This form of scabies should be suspected if the older person has:

  a. Widespread granular crusts in an area where you would expect burrows
  b. Multiple burrows close together that are excoriated
  c. Erythematous rash with a superimposed impetigo
  d. Red, papular lesions

ANSWERS AND RATIONALES

1. *Answer:* c (assessment/history/integumentary/NAS)
Rationale: Symptoms do not develop as soon as the mites start to burrow but usually occur in 4 to 6 weeks, the time it takes to initiate an immune reaction. (Cutter, 1996)

2. *Answer:* d (assessment/physical examination/integumentary/adult)
Rationale: A magnifying glass and good lighting are essential. (Uphold & Graham, 1994, p. 269)

3. *Answer:* a (plan/integumentary/NAS)
Rationale: Permethrin 5% cream (Elimite) is considered the treatment of choice because of its low toxicity and high efficacy. (Forsman, 1995, p. 99)

4. *Answer:* d (plan/evaluation/integumentary/NAS)
Rationale: The most important factor in the elimination of scabies is to be certain that all exposed individuals are treated, including all family members, nursing personnel, and occasional visitors, especially those who have hugged or touched the infested individual. (Elgart, 1993, p. 467)

5. *Answer:* c (evaluation/integumentary/adolescent)
Rationale: Clients are instructed to return for follow-up in 2 weeks after scabicidal treatment. If the client is completely clear at that time and no new lesions appear at 4 weeks after treatment, the therapy is considered successful. (Belkengren & Sapala, 1995, p. 164)

6. *Answer:* a (assessment/history/integumentary/adult)
Rationale: Scabies is transmitted from skin-to-skin contact, particularly from families and sexual partners. The rash is typically seen in sexually active young adults (Cutter, 1996; Reeves & Maibach, 1991, p. 243)

7. *Answer:* b (assessment/physical examination/integumentary/adult)
Rationale: Often a diagnosis may be made clinically and includes a history of severe itching and the presence of burrows, especially in the folds of the skin, between fingers, breast area, axilla, and genitalia. (Elgart, 1993, p. 465)

8. ***Answer:*** a (assessment/physical examination/integumentary/NAS)

Rationale: Microscopic identification of mites, ova, or feces proves the diagnosis. (Uphold & Graham, 1994, p. 269)

9. ***Answer:*** b (plan/integumentary/child)

Rationale: Total body treatment is required. Treatment in younger populations should include the head and neck because the mite tends to infest above the neck. (Elgart, 1993, pp. 465-467)

10. ***Answer:*** a (assessment/physical examination/integumentary/aging adult)

Rationale: Norwegian or crusted scabies has neither burrows nor excoriations, but rather granular crusts. (Hicks & Lewis, 1995, p. 231; Elgart, 1993, p. 465)

SKIN CANCER AND SUN-RELATED CONDITIONS

OVERVIEW
Definition

SCLEROTIC KERATOSIS. *Sclerotic keratosis* is proliferating immature keratinocytes and melanocytes.

NEVI. *Nevi* are hyperplasia and proliferation of melanocytes located in the epidermis, dermis, and occasionally subcutaneous tissue.

SOLAR LENTIGO. This is a localized proliferation of melanocytes as a result of chronic exposure to sunlight.

ACTINIC KERATOSIS. This condition involves damage to keratinocytes by sunlight or ultraviolet energy. It may develop into squamous cell carcinoma.

BASAL CELL CARCINOMA. This is a neoplastic lesion with rare metastasis caused by sun exposure.

MELANOMA. *Melanoma* arises from normal skin or from preexisting congenital nevocytic nevus. It causes 80% of deaths from skin cancer.

SQUAMOUS CELL CARCINOMA. This type of tumor arises from keratinocytes that have been damaged by exogenous agents acting as carcinogens, especially sun exposure. It can arise from an actinic keratosis lesion.

Incidence

- Seborrheic keratosis: Males 30 years old and older
- Nevi: More common in whites, with a hereditary pattern
- Solar lentigo: More common in males, whites, and those older than 40 years
- Actinic keratosis: More common in males, whites, and those older than 40 years
- Basal cell carcinoma: More common in males, whites, and those older than 40 years.

- Melanoma
  —Superficial spreading melanoma: An age of 47 years is average.
  —Nodular melanoma: Median age is 50 years.
  —Lentigo maligna melanoma: Median age is 70 years.
  —Acral lentigenous melanoma: Blacks and Asians, all ages
- Squamous cell carcinoma: It is more common in males older than 50 years with chronic wind or sun exposure.

Risk Factors

ALL SUN-RELATED CONDITIONS
- Outdoor workers
- Frequent sun exposure without sunscreen
- History of sunburn

MELANOMA. Intense intermittent sun exposure is a risk factor.

SQUAMOUS CELL CARCINOMA
- Smoking
- Immunosuppression
- Industrial carcinogen exposure

ASSESSMENT: SUBJECTIVE/HISTORY
Seborrheic Keratosis

Client reports "stuck on" brown spots over trunk. The condition is asymptomatic unless traumatized by clothing or picking.

Nevi

Asymptomatic "spots" catch clothing.

Solar Lentigo

Excessive lifelong sun exposure is reported.

Actinic Keratosis

Client usually reports multiple lesions.

Basal Cell Carcinoma

Client reports lesion that gets red, peels, or bleeds, then improves, only to repeat the cycle (Barker, Burton, & Zieve, 1995).

Melanoma

Client usually reports change in color, size, or border of lesion.

Squamous Cell Carcinoma

Client may report firm, hard, nodule.

ASSESSMENT: OBJECTIVE/ PHYSICAL EXAMINATION

Seborrheic Keratosis

PHYSICAL EXAMINATION. Size varies from 1 to 3 cm. The color may be skin color, tan, brown, or black. Usually the lesion is oval and has a warty, greasy feel. Distribution is on the face, neck, scalp, back, and upper chest. Less common distribution is on the arms, legs, and lower parts of the trunk.

DIAGNOSTIC PROCEDURES. Biopsy is performed.

Nevi

PHYSICAL EXAMINATION. The lesion is symmetric in color, skin color to brown, and may be flat or nodular.

DIAGNOSTIC PROCEDURES. Biopsy is performed.

Solar Lentigo

PHYSICAL EXAMINATION. Flat brown macules are reported as aging spots. They are frequently present on the hands.

DIAGNOSTIC PROCEDURES. Diagnosis is made on clinical grounds.

Actinic Keratosis

PHYSICAL EXAMINATION. Lesions are usually multiple, flat or slightly elevated, brownish or tan, scaly, and "stuck-on" in appearance. They measure ≤1.5 cm and feel like sandpaper.

DIAGNOSTIC PROCEDURES. Biopsy will yield definite diagnosis.

Basal Cell Carcinoma

PHYSICAL EXAMINATION. Many clinical forms are seen: noduloulcerative, pigmented, or superficial. Color is whitish, brown, or black, with ill-defined borders. Lesions are usually seen on the face or other exposed skin areas. The tumor is extremely slow growing.

DIAGNOSTIC PROCEDURES. Excise for histologic diagnosis; never use electrocautery or liquid nitrogen.

Melanoma

PHYSICAL EXAMINATION

- Superficial spreading melanoma: This is the most common type; it develops from an in situ lesion and is slow growing, flat, and usually dark, with variegated colors. It has a good prognosis.
- Nodular melanoma: This cancer is rapidly growing. Its raised nodule is usually dark, with variegated colors and a notched border. It has a poor prognosis.
- Lentigo maligna melanoma: This is the least aggressive form and may be present for 5 to 50 years before a nodule develops. Nodules are found mainly on the arms and legs; they are flat, usually dark, with variegated colors. The disease has a good prognosis.
- Acral lentiginous melanoma: Occurs on the palms, soles and around the nails; ulcerates and metastases rapidly; usually dark with variegated colors and notched border; has a poor prognosis.
- Hutchinson's sign: Pigment extends onto nail, with subungual pigmented lesion. Excise for histologic diagnosis; never use electrocautery or use liquid nitrogen.

DIAGNOSTIC PROCEDURES. Biopsy will yield definitive diagnosis.

Squamous Cell Carcinoma

PHYSICAL EXAMINATION. This is an isolated, keratotic, eroded, ulcerating lesion (papule, plaque, or nodule). A central ulcer and an indurated raised border on a red base develop on this rapidly growing nodule.

DIAGNOSTIC PROCEDURES. Excise for histologic diagnosis; never use electrocautery or use liquid nitrogen.

DIAGNOSIS

Differential diagnosis includes the following:
- Seborrheic keratosis: Warts, squamous cell carcinoma, basal cell carcinoma, nevi

- Nevi: Melanoma
- Solar lentigo: Nevi, melanoma
- Actinic keratosis: Dermatitis, tinea
- Basal cell carcinoma: Nevi, actinic and seborrheic keratosis, melanoma
- Melanoma: Nevi
- Squamous cell carcinoma; Actinic and seborrheic keratosis, dermatitis, warts

THERAPEUTIC PLAN

Seborrheic Keratosis

Treatment is nonpharmacologic. If the client believes that the lesions are interfering with self-image, the practitioner may remove lesions with a curette, electrosurgery, or cryotherapy. These therapies may scar.

Nevi

Treatment is nonpharmacologic. Excise for histologic diagnosis.

Solar Lentigo

Pharmacologic agents include sun blocks with *para*-aminobenzoic acid (PABA).

Actinic Keratosis

Treatment is nonpharmacologic. The lesion is treated by cryosurgery with liquid nitrogen.

Melanoma, Basal Cell Carcinoma, and Squamous Cell Carcinoma

Treatment is nonpharmacologic. Removal is the treatment of choice. Refer the client to dermatologist for immediate removal.

Client Education

ACTINIC KERATOSIS. Area may be hypopigmented after removal.

ALL SUN-RELATED DISORDERS. Have clients do a skin self-examination every month and report any sensations or changes in moles. Use sunblocks with PABA. Avoid sun exposure; wear long-sleeve shirts, long pants, and hats.

EVALUATION/FOLLOW-UP

Follow-up for actinic keratosis should be every 6 months because new lesions frequently occur.

REFERENCES

Barker, L. R., Burton, J. R., & Zieve, P. D. (1995). *Principles of ambulatory medicine* (4th ed.). Baltimore: Williams & Wilkins.

Boynton, R., Dunn, E., & Stephens, G. (1994). *Manual of ambulatory pediatrics* (3rd ed.). Philadelphia: J. B. Lippincott.

Fenstermacher, K., & Hudson, B. (1997). *Practice guidelines for family nurse practitioners.* Philadelphia: W. B. Saunders.

REVIEW QUESTIONS

1. Which of the following in a client's history would place the client most at risk for melanoma?

  a. Gender
  b. Age
  c. White ethnicity
  d. Intense intermittent sun exposure

2. When removing a lesion for biopsy purposes, which technique should be used?

  a. Electrocautery
  b. Liquid nitrogen
  c. Laser
  d. Knife or scalpel excision

3. When distinguishing between basal cell and squamous cell carcinoma, the nurse practitioner should focus on which of the following?

  a. Texture of the lesion
  b. Color of the lesion
  c. Borders of the lesion
  d. Location of the lesion

4. A client who had an actinic keratosis lesion removed returns with hypopigmentation at the site. The nurse practitioner recognizes this as:

  a. Normal
  b. Fungal infection
  c. Precancerous area
  d. Secondary bacterial infection

ANSWERS AND RATIONALES:

1. *Answer:* d (assessment/history/integumentary/NAS)

Rationale: Males in the 30- to 50-year-old range are most at risk for all sun-related skin conditions. Whites are also at higher risk. However, intense intermittent sun exposure is associated with melanoma.

2. *Answer:* d (assessment/management/diagnostics/integumentary/NAS)

Rationale: Accompanying skin should be included with excision for biopsy purposes. The other techniques destroy the histologic composition of the tissue.

3. *Answer:* c (diagnosis/integumentary/NAS)

Rationale: Both may be firm nodules and vary in color. Both may develop anywhere on the body. However, basal cell lesions tend to have a cycle of bleeding, peeling, and improvement with the borders ill defined. Squamous cell lesions have an indurated, raised border on a red base.

4. *Answer:* a (evaluation/integumentary/NAS)

Rationale: Hypopigmentation occurs frequently after removal.

TINEA INFECTIONS

OVERVIEW
Definition

Tinea is a fungal infection caused by an organism known as a dermatophyte, which is capable of colonizing keratinized tissues such as the epidermis, nails, hair, tissues of various animals, and feathers of birds. These dermatophytes rarely affect deep layers of tissue or cause systemic infections.

Pathophysiology

Infection begins when a fungal spore adheres to the skin under suitable conditions, such as trauma to tissue and moist, occlusive environment. The spore germinates within 4 to 6 hours. Hyphae develop and the germinated spores complete the life cycle by producing more spores. As the dermatophyte grows on the skin, there may be no clinical signs of infection. Some individuals may be symptom-free carriers. Dermatophyte colonizations are not highly infectious. Inflammation associated with the fungal growth is usually an allergic response to fungal antigens that have affected the epidermal layer composed of living cells. Common types of tineal infection are summarized in Table 12-1.

GENERAL CONSIDERATIONS FOR TINEA INFECTIONS
Diagnostic Procedures

KOH PREPARATION. Obtain several hair roots. The proximal 5 to 6 cm is the most important area. Scalp scrapings from the active margin of the suspected infection may be used. Place the scraping on a slide and add 10% aqueous KOH. Let the specimen sit for 5 to 10 minutes to clear the keratinous material. A drop of ink may be added to highlight the hyphae. Hyphae appear as long, translucent, branching filaments of uniform width. Septa may be visible as lines of separation at irregular intervals. Visualization of hyphae and spores under the standard light microscope should be suitable for diagnostic purposes.

FUNGAL CULTURE. Several hairs or scrapings from an infected area may be obtained and placed on the appropriate test medium. Dermatophyte test media have a color indicator that changes the medium from yellow to red in the presence of a dermatophyte. Although this yields a more precise diagnosis, the results take longer. Such precision is not usually necessary. For most clinical purposes, classification of fungal infection by anatomic site is preferred.

WOOD'S LAMP. Dermatophytes fluoresce a yellowish color. Not all strains causing tinea fluoresce.

Tinea Barbae

This condition is similar to tinea capitis, but it affects the beard and mustache. The organism is often transferred by animals and is common in rural areas and in men with exposure to animals (agricultural workers). Treat with griseofulvin 500 to 100 mg qd for 2 to 3 weeks after clinical resolution. Apply wet compresses, débride crusted areas.

Table 12-1 Common Types of Tineal Infection

	CAPITUS	CORPORIS
Definition	Infection of hair follicles and surrounding skin	Fungal infection of glabrous skin of trunk
Incidence and Spread	Worldwide; spread person to person or by fomites	Seen worldwide, both sexes, all ages; spread through direct contact or inanimate objects
Risk factors	Children 2 to 10 years old; more in males than females; more common in blacks; contact with infected persons; contact with infected animals; day care; sharing combs, brushes, and hats; family history of tinea capitis; living in confined quarters; poor hygiene; immunosuppression	Children; warm, humid climates; wearing occlusive clothing; day care centers; pets; immunosuppression; contact with infected person
Assessment: Subjective/history	Itching; exposure in day care; current treatments; animal contacts; history of shared combs or hats; recent travel	Mild pruritis, although may have intense itching
Assessment: Objective/physical examination	Noninflammatory: Areas of alopecia with characteristic black dots, caused by the breaking of the hair shaft at the level of the follicle; areas of hair loss are patchy and round; may have single or multiple erythematous plaques with follicular papules, nodules, crusting Inflammatory: A swollen, hairless, purulent area develops, accompanied by suppurative folliculitis; pus may be present at the site; scarring and permanent hair loss can occur	Annular plaque with scaling, vesicle formation, and papules seen in an advancing border with hypopigmented or light brown center; may occur singly or in groups of 3 to 4
Diagnostic procedures	KOH slide; culture	KOH slide; Wood's lamp
Diagnosis	Seborrheic dermatitis, atopic dermatitis, psoriasis, alopecia areata, impetigo, bacterial folliculitis	Nummular eczema, granuloma annular, psoriasis, lichen planus, seborrheic dermatitis, pityriasis rosea
Therapeutic plan	Best treated with oral and topical agents; oral agents penetrate the hair shaft and topical agents limit the spread of spores Oral medications: Griseofulvin, ketoconazole, 3.3 to 6.6 mg/kg/day, ≤200 mg qd for 6 to 8 weeks Topical medications: Adjunctive therapy, 2.5% selenium sulfide shampoo to prevent spread of infection, available by prescription only; 1% Selsun Blue shampoo can be purchased OTC	Topical agents usually are effective: Miconazole, clotrimazole; apply bid for 4 weeks or 2 weeks after symptoms have disappeared Oral: Only for widespread, inflammatory lesions
Client education	Clean environment of fomites; shampoo scalp daily; avoid sharing brushes, combs, and hats; search out infected pets or other animals and treat appropriately; all family members can use selenium sulfide shampoo to prevent recurrence by symptom-free carriers; children in day care do not need to be isolated once treatment has begun; no oils to hair or scalp; without treatment, lesions will spontaneously heal in 6 months, but client may have permanent hair loss and scarring	Apply topical in morning and afternoon; reapply after swimming, bathing, or exercising; isolation not needed after treatment has started
Evaluation/Follow-up	Follow-up visit in 2 weeks to evaluate progress; monitor CBC monthly during griseofulvin treatment; periodic monitoring of hepatic, renal, and hematopoietic function may be indicated; monitor other medications because some may react with antifungal agents	Follow up in 2 weeks; consult in 2 weeks if no improvement

VERSICOLOR	PEDIS	CRURIS
Fungal infection of skin	Fungal infection of feet; common name "athlete's foot"	Fungal infection of groin area; common name "jock itch"
Common in spring and summer, occurs after puberty, rare in older adults	Occurs more in men, most in 20 to 40 year age group, more in summer and in tropical or subtropical climates	Occurs more in men, children rarely affected; high incidence in summer and in warm, humid climates; transmitted from person to person and by nonliving objects
Humidity; warm temperatures; occlusive clothing; excessive sweating; immunosuppression; malnutrition	Athletes; communal showers or pools; occlusive footwear; excessive sweating	Occlusive or tight clothing; athletic supporters; obesity; wet swimsuits; immunosuppression; warm, humid climates
Reports are a not tanning, mild pruritis	Burning, itching, soreness of web between toes and plantar aspect of foot; history of being in communal shower or pool, wearing occlusive shoes; foot odor	Burning, pruritis, pain, rash
Hypopigmented or hyperpigmented macules, sharply marginated fine scale, visible only with scratching	Mild to moderate erythema between toes; macerated and scaly skin between toes and plantar and lateral surfaces of feet; vesicles or pustules in severe cases; foot odor	Annular formation with advancing, erythematous, raised well-marginated border; pigmented red to brown; rarely extends beyond genitocrural crease and medial upper thigh; first site is left medial thigh adjacent to scrotum
KOH; Wood's lamp	KOH	KOH; Wood's lamp
Pityriasis alba, seborrheic dermatitis, secondary syphilis, pitriasis rosea, vitiligo	Contact dermatitis, interdigital psoriasis, eczema	
Selenium sulfide lotion or miconazole or clotrimazole: Apply beyond borders of affected areas for 5 to 10 minutes daily for 2 weeks; ketoconazole, 200 to 400 mg, has been used 1 to 2 times month for prophylaxis	Antifungal creams: Clotrimazole, miconazole; apply creams bid to feet, apply for 2 weeks after feet have cleared up, use OTC powders to help keep feet dry	Antifungal topical cream, apply bid for 3 to 4 weeks
Recurrence common because organism occurs normally on skin; cleanliness may decrease risk of recurrence; whiteness may remain several months after treatment, treatment may be needed before tanning season	Wear absorbant, cotton socks; wear nonocclusive shoes; thoroughly dry feet between toes; may take 4 weeks to improve; wear shoes or sandals in communal areas; use powders to keep feet dry; recurrance is common	Good hygiene; loose-fitting, cotton undergarments; maintain dryness; use absorbent powder
None needed	Follow up in 2 weeks for improvement	Follow up in 2 weeks for response

Tinea Manuum

This is fungal infection of the palmar and interdigital area of the hand. It occurs on one hand and is usually associated with tinea pedis. Its appearance is similar to that of tinea pedis and the treatment is the same.

Tinea Unguium

This condition, also called *onychomycosis,* is superficial fungal infection of the nails. It more commonly affects the toenails than the fingernails. The affected nail loses its luster and becomes yellowed and opaque. It eventually thickens, lifting up the nailbed, and the distal edge becomes brittle and crumbles. This condition occurs worldwide. It is rarely found in children; incidence in the 40- to 60-year-old population is 15% to 20%. Older adults with chronic venous insufficiency, persons with diabetes, immunosuppressed populations, and those with trauma (athletes) are at risk. Treatment of fingernails may last 4 to 6 months. Treatment of toenails may last for 12 to 18 months. It is a resistant infection, and recurrence rate is high. Topical agents are of little value. Treatment is expensive and requires close monitoring of toxicity related to griseofulvin and ketoconazole. Newer agents, such as terbinafine (Lamisil) and itraconazole (Spornox), are more effective than older products. Clients may choose to ignore toenails and treat fingernails, because the latter are in view and therapy is more effective.

REFERENCES

Bergus, G. (1996). Tinea capitis. In H. Griffith & M. Dambro (Eds.), *Griffith's 5-minute clinical consult* (pp. 1054-1055). Baltimore: Williams & Wilkins.

Bergus, G. R., & Johnson, J. S. (1993). Superficial tinea infections. *American Family Physician, 48*(2), 259-267.

Fitzpatrick, T., Johnson, R., Wolff, K., Polano, M., & Suurmond, D. (1997). *Color atlas and synopsis of clinical dermatology* (3rd ed., pp. 688-710). New York: McGraw-Hill.

Hoffmann, T. J., & Schelkum, P. H. (1995). How I manage athlete's foot. *The Physician and Sportsmedicine, 23*(4), 29-32.

Lesher, J., Levine, N., & Treadwell, P. (1994). Fungal skin infections: Common but stubborn. *Patient Care, 28*(2), 16-30.

Martin, A. G., & Kobayashi, G. S. (1993). Yeast infections: Candidiasis, pityriasis (tinea) versicolor. In T. B. Fitzpatrick, A. Z. Eisen, K. Wolff, I. M. Freedberg, & K. F. Austen (Eds.), *Dermatology in general medicine* (pp. 2452-2467). New York: McGraw Hill.

Reilly, K. (1996). Tinea versicolor. In H. Griffith & M. Dambro (Eds.), *Griffith's 5-minute clinical consult* (pp. 1062-1063). Baltimore: Williams & Wilkins.

Stephenson, L., & Brooke, D. S. (1994). Tinea capitis: Practice guidelines. *Journal of Pediatric Health Care, 8*(4), 189-190.

Uphold, C. R., & Graham, M. V. (1994). *Clinical guidelines in family practice.* Gainesville, FL: Barmarrae Books.

Williams, W. C. (1996). Tinea corporis. In H. Griffith & M. Dambro (Eds.), *Griffith's 5-minute clinical consult* (pp. 1056-1057). Baltimore: Williams & Wilkins.

REVIEW QUESTIONS

1. James is an 8-year-old black male who comes to the clinic with a report of hair loss. You examine his head and observe a lesion that you know to be characteristic of tinea capitis. It is a(n):

   a. Round, erythematous plaque with black dots
   b. Erythematous macule with pustules in the center
   c. Red, raised area with white crusting and yellow exudate
   d. Circular area without hair, of normal skin color

2. The treatment of choice of tinea capitis is:

   a. Corticosteroid topical gel, qd
   b. OTC 1% selenium shampoo
   c. Ketoconazole, 5 to 10 mg/kg/day, and 2.5% selenium sulfide shampoo
   d. Griseofulvin, 10 to 20 mg/kg/day, and 2.5% selenium shampoo

3. Which of the following is most likely to cause a client to seek treatment for tinea versicolor?

   a. Intense pruritis
   b. Pain and tenderness, with range of motion to shoulder joints
   c. Cosmetic appearance
   d. Oozing of serous fluid from the pustule

4. Which of the following is an appropriate treatment for tinea pedis?

   a. Apply clotrimazole cream twice a day for 2 weeks.

   b. Apply clotrimazole cream twice a day until the feet have been free of lesions for 2 weeks.

   c. Administer griseofulvin, 1g every day in divided doses, for 4 weeks.

   d. Apply soaks of hydrogen peroxide and vinegar twice a day for 2 weeks.

5. Which of the following statements represents an accurate statement concerning tinea infections?

   a. Client should be reevaluated when treatment is complete.

   b. A follow-up appointment is not necessary unless there is a secondary bacterial infection.

   c. All tinea infections should be evaluated 2 weeks after therapy has been initiated.

   d. All tinea infections should be evaluated every 2 weeks until lesions have cleared.

6. You see a client with recurring rash in the groin area. You decide that the client has tinea cruris on the basis of the classic location of the lesions. They are located on the:

   a. Scrotum

   b. Glans penis

   c. Scrotum, glans penis, and around the rectum

   d. Medial aspect of the thigh bilaterally

7. To avoid recurrence of tinea pedis, you instruct Mark, a 19-year-old college student, to do all the following **except:**

   a. Avoid leather shoes

   b. Wear rubber sandals in communal areas

   c. Dry carefully between his toes

   d. Wear absorbent cotton socks

ANSWERS AND RATIONALES

1. *Answer:* a (assessment/physical examination/integumentary/child)

Rationale: Examination of the scalp will reveal areas of alopecia with characteristic black dots, caused by breaking of the hair shaft at the level of the follicle, leaving a spore-filled remnant of hair. (Lesher, Levine, & Treadwell, 1994, p. 30)

2. *Answer:* d (plan/integumentary/NAS)

Rationale: D-Griseofulvin is the drug of choice of tinea capitis in pediatric clients. In addition, the client should use a shampoo with 2.5% selenium sulfide to help prevent the spread of infection. (Lesher et al., 1994, p. 27)

3. *Answer:* c (assessment/history/integumentary/NAS)

Rationale: The presenting complaint is usually a cosmetic one, because lesions often fail to tan with sun exposure. Pruritis is often mild or absent. (Fitzpatrick, Johnson, Wolff, Polano, & Suurmond, 1997, p. 730)

4. *Answer:* b (plan/integumentary/NAS)

Rationale: Use clotrimazole cream until the infection clears and then for a few weeks or so afterward. (Hoffmann & Schelkum, 1995, p. 31)

5. *Answer:* c (evaluation/integumentary/NAS)

Rationale: Clients should be seen in 2 weeks to evaluate the effectiveness of treatment. (Uphold & Graham, 1994, p. 268)

6. *Answer:* d (diagnosis/integumentary/NAS)

Rationale: Infection involves the medial aspect of the upper thigh on one or both legs. (Lesher, Levine, & Treadwell, p. 20; Bergus & Johnson, 1993, p. 263)

7. *Answer:* a (plan/integumentary/adult)

Rationale: Treatment of tinea pedis begins by emphasizing hygiene, specifically thorough drying of the feet after bathing. Absorbent cotton socks may help to maintain dryness, and shoes should be made of leather to allow the feet to breathe. It would be prudent to wear sandals or other protective footwear in the locker room. (Lesher, Levine, & Treadwell, 1994, p. 30; Hoffmann & Schelkum, 1995, p. 32)

WARTS: GENITAL AND NONGENITAL

Genital Warts

OVERVIEW
Definition

Condylomata acuminata (or *genital warts*) are "pointed condylomas." They are considered an STD. The condition is the most common form of mucosal human papillomavirus (HPV) infection and the most common STD in developed countries. Certain HPV infections have a major etiologic role in the pathogenesis of in situ and also invasive squamous cell carcinoma of the anogenital epithelium. The maternal genital HPV infection can be transmitted to the fetus during delivery, which can result in anogenital warts or respiratory papillomatosis if the infant aspirates the virus into the upper respiratory tract.

Incidence

Young, sexually active adults are primarily affected. Incidence has increased during the last two decades. Prevalence of HPV infection in women ranges from 3% to 28%, depending on the population studied.

Pathophysiology

HPV is a DNA papovavirus that multiplies in the nuclei of infected epithelial cells and is strongly associated with genital dysplasia and carcinoma. It enters the body through epithelial defects.

FACTORS INCREASING SUSCEPTIBILITY
- Multiple sexual partners
- Not using condoms during intercourse
- The risk is greater in smoking women than nonsmokers.
- Long-term use of oral contraceptives may increase the risk of HPV infection.

Transmission

The condition is contagious, both nonsexually and sexually transmitted. Between 90% and 100% of male sex partners of infected females become infected with HPV, most subclinically. HPV infection probably persists throughout a client's lifetime in a dormant state and becomes infectious intermittently. In infants, HPV may be acquired during delivery.

ASSESSMENT: SUBJECTIVE/HISTORY
History of Present Illness

- Ask about location, onset, duration, and symptoms present.
- Ask about sexual partners with any similar complaint or presenting symptoms.
- Usually asymptomatic, except for cosmetic appearance
- Associated symptoms: Bleeding, pain

Past Medical History

Ask about other occurrences of warts and previous treatments.

Medication History

- Use of oral contraceptives, including duration
- Medications used previously and response

Family History

Positive family history may be present.

Psychosocial History

- Smoker
- Sexual history, use of condoms, STDs
- Children: In infants and children, the disease may indicate sexual abuse.

ASSESSMENT: OBJECTIVE/ PHYSICAL EXAMINATION
Physical Examination

Examine area for characteristic skin lesions.
- Type: Ranges from pinhead papules to cauliflower-like masses. Condition is subclinical on penis, vulva, or other genital skin; it is visible only after application of acetic acid, appearing as white patches.
- Color: Skin color, pink, or red
- Palpation: Soft
- Shape: Filiform, sessile (especially on penis)
- Distribution: Rarely a few isolated lesions, usually clusters
- Arrangement: Lesion may be solitary. Lesions are generally grouped into grapelike or cauliflower-like clusters. Perianal lesions may range in size from a walnut to an apple.
- Sites of predilection

—Male: Frenulum, corona, glans, prepuce, shaft, scrotum

—Female: Labia, clitoris, periurethral area, perineum, vagina, cervix

—Both sexes: Perineal, perianal, anal canal, rectal, urethral meatus, urethra, bladder, oropharynx

Diagnostic Procedures

• Acetowhitening: To visualize subclinical lesions, apply gauze soaked in 5% acetic acid for 5 minutes. Use colposcope or a 10× hand lens. Warts appear as tiny, white papules.
• Veneral Disease Research Laboratory (VDRL) test
• HIV testing offered
• Papanicolaou smear
• Biopsy

DIAGNOSIS

Differential diagnosis includes the following:
  • Condylomata lata
  • Intraepithelial neoplasia
  • Bowenoid papulosis
  • Squamous cell carcinoma
  • Molluscum contagiosum
  • Lichen planus
  • Normal sebaceous glands
  • Angiokeratoma
  • Pearly penile papules
  • Folliculitis
  • Moles
  • Seborrheic keratoses
  • Skin tags
  • Pilar cyst
  • Scabetic nodules
  • Herpes simplex
  • Syphilis

THERAPEUTIC PLAN

• Goal of treatment is to remove exophytic warts and ameliorate symptoms, not to eradicate HPV.
• Treatments for external and perianal warts: Cryosurgery, podophyllum resin 0.5% (contraindicated in pregnancy), podophyllum resin 10% to 25% in compound of tincture of benzoin, trichloroacetic acid 80% to 90%, electrocautery, intralesional interferon, laser treatment.

• Dysplasia must be ruled out before treatment is begun.

Client Education

• Use of condoms
• Communicability of warts
• Importance of yearly Papanicolaou smear

Referral

Referral is necessary for extensive lesions.

EVALUATION/FOLLOW-UP

Follow-up is determined by treatment of symptoms and monitoring for recurrence, with appropriate treatment. Annual Papanicolaou smear should be performed.

Nongenital Warts

OVERVIEW

Definition

Nongenital warts are virus-induced epidermal tumors caused by HPV. More than 70 HPV types have been identified. There are three types of the HPV infections that occur in the general population: *common wart, plantar wart,* and *flat wart.* Warts can last for many months to several years if not treated.

Incidence

The common wart occurs in approximately 70% of all cases of cutaneous warts, with 20% occurring in school-age children. Plantar warts are seen in older children and young adults, representing approximately 30% of cutaneous warts. Flat warts are also found in children and adults, representing 4% of cutaneous warts.

Pathophysiology

Human papillomavirus is a double-stranded DNA virus of the papovavirus class. Wart virus is located within epidermal cell nuclei. Cells proliferate to form a mass of the stratum granulosum and keratin layers of the epidermis.

FACTORS INCREASING SUSCEPTIBILITY. Immunocompromise by HIV disease or after organ transplantation increases the risk of widespread cutaneous warts. There is an occupational risk associated with butchers and meat packers.

Transmission. Transmission is by skin-to-skin contact. Minor trauma to skin facilitates infection. Medical personnel may be exposed to the virus from the plume arising from warts treated by laser or electrosurgery, resulting in a nosocomial infection. Heredity is a factor in epidermodysplasia verruciformis, most often autosomal recessive.

ASSESSMENT: SUBJECTIVE/HISTORY
History of Present Illness
- Ask about location, onset, duration, and symptoms present.
- Ask about treatments tried and their results.

Symptoms
- Cosmetic disfigurement
- Plantar warts can be painful
- Bleeding after shaving

Past Medical History
Past medical history may be significant.

Medication History
Medication history is noncontributory.

Family History
Positive family history is often significant.

Psychosocial History
Ask about occupational exposures (butcher/meat-packer, medical)

ASSESSMENT: OBJECTIVE/ PHYSICAL EXAMINATION
Physical Examination
- Examine the lesion, looking for characteristic appearance.
- Use hand lens to assist in visualizing surface characteristics.
- Perform physical examination with particular attention to any skin lesions.
  #### Verruca Vulgaris (Common Warts)
  - Firm papules, 1 to 10 mm, skin-color, round
  - Isolated or scattered discrete lesions
  - Typically at site of trauma, such as hands, fingers, or knees

Verruca Plantaris (Plantar Warts)
- Early stages are small, shiny papules; plaques with rough surface develop later.
- Skin-colored, they may have marked tenderness.
- Confluence of many small warts may result in a mosaic wart. Lesions may also occur on the two facing surfaces of toes.
- Lesions are often solitary (there may be more) and usually occur on pressure points, such as heads of metatarsal, heels, or toes.

Verruca Plana (Flat Warts)
- Flat papules, 1 to 5 mm on surface and 1 to 2 mm in thickness
- Skin-color, light brown
- Round, oval, polygonal, or linear if caused by traumatic inoculation
- Many discrete lesions, closely set
- Commonly on face, beard area, dorsa of hands, shins

Epidermodysplasia Verruciformis
- Flat, wartlike lesions
- Lesions may be large, numerous, and confluent
- Squamous cell carcinoma, in situ and invasive
- Skin-color, light brown, pink, hypopigmented
- Round or oval
- Confluent lesions, forming large, maplike areas or linear pattern if traumatic inoculation
- Occurring on face, trunk, extremities
- Premalignant and malignant lesions are most often seen on the face.

Diagnostic Procedures
No diagnostic tests are indicated.

DIAGNOSIS
Differential diagnosis includes the following:
- Verruca vulgaris: Molluscum contagiosum, seborrheic keratosis
- Verruca plantaris: Callus, corn (keratosis), exostosis
- Verruca plana: Syringoma (facial), molluscum contagiosum
- Epidermodysplasia verruciformis: Pityriasis versicolor, actinic keratoses, seborrheic ker-

atoses, squamous cell carcinoma, basal cell carcinoma

THERAPEUTIC PLAN

Conditions may resolve spontaneously in 12 to 24 months without treatment.

Common Wart

Topical salicylic acid preparations (Compound W gel), are applied bid for as long as 12 weeks.

Filiform Wart

Refer for removal with curette.

Flat Wart

Refer for removal. These warts are resistant to treatment and are usually located in cosmetically important areas.

Plantar Wart

Use 40% salicylic acid plasters (Mediplast). The plaster is cut to size, applied to the wart, and removed in 24 to 48 hours. This is repeated every 24 to 48 hours. Any pliable, dead, white keratin can be removed with a pumice stone. This process of plaster and pumice stone application can be continued as long as 4 to 6 weeks, until the wart is removed. Pain relief results in the first few days because a large part of the wart can be removed during that time. Aggressive therapies may be painful and can result in scarring. Surgical removal, cryosurgery, electrosurgery, or laser may be considered.

EVALUATION/FOLLOW-UP

- Evaluation is determined by clinical observation of the resolving lesion.
- If lesion is on fingertips, return of fingerprint indicates resolution of wart.
- Further follow-up may not be indicated.

REFERENCES

Berger, T. (1998). Skin and appendages. In Tierney, L., McPhee, S., & Papadakis, M. *Current medical diagnosis and treatment* (37th ed., pp. 111-180). Norwalk, CT: Appleton & Lange.

Decherney, A., & Pernoll, M. (1994). *Current obstetrics and gynecologic diagnosis and treatment* (8th ed.). Norwalk, CT: Appleton & Lange.

Fitzpatrick, T., Johnson, R., Wolff, K., Polano, M., & Suurmond, D. (1997). *Color atlas and synopsis of clinical dermatology* (3rd ed.). New York: McGraw-Hill.

REVIEW QUESTIONS

1. Workers who are **not** at risk of acquiring warts on the job are:

   a. Butchers
   b. Meat packers
   c. Fish handlers
   d. Teachers

2. The type of cutaneous wart that is often painful is:

   a. Common
   b. Flat
   c. Plantar
   d. Filiform

3. Women least likely to become infected with genital warts are those who:

   a. Smoke
   b. Use a diaphragm as a birth control method
   c. Have multiple sexual partners
   d. Have their sexual partners wear condoms consistently

4. Which of the following lesions are most characteristic of warts?

   a. Firm, skin-color papules
   b. Vesicles painful to touch
   c. Oval, erythematous lesion with fine, colliform edges
   d. Round, pearly white papules that are umbilicated

5. Which of the following is **not** an appropriate treatment for common warts?

   a. Do nothing; the warts may disappear on their own.
   b. Be aggressive with therapy, otherwise the warts will become painful.
   c. Use salicylic acid applications.
   d. Perform cryosurgery

6. What is the most important issue of follow-up for women who have genital warts?

    a. Always tell her partner of the warts.

    b. Never use vinegar douches because they make the warts more visible.

    c. Smoking will increase the reappearance of warts.

    d. Yearly Papanicolaou smears are vital.

ANSWERS AND RATIONALES

1. *Answer:* d (diagnosis/integumentary/NAS)

    Rationale: All of those listed except teachers are at risk of coming in contact with the viruses that cause warts. (Fitzpatrick, Johnson, Wolff, Polano, & Suurmond, 1997, p. 766; Berger, 1998, p. 111)

2. *Answer:* c (assessment/history/integumentary/ NAS)

    Rationale: Tenderness may occur with plantar warts, especially in area of pressure, such as over the metatarsal head. (Fitzpatrick, 1997, p. 767)

3. *Answer:* d (assessment/history/integumentary/ NAS)

    Rationale: Women who smoke have a higher risk of contracting genital warts. Not using a condom during intercourse and multiple partners also increase the risk of genital warts. (Decherney & Pernoll, 1994)

4. *Answer:* a (assessment/physical examination/ integumentary/NAS)

    Rationale: Warts are commonly firm, skin-color papules. Vesicles painful to touch are common of herpes; oval, erythematous lesions are characteristic of pityriasis; round, pearly papules are molluscum contagiosum. (Fitzpatrick, 1997, pp. 766-772)

5. *Answer:* b (plan/integumentary/NAS)

    Rationale: Most warts will spontaneously resolve. Aggressive therapies can cause scarring and pain. (Fitzpatrick, 1997, p. 768)

6. *Answer:* d (evaluation/integumentary/NAS)

    Rationale: Women who have cervical warts are at risk for the development of cervical cancer, so yearly Papanicolaou smears are essential. (Fitzpatrick, 1997, p. 766)

WOUND MANAGEMENT

OVERVIEW
Definition

A *wound* is a structural alteration that results when energy is imparted during an interaction with a physical or chemical agent. It involves alteration in skin integrity.

Incidence

Nearly 10 million wounds occur per year in the United States.

Types of Wounds

LACERATIONS

Shearing. Eighty percent of soft-tissue injuries are shearing injuries. A sharp force is applied to the tissue by glass, metal, or blades. This results in a linear wound. These wounds may be superficial, extending through the dermis, or deep, extending through the subcutaneous tissue. This type of wound is the most resistant to infection.

Stellate. Stellate wounds are caused by collision of two bodies, applying compression to soft tissue supported by bone. They are often associated with a hematoma. Most common are chin and eyebrow lacerations.

ABRASION. An abrasion is the rubbing away of the dermal layer of skin against a firm surface. There may or may not be embedded material. An abrasion is similar to a second-degree burn.

AVULSION. Avulsion is a full-thickness tearing away of the skin, exposing the underlying fat. It is the most common tissue injury in older adults.

PUNCTURE. A puncture is any penetration of the skin by a sharp or pointed object. This wound has minimal bleeding and can cause serious injury to underlying tissues and structures. It carries an extremely high risk for infection.

BITES. Bites include punctures and possible wounds of the skin. They may be of human or animal origin.

ASSESSMENT: SUBJECTIVE/HISTORY
History of Injury Event

- Mechanism of injury: If related to a fall, what caused the fall? If caused by a syncopal episode, this client must be evaluated further. Possible causes of syncope may include cardiac arrhythmias, dehydration, pregnancy, electrolyte imbalance, or anemia.
- Puncture wounds
  —What was the instrument that caused the puncture wound?
  —How long and wide was the instrument that caused the puncture wound?
  —What position was the body in when the puncture wound occurred?
  —This information will aid in determining what underlying tissues (organs, bones, nerves, etc.) may also be involved in this injury.
- Time of injury: Wounds older than 6 to 24 hours are more prone to infection and require special attention, such as antibiotic treatment, excessive irrigation, or delayed closure.
- First aid before arrival

Past Medical History

- Tetanus status
- Allergies, especially to lidocaine, povidone-iodine (Betadine), tetanus toxoid, and antibiotics
- Previous experiences with sutures
- Immune disorders
- Diabetes
- Last menstrual period (Be sure client is not pregnant before x-ray studies, antibiotic therapy, or tetanus toxoid injections.)

Medication History

Ask about current medications, especially cardiac, hypertension, and asthma medications, which may cause potential harmful side effects with the use of lidocaine with or without epinephrine. Side effects include elevation of heart rate or blood pressure.

Psychosocial History

Consider the possibility of abuse (child, elder, or spousal) as cause of injury.

ASSESSMENT: OBJECTIVE/ PHYSICAL EXAMINATION
Physical Examination

A problem-oriented examination should be conducted with particular attention to vital signs:

- Heart rate: Increase may be due to infection; decrease may be due to a cardiac dysrhythmia.
- Blood pressure: An indication of potential shock
- Temperature: An indication of infection

Diagnostic Procedures

RADIOLOGY

- X-ray examination of the site of injury to rule out foreign bodies or bone involvement
- Be aware that glass will only be visible on an x-ray film if it contains lead.
- Wood will not be visible on an x-ray film.
- If an infection is involved, an x-ray film may help to determine the depth and extent of the infection.

ELECTROCARDIOGRAPHY. This is especially important in the older adult with a wound caused by a fall or unexplained. The cause could possibly be related to cardiac dysrhythmias.

WOUND CULTURE. If the wound appears infected, a wound culture should be obtained before any débridement or cleansing.

DIAGNOSIS

- Type of wound
- Signs of infection
- Sensory, motor (including range of motion of the joints above and below the wound), and vascular assessment distal to the injury
- Presence of foreign bodies
- Palpation of bony area below and adjacent to injuries
- Children: If child is younger than 7 years, diphtheria, pertussis, and tetanus toxoids absorbed should be administered, or Td if pertussis is contraindicated.
- Tetanus-prone wounds include the following:
  —Older than 6 hours
  —Stellate wound configuration
  —Injuries caused by missile, crush, burn, or frostbite
  —Greater than 1 cm in depth

—Contaminated by debris (soil, feces, saliva, etc.)

—Devitalized or ischemic tissue

THERAPEUTIC PLAN

A plan for tetanus immunization is presented in Table 12-2.

Wound Cleansing

Irrigation under high pressure with normal saline solution is the most effective way to cleanse a wound. An inexpensive and easy method is the use of a 35 ml syringe and a 19-gauge needle to create high-flow irrigation. If povidone-iodine (Betadine) solution is used to cleanse the wound, it must be irrigated away completely to avoid tissue damage.

Hair Removal

- Hair should be clipped from around the wound with scissors.
- Hair in the wound acts like a foreign body and may delay the healing processes and potentiate the infectious process.
- Shaving the hair may cause injury to the hair follicle and increases the risk of infection.
- Eyebrows should never be shaved. Shaving will alter the landmarks, leading to possible misalignment of the wound edges. Eyebrows grow back very slowly, causing alteration in cosmetic appearance.

Analgesia

TOPICAL APPLICATION. This is an excellent choice for use in small children and anxious adults. These preparations are generally used on small, superficial lacerations.

TAC. This is a topical mixture of tetracaine 1%, topical epinephrine (adrenaline) 1:4000, and cocaine hydrochloride 4%. A cotton ball is soaked with 10 ml solution and then applied to the wound. Anesthesia is achieved in approximately 10 to 15 minutes. It should never be used on mucous membranes or areas with poor perfusion. The person holding the TAC to the wound should wear an examination glove to avoid absorption of the mixture through the skin.

LET. This is a topical mixture of lidocaine 2% to 4%, topical epinephrine 1:4000, and tetracaine 1%. LET is used in the same manner as TAC. Anesthesia is achieved within 20 to 25 minutes.

INFILTRATIVE ADMINISTRATION
- Lidocaine
  —Concentration: 0.5% to 2%
  —Onset: 3 to 5 minutes
  —Duration: 30 to 60 minutes
  —Maximum adult dose: 300 mg
  —Maximum pediatric dose: 4 mg/kg
- Bupivacaine (Marcaine)
  —Concentration: 0.25%
  —Onset: 5 to 10 minutes
  —Duration: 90 to 120 minutes
  —Maximum adult dose: 175 mg
  —Maximum pediatric dose: Not recommended for those younger than 12 years.
- Mepivacaine (Carbocaine)
  —Concentration: 0.5%
  —Onset: 5 to 10 minutes
  —Duration: 75 to 150 minutes
  —Maximum adult dose: 400 mg
  —Maximum pediatric dose: 5 mg/kg
- Epinephrine: A solution 1:1000 can be added to lidocaine and bupivacaine. It aids in hemostasis of the wound and prolongs the effects of the anesthetic. It should never be used on fingers, toes, noses, tips of the ears, nipples, penis, or the tarsal plate of the eye.
- Sodium bicarbonate: This may be added to lidocaine in a 1:10 ratio to neutralize the pH of the lidocaine. This reduces the burning sensation that is felt during the infiltra-

Table 12-2 Tetatunus Immunization

HISTORY OF Td	TETANUS PRONE		NOT TETANUS PRONE	
	Td	TIG	Td	TIG
Uncertain or <3	Yes	Yes	Yes	No
≥3 (last dose within 5 years)	No	No	No	No
≥3 (last dose within 6-10 years)	Yes	No	No (Yes if >10 years)	No

TIG, human tetanus immune globulin.

tion of the lidocaine. The shelf-life of the mixture is 1 week.
—0.5% = 5 mg/ml
—1% = 10 mg/ml
—2% = 20 mg/ml

Wound Closure

ABSORBABLE SUTURE. These are biodegraded, last 2 to 6 weeks, and are used for internal sutures.
- Gut: This is made from sheep submucosa or beef serosa and rapidly degraded.
  —Plain: This may cause inflammatory reaction in the wound. It lasts about 2 weeks.
  —Chromic: There is less tissue reactivity, but it may potentiate wound infections. It lasts about 4 weeks.
- Synthetic
  —Polyglycolic acid (Dexon), polyglactin 910 (Vicryl), polydioxanone suture (PDS)
  —Minimal tissue reaction
  —It is used for closures of dermal and subcutaneous layers and the ligation of blood vessels.

NONABSORBABLE SUTURES. These will not degrade or may degrade extremely slowly. They are generally used for external closure.
- Silk: This natural fiber is highly tissue reactive. It is a slow-absorbing suture.
- Polyethylene terephthalate fiber (Dacron): This synthetic polyester material is less reactive than silk. It is difficult to handle because of high friction.
- Nylon: This synthetic material is less reactive than Dacron suture. When used in contaminated wounds, there is a decreased risk of infection.
  —Monofilament: This type is difficult to tie.
  —Multifilament: This type is easy to tie.
- Polypropylene and polyester: These synthetics have the least tissue reactivity of all suture materials. They carry the least chance of infection when used in contaminated wounds and hold knots better than nylon.
- Staples: Staples are made of stainless steel. They are cumbersome and not to be used over moveable joints. Staples are excellent for scalp lacerations. Increased infection rates are seen when they are used in contaminated wounds.

Wound Care
- The wound should remain covered with a clean, dry dressing for 24 to 48 hours. It takes approximately 48 hours for a wound to become impermeable to bacteria.
- The suture line should then be cleaned with soap and water 2 to 3 times a day to remove exudate and crusted blood from the site. This will aid in reducing the scarring.
- An antibiotic ointment may be applied to the suture line.
- Note that neomycin may cause local reactions.
- Wounds that are likely to become contaminated should remain covered for 1 week.
- A joint should be immobilized for as long as the sutures remain in the position of function if movement of that joint will compromise the suture line integrity.

Suture Removal
- Face: 3 to 5 days
- Scalp: 5 to 7 days
- Neck: 4 to 6 days
- Hand and foot: 10 to 14 days
- Arm and leg: 10 to 14 days
- Chest, abdomen, and back: 6 to 12 days
- Nail bed: Use absorbable suture and allow to absorb.

Antibiotics

LACERATIONS. Use antibiotics against *S. aureus.*
- Amoxicillin-clavulanate (Augmentin), 250 to 500 mg PO tid
  —Pediatric: 20 to 40 mg/kg/day in 3 divided doses
- Cefuroxime (Ceftin), 250 to 500 mg PO bid
  —Pediatric: 125 mg PO bid
- Cephalexen (Keflex), 250 to 500 mg PO tid
- Erythromycin, 250 mg PO qid
  —Pediatric: 30 to 60 mg/kg/day PO in 4 divided doses

PUNCTURE WOUNDS. Use antibiotics for *S. aureus* and *P. aeruginosa.*
- Cefuroxime (Ceftin), 250 to 500 mg PO bid
  —Pediatric: 125 mg PO bid
- Amoxicillin-clavulanate (Augmentin), 250 to 500 mg PO tid
  —Pediatric: 20 to 40 mg/kg/day in 3 divided doses
- Erythromycin, 250 mg PO qid

—Pediatric: 30 to 60 mg/kg/day PO in 4 divided doses

HUMAN BITES. Use antibiotics for multiple aerobic and anaerobic organisms.

- Cefuroxime (Ceftin), 250 to 500 mg PO bid
  —Pediatric: 125 mg PO bid
- Amoxicillin-clavulanate (Augmentin) 250 to 500 mg PO tid
  —Pediatric: 20 to 40 mg/kg/day in 3 divided doses
- Ampicillin-sulbactam (Unasyn), 1.5 to 3.0 g IV q 6 hours
- Cefuroxime (Zinacef), 750 mg to 1.5 g IV q 8 hours
  —Pediatric: 50 to 100 mg/kg/day in 3 divided doses
- Penicillin G, 2.5 MU q 4 hours
  —Pediatric: 400,000 U/kg/day PO in 4 divided doses
- Erythromycin, 250 mg PO qid
  —Pediatric: 30 to 60 mg/kg/day PO in 4 divided doses

ANIMAL BITES

- Treat like human bites.
- Rabies prophylaxis should be administered if client was bitten by a wild animal or by a domestic animal that was unhealthy and unavailable to be observed for 10 days. The local public health department should have information on the incidence of rabies in your area.

Client Education

WOUND CARE INSTRUCTIONS

- Keep wound clean and dry.
- Keep dressing in place for 24 to 48 hours.
- Clean suture lines with soap and water. Removing crusted material from suture line will ensure proper healing of the wound.
- Apply antibiotic ointment if desired.
- Keep wound elevated above heart to decrease swelling.
- Watch for signs of infection—redness, red streaks, swelling, pus, and fever.

SIDE EFFECTS OF TETANUS IMMUNIZATION

- Common: Fever and body aches
- Treatment: Acetaminophen or ibuprofen at the time of immunization and q 4 hours as needed to relieve the symptoms

PREVENTION TECHNIQUES

- Home safety assessment
- Use of appropriate safety equipment

Referral

- Depending on the extent and site of the wound (multilayer, large area, etc.), client may need to be referred to a surgeon or plastic surgeon
- If infection occurs, client may need referral to infectious disease physician.
- Eyelid lacerations: Ophthalmologist
- Facial injuries: Plastic surgeon
- Hand injuries: Orthopedic surgeon, hand surgeon, or plastic surgeon
- Clients with human bites to the hand are usually admitted to the hospital for IV antibiotic therapy.

EVALUATION/FOLLOW-UP

- All suture lines should be evaluated within 2 to 3 days to ensure proper healing without complications of infection.
- Closely follow up any wound that becomes infected.
- All puncture wounds should be reevaluated within 2 to 5 days.
- Look for any loss of function, change of sensation, or change in color at or distal to wound.
- Watch for development of fever.

REFERENCES

Barkin, R. M., & Rosen, P. (1994). Bites. In R. M. Barkin & P. Rosen, *Emergency pediatrics: A guide to ambulatory care* (4th ed., pp. 284-292). St. Louis: Mosby.

Brokaw, A., & Ellwood, L. (1996). Planning for pediatric laceration repairs. *The Nurse Practitioner: The American Journal of Primary Health Care, 21*(3), 42-49.

Hoole, A. J., Pickard, C. G., Ouimette, R. M., Lohr, J. A., & Greenberg, R. A. (1995). Emergencies. In A. J. Hoole, C. G. Pickard, R. M. Ouimette, J. A. Lohr, & R. A. Greenberg, *Patient care guidelines for nurse practitioners* (4th ed., pp. 55-89). Philadelphia: J. B. Lippincott.

Kidd, P. S. (1993). Assessment of the trauma patient. In J. A. Neff & P. S. Kidd, *Trauma nursing: The art and science* (pp. 115-142). St. Louis: Mosby.

Larsen, J. L., & Wischman, J. (1993). Tissue integrity: Surface trauma. In J. A. Neff & P. S. Kidd, *Trauma nursing: The art and science* (pp. 413-475). St. Louis: Mosby.

MacPherson, K. (1993). Procedures involving the integumentary system. In L. M. Bernardo & M. Bove, *Pediatric emergency nursing procedures* (pp. 177-195). Boston: Jones & Bartlett.

Markovchick, V. J., & Cantrill, S. V. (1994). Soft tissue injuries. In R. M. Barkin & P. Rosen, *Emergency pediatrics: A guide to ambulatory care* (4th ed., pp. 463-474). St. Louis: Mosby.

Martin, D. R. (1996). Soft-tissue injuries and lacerations. In D. A. Rund, R. M. Barkin, P. Rosen, & G. L. Sternbach, *Essentials of emergency medicine* (2nd ed., pp. 283-293). St. Louis: Mosby.

Uphold, C. R., & Graham, M. V. (1994). Wounds. In C. R. Uphold & M. V. Graham, *Clinical guidelines in family practice* (2nd ed., pp. 834-840). Gainesville, FL: Barmarrae Books.

REVIEW QUESTIONS

1. Mrs. J.P., a 72-year-old woman, arrives at your clinic with a laceration to her forehead. She states that she fell earlier today but does not remember how. Your initial evaluation of Mrs. J.P. should include which of the following?

   a. ECG
   b. Stress test
   c. CT scan of her brain
   d. Skull x-ray film

2. P.J. states that she dropped a sharp knife on her foot while removing it from the dishwasher. She now has a laceration to her foot that will require stitches. P.J. states that her last Td shot was 7 years ago. You determine that P.J.:

   a. Requires a Td immunization because it has been longer than 5 years since her last immunization
   b. Does not require a Td immunization because the wound is considered a clean wound and her last immunization was less than 10 years ago.
   c. Requires Td immunization because all wounds to the feet should be considered dirty and must be protected with prophylactic immunization.
   d. Does not require a Td immunization because the wound is a clean wound, and clean wounds do not require Td immunization.

3. Tommy comes to your clinic with a long, linear laceration to his scalp. It is a clean, superficial wound without contamination. His past medical history is noncontributory. He is extremely anxious and impatient. The best way to close this wound would be the use of:

   a. Chromic gut sutures
   b. Silk sutures
   c. Staples
   d. Dacron sutures

4. J.W.'s puncture wound is at high risk for infection. You have decided to send him home with an antibiotic. He has no known allergies. Which of the following antibiotics would you use to treat this adult?

   a. Amoxicillin-clavulanate
   b. Cefuroxime
   c. Trimethoprim-sulfamethoxazole
   d. Bacitracin zinc–polymyxin B sulfate (Polysporin)

5. B.C. has had a laceration to the lower leg repaired. Discharge instructions for this client should include all the following **except:**

   a. The wound should be reevaluated in 2 days for possible signs of infection and to ensure that it is healing well.
   b. A topical antibiotic ointment can be applied to the suture line after cleaning.
   c. The sutures need to be removed in 5 to 7 days.
   d. The client should be seen immediately if the area becomes painful, red streaks develop, or drainage is noted from the wound.

6. D.K. states that he fell from his motorcycle earlier in the day. He is now reporting lacerations to his left outer thigh and left upper arm. You evaluate the wounds and determine that he has sustained multiple abrasions. You explain to D.K. that an abrasion is:

   a. Caused by shearing forces that tear away the full thickness of the skin and fat layers
   b. Caused by shearing forces that tear away the epidermis and the upper layer of the dermis, with dirt often embedded in the wound
   c. Caused by shearing or tearing forces that result in a linear wound that expands through the dermis
   d. Caused by compression of soft tissue

Answers and Rationales

1. *Answer:* a (assessment/management/diagnostics/integumentary/NAS)

Rationale: All clients must be examined for any life-threatening conditions. A high index of suspicion must be maintained when evaluating a mechanism of injury. A cardiac arrhythmia may have caused this client to fall. A stress test may be needed at a later time, but not yet. A CT scan or a skull x-ray film may be required after further evaluation of the wound. (Kidd, 1993)

2. *Answer:* b (plan/management/therapeutics/pharmacologic/integumentary/NAS)

Rationale: The wound is not considered a tetanus-prone wound, and the tetanus status is up to date within the past 10 years. If a wound is tetanus prone, then the immunization status should be within the past 5 years. (Hoole, Pickard, Ouimette, Lohr, & Greenberg, 1995)

3. *Answer:* c (plan/management/therapeutics/nonpharmacologic/integumentary/NAS)

Rationale: Staples are indicated for use on the scalp, trunk and extremities. They are especially useful when time is a factor. Chromic gut is an absorbable suture and is not indicated for skin closure. Silk and Dacron are associated with increased skin reactions. (Martin, 1996)

4. *Answer:* a (plan/management/therapeutics/pharmacologic/integumentary/NAS)

Rationale: The first choice of antibiotic is a penicillinase-resistant penicillin or a first-generation cephalosporin. Amoxicillin-clavulanate (Augmentin) is effective in the treatment of *S. aureus* and *P. aeruginosa,* both of which are common organisms associated with puncture wounds. Choice *b*, cefuroxime, is an IV antibiotic and is not needed for this client. Choice *c*, trimethoprim-sulfamethoxazole (Bactrim), is not effective against *P. aeruginosa.* Choice *d*, Polysporin, is a topical antibiotic ointment and is inappropriate for use with this type of wound. (Uphold & Graham, 1994; Martin, 1996)

5. *Answer:* c (plan/management/client education/integumentary/NAS)

Rationale: Sutures to the leg should remain for 10 to 14 days to ensure adequate scar formation. The remaining choices are important discharge instructions that should be given to all clients who come in for wound care. (Uphold & Graham, 1994)

6. *Answer:* b (diagnosis/integumentary/NAS)

Rationale: Abrasions are often treated like burn injuries. The wound must be débrided to remove the dirt embedded in it to avoid tattooing. Choice *a* describes an avulsion injury. Choice *c* describes a laceration. Choice *d* describes a crush injury, which is usually associated with a hematoma. (Larsen & Wischman, 1993)

13

Lymphatic System

LYMPHOMA

OVERVIEW
Definition

Lymphadenopathy is a condition involving a pain-less lymph node that is >10 mm in size (except epitrochlear [>5 mm] and inguinal [>15 mm]). *Adenitis* is inflammation of a lymph node, usually caused by staphylococci or streptococci. *Cat-scratch fever* also causes enlarged lymph nodes. Enlarged lymph nodes are common with viral in-fections in children. Some systemic illnesses, such as mononucleosis, AIDS, and Kawasaki syn-drome, can cause generalized lymphadenopathy.

Lymphoma is a malignant disease of the lym-phoid tissue, either Hodgkin's or non-Hodgkin's lymphoma. Usually it is a painless, unilateral, en-larging, firm, neck mass (70% of cases are located in the neck), often in the upper third of the neck. *Non-Hodgkin's lymphoma* is malignant disease of the lymphoid tissue with no Reed-Sternberg cells present.

Incidence

Hodgkin's lymphoma incidence is 3.5 cases/100,000 population. Approximately 7500 cases/year occur in the United States, more often in males than in females. Non-Hodgkin's lym-phoma has an incidence of 9 cases/100,000 pop-ulation, with peak incidence at 7 to 11 years.

CHILDREN
- Birth to 6 years: Lymphoma is one of the top four malignancies
- Younger than 12 years: Hodgkin's lym-phoma is one of the top two malignancies.

- Older than 12 years: Hodgkin's lymphoma is the most frequent malignancy of the head and neck.

Pathophysiology

Malignant transformation of an uncertain pro-genitor cell leads to the Reed-Sternberg cell or other malignant cell. Disease spreads to lym-phoid tissue and eventually to nonlymphoid tis-sue (Table 13-1).

RISK FACTORS
- Autoimmune disease
- Immunodeficiency
- Onset before 1 month of age

ASSESSMENT: SUBJECTIVE/HISTORY
Symptoms
- Painless, enlarged lymph nodes
- Fever
- Night sweats
- Weight loss
- Fatigue
- Anorexia

Past Medical History
- Ask about recent infections that may have caused enlarged lymph nodes and about ex-posure to someone who is ill.
- Ask about unusual exposure to animals, inges-tion of unpasteurized milk, travel to exotic lands.

Table 13-1 Staging of Hodgkin's Disease

STAGE	CHARACTERISTICS		SURVIVAL
Stage I	Single node group		90% at 5 yr
Stage II	Two or more groups on same side of diaphragm		90% at 5 yr
Stage III	Node groups on both sides of diaphragm		75% at 10 yr
Stage IV	Dissemination involving nonlymphatic organs		66% at 10 yr
Subclassification		A, Asymptomatic	Better prognosis
		B, Symptomatic	

- Ask about congenital/acquired dysfunction of the immune system.
- History of blood product use
- Risk factors for HIV

Medication History

Ask about chronic treatment with phenytoin (increased risk of lymphoma).

Family History

Ask about family history of lymphoma or other malignancies.

ASSESSMENT: OBJECTIVE/ PHYSICAL EXAMINATION

Physical Examination

A problem-oriented physical examination should be conducted with particular attention to vital signs, weight, general appearance, and growth parameters in children.

- Lymph: Check neck, axilla, and groin for enlarged nodes. Evaluate for size, shape, consistency, location, fixation, and duration and rate of change.
- Abdomen: Liver and spleen enlargement

DIAGNOSTIC PROCEDURES

Laboratory Tests

- Complete blood cell count with differential
- Chemistry
- Sedimentation rate

Special Tests/Diagnostic Procedures

- Liver and renal function tests
- Chest x-ray film (CXR)
- CT or MRI scan

- Lymph node biopsy: Excisional; Reed-Sternberg cell is diagnostic for Hodgkin's lymphoma.
- Lymphangiogram
- Exploratory laparotomy, with splenectomy in some people
- Bone marrow biopsy

DIAGNOSIS

Differential diagnosis includes the following:
- Other lymphomas
- Mononucleosis
- Sarcoidosis
- AIDS
- Autoimmune disease

THERAPEUTIC PLAN

Pharmacologic Treatment

Chemotherapeutic regimen is called *MOPP* (*m*echlorethamine [nitrogen mustard], vincristine [*O*ncovin], *P*rocarbazine, prednisone).

Nonpharmacologic Treatment

Subtotal or total nodal irradiation may be used.

Client Education

- Effect of therapy on gonads, consideration of sperm banking
- Risk of secondary malignancies

Referral

All clients should be referred to surgeon for excisional biopsy and then to oncologist if disease is malignant.

REFERENCES

Barker, L., Burton, J., & Zieve, P. (1995). *Principles of ambulatory medicine* (4th ed.). Baltimore: Williams & Wilkins.

Dershewitz, R. (1993). *Ambulatory pediatric care.* Philadelphia: J. B. Lippincott.

Ramsey, P., & Larson, E. (1993). *Medical therapeutics* (2nd ed.). Philadelphia: W. B. Saunders.

Uphold, C., & Graham, M. (1994). *Clinical guidelines in family practice.* Gainesville, FL: Barmarrae Books.

REVIEW QUESTIONS

1. All the following may cause generalized lymphadenopathy **except:**

   a. AIDS

   b. Mononucleosis

   c. Cat-scratch fever

   d. Streptococcal infection

2. The most frequent site of a palpable lesion in lymphoma is the:

   a. Neck

   b. Groin

   c. Extremity

   d. Abdomen

3. A client comes in with fever, weight loss, and fatigue. Differential diagnosis would include all the following **except:**

   a. Chronic fatigue syndrome

   b. Lymphoma

   c. AIDS

   d. Tuberculosis

4. A risk factor for lymphoma elicited in the past medical history would be:

   a. Lupus

   b. Mononucleosis

   c. Splenectomy

   d. Lyme disease

5. When an enlarged, painless, firm node is discovered in client's neck, the nurse practitioner should do which of the following?

   a. Order a soft-tissue film of the neck.

   b. Perform an incision and drainage of the lesion and culture the drainage.

   c. Refer the client to a surgeon for biopsy.

   d. Order a CXR.

ANSWERS AND RATIONALES

1. *Answer:* d (diagnosis/lymphatic/NAS)
Rationale: Streptococcal infection usually causes inflammation of a particular lymph node or nodes in a specific area related to a local infection. The other diagnoses are associated with generalized lymphadenopathy. (Barker, Burton, & Zieve, 1995)

2. *Answer:* a (assessment/physical examination/lymphatic/NAS)
  Rationale: About 70% of lymphomas are first seen as a painless, unilateral, enlarging, firm neck mass. (Barker, Burton, & Zieve, 1995)

3. *Answer:* a (diagnosis/diagnosis/lymphatic/NAS)
  Rationale: Chronic fatigue syndrome does not have fever or weight loss associated. The other choices have all three symptoms. (Barker, Burton, & Zieve, 1995)

4. *Answer:* a (assessment/history/lymphatic/NAS)
  Rationale: Autoimmune diseases increase the risk of lymphoma. Lupus is the only autoimmune disease listed. (Ramsey & Larson, 1993)

5. *Answer:* c (plan/management, consultation, and referral/NAS)
  Rationale: A soft-tissue film of the neck might give better parameters for the size of the lesion, but it will not help in diagnosing the source of the lesion. A firm lesion will not have drainage and should not be excised until it has been sampled for biopsy. Neither biopsy nor excision is within the normal nurse practitioner scope of practice. A CXR will be helpful when staging the disease or before surgery. (Barker, Burton, & Zieve, 1995)

14

Allergies

ASTHMA

OVERVIEW
Definition

Asthma is a chronic inflammatory disorder of the airways that causes airway hyperresponsiveness and obstruction. Airway obstruction may either reverse spontaneously or require treatment. Inflammation also increases existing bronchial hyperresponsiveness to a variety of stimuli. The syndrome of symptoms includes recurrent wheeze, cough (particularly at night), and mild to severe respiratory distress.

Incidence

- More than 15 million people in the United States have had asthma diagnosed.
- From 5% to 10% of all persons younger than 20 years are affected.
- Asthma is a major cause of outpatient visits and hospitalizations for all ages.
- Incidence is high among black adolescents and young adults.

Pathophysiology

- Bronchial obstruction results from acute airway constriction, airway edema, and mucus plug formation.
- Asthma is characterized by erosion of the airway epithelium, deposition of collagen beneath the basement membrane, edema, mast-cell activation, and infiltration by inflammatory cells.

Epidemiology

- Atopy is the strongest predisposing factor associated with asthma (immunoglobin E–mediated response to allergens manifested as rash, or upper respiratory tract symptoms).
- Development of asthma is also associated with sensitivity to nonsteroidal antiinflammatory drugs, presence of nasal polyps, or chronic sinusitis.
- Viral respiratory illness may act as a trigger.
- Environmental exposures are highly associated.
  - Children: Most common environmental triggers are cigarette smoke, animal proteins, and house dust mites
  - Adults: Occupational exposures include organic chemicals and wood dusts.

ASSESSMENT: SUBJECTIVE/HISTORY
History of Present Illness

- Cough (especially nocturnal)
- Recurrent wheeze
- Recurrent breathing trouble (dyspnea)
- Recurrent chest tightness

Symptoms

Symptoms occur or worsen in the presence of certain factors:

- Airborne dust or chemicals
- Animals with fur or feathers
- Weather changes
- Exercise
- House dust

- Mold
- Pollen
- Smoke (tobacco or wood)
- Stress/emotional response
- Viral infection

ASSESSMENT: OBJECTIVE/ PHYSICAL EXAMINATION
Physical Examination

The physical examination is targeted. Other systems are checked as individually indicated.

- General: Vital signs, responsiveness, signs of distress
- Eyes: Allergic shiners, injection, watery discharge
- Ears (children): Concurrent signs of otitis media (acute or with effusion)
- Nose: Polyps, congestion, discharge
- Mouth: Injection of throat, postnasal discharge
- Skin: Signs of atopy (i.e. eczema, dermatitis)
- Chest:
  - Observation: Use of accessory muscles, retractions, breathing effort
  - Auscultation: Wheeze (end-expiratory), air movement (decrease or absence a sign of a more severe condition)
  - Percussion: Resonance

Diagnostic Procedures

Test lung function. Peak expiratory flow rate (PEFR) is measured. A 20% variation between first morning measurement (before medications) and early afternoon measurement (after taking short-acting inhaled beta-adrenergic agonist) suggests an asthmatic state.

NOTE: Asthma diagnosis is also based on symptom history, identifiable triggers, and reversibility of airway obstruction.

DIAGNOSIS

See Table 14-1 for classification of severity of asthma. Differential diagnosis includes the following:

- Allergic rhinitis
- Heart disease
- Gastroesophageal reflux
- Sinusitis
- Vocal cord dysfunction

INFANTS AND CHILDREN
- Aspiration
- Bronchopulmonary dysplasia
- Cystic fibrosis
- Foreign body
- Laryngeotracheomalacia
- Tracheal stenosis
- Vascular rings

Table 14-1 Classification of Asthma Severity

CATEGORY	SYMPTOMS	NOCTURNAL SYMPTOMS	LUNG FUNCTION
Step 1 Mild intermittent	Symptoms <2×/wk No symptoms between exacerbations Brief exacerbations Exacerbations vary in intensity	≤2×/mo	PEFR at least 80% of predicted <20% variability Normal EPFR between exacerbations
Step 2 Mild persistent	Symptoms <1×/day but >2×/wk Exacerbations may affect activity	>2×/mo	PEFR 80% 20% to 30% variability
Step 3 Moderate persistent	Daily symptoms Daily use of inhaled short-acting beta-agonist Exacerbations affect activity Exacerbations >2×/wk	>1×/wk	PEFR 60% to 80% >30% variability
Step 4 Severe persistent	Continual symptoms Limited activity Frequent exacerbations	Frequent	PEFR ≤60% >30% variability

ADULTS
- Chronic obstructive pulmonary disease
- Congestive heart failure

THERAPEUTIC PLAN
Therapeutic Management
Management is done in conjunction with physician consultation (especially during the diagnostic phase).
1. Control acute exacerbation.
   a. Correct significant hypoxia.
   b. Reverse airway obstruction.
   c. Reduce inflammation and risk of recurrence by intensifying therapy.
2. Manage coexisting illness or disease.
3. Determine client's personal best PEFR once condition has stabilized.
   a. Record PEFR 2 to 4 times/day for 2 to 3 weeks to obtain a consistent pattern.
   b. Personal best measure is established as 100% PEFR; other parameters for identification of worsening symptoms and medication adjustments are based on this measure.
4. Establish an individualized written action plan in partnership with the client and family.
5. Consider allergy testing and immunotherapy once unavoidable allergens have been determined.

Pharmacologic Management
STEPPED CARE APPROACH (TABLE 14-2)
1. Step up (in number) if control is not maintained after confirmation of medication technique, compliance, and environmental control.
2. Step down (in number) gradually if review of status (Table 14-1) signifies that reduction of medications is possible.

TYPES OF MEDICATION
1. Long-term control: Medication is given on a daily basis. These agents are not to be given to relieve an attack. Benefit accrues over time. Agents include glucocorticoids (e.g., prednisone), cromolyn sodium (Intal), nedocromil sodium (Tilade), long-acting beta-agonists (e.g., salmeterol xinafoate [Servent]), leukotriene modifiers (e.g., Accolate) and possibly sustained-release the-

ophylline. Consider side effects, cost, and current practice.
   a. Side effects: Cromolyn sodium and nedocromil have fewer side effects than do glucocorticoids.
   b. Cost: Leukotriene modifiers and cromolyn sodium are more expensive than are other therapies.
   c. Current practice:. Theophylline has limited use only (nocturnal symptoms); it is not preferred therapy. The role of leukotriene modifiers is not well established.
2. Quick relief: Medication is given as needed for relief of exacerbations (acute symptoms) and prevention of exercise-induced bronchospasm. Agents include short-acting beta-agonists (e.g., albuterol), anticholinergics (e.g., metaproteranol sulfate [Alupent]) and systemic glucocorticoids.
   a. See Table 14-2 for a guide to stepped care.

Client Education
- Ongoing process
- Continuity of primary provider is important in developing accountability to partnership.
- Reinforce and confirm knowledge base at each visit.
- Basic asthma facts (overview)
- Role of medications, with emphasis on differences between quick relief and long-term control
- Medication administration: inhaler or spacer use, nebulizer use, cleaning of equipment
- Self-monitoring
  —Recognizing signs and symptoms of an attack
  —Lung function: PEFR
  —Tracking of condition with asthma diary
- Medication adjustment according to symptoms and response
- Emergency plan "rescue steps"
  —Give initial home treatment with quick-relief medication
  —Contact provider according to response:
    Good response, PEFR >80% (green): Call for follow-up.
    Incomplete response, PEFR 50% to 80% (yellow): Call today for appointment.
    Poor response, PEFR <50% (red): Go to emergency department (ED).

Table 14-2   Guide to Stepped Care*

	DAILY MEDICATIONS FOR LONG-TERM CONTROL	MEDICATIONS FOR QUICK RELIEF
Step 1 Mild intermittent	*No daily medications*	Short-acting inhaled beta-agonist; use more than 2×/wk may indicate the need to initiate long-term therapy†
Step 2 Mild persistent	*One daily medication* Anti-inflammatory agent (low-dose inhaled glucocorticoid, clocromolyn, or necromil) *or* Alternate therapies: Sustained-release theophylline, not preferred treatment; leukotriene modifiers (>12 years old, role in therapy not fully established)	Short-acting inhaled beta-agonist; daily use or increasing use indicates need for additional long-term therapy†
Step 3 Moderate persistent	*One or two daily medications* Antiinflammatory agent (medium dose) *and/or* Long-acting bronchodilator, especially for nocturnal symptoms (e.g., salmeterol or sustained-release theophylline) plus medium-dose inhaled glucocorticoid	Short-acting inhaled beta-agonist; daily use or increasing use indicates need for additional long-term therapy‡
Step 4 Severe persistent	*Two daily medications* Antiinflammatory agent (high dose) *and* Long-acting bronchodilator *and* Oral glucocorticoid	Short-acting inhaled beta agonist; daily use or increasing use indicates need for additional long-term therapy†

*Match to step number identified in classification of asthma severity (see Table 14-1).
†Referral to specialist.
‡Referral to specialist (children).

EVALUATION/FOLLOW-UP

- Initial follow-up depends on severity of exacerbation (1 day to 3 weeks).
- Schedule regular follow-up at 1- to 6-month intervals.
- Successful therapy is based on the following parameters:
  —Prevention of symptoms such as cough
  —Maintenance of nearly normal pulmonary function
  —Maintenance of regular activities
  —Prevention of exacerbations (no hospitalizations or visits to ED)

Referral

Refer to asthma specialist any client with severe persistent condition (step 4 care) or anyone whose asthma control can not be maintained.

CHILDREN (YOUNGER THAN 5 YEARS)

1. Do trials of inhaled bronchodilators and antiinflammatory medications for diagnostic purposes. Symptomatology is difficult in this age group because performance on spirometry is inconsistent or impossible to obtain.
2. Symptoms more frequent than 2 times per week require long-term control medication. Cromolyn and nedocromil are good

choices secondary because they have extremely limited side effects. Leukotriene modifiers are not indicated for children younger than 12 years.

3. Close monitoring is critical, especially until control of symptoms has been achieved.

   a. Asthma diaries should be kept, with symptom severity criteria for medication adjustments by parents (similar to the red/yellow/green stoplight categories used in diaries with PEFR measures).

   b. Require more frequent follow-up, especially during an exacerbation (days vs weeks).

4. Refer to specialist at step 3 (moderate, persistent); consider referral at step 2 level of care.

REFERENCES

Arvin, A. M., Behrman, R. E., Kliegman, R. M., & Nelson, W. E. (Eds.). (1996). *Nelson textbook of pediatrics* (15th ed.). Philadelphia: W. B. Saunders.

Boyton, R. W., Dunn, E. S., & Stephens, G. R., (Eds.). (1994). *Ambulatory pediatric care* (2nd ed.). Philadelphia: J. B. Lippincott.

Milgrom, H., Bender, B., Ackerson, L., Bowry, P., Smith, B., & Rand, C. (1996). Noncompliance and treatment failure in children with asthma. *Journal of Allergy and Clinical Immunology, 98*, 1051-1057.

National Asthma Education and Prevention Program. (1995). *Nurses: Partners in asthma care*. Bethesda, MD: National Heart, Lung and Blood Institute.

National Asthma Education and Prevention Program. (1997). *Expert panel report 2: Guidelines for the diagnosis and management of asthma*. Bethesda, MD: National Heart, Lung and Blood Institute.

Plaut, T. F. (1996). *One-minute asthma* (3rd ed.). Amherst, MA: Pedipress.

Suissa, S., Dennis, R., Ernst, P., Sheehy, O., & Wood-Dauphinee, S. (1997). Effectiveness of the leukotriene receptor antagonist Zafirlukast for mild to moderate asthma. *Annals of Internal Medicine, 126*, 177-183.

Uphold, C. R., & Graham, M. V. (1994a). *Clinical guidelines in child health*. Gainesville, FL: Barmarrae Books.

Uphold, C. R., & Graham, M. V. (1994b). *Clinical guidelines in family practice*. Gainesville, FL: Barmarrae Books.

Wise, R. A., & Liu, M. C. (1995). Obstructive airway diseases: Asthma and chronic pulmonary obstructive disease. In L. Barker, J. Burton, & P. Zieve (Eds.), *Principles of ambulatory medicine* (4th ed.). Baltimore: Williams & Wilkins.

REVIEW QUESTIONS

1. A 3-year-old girl comes in with a history of cough that "will not go away." What associated history would support a diagnosis of asthma?

   a. Smokers in the home
   b. Recurrent skin problems since infancy
   c. Older brother with seasonal allergies
   d. Chronic otitis media during the first 2 years of life

2. A 5-year-old child comes in with respiratory difficulty, respiratory rate (RR) of 48 breaths/min, mild intercostal retractions, and generalized wheezing. What further objective data would support a diagnosis of asthma?

   a. Wheezing improved after treatment with albuterol in normal saline solution per nebulizer.
   b. PEFR was 75% after treatment with albuterol in normal saline per nebulizer.
   c. Associated signs of concurrent upper respiratory tract infection are present.
   d. Barrel appearance of chest and clubbing of fingers are noted.

3. A 6-month-old infant comes to your office with a 3-day history of worsening respiratory symptoms. The condition began as "a cold," but the infant now is "breathing so fast he can hardly eat or sleep." There is an intermittent, nonproductive cough, paroxysmal at times. On examination, RR is 64 breaths/min, and there are marked intercostal retractions and generalized wheezing. Parents are worried because the father has asthma. On the basis of these data, what is the most likely diagnosis?

   a. Asthma
   b. Pneumonia
   c. Bronchopulmonary dysplasia
   d. Bronchiolitis

4. Appropriate management for a 6-month-old with generalized wheezing and moderate respiratory distress would include:

   a. Referral for hospitalization
   b. In-office nebulization treatment with 0.25 ml albuterol in 2 ml normal saline
   c. Education regarding PEFR monitoring
   d. Respiratory follow-up in 1 to 2 weeks

5. A 7-year-old with moderate persistent asthma uses an asthma diary to monitor the effectiveness of medications and the status of the disease. Which tool or technique below could be used in this process to serve as an indicator for treatment change?

    a. PEFR
    b. RR
    c. Tissue perfusion
    d. Frequency and duration of cough

6. A 34-year-old female athlete has asthma diagnosed. Sports activities tend to aggravate her condition, but she is able to participate successfully with additional medications. Daily control medication (nedocromil [Tilade] metered-dose inhaler [MDI]) and supplements with quick-relief medication (albuterol [Proventil] MDI) before sports activity are included in current management. According to this level of therapy, this case of asthma is classified as:

    a. Mild intermittent
    b. Severe persistent
    c. Moderate persistent
    d. Mild persistent

7. Of the medications used for ongoing asthma management, which displays **fewer** side effects?

    a. Albuterol
    b. Cromolyn (Intal)
    c. Theophylline
    d. Beclomethasone nasal spray

8. A 19-year-old male comes in for asthma follow-up. After many years of ED visits for acute attacks, the client expresses new interest in achieving control as he gets ready to go away to college. Current management involves daily PEFR monitoring and two long-term control medications. Evidence of effective treatment with this plan would include which of the following?

    a. No more than three "yellow" PEFR readings per week
    b. Only one ED visit since initiation of the new treatment plan
    c. Consistent PEFR measures at 90% or better, no ED visits in 3 months
    d. Daily use of beta-agonist inhaler in addition to long-term medications

ANSWERS AND RATIONALES

1. *Answer:* b (assessment/history/allergies/child)
    Rationale: Atopy is the strongest predisposing factor associated with the development of asthma. Irritants and illnesses can serve as triggers for allergy attacks. A family history of allergies is not as much a support as are the symptoms of the child herself. (National Asthma Education and Prevention Program, 1997)

2. *Answer:* a (assessment/physical examination/allergies/child)
    Rationale: Reversible airway obstruction would support the diagnosis of asthma. PEFR of 75% demonstrates a lack of response or incomplete response to beta-agonist (albuterol). A concurrent upper respiratory tract infection might serve as a trigger but is not diagnostic. The barrel chest and clubbing of fingers demonstrate a chronic hypoxic state, more indicative of chronic lung disease such as cystic fibrosis or bronchopulmonary dysplasia. (National Asthma Education and Prevention Program, 1997)

3. *Answer:* d (diagnosis/allergies/infant)
    Rationale: Bronchiolitis would be considered at the top of the list of differential diagnoses for a 6-month-old with wheezing. Assuming that this is the first episode of wheezing, a diagnosis of asthma would be premature, even with his family history of a father with asthma. The progression of upper respiratory tract infection symptoms to respiratory distress signs and symptoms is typical of bronchiolitis. (Boynton, Dunn, & Stephens, 1994)

4. *Answer:* b (plan/allergies/infant)
    Rationale: A trial of short-acting beta-agonist is indicated for children younger than 5 years with wheezing and may be diagnostic. (National Asthma Education and Prevention Program, 1997)

5. *Answer:* a (plan/allergies/child)
    Rationale: PEFR is used as an indicator of lung function. It provides an objective measure that can be used for assessment against a predicted value or personal best record. (Plaut, 1996)

6. *Answer:* d (diagnosis/allergies/NAS)

Rationale: According to the newest guidelines, this case of asthma would be classified as mild persistent. This woman uses one antiinflammatory agent and inhaled beta-agonists for quick relief related to physical exercise. (National Asthma Education and Prevention Program, 1997)

7. *Answer:* b (plan/allergies/NAS)

Rationale: Cromolyn (Intal) is known for having virtually no side effects. (Wise & Liu, 1995)

8. *Answer:* c (evaluation/allergies/NAS)

Rationale: Successful therapy for asthma is determined according to prevention of troublesome symptoms, maintenance of nearly normal pulmonary function, prevention of exacerbations, and subsequent visits to the ED. (National Asthma Education and Prevention Program, 1997; Wise & Liu, 1995)

15

Psychosocial Conditions

ABUSE

OVERVIEW
Definition

Abuse is nonaccidental injury as a result of commission or omission on the part of a parent, guardian, spouse, or other caretaker. Harm may also occur as a result of neglect or inattention to physical, emotional, medical, and financial needs in a dependent situation.

TYPES OF ABUSE

- Physical abuse: Inflicted injuries often a result of hitting, beating, shaking, or burning; may be unusual for age of victim or incompatible with history
- Sexual abuse: (Children and older adults) assault, incest, or exploitation for the sexual gratification of an adult caregiver; (women) forced sexual activity without the consent of the sexual partner
  —Nontouching offenses: Verbal sexual stimulation, exhibitionism, and invasions of privacy
  —Touching offenses: Fondling, masturbation, intercourse, sodomy, anal penetration, and/or oral genital contact
- Emotional/psychologic abuse: An attack on the person's sense of self and social competence; concurrent with other forms of abuse
  —Types: Ignoring, rejecting, isolating, terrorizing, corrupting, verbal assault, and overpressuring
- Financial abuse: Exploitation of resources through misrepresentation, coercion, or theft (most likely to older adults)

- Neglect: Failure of responsible person to provide adequate food, clothing, shelter, and/or medical care

Incidence

Numbers are known to be underreported/underrecognized in the United States:
- Children: More than 200,000 are abused; more than 800,000 are neglected each year.
- Women
  —Approximately 2 million are victims of domestic violence per year, and more than 12 million are abused at some time in their lives.
  —Forty-five percent of wives of men with alcoholism have been assaulted.
- Older adults: Up to 2 million are abused each year; problems are expected to worsen as the population ages.

Pathophysiology

- Often physical abuse is explained as an accident, but it is more likely the result of a stressful situation and a caretaker/partner with poor decision-making and/or coping skills.
- Families under chronic strain from financial and health problems are particularly at risk.
- Isolation/lack of social support may contribute.
- Strong association of history of psychopathology and/or substance abuse by the abuser.
- Vulnerable or powerless persons (children, women, older adults) tend to be victims of abuse.

415

ASSESSMENT: SUBJECTIVE/HISTORY

- Multiple health care providers and/or multiple emergency department visits
- Conflicting stories to how injuries occurred
- Information unknowingly revealed in the context of other questions, for example:

    NURSE PRACTITIONER: What was your last medicine for this condition?

    PARENT: I did not get that prescription filled, I thought she was better.

    OR

    OLDER ADULT: I don't have money in my checkbook anymore, so I didn't get it.

- Caretaker affect inappropriate for situation (e.g., laughter, anger, lack of concern)
- History of sleep disturbances, appetite changes, withdrawn behavior, aggressive behavior/violent outbursts, suicide attempts
- Children: Temper tantrums, poor school performance, accident described inconsistent with child's developmental ability, delinquent behavior, knowledge and use of sexual terms, excessive masturbation or sex play, suspicious of adults
- Women/older adults: Frequent requests for pain medication, frequent visits for somatic complaints, gastrointestinal disturbances, chronic pain of unclear origin

ASSESSMENT: OBJECTIVE/ PHYSICAL EXAMINATION

Physical Examination

A complete physical examination is warranted with particular focus on the following areas:

- General: Responsiveness/affect, hygiene, nutritional status, appropriateness of dress, presence of unattended physical problems
- HEENT: Head trauma, patchy hair loss, pupils
- Funduscopic: Retinal hemorrhage; hemorrhage of sclerae; bleeding from ears/nose; blood behind tympanic membrane
- Skin: Bruises in different stages of healing; burns; physical marks of an object (e.g., looped cord, belt buckle); restraint marks on extremities, neck, or mouth; human bite marks
- Abdomen: Tenderness, organomegaly, bruising
- Musculoskeletal: Tenderness or swelling of joints, signs of spiral fractures or dislocations
- Neurologic: Mental status, neurodevelopmental screening (children)
- Genitalia: Genital, urethral, vaginal, or anal bruising or bleeding; swollen, red vulva or perineum; presence of foreign body in genital area

Diagnostic Procedures

- Growth measures are plotted on appropriate growth charts (for children only).
    - Height, weight, head circumference (2 years and younger): Accurate/thorough descriptions of findings (photographs helpful); significant negatives are required.
    - Flattening weight curve may indicate early signs of neglect or nonorganic failure to thrive, whereas flattening of curves in all growth parameters is indicative of more serious condition.
- Employ other procedures such as radiographs and laboratory tests as indicated by subjective and objective data.

DIAGNOSIS

The differential diagnosis includes the following:

- Women/older adults
    - Unintended injury
    - Self-neglect
    - Poverty
- Children
    - Nonintentional injury
    - Normal skin variations (e.g., mongolian spots)
    - Organic failure to thrive
    - Blood dyscrasias (e.g., leukemia)
    - Osteogenesis imperfecta
    - Cultural practices (e.g., Asian—cupping)

THERAPEUTIC PLAN

Management

- Report any suspected abuse to the appropriate social service agency. NOTE: Nurse practitioners are considered mandated reporters and are required by law to report suspected cases of abuse. Nurse practitioners incur some form of legal immunity (varies by state) if they make a good faith report but are also subject to criminal charges if they fail to make a report in a case of suspected abuse.

- Treat/refer identified medical conditions.
- Ensure that victim does not return to hostile environment in case of life-threatening situations (rare).
- Initiate team approach including medical, social services, and law enforcement members as appropriate.

Prevention

Incorporate screenings into practice that would identify families at risk.

Client Education

Client education is most appropriate as a preventive measure.

Children

- Negative attitudes toward child/pregnancy may contribute to later abuse.
- Explain behavioral expectations by developmental level.
- Discuss parenting strategies for specific behaviors.
- Address further knowlege deficits regarding child behavior and parenting as identified.
- Parents need time away from their children.

Women/Older Adults

- Risk factors for abuse
- Resources available to families at risk
- Shelters/referral sources if abuse does occur

EVALUATION/FOLLOW-UP

- Same-day phone follow-up if returning to same environment.
- Confirm social services investigation once a report is made (within 24 hours).
- Monitor progress of case until resolution.

REFERENCES

Arvin, A. M., Behrman, R. E., Kliegman, R. M., & Nelson, W. E. (1996). *Nelson textbook of pediatrics* (15th ed.). Philadelphia: W. B. Saunders.

Boyton, R. W., Dunn, E. S., & Stephens, G. R. (Eds.), (1994). *Ambulatory pediatric care* (2nd ed.). Philadelphia: J. B. Lippincott.

Fingerhood, M. I., & Barker, L. R. (1995). Alcoholism and associated problems. In L. Barker, J. Burton, & P. Zieve (Eds.), *Principles of ambulatory medicine* (4th ed.). Baltimore: Williams & Wilkins.

Finucane, T. E., & Burton, J. R. (1995). Geriatric medicine: Special considerations. In L. Barker, J. Burton, & P. Zieve (Eds.), *Principles of ambulatory medicine* (4th ed.). Baltimore: Williams & Wilkins.

Lynch, S. H. (1997). Elder abuse: What to look for, how to intervene. *American Journal of Nursing, 97*(1), 26-32.

Monteleone, J. A. (1994). *Recognition of child abuse for the mandated reporter.* St. Louis: Green-Warren Medical Publishing.

Schmitt, B. D. (1987). Seven deadly sins of childhood: Advising parents about difficult developmental phases. *Child Abuse & Neglect, 11,* 421-432.

Uphold, C. R., & Graham, M. V. (1994a). *Clinical guidelines in child health.* Gainesville, FL: Barmarrae Books.

Uphold, C. R., & Graham, M. V. (1994b). *Clinical guidelines on family practice.* Gainesville, FL: Barmarrae Books.

REVIEW QUESTIONS

1. Which aspect of an episodic history for a broken arm in an older man would be most indicative of abuse?

  a. The client lives alone.
  b. The client states he fell off a chair while changing a lightbulb, but an accompanying family member states he fell down the steps.
  c. The client's wife died 6 months ago.
  d. The client has a poor health and nutritional status.

2. The nurse practitioner suspects abuse after completing a history and physical examination. Which finding most likely raised the red flag?

  a. Purulent nasal discharge with postnasal drainage
  b. Flat affect
  c. Multiple bruises on extremities and face ranging in color from purple to brown
  d. 3-cm scar in the right lower quadrant of the abdomen

3. Which type of fracture is most often the result of abuse?

a. Spiral
b. Compound
c. Simple
d. Avulsion

4. The best intervention for the nurse practitioner trying to prevent child abuse is to:

a. Refer the child for ADHD testing.
b. Encourage parents to have time away from their children.
c. Educate parents regarding appropriate developmental expectations.
d. Screen families for child abuse potential.

5. A 24-year-old woman is seen for multiple contusions secondary to physical abuse. She refuses recommendations to seek shelter other than her home while the case is under investigation. Appropriate follow-up by the nurse practitioner would be:

a. Contact the client's social worker within 2 days of abuse report.
b. Follow-up via phone that same day.
c. Call within 1 week to check healing of contusions.
d. Schedule clinic follow-up in 1 week for reevaluation.

6. A 35-year-old woman complains of shoulder trauma secondary to a fall. This is her fourth visit in 2 months for relatively minor complaints. What data would motivate the nurse practitioner to consider abuse?

a. A large contusion on the upper arm and a statement like "I tripped over a chair and hit the coffee table"
b. Poor nutritional status (emaciated appearance)
c. A statement like "I can't seem to do anything right"
d. Multiple visits for vague or minor complaints

7. A 4-year-old boy comes to the clinic for a behavior problem. The mother reports problems at day care with sexual play and recent use of slang words for genital parts. The mother explains, "I don't know where he heard it. We don't use those words at home." The physical examination is normal. Although more data would be helpful, the first consideration for diagnosis is:

a. Physical abuse
b. Emotional abuse

c. Behavior problem
d. Sexual abuse

8. A child was placed in foster care 6 weeks ago after being physically abused. He visits the clinic today for a preschool physical examination. The child is withdrawn with minimal verbalization. The physical examination is significant for an erythematous loop-shaped mark on his back. The foster parents deny knowledge of the mark. Evaluation of management of this child for physical abuse includes:

a. Physical marks are likely a result of abuse before foster care placement.
b. Further investigation is needed to evaluate the situation.
c. Physical abuse is still occurring; call the case worker immediately.
d. Referral is needed to another foster care placement.

Answers and Rationales

1. *Answer:* b (assessment/history/psychosocial/aging adult)
   Rationale: Inconsistency in history, especially between family members should be highly suggestive of abuse. Poor health and isolation are risk factors rather than indicators. (Lynch, 1997; Uphold & Graham, 1994b)

2. *Answer:* c (assessment/physical examination/psychosocial/NAS)
   Rationale: Bruises in different stages of healing indicate multiple episodes of trauma over time, a key indicator of abuse. (Monteleone, 1994)

3. *Answer:* a (diagnosis/psychosocial/NAS)
   Rationale: Spiral fractures, associated with a twisting motion, are the most common type of fracture associated with abuse. (Lynch, 1997; Monteleone, 1994)

4. *Answer:* c (plan/psychosocial/child)
   Rationale: Parenting is difficult. Developmental issues such as colic and toilet training have high associations with abuse. All children are at risk during certain time periods. For this reason, proper education regarding developmental expectations is likely to prevent more cases of abuse (Schmitt, 1987). Referral for ADHD evaluation, respite for parents, and screening families for child abuse potential may also

be helpful, but not the best action for the nurse practitioner from the options offered.

5. *Answer:* b (plan/psychosocial/NAS)

Rationale: Same-day phone follow-up is the best option considering the client's safety may be at risk. It is especially important in cases where victims refuse to seek alternative shelter to document that such a recommendation was made. It is the role of the nurse practitioner to closely monitor all ongoing cases of abuse, although the responsibility to investigate the case is that of Adult Protective Services and the responsibility to provide for her safety is that of law enforcement officials. (Monteleone, 1994; Uphold & Graham, 1994b)

6. *Answer:* d (assessment/physical examination/psychosocial/NAS)

Rationale: Clinical signs and symptoms of domestic violence include frequent medical contacts/visits with vague, somatic complaints. (Fingerhood & Barker, 1995)

7. *Answer:* d (diagnosis/psychosocial/child)

Rationale: Behavioral signs of sexual abuse include the child that knows and uses sexual terms, excessive sexual play, and excessive masturbation. (Boynton, Dunn, & Stephens, 1994)

8. *Answer:* c (evaluation/psychosocial/child)

Rationale: A loop mark (red, indicating a more recent infliction) is indicative of abuse. Abuse does occur in foster home placements. Reporting of this case is warranted. (Monteleone, 1994)

ANANXIETY

OVERVIEW
Definition

Anxiety is the fundamental emotion that is thought to be the motivating factor from which other emotions, such as anger and guilt, flow. It is an uncomfortable feeling of apprehension and/or fear usually accompanied by psychologic, physiologic, and behavioral symptoms. The symptoms of anxiety alert the individual to real or perceived threats to self or significant others and motivates the individual to take action to relieve the unpleasant feelings. The source of the anxiety is frequently unknown to the person who is experiencing it and is referred to as generalized or diffuse. Although anxiety is essential for human survival, excessive high and persistent levels interfere with health and life.

Incidence

Anxiety is a pervasive human emotion. Individuals respond very differently with related symptoms and in their use of coping skills. What may result in a moderate level of anxiety for one individual may cause panic in another. To be therapeutic, it is essential that the nurse practitioner understand the meaning this subjective experience has for the individual. Anxiety disorders are more common in women than in men and represent one of the most prevalent mental health problems in the United States today. Cardiac problems, hypoglycemia, and seizure disorders have been associated more with individuals who suffer from anxiety than with the general population.

Etiology

There are four basic theoretic perspectives to understanding anxiety:

- In psychoanalytic (Freudian) theory, anxiety reflects a conflict between the demands of one's instinctual drives (the id), the realistic perception of the specific situation (the ego), and the moralistic controlling conscience (the superego). Anxiety signals the ego of an unconscious impulse reflecting hidden psychologic conflict.
- According to learning-behavioral theory, anxiety is a learned response to a stimulus that is perceived as painful or uncomfortable. The individual learns to reduce anxiety by avoiding the uncomfortable stimulus.
- The biochemical theory states that anxiety is the uncomfortable feeling caused by a perceived danger and accompanied by physiologic symptoms that prepares the individual for the "fight or flight" response. Primarily these symptoms are due to car-

diovascular and neuroendocrine system stimulation. As the production of norepinephrine increases in humans, so does the level of anxiety.

- Interpersonal theory views all human behavior as a response to our relationship with significant others in our life. Anxiety is the emotional discomfort that results when our expectations of others are not met and our interpersonal security is threatened. Coping mechanisms are learned as a child and then become integrated into the personality of the adult.

Pathophysiology

PROTECTIVE FACTORS. Defense mechanisms and coping behaviors learned early in life relieve the discomfort of anxiety and provide a sense of protection.

Examples of individual coping behaviors include the following:

ADAPTIVE	MALADAPTIVE
Prayer	Drugs and/or alcohol
Exercise	abuse
Relaxation techniques	Excessive eating
Problem solving	Social isolation
	Self-injury

As the level of anxiety increases, the use of the following ego defense mechanisms may become necessary:

- Compensation: Emphasizing a perceived asset in an attempt to overcome feelings of insecurity
- Denial: Refusal to accept an unpleasant situation as reality based
- Displacement: Transferring a feeling from an original person or experience to a more neutral one
- Dissociation: Breaking off of certain aspects of one's personality from one's consciousness
- Identification: Transferring to oneself the attributes of another person
- Intellectualization: Separation of a painful feeling from the experience by the use of excessive reasoning
- Projection: Transferring one's unacceptable ideas or feelings to another person

- Rationalization: Using excuses or substituting acceptable reasons to justify unacceptable thoughts or behavior
- Reaction formation: Behavior that is the opposite of one's true, unacceptable feelings
- Regression: Reverting to an earlier personality developmental level of functioning
- Repression: Dismissing any undesirable thoughts, feelings, or desires from conscious awareness
- Sublimation: Expressing unacceptable desires in a more socially acceptable manner

Coping resources include individual abilities, social support, economic resources, motivation, defensive techniques, health, and high self-esteem.

FACTORS INCREASING SUSCEPTIBILITY
- Anxiety levels exceed coping abilities.
- Coping mechanisms are maladaptive.
- Abnormal levels of norepinephrine and blood lactate are thought to be etiologic factors.
- Anxiety is considered pathologic when any of the following occur:
  —The anxiety reaction exceeds the severity or the duration of the threat.
  —Impairment in social or intellectual functioning occurs.
  —Concurrent psychosomatic problems, such as colitis, exist.

COMMON CAUSAL FACTORS
- Developmental crisis
  —Separation of a child from the parent to attend school
  —Growth and sexual development
  —Changes in relationships and roles
  —Aging
- Threats to safety and security
  —Assault and abuse
  —Natural disasters
- Loss
  —Death of loved one
  —Divorce
  —Major illness and disability
  —Retirement
- Threats to self-esteem and integrity
- Guilt

ASSESSMENT: SUBJECTIVE/HISTORY
Characteristics of Anxiety by Level

1 Mild anxiety/normal state of alertness
—Enhanced perception and concentration
—Increased motivation and problem solving
2 Moderate anxiety/narrowed focus of perception
—Selective inattention and hesitation
—Diminished problem solving
—Rapid speech with frequent change of topic
—Muscle tension and restlessness
3 Severe anxiety/severely limited cognitive and perceptual ability
—Loss of ability to concentrate or problem solve
—Fear of loss of control and impending doom
—Continued increase in vital signs with hyperventilation and tachycardia
—Headache, dizziness
—Trembling and purposeless movement
—Urinary frequency, nausea
4 Panic anxiety/greatly impaired perception
—Inability to reason or problem solve
—Inability to function safely by self
—Incoherent speech
—Chest pain and feeling of choking
—Incontinence
—Fear of dying
—Restlessness and irritability

Other Symptoms

- Difficulty sleeping (awakening frequently during the night or awakening in the early morning)
- Significant changes in eating (anorexia, overeating)
- Chronic fatigue
- Feelings of apprehension, guilt, dread
- Acting out behaviors (anger that may be directly or indirectly expressed, violence, truancy, alcohol and drug abuse)
- Somatic complaints (stomach ache, nausea and vomiting, headache)

Mental Health Evaluation

- Attempt to identify the precipitating factor or event as perceived by the client.
- Determine the client's perception of when the problem started and its duration.
- Determine the client's coping behaviors and support systems.
- Obtain a history: social, medical, psychiatric, family.

ASSESSMENT: OBJECTIVE/ PHYSICAL EXAMINATION
Physical Examination

A complete physical examination should be made with particular attention to the cardiovascular and neuroendocrine systems. It is essential to rule out medical problems that cause similar symptoms of anxiety and/or that include anxiety as a symptom, such as the following:

- Cerebral vascular problems
- Impending myocardial infarction
- Hyperthyroidism
- Hypoglycemia
- Pituitary disorder
- Use of certain medications (caffeine, amphetamine)
- Withdrawal from alcohol or sedatives

Complete a mental status examination, observing for the following:

- Behavior and appearance
- Level of consciousness, cognitive functioning, and memory
- Thought processes, speech patterns
- Insight
- Suicidal or homicidal ideation

Several assessment tools exist to assist in this examination. They include the Mini-Mental State Examination and the Short Portable Mental Status Questionnaire.

Diagnostic Procedures

Laboratory tests primarily ordered to rule out physiologic causes for the presenting symptoms usually include the following:

- ECG
- CBC with differential and electrolytes
- Thyroid function profile (blood)
- Liver function profile
- Urinalysis with drug screen
- Chest x-ray examination

DIAGNOSIS

- Establish the level of anxiety as mild, moderate, severe, or panic.
- At this point several other abnormal anxiety syndromes must be ruled out:

—Panic disorder is characterized by sudden intense, unpredictable anxiety attacks and manifested by severe debilitating physical and emotional symptoms associated with a sense of fear and impending doom.

—Posttraumatic stress disorder is the recurrent reexperiencing of a traumatic event and the feelings associated with that previous experience. Examples include natural disasters, rape, major injury events, and military combat. Beside the symptoms of severe anxiety, substance abuse and depression are frequently seen as a means of dealing with the emotional pain.

—Phobia is an anxiety disorder characterized by irrational fear of specific places or situations (agoraphobia), appearing inept in the company of others (social phobia), or fear of a specific object or thing (specific phobia).

THERAPEUTIC PLAN
Pharmacologic Treatment

Antianxiety agents such as the benzodiazepines (lorazepam [Ativan], alprazolam [Xanax]) and the nonbenzodiazepine antianxiety agent (buspirone [BuSpar]).

It is important to remember that the benzodiazepines are both psychologically and physiologically addicting; if benzodiazepines are given for long periods of time, increasingly higher doses are required. Also if benzodiazepines are discontinued abruptly, withdrawal symptoms can occur, which may not appear for a week following the last dose. Buspirone (BuSpar) is not effective for acute crises because of its delayed onset of action.

Sedatives (e.g., zolpidem [Ambien]) may be ordered to relieve the insomnia that frequently occurs in anxiety.

Antidepressants are sometimes prescribed when depression is an intregral factor in the anxiety.

Psychologic Modalities

For generalized moderate anxiety, assist the client in problem solving to facilitate the identification of stressors and effective coping skills.

Various relaxation techniques, such as exercise and rest, guided imagery, and other stress reduction techniques, can be used in combination with medication or alone.

If the client is experiencing a higher level of anxiety (severe or panic), crisis intervention techniques are used. The initial focus is to relieve symptoms and ensure safety:

- The client must not be left alone.
- Provide a quiet safe environment.
- Assess for suicidal or homicidal ideation.
- Permit expression of feelings but do not ask for detailed explanations.
- Assess support systems and coping mechanisms.
- Evaluate the need for medication and/or hospitalization.

The broad treatment modalities for anxiety include cognitive therapy, individual psychotherapy, behavior therapy, and group/family therapy.

Client Education

- Stress reduction exercises
- Effective coping behaviors
- Appropriate use of medication
- Availability of various treatment resources

Referral

Seek consultation with a mental health specialist when any of the following occur:

- Psychotic paranoid thought processes
- Panic level of anxiety
- Suicidal/homicidal ideation
- Escalation of symptoms to the point of refusal of treatment

Refer to Alcoholics Anonymous or Narcotics Anonymous if alcohol or drug abuse is a contributing factor.

EVALUATION/FOLLOW-UP

Follow-up should be weekly to evaluate the client's response. Progress is made when the client accomplishes the following:

- Is compliant with the treatment plan
- Is able to recognize early signs of own anxiety response
- Is able to recognize current life stressors that trigger an anxiety response
- Attempts to eliminate maladaptive coping behaviors
- Implements adaptive coping behaviors

REFERENCES

American Psychiatric Association (1994). *Diagnostic and statistical manual of mental disorders (DSM-IV)* (4th ed.). Washington, DC: Author.

Anxiety and antidepressant drugs. (1993, January). *The Harvard Mental Health Letter*, p. 6.

Aquilera, D. C., & Messick, J. M. (1990). *Crisis intervention theory and methodology.* St. Louis: Mosby.

Aromando, L. (1995). *Mental health and psychiatric nursing* (2nd ed., pp. 18-25). Springhouse, PA: Springhouse.

Burgess, A. N. (1997). *Psychiatric nursing promoting mental health* (pp. 78-89, 202-221). Norwalk, CT: Appleton & Lange.

Copel, L. C. (1996). *Nurse's clinical guide. Psychiatric and mental health care* (pp. 154-189). Springhouse, PA: Springhouse.

Randolph, N. (1993). *American nursing review for psychiatric and mental health nursing certification* (pp. 8-16). Springhouse, PA: Springhouse.

Wilson, B. A., Shannon, M. T., & Stang, C. L. (1997). *Nurses drug book.* Norwalk, CT: Appleton & Lange.

REVIEW QUESTIONS

1. You explain to Mrs. Jones that she may need a lung biopsy as part of her diagnostic workup. As you continue to explain the diagnostic process, you notice that Mrs. Jones seems to be having difficulty understanding. She frequently interrupts with questions like: "Am I going to lose my hair? Am I going to need surgery?" Her respirations have increased to 26 breaths/min, with a pulse of 106 beats/min, and she is restless. You assess her level of anxiety to be:

    a. Mild
    b. Moderate
    c. Severe
    d. Panic

2. Ruth is a 25-year-old college student who reports that when she must take an examination, she experiences inability to problem solve, urinary frequency, rapid heartbeat, and respirations. You assess her as having:

    a. Severe anxiety attacks
    b. Attention-seeking behavior
    c. Moderate anxiety
    d. Hypoglycemia

3. To decrease the severe anxiety level being manifested by Martha who was in an automobile crash with her boyfriend, Bill, the nurse practitioner should:

    a. Remain with Martha.
    b. Question Martha about the automobile crash.

    c. Reassure Martha that Bill is going to be OK.
    d. Tell Martha that her family is on their way to the hospital.

4. A client's stage of anxiety is between 3 and 4. What is the primary gain or purpose of these symptoms?

    a. Gain sympathy
    b. Relief of the tension and anxiety
    c. Express dependency needs
    d. Express concern

5. Which medication should be ordered for someone manifesting moderate-to-severe anxiety?

    a. Haloperidol (Haldol)
    b. Imipramine (Tofranil)
    c. Fluphenazine (Prolixin)
    d. Lorazepam (Ativan)

6. A client who has been treated for 2 months with a benzodiazepine telephones and complains of sweating, tremors, and inability to sleep. Based on an evaluation of the symptoms, the client:

    a. Probably stopped taking the medication abruptly and is having withdrawal symptoms
    b. Requires an increase in medication dosage because of exacerbation in anxiety symptoms
    c. Has built up a tolerance to the medication and needs an increase in the dosage
    d. Is experiencing common side effects of the drug and needs the dosage slightly altered

7. When evaluating a client's coping skills, which of the following would be considered a maladaptive coping behavior?

    a. Daily prayer
    b. Social isolation
    c. Exercise
    d. Relaxation techniques

8. The defense mechanism of emphasizing a perceived asset in an attempt to overcome feelings of insecurity is called:

    a. Compensation
    b. Denial
    c. Displacement
    d. Dissociation

9. Martha, a 17-year-old, and her 20-year-old boyfriend, Bill, were brought to the emergency department following an automobile crash. Bill is in critical condition but Martha has no physical injury. However, Martha seems to be in a daze, walking about aimlessly, and complaining of nausea. When attempts are made to discuss the crash she begins to hyperventilate. You would assess Martha's anxiety level to be:

    a. Mild
    b. Moderate
    c. Severe
    d. Panic

ANSWERS AND RATIONALES

1. *Answer:* b (diagnosis/psychosocial/adult)
    Rationale: Moderate anxiety results in selective inattention with frequent changes in topic of conversation. Muscle tension, restlessness, and increased vital signs also occur at this stage. (Aquilera & Messick, 1990)

2. *Answer:* a (diagnosis/psychosocial/adult)
    Rationale: The symptoms listed are characteristic severe anxiety. (American Psychiatric Association [APA], 1994)

3. *Answer:* a (plan/psychosocial/NAS)
    Rationale: The presence of the nurse practitioner can provide a sense of security and a link with reality. (Aromando, 1995)

4. *Answer:* b (assessment/physical examination/psychosocial/NAS)
    Rationale: The manifestations of anxiety alert the individual to perceived threats and motivates the individual to take action to relieve the unpleasant feelings. (Burgess, 1997)

5. *Answer:* d (plan/psychosocial/NAS)
    Rationale: The only antianxiety agent listed is lorazepam (Ativan). (Wilson, 1997)

6. *Answer:* a (diagnosis/psychosocial/NAS)
    Rationale: Benzodiazepines are addicting; if benzodiazepines are discontinued abruptly, withdrawal can occur. (Wilson, Shannon, & Stang, 1997)

7. *Answer:* b (evaluation/psychosocial/NAS)
    Rationale: Social isolation does not relieve the discomfort of anxiety or provide a sense of protection. (Burgess, 1997)

8. *Answer:* a (history/psychosocial/NAS)
    Rationale: Definition. (Randolph, 1993)

9. *Answer:* c (diagnosis/psychosocial/adolescent)
    Rationale: In severe anxiety the person frequently experiences impaired cognitive and perceptual ability, restlessness, and somatic symptoms. If the person was in a panic state, the individual's behavior would be more disturbed and not reality based. (Aquilera & Messick, 1990)

ATTENTION-DEFICIT/HYPERACTIVITY DISORDER

OVERVIEW
Definition

Attention-deficit/hyperactivity disorder (ADHD) is the current term applied to specific developmental disorders of both children and adults that are characterized by deficits in sustained attention, impulse control, and the regulation of activity level to situational demands. ADHD has had a variety of labels including hyperkinetic disorder of childhood, minimal brain dysfunction, and attention deficit disorder (with or without hyperactivity).

Incidence

- ADHD is one of the most common disorders of childhood, affecting 3% to 5% of children in the United States.
- ADHD is much more frequent in males than in females in the United States. The fourth edition of the *Diagnostic and Statistical Manual of Mental Disorders (DSM-IV)* states the male-to-female ratio to range from 4:1 to 9:1 depending on the setting (i.e., general population or clinics).
- It is estimated that one child in every classroom in the United States needs help for the disorder.

Pathophysiology

There are many different theories about the cause of ADHD. There may be a biologic basis, imbalance in brain chemistry, especially neurotransmitters such as dopamine, norepinephrine, and serotonin. ADHD has a genetic component in that 30% to 40% of children diagnosed with ADHD have relatives with similar difficulties.

Studies of parent-child interactions of hyperactive children compared to normal children show the parents of the hyperactive child to be more likely to give commands to their children, more negative toward the child, and less likely to respond to the social initiatives of the child toward them. Hyperactive children compared to normal children are shown by these studies to be less compliant, more negative, and less able to sustain compliance to parental commands.

There is no scientific proof to render the following toxins responsible for the development of ADHD:

- Food additives
- Food dyes
- Preservatives
- Salicylates
- Refined sugar
- Florescent lighting

FACTORS INCREASING SUSCEPTIBILITY. Higher rates of psychopathology are demonstrated among the biologic relatives of children with ADHD vs normal children. The heritability for the traits of ADHD is 30% to 50%. Between 20% and 32% of parents and siblings of children with ADHD also have the disorder. Susceptibility to ADHD is increased with the following:

- Prenatal and postnatal exposure to lead
- Cigarette smoking during pregnancy
- Alcohol consumption during pregnancy
- Drug abuse during pregnancy
- Poor maternal prenatal nutrition
- Brain injuries during and after birth
- Infections
- Possible side effects of sedatives or anticonvulsants

ASSESSMENT: SUBJECTIVE/HISTORY

History of Present Illness/ Developmental Factors

Determine the client's prenatal history, perinatal history, postnatal period and infancy history, and developmental milestones.

Children with ADHD demonstrate characteristic behaviors during developmental stages:

- Infancy: Sleep problems, crying, feeding problems
- Preschool: Gross motor activity (running, etc.) rather than small muscle activities (coloring, etc.)
- School: Restlessness, inattention, impulsiveness
- Adolescence: Rebelliousness and antisocial behaviors

Symptoms

- Uninhibited behavior, demonstrated by lack of ability to regulate behavior by awareness of rules and consequences
- Inability to sustain attention; easily bored with repetitive tasks, loss of concentration during lengthy tasks, and failure to complete tasks or activities without supervision
- Impaired impulse control; inability to stop and think about consequences before acting, interrupting conversations, not able to wait one's turn, needing immediate rewards rather than being able to wait for a long-term reward
- Excessive movements; typically "on the move," fidgeting, restlessness, cannot sit still, "bouncing off the walls"

Past Medical History

- Ask questions relevant to risk factors.
- Are there chronic health problems (e.g., asthma, diabetes, heart condition)?
- Is there a history of injury events?

Medication History

Has the child ever taken or is the child currently taking any of the following?

- Methylphenidate (Ritalin)
- Dextroamphetamine (Dexedrine)
- Pemoline (Cylert)
- Tranquilizers
- Anticonvulsants
- Antihistamines
- Other prescription drugs

Family History

Identify parents or siblings with ADHD or similar symptoms.

Psychosocial History

Ask about relationships with siblings and friends.

ASSESSMENT: OBJECTIVE/ PHYSICAL EXAMINATION

Physical Examination

- Conduct a full physical examination, including a thorough neurologic examination and hearing and vision testing.
- Determine if the child has any developmental difficulties such as problems with motor skills, motor coordination, memory, remembering sequences, listening and speaking, and recognizing and reproducing pictures and symbols.

Behavioral Assessment

- Obtain information about the child's behavior in a variety of settings: school, play, at home, organized sports, youth organizations, and after school programs.
- Use the DSM-IV criteria to make the diagnosis.
- Use any of the available "checklists" or behavior rating scales to have teachers and others who observe the child's behavior assess the child's behavior in different environments.

Diagnostic Procedures

There are currently no laboratory tests available to assist in the diagnosis of ADHD.

DIAGNOSIS

The differential diagnosis includes the following:
- Oppositional defiant disorder (ODD)
- Conduct disorder (CD)
- Generalized anxiety disorder
- Learning disability
- Mental retardation
- Understimulating environment
- Developmentally appropriate behaviors in active children

Comorbidity frequently occurs (ADHD+ODD, ADHD+CD, ADHD+depression, and ADHD+ anxiety disorders).

DSM-IV Criteria

1. Either *(a)* or *(b)*:
    a. Six (or more) of the following symptoms of inattention have persisted for at least 6 months to a degree that is maladaptive and inconsistent with developmental level:
      (1) Fails to give close attention to details or makes careless mistakes in schoolwork, work, or other activities
      (2) Has difficulty sustaining attention in tasks or play activities
      (3) Does not seem to listen when spoken to directly
      (4) Does not follow through on instructions and fails to finish schoolwork, chores, or duties in the workplace (not as a result of oppositional behavior or failure to understand instructions)
      (5) Has difficulty organizing tasks and activities
      (6) Avoids, dislikes, or is reluctant to engage in tasks that require sustained mental effort (such as schoolwork or homework)
      (7) Loses things necessary for tasks or activities (e.g., toys, school assignments, pencils, books, or tools)
      (8) Is easily distracted by extraneous stimuli
      (9) Is forgetful in daily activities
    b. Six (or more) of the following symptoms of hyperactivity-impulsivity have persisted for at least 6 months to a degree that is maladaptive and inconsistent with developmental level:
      (1) Fidgets with hands or feet or squirms in seat
      (2) Leaves seat in classroom or in other situations in which remaining seated is expected
      (3) Runs about or climbs excessively in situations in which it is inappropriate (in adolescents or adults, may be limited to subjective feelings of restlessness)
      (4) Has difficulty playing or engaging in leisure activities quietly
      (5) Is "on the go" or often acts as if "driven by a motor"
      (6) Talks excessively
      (7) Blurts out answers before questions have been completed
      (8) Has difficulty awaiting turn
      (9) Interrupts or intrudes on others (e.g., butts into conversations or games)

2. Some hyperactive-impulsive or inattentive symptoms that caused impairment were present before age 7 years.
3. Some impairment from the symptoms is present in two or more settings (e.g., at school [or work] and at home).
4. There must be clear evidence of clinically significant impairment in social, academic, or occupational functioning.
5. The symptoms do not occur exclusively during the course of a pervasive developmental disorder, schizophrenia, or other psychotic disorder and are not better accounted for by another mental disorder (e.g., mood disorder, anxiety disorder, dissociative disorder, or personality disorder).

THERAPEUTIC PLAN

- The best approach is via a multidisciplinary team.
- A consistent primary provider is essential.
- The nurse practitioner may serve as the case manager.

Pharmacologic Treatment

CNS stimulants are very effective for the management of symptoms, primarily attention span and impulse control. Changes in other behaviors are most likely the result of the improvement in attention span and impulse control. School performance also shows improvement as a result of medication.

- Methylphenidate (Ritalin) (77% positive response)
  —Dosage 5 to 20 mg (0.3 to 0.7 mg/kg)
  —bid dose given early morning and midday
  —tid dose given early morning, midday, after school
  —Maximum dose not to exceed 60 mg daily
- Methylphenidate (Ritalin-SR) (1 dose/day; effect lasts 8 hours)
- Dextroamphetamine (Dexedrine) (74% positive response)
  —Dosage 2.5 to 10 mg bid/tid
  —Dosage intervals as for Ritalin
- Dextroamphetamine (Dexedrine Spansules) (1 dose/day)

Nonpharmacologic Treatment

- Provide parent education on ADHD including a review of symptoms, course, and what is known about the causative factors.
- Training the parents in the use of techniques for dealing with the child's behavior is one of the best therapeutic approaches when done properly. Behavior management skills help the parents to reduce negative behaviors and promote positive behaviors.
- Parents need guidance on modifying the environment rather than the child. The child with ADHD functions best in a highly structured environment with clear rules/limits and consequences.
- Parents benefit from counseling in the areas of acceptance of ADHD and the potential for grief reaction.
- Psychotherapy may be needed to help some children with ADHD cope with the anxiety, depression, and self-esteem issues they are experiencing.
- Family therapy is helpful to improve communication within the family and help siblings deal with their concerns.
- Social skills training and peer relationship training may be beneficial to children with ADHD since they demonstrate problems in social situations and are at high risk for peer rejection.

Client Education/School Intervention

- Provide teacher and staff education on ADHD.
- Provide teacher training in classroom management of ADHD.
- Work with the teacher to develop educational approaches.

EVALUATION/FOLLOW-UP

- Referral and/or consultation may be necessary.
- The family should be involved in the development of the treatment plan.
- A multidisciplinary approach is most successful.
- Treatment of ADHD is long term.
  —Adjustments in medications must be made as the child grows.
  —The interaction and plan developed with the child and the family will change as the child and family changes.

- It was previously thought that children "outgrow" ADHD, now it is more widely accepted that ADHD has an inborn biologic basis and that parents and children can learn how to cope with the behavioral difficulties rather than cure them. The core symptoms of ADHD are carried into adulthood by 50% to 80% of the children diagnosed with ADHD.

REFERENCES

American Psychiatric Association (1994). *Diagnostic and statistical manual of mental disorders (DSM-IV)* (4th ed.). Washington, DC: Author.

Barkley, R. A. (1991). *Attention-deficit hyperactivity disorder: A clinical workbook.* New York: Guilford Press.

Barkley, R. A. (1990). *Attention-deficit hyperactivity disorder: A handbook for diagnosis and treatment.* New York: Guilford Press.

Biederman, J., et al. (1996a). A prospective 4-year follow-up study of attention-deficit hyperactivity and related disorders. *Archives of General Psychiatry, 53* (5), 437-446.

Biederman, J., et al. (1996b). Is childhood oppositional defiant disorder a precursor to adolescent conduct disorder? Findings from a four-year follow-up study of children with ADHD. *Journal of the American Academy of Child and Adolescent Psychiatry, 35*(9), 1193-1204.

Biederman, J., et al. (1996c). Predictors of persistence and remission of ADHD into adolescence: Results from a four-year prospective follow-up study. *Journal of the American Academy of Child and Adolescent Psychiatry, 35*(3), 343-351.

Burns, C., & Shelton, K. (1996). Cognitive-perceptual patterns. In C. Burns, N. Barber, M. Brady, & A. Dunn (Eds.), *Pediatric primary care: A handbook for nurse practitioners.* Philadelphia: W. B. Saunders.

Dahl, R. E. (1996). The impact of inadequate sleep on children's daytime cognitive function. *Seminars in Pediatric Neurology, 3*(1), 44-50.

Javorsky, J. (1996). An examination of youth with attention-deficit/hyperactivity disorder and language learning disabilities: A clinical study. *Journal of Learning Disabilities, 29*(3), 247-258.

MacDonald, V. M., & Achenback, T. M. (1996). Attention problems versus conduct problems as six-year predictors of problem scores in a national sample. *Journal of the American Academy of Child and Adolescent Psychiatry, 35*(9), 1237-1246.

Murphy, K. R., & Barkley, R. A. (1996). Parents of children with attention-deficit/hyperactivity disorder: Psychological and attentional impairment. *American Journal of Orthopsychiatry, 66*(1), 93-102.

Taylor, E., Chadwick, O., Heptenstall, E., Danckaerts, M. (1996). Hyperactivity and conduct problems as risk factors for adolescent development. *Journal of the American Academy of Child and Adolescent Psychiatry, 35*(9), 1213-1226.

REVIEW QUESTIONS

1. Which of the following symptoms best describes the child with ADHD inattentive type?

a. Makes careless mistakes in schoolwork, does not seem to listen when spoken to directly, has difficulty sustaining attention
b. Has difficulty organizing tasks, fidgets with hands, has difficulty waiting turn
c. Makes careless mistakes in schoolwork, has difficulty waiting turn, talks excessively
d. Interrupts others, talks excessively, does not seem to listen when spoken to directly

2. Researchers have linked the development of ADHD to which of the following factors?

a. Refined sugar, drug abuse during pregnancy, brain injuries after birth
b. Food additives, fluorescent lighting, cigarette smoking during pregnancy
c. Food additives, prenatal exposure to lead, poor maternal nutrition
d. Cigarette smoking during pregnancy, prenatal exposure to lead, poor maternal nutrition

3. When a behavioral assessment is conducted, it is necessary to obtain information about the child's behavior in a variety of settings. Which of the following best describes the areas that must be assessed with all children?

a. School, organized sports, after school programs
b. Organized sports, after school programs, youth organizations
c. School, home, at play
d. School, home, organized sports

4. Which of the following statements about conducting a physical examination on a child being evaluated for ADHD is correct?

a. A physical examination is not necessary.
b. Testing motor skills is not necessary.
c. Testing memory is important.
d. Testing motor coordination, hearing, and vision is necessary.

5. The differential diagnosis for ADHD includes which of the following?

   a. ODD, CD, learning disability
   b. CD, learning disability, depression
   c. Learning disability, depression, ODD
   d. ODD, CD, depression

6. The parents of a 9-year-old boy with ADHD report that his behavior has improved at school, but they see no change in his behavior at home. The parents should be encouraged to:

   a. See a therapist who can teach them behavior management skills.
   b. Double check with the school to make sure he is taking his midday dose of methylphenidate (Ritalin) as prescribed.
   c. Do away with any rules or limits they set at home; he is not able to follow rules all day.
   d. Enroll the child in a social skills training program to improve his behavior in social situations.

7. Working with the school is an important part of the treatment of a child with ADHD. The therapist can be most helpful to the teacher by providing which of the following services?

   a. Meet monthly with the principal and school counselor.
   b. Meet weekly with parents and teacher to establish behavior management programs.
   c. Meet weekly with parents and teacher to establish system of punishments.
   d. Meet monthly with the principal to plan an individualized educational program (IEP).

8. Treatment of ADHD is multifaceted. For the best possible outcomes, which of the following are necessary components of treatment?

   a. Medication, psychologic and behavioral approaches, school intervention
   b. Medication, psychologic and behavioral approaches, family therapy
   c. Psychologic and behavioral approaches, family therapy, school intervention
   d. Family therapy, school intervention, medication

9. When a child is being treated for ADHD, the child and parents must understand that:

   a. Treatment is short term; once the medication dose is stable, the child will need no further treatment.
   b. With the combination of medication and behavior management programs, the treatment will be complete in 1 year with no additional follow-up needed.
   c. The child will eventually "outgrow" ADHD in adolescence.
   d. Comprehensive treatment is long term; medication and behavior management techniques will change as the child and family change.

10. Which of the following is a proven treatment for ADHD?

   a. Dietary management
   b. Traditional play therapy
   c. Social skills training in clinics
   d. Parent problem solving and communication training

ANSWERS AND RATIONALES

1. *Answer:* a (assessment/history/psychosocial/child)
   Rationale: Fidgeting, not waiting turn, talking excessively, and interrupting others are hyperactive behaviors. (American Psychiatric Association, 1994)

2. *Answer:* d (assessment/history/psychosocial/NAS)
   Rationale: There is no research to back up the theories about refined sugar, food additives, and fluorescent lighting being causes of ADHD. (Barkley, 1990)

3. *Answer:* c (assessment/physical examination/psychosocial/child)
   Rationale: The parent will come with information about the child's functioning in these three areas. Many children with ADHD have difficulty with sport teams and do not participate in them. Not all children participate in after school programs. (Barkley, 1990)

4. *Answer:* d (assessment/physical examination/psychosocial/child)

Rationale: A thorough physical examination is necessary to rule out a developmental disorder, visual deficiencies, impaired hearing, and neurologic deficits. (Barkley, 1990)

5. *Answer:* a (diagnosis/psychosocial/NAS)

Rationale: Depression may be present with ADHD, but the symptoms of depression are easily separated from the symptoms of ADHD. (Barkley, 1990)

6. *Answer:* a (plan/psychosocial/child)

Rationale: Many children demonstrate this phenomenon since the school often is a more structured environment than the home. When the parents and child begin to work with a therapist on behavior management skills, the behavior at home will improve. (Barkley, 1990)

7. *Answer:* b (plan/psychosocial/child)

Rationale: It is important to meet with parents and teachers frequently to establish the behavior management program. The program is highly individualized and must be consistent at home and at school. After the program is well established, less frequent contact with the school is necessary. (Barkley, 1990)

8. *Answer:* a (evaluation/psychosocial/child)

Rationale: Family therapy is only indicated when there are family issues such as sibling issues, divorce, losses. (Barkley, 1990)

9. *Answer:* d (evaluation/psychosocial/child)

Rationale: Treatment of ADHD is long term, and 50% to 80% of children treated carry symptoms into adulthood. Adjustments in medication and behavior management are made as the child grows and develops. (Barkley, 1990)

10. *Answer:* d (diagnosis/psychosocial/NAS)

Rationale: Problem solving and communication training for the parents and the child will provide new techniques to approach situations in a positive manner. (Barkley, 1990)

BEHAVIOR PROBLEMS

OVERVIEW
Definition

Behavior problems exist when a child's behavior is perceived by a supervising adult to deviate from acceptable norms. The problems may be specific to a situation or a person. Common behavior problems include temper tantrums, hitting, kicking, biting, noncompliance, back-talk, fighting, arguing, yelling, and refusing to go to bed.

Incidence

- Most children display one or more problematic behaviors during the first years of life through adolescence.
- The incidence is highest during preschool years, with 90% of mothers reporting at least mild concern.
- Behavior problems are often undiagnosed.

Pathophysiology

- Unclear and irregular enforcement of parental expectations for behavior is the primary cause.
- The temperament of the child and parenting skills of the parents also contribute.
- Research has demonstrated associations of maternal smoking, increased family stress, increased family size, illness in family, socioeconomic status, and maternal marital status.

ASSESSMENT: SUBJECTIVE/HISTORY

- Obtain a pertinent history: Birth order, family composition, family dynamics, discipline techniques, illness, developmental milestones, family history of behavior problems.
- Obtain a description of misbehavior(s), and parental response and its effectiveness.
- Consider the following:
  —Age and sex appropriateness
  —Persistence
  —Life circumstance and precipitating events
  —Setting/situation specificity
  —Extent of disturbance
  —Type, severity, and frequency of symptoms
  —Change in behavior

ASSESSMENT: OBJECTIVE/ PHYSICAL EXAMINATION
Physical Examination

- Complete a physical examination to rule out illness or other physical cause for the behavior change.
- Focus on the following areas:
  - General: Observation of parent-child interaction; child's response to direction and correction; child's affect and behavior during play
  - Neurologic: Neurodevelopmental screen, vision and hearing screen

Diagnostic Procedures

BEHAVIOR RATING SCALE
- Select scale according to age and complaint.
- Scales may be completed by supervising adults other than parents (e.g., teachers).
- A scale is helpful to differentiate the psychologically disturbed child.

DIAGNOSIS

The differential diagnosis for a common (minor) behavior problem includes the following:
- Normal behavior of childhood
- Major behavior problem
- Psychologic disturbance
- Learning disorder

- Ineffective parenting
- Dysfunctional parenting
- Child abuse

THERAPEUTIC PLAN

- Establish a relationship with the family.
- Acknowledge the difficulty of developmental issues.
- Initiate a behavior management system as appropriate.
- Refer for parenting classes, parent support groups, and/or social services as needed.
- Maintain open communication and support during the process of implementing the behavior management system; it may take weeks to notice a consistent change.

Client Education

- Consider developmental stages.
  - Outline the expected behaviors according to the child's developmental level.
  - Parents must discuss and agree early in the child's life what constitutes misbehavior; what is cute to some is misbehaving to others.
- Discuss appropriate parenting strategies, including a system for behavior modification.
  - Present clear expectations.
  - Discuss consequences (punishment) for misbehavior (Table 15-1).

Table 15-1 Comparison of Mild Punishments

METHOD	DESCRIPTION	APPLICABLE AGES
Distraction	Removal from situation by providing alternative site for attention (i.e., another toy if one is in dispute)	Infant and toddlers
Time-out	Interruption of disruptive or aggressive behavior by immediate isolation at onset; few words; boring place; timed for a minute per year of age	2-12 yr
Scolding/disapproval	Naming misbehavior (stern voice) and expressing dissatisfaction	All ages
Natural consequences	Allowing result to occur without intervention from parent only if does not jeopardize safety (e.g., play too roughly with cat, get scratched)	All ages
Logical consequences	Punishment determined by parent and logically connected to misbehavior (e.g., ride bike without helmet, no bike riding for 1 week)	3 yr to adolescence
Behavioral penalty	Loss of privileges for misbehavior that has no clear consequence (e.g., refusal to do chores, "grounded" for the weekend)	5 yr to adolescence

—Use positive reinforcement of appropriate behavior.

- Reinforce consistency as the key to a successful system.
  —Consistency between parents and all caretakers is important.
  —It must be applicable across circumstances.
- Identify parents as role models. Encourage a consciousness for their own behavior in all situations.

Guidelines for Using Punishment

- Use punishment sparingly.
- Use mild punishment. Avoid physical punishment.
- Punish quickly after misbehavior.
- Punish only if in control of self.
- Provide a brief reason for the punishment.

EVALUATION/FOLLOW-UP

- Follow up by phone in 1 to 2 weeks: Encourage the parent to call sooner with questions/difficulties with implementing the behavior management system.
- Schedule a return visit in 4 to 6 weeks.
  —Repeat the neurodevelopmental screen if there are any developmental lags/deficits.
  —If misbehavior is still unmanaged after 4 weeks of implementing a behavior management system, consider another behavior management strategy or referral to psychologist or physician for possible psychiatric evaluation.
- Consider a 6-month interval between well-child visits until stability is maintained.

Referral

- Consult with a physician regarding aggressive or self-destructive behaviors.
- Report any suspected cases of child abuse to the appropriate authorities.
- Refer complicated (multiple types) and/or major behavior problems (persistent, inappropriate for age/sex, increasing severity or frequency of symptoms) for evaluation by a physician and possible psychiatric evaluation.

REFERENCES

Arvin, A. M., Behrman, R. E., Kliegman, R. M., & Nelson, W. E. (1996). *Nelson textbook of pediatrics* (15th ed.). Philadelphia: W. B. Saunders.

Boyton, R. W., Dunn, E. S., & Stephens, G. R., (Eds.). (1994). *Ambulatory pediatric care* (2nd ed.). Philadelphia: J. B. Lippincott.

Clark, L. (1985). *SOS! Help for parents.* Bowling Green, KY: Parents Press.

Herman-Staab, B. (1994). Screening, management and appropriate referral for pediatric behavior problems. *Nurse Practitioner, 19*(7), 40-49.

Schmitt, B. D. (1987). Seven deadly sins of childhood: Advising parents about difficult developmental phases. *Child Abuse and Neglect, 11*, 421-432.

Schmitt, B. D. (1993). Time-out: Intervention of choice for the irrational years. *Contemporary Pediatrics, 10*, 64-71.

REVIEW QUESTIONS

1. Ineffective behavior management is best reflected in which of the following reports?

a. "I use distraction when my 15-month-old gets into things he shouldn't."
b. "I've tried putting my child in time-out, but he just gets up. I warn him and warn him, but nothing seems to work."
c. "We put the toy in time-out if the children fight over it."
d. "Sally used to refuse to eat. After a few times going to bed with a growling tummy, however, she is more willing to try new foods."

2. A 3-year-old with minor behavior problems is likely to have what physical findings?

a. Personal/social developmental delay
b. Signs of acute otitis media
c. Failed vision screen
d. Normal findings from physical examination

3. Billy pushes his older brother who is picking on him. Both are placed in time-out by the mother for 8 minutes (their average ages). Another day, the father cheers Billy on for "standing up for himself" when he pushes his older brother for picking on him. What is the most accurate assessment of the situation?

a. Birth order intensifies the misbehavior.
b. Inconsistency of parental response sends mixed messages regarding expectations.
c. Time out would be more effective for one child at a time.
d. Family stress and tension may contribute to the boy's misbehavior.

4. Important components for a behavior management system include all the following **except:**

  a. Clear expectations
  b. Consequences (punishment) for misbehavior
  c. Positive reinforcement of appropriate behavior
  d. Variation of system according to child's temperament

5. Phone follow-up for a minor behavior problem should be initiated in what time period?

  a. 24 hours
  b. 1 to 2 days
  c. 1 to 2 weeks
  d. 4 to 6 weeks

6. A harried parent brings his child in for an ear infection follow-up. "Oh, by the way, do you have any suggestions for dealing with biting?" the parent asks. "This is a new occurrence for my 2-year-old. They are threatening to throw him out of day care." The best response for the nurse practitioner is which of the following?

  a. "Check to see if he is teething. He might be cutting molars."
  b. "Tell me a little more about the biting. How long has it been going on? What is your response?"
  c. "This is common for a 2-year-old. He'll grow out of it."
  d. "You might offer a chew-cloth for your son to bite instead of another child."

7. A 3-year-old is accompanied by her mother for a well-child check. The only concern reported by the mother is the child's "horrible behavior over the past week." The child will not stay in bed and is combative at times. She whines and constantly wants attention. The history is significant for mild cold symptoms that occurred in the family 2 weeks ago. Which physical findings are likely in this case?

  a. Personal/social developmental delay
  b. Signs of acute otitis media
  c. Failed vision screen
  d. Normal findings from physical examination

8. A previously well-behaved 5-year-old enters kindergarten and displays behavior problems during the first weeks of school. A note is sent home about the child's difficulty in sharing and noncompliance with ending free play. The most likely assessment is:

  a. Mild behavior problem secondary to developmental transition
  b. Normal behavior of childhood
  c. Major behavior problem as a result of multiple disturbances
  d. Mild behavior problem specific to school situation

ANSWERS AND RATIONALES

1. *Answer:* b (assessment/history/psychosocial/child)
  Rationale: Warning that a time-out will occur is ineffective use of this method. Successful use of time-out serves to interrupt and stop misbehavior at its onset. Warnings simply teach children they can misbehave without consequence. Other options are examples of age- and situation-appropriate behavior management. (Schmitt, 1993)

2. *Answer:* d (assessment/physical examination/psychosocial/child)
  Rationale: The most common cause of minor behavior problems during childhood is ineffective parenting, thus a 3-year-old is likely to have no underlying physical complaint for minor behavior problems. Developmental delays, acute illness, and visual deficits may also contribute to behavior problems but are less common causes. (Herman-Staab, 1994; Schmitt, 1987)

3. *Answer:* b (diagnosis/psychosocial/child)
  Rationale: Consistency of enforcing established guidelines/rules across situations and between parents is key to discipline or behavior management. Birth order and family stress may contribute to misbehavior as well but are of less importance if there is a flaw in the management system. Ineffective parenting is the primary cause of behavior problems in children. Time-out technique can be effectively used with two children at once under the parameters this mother used. (Boyton, Dunn, & Stephens, 1994; Clark, 1985; Herman-Staab, 1994)

4. *Answer:* d (plan/psychosocial/child)
  Rationale: Key components of a behavior management system are clear expectations, enforced consequences for misbehavior, and positive reinforcement of appropriate behavior. Systems may vary across families but must be consistently implemented with all children, despite differing temperaments, to avoid mixed messages and sibling conflict. (Schmitt, 1987)

5. *Answer:* c (evaluation/psychosocial/child)

Rationale: Minor behavior problems warrant ongoing communication (1 to 2 weeks), but the immediate follow-up periods (24 hours, 1 to 2 days) would be more appropriate for the more complex situations. For instance, a child with a major behavior problem may be waiting for an available appointment for a psychiatric evaluation. Ongoing contact until that appointment is made provides support for the parents and provides an opportunity to monitor a situation that may worsen and require further intervention. Waiting 4 to 6 weeks to follow up would delay identification of unmanaged behavior. (Schmitt, 1987)

6. *Answer:* b (plan/psychosocial/child)

Rationale: Information about severity and frequency of symptoms, precipitating events, and situation specificity are important to ascertain before making recommendations for dealing with biting. The problem must be understood before reassuring the parent (which may be appropriate at a later time). (Herman-Staab, 1994)

7. *Answer:* b (assessment/physical examination/child)

Rationale: A sudden change in behavior is more likely to be a manifestation of a physical etiologic factor. Behavior, sleep, activity, and appetite changes are major indicators of acute illness in young children. This child is not likely to have normal findings from physical examination. The developmental issues would likely demonstrate a more insidious onset. (Boyton, Dunn, & Stephens, 1994)

8. *Answer:* a (diagnosis/pyschosocial/child)

Rationale: Because of the timing (behavior change with developmental transition) assessment would be minor behavior problem. If the problem persisted or worsened, consider more in-depth evaluation (possibly behavior rating scale to parents and teacher). The behavior may be anticipated because of the transition to kindergarten but would not be considered normal for this child. (Herman-Staab, 1994)

DEPRESSION

OVERVIEW
Definition

Depression is a disturbance in mood or affect. According to the *DSM-IV*, depressive disorders are classified as major depressive disorder, single episode, major depressive disorder, recurrent, dysthymic disorder, depressive disorder not otherwise specified, and then the bipolar disorders. The reader is referred to the DSM-IV for the specific sets of criteria for each disorder.

A major depressive disorder is characterized by two or more episodes of a depressed mood or loss of interest lasting at least 2 weeks and consisting of five or more of the symptoms listed under Symptoms.

Incidence

- Depression is twice as common in women than in men, except in persons with bipolar disorder, where the incidence is about equal. It is believed that 8% to 12% of men and 18% to 25% of women suffer a major depression in their lifetime. At any given time 10 to 14 million Americans are suffering from some form of a mood disorder.
- Depression is the most common reason for seeking mental health treatment. It accounts for 75% of the hospitalized psychiatric clients and 6% to 8% of all outpatients in a primary care setting.
- There is an increased incidence of depression in older adults who are living in long-term facilities.
- Depression is more common in young women and tends to decrease with age. However, the incidence increases in women older than 50 with hypothyroidism. In men, the incidence tends to increase with age. Older adults are at a high risk for depression because of the multiple losses and health problems that frequently occur at this stage of life.

- Marital status: Depression is more common in divorced and single persons than in those who are married.
- Seasonal: Mood disorders are more common in the spring and fall.
- Race: No significant relationship has been found between race and mood disorders.
- Recurrence: The incidence increases once a person has experienced a depressive episode (50% after the first, 70% to 80% after the second).
- Suicide: Suicide is a risk for all clients with a mood disorder. It is the eighth leading cause of death in the United States across all age groups and the third for adolescents and young adults. Suicide is also a leading cause of preventable death for adults older than 60.
  RISK FACTORS FOR SUICIDE
  - White
  - Physical illness
  - Substance abuse
  - Male
  - Increasing age
  - Living alone

Pathophysiology

Various theories have been formulated to explain the cause and dynamics of mood/affective disorders. It is believed that these disorders are a syndrome with common features and a variety of causative factors. Several of the most common theoretical perspectives follow:

- Biochemical/neurobiologic: Research indicates that there is a genetic predisposition. There is a functional deficiency of the neurotransmitters: serotonin (5-HT), dopamine, norepinephrine, and acetylcholine.
- Psychodynamic: The psychodynamic theory focuses on the perceived loss and the unresolved grieving that occurred in the early child-parent relationship. The unresolved grieving is accompanied with repressed anger. The result is that the anger is turned against the self, which results in depressive episodes.
- Cognitive: Schemas direct the way people experience others and themselves. Those who are depressed ignore the positive and focus on the negative messages, thus contributing to a view of self as unworthy, incompetent, and unlovable. When this occurs, cognitive distortions result.

ASSESSMENT: SUBJECTIVE/HISTORY
History of Present Illness

- Obtain a complete personal and family history of panic attacks, depression, and/or suicide attempts.
- Discuss the client's support systems and coping techniques.
- Determine whether there is substance abuse. Illegal or legal drug use and alcohol can complicate or cause depression. It is essential that the clinician obtain a complete list of all substances used by the client.
- Ascertain the client's perceived losses and current stressors.
- Obtain a history of cerebral vascular accident, myocardial infarction, or other chronic debilitating illness.
- Determine the level of anxiety and severity of symptoms.
- Suicide risk must be critically assessed. Specific and clear questions should be asked by the nurse practitioner regarding the following:
  —Suicidal thoughts and history of past attempts
  —Presence of a plan for suicide
  —Access to a means or weapon for suicide
  —The more specific and structured the plan, the greater the risk for suicide

Symptoms

Symptoms most frequently associated with depression include the following:

- Feelings of sadness, guilt, low self-esteem
- Pessimistic thoughts
- Suicidal thoughts, gestures, attempts
- Tearfulness, anxiety, irritability
- Anhedonia (loss of interest or pleasure in activities that were previously enjoyed)
- Sleep disturbances
- Changes in appetite, with either weight gain or loss
- Decreased libido
- Impaired cognitive reasoning (all-or-nothing thinking, jumping to conclusions, mental filtering, personalization, and "should" statements)
- Physiologic symptoms
  —Fatigue
  —Headache
  —Chest pain
  —Alteration in bowel and bladder function

—Amenorrhea
—Nausea and vomiting
—Psychomotor agitation or retardation

In children the symptoms frequently seen include the following:

- Loss of appetite
- Fatigue
- Conduct problems
- Aggression
- Anhedonia
- Fear of separation from caregiver or fear of caregiver
- Failure to achieve developmental tasks

Adolescents may demonstrate the following:

- Isolation
- Self-destructive behavior
- Sexual promiscuity
- Antisocial behavior
- Negative thinking

Many of the physical symptoms of depression, such as fatigue, anorexia, bowel and bladder problems are often attributed to "old age." Older adults may also manifest symptoms that must be differentiated from those of dementia:

- Disorientation
- Impaired memory
- Inability to concentrate
- Anhedonia

Medication History

- Reserpine
- Oral contraceptive pills
- Steroids
- Amphetamine/cocaine withdrawal

Summary

Depression is manifested by impaired responses in four areas:

1. Emotional: Sadness, worthlessness, apathy, guilt and anger, suicidal ideation or gestures
2. Behavioral: Anhedonia, poor hygiene, psychomotor retardation
3. Cognitive: Impaired concentration, obsessive thoughts, indecisiveness
4. Physical: Fatigue, appetite, sleep, constipation

ASSESSMENT: OBJECTIVE/ PHYSICAL EXAMINATION

Physical Examination

The physical examination should be thorough with particular attention given to the following:

- Thyroid enlargement
- Cardiovascular status
- Neurologic status

Diagnostic Procedures

Currently there are no conclusive diagnostic physical examination findings or laboratory tests for depression. However, certain abnormal results have been noted in a few tests:

- Abnormal sleep EEG are seen in about 50% of all outpatients with depression.
- The dexamethasone-suppression test (DST) is sometimes employed to help establish a diagnosis of depression:
  —In a nondepressed person, the production and secretion of cortisol by the adrenal gland is suppressed.
  —If the person is depressed, the suppression of cortisol is slight and/or the recovery from the effects of the DST is quite rapid.
- Thyroid function studies are frequently done to rule out hypothyroid disorder.
- Many clinicians use various rating scale instruments designed to measure the client's mood to aid in the diagnosis of depression.

DIAGNOSIS

The differential diagnosis includes the following:

- Organic mood disorder
- Schizophrenia
- Grief
- Delirium
- Dementia
- Substance abuse
- Endocrine disorders
- Liver failure
- Chronic fatigue
- Renal failure

THERAPEUTIC PLAN

- The initial and primary goal is to provide for the safety of the client. Determine the lethality of the client's suicidal ideation/plan. Remember that suicide is most likely when a client is going into or emerging from depression.
- Avoid excessive cheerfulness, which might diminish the significance of the client's feelings.
- Establish a no-suicide contract with the client.
- Assist the client in contacting immediate support systems. If the client is clearly suicidal and unwilling to contract not to harm self, immediate hospitalization must be considered.
- Exercise appears to be beneficial. Initially a 10-minute walk is suggested.

Pharmacologic Treatment

Antidepressants are effective in the treatment of depression, ranging from dysthymia to severe depression. Appropriate agents include the tricyclic antidepressants, monoamine oxidase inhibitors (MAOIs), and the selective serotonin reuptake inhibitors (SSRIs). The choice of medication is based on the following:

- Client history of prior treatment and response
- Type of depression
- Side effects of the medication
- Other medications the client may be taking

Most antidepressant medications take 4 to 6 weeks before any significant results are obtained, although benefits may be seen in as little as 2 weeks. Anticholinergic side effects may be a problem with tricyclics and MAOIs more than with SSRIs. If the client is experiencing other symptoms, such as delusions, anxiety, or hallucinations, other psychotropic medications may be required.

Nonpharmacologic Treatment

Psychotherapy is recommended for the treatment of depression, either alone or in combination with medication. Individual or group therapy are both effective modalities.

Electroconvulsive therapy (ECT) is recommended for treatment of the most severe forms of psychotic depression that are not responsive to other forms of therapy.

Client Education

- Inform the client and family of medication side effects, with special emphasis on those effects that must be reported. Include dietary and activity restrictions related to the medication.
- Instruct the client and family when to seek professional help. Teach the client and family to report increasing signs of depression or suicidal thoughts.
- Reinforce effective coping behaviors, nutrition, exercise, rest, and socialization.

Referral

Referral to a mental health specialist for the treatment of any major depression should be seriously considered.

EVALUATION/FOLLOW-UP

Clients who are depressed and receiving antidepressant medications should return weekly for evaluation. After 5 to 6 weeks when improvement is seen, the follow-up can go to 2 times a month, then monthly, etc. Counseling combined with antidepressant therapy is critical to see the most improvement. Improvement is seen when the client accomplishes the following:

- Verbalizes and demonstrates compliance with treatment plan
- Experiences no suicidal thoughts and does not have a plan
- Verbalizes positive feelings about the future
- Demonstrates resolution of presenting symptoms

REFERENCES

American Psychiatric Association (1994). *Diagnostic and statistical manual of mental disorders (DSM-IV)* (4th ed.). Washington, DC: Author.

Flowers, M. E. (1997). Recognition and psychopharmacologic treatment of geriatric depression. *Journal of the American Psychiatric Nurses Association, 3*(2), 32-39.

The Harvard Mental Health Letter. (1994, December). Update on mood disorders. Part 1. pp. 1-4.

The Harvard Mental Health Letter. (1995, January). Update on Mood Disorders. Part 2. pp. 1-4.

The Harvard Mental Health Letter. (1996, November). Suicide. Part 1. pp. 1-4.

Rush, A., Golden, W., Hall, G., et al. (1993, April). *Depression in primary care: Volume 1 and 2, Clinical practice guidelines, No. 5* (AHCPR Publication No. 93-0550). Rockville, MD: U.S. Department of Health and Human Services, Public Health Service, Agency for Health Care Policy and Research.

Wilson, H., & Kneisl, C. (1996). *Psychiatric nursing* (5th ed., pp. 324-359, 793-802). Menlo Park, CA: Addison-Wesley.

REVIEW QUESTIONS

1. Which theory of depression states that the individual focuses on negative ideas and messages about the environment and self?

    a. Biochemical theory
    b. Psychodynamic theory
    c. Transactional theory
    d. Cognitive theory

2. Depression, dysthymia, and bipolar disorder are alike in that:

    a. They are considered affective/mood disorders.
    b. They are more common in men than in women.
    c. The incidence tends to decrease with age for both men and women.
    d. They are seldom seen in blacks.

3. A client complains of severe anticholinergic side effects following 4 weeks of treatment on a tricyclic antidepressant (imipramine [Tofranil]). Which of the following drugs should be prescribed next?

    a. SSRI (sertraline [Zoloft])
    b. Tricyclic (nortriptyline [Pamelor])
    c. MAOI (phenelzine [Nardil])
    d. Antianxiety/sedative (alprazolam [Xanax])

4. A client with severe clinical depression who has been treated for 3 weeks is starting to show signs of improvement. During this recovery period, the client:

    a. Is no longer at risk for suicide
    b. Is at a greater risk for suicide than when severely depressed
    c. Is less of a risk for suicide than when severely depressed
    d. Will always be at a high risk for suicide

5. A middle-aged married couple comes to the clinic. During the interview assessment the wife verbalizes concern about her husband's major mood swings and not knowing what to expect from him. What information should the nurse practitioner focus on first?

    a. Family history of mental illness
    b. Information about their sexual relationship
    c. Information about any stresses or losses that have occurred within the past year
    d. More detailed information about the symptoms and what impact they have on the couple's daily life

6. In the evaluation of a client with clinical depression, the **least** important factor would be the client's:

    a. Thinking process
    b. Physical manifestations
    c. Basic personality type
    d. Potential for suicide

7. Subjective symptoms of clinical depression include all the following **except:**

    a. Grandiosity
    b. A sense of worthlessness
    c. Fatigue
    d. Anhedonia

8. Which of the following interventions would **not** be appropriate in treating a client with clinical depression?

    a. Convey unconditional acceptance and respect.
    b. Assist in the identification of real achievements to promote self-esteem.
    c. Consistently maintain a very cheerful attitude when interacting with the client.
    d. Keep all commitments to build trust.

9. What should the nurse practitioner teach the family of a client with clinical depression?

    a. It is important that the client feel a sense of being a useful and valued member of the family.
    b. The family should hide any of their negative feelings from the client.
    c. The family needs family therapy to prevent a relapse in the client.
    d. Depression will be a constant problem throughout the client's life.

ANSWERS AND RATIONALES

1. *Answer:* d (assessment/history/psychosocial/NAS)
Rationale: The cognitive theory states that schemas direct the way people see the world and themselves. Depressed individuals tend to focus on negative messages. (Wilson & Kneisl, 1996)

2. *Answer:* a (assessment/physical examination/psychosocial/NAS)
Rationale: All are classified as affective/mood disorders. (American Psychiatric Association, 1994)

3. *Answer:* a (plan/psychosocial/NAS)
Rationale: SSRIs are thought to have less anticholinergic effects than the tricyclic drugs. (Wilson & Kneisl, 1996)

4. *Answer:* b (evaluation/psychosocial/NAS)
Rationale: Individuals are at a greater risk for suicide when going into or emerging from depression. (*Harvard Mental Health Letter,* 1996, November)

5. *Answer:* d (diagnosis/psychosocial/adult)
Rationale: Although all the information may be essential, the nurse practitioner first needs accurate information about the symptoms to complete a comprehensive assessment. (Wilson & Kneisl, 1996)

6. *Answer:* c (evaluation/psychosocial/NAS)
Rationale: Depression is manifested by changes in choices *a, c,* and *d.* Although depression and stress may exacerbate symptoms of a personality disorder, the basic personality type has been established in early life and is not the focus of therapy for depression. (American Psychiatric Association, 1994)

7. *Answer:* a (assessment/history/psychosocial/NAS)
Rationale: Grandiosity implies feelings of self-importance, which is more characteristic in mania. (Wilson & Kneisl, 1996)

8. *Answer:* c (plan/psychosocial/NAS)
Rationale: Excessive cheerfulness can diminish the significance of the depressed person's feelings. (Wilson & Kneisl, 1996)

9. *Answer:* a (plan/psychosocial/NAS)
Rationale: A major emotional symptom seen in depression is a sense of worthlessness. (American Psychiatric Association, 1994)

EATING DISORDERS

Anorexia Nervosa and Bulimia Nervosa

OVERVIEW
Definition

Anorexia nervosa (AN) is a life-threatening eating disorder in which there is a severe disturbance in eating with self-starvation and excessive weight loss.

There are four criteria for diagnosis and according to the *Diagnostic and Statistical Manual of Mental Disorders (DSM-IV):*

1. Refusal to maintain body weight at or above minimally normal weight for age and height (body weight <85% of expected body weight)
2. Intense fear of gaining weight or becoming fat, even though underweight
3. Disturbance in the way in which one's body weight or shape is experienced, undue influence on body weight or shape on self-evaluation, or denial of the seriousness of the current low body weight
4. In postmenarcheal females, amenorrhea (i.e., the absence of at least three consecutive menstrual cycles)

There are two types of AN according to the *DSM-IV:*

1. Restricting: During the current episode of AN, the person has not regularly engaged in binge eating or purging behaviors (i.e., self-induced vomiting or the misuse of laxatives, diuretics, or enemas).
2. Binge-eating/purging type: During the current episode of AN, the person has regularly engaged in binge eating or purging behaviors (i.e., self-induced vomiting or the misuse of laxatives, diuretics, or enemas).

Bulimia nervosa (BN) is an eating disorder characterized by binge eating and inappropriate compensatory acts to prevent weight gain.

The criteria and types of BN according to the *DSM-IV* are as follows:

1. A recurrent episode of binge eating is characterized by both of the following:
   a. Eating in a discrete period of time (e.g., within any 2-hour period) an amount of food that is definitely larger than most people would eat during a similar period of time and under similar circumstances
   b. A sense of lack of control over eating during an episode (e.g., a feeling that one cannot stop eating or control what or how much one is eating)
2. Recurrent inappropriate compensatory behaviors are used to prevent weight gain, such as self-induced vomiting; misuse of laxatives, diuretics, enemas, or other medications; fasting; or excessive exercise.
3. The binge eating and inappropriate compensatory behaviors both occur, on average, at least twice a week for 3 months.
4. Self-evaluation is unduly influenced by body and weight.
5. The disturbance does not occur exclusively during an episode of AN.

There are two types of BN, according to the *DSM-IV.*

1. Purging type: During the current episode of BN, the person has regularly engaged in self-induced vomiting or misuse of laxatives, diuretics, or enemas.
2. Nonpurging type: During the current episode of BN, the person has used other inappropriate compensatory behaviors, such as fasting or excessive exercise, but has not regularly engaged in self-induced vomiting or the misuse of laxatives, diuretics, or enemas.

It has been estimated 75% to 94% of persons with BN use vomiting at least once per day.

Incidence

ANOREXIA

- AN occurs typically in young, white middle to upper middle class females (90% to 95%), estimated 0.5% to 1% of young female population in the United States. However, an increase in all socioeconomic classes and other ethnic groups has been noted.
- There is a higher risk of AN if first-degree biologic relatives have an eating disorder.
- Age of onset of AN is concentrated between 12 and 25 years. Bimodal peak of AN is 14 and 18 years.
- AN usually occurs after puberty begins and rarely occurs after 40 years.

BULIMIA

- The incidence of BN is estimated at 1% to 3% of adolescent and young adult females in the United States.
- Age of onset of BN is usually late adolescent or early adult life. Binge eating usually begins after a diet.
- Most persons with BN are average weight, slightly underweight, or slightly overweight.
- One third to one half of cases have a history of being overweight.

GENERAL

- It is not unusual for persons with eating disorder to slide from AN to BN and vice versa.
- An estimated 5% to 10% of persons with AN are male. An estimated 1 out of 10 or 1% to 3% of persons with BN are male. An increased incidence of AN and BN are noted in the homosexual population.
- Persons involved in sports with emphasis on weight and shape such as wrestling, gymnastics, swimming, and long-distance running or persons involved in activities such as modeling or ballet are at higher risk for AN and BN. Eating disorder develops after participation in these sports and/or activities is initiated.
- About 10% of all persons with AN hospitalized in university settings die. Death is related to complications associated with starvation or suicide. Mortality figures for persons with BN are unknown.

Pathophysiology

It is difficult to identify what causes AN/BN because the disorders are multidetermined. Persons with AN/BN share many of the same characteristics/factors. These factors include individual, family, sociocultural, and biologic ones.

INDIVIDUAL FACTORS

- Weight disturbance as child/adolescent
- Low self-esteem

- Sense of ineffectiveness/lack of control/powerlessness
- Need for approval
- Perfectionism
- Fear of growing up
- Self-criticism
- Inability to identify/tolerate feelings
- Dependence
- High value placed on self-control and self-discipline
- For males, sexual identity issues
- Impulsivity in persons with BN
- Obsessive traits in persons with AN
- Difficulty developing a sense of "self"/problems with being able to separate from family and individuate

FAMILY FACTORS
- Lack of conflict resolution
- Parental overprotectiveness
- Disengagement/emeshment rigidity
- Unbearable rules
- No compromises
- Blurring of generational boundaries (the child acts as the parent)
- High parental expectations
- Overly concerned with appearance/achievement
- Affective and substance abuse disorders

SOCIOCULTURAL FACTORS
- Pressure to be thin in society
- Mixed messages about women's worth in relation to their bodies/"appearance is your worth"
- Changing roles of women and role destabilization
- Prejudice against obesity/"fat phobias"
- Emphasis on achievement and perfection

POSSIBLE BIOLOGIC FACTORS
- AN may have genetic predisposition based on twin studies in which concordance rates of 50% monozygotic twins vs 10% for dizygotic.
- Higher incidences of affective disorders in family members of eating disordered person may indicate genetic predisposition.

ASSESSMENT: SUBJECTIVE/HISTORY

Symptoms

- Denial of any problems especially in persons with AN
- Feelings of guilt or shame in persons with BN

- Body distortion (i.e., feel "too fat" although emaciated)
- Dizziness
- Menstrual irregularities
- Complaints of being cold
- Decreased energy/fatigue
- Complaints of increased sensitivity to heat, cold, acid substances in teeth/mouth
- Gastrointestinal disorders, including constipation, diarrhea, nausea, vomiting, bloating, and heartburn
- Social withdrawal, anhedonia

Past Medical History

Include questions pertaining to the Associated Symptoms, as well as to the following:
- Substance abuse (especially in males and persons with BN)
- Use of ipecac (extremely dangerous, cardiotoxic), laxatives, diuretics, enemas, purging
- Swelling in extremities
- Seizures
- Activity level especially exercise history (type, frequency, duration, compulsiveness), increased restlessness, changes in strength and endurance

Family History

- Parents' ages, careers, general health, relationship with client, attitudes toward food, physical appearance
- Age and sex of siblings and their relationships
- History of psychiatric illnesses in the family, especially incidence of eating disorders, substance abuse, affective disorders

Psychosocial History

- Involvement in activities and educational history
- Ways the client views self (especially looking for perfectionism and self-criticism and body distortions)
- Relationships outside family
- Physical and sexual abuse
- Mood fluctuations, inability to describe feelings, suicidal ideation, past psychiatric history and treatment
- High co-morbidity of affective, obsessive, compulsive, anxiety, and personality disorders in persons with AN.

- In persons with BN possible co-morbidity of affective, anxiety, or personality disorders and substance abuse and impulsivity (e.g., promiscuity, shoplifting)

Dietary History

- Onset of weight loss
- Highest and lowest weights
- Fluctuations in weights
- Changes in appetite
- Typical pattern of eating
- Binge-purge episodes
- Habits of hiding/throwing away food
- Preoccupation with food
- Unusual handling of food (e.g., cutting into small pieces)
- Guilt after eating

Sexual History

- Ask about development of second sexual characteristics, menstrual history, preparation for puberty, sexual orientation, attitudes toward sexual development/sexuality, and history of STDs.
- Inquire about sexual activity.
  —Adolescents/young adults with AN report no to little sexual activity
  —Older persons with AN usually report decreased sexual interest.
  —Persons with BN may report multiple partners and high-risk sexual activity.

ASSESSMENT: OBJECTIVE/ PHYSICAL EXAMINATION

Physical Examination

Perform a problem-oriented physical examination with particular attention to the following:

- Vital signs: Assess for orthostatic hypotension, decreased temperature (may be decreased to 95° F [35° C] or below), bradycardia, and arrhythmias.
- Weight/height: Compare to expected weight charts.
- General appearance: Look for yellowing of skin (hypercarotenemia), jaundice (may be present in older persons with AN), lanugo hair, and parotid salivary gland tenderness and enlargement.

- General hydration status: Look for signs of dehydration secondary to purging or restricting.
- Mouth and teeth: Assess for discolored tooth enamel and excessive caries, hallitosis, and sore oral and esophageal mucosa.
- Extremities: Look for acrocyanosis, pedal edema, and scarring on the dorsum of hands from self-induced vomiting.
- Note delayed development of secondary sexual characteristics in persons with AN.
- Neurologic/mental status: Assess for alterations in state of consciousness related to starvation, suicidal thoughts and intentions, obsessions, compulsions, and anxieties and fears related to food, getting fat, and growing up.
- Musculoskeletal: Observe for loss of muscle mass and subcutaneous fat, muscle weakness, and tetany.
- Anal: Determine presence of bleeding or hemorrhoids.

There may be a lack of physical signs/symptoms in persons with BN.

Diagnostic Procedures

Abnormalities in laboratory and diagnostic test results are related to the severity of the restricting or purging activities of the person with eating disorder.

- Renal/electrolytes: Increased BUN, hypokalemia, hypochloremia, hypoglycemia, hyponatremia, hypomagnesemia, hypocalcemia
- SMA-12/60: Hypercholesterolemia
- Decreased phosphorus: Must be monitored carefully when refeeding a person with AN to avoid "refeeding syndrome" (edema in lower extremities and possible congestive heart failure)
- CBC with differential: Leukopenia and mild anemia
- Thyroid function studies: Thyroxine (T_4) low-normal, triiodothyronine (T_3) subclinical
- Liver function tests: Abnormalities (elevations) possible in chronically starved or older persons with AN or in persons with significant substance abuse
- pH balance: Possible signs of metabolic acidosis or metabolic alkalosis (related to hypochloremia and hypokalemia).

- Urine/stool: May show evidence of diuretic or laxative abuse (e.g., occult blood in stool)
- Endocrine studies in persons with AN: Female—decreased luteinizing hormone, follicle-stimulating hormone, and estrogen; males—decreased testosterone
- ECG: Sinus bradycardia and rarely arrhythmias
- Gynecologic: Referral for examination as indicated for possible STDs
- Psychologic/psychiatric evaluation: Referral for diagnostic evaluation

DIAGNOSIS

The differential diagnosis for AN includes the following disorders since they may have significant weight loss and should be ruled out. However, none of the disorders includes the intense body distortions or the desire for weight loss that is present in persons with eating disorders.
- Thyroid disease
- Diabetes
- AIDS
- Inflammatory bowel disease
- Malignancy
- Major depressive disorder
- Schizophrenia

The differential diagnosis for BN includes the following:
- AN binge-eating/purging type
- Neurologic or medical conditions such as Kleine-Levin syndrome
- Major depression with atypical features
- Borderline personality disorder

THERAPEUTIC PLAN
Nonpharmacologic Treatment
- The severity of the orthostasis/cardiac and hydration status including hypokalemia determines if hospitalization is warranted. The stabilization of homeostasis is paramount before any psychiatric/psychologic treatment can occur.
- Suicidal tendency should also be assessed, and hospitalization should occur if it is felt that the client is at imminent risk.
- Development of therapeutic rapport between caregivers and client and family is important.

Referral/Consultation
- The treatment of eating disorders must be of a collaborative "team" nature. A referral for a psychiatric/psychologic evaluation must be made in assisting with the diagnosis.
- It is also important that an agreement be made between the primary health provider, the client and family, and the client's therapist about the manner in which vital signs, weight, and pertinent laboratory data will be monitored. Within the agreement, the parameters for when hospitalization will occur if necessary should be set.
- A dietitian to assist with nutritional counseling and any medical specialist(s) needed to manage medical complications should also be members of the treatment team.
- The client will need ongoing medical as well as psychiatric/psychologic treatment.

Pharmacologic Treatment
Pharmacologic treatment should be initiated by a psychiatrist or advanced practice psychiatric nurse.
- Antidepressants: It is estimated that at least 50% of persons with eating disorder are depressed. There is controversy on how effective antidepressants are in persons with AN since many show a decrease in depression once starvation has been addressed. It is estimated however that 40% to 60% may benefit from antidepressants.
- SSRI (first-line choice): Fluoxetine (Prozac) and other SSRIs are used since these medications do not cause orthostasis and have minimal effects on cardiac rhythms unlike the tricyclic antidepressants impiramine, desipramine, and amitriptyline, which have been used but have significant cardiac effects.
- Benzodiazepines: Benzodiazepines are sometimes used in hospitalized clients for short intervals to decrease anxiety before meals.
- Other medications may be needed to address associated medical conditions related to the effects of eating disorders (i.e., potassium/phosphorus supplements, estrogen replacement for decreasing bone loss, etc.).

Client Education

Discuss with client:
- Disease process and possible results
- Nutritionally sound diet
- Need for counseling
- Long-term commitment
- Keeping a food and exercise diary

EVALUATION/FOLLOW-UP

Monitor client's weight weekly until stable, then monthly.

REFERENCES

American Psychiatric Association (1994). *Diagnostic and statistical manual of mental disorders (DSM-IV)* (4th ed.). Washington, DC: Author.

Eckert, E. D. (1985). Characteristics of anorexia nervosa. In *Anorexia and bulimia: diagnosis and treatment.* Minneapolis: University of Minnesota Press.

Garfinkle, P. E., & Kennedy, S. H. (1992). Advances in diagnosis and treatment of anorexia nervosa and bulimia nervosa. *Canadian Journal of Psychiatry, 37,* 309-315.

Harper-Guiffre, J., & MacKenzie, K. R. (1992). *Group psychotherapy for eating disorders.* Washington, DC: American Psychiatric Press.

Hofland, S. L., & Dardis, P. O. (1992). Bulimia nervosa. Associated physical problems. *Journal of Psychosocial Nursing, 30*(2), 23-27.

Ignataricius, D. D., & Bayne, M. V. (1991). *Medical-surgical nursing: A nursing process approach.* Philadelphia: W. B. Saunders.

Maxmen, J. S., & Ward, N. G. (1995). Eating disorders. *Essential psychopathology and its treatment* (2nd ed.). New York: W. W. Norton.

Muscari, M. E. (1996). Primary care of adolescents with bulimia nervosa. *Journal of Pediatric Health Care, 10*(1), 17-25.

Wachsmuth, J. R., & Garfinkel, P. E. (1993). Treatment of anorexia nervosa in young adults. *Child and Adolescent Psychiatry Clinics of North America, 2,* 145-160.

Zerbe, K. J. (1996). Anorexia nervosa and bulimia nervosa. *Postgraduate Medicine, 99*(1), 161-169.

REVIEW QUESTIONS

1. Lisa Evans, 21 years old, has a history of BN for the past 3 years. When obtaining a history, the nurse practitioner could expect to find:

- a. History of maternal depression and substance abuse in paternal family
- b. Strong sense of self-esteem
- c. Several school failures
- d. No weight disturbances in childhood and adolescence

2. Ms. Evans describes a "binge" episode. The description will probably include:

- a. A feeling of being in control of type and amount of food consumed
- b. The intake of an extra ice cream cone when out with friends
- c. Eating two 13-ounce bags of potato chips in less than 45 minutes
- d. Consuming two pieces of pizza and a salad for dinner

3. While talking with a mother and her 15-year-old daughter with AN, the nurse practitioner may observe which of the following interactional patterns?

- a. Mother and daughter do not interact.
- b. Mother and daughter are openly hostile to each other.
- c. Mother and daughter sit close, and mother answers all the questions.
- d. Mother and daughter equally interact.

4. When considering a diagnosis of AN, the nurse practitioner should consider which of the following differential diagnosis?

- a. Major depressive disorder with atypical features and thyroid disease
- b. Kleine-Levin syndrome and AIDS
- c. Diabetes and borderline personality disorder
- d. Malignancy and thyroid disease

5. Because of the complex medical and psycho-logic components of AN, treatment must include:

    a. Providing educational opportunities for clients and families to learn about AN

    b. Development of a "team" approach with the health care professionals, client, and family members involved

    c. Starting antidepressant medications

    d. Hospitalization

6. Participation in which of the following activities could indicate improvement in a person with BN?

    a. Exercise group

    b. Drama club

    c. Substance abuse program

    d. Taking classes at a community college

7. While interviewing a 14-year-old suspected of being anorexic, the nurse practitioner may observe the following psychiatric symptoms?

    a. Anxiety and irritability

    b. Delusions of grandeur

    c. Paranoia

    d. Hallucinations

8. Which laboratory result would **not** be expected in AN, purging type?

    a. Hypokalemia

    b. Hyponatremia

    c. Decreased BUN

    d. Hypochloremia

9. A family of a child with eating disorder should remove which of the following from their home secondary to possible abuse and cardiotoxic effects?

    a. Laxatives

    b. Diuretics

    c. Syrup of ipecac

    d. OTC diet pills

10. Improvements in interactions in families of anorexic persons can be seen by:

    a. Setting high family goals

    b. Loosening of rules

    c. Disengagement

    d. Parentalization of the anorexic person

ANSWERS AND RATIONALES

1. *Answer:* a (assessment/history/psychosocial/adult)

  Rationale: It has been noted that there is higher likelihood of affective disorders and substance abuse in families of persons with BN. Low self-esteem is usually present. Persons with BN tend to be perfectionist and "overachievers" and are not likely to have school failures. They often have histories of weight disturbances. (Harper-Guiffre & MacKenzie, 1992)

2. *Answer:* c (assessment/history/psychosocial/adult)

  Rationale: A "binge" is defined as eating a larger amount of food than most people would eat during a similar period of time and under similar circumstances. Options *b* and *d* do not meet this definition; there is a sense of loss of control over eating not a sense of control. (American Psychiatric Association, 1994)

3. *Answer:* c (assessment/physical examination/psychosocial/NAS)

  Rationale: Often in families of anorexic persons there is enmeshment in which the individuals of the family are "lost" and separation is not allowed to occur. (Harper-Guiffre & MacKenzie, 1992)

4. *Answer:* b (diagnosis/psychosocial/NAS)

  Rationale: Because of the significant weight loss often associated with this disease process, one should consider Kleine-Levin syndrome and AIDS when assessing an individual. The other options include a differential diagnosis for BN. (American Psychiatric Association, 1994)

5. *Answer:* b (plan/psychosocial/NAS)

  Rationale: The coordination of the treatment plan for AN is extremely important because of the serious and complex nature of the illness. A "team" approach in which the professional caregivers, family, and client work together is essential. The other options presented may or may not be part of the treatment plan. (Wachsmuth & Garfinkel, 1993)

6. *Answer:* c (evaluation/psychosocial/NAS)

  Rationale: Because of the increased incidence of substance abuse in persons with BN, involvement in a substance abuse group could indicate improvement. (Harper-Guiffre & MacKenzie, 1992)

7. *Answer:* a (assessment/physical examination/psychosocial/adolescent)

Rationale: Irritability and anxiety are symptoms associated with depression, which anorexic persons are known to often have as a co-morbid diagnosis. The other symptoms are usually associated with thought disorders. (Harper-Guiffre & MacKenzie, 1992)

8. *Answer:* c (diagnosis/psychosocial/NAS)

Rationale: One could expect that there would be a decrease in potassium chloride, sodium, and chloride if the client is purging through diuretic and or laxative use/vomiting and an increase in BUN related to volume depletion. (Hofland & Dardis, 1992)

9. *Answer:* c (plan/psychosocial/child)

Rationale: Abuse of syrup of ipecac can be life-threatening secondary to cardiotoxicity. The other substances can affect cardiac function. (Ignataricius & Bayne, 1991)

10. *Answer:* b (evaluative/psychosocial/NAS)

Rationale: Because of the rigidity and noncompromising patterns often noted in families of anorexic persons, a loosening of rules could be seen as improvement. The other options are often symptoms of the family's dysfunction. (Harper-Guiffre & MacKenzie, 1992)

SUBSTANCE ABUSE

OVERVIEW
Definition

- Substance: Drug of abuse, a medication or toxin
- Classes: Most common alcohol and other sedative-hypnotics, stimulants, opioids (Grinspoon, 1995)
- Schedules: Schedule I—strong potential for abuse, most strongly regulated; schedules II through V—decreasing potential for abuse
- Substance abuse: Recurrent use resulting in failure to fulfill obligations, use in hazardous situations, legal problems
- Substance dependence: Recurrent use for more than 12 months leading to three or more of following:
  - Tolerance: Need more of the substance for the same effect or less effect from the same amount
  - Withdrawal: Symptoms typical for the substance
  - Unsuccessful efforts to cut back use
  - Much time spent obtaining or recovering from effects of the substance
  - Continued use despite adverse physical or psychologic effects

Meeting the definition of substance dependence supersedes the definition of substance abuse (American Psychiatric Association, 1994).

Incidence*

- Problem drinking: 8% to 20% of primary care clients (abuse or dependence) in the United States; male-to-female ratio 5:1
  - Men

AGE	PERCENT
18-29	17-24%
30-44	11-14%
45-64	6-8%
Older than 65	1-2%

  - Women

AGE	PERCENT
18-29	4-10%
30-44	2-4%
45-64	1-2%
Older than 65	<1%

- Pregnant women: Fetal alcohol syndrome (FAS) in 3% to 40% of infants of alcohol-dependent women
- Adolescents (ages 12-17): 18% used alcohol in past month, 35% in past year
- Older adults: 70% abuse/dependence chronic, long-standing; 30% late onset (Chenitz, Stone, & Salisbury, 1991)

---

*Data from U.S. Preventive Services Task Force, 1996.

- Other drugs: More common use in teens and young adults, men, unemployed, urban area, those who have not completed high school
  - Marijuana: 5 million used in past week
  - Heroin/injection drugs: 1 to 1.6 million dependent users
  - Young adults: 14% ages 18 to 25 used drugs in past month
  - Pregnant women: 5.5% illicit drug use at least once, 2.9% marijuana, 1.1% cocaine

Etiology

Substance dependence: Positive family history, genetics, cultural attitudes, availability, personal experience with the substance, stress (American Psychiatric Association, 1994).

Pathophysiology

- Alcohol
  - **Depresses CNS:** Sedation, lack of coordination, unconsciousness; absorbed from small intestine, accumulated in blood, oxidized in liver
  - Intoxication: Blood alcohol level 150 to 200 mg/dl; legal driving level most states 80 mg/dl
  - Organ damage: Cirrhosis, peripheral neuropathy, brain damage, cardiomyopathy, congestive heart failure, arrhythmia, gastritis, pancreatitis, thiamine deficiency
  - Withdrawal: Occurs 12 to 48 hours after use stops; tremor, weakness, sweating, hyperreflexia, gastrointestinal symptoms, seizures, hallucinosis, delirium tremens (Berkow, 1992)
  - *Women:* Adverse health affects developing sooner with less consumption than men
  - Pregnant women: FAS with 7 to 14 drinks/wk; more risk early in pregnancy or with binge drinking; FAS— fetal growth retardation, facial deformities, CNS dysfunction (microcephaly, mental retardation, behavior problems); possible risk with any alcohol
  - *Adolescents and young adults:* Contributes to leading causes of death (motor vehicle crashes, injuries, homicides, suicides), problems with school, unsafe sex, legal problems
  - Older adults: Slowed metabolism; elevated blood alcohol levels with less alcohol; isolation, falls, malnutrition, dementia, self-neglect, suicide (Chenitz, Stone, & Salisbury, 1991)

- Substances/drugs other than alcohol
  - Pregnancy: Substance/drug use during pregnancy associated with use of alcohol, cigarettes, poverty, poor nutrition, and inadequate prenatal care, all of which can adversely affect the fetus; difficulty in separating long-term developmental effects caused by the substance or associated risk factors (U.S. Preventive Services Task Force, 1996)
  - Children and adolescents: Poor school performance, injuries, unsafe sex, progression to regular drug use
  - Older adults: Suicide (Chenitz, Stone, & Salisbury, 1991)
  - Inhalants: Asphyxiation, arrhythmia, central and peripheral neurologic damage
  - Steroids: Psychiatric symptoms; liver, endocrine, and cardiovascular problems (U.S. Preventive Services Task Force, 1996)
  - Injection drug use (IDU): Shared needles; hepatitis B and C, HIV, septicemia, bacterial endocarditis, cellulitis
- Cocaine: Powder injected or snorted, crack smoked
  - Stimulates CNS: Euphoria, hyperactivity, alertness, grandiosity, anger, impaired judgment; short-acting drug, rapid dependence
  - Chronic use: Fatigue and social withdrawal, weight loss; with snorting-irritation of nasal mucosa, perforated septum; with intoxication-altered pulse rate and agitation, chest pain, cardiac arrhythmia, seizures
  - Withdrawal: Fatigue, unpleasant dreams, psychomotor agitation or retardation, increased appetite; with acute withdrawal depression, suicidal ideation.
  - Dependence: Large amounts of money for repetitive use leading to criminal behavior, prostitution (American Psychiatric Association, 1994)
- Opioids: Taken by mouth, snorted, smoked, injected
  - CNS depressant: Euphoria, flushing, itching of skin, drowsiness, decreased respiration and body temperature; hypotension, bradycardia, dry mouth, constipation; tolerance 2 to 3 days after prescribed use
  - Withdrawal: Within 4 to 6 hours; CNS hyperactivity, anxiety, increased respirations, yawning, perspiration, lacrimation, rhinorrhea

—Dependence: Associated with high death rate from overdose, injuries, violence

—Men: Erectile dysfunction

—Women: Irregular menses (American Psychiatric Association, 1994)

—Pregnant women: Withdrawal in newborn

ASSESSMENT: SUBJECTIVE/HISTORY

Screening Tests for Alcohol Abuse

- Screen all adolescent and adult primary care clients and pregnant women: Note quantity, frequency; consider if the client is underreporting (common).
- CAGE (felt you should Cut down, have Annoyed others, felt Guilty, had morning drink Eye opener): Easy to administer, useful in primary care setting; less sensitive for early problem drinking or heavy drinking.
- MAST (Michigan Alcoholism Screening Test): 25 questions; good at uncovering abuse and independence, but too lengthy for routine screening; shortened version less sensitive.
- AUDIT (Alcohol Use Disorders Identification Test): 10 items; good for current hazardous drinking; less sensitive for past drinking problems.
- POSIT (Problem-Oriented Screening Instrument for Teenagers).
- Pregnant women: Include questions of tolerance (How many drinks does it take to feel high? [or] How many drinks can you hold?) Tolerance: Three or more drinks to feel high or ability to drink five drinks at a time. Two drinks per day or binge drinking: Risk drinking for pregnant women. Any alcohol use may cause risk.

Screening Tests for Other Substances/Drugs

- All adolescents and pregnant women
- Quantity, frequency, pattern of other drug use, adverse effects of work, health and social relationships
- Screening tests not as accurate
- Barriers: Distrust, fear, denial (U.S. Preventive Services Task Force, 1996)

Symptoms

- Anxiety
- Depression
- Fatigue
- Weight loss
- Insomnia
- Headaches
- Rhinorrhea
- Hoarseness
- Dysphagia
- Cough
- Shortness of breath
- Chest pain
- Edema
- Indigestion
- Abdominal pain
- Dysuria
- Genital discharge or discomfort
- Rectal bleeding
- Constipation
- Diarrhea
- Rash
- Paresthesia

Past Medical History

- Substance abuse or dependence, age of onset each substance, amounts and patterns of use, routes of use (oral, nasal, IDU), treatment, length of substance-free periods (remission), circumstances of remission (incarceration, inpatient unit).
- Head injury, seizures, learning disorders, high blood pressure, cardiovascular disease, pneumonia, emphysema, tuberculosis, gastritis, hepatitis (alcoholic or viral), cirrhosis, pancreatitis, cancer, sexual dysfunction, sexually transmitted infection, motor vehicle crashes, other injuries/fractures

Medication History

- Current medications
- Psychotropics
- Prescription drug of abuse (opioids, benzodiazepines, barbiturates, stimulants)

Family History

- Substance abuse or dependence and effect on family
- Physical, emotional, sexual abuse

Psychosocial History

- Marital history, ages of children, occupation, financial status, legal problems, homelessness
- Psychiatric disorders in client or family (depression, suicide attempts, suicidal ideation,

schizophrenia, anxiety, manic depressive illness, hyperactivity)
- Sexual preferences, contacts

ASSESSMENT: OBJECTIVE/ PHYSICAL EXAMINATION
Physical Examination

- Problem-oriented, guided by substance of abuse, symptoms, risk behaviors
- General appearance, hygiene
- Mental status: Affect (full, flat, blunted, inappropriate, labile, restricted) (American Psychiatric Association, 1994)
- Coherence, orientation
- Vital signs: Blood pressure, pulse, respiration, weight; temperature if infection suspected
- Eyes: PERRLA; EOM: Intact, nystagmus; Pupils: Constriction, dilation
- Sclera: Jaundice, clear
- Fundoscopy: If blood pressure elevated
- Nares/nasal mucosa: Rhinorrhea; septum intact, perforated
- Mouth and pharynx: Dentition, lesions
- Neck: Thyroid size, symmetry, mass; Carotid: Bruit if blood pressure elevated
- Chest: Diameter, breath sounds, dullness, hyperresonance
- Heart: Rate, rhythm, murmurs, rubs
- Abdomen: Hepatosplenomegaly, pain, mass, bruit, bowel sounds
- Neurologic: Tremors, coordination and reflexes if intoxicated, sensation if symptoms of peripheral neuropathy
- Skin: Lesions, scars, tracks, jaundice, ecchymosis, petechiae
- Genital/rectal: Examine if symptomatic, risk behaviors

Diagnostic Procedures

- Liver function tests: Alcohol abuse (Aud, 1997)
- Isolated elevated gamma-glutamyltransferase (GGT): Alcohol abuse >20 g/day, drugs (anticonvulsants, tranquilizers) or metabolic disease (diabetes, hyperlipidemia); discontinue alcohol and repeat GGT in 2 to 3 months; if normal, alcohol abuse cause
- Alanine aminotransferase/aspartate aminotransferase (ALT/AST) ratio of <1: Alcohol abuse; alcohol suppresses ALT: Nonviral hepatitis

- CBC with elevated mean corpuscular volume (MCV): Closet alcoholic; hypersplenism destroys RBCs
- Advanced disease (alcohol): Low WBC, low platelets (bone marrow depression), low albumin, prolonged prothrombin time
- Low hemoglobin, hematocrit: Alcoholic gastritis
- Elevated uric acid
- Toxicology tests: Alcohol and other substances/drugs: Radioimmune assay (RIA), enzymatic immunoassay (EIA), fluorescence polarization immunoassay (FPI), thin layer chromatography (TLC); prevent false-positives with confirmatory tests (gas chromatography, mass spectroscopy); excretion rates vary; positive 1 to 4 days after use (several weeks for long-term marijuana use) (Warner, 1996)
- Newborn meconium toxicology test: Recent maternal use (research) (U.S. Preventive Services Task Force, 1996)
- Risk behaviors: HIV, hepatitis B or C, RPR
- Psychiatric disorders: Thyroid-stimulating hormone, T_4
- Radiographic: Chest x-ray for adult smokers

DIAGNOSIS

The differential diagnosis includes the following:
- Substance abuse (specify substance)
- Substance dependence (specify): For example, alcohol abuse, cocaine dependence

THERAPEUTIC PLAN

- No "quick fixes" (Substance Abuse, 1994)
- Goal: Complete abstinence for abuse or dependence (Uphold & Graham, 1994); mutually acceptable goals for patient and provider
- Federal law: Protects the confidentiality of persons receiving alcohol and drug abuse prevention and treatment services; signed consent for release of information. Minors: Check state laws. Exceptions: Medical emergencies, court orders, client crime against program or staff, approved research, initial child abuse reports (Substance Abuse, 1994)
- Level of treatment: Match personality, background, mental condition, duration and extent of drug use, and type of substance, with level of treatment (Substance Abuse, 1994)

- Nondependent, problem drinkers (alcohol abuse)
  —Brief counseling with regular follow-up: Reduces alcohol consumption, risk behaviors, adverse outcomes; improves laboratory study results
  —Counseling of all primary care clients regarding risk of drinking and driving (U.S. Preventive Services Task Force, 1996)
- Substance/drug dependent clients
  —Detoxification inpatient or outpatient
  —Intensive treatment (intensive outpatient, inpatient, community support groups such as 12-step programs, Alcoholics Anonymous, Narcotics Anonymous, Al-Anon, Rational Recovery); family therapy; no single method superior for all clients; success linked to client motivation, quality of program, family support, posttreatment environment, level of stress (U.S. Preventive Services Task Force, 1996)

Pharmacologic Treatment

ALCOHOL
- Acute detoxification: Short-term use of carbamazepine or benzodiazepine
- Long-term maintenance: Disulfiram
OPIOIDS
- Acute detoxification: Clonidine
- Long-term maintenance: Methadone or naltrexone (Substance Abuse, 1994)

Additional Therapies

WOMEN. Address unique issue, (i.e., co-dependence, incest, abuse victimization, sexuality, problems with significant other, gynecologic health, single parenthood, limited income, low self-esteem, lack of assertiveness) (Substance Abuse, 1994)

PREGNANT WOMEN
- All pregnant women should be told to abstain from all alcohol and illicit drugs. There are no known safe levels of these substances.
- Increase number of prenatal visits to decrease risk for women who use alcohol or other drugs.
- Less cocaine reduces risk.
- Methadone maintenance reduces risk if opioid dependency. (U.S. Preventive Services Task Force, 1996)

- Provide prenatal care; improve nutrition; inform regarding child care, financial support, vocational services, educational services, inpatient drug treatment, drug-free transitional housing for women and children.

INFANTS AND CHILDREN. Infants and children may need alternative care if parents and relatives are unable to provide care (foster home, special health care facilities) (Substance Abuse, 1994).

ADOLESCENTS*
- Parental involvement
- Address developmental levels
- Preventive education grades 7 through 9 to reduce alcohol and tobacco use
- School-based prevention
- Drug education classes
- Outpatient treatment
- Partial hospitalization
- Residential treatment

Co-existing Mental Disorders*

- Treatment for both disorders
- Crisis intervention, psychiatric stabilization, detoxification
- Long-term residential treatment
- Relapse prevention
- Community case management
- Assistance with housing, education, vocational rehabilitation

EVALUATION/FOLLOW-UP*

- Laboratory tests improved
- Target signs and symptoms improved (blood glucose in diabetes, blood pressure in hypertension)
- Treatment goals met
- Participation in treatment for at least 3 months
- Criminal behavior declines
- Employment level 6 months after treatment
- Abstinence from alcohol and other drugs

REFERENCES

American Psychiatric Association (1994). *Diagnostic and statistical manual of mental disorders (DSM-IV)* (4th ed.). Washington, DC: Author.

---

*Substance Abuse, 1994.

Aud, R. E. (1997). *Case approach to interpretation of laboratory data.* Presentation at The Ninth Annual Conference Towards Excellence in Primary Care and Midwifery. Louisville, KY.

Berkow, R. (1992). *The Merck manual.* Rathway, NJ: Merck.

Chenitz, W. C., Stone, J. T., & Salisbury, S. A. (1991). *Clinical gerontological nursing: A guide to advanced practice.* Philadelphia: W. B. Saunders.

Grinspoon, L. (1995). Treatment of drug abuse and addiction. Part I. *The Harvard Mental Health Letter, 12* (2).

Substance Abuse and Mental Health Services Administration (1994). *Treatment for alcohol and other drug abuse: Opportunities for coordination.* Technical Assistance Publication Series: 11. (DHHS Publication No. (SMA) 94-2075). Rockville, MD: U.S. Government Printing Office.

Uphold, C. R., & Graham, M. V. (1994). *Clinical guidelines in family practice.* Gainesville, FL: Barmarrae Books.

U.S. Preventive Services Task Force (1996). *Guide to clinical preventive services* (2nd ed.). Baltimore: Williams & Wilkins.

Warner, A. (1996). *Drug testing—Practices and pitfalls* [Unpublished handout]. Cincinnati, OH: University of Cincinnati Medical Center Division of Toxicology.

REVIEW QUESTIONS

1. Which of the screening techniques is most sensitive for risky drinking practices in pregnant women?

    a. CAGE screening

    b. Items about alcohol use on a questionnaire

    c. Questions about tolerance in history

    d. Direct questions about amount of alcohol consumed

2. Careful routine screening for drug use other than alcohol is especially indicated for:

    a. Female clients

    b. Clients older than 65

    c. Adolescents and pregnant women

    d. Clients younger than 65

3. Which test results are highly suggestive of alcohol abuse?

    a. Elevated GGT, elevated MCV, and ALT/AST ratio of <1

    b. Elevated GGT, decreased MCV, and elevated sodium

    c. Low HDL, elevated WBC, and elevated total bilirubin

    d. Decreased MCHC, elevated GGT, elevated potassium

4. What is the best way to prevent false-positive urine drug tests?

    a. Have a trained laboratory technician collect the specimen.

    b. Send the report to the primary provider.

    c. Run confirmatory tests on a positive sample.

    d. Send a list of the prescribed drugs with the specimen.

5. Meeting the definition of substance dependence does **not** include:

    a. Headaches

    b. Tolerance

    c. Much time spent obtaining or recovering from the substance

    d. Withdrawal

6. How many specific criteria must exist to meet the definition of substance dependence according to *DSM-IV?*

    a. One

    b. Two

    c. Three

    d. Four or more

7. Pregnant women who are opioid dependent have improved outcomes with:

    a. Detoxification with benzodiazepine

    b. Direct confrontation at each visit about harmful effect of drug on fetus

    c. Examination for needle marks (tracks) at each visit

    d. Methadone maintenance

8. A 44-year-old man with elevated GGT and other serum liver test results normal agrees to discontinue alcohol use. When should he be told to return for a follow-up GGT to determine if his alcohol consumption is affecting his liver?

    a. In 1 month

    b. In 2 to 3 months

    c. In 1 week

    d. Every 4 months for 1 year

9. A pregnant 25-year-old diagnosed with cocaine dependence should be instructed to return for follow-up prenatal visits:

   a. According to the number of weeks' gestation (standard schedule) as long as she agrees to enter a treatment program

   b. More frequently than the standard schedule

   c. With regular psychiatric evaluations scheduled throughout pregnancy

   d. With AUDIT questionnaire administered at each visit

ANSWERS AND RATIONALES

1. *Answer:* c (assessment/history/psychosocial/childbearing female)

Rationale: Light drinking in pregnant women is hazardous and may not be uncovered by direct questioning or screening questionnaires. Questions about tolerance are more revealing. Two drinks per day or binge drinking is most risky during pregnancy. Women who drink three or more drinks to feel high or who can drink five drinks at a time demonstrate tolerance. (U.S. Preventive Services Task Force, 1996)

2. *Answer:* c (assessment/history/psychosocial/adolescent)

Rationale: Drug abuse has increased among adolescents. Drug use during pregnancy is associated with adverse outcomes, with the potential for developmental delay. (U.S. Preventive Services Task Force, 1996)

3. *Answer:* a (assessment/physical examination/psychosocial/NAS)

Rationale: Alcohol causes elevated GGT by microsomal enzyme induction, elevated MCV from RBCs destroyed by hypersplenism, and ALT/AST ratio of <1 with suppressed ALT from nonviral hepatitis. (Aud, 1997)

4. *Answer:* c (assessment/physical examination/psychosocial/NAS)

Rationale: False-positive results can be reduced by performing a second, more specific confirmatory test. (U.S. Preventive Services Task Force, 1996)

5. *Answer:* a (diagnosis/psychosocial/NAS)

Rationale: The definition of substance dependence includes three of the following in the same 12 months: tolerance, withdrawal, inability to cut down use, much time spent obtaining the substance or recovering from its effects, continued use despite adverse effects. (American Psychiatric Association, 1994)

6. *Answer:* c (diagnosis/psychosocial/NAS)

Rationale: Three specific criteria must exist to meet the definition of substance dependence. (American Psychiatric Association, 1994)

7. *Answer:* d (plan/management/therapeutics/psychosocial/childbearing female)

Rationale: Methadone maintenance improves outcomes in pregnant, opioid-dependent women. Opiate withdrawal is dangerous during pregnancy. Regular contact to obtain methadone can improve prenatal care. (U.S. Preventive Services Task Force, 1996)

8. *Answer:* b (evaluation/psychosocial/adult)

Rationale: GGT should return to normal within 2 to 3 months after cessation of alcohol use. (Aud, 1997)

9. *Answer:* b (evaluation/psychosocial/adult/childbearing female)

Rationale: Outcomes are improved in substance-dependent pregnant women with more frequent prenatal visits. (U.S. Preventive Services Task Force, 1996)

16

Multisystem Disorders

DEVELOPMENTAL DELAYS AND DISABILITIES

OVERVIEW
Definition

Developmental delays and disabilities constitute a spectrum characterized by deficits in cognitive, social, and emotional functioning.

Pathophysiology

The common factor in these disorders is a dysfunction resulting from a central nervous system (CNS) disorder that manifests in childhood and results in a chronic course with a high likelihood of functional limitation. Classification is difficult because CNS lesions are diffuse in children, and multiple disorders may exist. These disorders include cerebral palsy, mental retardation, blindness and deafness, central processing disorders, and pervasive developmental delay, such as autism, Asperger's syndrome, Down syndrome, fragile X syndrome, or childhood schizophrenia.

ASSESSMENT: SUBJECTIVE/HISTORY

Developmental disabilities usually are seen as a result of the child's failure to meet developmental milestones or age-related expectations. Other disabilities may be seen as being related to failure to establish feeding or poor interaction with caregivers. Gross motor failures, such as failure to sit, predominate after 9 months, whereas language delay becomes the major reason for referral between 21 and 30 months (Dershewitz, 1993). If there is concern, an assessment should be performed.

History

History taking includes the following areas:
- Family history
- Prenatal history
- Perinatal history
- Past medical history
- Current functioning
- Behavioral functioning
- Environmental exposures: lead, alcohol, and others

ASSESSMENT: OBJECTIVE/ PHYSICAL EXAMINATION
Physical Examination

A comprehensive physical examination is performed with particular attention to the following:
- Dysmorphism
- Pigmentary abnormalities
- Expanded neurologic examination
- Evaluation of the four milestones:
  1. Gross motor milestone: Independent locomotion
  2. Language milestones (best predictor of later cognition)
     —Reception
     —Expression
     —Visual language
  3. Fine motor and problem-solving milestones (these form basis for most infant intelligence scales):
     —Hand function
     —Problem solving
     —Visual motor abilities

4. Personal social abilities: Mastery of child over environment; feeding, dressing, hygiene

DIAGNOSIS

Diagnosis includes the three levels of developmental delay:

1. Delay: This is the most common reason, usually <75% normal rate of development. Infants and toddlers with ≥25% deficit in development are eligible for early intervention services.
2. Dissociation: This is a state in which one phase of development is out of synchrony with others.
3. Deviance: This nonsequential development is most commonly seen in processing disorders, for example, a child who walks without crawling (Dershewitz, 1993).

THERAPEUTIC PLAN

These disorders are complex cases because they often require inpatient or residential placement for stabilization and medication management. Self-help skills are delayed, and normal socialization skills may be absent. The disorders are chronic, placing a strain on normal family resources. Family dysfunction is common (Pearson, 1995).

EVALUATION/FOLLOW-UP

All clients who may have a developmental delay or disability should be quickly referred to a professional or center (preferably multispecialty) who can conduct a thorough examination and follow through with the needed treatment plan. A center for developmental disabilities is usually part of a children's hospital medical center.

REFERENCES

Dershewitz, R. (1993). *Ambulatory pediatric care*. Philadelphia: J. B. Lippincott.

Pearson, G. (1995). Pervasive developmental disorders. In B. Johnson (Ed.), *Child, adolescent, and family psychiatric nursing*. Philadelphia: J. B. Lippincott.

REVIEW QUESTIONS

1. Maggie is a 12-month-old infant who is unable to sit without assistance. The nurse practitioner should do which of the following?

a. Suspect abuse.
b. Encourage the family to stimulate Maggie more.
c. Refer Maggie for developmental delay.
d. Recheck Maggie in 1 month to assess progress.

2. To appropriately refer a client with a developmental disability, the nurse practitioner must first assess all the following **except:**

a. Gross motor function
b. Language use
c. Social abilities
d. Height and weight

ANSWERS AND RATIONALES

1. *Answer:* c (assessment/history/multisystem/infant)

Rationale: Gross motor failures are the major reason for referral in infants and toddlers. At 12 months, Maggie needs to be sitting alone and standing at least with assistance. Earlier intervention carries better outcomes. (Pearson, 1995)

2. *Answer:* d (assessment/physical examination/multisystem/child)

Rationale: Height and weight should be recorded for every client, not just a client with a developmental disability. However, the absence of this assessment will not interfere with the referral. Baseline language, fine motor, gross motor, and social skills must be assessed. (Pearson, 1995)

EDEMA

OVERVIEW
Definition

Edema is an abnormal accumulation of fluid in the interstitial space. It can be localized or generalized.

LOCALIZED EDEMA. Localized edema is produced by regional obstruction to venous flow, lymphatic flow, or both.

- Loss of vascular integrity occurs with urticaria and angioneurotic edema.
- Increase in tissue osmotic pressure may occur, for example from surgical trauma, such as edema of the arm after a radical mastectomy (occurs in 10% to 30% of clients).
- Increase in hydrostatic pressure results from increase in venous resistance.

GENERALIZED EDEMA. Generalized edema is soft-tissue swelling of most or all regions of the body. It indicates an increase in the interstitial fluid but also in the sodium content of the extracellular compartment and signifies potentially serious disease.

- Renal disease (acute and chronic)
- Liver disease
- Cardiac and pulmonary disease (congestive heart failure [CHF] or CHF coexisting with chronic obstructive pulmonary disease); edema is a late feature of heart failure
- Nutritional disease (insufficient protein or malnutrition)
- Gastrointestinal (GI) disease

OTHER CAUSES
- Idiopathic edema
- Orthostatic sodium retention (an abnormal capillary leak of protein resulting in a reduction in blood volume, most pronounced in the upright posture)
- Diuretic and laxative abuse
- Carbohydrate loading
- Heat edema
- Altitude edema
- Drugs: Pharmacologic agents such as nonsteroidal antiinflammatory drugs (NSAIDs), vasodilators, adrenal steroids, and estrogens can cause sodium and water retention. Calcium agonist may cause peripheral edema.

Incidence

Sixteen percent of persons 65 years old have swelling of ankles and lower calves, with pitting to 1 cm depth or more in response to firm pressure from examiner's finger.

ASSESSMENT: SUBJECTIVE/HISTORY
History of Present Illness

- Distribution of edema
- How quickly edema developed
- Associated trauma, shortness of breath (SOB), or pain
- Urinary output
- Weight gain

Edema that develops quickly excludes lymphedema and lipedema. Generalized edema involving the face or sacrum or associated with abdominal swelling or SOB suggests cardiac, renal, or hepatic disease.

Idiopathic edema occurs most commonly in young women. They need to be asked about the periodic or cyclic nature of the edema formation and any apparent relationship to the menstrual cycle.

Symptoms

- Unexplained weight gain
- Tightness of a ring
- Puffiness of the face
- Swollen extremities
- Enlarged abdominal girth
- Persistence of indentation of the skin after pressure

Past Medical History

- Trauma
- History of deep venous thrombosis
- Thrombophlebitis
- Venous insufficiency
- Ethanol abuse
- Coronary artery disease
- Renal disease
- Diabetes mellitus (DM)
- Systemic lupus erythematosus (SLE)
- Jaundice
- Dyspnea
- Orthopnea

- Cough
- Fatigue
- Weakness
- Abdominal distention
- Paroxysmal nocturnal dyspnea
- Anorexia
- Weight loss or gain

Medication History

Any drugs that cause sodium retention (antihypertensives, corticosteroids, androgenic and anabolic steroids, estrogens, and NSAIDs) may aggravate or cause generalized edema. Localized edema of the face may characterize both local allergic reactions and anaphylaxis.

Family History

A family history of chronic health problems should be elicited.

Psychosocial History

- Work history (how much time spent standing)
- Past or current substance abuse
- Smoking history
- Ethanol use history
- Support networks (who cooks and cleans)
- Exercise and recreational activities
- Inactivity (especially in the older adult).

Dietary History

- Salt intake
- Protein intake
- Fluid intake

ASSESSMENT: OBJECTIVE/ PHYSICAL EXAMINATION

Physical Examination

- General appearance: Vital signs, weight (In pregnancy, ≥5-pound weight gain in 1 week with hypertension and proteinuria is indicative of preeclampsia.)
- HEENT: Jugular venous distention, carotid pulse
- Cardiovascular: Cardiomegaly, displacement of point of maximal impulse, atrial fibrillation, S_3 gallop (left ventricular dilation), rubs
- Chest: Breath sounds, crackles, wheeze, dullness to percussion, bibasilar rales
- Abdomen: Hepatomegaly, ascites, splenomegaly

- Extremities
  - —Pitting or nonpitting edema with firm pressure of examiner's finger
  - —Varicose veins
  - —Redness
  - —Warmth
  - —Mottled, brown discoloration of ankle skin (venous insufficiency)
  - —Leg circumference
  - —Tenderness
  - —Homans' sign (dorsiflexion elicits pain in thrombosis)
  - —Pulses
  - —Cyanosis
  - —Clubbing
  - —Decreased hair on lower extremities

Diagnostic Procedures

- Complete blood cell count (CBC)
- Urinalysis
- Chest x-ray film (CXR)
- Echocardiogram
- Liver function test
- Thyroid panel
- Thyroid-stimulating hormone (TSH)

DIAGNOSIS

Differential diagnosis includes the following:
- Venous or lymphatic obstruction
- Chronic venous insufficiency
- CHF
- Cirrhosis
- Renal disease
- Nephrotic syndrome
- Hypothyroidism
- Drug-associated edema
- Hypoalbuminemia (malnutrition, enteropathies)
- Anemia
- Angioedema
- Cellulitis
- Renal failure in children usually causes generalized edema.

THERAPEUTIC PLAN

Primary management is to identify and treat the underlying cause of edema.

Pharmacologic Treatment

Diuretics are indicated for marked peripheral edema, pulmonary edema, CHF, and inadequate dietary salt restriction.

MILD FLUID RETENTION (PERIPHERAL)

- Potassium losing (hydrochlorothiazide, chlorthalidone, metolazone)
- Potassium sparing (spironolactone, amiloride, triamterene)

MORE SEVERE HEART FAILURE: Use loop diuretics (furosemide, bumetanide, ethacrynic acid). Refractory edema may respond to combination of loop diuretics and thiazide-like agents. Diuretics are most effective for symptomatic relief. Excessive diuresis can lead to electrolyte imbalance and may cause a fall in cardiac output and prerenal azotemia. A combination of a loop diuretic and an angiotensin-converting enzyme inhibitor should be the initial treatment in most clients with symptoms.

Nonpharmacologic Treatment

DIET. Sodium restriction to <500 mg/day may prevent further edema.

ACTIVITY

- Bed rest enhances response to salt restriction in CHF and cirrhosis. It reduces cardiac workload and also promotes diuresis.
- The use of support stockings and elevation of edematous lower extremities will help mobilize interstitial fluid and reduce dependent edema.
- If severe hyponatremia is present, water intake should be reduced.
- Monitor for and treat cellulitis or ulcerations.
- Avoid offending medications if possible.
- Chronic venous insufficiency: Bed rest, avoidance of long periods of standing, and use of well-fitting, heavy-duty elastic support stockings.

EVALUATION/FOLLOW-UP
Congestive Heart Failure

- Contact the client within 24 hours after a clinic visit to determine whether condition is stable or improving.

- Schedule return visit every 1 to 2 weeks until the client is free of symptoms, after which schedule visits for every 3 to 6 months.
- See the chapter on CHF regarding laboratory monitoring.

Nephrotic Syndrome

Refer to renal specialist.

Liver Disease

Refer to GI specialist.

Venous Insufficiency

See the client 1 week after initiating treatment with a diuretic to recheck electrolytes, vital signs, and weight. Recheck may be performed after 2 weeks. Clients tend to have recurrent problems, especially if treatment measures are not followed. Stasis dermatitis, ulcerations, or secondary varicosities may develop. Prevention includes early and energetic treatment of acute thrombophlebitis with anticoagulants. This may minimize occlusive and valve damage.

REFERENCES

Dornbrand, L., Hoole, A., & Pickard, C. (1992). *Manual of clinical problems in adult ambulatory care* (pp. 658-662). Boston: Little, Brown.

Friedman, H. (1996). *Problem-oriented medical diagnosis* (pp. 1-4). Boston: Little, Brown.

Isselbacher, K., Braunwald, E., Wilson, J., Martin, J., Fauci, A., & Kasper, D. (1994). *Harrison's principles of internal medicine* (pp. 50-54). New York: McGraw-Hill.

Kochan, M., & Kutty, K. (1990). *Concise textbook of medicine* (pp. 28-29). New York: Elsevier.

Tierney, L., McPhee, S., & Papadakis, M. (1996). *Current medical diagnosis and treatment.* Norwalk, CT: Appleton & Lange.

Uphold, C., & Graham, M. (1994). *Clinical guidelines in family practice.* Gainesville, FL: Barmarrae Books.

REVIEW QUESTIONS

1. Which of the following medications may produce edema?

   a. NSAIDs
   b. Furosemide (Lasix)
   c. Hydrochlorothiazide
   d. Vitamins

2. Which of the following findings suggests that the edema is related to venous insufficiency?

   a. Unilateral edema
   b. Brawny shins
   c. SOB
   d. Displaced maximum point of impulse (PMI)

3. In assessing edema, which system is **least** important to include in the examination?

   a. Neurologic
   b. Cardiovascular
   c. Respiratory
   d. Extremities

4. Common differential diagnoses for generalized edema include all the following **except:**

   a. Chronic venous insufficiency
   b. CHF
   c. Pneumonia
   d. Renal disease

5. All the following may be ordered for chronic venous insufficiency **except:**

   a. Bed rest
   b. NSAIDs
   c. Intermittent elevation of the legs
   d. Use of well-fitting, heavy-duty elastic support hose

6. Clients with CHF need to be seen for follow-up:

   a. 24 hours after starting diuretics
   b. Every 1 to 2 weeks
   c. Every 1 to 2 weeks until free of symptoms, then every 3 to 6 months
   d. Every year

7. Prevention of chronic venous insufficiency includes all the following **except:**

   a. Early and energetic treatment of acute thrombophlebitis with anticoagulants
   b. Bed rest with legs elevated
   c. Long periods of standing or sitting
   d. Use of support stockings

ANSWERS AND RATIONALES

1. *Answer:* a (assessment/history/multisystem/NAS)
   Rationale: NSAIDs, vasodilators, adrenal steroids, and estrogens may cause sodium and water retention. (Friedman, 1996)

2. *Answer:* b (assessment/physical examination/ multisystem/NAS)
   Rationale: Lymphedema is associated with brawny thickening in the subcutaneous tissue. Brownish pigment of the skin (brawny shins) is a classic sign of venous insufficiency. (Isselbacher et al., 1994)

3. *Answer:* a (assessment, physical examination/ multisystem/NAS)
   Rationale: It is extremely important to look for cardiomegaly, displacement of the MPI, and S_3 gallop; to evaluate breath sounds; and to determine whether there is any extremity edema. (Dorbrand, Hoole, & Pickard, 1992)

4. *Answer:* c (diagnosis/multisystem/NAS)
   Rationale: Pneumonia is not a common differential diagnosis for generalized edema. (Uphold & Graham, 1994)

5. *Answer:* b (plan/multisystem/NAS)
   Rationale: NSAIDs may cause edema.

6. *Answer:* c (evaluation/multisystem/NAS)
   Rationale: Clients with CHF need to be seen for follow-up every 1 to 2 weeks until free of symptoms, then every 3 to 6 months. (Tierney, McPhee, & Papadakis, 1996)

7. *Answer:* c (plan/multisystem/NAS)
   Rationale: Measures to control edema include intermittent elevation of legs during the day and elevation of the legs at night (above heart level), *avoidance* of long periods of sitting or standing, and wearing well-fitting, heavy-duty elastic support stockings from the midfoot to just below the knee during the day. (Tierney, McPhee, & Papadakis, 1996)

FATIGUE

OVERVIEW
Definition

Fatigue can be classified as acute or chronic.

ACUTE FATIGUE. *Acute fatigue* is defined as normal or expected tiredness that is intermittent in nature and serves a protective function. Symptoms are localized, rapid in onset, and short in duration.

CHRONIC FATIGUE. *Chronic fatigue* is unusual and extreme tiredness with an physiologic unknown function. It has a cumulative effect and lasts longer than 1 month.

OTHER. Fatigue can also result from hypermetabolic causes, such as cancer, hyperthyroidism, and Cushing's disease, or from hypometabolic diseases, such as Addison's disease and hypothyroidism.

ASSESSMENT: SUBJECTIVE/HISTORY
History of Present Illness

Ask about duration. Persistent fatigue lasting longer than a month needs a more comprehensive workup.

WOMEN. In women of childbearing age, ask about date of last menstrual period and method of contraceptive use. Fatigue may be among the first indicators of pregnancy. Postpartum fatigue is common for at least 6 weeks after delivery.

CHILDREN. Children often show changes in activity level.

Symptoms

Systemic diseases also manifest other symptoms, rather than just fatigue. If a client reports SOB, consider a renal, hematologic, or cardiac origin. If a client reports weight loss, consider infection, tumor, or hypermetabolism. If weight gain has occurred, consider hypothyroidism and renal disease. Bleeding may indicate a hematologic or GI origin.

Past Medical History

Sleep disorders may produce fatigue. Insomnia may indicate substance abuse, and further questioning may be needed.

Repeated infections in conjunction with sexual history (or parental sexual or drug use history in relation to children) may suggest the need for HIV testing. AIDS symptoms appear an average of 18 months after infection, but dormant periods of 1.9 years are seen in children younger than 4 years. Previous treatment for hyperthyroidism may produce fatigue from hypothyroidism.

Medication History

Antihypertensive agents, drugs with anticholinergic effects, antidepressants, and antihistamine drugs may cause fatigue.

Family History

A family history of chronic health problems should be elicited. Certain anemias (e.g., sickle cell anemia) and autoimmune diseases (e.g., lupus) have familial tendencies.

Psychosocial History

Depression is associated with fatigue and may be triggered by the loss of a job, a friend, a family member, or self-esteem. Psychosocial assessment should include the following:

- Work history
- Past or current substance abuse
- Psychiatric disorders
- Support networks
- Sexual activity and function
- Exercise and recreational activities
- Coping skills
- Relaxation techniques used
- Significant life changes

Dietary History

Poor nutrition or inadequate protein intake can lead to muscular fatigue with activity.

ASSESSMENT: OBJECTIVE/ PHYSICAL EXAMINATION
Physical Examination

- A complete physical examination is indicated for a chief complaint of fatigue. Particular attention should be given to assessment of the thyroid gland, lymphatic system, heart, lungs, neurologic system, and abdomen.
- Baseline vital signs, including weight, height, and temperature, should be obtained.

Diagnostic Procedures

- First-level tests should include CBC, TSH or thyroxine, urinalysis, serum or urine pregnancy test (if indicated), Epstein-Barr virus serologic studies, and blood glucose level.
- Clients at high risk should have syphilis, HIV, and tuberculosis tests. If client is at geographic risk, a Lyme titer may be helpful.
- If the fatigue is severe, the following tests should be ordered: CXR, electrolytes, ECG, calcium, blood urea nitrogen, creatinine, and liver function tests.
- Perform mammogram, Papanicolaou smear, fecal occult blood test, and sigmoidoscopy if these tests have not been performed recently and are appropriate to the age of the client.

DIAGNOSIS

Differential diagnosis includes the following:
- Anemia
- Thyroid dysfunction
- Adrenal gland dysfunction
- Heart or lung disease
- Liver disease
- DM
- Tuberculosis
- Opportunistic infection
- Autoimmune disease (rheumatoid arthritis, SLE)
- Multiple sclerosis
- Myasthenia gravis
- Chronic fatigue syndrome (CFS)
- HIV infection

Chronic Fatigue Syndrome

MAJOR CRITERIA
- Fatigue lasting at least 6 months that is unrelieved with bed rest
- Fatigue severe enough to reduce average daily activity by at least 50%

MINOR CRITERIA
- Mild fever or chills
- Sore throat
- Lymph node pain in anterior or posterior cervical or axillary nodes
- Unexplained general muscle weakness
- Myalgia
- Prolonged fatigue (longer than 24 hours) after previously tolerable levels of exercise
- New generalized headaches
- Migratory noninflammatory arthralgia
- Sleep disturbance
- Neuropsychologic symptoms (photophobia, transient visual scotomata, forgetfulness, excessive irritability, confusion, difficulty thinking, inability to concentrate, depression)

PHYSICAL CRITERIA
These must be documented on at least two occasions 1 month apart.
- Low-grade fever
- Nonexudative pharyngitis
- Palpable or tender anterior or posterior lymph nodes

For a diagnosis of CFS, the client must have the two major criteria and eight minor criteria or two major criteria, six minor criteria, and two physical criteria.

THERAPEUTIC PLAN

- Treatment depends on the selected diagnosis. Appropriate referrals for the fatigued client may include a psychiatrist or counselor for depression, substance abuse, or somatization. Sleep testing may be indicated.
- Consider ordering an antidepressant medication.
- Regular exercise, with gradual increase in intensity according to symptoms
- Massage therapy for comfort and muscular fatigue

EVALUATION/FOLLOW-UP

- Suggest that the person bring a significant other to the next visit for another's appraisal of how fatigue is affecting the person.
- Schedule a return visit for 2 to 3 weeks.
- If CFS is diagnosed, stress to the client that it is not fatal, that symptoms will improve with time, and to expect relapses and remissions.
- Have the client keep a diary of symptoms and bring it to the next visit. Documentation should include the effects of fatigue on daily activities, sleep patterns, and diet. Fatigue should be rated on a standardized scale each day. Fatigue can be measured with standardized scales. Commonly used scales include the following:
  —Pearson Byars Fatigue Feeling Checklist

—Rhoten 10-point fatigue scale
—Piper's fatigue scale
—Visual analog fatigue scale
—Fatigue Relief Scale

REFERENCES

Bombardier, C., & Buchwald, D. (1995). Outcome and prognosis of patients with chronic fatigue versus chronic fatigue syndrome. *Archives of Internal Medicine, 155,* 2109.

Boynton, R., Dunn, E., & Stephans, G. (1994). *Manual of ambulatory pediatrics.* Philadelphia, J. B. Lippincott.

Farrar, D., Locke, S., & Kantrowitz, F. (1995). Chronic fatigue syndrome 1: Etiology and pathogenesis. *Behavioral Medicine, 21,* 5-16.

Kantrowitz, F., Farrar, D., & Locke, S. (1995). Chronic fatigue syndrome 2: Treatment and future research. *Behavioral Medicine, 21,* 17-24.

Kroenke, K., Schultz, A., & Yager, J. (1993, October 15). When fatigue is the major complaint. *Patient Care, 27*(16), 157-167.

Ruffin, M., & Cohen, M. (1994). Evaluation and management of fatigue. *American Family Physician, 50,* 625-632.

Siegel, R., & Melby, J. (1994, July 15). Fatigue: The role of adrenal insufficiency. *Hospital Practice,* 59-71.

REVIEW QUESTIONS

1. Which of the following medications may produce fatigue?

a. Antihistamines
b. Antacids
c. NSAIDs
d. Antitussives

2. Which of the following should be performed if recent results are not available?

a. Visual acuity screening
b. Weber's test
c. Pregnancy test
d. Fecal occult blood test

3. CSF is characterized by:

a. Fatigue unrelieved by bed rest for longer than 4 months
b. Intermittent nature, serving a protective function
c. Reduction in daily activity ≥50%
d. Localized symptoms

4. Why would the practitioner suggest that the client bring a friend or family member along on the next visit?

a. To keep the client from depleting energy stores from driving
b. To transport the client home after extensive diagnostic testing
c. To get another person's appraisal of how fatigue is affecting the client
d. To validate that the client is ill by explaining the client's diagnostic data to the friend or family member

5. Sleep testing is:

a. Always indicated with fatigue lasting longer than 2 weeks
b. Potentially helpful in diagnosing problems
c. Costly and not warranted
d. Useful in diagnosing substance abuse as a source of fatigue

6. In CFS the:

a. Symptoms will not improve with time
b. Client will eventually have associated disease
c. Client will have relapses
d. Symptoms will improve in 6 months

ANSWERS AND RATIONALES

1. *Answer:* a (assessment/history/multisystem/NAS)
Rationale: Antihypertensives, anticholinergics, psychotropic medications, and antihistamines produce fatigue. (Kroenke, Schultz, & Yager, 1993, p. 158)

2. *Answer:* d (assessment/plan/multisystem/NAS)
Rationale: Regular screening procedures and examinations for cancer should be performed, including mammography, Papanicolaou smear, fecal occult blood test, and sigmoidoscopy. (Kroenke, Schultz, & Yager, 1993, p. 161)

3. *Answer:* c (assessment/history/multisystem/NAS)
Rationale: CFS is fatigue lasting longer than 6 months that does not serve a protective function and may or may not be associated with localized symptoms. It is associated with a reduction in daily activity by at least 50%. (Ruffin & Cohen, 1994, p. 626)

4. *Answer:* c (plan/multisystem/NAS)

Rationale: This third party may provide additional information regarding how fatigue is affecting the client, particularly if fatigue is interfering with cognitive function or memory. (Ruffin & Cohen, 1994, p. 629)

5. *Answer:* b (assessment/plan/multisystem/NAS)

Rationale: If the client reports abnormal snoring, daytime napping, or falling asleep suddenly, sleep

testing is warranted (Kroenke, Schultz, & Yager, 1993, p. 162)

6. *Answer:* c (evaluation/multisystem/NAS)

Rationale: Although there is no cure for CFS, improvement occurs with time, an average of 1 to 2 years after diagnosis. However, the client's course is marked by remissions and relapses. (Kantrowitz, Farrar, & Locke, 1995, p. 17; Bombardier & Buchwald, 1995)

FEVER

OVERVIEW
Definition

Fever is a symptom and is a nonspecific response to an infectious or noninfectious disease process. Fever is defined as follows:

- Rectal or aural temperature >100.4° F (38° C)
- Oral temperature >99.5° F (37.5° C)
- Axillary temperature >98.6° F (37° C)
- *Fever of unknown origin* is defined as fever with temperature >100.9° F (38.3° C) for 3 weeks in which the diagnosis is not apparent after one week or more of studies.
- Low fever: Oral reading of 99° to 100.4 ° F (38° C).
- Moderate fever: oral reading of 100.5 to 104° F (38 to 40° C)
- High fever: Oral reading ≥104° F (40° C)
- Fever with temperature >108° F (42.2° C) produces unconsciousness and brain damage if sustained.

Pathophysiology

Fever occurs when bacteria, viruses, or toxins are phagocytosed by leukocytes and cytokines are released. Shivering increases heat production. Peripheral vasoconstriction prevents heat loss.

ETIOLOGY

Usually a viral organism initiates phagocytosis, but fevers can also be bacterial, rickettsial, fungal, or parasitic in origin.

ASSESSMENT: SUBJECTIVE/HISTORY
History of Present Illness

- Ask about onset, duration, and pattern of fever.
- Ask how the temperature was determined. Was a thermometer used. If so, by what route? Was the temperature determined by touch?
- Ask about hydration status, including fluid intake, urination, vomiting, and diarrhea.
- Ask about level of discomfort.
- Ask about recent immunizations or new medications.
- Ask whether family members are ill or have recently traveled.
- Ask about last dose of antipyretic or other self-care measures.

  CHILDREN

- Ask parent about the child's activity and whether child seems irritable, more drowsy, or not playing as usual.
- Inquire about previous episodes of febrile seizures, which affect approximately 4% of children.
- Children tend to have greater febrile responses than do adults. Teething does not cause fever with temperature >101.1° F (38.4° C).

Symptoms

- Changes in activity
- Appetite
- Chills
- Headache
- Nasal congestion
- Earache

- Sore throat
- Cough
- Abdominal pain
- Vomiting
- Diarrhea
- Painful urination

Past Medical History

- Current medications
- Previous illnesses and diseases, particularly any cardiac or chronic debilitating disorders, especially immunosuppressive treatments or disorders
- Infections
- Trauma
- Surgery
- Diagnostic testing
- Use of anesthesia
- Older persons, neonates, and those receiving medications such as NSAIDs and corticosteroids may have a less marked or even absent febrile response, even in the presence of bacteremia.

ASSESSMENT: OBJECTIVE/ PHYSICAL EXAMINATION

Physical Examination

- Measure temperature.
  - —Rectal or aural temperature is 0.5° C higher than oral temperature
  - —Axillary temperature is 0.5° C lower than oral temperature
  - —Record rectal temperature in infant younger than 3 months.
- Measure vital signs, including respirations, pulse, and blood pressure.
- Observe the general appearance and mental alertness of both adults and children.
- Assess the quality of the cry of an infant.
- Assess skin for color rash, petechiae, purpura, dryness, turgor, capillary refill, redness, and warmth.
- Assess for nuchal rigidity.
- Assess for both upper and lower respiratory involvement.
- Assess for lymphadenopathy.
- Assess for swollen joints.

A complete examination may be indicated, depending on the presenting complaint and the age of the client to find a localized infection such as otitis media, pharyngitis, sinusitis, meningitis, or pneumonia. See specific chapters for more information about individual diagnoses.

Diagnostic Procedures

Usually the history and physical examination will uncover the source of the fever.

For the following clients:

- Younger than 3 months
- Looking toxic
- Immunocompromised
- With underlying chronic disease
- With extremely elevated temperature

Consider ordering the following tests:

- Urinalysis and culture
- CBC with differential, erythrocyte sedimentation rate, and blood cultures
- CXR
- Cerebrospinal fluid for culture, cell count and differential, and chemistries

Physician consultation is indicated for any infant younger than 3 months. In most cases, hospitalization is necessary even if the source of the fever is identified because of the risks of dehydration, sepsis, meningitis, and pneumonia.

DIAGNOSIS

Infection is the most common cause of fever and may be viral, bacterial, rickettsial, fungal, or parasitic. Differential diagnosis includes the following:

- Autoimmune disease
- Malignant neoplastic disease
- Hematologic disease
- Cardiovascular disease
- GI disease
- Endocrine disease
- Drug reactions, including serum sickness, neuroleptic malignant syndrome, and malignant hyperthermia of anesthesia, are diseases that cause fever as a result of chemical agents. CNS disease interferes with the thermal regulatory process and is seen with fever.

THERAPEUTIC PLAN

Clients with fever who are disoriented or delirious, or who have meningismus, petechiae, or purpura should be transported to the emergency department immediately by another responsible person or by ambulance.

Clients who are immunodeficient, have cardiac disease, or have another serious disease also need immediate evaluation because the heart rate increases about 10 beats/min for every degree Fahrenheit. Respiration rate also increases.

The following children with fever need immediate evaluation (Hay, 1995):

- Younger than 3 months
- With temperature >104.2° F (40.1° C)
- Crying inconsolably or whimpering
- Crying when moved or touched
- Difficult to awaken
- With stiff neck
- With purple spots on the skin
- With difficulty breathing
- Drooling saliva and unable to swallow food or fluids
- With history of convulsion
- Looking or acting extremely sick

Children between 3 months and 2 years of age with fever can be treated on an outpatient basis in the presence of a localized, nonserious infection, as long as they are playful, drinking, and voiding and they do not appear toxic. Bacteremia is more likely in a child with a temperature >105° F (40.6° C) and should be considered even if a localized infection is found.

Pharmacologic Treatment

ANTIPYRETIC INDICATIONS

- Fevers with temperature ≥103° F (39.4° C)
- Children with a history of febrile seizures
- Clients who have compensated cardiac disease or chronic debilitating disorders, who become dehydrated easily, or who are alcoholics
- Clients who are uncomfortable and cannot rest
- Considerations for not treating low to moderate fevers include the fact that antipyretics may mask the signs or symptoms of a serious disease and possibly confuse the clinical picture.

MEDICATIONS

- Acetaminophen, PO or rectal q 4 to 6 hours, for adults and for children older than 2 months
- Ibuprofen, PO q 6 to 8 hours, for adults and for children older than 6 months

- Aspirin, PO q 4 to 6 hours, may be used for adults only

Client Education

- Teach parents the proper method of assessing temperature. If child is younger than 3 months, use a rectal thermometer. Oral thermometers can be used for children older than 3 years.
- Avoid OTC medications that contain aspirin, such as Pepto-Bismol.
- Keep the child well hydrated by offering fluids q 15 to 30 minutes. Use oral rehydration solution in cases of vomiting. Consume extra fluids during a fever.
- Avoid overdressing when febrile.
- Avoid strenuous activity. Rest.
- Use lukewarm water sponge baths in the following cases:
  —Fever with temperature level >106.2° F (41.2° C)
  —Clients with liver disease who cannot take acetaminophen
  —Clients with neurologic problems in which temperature regulation is impaired
- Alcohol is never used for sponging.
- Sponging should not cause the client to shiver.

EVALUATION/FOLLOW-UP

- Recheck infants, young children, older adults, and clients with chronic conditions in 24 hours in person or by phone.
- Have the client return if fever persists for 2 to 3 days.

REFERENCES

Grimes, D. (1991). *Infectious diseases* (p. 26). St. Louis: Mosby.

Hay, W., Groothies, J., Hayward, A., & Levin, M. (1995). *Current pediatric diagnosis and treatment* (12th ed., pp. 308-314). Norwalk, CT: Appleton & Lange.

Professional guide to signs and symptoms (2nd ed., pp. 317-318). (1996). Springhouse, PA: Springhouse.

Tierney, L. M., McPhee, S. J., & Papadakis, M. A. (1996). *Current medical diagnosis and treatment* (35th ed., pp. 21-22). Norwalk, CT: Appleton & Lange.

Uphold, C., & Graham, M. (1994). *Clinical guidelines in family practice* (pp. 59-65). Gainesville, FL: Barmarrae Books.

Wells, N., King, J., Hedstrom, C., & Youngkins, J. (1995). Does tympanic temperature measure up? *American Journal of Maternal/Child Nursing, 20* (1), 95-100.

REVIEW QUESTIONS

1. Which of the following symptoms associated with fever indicates a serious illness?

    a. Degree of the temperature

    b. Concurrent nasal congestion, cough

    c. Other family members with similar symptoms

    d. Change in behavior, such as irritability or lethargy

2. Which of the following measurements of temperature with a mercury thermometer is most reliable for a 2-year-old?

    a. Oral temperature, left in place for 2 minutes

    b. Rectal temperature, left in place for 2 minutes

    c. Axillary temperature, left in place for 2 mintures

    d. Ear temperature, left in place for 2 minutes

3. The most common cause of fever in both adults and children is:

    a. Bacterial infection, such as otitis and sinusitis

    b. Autoimmune illness, such as rheumatic fever and rheumatoid arthritis

    c. Viral illness, such as enteroviruses and adenoviruses

    d. Drug reaction

4. Children should be evaluated immediately in which of the following cases?

    a. Temperature is >101° F.

    b. Child is sleeping more but is easily awakened.

    c. Child looks or acts sick.

    d. Child is drinking but not eating.

5. Follow-up and evaluation of the client with fever depend on all the following **except:**

    a. Current medications

    b. Diagnosis and clinical presentation

    c. Age

    d. Support systems

6. The medication of choice for moderate fever in adults and children is:

    a. Acetaminophen

    b. Aspirin

    c. Ibuprofen

    d. None

ANSWERS AND RATIONALES

1. *Answer:* d (assessment/history/multisystem/NAS)

    Rationale: The degree of the temperature does not correlate well with the severity of the illness. Clients with viral infections may have upper respiratory symptoms and may have household contacts with similar symptoms. CNS involvement may show irritability, as with meningitis, and lethargy may be seen with bacteremia, both of which are serious. (Hay, 1995)

2. *Answer:* b (assessment/physical examination/multisystem/child)

    Rationale: With a mercury thermometer, rectal temperatures are most accurate. Oral temperatures are also reliable if done properly but are reserved for older children. Axillary temperatures are the least accurate, but they are better than no measurement. The thermometer must be left in place 2 minutes for a rectal temperature, 3 minutes for an oral temperature, and 5 to 6 minutes for an axillary temperature. A mercury thermometer is not placed in the ear.

3. *Answer:* c (pathophysiology/multisystem/NAS)

    Rationale: Infection is the most common cause of fever in both adults and children. Most infections are viral in etiology. (Uphold & Graham, 1994)

4. *Answer:* c (plan/management/consult, referral/multisystem/child)

    Rationale: Children should be evaluated immediately if the temperature is >104° F, if the child is difficult to awaken, or if the child is not drinking or eating, the last because of the risk of dehydration (Hay, 1995). The behavior and appearance of the child are important determinants, and a child who looks or acts ill should be seen immediately.

5. *Answer:* a (evaluation/multisystem/NAS)

    Rationale: Current medications are important in terms of history and management, but follow-up depends primarily on age, diagnosis, clinical presentation, and support systems.

6. *Answer:* a (plan/management/therapeutic/pharmacologic/multisystem/NAS)

Rationale: Acetaminophen is the drug of choice for fever for adults and children older than 2 months. Ibuprofen is an alternative for adults and children older than 6 months. Aspirin can be used in adults, not children, for the management of fever. At times, it is appropriate not to use antipyretics for low-grade fevers.

FUNCTIONAL LIMITATIONS

OVERVIEW
Definition

Functional limitations include recent or progressive difficulties in performing or inability to perform various tasks that are necessary or highly desirable for independent living (Lachs, 1996). The impairments are relatively new, and the tasks were at one time within the capabilities of the older client.

Incidence

The incidence is unknown. The condition is frequently missed by clinicians and may be falsely attributed to normal aging.

Pathophysiology

The condition seldom occurs in isolation. Functional limitations may be signs and symptoms of a new underlying medical illness or of decompensating chronic disease. They may also suggest a change in environment. For example, incontinence may occur as a result of staying in a new home and having further to go to reach the bathroom.

FACTORS INCREASING SUSCEPTIBILITY
- New environment
- New drug
- Disruptions in usual routine

ASSESSMENT: SUBJECTIVE/HISTORY
History of Present Illness

NOTE: The history is *the* most important tool in assessing functional limitations.
- Track limitations according to landmarks, such as holidays. This helps family assess when and for how long a functional limitation has been present, particularly in situations of gradual decline. Acute onset suggests an acute underlying medical condition. If the client and family cannot reach consensus concerning onset, most likely the limitation is due to the natural history of a chronic disease.
- When multiple limitations are present, assess the chronology of onset. These usually appear in the following order (1) bathing, (2) dressing, (3) toileting, (4) transferring, and (5) feeding. Impairments in activities of daily living (ADLs) with normal instrumental activities of daily living (IADLS) suggest specific local problems (e.g., incontinence related to enlarged prostate).
- Distinguish capability from ability. Is the client unmotivated or depressed, rather than truly experiencing a functional limitation?

Past Medical History

Review all chronic diseases with the client. Functional limitations may appear in place of typical dyspnea or pain. Consider multiple coexisting conditions. The addition of a new condition to a chronic disorder may cause decompensation of the client.

Medications, particularly drugs that produce vasodilatation or anorexia, may cause functional decline. Diuretics increase the need to go to the bathroom, which may result in incontinence.

Psychosocial History

Consider environmental factors as the basis for any limitations. Examples include obstacles in the home, a new dwelling, and change in caregiver or social services.

ASSESSMENT: OBJECTIVE/
PHYSICAL EXAMINATION
Physical Examination

NOTE: Because clients tend to rate self-function higher than do family members, performance measures are more reliable.

The use of standardized tools allows measurement of changes from normal abilities and of treatment effectiveness. Examples include Katz ADLs, which assess toileting, bathing, dressing, and feeding abilities; and Lawton IADLs, which assess higher order functions necessary for managing a home and household, such as shopping, balancing a checkbook, and telephone use.

- Personal performance tests allow the nurse practitioner to assess psychomotor skills. For example, ask the client to put on a lab coat or to get up and go from a sitting position.
- Assess sources of pain that may be overlooked, such as mouth (dental problems), perineum (abscess), and feet (bunions).
- Assess general hygiene, dress, and nutritional status.
- Assess cognitive status with a formal tool (e.g., Mini-Mental State Exam) because functional limitations may represent disorientation or cognitive impairment.

Diagnostic Procedures

Electrolyte profiles, urinalysis, and CBC will help rule out infection, anemia, and electrolyte shifts as a source of the decline. Radiographic films may help in assessing infection or abscesses as possible causes of decline.

DIAGNOSIS

Depression, infection, angina, diabetes, and arthritis are all frequent causes of functional decline and should be considered as precipitating factors. Drug side effects should also be considered in the differential diagnosis.

THERAPEUTIC PLAN
Nonpharmacologic Treatment

If no cause can be found and the client has decompensated to the state that assistance with caregiving is necessary, hospital admission may be necessary, until social services can be obtained, particularly when family is not physically present.

Pharmacologic Treatment

As indicated, treat the precipitating cause of the decline (e.g., infection).

Client Education

Caregiver may need information about the precipitating factors and immediate and long-term needs of the client.

Referral

A referral to and consultation with a physician or gerontologist and geriatric assessment team should always be made when no basis for the functional limitations can be identified.

EVALUATION/FOLLOW-UP

Follow-up phone calls should be placed at 24 and 48 hours after the client visit to see whether improvements have occurred after treatment. If so, 2-week follow-up is indicated to prevent recurrence of the precipitating factor.

REFERENCES

Bernstein, E. (1996). Functional assessment, mental status, and case finding. In A. Sanders (Ed.), *Emergency care of the elder person*. St. Louis: Mosby.

Lachs, M. (1996). Functional decline. In A. Sanders (Ed.), *Emergency care of the elder person*. St. Louis: Mosby.

REVIEW QUESTIONS

1. A daughter brings her mother to the nurse practitioner because the mother is not able "to keep up anymore." To help assess the scope of this problem, the nurse practitioner should do all the following **except:**

- a. Try to determine whether one or multiple impairments are present.
- b. Have the client rate herself with respect to ADLS.
- c. Determine the landmark time around when these changes began.
- d. Make sure that the client was able to perform the activities before.

2. When examining a client with functional limitations, the nurse practitioner notes that IADLs are intact but toileting is impaired. This suggests:

- a. More ADLs are disrupted.
- b. The problem's cause is local.
- c. Cognitive impairments may exist.
- d. Motivation is the problem.

3. In the differential diagnosis of functional limitations, which of the following should be considered?

    a. Mental health problems

    b. Sexually transmitted diseases

    c. Occupational-related disorder

    d. Biologic aging

4. When planning care for a client with functional limitations of unknown etiology, the nurse practitioner should do which of the following?

    a. Consult with a physician.

    b. Admit the client or arrange for hospital admission.

    c. Refer the client to psychiatry.

    d. Contact home health care.

5. Initial evaluation of a client with functional limitations should be done:

    a. In the office within 24 hours

    b. By phone within 1 week

    c. By phone within 24 hours

    d. Within 1 month

ANSWERS AND RATIONALES

1. *Answer:* b (assessment/history/functional limitation/aging adult)

    Rationale: Clients tend to overrate their abilities, and self-assessment is not reliable. Understanding the number of impairments and their onset, duration, and severity is important. If the client was never able to perform a task, the inability to perform it now may not be related to functional limitations.

2. *Answer:* b (assessment/physical examination/functional limitation/aging adult)

    Rationale: If higher order function is preserved, there is no cognitive impairment. This also suggests that a specific structural cause may be present. Motivation level should be assessed, but there is no reason yet to believe that it is the problem.

3. *Answer:* a (diagnosis/functional limitation/aging adult)

    Rationale: Depression may be a source of functional decline because of the lack of energy to perform ADLs. No specific occupational illnesses have been associated with functional limitations as initial presenting symptoms. Aging does not in itself produce functional limitations. Sexually transmitted diseases do not induce changes in ADLs. Only syphilis may produce neurologic symptoms and possible deterioration of IADLs.

4. *Answer:* a (plan/therapeutics/nonpharmacologic/functional limitation/aging adult)

    Rationale: Functional limitations of unknown etiology need further evaluation to ensure that an acute or chronic illness is not being missed. This evaluation may be done on an outpatient basis, depending on client status. Psychiatry is not needed initially unless a diagnosis of a mental health problem has been made. Home health care may not be necessary if adequate caregiving can be provided by the family or if functional changes are minor.

5. *Answer:* c (evaluation/functional limitation/aging adult)

    Rationale: Follow-up within 24 hours of the visit is necessary to assess whether severity has increased, perhaps as the result of an acute process. An office visit is not necessary, however, if the family's reports are reliable.

LYME DISEASE

OVERVIEW
Definition

Lyme disease is an infection caused by *Borrelia burgdorferi*, a spirochete. It is the most common arthropod-borne disease in the United States.

Incidence

The highest incidences are in the northeast, the upper Midwest, and northern California; however, cases have been reported in all 50 states.

Prevalence is associated with increased deer population in endemic areas. Most infections occur between the months of May to August in the United States, except in the Pacific Northwest, where they peak January through May.

Pathophysiology

The *B. burgdorferi* spirochete is transmitted by prolonged attachment, of 2 days or more of an infected tick. The vector is *Ixodes dammini* (deer tick) in the northeast and Midwest, *Ixodes pacifica* in the far west, and *Ixodes ricinus* in Europe. The incubation period is 2 to 36 days, median 9 days

ASSESSMENT: SUBJECTIVE/HISTORY
History of Present Illness

- Ask about possible exposure to tick bites, such as a recent camping trip, hiking, or working in the yard.
- Ask the client to describe the duration and characteristics of any skin lesions. Question the client about recent headaches, fatigue, fever, and myalgias.
- Fewer than 50% of clients with Lyme disease recall the precipitating tick bite.

Symptoms

Symptoms include malaise, fatigue, headache, fever, chills, stiff neck, muscle and joint pain, lymphadenopathy, and erythema migrans: a skin lesion at the sight of tick bite that begins as a red bull's-eye with central clearing and enlarges during a course of days to weeks. Lesions >5 cm in diameter are most specific for a diagnosis of Lyme disease. Erythema migrans does not occur in all cases; in some clients, arthritis is the first and only sign.

Past Medical History

- Any history of arthritis, SLE, or recent viral syndrome
- Previous history of Lyme disease or treatment

Medication History

Examine current and recent medication therapy to rule out any recent infections, such as syphilis, or any chronic problems, such as arthritis or SLE, that the client may not have included in the past medical history.

Family History

- Ask about any other family members with similar symptoms.
- Ask about family history of rheumatoid arthritis.

Dietary History

Ask about recent ingestion of inadequately cooked meat or possibly contaminated water to rule out tularemia.

ASSESSMENT: OBJECTIVE/ PHYSICAL EXAMINATION
Physical Examination

- Carefully inspect the skin for lesions.
- Palpate for lymphadenopathy.
- Perform a thorough cardiac examination for secondary carditis, which occurs in 6% to 10% of untreated cases. It is manifested by atrioventricular conduction abnormalities and left ventricular dysfunction.
- Inspect the joints, particularly the knees, shoulders, hips, elbows, and ankles for swelling, tenderness, or erythema.
- Perform a neurologic examination. From 10% to 20% of untreated cases result in neurologic complications, including meningitis (headache and neck pain), encephalitis (sleep disturbances, poor memory, irritability, and dementia), and cranial neuropathies (Bell's palsy, decreased sensation, weakness, and loss of reflexes).

Diagnostic Procedures

- Indirect fluorescent antibody: Not specific, poor diagnostic tool
- Enzyme-linked immunosorbent assy (ELISA): Usual method (high false-positive rates with viral infections, SLE, rheumatoid arthritis)
- Western blot assay: Confirmatory, helps identify false-positive ELISA results
  Diagnostic tests identify 50% of early Lyme disease and discern 100% of clients with later complications of carditis, neuritis, and arthritis.

DIAGNOSIS

Differential diagnosis includes the following:
- Syphilis
- Rheumatoid arthritis
- Meningitis or encephalitis
- Viral syndrome
- SLE
- Rocky Mountain spotted fever
- Tularemia
- Bell's palsy

THERAPEUTIC PLAN
Pharmacologic Treatment

ADULTS. The following are used for adults (including nonpregnant, nonlactating females and children older than 8 years)

- Doxycycline, 100 mg bid for 10 to 21 days
- Tetracycline, 250 to 500 mg qid for 10 to 21 days
- Erythromycin, 250 mg qid for 10 to 21 days (for those allergic to penicillin or tetracycline)

CHILDREN AND PREGNANT OR LACTATING WOMEN. Amoxicillin, 250 to 500 mg tid for 10 to 21 days, is the preferred treatment for pregnant or lactating women and for children younger than 8 years

CLIENTS WITH CARDIAC OR NEUROLOGIC CONDITIONS. Consult physician about treatment of clients with cardiac or neurologic manifestations. IV therapy with penicillin, 20 MU/day, or ceftriaxone, 2 g/day, for 14 days is recommended. Doxycycline bid or amoxicillin tid for 30 days is effective for clients with arthritis.

Client Education

- Avoid exposure to ticks by wearing light-colored clothes, so that ticks are easily detected.
- Wear long pants tucked into socks and a long-sleeved shirt tucked in at the waist.
- Use insect repellent (DEET) that is safe for all ages. Read the precautions on the container.
- Avoid tick-infested areas during May through August.
- Keep areas around the house and yard free of brush and tall grass.
- Inspect the entire body after potential exposure.
- Use tweezers to remove an attached tick.
- Most ticks removed are not infected with *B. burgdorferi*. Prophylactic antimicrobial therapy is therefore not recommended.
- No data exist to document resistance to reinfection after treatment.
- Reinfection is difficult to distinguish from recurrence in endemic regions.

Referral

Any clients with cardiac or neurologic manifestations should be referred to a physician. Follow-up by a cardiologist or neurologist may be indicated.

EVALUATION/FOLLOW-UP

Follow-up evaluation at end of treatment is adequate in uncomplicated cases. Clients with more severe symptoms, such as cardiac or neurologic manifestations, should be seen more frequently.

REFERENCES

Bartlett, C. R., & Brown, J. W. (1996). New and emerging pathogens, part 2: Tick, tick, tick, tick, . . . boom! The explosion of tick borne diseases. *Medical Laboratory Observer, 28*(3), 44-52.

Deltombe, T., Hanson, P., Boutsen, Y., Laloux, P., & Clerin, M. (1996). Lyme borreliosus neuropathy: A case report. *American Journal of Physical Medicine and Rehabilitation, 75*(4), 314-316.

Fitzpatrick, T. B., Johnson, R. A., Polana, M. K., Suurmond, D., & Wolff, K. (1994). *Color atlas and synopsis of clinical dermatology* (15th ed., pp 360-69). New York: McGraw-Hill.

Herman, L., Robinson, T. T., & Birrer, R. B. (1996). Lyme disease: Ready cure, but a challenging diagnosis. *Journal of the American Academy of Physician Assistants, 9*(10), 39-40, 43-44, & 47-48.

Masters, E. J. (1993). Erythema migrans: Rash as key to early diagnosis of Lyme disease. *Postgraduate Medicine, 94*(1), 133-134 & 137-138.

Newland, J. A. (1995). Nurse practitioner extra. Primary care protocol, Lyme disease. *American Journal of Nursing, 95*(7), 16.

Schneiderman, H. (1995). What's your diagnosis? Erythema migrans of Lyme disease. *Consultant, 35*(5), 677-678 & 680.

REVIEW QUESTIONS

1. Which of the following sets of symptoms is most indicative of Lyme disease?

- a. Fatigue and headache
- b. Fever and stiff neck
- c. Joint stiffness and erythematous skin lesions
- d. Lymphadenopathy and malaise

2. Which of the following diseases results in false-positive results of the ELISA test for Lyme disease?

- a. Meningitis
- b. Tularemia
- c. SLE
- d. Rocky Mountain spotted fever

3. Which sign or symptom is most specific for the diagnosis of Lyme disease?

- a. Erythematous macular lesion with central clearing
- b. Positive indirect fluorescent antibody test result
- c. Persistent fatigue
- d. Adenopathy and pharyngitis

4. Which differential diagnosis may result in a false-positive ELISA result for Lyme disease?

   a. Meningitis
   b. Rheumatoid arthritis
   c. Rocky Mountain spotted fever
   d. CFS

5. Treatment of choice for an 11-year-old boy with a presenting symptom of a 5 cm erythema migrans lesion and a positive ELISA test result would be which of the following?

   a. Doxycycline, 100 mg bid for 14 days
   b. Erythromycin, 250 mg qid for 14 days
   c. Amoxicillin, 500 mg tid for 14 days
   d. Trimethoprim-sulfamethoazole (Bactrim), 1 tablet bid for 14 days

6. Kevin Jones, a 14-year-old, from Coon Rapids, Minnesota, has doxycycline, 100 mg bid for 10 days prescribed. He should be instructed to return for follow-up:

   a. After 3 days of antibiotic therapy
   b. At the end of treatment
   c. One month after completion to ensure that symptoms have resolved
   d. Follow-up is not necessary.

ANSWERS AND RATIONALES

1. *Answer:* c (assessment/history/multisystem/NAS)
   Rationale: Erythema migrans is the most specific symptom for Lyme disease; however, it does not occur in all cases. Many clients have arthritic symptoms as the first and only sign.

2. *Answer:* c (assessment/plan/multisystem/NAS)
   Rationale: SLE, viral infections, and rheumatoid arthritis may also result in a positive ELISA result.

3. *Answer:* a (assessment/physical examination/multisystem/NAS)
   Rationale: Fatigue, adenopathy, and pharyngitis are nonspecific symptoms of numerous disease processes; erythema migrans is most specific for Lyme disease.

4. *Answer:* b (assessment/plan/multisystem/NAS)
   Rationale: Viral infections, syphilis, SLE, and rheumatoid arthritis may also result in a false-positive ELISA result.

5. *Answer:* a (plan/multisystem/child)
   Rationale: Doxycycline is the drug of choice for all adults who are not pregnant or lactating and for children older than 8 years.

6. *Answer:* b (evaluation/multisystem/child)
   Rationale: For first-time cases or those without severe secondary symptoms, follow-up is recommended at the end of treatment.

Communicable Diseases

INFECTIOUS DISEASES

OVERVIEW

Definition

ROSEOLA. *Roseola* is an infection of the Herpesviridae family.

ERYTHEMA INFECTIOSUM (FIFTH DISEASE). *Fifth disease* is a viral infection (human parvovirus B19 [HPV-B19]).

SCARLET FEVER. Disease produced by group A beta-hemolytic streptococci.

VARICELLA-ZOSTER (CHICKENPOX, SHINGLES). *Varicella zoster* is a viral infection of the Herpesviridae family.

MUMPS. *Mumps* is a systemic viral disease characterized by swelling of the salivary glands, but it can involve multiple organs and be moderately debilitating.

MEASLES (RUBEOLA). *Measles* is an acute viral epidemic disease.

RUBELLA. *Rubella* is a mild viral disease; it is mainly of importance because of its teratogenicity.

PERTUSSIS (WHOOPING COUGH). *Pertussis* is an acute viral disease with an insidious onset.

MENINGOCOCCAL INFECTION. This is usually an acute bacterial infection, with rapid onset and progression if untreated.

Incidence

ROSEOLA. Incidence peaks in spring and fall. Incubation period is 5 to 15 days. The disease is contagious before and during the febrile period. Roseola is rare before 3 months and after 4 years of age.

ERYTHEMA INFECTIOSUM. Peak incidence is in the spring. Incubation period is 4 to 14 days. It is contagious before onset of illness but not after onset of rash. The infection is common in children 5 to 15 years old.

SCARLET FEVER. Incubation period is 2 to 5 days. Scarlet fever is contagious for 24 hours before symptoms develop until 48 hours after treatment with penicillin. The disease usually occurs in children between 2 and 10 years old.

VARICELLA-ZOSTER. Peak incidence is in the late winter and early spring. Incubation period is 14 to 16 days. Varicella-zoster is contagious for 1 to 2 days before and 5 days after the development of lesions. The disease is common in children between 5 to 10 years old. Immunity is lifelong.

MUMPS. Peak incidence is in the late winter and spring. Incubation period is 16 to 18 days. Mumps is contagious 1 to 2 days before and 3 to 7 days after the development of swelling. Complications are worse in adults (50% of all deaths occur in this group). Vaccine and illness confer lifelong immunity.

MEASLES. Peak incidence is in the winter and spring. Incubation period is 8 to 12 days. Measles is contagious 1 to 2 days before any symptoms and until 4 days after the rash clears. Measles is more common now in 10- to 19-year-olds.

RUBELLA. Peak incidence is in the late winter and early spring. Incubation period is 14 to 21 days. Rubella is contagious a few days before rash development and 5 to 7 days after the rash develops. Clients with congenital rubella can shed the virus in urine and nasopharyngeal fluids for 1 year.

PERTUSSIS. Every 3 to 4 years, there is increased incidence in the United States. Incubation period is 7 to 13 days. Pertussis affects females more frequently than males. Infants 1 to 2 months old are highly susceptible.

MENINGOCOCCAL INFECTION. This disease mainly affects children.

Pathophysiology

ROSEOLA. There are antibodies to human herpesvirus 6 in cord blood. By the age of 4 years, almost all persons are seropositive, indicating infection, in many cases without symptoms.

ERYTHEMA INFECTIOSUM. Humans are the only known host of HPV-B19. Spread is by respiratory and blood routes. Children of adults with chronic hemolytic anemia may have an aplastic crisis. They are also more contagious.

SCARLET FEVER. Spread is by direct contact and the respiratory route. Potential complications include glomerulonephritis and rheumatic fever.

VARICELLA-ZOSTER. Person-to-person spread is by direct contact and airborne droplets. Complications include bacterial superinfections (pneumonia in adults), thrombocytopenia, arthritis, hepatitis, encephalitis, meningitis, and glomerulonephritis. Reye's syndrome may occur, especially if aspirin is used to control fever. Exposure during pregnancy in the first or early second trimester may result in fetal deformity. Infection within 2 to 5 days before delivery may result in fetal death.

MUMPS. Spread is by direct contact and the respiratory route. Aseptic meningitis occurs in 50% of cases. Orchitis and epididymitis occur in 15% to 35% of adults. Infertility is rare. Pancreatitis may occur because salivary gland secretion elevates serum amylase level.

MEASLES. Measles is spread by direct contact and the respiratory route.

RUBELLA. Spread is by direct contact and the respiratory route.

PERTUSSIS. Pertussis is spread by respiratory secretions.

MENINGOCOCCAL INFECTION. This infection is transmitted by nasopharyngeal droplets. If it progresses to disease (meningococcemia), disseminated intravascular coagulation occurs, with septic shock.

ASSESSMENT: SUBJECTIVE/HISTORY
History of Present Illness

ROSEOLA. Fever (as high as 106° F) of abrupt onset occurs in a well child. Child may be mildly lethargic and irritable (occasionally pharynx, tonsils, and tympanic membranes are injected). No other symptoms are present. Fever lasts as long as 5 days (4 days is average duration and disappears as abruptly as it started). As the fever disappears, rash occurs, first on the trunk and then spreading to the arms and neck. The rash, which may also involve the face and legs, fades within 24 hours.

ERYTHEMA INFECTIOSUM. Approximately 50% of children have mild systemic symptoms, which include low-grade fever (100.4° F to 101.3° F [38° to 38.5° C]), mild malaise, sore throat, cough, and conjunctivitis. A rash may be the first symptom or sign. Adolescents have similar presenting symptoms as those seen in children; they may also have symptoms of arthritis lasting for 2 to 3 weeks.

SCARLET FEVER. Rash occurs 3 to 5 days after onset of sore throat.

VARICELLA-ZOSTER. History is usually 1 to 3 days of fever, upper respiratory tract infection (URI) symptoms, anorexia, and pruritis.

MUMPS. History is usually 1 to 2 days of fever, headache, malaise, and swelling of the "jaw area." Sour foods cause pain as a result of stimulation of salivary flow.

MEASLES. URI symptoms, conjunctivitis, cough, and photophobia are present.

RUBELLA. Nonspecific URI symptoms are seen about 24 hours before onset of rash.

PERTUSSIS. History is of a cough lasting more than 7 days or a loud cough with cough-induced vomiting.

MENINGOCOCCEMIA. Fever, stiff, painful neck, changes in level of consciousness, rash, and photophobia are seen.

General Historical Data

The following are pertinent to all infectious diseases:
- Immunization history
- Environmental exposure (illness at home, work, school, day care)
- Travel (to area with high incidence)
- Communicable disease history

ASSESSMENT: OBJECTIVE/ PHYSICAL EXAMINATION
Physical Examination

ROSEOLA. Rash is maculopapular, rose to pink, pinpoint, and nonpruritic.

ERYTHEMA INFECTIOSUM
Stage 1. Erythematous cheeks have appearance

of "slapped cheeks" because of redness. They may be warm and nontender, and they may itch. Rash may also be present on chin, forehead, and postauricular areas, but the area around the mouth is spared.

Stage 2 (1 to 2 days later). An erythematous, symmetric, maculopapular rash occurs on the trunk, neck, buttocks, or all three.

Stage 3. This rash fades with central clearing, leaving a distinctive lacy, reticulated rash that can last 2 to 40 days (average 2 weeks). Rash will recur with heat, exercise, bathing, or stress.

SCARLET FEVER. Rash is bright red and maculopapular, with a fine sandpaper-like texture. It will blanch on pressure. It is less intense on the face (sparing the mouth), usually beginning on the neck, and more prevalent under axillar and genital areas. *Pastia's sign* is when the antecubital folds of elbows become dark red with fine, linear petechiae. Beefy red tonsils are seen, with a coated tongue.

VARICELLA ZOSTER. Rash appears initially as small red papules that rapidly change to nonumbilicated oval "teardrop" vesicles on an erythematous base. Fluid changes from clear to cloudy; vesicles rupture, crust over, and heal. New crops appear for 3 to 4 days (longer in immunosuppressed persons). Lesions first appear on the trunk, head, face, and legs. Rash and systemic symptoms vary considerably.

MUMPS. Swelling occurs in the parotid gland, which obscures the angle of mandible, pushes the earlobe upward and outward, and causes pain with pressure on the gland. There are swelling and redness of Stensen's duct (yellow drainage with no pus). The submandibular or sublingual gland may be involved. Rarely, one of these glands is swollen and not the parotid.

MEASLES. Koplik's spots are gray or white, sand grain–sized dots on red base on the buccal mucosa opposite the lower molars. The rash is a discrete maculopapular rash that starts on the face and quickly spreads down the body. It coalesces to a bright red. The rash fades from the face down and is completely gone within 6 to 10 days. Fever falls within 2 to 3 days after onset of rash. Complications include otitis, bronchopneumonia, and encephalitis, the last of which usually results in permanent brain damage.

RUBELLA. A maculopapular rash starts on the face and spreads downward. It disappears by the third or fourth day. There are extremely few systemic symptoms. Postauricular and occipital adenopathy are seen.

PERTUSSIS. Nasal congestion is present.

MENINGOCOCCEMIA. Petechiae and purpura are present, with a macular rash on the extremities and trunk. Hypotension and signs of congestive heart failure or pulmonary edema are seen.

Diagnostic Procedures

ROSEOLA. None are necessary. Initially, elevated leukocytosis is seen, then leukopenia with relative lymphocytosis is seen by the second and third days.

ERYTHEMA INFECTIOSUM. No diagnostic tests are necessary.

SCARLET FEVER. Streptococcal screen or throat culture is done; diagnosis also may be made on clinical grounds.

VARICELLA-ZOSTER. Diagnosis is made on clinical grounds; virus can be isolated from vesicular lesions.

MUMPS. Diagnosis is made on clinical grounds.

MEASLES. Diagnosis is made on clinical grounds; the disease course can be followed with titers.

RUBELLA. Diagnosis is made on clinical grounds; the disease course can be followed with titers.

PERTUSSIS. Diagnosis is made on clinical grounds; the disease course can be followed with titers. Cough history may be relevant.

MENINGOCOCCEMIA. Diagnosis is made by clinical presentation and cultures of lesions, blood, and cerebrospinal fluid (CSF).

DIAGNOSIS
Mumps

- Cervical adenitis: The angle of the jaw may be obscured, but the earlobe is not displaced and Stensen's duct is normal.
- Bacterial parotitis: Pus is present in Stensen's duct, systemic toxicity is seen.

Most Infectious Diseases

Differential diagnosis includes impetigo, scabies, and tinea.

THERAPEUTIC PLAN
Roseola

Pharmacologic treatment is fever control for children at risk for febrile seizures.

Erythema Infectiosum

Nonpharmacologic treatment is supportive. Isolation is used for children with aplastic crisis. Pregnant women should not be excluded from the workplace and children should not be excluded from school because once rash is present, children are not contagious.

Scarlet Fever

Pharmacologic treatment includes the following:
- Benzathine penicillin G, 600,000 U IM (<60 pounds)
- Benzathine penicillin G, 1.2 MU IM (>60 pounds and adults)
- Penicillin V, 125 mg qid for 10 days (>60 pounds)
- Penicillin V, 250 mg qid for 10 days (>60 pounds)
- Erythromycin as alternative (estolate 20 to 30 mg/kg/day or ethyl succinate 40 to 50 mg/kg/day tid or qid for 10 days)

Varicella-Zoster

PHARMACOLOGIC TREATMENT
- Antipruritics for itching (diphenhydramine or hydroxizine)
- Acyclovir, 40 to 80 mg/kg/day, will shorten illness when given within first 24 hours. Advise only for children older than 14 years.
- Immunoglobulin can be given within 6 hours of exposure to prevent or modify illness.

NONPHARMACOLOGIC TREATMENT
- Supportive
- Fluids
- Analgesics
- Rest
- Cool baths
- Careful hygiene

Mumps

Nonpharmacologic treatment is supportive, with fluids, analgesics, and scrotal support for orchitis.

Measles

PHARMACOLOGIC TREATMENT. Vaccine, if given within 72 hours of measles exposure, can offer protection. Immunoglobulin within 6 days of exposure will prevent or alter severity.

NONPHARMACOLOGIC TREATMENT. Supportive treatment includes fluids, analgesics, and rest.

Rubella

Nonpharmacologic treatment is supportive, with fluids, analgesics, rest, and darkened room.

Pertussis

Nonpharmacologic treatment is supportive, with fluids and antipyretics.

Meningococcemia

Pharmacologic treatment is penicillin, 300,000 mg/kg/day IV.

Client Education

SCARLET FEVER
- The disease is no longer contagious after 48 hours of treatment.
- Stress the need to complete the course of antibiotics.

VARICELLA ZOSTER
- The child should be excluded from school for 6 days after onset of rash and may return when lesions crust over.
- Varicella vaccine may be given to those older than 1 year.

MUMPS

Exclude an affected child from school for 9 days after onset of swelling.

Vaccine given after exposure will not prevent illness.

MEASLES

Client should be excluded from school or workplace until 7 days after onset of rash.

RUBELLA

Affected children are excluded from school for 7 days after onset of rash.

MENINGOCOCCAL INFECTION

Immediate referral and hospitalization are necessary.

EVALUATION/FOLLOW-UP

Male adult clients with mumps should be seen in 1 to 2 weeks for genital examination. Clients with diseases that feature pruritic rashes (e.g., varicella) are more likely to become infected with *Staphylococcus aureus* and require antibiotic therapy. They should be reexamined in 1 week.

REFERENCES

Bartlett, J. G. (1996). *Pocket book of infectious disease therapy.* Baltimore: Williams & Wilkins.

Benenson, A. (1995). *Control of communicable diseases manual* (16th ed.). Washington, DC: American Public Health Association.

Burns, C. E., Barber, N., Brady, M. A., & Dunn, A. M. (1996). *Pediatric primary care: A handbook for nurse practitioners.* Philadelphia: W. B. Saunders.

Committee on Infectious Diseases, American Academy of Pediatrics (1997). In *1997 Red book: Report of the committee on infectious diseases* (24th ed.). Elk Grove Village, IL: Author.

Hay, W. W., Groothuis, J. R., Hayward, A. R., & Levin, M. J. (1997). *Current pediatric diagnosis and treatment* (13th ed.). Norwalk, CT: Appleton & Lange.

Merenstein, G. B., Kaplan, D. W., & Rosenberg, A. A. (1997). *Handbook of pediatrics* (18th ed.). Norwalk, CT: Appleton & Lange.

REVIEW QUESTIONS

1. A mother asks the nurse practitioner how long her daughter should remain home from school after being treated for scarlet fever. The correct response is:

   a. 1 week
   b. 2 days
   c. 1 day
   d. She can return immediately after treatment.

2. A child has varicella-zoster diagnosed. Which of the following should be reinforced with the parents?

   a. Need for immunization with varicella vaccine
   b. Avoidance of aspirin products
   c. Avoidance of antihistamines
   d. Need for possible plastic surgery follow-up to deal with scarring

3. The rash of roseola differs from that of measles in which of the following ways?

   a. Roseola rash starts on the trunk.
   b. Measles is a maculopapular rash.
   c. Roseola is pink.
   d. Measles is a nonpruritic rash.

4. The nurse practitioner suspects meningococcemia in a child. The treatment plan should include:

   a. Erythromycin
   b. Acyclovir
   c. Immediate physician consultation
   d. Immunoglobulin administration

5. A client with a pruritic rash should be followed up within 1 week of onset because of:

   a. Susceptibility to scarring
   b. Susceptibility to secondary bacterial infection
   c. Need for topical antihistamine
   d. Susceptibility to systemic complications

ANSWERS AND RATIONALES

1. *Answer:* b (plan/management/client education/communicable disease/child)

   Rationale: The child was contagious for 24 hours before the onset of symptoms and until 48 hours after treatment with penicillin.

2. *Answer:* b (plan/management/client education/communicable disease/child)

   Rationale: Immunoglobulin may be given within 6 hours of exposure to prevent or modify illness. Lifelong immunity usually occurs after infection, negating the need for vaccination. Reye's syndrome has been associated with varicella and aspirin use. Antihistamines are used to prevent itching. Scarring is usually minimal.

3. *Answer:* a (assessment/physical examination/communicable disease/child)

   Rationale: Both measles and roseola are pink to red, maculopapular, nonpruritic rashes. Roseola starts on the trunk, whereas measles usually starts on the face.

4. *Answer:* c (plan/management/nonpharmacologic/communicable disease/child)

   Rationale: Meningococcemia is a medical emergency and requires IV antibiotics with hospital admission.

5. *Answer:* b (evaluation/communicable disease/child)

   Rationale: Scratching increases the likelihood of a staphylococcal infection and the need for antibiotic therapy. Itching does not usually last as long as 1 week. Scarring is usually minimal.

LICE

OVERVIEW

Definition

Pedicular infestation of the skin or hair is caused by a species of blood-sucking lice capable of living as external parasites on the human host. There are three types of lice that inhabit the human host.

PEDICULUS HUMANIS CORPORIS. The body louse infests the body but actually emerges from the lining or seams of infested clothing, upholstery, or bedding to bite the human host.

PEDICULUS HUMANIS CAPITIS. The head louse infests the scalp and head hair.

PHTHIRUS PUBIS. The crab louse infests the genital region. Referred to as pediculosis pubis, *P. pubis* infestation may also affect the hair of the axilla, chest, abdomen, thighs, and eyelashes.

Incidence

- From 6 to 12 million cases occur annually in the United States.
- 50% to 75% in children younger than 12 years old.
- Can be epidemic in day care, kindergartens, and schools.
- Occurs in all ages, races, and socioeconomic groups and in all geographic regions.
- Can occur in any season but is most common August through November.

PEDICULOSIS CAPITIS. Infestation occurs most commonly in 5 to 12-year-olds, more often in girls. It may spread to other family members. Occurs in <1% of blacks because the structure of their hair shaft is less conducive. Head lice are acquired through personal contact.

PEDICULOSIS CORPORIS. Infestation occurs most commonly in crowded living conditions, situations of poverty, and where laundering is limited, such as in the homeless population.

PEDICULOSIS PUBIS. Infestation is highly contagious (90% acquisition rate per contact). Transmission occurs during intimate personal or sexual contact. Infestation can occur in children who have been sexually abused.

Pathophysiology

Lice are ectoparasites that, when spread by direct or fomite contact, pierce the skin to feed. When they bite, they infuse saliva to prevent clotting and probe for a vessel. The louse lays 100 to 300 eggs (nits) during a lifetime. Nits are attached to the hair shaft by a cementlike structure, which makes them difficult to remove. Lice cannot live away from a human host for more than 48 hours. It is the saliva of the louse that creates symptoms through a histamine response.

FACTORS INCREASING SUSCEPTIBILITY

Pediculosis Capitis

- Childhood, especially with enrollment in day care, school, or camp
- Family member with infestation
- Sharing of combs, brushes, hair decorations, and other objects that touch the head where lice are present

Pediculosis Corporis

- Homelessness
- Poor hygiene
- Infrequent laundering
- Close contact in crowded situations with individuals who are infested with lice
- Sharing of clothing or bedding that is contaminated

Pediculosis Pubis. Sexual contact with individual infected with pubic lice increases transmission chance.

PROTECTIVE FACTORS

- Clean hair and good hygiene do not prevent infestation with lice.
- Lifestyle that does not include behaviors and situations that provide exposure
- Black race

ASSESSMENT: SUBJECTIVE/HISTORY

History of Present Illness

- Intense itching, often worse at night
- With *P. capitis,* itching at the occipital hairline and the postauricular area is common.
- Known exposure

Symptoms

- Sleeplessness
- Irritability
- Difficulty concentrating in school because of itching

Family History

Inquire about infestation in family member.

Psychosocial History

PEDICULOSIS CAPITIS
- Child enrolled in day care, kindergarten, school, or camp
- Sharing of clothing or hairbrushes, combs, barrettes, and other hair care items
- Participation in sports in which equipment is shared
- Participation in theater activities in which wigs and borrowed clothes are shared

PEDICULOSIS CORPORIS
- Living in crowded environment, being homeless, or otherwise being unable to bathe, shampoo, and launder clothing as needed
- Sharing clothing, pillows, and bedding
- Purchasing clothing (and not laundering it before use) from yard sales or thrift shops
- Wearing clothing found on street or from lost and found sites

PEDICULOSIS PUBIS
- Multiple sexual partners
- Child: Sexual abuse by an adult or older child with lice infestation

GENERAL. It is important to assess client, parent, and family perceptions of the problem of lice because there are many misconceptions about infestation. A stigma exists concerning lice infestations.

ASSESSMENT: OBJECTIVE/ PHYSICAL EXAMINATION

Physical Examination

Strong lighting and a magnifying lens facilitate identification of lice and nits. The examiner should always wear gloves when examining for lice.

SKIN AND HAIR
- Visualize lice on hair shaft. Lice are smaller than a sesame seed, 3 to 4 mm, and gray-brown; they quickly move away from light and hide.
- Identify nits. Nits are teardrop shaped, 0.8 mm, and cream colored; empty ova shells are white. They are attached near the base of hair shafts at the scalp or pubic area. Dandruff and hair product artifacts usually blow or fall away, whereas a nit must be pulled along the hair shaft.
- Pinpoint red bites or black specks (lice feces) may be noted.
- Erythema at the nape of the neck and postauricular areas

LYMPH AND FEMORAL LYMPHADENOPATHY
- Lesions of secondary infection from scratching
- Cervical lymphadenopathy may occur with secondary infections associated with head lice
- Symptoms of other sexually transmitted diseases (STDs) may coexist with pediculosis pubis

Diagnostic Procedures

- A louse may be removed for examination under a microscope for confirmation if desired.
- Wood's lamp may be used because lice fluoresce. This is normally not necessary for diagnosis.

DIAGNOSIS

Confirm the type of lice infestation. Rule out hair artifacts (spray, gel), dandruff, seborrhea, psoriasis, and tinea capitis.

THERAPEUTIC PLAN

Pharmacologic Treatment

Pediculicides are required to kill lice and nits. Most are contraindicated in children younger than 2 years and in pregnant and lactating women. During use the client's eyes should be covered and shut.

TYPES OF PEDICULICIDES
- Pyrethrins (with piperonyl butoxide) 0.3% (A200, RID, Triple X): Leave shampoo on for 10 minutes, then rinse thoroughly. Reapplication may be needed in 7 to 10 days. Products are available OTC.
- Permethrin 1% cream rinse (Nix, Elimite): This is the drug of choice because it has a 97% to 99% cure rate and minimal side effects. Apply after shampooing hair, leave on for 10 minutes, and rinse thoroughly. Do not shampoo for 24 hours after use. Reapplication is not usually necessary. These products are available OTC.

- Lindane (Kwell): Prescription is required. Product comes as 1% lotion, 1% cream, and 1% shampoo. Shampoo, leave on for 4 minutes, then rinse. Repeat in 1 week. Product must be used with caution because it may cause neurotoxicity. Lindane should not be used on acutely inflamed skin or scalp.

Nonpharmacologic Treatment

NOTE: No pediculicide is 100% ovicidal. Nit removal is essential.

There are commercial preparations, such as Step 2, that assist in nit removal. A 50/50 white vinegar–water solution may also be used to loosen nits. A nit comb (metal ones work better) is used to remove all nits from the hair shafts. This can be a time-consuming process.

To treat lice-infested eyelashes, apply petrolatum 2 times a day for 10 days.

Client Education

- Reassure the client and family that pediculosis is curable, does not cause long-term effects, and is a common problem in all socioeconomic groups.
- Because person-to-person transmission occurs, educate children and parents about mode of transmission and preventive measures, such as not sharing combs, brushes, hair decorations, hats, scarves, helmets, headphones, bedding, and sleeping bags. Coats and hats should be hung separately, not touching those of others. Sleeping mats should be individually labeled and kept separately in plastic bags, not stacked.
- Teach how to disinfect the personal articles of the infested individual and how to clean the environment, reinforcing that lice do not jump or fly but spread through crawling.
  —Machine wash all washable clothing and bedding used within the last 48 hours with hot water and detergent (water should be >125° F).
  —Dry clothing and bedding on as high heat as possible in a clothes dryer for at least 20 minutes.
  —Dry clean clothing and personal items that cannot be washed. Upholstered furniture, pillows, and stuffed animals may be ironed with a hot iron.
  —Soak brushes, combs, barrettes, and similar hair items in 2% disinfectant or pediculicide for 1 hour (items can be boiled on stove for 10 minutes if they are not plastic).
  —Clean other objects that have been in contact with infested hair within the last 48 hours, such as curlers, headphones, earpieces or glasses, helmets, and car seats.
  —Place other items that have been exposed to infestation in a plastic bag and keep it closed for 2 weeks; lice will die of starvation.
- Recommend that all family members and close contacts be examined for presence of infestation and treated at the same time as the identified client.
- Advise parents to inform school authorities about infested children.
- Reinforce the importance of exposing all lice and nits to pediculicide and destroying or removing all nits from infested hair. Hair should be separated into multiple sections, with each part of the scalp exposed, examined, and methodically treated. Nits are removed with a nit comb. A different comb should be used for each infested person, and combs should be cleaned frequently during the removal process. Vinegar or a nit removal product may be used to loosen nits from the hair shaft for easier removal.

Referral

Referral to a physician is necessary for the following:

- Children younger than 2 years of age
- Pregnant and lactating women
- Treatment failures
- Lice in eyelashes that persist despite treatment
- Coexisting dermatologic conditions

If pediculosis pubis is seen in a child, appropriate authorities should be notified regarding the potential for child sexual abuse.

EVALUATION/FOLLOW-UP

During lice season, the parent should check the child's hair every 3 days. Once treated for lice, the individual should be reexamined at least by a family member several days after treatment. Reapplication of pediculicide 7 to 10 days after the initial treatment is often necessary. In the case of pediculosis pubis, all sexual contacts for the past month should receive treatment.

REFERENCES

Copeland, L. (1995). *The lice-buster book.* New York: Warner Books.

Crain, E. F., & Gershel, J. C. (1997). *Clinical manual of emergency pediatrics.* New York: McGraw-Hill.

Fenstermacher, K., & Hudson, B. T. (1997). *Practice guidelines for family nurse practitioners.* Philadelphia: W. B. Saunders.

Fitzpatrick, T. B., Johnson, R. A., Polano, M. K., Suurmond, D., & Wolff, K. (1992). *Color atlas and synopsis of clinical dermatology.* New York: McGraw-Hill.

Forsman, K. E. (1995). Pediculosis and scabies: What to look for in patients who are crawling with clues. *Postgraduate Medicine, 98*(6), 89-100.

Hawkins, J. W., Roberto-Nichols, D. M., & Stanley-Haney, J. L. (1995). *Protocols for nurse practitioners.* New York: Tiresias Press.

Lichtman, R., & Papera, S. (1990). *Gynecology–well woman care.* Norwalk, CT: Appleton & Lange.

Millonig, V. L. (1991). Back to school signals "head lice season." *Journal of the American Academy of Nurse Practitioners, 3*(3), 136-137.

Sokoloff, F. (1994). Identification and management of pediculosis. *Nurse Practitioner, 19*(8), 62-64.

Star, W. L., Lommel, L. L., & Shannon, M. T. (1995). *Women's primary health care: Protocols for practice.* Washington, DC: American Nurses Publishing.

Uphold, C. R., & Graham, M. V. (1994). *Clinical guidelines in family practice.* Gainesville, FL: Barmarrae Books.

Wong, D. (1995). *Nursing care of infants and children* (5th ed.). St. Louis: Mosby.

Youngkin, E. O., & Davis, M. S. (1994). *Women's health: A primary care clinical guide.* Norwalk, CT: Appleton & Lange.

REVIEW QUESTIONS

1. Which symptom associated with pediculosis capitis would be **least** likely to be reported by Megan, a 7-year-old female, or her mother?

a. Difficulty sleeping
b. Problems concentrating on school work
c. Headache
d. Irritability

2. The nurse practitioner suspects that Megan has pediculosis capitis. What diagnostic measure can provide additional supportive evidence?

a. Use of Wood's lamp
b. Eosinophil count
c. Sedimentation rate
d. WBC count

3. Which of the following individuals is most likely to have pediculosis corporis?

a. Older, homeless woman
b. Black transportation executive
c. Middle-aged wheat farmer
d. Hispanic high-school librarian

4. In cases of pediculosis capitis, in what area of the head are findings most evident?

a. Frontal hair, such as bangs
b. Crown of head
c. Occipital hairline
d. Preauricular region

5. How can lice and nits in the eyelashes be treated?

a. Soak lashes bid in permethrin for 3 days.
b. Coat lashes with petrolatum bid for 1 week.
c. Apply hot, moist cloths tid for 7 days.
d. Brush lashes with a gauze dipped in disinfectant.

6. What is the appropriate approach in the event of initial treatment failure for pediculosis capitis?

a. Reapply pediculicide daily for 1 week.
b. Shave the hair.
c. Initiate oral pediculicide.
d. Reapply pediculicide 7 to 10 days after initial treatment.

7. Mr. Ludlum is a 33-year-old male with pediculosis pubis. Which additional associated diagnosis does **not** need to be considered?

a. Gonorrhea
b. HIV infection
c. Chlamydial infection
d. Orchitis

8. Which follow-up is essential for Sherry, a 15-year-old with pediculosis pubis?

a. Are her menses heavier than before?
b. Has she been sexually abused?
c. Is she allergic to iodine?
d. Does she use sanitary napkins or tampons?

9. A kindergarten teacher has followed instructions for cleaning her room after a lice infestation. She calls the clinic for advice about how to care for several stuffed animals. Which is appropriate advice?

a. Discard the stuffed animals because they cannot be properly cleaned.

b. Seal the stuffed animals in plastic bags for 2 weeks.

c. Spray the stuffed animals with a dilute solution of chlorine bleach and water.

d. Brush the stuffed animals vigorously with a clothes brush.

ANSWERS AND RATIONALES

1. *Answer:* c (assessment/history/communicable disease/child)

Rationale: Sleeplessness, difficulty concentrating, and irritability are commonly associated with lice infestation. (Sokoloff, 1994)

2. *Answer:* a (diagnosis/communicable disease/child)

Rationale: Lice fluoresce under the Wood's lamp. (Millonig, 1991)

3. *Answer:* a (diagnosis/communicable disease/adult)

Rationale: Homeless populations are at particular risk for body lice infestations because of compromised hygiene and laundering. (Forsman, 1995)

4. *Answer:* c (assessment/physical examination/communicable disease/NAS)

Rationale: Although any part of the head may itch and have lice present, the occipital hairline and postauricular area are generally most affected. (Millonig, 1991)

5. *Answer:* b (plan/communicable disease/NAS)

Rationale: Petrolatum applied to lashes two times daily for 7 to 10 days will effectively remove lice and nits. (Uphold & Graham, 1994)

6. *Answer:* d (plan/communicable disease/NAS)

Rationale: Ovicides may need to be reapplied in 7 to 10 days to kill nits. (Forsman, 1995)

7. *Answer:* d (diagnosis/communicable disease/adult)

Rationale: In the presence of pediculosis pubis, other STDs must be considered as possible coexisting diagnoses. (Fitzpatrick, Johnson, Polano, Suurmond, & Wolff, 1992)

8. *Answer:* b (evaluation/communicable disease/adolescent)

Rationale: Children with pediculosis pubis need to be evaluated for the possibility of sexual abuse. (Uphold & Graham, 1994)

9. *Answer:* b (evaluation/communicable disease/adult)

Rationale: Items that cannot be washed or dry cleaned can be sealed in plastic bags for 2 weeks. This will cause lice to die of starvation. (Sokoloff, 1994)

MONONUCLEOSIS (INFECTIOUS)

OVERVIEW
Definition

Infectious mononucleosis (IM) refers to the presence of an abnormally high number of mononuclear leukocytes in the body.

Incidence

- Approximately 12% to 30% of the total cases of IM occur among university students and military cadets.

- By adulthood, most individuals have had at least one infection with Epstein-Barr virus (EBV).
- IM occurs most often in adolescents from higher socioeconomic groups and college students.
- The peak incidence in boys is ages 16 to 18 years old and that in girls is 14 to 16 years old.
- Children: IM is rare in children younger than 5 years, but infection occurs early in life among

lower socioeconomic groups and in developing countries.

Pathophysiology

IM results from a viral syndrome caused by EBV. The virus is introduced when the prospective host comes into close contact with an individual who is shedding EBV in the oropharynx. IM is frequently called the "kissing disease" because of the close contact needed for transmission. The virus replicates in epithelial cells of the pharynx and salivary glands. A localized inflammatory response produces the pharyngeal exudate. The virus is then carried through the lymphatics to the lymph nodes. Local and generalized lymphadenopathy develop. Incubation period is 30 to 50 days.

ASSESSMENT: SUBJECTIVE/HISTORY
Most Common Symptoms

- Fever and fatigue for 1 week
- Sore throat (may be described as the worst the client has ever had)
- Dysphagia
- Swelling of lymph nodes, especially of posterior cervical lymph nodes
- Clients younger than 10 years and clients older than 50 years may have atypical presenting symptoms of rash and nonspecific gastrointestinal complaints.

Associated Symptoms

- Anorexia
- Headache
- Abdominal pain
- Jaundice (rare)

Past Medical History

- Exposure to person with IM, history of URI in past
- History of recent streptococcal sore throat (coexists in approximately 26%)
- Last menstrual period (LMP) for females
- Allergies

Medication History

Inquire about recent use of antibiotics and any other medications.

Family History

Ask about other family members who may be sick.

Psychosocial History

- Smoking history
- Ability to perform normal activities; extent to which fatigue has interfered with work or school expectations
- Assess ability to cope with interference with activities of daily living

Dietary History

Ask about the type of diet the client usually eats.

ASSESSMENT: OBJECTIVE/ PHYSICAL EXAMINATION
Physical Examination

A problem-oriented physical examination should be conducted with particular attention to the following:

- Vital signs, weight, and general appearance
- Skin: Check for maculopapular rash.
- HEENT: Assess for erythema of pharynx and exudate.
  —Petechiae at the junction of hard and soft palate occur in 25%.
  —Facial edema, especially eyelid edema, is rarely encountered in young adults and is suggestive of IM.
- Lymph nodes: Significant lymphadenopathy is almost always present in the cervical and epitrochlear nodes; if not question diagnosis.
- Abdominal: Hepatomegaly (50%), and splenomegaly (75%)
- Children: Assess for dehydration and activity level.

Diagnostic Procedures

- Complete blood cell count with differential (>10,000 to 20,000); lymphocytes >50% with numerous atypical lymphocytes and monocytes
- Immunoglobin M antibodies
- Monospot result positive after 7 to 10 days of illness
- Streptococcal screen
- Liver function tests: Mild elevation

DIAGNOSIS

Differential diagnosis includes the following:
- Streptococcal pharyngitis
- Measles
- Viral exanthems
- Viral hepatitis
- Cytomegalovirus (CMV)

THERAPEUTIC PLAN
Pharmacologic Treatment

Symptomatic treatment only includes acetaminophen for fever and pain relief. About 20% of clients may also need antibiotics for concomitant streptococcal pharyngitis. Avoid ampicillin because it causes a rash in 80% of clients treated.

Nonpharmacologic Treatment
- Bed rest for fatigue
- Maintenance of adequate fluid intake
- Anesthetic lozenges for pain relief
- Salt water gargles
- Soft diet

Client Education
- Teach the client to prevent splenic rupture by avoidance of minor trauma, heavy lifting, overexertion, and contact sports for 1 to 2 months.
- Teach the client strategies to avoid constipation because this causes increased pressure on the spleen.
- Illness is self-limiting and isolation is unnecessary.

Referral
- Marked splenomegaly
- Respiratory compromise
- Excessively enlarged tonsils and difficulty swallowing
- Jaundice
- Hyperbilirubinemia

EVALUATION/FOLLOW-UP
- Promptly report abdominal pain and upper quadrant pain radiating to the shoulder.
- If the client experiences shortness of breath or inability to swallow, emergency services should be accessed immediately.
- Assess splenomegaly weekly until it no longer persists.

REFERENCES

Boynton, R., Dunn, E., & Stephens, G. (1994). *Manual of ambulatory pediatrics.* (3rd ed.). Philadelphia: J. B. Lippincott.

Hoole, A., Pickard, C. Ouimette, R., Lohr, J., & Greenberg, J. (1996). *Patient care guidelines for nurse practitioners* (4th ed.). Philadelphia: J.B. Lippincott.

McCue, J. (1992). Infectious mononucleosis. In L. Dornbrand, A. Hoole, & C. Pickard (Eds.). *Manual of clinical problems in adult ambulatory care* (pp. 563-566). Boston: Little, Brown.

Robinson, D. (1996). Mononucleosis. In M. Sommers & S. Johnson (Eds.). *Davis's manual of nursing therapeutics for diseases and disorders* (pp. 696-699). Philadelphia: F.A. Davis.

REVIEW QUESTIONS

1. What symptoms would make you most suspicious of IM in a 21-year-old college student?

  a. Sore throat, fatigue, and cough
  b. Abdominal pain and sore throat
  c. Rash, sore throat, and fever
  d. Headache, jaundice, and sore throat

2. Which of the following objective findings if **not** present would make you reconsider the diagnosis of IM?

  a. Throat erythematous, no exudate
  b. Maculopapular rash
  c. Facial edema
  d. Lymphadenopathy

3. Sarah is a 20-year-old college student. She reports a sore throat for 2 weeks, enlarged glands in her neck, and a fever. In addition to IM, what diagnosis needs to be considered?

  a. Rubella
  b. Streptococcal pharyngitis
  c. Viral hepatitis
  d. CMV

4. Treatment for mononucleosis should include:

  a. Ampicillin, 250 mg bid for 10 days
  b. Symptomatic treatment
  c. Interferon
  d. Acyclovir

5. Sarah, a 20-year-old college student, had IM diagnosed 2 weeks ago. She is now reporting abdominal pain. When should she be seen for follow-up?

   a. Sarah should be seen as soon as possible.

   b. Sarah should be followed up in 1 week.

   c. She should return for follow-up in 1 month.

   d. Follow-up is not needed because she has been feeling better.

ANSWERS AND RATIONALES

1. Answer: c (assessment/history/communicable disease/adult)

Rationale: Jaundice and cough are not usual in IM. Abdominal pain may occur; however, it would not lead you to suspect IM. A rash occurs in 25% of clients. (Hoole, 1996)

2. Answer: d (assessment/physical examination/communicable disease/NAS)

Rationale: The localized inflammatory response produces the lymphadenopathy that is almost always present in IM. Although usually present in IM, the rash, facial edema, and sore throat could also occur with other illnesses. Their absence does not make one question the diagnosis. (Robinson, 1996)

3. Answer: b (diagnosis/communicable disease/adult)

Rationale: Sarah's symptoms are those commonly encountered with streptococcal pharyngitis. This occurs in approximately 20% of clients with IM. (Boynton, Dunn, & Stephens, 1994)

4. Answer: b (plan/communicable disease/NAS)

Rationale: The treatment for IM is rest and fluids along with symptomatic care, such as antipyretics for fever or pain. Ampicillin commonly causes a rash when given to clients with IM. Interferon and acyclovir have no place in the treatment of IM. (Hoole, 1996)

5. Answer: a (evaluation/communicable disease/adult)

Rationale: Because splenic rupture is a possibility, as a result of splenomegaly during IM, Sarah should be seen as soon as possible to rule out it out. (Robinson, 1996)

SYHILIS

OVERVIEW
Definition

Syphilis is a complex multisystem disease caused by the spirochete *Treponema pallidum*. This disease has been known throughout history as the "great imitator" or the "great imposter" because of its variety of presentations (Tramont, 1995).

Incidence

The incidence of syphilis varies greatly from country to country. Developing countries have a higher incidence, even considering that the completeness and accuracy of reporting are questionable.

The United States has noted fluctuations in the incidence of syphilis with time. There was an 88% decrease in annual reported cases of syphilis between 1943 and 1977. Between 1986 and 1990, there was a 97% increase. In 1990, there were 50,223 reported cases of primary and secondary syphilis and 55,132 cases yearly of latent syphilis. The number of undiagnosed cases is estimated to be much higher (Lukehart & Holmes, 1997, p. 727).

Pathology

PATHOGENESIS. Exposure to *T. pallidum* results in its rapid penetration through intact mucous membranes or abraded skin to the blood and lymphatics, where it then causes a systemic infection. The median incubation period in humans is 21 days. A primary lesion then develops at the site of inoculation. This lesion remains for 2 to 6 weeks and heals spontaneously.

The generalized lesions, lymphadenopathy, and malaise of secondary syphilis usually appear 6 to 8 weeks after the healing of the primary lesion (chancre). These lesions subside spontaneously in 2 to 6 weeks, and the affected person then enters the latent phase.

The latent phase may be undetectable except by serologic examination. Untreated syphilis can develop into tertiary syphilis, with manifestations such as cardiovascular syphilis, neurovascular syphilis, and gummas (Lukehart & Holmes, 1997).

CLASSIFICATION. Syphilis is classified into groups primarily on the basis of presenting clinical manifestations of the disease.

Primary Syphilis. After exposure to an infected individual, a primary lesion develops at the site of inoculation. This is a painless, indurated lesion that may not be noticed, depending on its location. Common sites of this primary lesion, known as a *chancre,* include the penis, anus, cervix, vulva, and vagina.

Secondary State. The secondary stage is characterized by a generalized, hyperpigmented, papular rash that includes palmar and plantar surfaces. This rash develops within 6 weeks of the healing of the primary lesion. Concomitant symptoms include sore throat, fever, malaise, generalized, nontender lymphadenopathy, and patchy alopecia including scalp hair, eyebrows, and beard. Rarely, hepatitis and meningitis may also be seen. The secondary lesions of syphilis resolve within 2 to 10 weeks with or without treatment.

Latency. The period of untreated resolution of symptoms of secondary syphilis is called *latency.* Latency is subdivided into early and late latency. *Early latency* is within 1 year of the initial infection. *Late latency* is longer than 1 year after the initial infection.

Tertiary Stage. Tertiary syphilis develops after a variable period of latency in untreated or undertreated persons. This stage is characterized by further involvement of multiple systems.

Central Nervous System (CNS). Neurosyphilis may be symptomatic or asymptomatic. The CNS involvement in syphilis includes but is not limited to the tertiary stage. Examples of CNS involvement include meningeal syphilis, cranial nerve involvement, meningomyelitis, focal CNS lesions or stroke, dementia, ataxia, and optic atrophy (Hook & Marra, 1992).

Cardiovascular Syphilis. This involves aortitis with an aortic dissection that most frequently involves the ascending aorta, followed in frequency by the transverse segment of the aorta. The aorta below the renal arteries is rarely involved. Symp-tomatic syphilitic aortitis should be suspected whenever linear calcifications are noted on chest radiographs of the ascending aorta. Syphilitic aneurysms rarely dissect. Other large arteries may also be involved, such as the temporal artery. Cardiovascular syphilis is extremely rare in the United States because of antibiotic treatment (Tramont, 1995).

Benign Late Syphilis. This is characterized by lesions called *gummas.* The gumma is rarely seen today. These lesions, which can occur in the skin, bone, mucus, or any organ system, resemble the granulomas of tuberculosis. These lesions may develop from 2 to more than 40 years after the initial infection.

Congenital Syphilis. Congenital syphilis is syphilis transmitted from an infected mother to her unborn child transplacentally. In 1989, the definition of congenital syphilis was broadened to include all stillborn infants delivered to women with untreated or inadequately treated syphilis at delivery (Lukehart & Holmes, 1997, p. 728).

RISK GROUPS

- The populations at highest risk for contracting this disease have also changed with time. Between 1977 and 1982, approximately half of all clients with early syphilis in the United States were men who had sex with other men. Because of the changes in sexual practices among bisexual men and homosexual men since the AIDS epidemic, the incidence in this group of men has decreased.
- The current epidemic involves men and women of black descent living in urban areas. In some cities, infectious syphilis is highly correlated with the exchange of sex for drugs, especially crack cocaine.
- The age group of peak incidence of syphilis is 15 to 34 years.
- The incidence of congenital syphilis is related to the incidence of women with syphilis. In 1990, there were 2899 infants with diagnosed cases of congenital syphilis.

INFECTIVITY. Approximately 50% of named contacts of primary and secondary syphilis become infected. The actual risk from a single exposure is probably lower.

ASSESSMENT: SUBJECTIVE/HISTORY

Symptoms

PRIMARY SYPHILIS
- Chancre sore
- Painless, rubbery lymphadenopathy, usually in the groin

SECONDARY SYPHILIS
- Rash, especially on palms of hands and soles of feet
- Painless lymphadenopathy
- Fever, sore throat, and malaise
- Hair loss
- Symptoms of meningitis or hepatitis

TERTIARY SYPHILIS
- Subjective symptoms depend on the organ system or systems involved.
- Tertiary syphilis is usually found during extensive workup on inpatient basis.

CONGENITAL SYPHILIS
- Snuffles (rhinitis)
- Maculopapular rash with desquamation and sloughing of the epithelium, particularly palms and soles
- Vesicular rash and bullae
- Congenital syphilis may be seen as saddle nose or anterior bowing of lower extremities.
- Abdominal organomegaly
- Anemia, thrombocytopenia

History

If a client has vague complaints that do not immediately direct the health care provider to suspect STD, then a complete history and physical would be indicated, especially if problem-oriented examination and treatment do not resolve the problem. On the other hand, if the client arrives with symptoms or a history that leads the provider to suspect STD, then a problem-oriented history and physical examination should be performed.

Chief Complaint (Reason for Visit)

Ask about contact with infected individual (specify what sort of contact, be specific).

History of Present Illness

SYMPTOMS. When did symptoms begin? Was onset acute or gradual? How many days, weeks, or months have symptoms persisted (be specific)?

ASSOCIATED SYMPTOMS. Ask about discharge, odor, dysuria, lesion, genital itch, abdominal rash, or scrotal pain.

PRECIPITATING FACTORS. Has the client had unprotected sex?

RELIEVING FACTORS. Does any thing make the client feel better?

TREATMENT. What kinds of treatments have been used so far?

Past Medical History

PREVIOUS STDS
- When did the client have a previous STD?
- What type of STD was it: syphilis, nongonococcal urethritis, trichomoniasis, chlamydial infection, herpes, pelvic inflammatory disease, genital warts, other?
- What type of treatment did the client receive? For how long? Did the client take it all?

SEXUAL HISTORY
- Last exposure (sexual act)
- Number of partners in the last month and the last year
- Number of lifetime partners (fewer than 5, 5 to 10, more than 10)
- Sexual preference: Male, female, or both
- Sexual interaction with a bisexual
- Exposure site: Genital, rectal, oral
- Use of barrier protection (condom, dental dam): Never, sometimes, always
- Use of sex to obtain drugs or money

GYNECOLOGIC HISTORY
- LMP (normal?)
- Para and gravida status
- Ectopic pregnancy
- Infertility
- Hysterectomy
- Last Papanicolau smear (results?)
- Pregnancy status (yes, no, or unknown; if yes, which trimester?)

Medication History

CONTRACEPTIVE HISTORY
- None
- Condom
- Intrauterine device
- Oral contraceptives
- Sterilization
- Frequency of use

PRESENT MEDICATIONS
- Prescribed (watch for macrolide and terfenadine [seldane] combination)
- Antibiotics used in last 2 weeks
- Use of street drugs

Allergies
- Medications
- Latex
- Foods

Psychosocial History
- Economic factors: Can the client afford medications?
- Transportation: Access for follow-up
- Who lives with the client?
- Spouse or partner relationship
- Alcohol or drug history
- IV or IM drug use

TRAVEL. *Yaws, endemic syphilis,* and *pinta* are three nonvenereal trepomenatoses. These must be considered in clients who have traveled to third-world countries.

ASSESSMENT: OBJECTIVE/ PHYSICAL EXAMINATION
Physical Examination
A problem-oriented examination is done with particular attention to the following:
- Hair: Patchy alopecia in a pattern opposite to that of male pattern baldness progresses from occiput to temples, with loss of eyelashes and lateral third of eyebrows.
- Oropharynx: Ulcer, exudate, patches, pharyngitis, other
- Mucous membranes: Pink to gray mucus patches, painless, dull erythematous patches of grayish-white erosion
- Neck: Lymphadenopathy
- Skin: Folliculitis, rash (especially of soles and palms), chancre, painless, nonpruritic lesions (asymmetric distribution in secondary syphilis)
- Lymph nodes: Inguinal and cervical; firm, movable, discrete, rubbery, nonfluctuant, painless, unilateral or bilateral nodes
- Pubic hair: Patchy hair loss
- Penis: Ulcer, chancre
- Scrotum: Edema, lesion
- Vulva and vagina: Ulcer, rash

- Cervix: Lesion
- Bimanual: Mass, tenderness
- Perianal: Ulcer

Diagnostic Procedures
One STD may be superimposed on another. Other physical findings may indicate multiple STDs. Other tests may need to be performed, depending on findings of the history and physical examination. This section will concentrate only on the diagnostic procedures for syphilis.

PREGNANCY SCREENING. Congenital syphilis is preventable if maternal syphilis is treated in early pregnancy. Nontreponemal tests should be used for screening, and positive results should be confirmed with treponemal testing.

PRIMARY SYPHILIS
- Dark-field microscopy or fluorescent antibody (FA): This technique is used for examination of a genital or oral chancre or other suspected ulcer to look for *T. pallidum.*
- Reagin test for syphilis (nontreponemal). As many as 28% of clients with early syphilis may have nonreactive nontreponemal test results on the initial visit. If the test result is negative with suspect symptoms, then do a series of tests (first visit and repeat at 1 week, 1 month, and 3 months).
  —Venereal Disease Research Laboratory (VDRL) test
  —Rapid Plasma Reagin (RPR) test: Three negative reagin test results rule out syphilis as the cause of symptoms.
- Treponemal test: Use this test if a nontreponemal test result is positive with unknown infection history.

SECONDARY SYPHILIS
- Dark-field microscopy or FA: Material collected from lesions or lymph nodes
- Reagin test (blood test): Titer ≥1:16 is positive.
  —VDRL
  —RPR

LATENT SYPHILIS
- Reagin test (blood test): As many as 30% may have false negative results.
  —VDRL
  —RPR
- Treponemal test (confirmatory blood test): This is not indicated unless late syphilis is suspected on clinical grounds.

—Fluorescent treponemal antibody, absorbed, test

—Microhemagglutination *T. pallidum*

- Lumbar puncture: For CSF examination

CLIENTS PREVIOUSLY TREATED FOR SYPHILIS

- Reagin test: Must have a fourfold increase of the quantitative titer
- Dark-field examination

CONGENITAL SYPHILIS

- Direct examination of nasal discharge or material from lesions
- Reagin test (blood test)
- CSF examination

DIAGNOSIS

Differential diagnosis includes the following:
- Primary syphilis
- Secondary syphilis
- Tertiary or late syphilis
- Congenital syphilis
- Other

THERAPEUTIC PLAN
Pharmacologic Treatment

PRIMARY AND SECONDARY SYPHILIS OF LESS THAN 1 YEAR DURATION (ADULT)
- Benzathine penicillin G, 2.4 MU IM
- Only use alternative if client is allergic to penicillin and not pregnant (may refer for desensitization).
- Doxycycline, 100 mg PO bid for 14 days
- Tetracycline, 500 mg qid for 14 days
- Erythromycin, 500 mg PO qid for 14 days

PRIMARY AND SECONDARY SYPHILIS OF LESS THAN 1 YEAR DURATION (CHILD). Give benzathine penicillin, G 50,000 U/kg IM, total ≤2.4 MU.

LATE LATENT AND TERTIARY SYPHILIS. Give benzathine penicillin G, 2.4 MU IM every week for 3 weeks.

SYPHILIS IN PREGNANCY
- Penicillin, 2.4 MU IM (dosage and type of penicillin are debatable)
- No alternative is available in pregnancy. All the traditional alternatives have unacceptable side effects.

Client Education

- *Jarisch-Herxheimer reaction* is thought to be a reaction to lysis of treponemes. It occurs in approximately 30% of clients treated for primary syphilis and 70% of those treated for secondary syphilis. Usually, presenting symptoms are fever, chills, myalgia, headache, palpations, flushing, and so on, but it can be severe enough to cause hypotension. Mild forms can be treated with aspirin. More severe forms require emergency care to prevent end-organ damage.
- Importance of compliance with medication if one of the multidose, multiday therapies is initiated
- Barrier protection, including correct use of condoms
- Informing partner of STDs
- Abstinence during treatment and until symptoms resolve
- Identification of chancre and other signs of STDs in partners
- Limit partners
- Risk of other STDs
- Possible HIV testing and counseling

Referral

- Pregnancy
- Penicillin allergy
- HIV positivity
- Persistent elevation of titer
- Late latent syphilis
- Gummas
- Neurosyphilis
- Cardiovascular syphilis

EVALUATION/FOLLOW-UP

Nontreponemal tests at 1 month after treatment and then every 3 months for at least 1 year are required for evaluation. Adequate treatment of primary or secondary syphilis is indicated by a fourfold decrease in the titer by 3 months and by 6 months in latent syphilis. Some clients have a VDRL result that will remain unchanged on subsequent testing after treatment. These clients are considered "serofast" or "seroresistant." For most clients, the titer continues to decrease until it is nonreactive. A fourfold increase in the titer indicates a reinfection that requires further treatment.

A VDRL result obtained from cord blood of a neonate may be reactive as a result of the passive transfer of antibodies from the mother. A VDRL should be performed every month for 3 or 4 months to determine whether the titer is rising or falling. If the titer falls or becomes nonreactive, then the infant had maternal transfer and not congenital syphilis.

REFERENCES

Center for Prevention Services, Venereal Disease Control Division (1988). *Criteria and techniques for the diagnosis of early syphilis.* Atlanta, GA: U.S. Department of Health and Human Services, Public Health Service Centers for Disease Control and Prevention.

Cherniak, D. (1995). *STD handbook.* Montreal, Canada: Montreal Health Press.

Hook, E. W., & Marra, C. M. (1992). Acquired syphilis in adults. *New England Journal of Medicine, 326,* 1060-1067.

Koff, A. B., & Rosen, T. (1993). Nonvenereal treponematoses: Yaws, endemic syphilis and pinta. *Journal of the American Academy of Dermatology, 29*(4), 536-558.

Larsen, S. A., & Beck-Sagué, C. M. (1988). Syphilis. In A. Balows, W. J. Hausler, M. Ohashi, & A. Turano (Eds.), *Laboratory diagnosis of infectious diseases: Principles and practice* (Vol. 1, pp. 490-503). New York: Springer-Verlag.

Lukehart, S. A., & Holmes, K. K. Syphilis. In K. Isselbacher, E. Braunwald, J. Wilson, J. Martin, A. Fauci, & D. Karper (Eds.), *Harrison's principles of internal medicine* (13th ed., pp. 726-737). New York: McGraw-Hill.

Rolfs, R. T. (1995). Treatment of syphilis. *Clinical Infectious Diseases, 20* (Suppl. 1), S23-S38.

Sexually transmitted diseases: Syphilis—Epidemiology and laboratory examinations (1988). Cincinnati, OH: STD Training Center.

Tramont, E. C. (1995). *Treponema pallidum* (syphilis). In G. Mandell, J. Bennett, & R. Dohn (Eds.), *Principles and practice of infectious disease* (4th ed., pp. 2117-2131). New York: Churchill Livingstone.

Zenker, P. N., & Rolfs, R. T. (1989). Treatment of syphilis, 1989. *Review of Infectious Diseases, 12* (Suppl. 6), S590-S609.

REVIEW QUESTIONS

1. Tia is a 20-year-old Hispanic woman who comes to your clinic with a generalized maculopapular rash that includes her palmar and plantar surfaces. She has been living in a metropolitan area, has no regular source of income, and has a history of crack cocaine use. She has syphilis diagnosed. What stage of syphilis does she have?

   a. Primary
   b. Secondary
   c. Tertiary
   d. Late latent

2. Mark is a 25-year-old marketing executive. He is married and has two children. Mark has made an appointment to discuss a penile lesion. Several weeks ago on a business trip, he had unprotected intercourse with a woman he met at the hotel bar. Since returning home, he has had unprotected intercourse with his wife. If this is syphilis, the lesion would be:

   a. A painful erosion associated with tender inguinal lymph nodes
   b. Painless, indurated lesion associated with rubbery inguinal lymph nodes
   c. An indication of an early stage that is too early to be transmitted to his wife
   d. A sign of irreversible damage associated with syphilis

3. To determine the efficacy of treatment for syphilis, the following quantitative testing should be done:

   a. Microscopic examination
   b. Dark-field examination
   c. VDRL
   d. Scraping of the lesion

4. One diagnostic test for syphilis is examination of a scraping from a suspected chancre under a dark-field microscope. A positive test result would show:

   a. A gram-positive diplococcus
   b. Clue cells and many WBCs
   c. Giant cells
   d. A corkscrew-shaped organism

5. A 15-year-old anonymous female client arrives at the STD clinic after being told by her boyfriend that she needs to go to the clinic because he had syphilis. She is anxious, hostile, and angry. The best way to treat her exposure to syphilis and to ensure compliance is to treat her with:

   a. Rocephen, 250 mg IM × 1
   b. Benzathine penicillin G, 2.4 MU IM × 1
   c. Nothing, wait until serology returns before treatment.
   d. Erythromycin 500 mg PO qid for 14 days

ANSWERS AND RATIONALES

1. *Answer:* b (diagnosis/communicable disease/adult)

Rationale: The manifestations of secondary syphilis include a maculopapular rash that involves the plantar and palmar surfaces. The manifestations of primary, tertiary, and late latent syphilis do not include rashes. (Lukehart & Holmes, 1997)

2. *Answer:* b (assessment/history/communicable disease/adult)

Rationale: The typical syphilitic lesion is a painless lesion that may be indurated and associated with rubbery lymph nodes. *T. pallidum* is demonstrated in this primary lesion and can be transmitted at this time. This is also an opportune time to successfully treat syphilis. (Lukehart & Holmes, 1997)

3. *Answer:* c (evaluation/communicable disease/NAS)

Rationale: The VDRL is a quantitative serologic examination that provides a titer to evaluate the efficacy of the treatment. In some instances, the test result does not become negative but does become serofast. A serofast test result may also indicate an effective treatment. (Lukehart & Holmes, 1997)

4. *Answer:* d (assessment/physical examination/communicable disease/NAS)

Rationale: *T. pallidum,* the causative organism of syphilis, is visualized under dark-field microscopy as having a corkscrew appearance and a spiraling motion. (Tramont, 1995)

5. *Answer:* b (plan/communicable disease/adolescent)

Rationale: Benzathine penicillin G, 2.4 MU IM × 1, cures >95% of cases of primary syphilis. (Lukehart & Holmes, 1997)

18

Emergencies

URTICARIA AND ANAPHYLAXIS

OVERVIEW
Definition

There are two types of generalized allergic reactions:

- Urticaria/angioedema (usually not life threatening)
- Anaphylaxis (life threatening)

Urticaria/angioedema consists of lesions (extravascular accumulation of fluid in the dermis) resulting from exposure to an inciting substance.

Anaphylaxis is an acute systemic reaction manifested by sudden onset of pruritus, generalized flush, urticaria, respiratory distress, and vascular collapse (Griffith & Dambro, 1997). It results from an antigen exposure in a sensitized person.

Incidence

- Urticaria occurs at some time in one fifth of the population.
- Anaphylaxis occurs in 1 of 2700 hospitalized clients.
- Hymenoptera (stinging insects) causes allergic reactions in 0.4% of the U.S. population.
- Males and females are affected equally; allergic reactions occur in all age groups.
- Food allergies are much more common in children.

Pathophysiology

The underlying mechanism for both urticaria and anaphylaxis is a classic IgE-mediated allergy, causing an immune response in which chemical mediators (histamine and kinins) are released.

FACTORS INCREASING SUSCEPTIBILITY
- Family history of allergies
- Past history of allergic reaction
- History of asthma, hay fever, or other allergic disorders

COMMON CAUSES OF ALLERGIC REACTIONS
- Beta-lactam antimicrobials: Penicillin most common
- Insect stings: Honeybees/wasps
- Foreign serum
- Vaccines
- Blood products
- Hormones: Adrenocorticotropic hormone (ACTH), insulin, estradiol
- Diagnostic chemicals: Iodine
- Foods: Peanuts, eggs, legumes, popcorn, seafood; in children—milk, chocolate
- NSAIDs, aspirin
- Snake venom
- Animal dander
- Latex
- Exercise

ASSESSMENT: SUBJECTIVE/HISTORY
History of Present Illness

- Determine type of bite, sting, or antigen.
- Determine location of antigen.
- Inquire about time of occurrence.

Most Common Symptoms

- May need to treat quickly if respirations are compromised (given signs and symptoms and past history).

- Urticaria: Itching, transient hives on any part of the body, exposure preceding symptoms, dysphagia; edema
- Anaphylaxis: Generalized itching, erythema of skin followed by sense of warmth and then generalized hives; rapidly progressive respiratory distress; edema

Associated Symptoms

- Presence of systemic symptoms such as fever, chills, nausea, vomiting, and weakness
- Shortness of breath, chest tightness, or facial swelling, throat tightness

Past Medical History

- Hives/urticaria/anaphylaxis
- Hay fever or asthma

Family History

Ask about allergies or allergic reactions.

ASSESSMENT: OBJECTIVE/ PHYSICAL EXAMINATION

Physical Examination

A problem-oriented physical examination should be conducted with particular attention to the following:

- Vital signs: Hypotension
- Skin: Urticaria, cutaneous erythema
- HEENT: Eyelid edema, facial edema, throat swelling
- Respiratory status: Dyspnea, wheezing, shallow respirations
- Cardiovascular status: Tachycardia

Diagnostic Procedures

No diagnostic tests are recommended.

DIAGNOSIS

The differential diagnosis includes the following:

- Urticaria vs anaphylactoid reactions
- Vasovagal reaction
- Hyperventilation episode

THERAPEUTIC PLAN

Treatment depends on the severity of the reaction. If a life-threatening systemic reaction has occurred, follow the ABCs: airway, breathing, and circulation.

Life-Threatening Situation

- Initiate emergency transport service (call 911).
- Administer oxygen; assess the need for intubation.
- Administer epinephrine (1:1000 solution) 0.5 mg SC or IV repeated every 5 to 10 minutes prn. It can also be given via endotracheal tube.
- IV fluids: Administer normal saline or lactated Ringer's solution.
- Aminophylline: For bronchospasm administer 6 mg/kg IV during a period of 10 to 20 minutes.

Non–Life-Threatening Situation

- Administer epinephrine (1:1000 solution; 0.01 ml/kg) 0.3 to 0.5 ml SC every 20 to 30 minutes for up to 3 doses.
- Follow epinephrine with a long-acting agent (Sus-Phrine as a single dose 0.150 to 0.250 ml *SC*).
- Administer diphenhydramine (Benadryl) 25 mg to 50 mg; it may help shorten the duration of the reaction.
- If extensive swelling is present in a local reaction, consider adding a short course of prednisone.

Client Education

- Emphasize the need to have antihistamine or epinephrine (Epi-jet or Epi-pen [spring-loaded automatic injector of epinephrine] or Ana-Kit [contains a preloaded syringe of epinephrine and a chewable antihistamine]) on hand for self-treatment for all people at risk for anaphylaxis from stings.
- Caution the client to avoid insects, food, or drugs that cause reaction.
- Advise the client to wear a medical alert tag identifying the allergy.
- Alert client to beware of taking medications (especially OTC) if he or she has a history of allergic disorders, hay fever, or asthma.
- Warn the client that an acute generalized reaction means there is a potential for a life-threatening reaction in the future.
- Instruct the client that wearing shoes at all times is the single most important safeguard.

Referral

- Refer for allergy testing to identify the sensitizing agent if unknown.
- Immunotherapy reduces the likelihood of a similar reaction from 50% to 5%.

EVALUATION/FOLLOW-UP

- Clients who experience a moderate local reaction or mild allergic reaction: Follow up via phone in 24 hours.
- Clients who experience an anaphylactic reaction: Closely monitor for 12 to 24 hours afterward.

REFERENCES

Griffith, H., & Dambro, M. (1997). *The 5-minute clinical consultant.* Philadelphia: Lea & Febiger.
Kidd, P., & Sturt, P. (1996). *Mosby's emergency nursing reference.* St. Louis: Mosby.
Uphold, C., & Graham, M. (1994). *Clinical guidelines in family health.* Gainesville, FL: Barmarrae Books.
Valentine, M. (1995). Allergy and related conditions. In L. Barker, J. Burton, & P. Zieve (Eds.), *Principles of ambulatory medicine* (4th ed., pp. 277-294). Baltimore: Williams & Wilkins.

REVIEW QUESTIONS

1. Which of the following allergies are more common in children?

   a. Medicine
   b. Pet
   c. Food
   d. Environmental

2. When giving a penicillin injection to a child for the first time, which of the following children would be most likely to have an allergic reaction?

   a. An asthmatic child
   b. A child with an allergy to sulfa
   c. A boy
   d. A child being treated for a rash

3. When assessing a client for a life-threatening allergic reaction, the nurse practitioner should:

   a. Determine the distribution of hives.
   b. Assess the severity of itching.
   c. Ask about shortness of breath.
   d. Check for the presence of edema.

4. When treating a client with anaphylaxis, the nurse practitioner should first:

   a. Call 911.
   b. Administer oxygen.
   c. Administer epinephrine.
   d. Start an IV line.

5. When treating a client with a non–life-threatening allergic reaction, which of the following drugs may be used?

   a. Aminophylline
   b. Prednisone
   c. Ibuprofen
   d. Metaproterenol (Alupent)

ANSWERS AND RATIONALES

1. *Answer:* c (assessment/history/allergies/child)
   Rationale: Food allergies are much more common in children. There are no age distinctions in the other three.

2. *Answer:* a (assessment/history/allergies/child)
   Rationale: Children with an allergic disorder have an increased susceptibility for an allergic reaction. An allergy to sulfa does not indicate the child has an allergy disorder. Boys and girls are equally affected with allergic reactions. A rash may be related to a contagious disease or a nonallergenic source.

3. *Answer:* c (assessment/history/allergies/NAS)
   Rationale: Itching, hives, and edema may be present in both anaphylaxis and urticaria/local allergic reaction. Respiratory distress is associated with anaphylaxis.

4. *Answer:* c (plan/management/therapeutics/pharmacologic/allergies/NAS)
   Rationale: Although the client will need emergency transport and follow-up, initially the client needs epinephrine to counteract the effects of histamine release. Oxygen is necessary but it alone will not help. Epinephrine can be given subcutaneously.

5. *Answer:* b (plan/management/therapeutics/pharmacologic/allergies/NAS)
   Rationale: A life-threatening reaction may be treated with aminophylline, but it would not be the first-line drug. Ibuprofen and metaproterenol (Alupent) are not used. A non–life-threatening reaction is usually treated with epinephrine, antihistamine, and in cases of extensive swelling, prednisone.

PART **II**

Client Wellness

19

Wellness Across the Lifespan

The purpose of well care is to provide individualized care to healthy clients. Identification of risks for preventable illnesses, injuries, and deaths should be incorporated into wellness care. Evidence is abundant that the majority of deaths among Americans younger than age 65 are preventable, often through interventions introduced in the primary care office. Primary care providers have a key role in screening for many of these preventable problems. Equally important is the role of the provider in counseling clients to improve lifestyle behaviors, such as diet, smoking, alcohol use, exercise, injuries, and sexually transmitted diseases.

Although immunizations and screening tests are important, the most promising arena for prevention lies in changing the personal health behaviors of clients long before a clinical disease develops. Smoking contributes to one of every five deaths in the United States, including coronary artery disease, chronic obstructive pulmonary disease, and cerebrovascular disease. Motor vehicle crashes and injuries are compounded by failure to use seat belts and by the use of alcohol. Physical activity and dietary factors contribute to atherosclerosis, cancer, diabetes, and osteoporosis. High-risk sexual behaviors result in unintended pregnancy and various sexually transmitted diseases, including AIDS. Approximately one half of all deaths in the United States can be attributed to the above factors and have the potential for reduction through changes in personal behaviors (McGinnis & Foege, 1993).

Clinical preventive care can be defined as "an integral part of preventive health care concerned with the maintenance and promotion of health and the reduction of risk factors which result in injury and disease" (*ACPM News*, 1989). Components of clinical preventive care include:

- Assessment of individuals' risk for disease
- Implementation of interventions to modify or eliminate risk for disease/injury
- Integration and monitoring of personal prevention behaviors

Barriers to preventive care include:

- Failure of clinician to provide recommended clinical preventive services
- Inadequate reimbursement for preventive care
- Fragmentation of health care delivery
- Insufficient time during appointment
- Recommendations from multiple sources, sometimes contradictory
- Uncertainty as to effectiveness of preventive services

The U.S. Preventive Services Task Force was established in 1984 to address the issues of preventive care. This panel was charged with the task of developing preventive recommendations based on a systemic review of evidence of clinical effectiveness. Its findings include:

- Interventions that address personal health practices are vitally important.
- The provider and the client should share decision making.
- Clinicians should be selective in ordering tests and providing preventive services.
- Every opportunity must be taken to deliver preventive services, especially in those clients with limited access to care.
- For some health problems, community level interventions may be more effective than clinical preventive services (U.S. Preventive Services Task Force, 1996).

This chapter reviews the recommendations for health prevention and health promotion for all age groups.

INFANT 0 TO 12 MONTHS

Table 19-1   Growth and Development: 0 to 12 Months

SYSTEM	0-3 MONTHS	4-6 MONTHS	7-12 MONTHS
Neurologic	Turns head side to side by 1 mo. Head lag when pulled from supine to sitting until 2-3 mo. Upright head control should be obtained. Landau (ventral suspension): Flexion position Reaching/grasping; palmar grasp at birth until about 2 mo By 3 mo, growing hand-eye coordination and infant attempts contact with objects and holds briefly.	Raises head and chest with arms extended. Raises head on vertical axis and turns head from side to side. Pulled from supine to sitting with no head lag. In a sitting position, head may tilt a little forward but no head bobbing. Head is erect by 5 mo. By 5-6 mo, infant is purposefully rolling over, first front to back and then back to front. By 4 mo, infant loses tonic neck reflex and head stays midline with extensors in more of a symmetric position. Infant regards hands, brings them to midline and mouth (symmetrotonic posture). Infant bears the weight of an erect head and enjoys being supported in upright position. At 4 mo, infant has increased attention for various objects. By 6 mo, infant reaches out for, retrieves, and transfers object from hand to hand. After discovering hands, discovers rest of body: face, head, trunk, lower extremities, and genitals. At 4 mo, enjoys standing erect. By 5-6 mo, can pull from sitting to a standing position and can bear weight by holding hands. By 6½ mo, can do this and then flex their knees momentarily. Infant sits alone with head erect.	By 7 mo, is able to pivot in pursuit of an object. By 8-9 mo, many infants stand for a few seconds independently, cruising by 9 mo. By 9-10 mo, takes a few steps with hands held. Between 6-9 mo, radial-palmar grasp moves to thumb and forefinger (pincher) grasp; by 12 mo, pincher grasp is used without the ulnar surface. At 9 mo, uses finger to poke at objects. By 9 mo, is able to release an object by request; looks for objects (object permanency) and finds hidden objects if in sight. By 12 mo, is able to release object into hand.

Vision	Neonates fixate and track an object to midline. By 2 mo, objects are followed past midline. By 3 mo, objects are tracked 180 degrees; peripheral vision is 180 degrees by 2 mo. By 6 wk, binocular vision begins, and it is well established by 4 mo. Acuity at birth is 200/200-200/400; by 3-4 mo, it is 20/200-20/300.	Visual accommodation equals that of adults; infant follows objects 180 degrees; perceives the color spectrum similar to adults; visual acuity 20/200 to 20/300. Infant prefers moving objects. By 5-6 mo, visual acuity is 20/40-20/60. EOMI, cover-uncover test WNL.	Equal tracking; EOMI, improving eye-hand coordination
Hearing	Responds to human voice; positive startle reflex with loud noises. By 2 mo, turns head to side when sound is made at ear level. By 3 mo, makes initiative to look toward sounds; can discriminate between pitch.	Turns to sound; responds to human voice, discriminates between pitch sounds.	Infants can locate sounds, recognize their name, understand commands, but usually do not obey. By 12 mo, will follow some simple commands
Dental	There is increase in salivation at 3 mo. May begin teething as early as 3-4 mo.	Infant may begin teething; teeth eruption.	Lower and upper incisors usually are present; lateral incisors should be erupting or present.
Nutrition	Intake of 110 kcal/kg/day is needed.	Intake of 110 kcal/kg/day is needed, with feeding 4-6 times per day, 4-6 oz q 4-6 hr (24-32 oz).	Eating time is a socialization process at 9-12 mo. Infants want to be a part of family meal times.
Breast-feeding	Neonate: Feeds q 1-2 hr; 2 wk to 1 mo: Feeds q 2-4 hr; 1-2 mo: Feeds q 4-6 hr	By 4 mo, tongue thrusting diminishes and infants turn their heads if full.	Infant shows interest in drinking from a cup, attempts to feed self.
Formula	Neonate: Feeds 2-3 oz q 2-3 hr; 2 wk-1 mo: Feeds 3-4 oz q 3-4 hr; 2-3 mo: Feeds 4-6 oz q 4-6 hr		By 12 mo, drinks from a cup; feeds self. Needs approximately 12-16 oz milk/day. By 12 mo, infant is self-feeder, there is decrease in growth demands, therefore decrease in appetite. May be picky eater.

Continued

EOMI, Extraocular movements intact; *WNL,* within normal limits.

Table 19-1   Growth and Development: 0 to 12 Months—cont'd

SYSTEM	0-3 MONTHS	4-6 MONTHS	7-12 MONTHS
Sleep	Neonates alert 1 hr/10 hr. Neonates are awake 3-4 hr/24 hr. By 2 mo, infants may be awake as long as 10 hr/day. Usually infant sleeps 4-6 hr at night. By 3 mo, infant should be sleeping 3-8 hr at night.	Infant sleeps in own bed, own room; sleeps 6-8 hr; by 5-6 mo, sleeps 8-10 hr, 1-2 naps, begins to resist separation; begins to experience night awakening (does not need nighttime bottle) by 5-6 mo.	Infants may have decreased naps to 1 per day. They have more wakeful periods at night. A bedtime routine should be established.
Elimination	Stools begin as loose and watery; as infant matures, stools become more formed. Breast-fed infants: Stools with every feeding, UOP 6-8 wet diapers Formula-fed infant: Stools 1x/day, 1 every other day or 1 every 3rd day; UOP 6-8 wet diapers	Stools are formed; color changes are related to solids; bladder capacity is increasing, urination decreasing.	Stools are formed, 1-2 per day. UOP is same as at 4-6 mo.
Speech/Language	By 4 wk, makes throaty noises. Infant focuses on significant other and imitates. By 2 mo, makes vowel sounds and cooing. By 3 mo, infant attempts to make sounds in relation to socialization.	Infant continues to imitate; coos, babbles, squeals, laughs, vocalizes to mirror.	By 6½ mo, infant produces repetitive vowel sounds. By 9 mo, infant enjoys imitating sounds like "Mama" and "Dada" with babbling. Infant recognizes words said by others (mom, dog, etc.). By 8-9 mo, infant responds to own name. By 1 yr, infant says 1-3 words related to object.
Psychosocial	Social smile is fully developed by 3-5 wk. (Infants who do not develop social smile by 3 mo may be an early identification of problems). Neonate makes eye-to-eye contact and focuses on faces. By 3 mo, infant can recognize familar faces.	Infants 4 mo old begin to laugh, squeal, or blow bubbles as part of social exchange; they are able to show displeasure by facial expressions. By 4-7 mo, infant responds to emotional tones of social contacts. By 6 mo, demonstrated social preference to caregivers; when mom is around, can display stranger anxiety. Development of separation anxieties may depend on infant's comfort with communication and emotional exchange.	Infant is developing into very social being; plays games and enjoys books and being read to for very short periods. Infant tries to figure out how things work, likes to manipulate objects. Infant imitates activities of caregiver; interacts with others; parallel play, separation anxiety, stranger anxiety are seen.

UOP, Urinary output.

Table 19-2   Well-Child Care: 0 to 12 Months

	0-3 MONTHS	4-6 MONTHS	7-12 MONTHS
S	History: Determine any problems or changes since last seen. Ask about sleeping, elimination, immunizations, concerns of parents, birth history if has never been seen before. Nutrition: How often, how much formula or breast milk, feeding problems. Development: Infant cuddles, follows to midline, responds to sound, smiles with parent-child interaction. Family: Mom's health and rest, family adjustment to baby, child care issues, dad's involvement, support system, parents getting out and getting rest.	History: Determine any problems or changes since last seen. Ask about sleeping, elimination, immunization reactions and what immunizations have been completed, birth history if never seen before, parents' concerns. Nutrition: How often, how much formula or breast milk, feeding problems, solids Development: Infant follows 180 degrees, responds to voice, grasps rattle, rolls over one way, lifts head to 90 degrees, babbles, no head lag, coos, transfers, rolls over, sits up with minimal support. Family: Mom's health, dad's involvement, sibling adjustment.	History: Determine any problems or changes since last seen. Ask about sleeping, elimination, immunization reactions and what immunizations have been completed, birth history if never seen before, parents' concerns. Nutrition: How often, how much formula or breast milk, feeding problems, solids, feeding self with finger foods, fluoride Development: Infant plays peek-a-boo, looks for fallen object, pincher grasp, "mama, dada," crawls, sits without support, stands holding on, pat-a-cake, bangs 2 blocks together, imitates sounds, understands "no," cruises, stands alone 2-3 sec. Family: Family schedule, outside supports.
O	Physical examination (child is usually not fearful of strangers): 2 weeks: Infant gains 15-30 g, back to birth weight. Height, weight, HC. Skin, nodes, head, fontanelles, (flat, soft), eye (red reflex), ears, nose, oropharynx, neck, chest/breast, lungs, heart, abdomen, umbilicus: cord off, genitalia (testes descended), femoral pulse, musculoskeletal, hips (clicks/clunks), Moro's reflex, palmar reflex, plantar grasp, spine 2 months: Weight gain 15-30 g (1 oz/day), 1 inch/mo. Skin, nodes, head, fontanelles (posterior fused), eye (red reflex), ears, nose, oropharynx, neck, chest/breast, lungs, heart, abdomen, umbilicus (cord off), genitalia (testes descended), femoral pulse, musculoskeletal, hips (clicks/clunks), Moro's reflex, plantar grasp (less intense).	Physical examination (child is usually fearful of strangers): Height, weight, HC. Skin, nodes, head, fontanelles (flat, soft), eye (red reflex), visual tracking (cover-uncover at 6 mo), ears, nose, oropharynx, teeth and gums, neck, chest/breast, lungs, heart, abdomen, genitalia (testes descended), femoral pulse, musculoskeletal, hips (clicks/clunks), Moro's and tonic neck reflexes (disappear by 6 mo), plantar grasp	Physical examination (child is usually fearful of strangers): Height, weight, HC. Skin, nodes, head, fontanelles (flat, soft), eye (cover-uncover), ears, nose, oropharynx, neck, chest/breast, lungs, heart, abdomen, genitalia (testes descended), femoral pulse, musculoskeletal, plantar grasp (disappears by 8 mo), positive pincher, positive parachute reflex

Continued

HC, Head circumference.

Table 19-2 Well-Child Care: 0 to 12 Months—cont'd

	0-3 MONTHS	4-6 MONTHS	7-12 MONTHS
Dx	WCC Possible problems: Metabolic disorders, intestinal obstruction, cardiac anomalies, congenital defects, apnea, gastroesophageal reflux, FTT, STD (congenital syphilis, HIV, *Chlamydia*), abuse	WCC Possible problems: FTT, URI, OM, viral exanthem, diaper dermatitis, candidiasis diaper rash, atopic dermatitis, gastroenteritis, dacryostenosis, conjunctivitis, abuse	WCC Possible problems: OM, diaper dermatitis, URI, amblyopia, tibial torsion, genu varum; developmental delay, trained night feeders, undescended testicles, hypospadias, abuse
P	Immunizations DPT 1, HIB 1, IPV 1, HBV 2 Check neonatal screening results at 2 wk.	Immunizations 4 mo: DPT 2, HIB 2, IPV 2 6 mo: DPT 3, HIB 3, HBV 3 Sickle preparation if indicated	Immunizations 9 mo: Up to date 12 mo: DPT 4, HIB 4, oral polio vaccine 4, MMR 1; can offer varicella. Screen for lead level and CBC (or Hct) TB if indicated
E Guidance	Follow-up: 2 mo; next visit at 4 mo Assess parental ability to learn, previous experience as parent, educational level. Development: Review expected developmental changes, basic trust vs mistrust. Nutrition: Continue formula/breast, (25 oz formula/day 4-6 oz/time). Safety: Car, crib, falls, smoke alarm Parenting: Cuddling, talking to baby, music Potential problems: Possible diaper rash, spitting up, colic and crying	Follow-up: 6 mo, 9 mo Assess parental ability to learn, previous experience as parent, educational level. Development: Review expected developmental changes, basic trust vs mistrust. Nutrition: Continue formula/breast (5 feedings, 6-8 oz/time), can offer water especially during hot weather. At 6 mo, add 1 new food at a time/week for allergies. Can begin cereal* with iron (1-2 tbsp 1 time/day) increasing up to 1/3-1/2 cup (2 times/day), then add fruits and vegetables (1 tsp at a time) Safety: Car, crib, falls, smoke alarm, babyproof house, all objects go into mouth, choking, bathing, Poison Control number Parenting: Call child by name, use soft music, touching games such as "little piggy." Potential problems: Possible diaper rash, teething, susceptible to infections, sleep patterns (night awakening), dental hygiene (no bottle in bed)	Follow-up: 12 mo, 15-18 mo Assess parental ability to learn, prior experience as parent, educational level. Development: Review expected developmental changes, basic trust vs mistrust. Nutrition: Decrease in formula to 12-16 oz/day (8 mo), introduce cup, tolerance and acceptance of new foods. Introduce meat, breads, rice, macaroni, soft cheese, and egg yolks; decrease calorie intake, child will eat if hungry. Balanced diet, uses cup; use high chair to make child part of family mealtime. Safety: Check lead risks, gates on stairs, electrical outlets capped, car seat, playpen or crib for safe place, constant watching, falls and burns, poison (ipecac). Parenting: Reinforce positive behavior, stimulation (toy phone, name body parts, blowing games, noisy push/pulls, hugs/kisses), discipline, bedtime routine, separation and stranger anxiety, reading, dental care (no toothpaste). Prevention: Dental hygiene, weaning from bottle, pacifier

WCC, well-child check; *FTT*, failure to thrive; *STD*, sexually transmitted disease; *URI*, upper respiratory tract infection; *OM*, otitis media; *DPT*, diphtheria-pertussis-tetanus vaccine; *HIB*, *Haemophilus influenzae* B vaccine; *IPV*, inactivated poliomyelitis vaccine; *MMR*, measles-mumps-rubella vaccine; *CBC*, complete blood cell count; *Hct*, hematocrit; *TB*, tuberculosis.

*Rice cereal is less allergenic.

CHILD 1 TO 10 YEARS

Table 19-3 Growth and Development: 1 to 10 Years

SYSTEM	12-24 MONTHS	24-35 MONTHS	3-5 YEARS	5-10 YEARS
Neurologic	By 12 mo, infant moves to an upright stance, takes a few independent steps or should be walking; walking should be accomplished by no later than 15-18 mo. By 15 mo, gait is ataxic but symmetric stoops and recovers. By 18 mo, infant walks up stairs holding on; runs; walks backward. By 20 mo, goes down stairs. At 24 mo, able to run about; kicks ball. By 12 mo, infant can release object into hand. By 15 mo, can place raisin into bottle. By 18 mo, infant can remove raisin by dumping it out. Infant can make a tower of blocks of 2 cubes at 15 mo; at 18 mo, can make a tower of 4 cubes; by 24 mo, makes a tower of 6 cubes.	At 2 yr, child is able to kick a ball without falling. Child progresses to being able to kick a ball 10 feet at 3 yr. Child runs and jumps with both feet, jumps from chair or step, rides a push toy to pedaling a tricycle at 3 yr. By 3 yr, fine and gross motor skills are becoming more refined, smoother, and more coordinated. Child enjoys physical play. Child is able to walk upstairs and downstairs holding onto railing with 2 feet on step. Child begins to scribble at 2 yr. Child draws a circle, matches colors; crosses midline; can use scissors by age 3 yr. By 3 yr, child can make a tower of 8 blocks; makes a bridge after demonstration.	Preschooler is slender but sturdy, graceful, and agile, with erect posture. Hops, skips and climbs. Child advances with fine motor skills; copies figures and draws recognizable pictures.	At 6-8 yr, gross and fine motor skills become more controlled, with improved eye-hand coordination; child prints, colors in lines, ties bow; rides bike, hops, jumps. By 10 yr, gross and fine motor skills are more precise; child does tricks with bicycle, cursive writing, makes crafts, organized sports.
Vision	Smooth ocular movements; depth perception, good eye-hand coordination; intense interest in bright colors and different shapes.	Visual acuity is 20/80, with depth perception. Child copies a vertical line; color recognition not until 3 1/2 to 4 yr.	Visual capabilities continue to undergo refinement during preschool period. Color vision and depth perception are fully established. Visual acuity: 3 yr—20/50; 4 yr—20/40; 5 yr—20/30; hyperopic	At 6-8 yr, visual acuity 20/20; no color blindness

Continued

Table 19-3 Growth and Development: 1 to 10 Years—cont'd

SYSTEM	12-24 MONTHS	24-35 MONTHS	3-5 YEARS	5-10 YEARS
Hearing	Infant is reactive to whispering, localizes sounds well, understands most commands, recognizes name readily, and recognizes familiar words.	By 3 yr, acuity is at adult level; child is aware of pitch and tone.	Hearing develops to adult level; child is able to make fine discriminations among similar speech sounds, such as the differences between f, th, and s.	Normal
Dental	Infant may have as many as 6 teeth; during second year, 8 more teeth should erupt. First-year molars, cuspids, then second-year molars come in. Brush teeth bid with a washcloth until infant is able to spit. Infant no longer uses bottle by 15-18 mo.	Between 24-36 mo, dentition is completed.	Twenty deciduous teeth are present; primary teeth are important for chewing, speech, and to hold spaces for secondary teeth. Older preschoolers can be responsible for brushing with gentle reminding from parents.	Permanent teeth continue to erupt; continue brushing and flossing with regular dental visits.
Nutrition	By 1 yr, change to whole milk until 2 yr. Give soft table foods, with more textured foods by 15-18 mo. Infant usually eats one balanced meal, with decreased food intake related to decreased growth rate.	Average need at 2-3 yr is 100 kcal/kg/day. Fat should be approximately 30% or less. Calcium needs to be approximately 700 mg/day.	Average preschooler needs 95 kcal/kg/day. Child has definite food preferences; is likely to refuse new foods.	At 5-8 yr, child needs approximately 80 kcal/kg/day. Increased appetite, 3 meals/day plus 1-2 snacks. At 8-10 yr, nutrition is still under primary control of parent, but child is eating away from home more and more and influenced by peers and TV. Child likes a variety of foods, especially fast foods and snacks.
Sleep	Sleep is fitful at night; more REM periods. Increased tension; infant may have fits or energy bursts at night, rock crib, bang head. Infant naps, usually once per day. Infant sleeps 10-12 hr/day.	Child usually sleeps 10-12 hr; may still take afternoon naps; sleeps all night; enjoys sleeping with favorite toy or blanket; begins to be afraid of the dark. Bed should have side rails.	Average sleep is 8-12 hr/night. Bedtime rituals are still important; nightmares and night terrors can be common in this age group because of active imaginations.	Average sleep is 8-10 hr/night. Child usually resists bedtime, develops stall tactics.

REM, Rapid eye movement.

Elimination	Stools are formed, urine more concentrated; infant may show interest in potty.	Maturation of cortex layers is seen; sensory development for bladder and bowel control; elimination, especially of stool, is expression of pleasure in what a child of 2-3 yr has to produce. Nighttime wetting is not expected to end until 3-6 yr.	Child should have established daytime bowel and bladder control. Nighttime bladder control is usually accomplished by 3-6 yr. Around 5 yr, child should be able to manage toileting independently.	Normal patterns are established.
Speech and language	By 18 mo, vocabulary is about 10 words. Rapid learning of words and meanings usually develops by this time.	By 2 yr, >50 words is common vocabulary; child uses 2 word sentences, knows 5-6 body parts. Dysfluencies are common, child uses plurals, present verb tense; recognizes 3 colors. By 3 yr, child speaks in 3-4 word sentences; speech is clear. Child uses pronouns, negatives, past tense, understands some adjectives (e.g., big or little).	Language is sophisticated and complex; 3-4 yr, 3-4 word sentences; 4-5 yr, 4-5 word sentences with lots of why questions. Speech often has hesitations, repetitions, and revisions. Stuttering and stammering should be evaluated if lasting longer than 6 mo. Quality and quantity of language in home have the most important impact on the child's language development.	At 5 to 8 yr, child uses all parts of speech; learns to read; arranges story in sequence; composes stories; defines words according to related action. By 10 yr, uses metaphors; personifications; speech understable. Quick to use slang; loves jokes and humor.
Psycho-social	Toddlers develop sense of control over their bodies and expressively demonstrate this (temper tantrums, breath-holding spells, and biting). Infant is developing sense of self separate from others, striving for independence by taking initiative in making choices about behaviors.	Child is egocentric, has better sense of time, anticipates consequences from parents to form more careful actions, pretends, with magical thinking, dramatic-imitation play. Child moves from sensory to intuitive learning, with development of memory, symbolic play, global organization.	Child separates with some apprehension at 3 yr. By 4-5 yr, child relates to unfamiliar people easily, tolerates periods of separation. Child enjoys playing and interacting with other children. Child progresses from associative play to cooperative play. Egocentric behaviors are still present; role play, make-believe, or fantasy play.	Child is very sociable, group play increases, becomes competitive, learns to share, cooperates in organized manner. By 8-10 yr, child enjoys team sports, parties, sleepovers. Child needs time for free play; do not overschedule.

Table 19-4   Well-Child Care: 1 to 10 Years

	12-24 MONTHS	24-36 MONTHS	3-5 YEARS	5-10 YEARS
S	History: Determine any problems since last seen, any parental concerns. Ask about sleeping, elimination, illnesses, injuries, immunizations, birth history if never seen before. Nutrition: Number of meals/day, varied diet, balanced diet, fluoride, mealtime problems Development: Child drinks from cup, crawls up stairs, throws ball, walks well, removes clothes, stacks 2-3 blocks, walks up steps with help, knows body parts, uses 2-3 word sentences, handles spoon well. Family: Parents agree on discipline, child care, sibling rivalry.	History: Determine any problems since last seen, any parental concerns. Ask about sleeping, elimination, illnesses, injuries, immunizations, birth history if never seen before. Nutrition: Number of meals/day, varied diet, balanced diet, fluoride, mealtime problems. Development: Child follows simple directions, knows full name, sex, knows 1 color, uses plurals, rides tricycle. Family: Discipline, child care, sibling rivalry, playmates, family activities, FH of early MI, high cholesterol Ask child questions and have him or her follow directions to test hearing.	History: Determine any problems since last seen, any parental concerns. Ask about sleeping, elimination, illnesses, injuries, immunizations, birth history if never seen before. Nutrition: Number of meals/day, varied diet, balanced diet, fluoride, mealtime problems; child enjoys helping prepare meals. Development: Child puts toys away, knows prepositions, knows 3-4 colors, uses verbs and full sentences, hops on 1 foot, dresses alone, understands opposites, copies square and triangle, draws man (3-6 parts), uses heel-to-toe walk. Assess school readiness. Family: Mom and dad's work, family happy, discipline, any new family members, smokers or alcohol or drug use	History: Determine any problems since last seen, any parental concerns. Ask about sleeping, elimination, illnesses, injuries, immunizations, birth history if never seen before. Ask about menses for girl, sexual activity. Nutrition: Number of meals/day, varied diet, balanced diet, fluoride, mealtime problems Developmental: Behavior includes chores, outside activities, reading for pleasure. Child knows days of week, skips rope, tells time, peer interaction and organized sports. Family: Family schedule, family activities, discipline, new family members, any smokers or alcohol or drug use, after-school care, firearms at home, sibling problems or rivalry
O	Physical examination (fear of strangers): Height, weight, HC	Physical examination (fear of strangers): Height, weight (3 inches of height, 5 lb of weight per yr), HC	Physical examination (may be cooperative; parents close): Height (±3 inches per yr), weight, vital signs, vision screening, hearing	Physical examination (usually cooperative, older child may want privacy): Height, weight, vital signs, vision and hearing screening

FH, Family history; *MI,* myocardial infarction; *HBV,* hepatitis B virus.

	Skin, nodes, head, fontanelles, eye (cover-uncover), ears, nose, oropharynx, teeth and gums, neck, chest/breast, lungs, heart, abdomen, genitalia, musculoskeletal, neurologic	Skin, nodes, head, eye (fundi, cover-uncover), ears (whisper test), nose, oropharynx, teeth and gums, neck, chest/breast, lungs, heart, abdomen, genitalia	Skin, nodes, head, eye (fundi, cover-uncover), ears, nose, oropharynx, teeth and gums, neck, chest/breast, lungs, heart, abdomen, genitalia	Skin, nodes, head, eye (fundi cover-uncover), ears, nose, oropharynx, teeth and gums, neck, chest/breast, lungs, heart, abdomen, genitalia, Tanner staging, scoliosis screening
Dx	WCC Possible problems: Dental caries, developmental delays, intoeing, chronic OM, conductive hearing loss, croup, pica, impetigo	WCC Possible problems: Speech delays, tibial torsion, nursemaid elbow, encopresis, sexual abuse, stomatitis, pinworms, septic arthritis	WCC Possible problems: Hypertension, primary enuresis, masturbation, night terrors, coxsackievirus, varicella, osteomyelitis, dental caries	WCC Possible problems: Enuresis, poor school performance, sibling rivalry, abuse, dental caries, vision or hearing problems, eating disorders
P	MMR 1; offer varicella vaccine if child has not had chickenpox. Start HBV series if child has not gotten. Screen for TB exposure. Do lead screen if not already done.	Screen for TB exposure. Offer varicella vaccine if child has not had chickenpox.	Offer varicella vaccine if child has not had chickenpox. Immunizations (5 yr): DP at 5, OPV 4, MMR 2	Offer varicella vaccine if child has not had chickenpox. Assess for TB. Assess for HBV.
E Guidance	Follow-up: 15-18 mo, 2 yr Assess parental ability to learn, previous experience as parent, educational level. Development: Review expected developmental changes, autonomy vs shame.	Follow-up: 3 yr Assess parental ability to learn, previous experience as parent, educational level. Development: Review expected developmental changes, autonomy vs shame.	Follow-up: Yearly check Assess parental ability to learn, previous experience as parent, educational level. Development: Review expected developmental changes, initiative vs guilt.	Follow-up: Yearly check Assess parental ability to learn, previous experience as parent, educational level. Development: Review expected developmental changes, industry vs inferiority. Child goes from learning through intuition to learning through concrete experiences; discuss expected pubertal changes, body odor.

Continued

Table 19-4   Well-Child Care: 1 to 10 Years—cont'd

12-24 MONTHS	24-36 MONTHS	3-5 YEARS	5-10 YEARS
Nutrition: Stress need for balanced diet, milk intake 12-16 oz; decreased growth so decreased intake. Avoid soda, give fruit juice, not fruit drinks, discontinue bottle; decrease junk food.	Nutrition: Stress need for balanced diet, milk intake 12-16 oz; decreased growth so decreased intake. Avoid soda, give fruit juice, not fruit drinks, discontinue bottle; decrease junk food; no potato chips, coconut, nuts, whole kernel corn, hot dogs, raw carrots (aspiration).	Nutrition: Stress need for balanced diet, milk intake 12-16 oz. Offer raw vegetables during day; avoid soda, give fruit juice, not fruit drinks, discontinue bottle; decrease junk food.	Nutrition: Stress need for balanced diet. Avoid soda, give fruit juice, not fruit drinks; decrease junk food.
Safety: Aspiration, pets, plastic bags, outdoors, climbing out of crib, poison (ipecac), drowning	Safety: Aspiration, pets, plastic bags, outdoors, climbing out of crib, poison (ipecac), drowning	Safety: Pets, plastic bags, outdoors, poison (ipecac), strangers, tricycle/bike (helmets), drowning, matches, guns	Safety: Outdoors, bike (helmet), strangers, car, drowning, guns
Parenting: Consistent discipline; reinforce positive behavior, set limits; let child problem solve, play; read to child. Issues may include thumb sucking; dental care; naps.	Parenting: Toilet training, dental care, play; reading books, TV limits, 1 long nap/day, need for large-muscle use activity, anticipating consequences, dramatic play, discipline (limit setting), positive role model	Parenting: Ignore stuttering, provide positive role model for speech, provide a listener to allow child to express ideas and feelings, set TV limits, use consistent schedule, positive reinforcement, develop and enforce family rules, give chores; at 5 yr, child should learn/know telephone number and address.	Parenting: Consistent schedule, positive reinforcement, family rules developed and enforced, chores, positive role model, participation in school activities, limit on TV, time to talk with child, new responsibilities given with appropriate supervision, allowance, respect, communication
		Nightmares: Need lots of reassurance, explain difference between real and pretend; monitor TV viewing.	
		Preventive: Dental appointment, brushing at least bid	Preventive: Dental appointment, brushing teeth at least bid, emergency plan developed, discussion of drugs, alcohol, and smoking

REFERENCES

ACPM News, The Newsletter of the American College of Preventive Medicine 1, 3, 1989.

American Academy of Pediatrics (1997). Active and passive immunizations. In G. Peter (Ed.), *1997 Red book: Report of the Committee on Infectious Disease* (24th ed., pp. 1-71). Elk Grove Village, IL: Author.

Baker, R. (1996). *Handbook of pediatric primary care.* Boston: Little, Brown.

Barkauskas, V., Stoltenberg-Allen, K., Baumann, L., & Darling-Fisher, C. (1994). *Health and physical assessment.* St. Louis: Mosby.

Behrman, R. E., & Kleigman, R. (1992). *Nelson essentials of pediatrics* (14th ed.). Philadelphia: W. B. Saunders.

Brady, M. (1994). Patient management exchange: Educating youths and their parents about the prevention of firearm injury. *Journal of Pediatric Health Care, 8*(3), 127-129.

Hoekelman, R. A., Friedman, S., Nelson, N., & Seidel, H. (1992). *Primary pediatric care.* (2nd ed.). St. Louis: Mosby.

McGinnis, J., & Foege, W. (1993). Actual causes of death in the US. *JAMA, 270,* 2207-2212.

Ramos A. G., & Tuchman D. N. (1994). Persistent vomiting. *Pediatrics in Review, 5*(1), 24-31.

Schmitt, B. (1987). *Your child's health.* New York: Bantam.

U.S. Preventive Services Task Force (1996). *Guide to clinical preventive services* (2nd ed.). Baltimore: Williams & Wilkins.

WELL ADOLESCENT

Pubertal changes occur in a predictable sequence for all adolescents. The ages at which changes begin vary according to genetic, socioeconomic, and nutritional factors. The rate at which the changes occur is regarded as the *tempo*. There may be individual variances in tempo as well. The most prominent changes are in terms of the secondary sexual characteristics; however, changes in the endocrine glands, lymphatic system, brain, and body fat composition occur as well.

Table 19-5 Growth and Development: 11 to 21 Years

MAJOR EVENTS OF PUBERTY	SKELETAL GROWTH	SECONDARY SEX CHARACTERISTICS	SEQUENCE OF EVENTS: MALE	SEQUENCE OF EVENTS: FEMALE
Typical ages to begin puberty: Males, 11-12 yr, normal range 9-14 yr Females, 10-11 yr, range 8-13 yr	Body attains one fourth total adult height, with growth occurring in distal portions of limbs before proximal portions and trunk.	Females enter puberty earlier than males and take longer to complete the process. Average length of pubertal events for males is 3-4 yr; that for females is 4-5 yr.	Growth of testicles Pubic hair appears. Growth of penis and scrotum Axillary hair First ejaculations (average 13-14 yr) Growth spurt Facial hair Adult height	Ovaries increase in size. Breast buds appear, and/or pubic hair appears. Growth spurt Pubic hair matures. Breasts mature. Axillary hair Menarche (range 10-16 yr) Adult height

Table 19-6 Tanner Staging: Female

TANNER 1	TANNER 2	TANNER 3	TANNER 4	TANNER 5
Tanner stage 1 is prepubertal; there is no observable change.	Small, raised breast bud; sparse growth of fine downy hair, usually along sides of labia	There is general enlargement of breast, with elevation of entire breast and areola from general chest contour. Breast development is best assessed from a side view. Pubic hair is darker, coarser, and curlier; it extends over the middle of the pubic bone. This is usually period of most rapid growth.	Areola and papilla form a contour separate from rest of breast. Pubic hair has adult characteristics but does not extend to medial thigh. Menarche generally occurs during this stage.	Areola has same contour as rest of the breast, with an increase in overall size of breast. Pubic hair extends from thigh to thigh; some females may have additional growth at midline to form triangle.

Table 19-7 Tanner Staging: Male

TANNER 1	TANNER 2	TANNER 3	TANNER 4	TANNER 5
There is no pubic hair growth; child is prepubertal in appearance. Testes 1 cm	Sparse growth of fine, downy hair along base of penis. Slight enlargement, increased texture of scrotum. Testes 2-3.2 cm.	Hair becomes darker, coarser, and curlier and spreads over middle of pubic bone. Further growth and enlargement occurs. Testes 3.3-4 cm	Hair takes on adultlike characteristics but does not extend to thighs. Penis is significantly enlarged in length and circumference. Size of testes increases (4-4.9 cm), with darkening of scrotal skin.	Hair is distributed from thigh to thigh and may extend up to navel. Adult-sized genitalia (testes 5 cm)

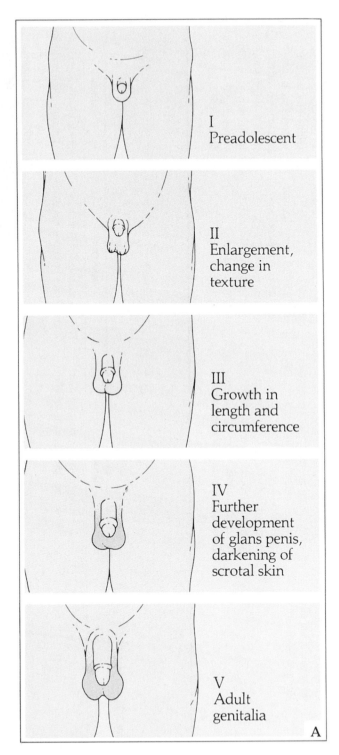

Figure 19-1 Schematic drawings of male and female Tanner stages. **A,** Male genital development. (Modified from Johnson, T.R., Moore, W.M., & Jefferies, J.E. [1978]. *Children are different: Development physiology* [2nd ed., pp. 26-29]. Columbus, OH: Ross Laboratories.)

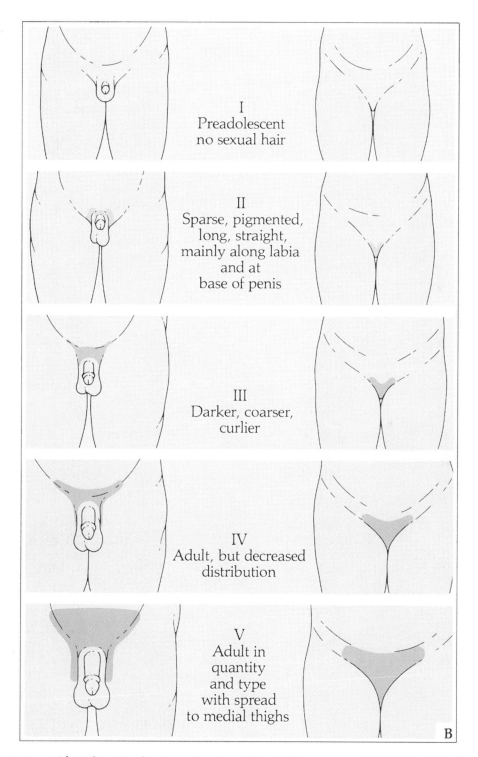

Figure 19-1, cont'd Schematic drawings of male and female Tanner stages. **B,** Pubic hair development.

Continued

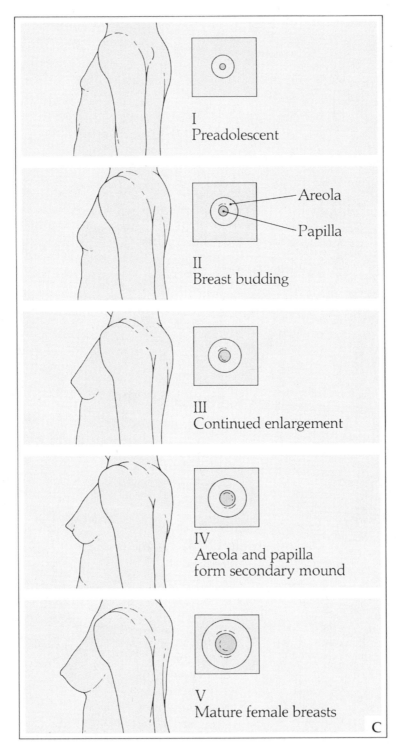

Figure 19-1, cont'd Schematic drawings of male and female Tanner stages. **C,** Breast development. (Modified from Johnson, T.R., Moore, W.M., & Jefferies, J.E. [1978]. *Children are different: Development physiology* [2nd ed., pp. 26-29]. Columbus, OH: Ross Laboratories.)

Table 19-8 Well Adolescent: 11 to 21 Years

	EARLY ADOLESCENT (11-14 YR)	MIDDLE ADOLESCENT (15-17 YR)	LATE ADOLESCENT (18-21 YR)
S	*Review of Systems* **Lifestyle** Family relationships, school, peer group activities, tobacco, drug and alcohol use, sexual involvement, legal history **Parent/Guardian** Home setting: Who lives with client, own room, relationships at home, what do parents do for a living, recent moves, running away, new people in home? Education/employment: School grade performance/changes, favorite/worst subjects, repeated classes, suspension, dropping out, future education plans, relations with teachers or employers, attendance Activities: Activities for fun—with whom, when, where, sports, church attendance, clubs, hobbies, TV, have car (seat belts), history of arrests, acting out Drugs: Use by peers, client, or family members, amounts, frequency, patterns, driving car while using, source (how paid for) Sexuality: Menarche, spermarche, sexual orientation, degree and type of sexual experience, number of partners, abortion, STD, contraception, comfort with sexual activity, history of sexual or physical abuse. *Nutrition* Body image, screen for eating disorders, typical daily intake.	*Review of Systems* **Lifestyle** Family relationships, employment, school, peer activities, substance use, sexual involvement, sexual orientation, weapon use, legal history **Parent/Guardian** Home setting: Who lives with client, own room, relationships at home, what do parents do for a living, recent moves, running away, new people in home? Education/employment: School grade performance/changes, favorite/worst subjects, repeated classes, suspension, dropping out, future education plans, relations with teachers or employers, attendance Activities: Activities for fun—with whom, when, where, sports, church attendance, clubs, hobbies, TV, have car (seat belts), history of arrests, acting out Drugs: Use by peers, client, or family members, amounts, frequency, patterns, driving car while using, source (how paid for) Sexuality: Orientation, degree and type of sexual experience, number of partners, masturbation (normalize), history of pregnancy, abortion, STD, contraception, comfort with sexual activity, history of sexual or physical abuse *Nutrition* Screen for eating disorders, body image, typical daily intake.	*Review of Systems* **Lifestyle** Family relationships, career plans, peer activities, substance use, sexual involvement, sexual orientation, weapon use, legal history **Parent/Guardian** Home setting: Who lives with client, own room, relationships at home, what do parents do for a living, recent moves, new people in home? Education/employment: School grade performance/changes, favorite/worst subjects, repeated classes, suspension, dropping out, future education plans, relations with teachers or employers, attendance Activities: Activities for fun—with whom, when, where, sports, church attendance, clubs, hobbies, TV, have car (seat belts), history of arrests, acting out Drugs: Use by peers, client, or family members, amounts, frequency, patterns, driving car while using, source (how paid for) Sexuality: Orientation, degree and type of sexual experience, number of partners, masturbation (normalize), history of pregnancy, abortion, STD, contraception, comfort with sexual activity, history of sexual and physical abuse, violence in dating relationships *Nutrition* Screen for eating disorders, especially bulimia, body image, typical daily intake.

Continued

Table 19-8 Well Adolescent: 11 to 21 Years—cont'd

	EARLY ADOLESCENT (11-14 YR)	MIDDLE ADOLESCENT (15-17 YR)	LATE ADOLESCENT (18-21 YR)
O	*Mental Health* Suicide assessment One complete physical examination during early adolescence BP, BMI Vision and hearing screens Dental screen Scoliosis screen Assess pubertal development, Tanner stage. Screen for STDs if sexually experienced, including Papanicolaou smear. Screen for TB if risk factors present. Do cholesterol screen if FH positive for early cardiovascular disease or hyperlipidemia.	*Mental Health* Depression, suicide assessment One complete physical examination during middle adolescence BP, BMI Vision and hearing screens Dental screen Scoliosis screen Assess pubertal development, Tanner stage. Screen for STDs if sexually experienced, including Papanicolaou smear; screen for HIV if risk factors Screen for TB if risk factors present. Do cholesterol screen if FH positive for early cardiovascular disease or hyperlipidemia.	*Mental Health* Depression, suicide assessment One complete physical examination during late adolescence. Papanicolaou smear for all females, regardless of sexual experience BP, BMI Vision and hearing screen Dental screen Screen for STDs if sexually experienced; screen for HIV if risk factors. Screen for TB if risk factors present. Do cholesterol screen if FH positive.
A	Well adolescent Possible findings: Gynecomastia, irregular menses, decreased school performance in junior high, myopia	Well adolescent Possible findings: Acne, dysmenorrhea, sports injuries, increased conflict at home	Well adolescent Possible findings: Acne, *Chlamydia*, obesity
P	Immunizations: Td, HBV series, if not given in childhood; varicella, if no reliable history of chickenpox or not given in routine childhood schedule; MMR, if 2 vaccinations not documented earlier in childhood Gynecomastia: Reassurance Irregular menses: Education about anovulatory cycles, reassurance, hormonal treatment if disruptive	Immunizations: None if updated at early adolescent visit Acne treatment: Begin with topical medications. Dysmenorrhea: Nonsteroidal antiinflammatory drugs before onset of menses and every 6-8 hr for first 2 days of menses Rehabilitate all sports injuries before return to play.	Immunizations: None if updated at early adolescent visit Acne treatment: Consider combination therapies. *Chlamydia*: Single-dose therapy, partner notification Obesity: Low-fat dietary education, increased exercise
Education	Educational approach is for concrete thinker. Development: Review normal physical changes, timing of menarche for females, peer pressure.	Educational approach is for early abstract thinking style. Development: Skin care for acne, menstrual calendar, beginning career planning	Educational approach for abstract thinking Development: Skin care, job/school/college search, leaving nest

BP, Blood pressure; *BMI,* body mass index; *Td,* tetanus-diphtheria toxoid; *BSE,* breast self-examination.

	Injury prevention: Bike helmet use, protective equipment with sports, seat belt use	Injury prevention: Stretching before physical activity, seat belts, no driving while intoxicated or riding with intoxicated driver, violence prevention and conflict resolution	Injury prevention: Occupational safety, seat belts, no driving while intoxicated or riding with intoxicated driver, conflict resolution
	Diet and physical activity: Calcium, iron sources in diet	Diet and physical activity: Calcium sources, fast food choices, adequate exercise levels	Diet and physical health: Folic acid before planned pregnancy, calcium requirements, low-fat, high-fiber diet, exercise
	Healthy lifestyle: Postponing sexual involvement—abstinence, contraception and condoms if sexually experienced; substance use risks	Healthy lifestyle: Postponing sexual involvement, contraception and condoms if sexually experienced, methods to avoid substance use, instruction in BSE, testicular self-examination	Healthy lifestyle: Contraception and condom use, obtaining partner's sexual activity to decrease risk, moderation with alcohol, smoking cessation, substance use avoidance, instruction in BSE, testicular self-examination
	Suggestions for client's parents: Normative adolescent development, both physical and emotional; role modeling health-related behaviors, monitoring social activities	Suggestions for client's parents: Communication, signs of emotional distress, monitoring use of motor vehicles, avoidance of weapons in home, monitoring social activities	Suggestions for client's parents: Separation from adult child, role model for health-related behavior
Follow-up	Return in 3 mo if menses remain irregular. Return in 1 mo for HBV 2	Return in 2 mo to evaluate dysmenorrhea resolution. Consider oral contraceptive pills if dysmenorrhea continues. Return in 2 mo for acne follow-up; if pustules continue begin combination treatment.	Return in 3 mo to rescreen for STDs and reevaluate acne. Return in 1 mo for further nutrition education; refer to dietitian if client is interested.

REFERENCES

American Medical Association (1994). *Guidelines for adolescent preventive services (GAPS).* Chicago: Author.

American Psychiatric Association (1994). *Diagnostic and statistical manual of mental disorders* (4th ed.). Washington, DC: Author.

Bienfang, D. C., Kelly, L. D., Nicholson, D. H., et al. (1990). Ophthalmology. *New England Journal of Medicine, 323,* 956-959.

Bright Futures. (1994). *Guidelines for health supervision of infants, children and adolescents.* National Center for Education in Maternal and Child Health.

Dawood, M. Y. (1990). Dysmenorrhea. *Clinical Obstetrics and Gynecology, 33*(1), 168-178.

Draelos, Z. K. (1995). Patient compliance: Enhancing clinician abilities and strategies. *Journal of the American Academy of Dermatology, 32,* S42-S48.

Glass, A. P. (1994). Gynecomastia. *Endocrinology and Metabolism Clinics of North America, 23*(4), 825-837.

Hurwitz, S. (1995). Acne treatment for the '90s. *Contemporary Pediatrics 12*(8), 19-32.

Centers for Disease Control and Prevention (1996). Immunization of adolescents. *MMWR Morbidity Mortality Weekly Report, 45* RR-13.

Neistein, L. S. (1996). *Adolescent health care: A practical guide* (3rd ed.). Baltimore: Urban & Schwarzenberg.

Tanner, M. M. (1987). Issues and advances in adolescent growth and development. *Journal of Adolescent Health Care, 8,* 470-478.

Wheeler, M. D. (1991). Physical changes of puberty. *Endocrinology and Metabolism Clinics of North America, 20,* 1-14.

WELL WOMAN

Table 19-9 Well-Woman Care: 18 to 64 Years

	18-39 YEARS	40-64 YEARS
S	**History:** FH; PMH, PSH; menstrual, gynecologic, obstetric, contraceptive histories; immunization and infectious disease history; allergies; blood transfusion 1978-1985, IVDU, occupational blood and body fluid exposure; dental care **Current:** Medications, dietary intake, physical activity, contraception, sexual practices (high risk for STDs) **Safety:** Abuse, smoke detectors, seat-belt use, safety gear for hobbies **Habits:** Alcohol, tobacco or illicit drug use **Erikson's developmental task:** Intimacy vs isolation or self-absorption	**History:** FH; PMH, PSH; menstrual, gynecologic, obstetric, contraceptive histories; immunization and infectious disease history; allegies; blood transfusion 1978-1985, IVDU, occupational blood and body fluid exposure; dental care **Current:** Medications, dietary intake, physical activity, contraception, sexual practices (high risk for STDs) **Safety:** Abuse, smoke detectors, seat-belt use, safety gear for hobbies **Habits:** Alcohol, tobacco, or illicit drug use **Erikson's developmental task:** Generativity vs stagnation
O	**Physical examination:** Height, weight, BP, adenopathy, skin, thyroid, lungs, heart, abdomen, breast and pelvic examinations, DRE **High-risk groups:** Oral cavity, thyroid, skin, osteoporosis screen **Laboratory and diagnostic procedures** *Screening:* Pap smear; cholesterol **High-risk groups:** PPD, FPG, rubella antibodies, urinalysis for bacteriuria, HIV, RPR, gonococcus/*Chlamydia,* hearing, mammogram, colonoscopy	**Physical examination:** Height, weight, BP, adenopathy, skin, thyroid, lungs, heart, abdomen, breast and pelvic examinations, DRE **High-risk groups:** Skin, oral cavity, thyroid, carotid bruits, osteoporosis screen **Laboratory and diagnostic procedures** *Screening:* Pap smear, mammogram, cholesterol **High-risk groups:** PPD, FPG, rubella antibodies, urinalysis for bacteruria, HIV, RPR, gonococcus/*Chlamydia,* hearing, FOB and sigmoidoscopy, colonoscopy, bone mineral content
Dx	**Well female** *Leading medical problems:* Nose, throat, and URIs; injuries; viral, bacterial, and parasitic infections; acute urinary tract infections; eating disorders; violence, rape; substance abuse	**Well female** *Leading medical problems:* Osteoporosis and arthritis; nose, throat, and URIs; orthopedic deformities and impairments of back, arms, and legs; cardiovascular diseases; hearing and vision impairments
P	**Immunizations:** Td booster **High-risk groups:** HBV, influenza, MMR, pneumococcus **Counseling:** Diet related to fat, cholesterol, complex carbohydrate, fiber, sodium, iron, and calcium intake; exercise program; smoking cessation; limited alcohol consumption, treatment for abuse; contraceptive options and safer sex practices; BSE, skin protection from ultraviolet light	**Immunizations:** Td booster **High-risk groups:** HBV, influenza, pneumococcus **Counseling:** Diet related to fat, cholesterol, complex carbohydrate, fiber, sodium, and calcium intake; exercise program; smoking cessation; limited alcohol consumption, treatment for abuse; contraceptive options and safer sex practices; BSE; HRT
E	**Follow-up:** Depends on risk factors and illness. **Leading causes of death:** MVC; cardiovascular diseases; homicide; CAD; AIDS; breast cancer; cerebrovascular diseases; cervical and other uterine cancers	**Follow-up:** Depends on risk factors and illness. **Leading causes of death:** Cardiovascular diseases; CAD; breast cancer; lung cancer; cerebrovascular diseases, colorectal cancer; COPD; ovarian cancer; diabetes

CAD, Coronary artery disease; *COPD,* chronic obstructive pulmonary disease; *DRE,* digital rectal examination; *FH,* family history; *FOB,* fecal occult blood; *FPG,* fasting plasma glucose; *HRT,* hormone replacement therapy; *IVDU,* IV drug user; *MVC,* motor vehicle crash; *PMH,* past medical history; *PPD,* purified protein derivative of tuberculin; *PSH,* past surgical history; *RPR,* rapid plasma reagin test; *URI,* upper respiratory tract infection.

SCREENING AND IMMUNIZATION

Indications and Frequencies for Screening

Blood Glucose. Baseline is at 18 to 39 years, then do every 2 years.

Cholesterol. Baseline is at 18 to 39 years, then do every 5 years. After 40 years, do every 3 to 5 years.

Dental Examination. Do every year.

Eye Examination with Tonometry. Get baseline at 18 to 39 years, then do every 3 to 5 years or more frequently if risk factors are present.

Gonococcus and *Chlamydia*. Screen if client engages in or has any partner who engages in high-risk sexual behavior, or if client has contact with a person with diagnosed *Chlamydia*. Screen anyone in a nonmonogamous relationship.

Hearing. Screen clients with regular exposure to excessive noise; establish baseline at 40 years, repeat at 50 years. After 60 years, do every year.

Hct/Hemoglobin. Check every 2 years from 18 to 50 years, then every 5 years.

HIV. Screen if client engages in or has any partner who engages in high-risk sexual behavior or if client has contact with HIV-seropositive person. Screen IVDUs. Screen women who have male partners who (a) have had sex with men, (b) are IVDUs, (c) have long-term residence or birth in an area with high prevalence of HIV infection, or (d) have a history of transfusion between 1978 and 1985.

Mammography. Obtain baseline at 35 to 40 years, then repeat every 1 to 2 years from 40 to 59 years, every year after 60 years. Women with FH of breast cancer should receive mammograms 5 years earlier than the age at which breast cancer was diagnosed in a first-degree relative.

Pelvic Examination and Papanicolaou Smear. Do every year until 60 years, then every 1 to 2 years.

Proctoscopy and Sigmoidoscopy. Screen those with FH of familial polyposis coli or cancer familial syndrome; screen those without FH starting at 40 years. Repeat every 3 to 5 years. Obtain two consecutive yearly negative examination results before switching to intervals of every 3 to 5 years.

Purified Protein Derivative of Tuberculin. Screen household members of persons with diagnosis of TB and those with other close contacts with known or suspected TB. Screen health care workers. Screen those with risk factors associated with TB (HIV seropositivity), immigrants from country with high TB prevalence, clients from medically underserved low-income population, those with history of alcoholism, IVDUs, and residents of long-term care facilities.

Rapid Plasma Reagin Test. Screen client who engage in or have any partner who engages in high-risk sexual behavior. Screen clients with contact with any person with a diagnosis of active syphilis.

Rectal Examination. Do every year.

Rubella Antibodies. Screen anyone without evidence of immunity.

Fecal Occult Blood. Check every year.

Thyroid Function. Check starting at 60 years; repeat every 3 to 5 years.

Indications for Immunizations

Influenza. Annually vaccinate residents of chronic care facilities; persons with chronic cardiopulmonary disorders, metabolic diseases, hemoglobinopathies, immunosuppression, or renal dysfunction; and health care providers for high-risk clients.

Hepatitis A. Vaccinate those who reside in, travel to, or work in areas where the disease is endemic and where periodic outbreaks occur (e.g., countries with high or intermediate endemicity, certain Alaskan Native, Pacific Islander, Native American, and religious communities). Vaccinate women who have male partners who have had sex with men or are IVDUs. Consider vaccination for institutionalized persons and workers in these institutions, for military personnel, and for daycare, hospital, and laboratory workers.

Hepatitis B Virus. Vaccinate against HBV blood product recipients (including hemodialysis clients), persons with frequent occupational exposure to blood or blood products, persons traveling to countries with endemic HBV, household and sexual contacts of HBV carriers, those with multiple recent sex partners or recent sex partners with diagnosis of other recently acquired STDs, prostitutes, and women who have male partners who have had sex with men or are IVDUs.

Measles-Mumps-Rubella. Vaccinate clients born after 1956 who lack evidence of immunity to measles (e.g., documented administration of live vaccine on or after the first birthday, laboratory evidence of immunity, or a history of diagnosed measles).

PNEUMOCOCCAL VACCINE. Vaccinate clients with medical conditions that increase the risk of pneumococcal infection (e.g., diabetes mellitus, sickle cell disease, nephrotic syndrome, chronic cardiac or pulmonary disease, Hodgkin's disease, anatomic asplenia, alcoholism, cirrhosis, multiple myeloma, renal disease, and conditions associated with immunosuppression). Vaccinate immunocompetent institutionalized persons older than 50 years. Vaccinate immunocompetent persons who live in high-risk environments or social settings (e.g., certain Native American and Alaskan Native populations). Vaccinate all those older than 65 years.

TETANUS-DIPHTHERIA. Administer Td every 10 years.

VARICELLA. Vaccinate healthy adults without a history of chickenpox or previous immunization. Consider serologic testing for presumed susceptible adults.

REFERENCES

American Academy of Family Physicians (1997). American Academy of Family Physicians age charts for periodic health examination. In R. B. Murray & J. P. Zentner (Eds.), *Health assessment and promotion strategies* (6th ed., pp. 853-867). Norwalk, CT: Appleton & Lange.

Estes, M. (1998). *Health assessment and physical examination.* New York: Delmar.

Murray, R. B., Zentner, J. P., Pinnell, N. N., & Boland, M. H. (1997). Assessment and health promotion for the person in later maturity. In R. B. Murray & J. P. Zentner (Eds.), *Health assessment and promotion strategies* (6th ed., pp. 693-774). Norwalk, CT: Appleton & Lange.

Prevention (1997). *Harvard Women's Health Watch,* 2-4.

Youngkin, E. Q., & Davis, M. S. (1994). Assessing women's health. In E. Q. Youngkin & M. S. Davis (Eds.), *Women's health: A primary care clinical guide* (pp. 33-59). Norwalk, CT: Appleton & Lange.

WELL MALE

Table 19-10 Well-Male Care: 18 to 64 Years

		18-24 YEARS	25-64 YEARS
S		**History:** PMH, PSH; immunization history, FH; medications; allergies	**History:** PMH, PSH; immunization history; FH; medications, allergies; after 45 yr, BPH symptoms
		Lifestyle: Healthy diet and exercise; high risk for STD; contraception method; dental care; fluoridated water	**Lifestyle:** Healthy diet and exercise; high risk for STD, contraception method; dental care, fluoridated water
		Habits: Alcohol, tobacco, or illicit drugs; IVDU	**Habits:** Alcohol, tobacco, or illicit drugs; IVDU
		Safety: Lap and shoulder belts, bicycle, motorcycle, or ATV helmet; smoke detector; safe storage and removal of firearms; blood transfusion 1978-1985 or occupational blood and body fluid exposure	**Safety:** Lap and shoulder belts; bicycle, motorcycle, or ATV helmet; smoke detector, safe storage and removal of firearms; alcohol or drug use while driving, swimming, or boating; blood transfusion 1978-1985 or occupational blood and body fluid exposure
		Ethnic background: Native American, Alaskan Native, black	**Ethnic background:** Native American, Alaskan Native, black
			Health maintenance: Last vision, hearing, and dental examination, pneumococcal or influenza vaccine
		Eriskon's developmental task: Identity vs role confusion (adolescence)	**Erikson's developmental tasks:** Intimacy vs isolation (early adulthood), generativity vs stagnation (middle adulthood)
O		**Physical examination:** Height, weight, and BP; adenopathy; skin; lungs; heart; abdomen; testes	**Physical examination:** Height, weight and BP; adenopathy; skin; lungs; heart; abdomen; DRE; FOB; testes; oral cavity
Dx		Well male	Well male
P		**Screening:** PPD, HIV, RPR, gonococcus/*Chlamydia*	**Screening:** Total cholesterol, DRE, PSA, FOB, sigmoidoscopy, HIV, PPD, RPR, glaucoma
		Immunization: Td, HBV, MMR, varicella, hepatitis A, influenza	**Immunizations:** Td, HBV, hepatitis A, influenza, MMR, varicella
		Counseling: Problem drinking and illicit drug use; lap and shoulder belts; bicycle, motorcycle and ATV helmets; smoke detector; safe storage and removal of firearms; smoking cessation; alcohol or drug use while driving, swimming, or boating; STD protection; contraception; healthy diet and exercise, regular dental visits and care, sun exposure, fluoride supplement for those with inadequate water fluoridation	**Counseling:** Problem drinking and illicit drug use; smoking cessation; healthy diet and exercise; lap and shoulder belts, motorcycle, bicycle, and ATV helmets; smoke detectors; firearm safety; STD prevention; contraception; regular dental care and visits, skin cancer prevention
E		**Leading causes of death:** MVC and other unintentional injuries; homicide, suicide, malignant neoplasms, heart diseases	**Leading causes of death:** Malignant neoplasms; heart diseases; MVC and other unintentional injuries; HIV; suicide and homicide

ATV, All-terrain vehicle; *BPH,* benign prostatic hyperplasia; *CAD,* coronary artery disease; *COPD,* chronic obstructive pulmonary disease; *DRE,* digital rectal examination; *FH,* family history; *FOB,* fecal occult blood; *FPG,* fasting plasma glucose; *HRT,* hormone replacement therapy; *IVDU,* IV drug user; *MVC,* motor vehicle crash; *PMH,* past medical history; *PPD,* purified protein derivative of tuberculin; *PSA,* prostate-specific antigen; *PSH,* past surgical history; *RPR,* rapid plasma reagin test; *URI,* upper respiratory tract infection.

SCREENING AND IMMUNIZATION

Indications for Screening

PURIFIED PROTEIN DERIVATIVE OF TUBERCULIN. Screen HIV-seropositive clients, close contacts of persons with known or suspected TB, health care workers, persons with medical risk factors associated with TB, immigrants from countries with high TB prevalence, medically underserved low-income populations (including homeless persons), alcoholics, IVDUs, and residents of long-term care facilities.

HIV INFECTION. Screen clients who engage in or have partners who engage in high-risk sexual behavior, or who have contact with any person who is HIV seropositive; IVDUs; men whose male partners have had sex with men, are IVDUs, or both; those with long-term residence or birth in an area with high prevalence of HIV infection; and clients with history of transfusion between 1978 and 1985.

RAPID PLASMA REAGIN TEST. Screen clients who engage in or have partners who engage in high-risk sexual behavior, or who have contact with a person with a diagnosis of active syphilis.

GONOCOCCUS AND *CHLAMYDIA*. Screen if high-risk sexual behavior is present.

TOTAL CHOLESTEROL. Screen every 5 years, starting at 25 years.

DIGITAL RECTAL EXAMINATION. Perform annually for prostate and colorectal cancer, starting at 50 years.

PROSTATE-SPECIFIC ANTIGEN. Screen annually, starting at 40 years for blacks and those with FH of prostate cancer and at 50 years for others.

FECAL OCCULT BLOOD. Screen for colon cancer annually, starting at 50 years.

SIGMOIDOSCOPY. Perform every 5 years, starting at 50 years, to screen for colon cancer.

GLAUCOMA. Screening should be done by eye specialist for blacks older than 40 years, whites older than 65 years, those with a positive FH, and those with severe myopia.

TESTICLES. Examine every 3 years in 25- to 39-year olds and every year in those older than 40 years with history of cryptorchidism or atrophic testes.

ORAL CAVITY. Examine in those older than 60 years, tobacco users, and those who drink alcohol regularly.

Indications for Immunizations

HEPATITIS B VIRUS. Vaccinate against HBV blood product recipients (including hemodialysis clients), persons with frequent occupational exposure to blood or blood products, men who have sex with men, IVDUs and their sex partners, persons with multiple recent sex partners, persons with other STDs (including HIV), and travelers to countries with endemic HBV.

MEASLES-MUMPS-RUBELLA. Vaccinate persons born after 1956 who lack evidence of immunity to measles or mumps (e.g., documented receipt of live vaccine on or after the first birthday, laboratory evidence of immunity, or a history of physician-diagnosed measles or mumps).

VARICELLA. Vaccinate healthy adults without a history of chickenpox or previous immunization. Consider serologic testing for presumed susceptible adults.

HEPATITIS A. Vaccinate persons living in, traveling to, or working in areas where the disease is endemic and where periodic outbreaks occur (e.g., countries with high or intermediate endemicity; certain Alaskan Native, Pacific Islander, Native American, and religious communities); men who have sex with men; and IVDUs or street drug users. Consider vaccination for institutionalized persons and workers in these institutions, military personnel, and day-care, hospital, and laboratory workers.

INFLUENZA. Annual vaccination is appropriate for residents of chronic care facilities; persons with chronic cardiopulmonary disorders, metabolic diseases (including diabetes mellitus), hemoglobinopathies, immunosuppression, or renal dysfunction; and health care providers for high-risk clients.

PNEUMOCOCCAL VACCINE. Vaccinate immunocompetent institutionalized persons older than 50 years and immunocompetent persons with certain medical conditions, including chronic cardiac or pulmonary disease, diabetes mellitus, and anatomic asplenia. Also vaccinate immunocompetent persons who live in high-risk environments or social settings (e.g., certain Native American and Alaskan Native populations). Vaccinate all those older than 65 years.

REFERENCE

U. S. Preventive Services Task Force (1996). *Guide to clinical preventive services* (2nd ed.). Baltimore: Williams & Wilkins.

WELL ADULT 65 YEARS AND OLDER

Table 19-11 Growth and Development: 65 Years and Older

SYSTEM	OVERVIEW OF DEVELOPMENTAL CHANGES
Heart and circulatory	Heart weight remains relatively constant after 25 yr. CO decreases 30%-40%. Cardiac power is decreased. Capacity to increase rate and strength is diminished. Women have a slightly higher resting HR than men. Maximal HR decreases. There is increased calcification and fibrosis of the aortic valve cusps.
Renal	Glomerular filtration rate decreases about 30%-47% from 20 to 90 yr. Renal mass decreases with age. Renal flow decreases 53% (perhaps to compensate for decreased CO). Urinary incontinence affects 15%-30% of ambulatory older adults, more women than men. Decreased muscle tone of ureters, bladder and urethra may contribute to incidence of incontinence. Bladder capacity decreases as much as 50%. Prostate increases in size.
Gastrointestinal	Salivary gland secretion decreases; saliva is more alkaline. Esophageal motility is decreased. Generalized atrophy of gastrointestinal tract is seen with advancing age. Acidity of gastric juices decreases with age, taste is also diminished. Hepatic blood flow is decreased. Abdomen is more protruberant. Abdominal wall is thinner and less taut. Sphincter control is decreased, with relaxation of perineal musculature.
Eyes	Approximately 95% of those older than 60 yr have some opacification of lens. Decreased visual acuity occurs in 50% of those older than 75 yr as a result of cateracts. There is decreased ability to accommodate (presbyopia). Cells responsible for lubricating conjunctiva decrease (dry eye syndrome). Arus senilus is common. Pupils decrease in size, react more slowly to light, and dilate more slowly in dark. Loss of fat pads from orbit of eye gives sunken appearance.
Ears	Skin of ear becomes dry and less resilient. Cerumen production is decreased. Hair growth increases, pinna increases in length. Presbycusis may result from degeneration of organ of Corti (loss of high frequency sounds).
Nose/mouth	Olfactory function decreases; with no loss or change in taste buds; there is decrease in salt/sweet taste perception.
Adipose tissue	There is increase of body fat, with corresponding decrease of lean muscle mass. Sharpness of contours increases, with increasingly bony landmarks. Adipose tissue is redistributed from extremities to hips and abdomen.
Lymphoid tissue	Only very small changes occur.
Respiratory	Lung size and weight decrease. Basal metabolic rate decreases (ratio higher in men than women). Chest wall becomes less compliant.
Skeletal	Vertebral disks thin, spinal column shortens, kyphosis is seen with spinal column compression, osteoporosis increases. Loss of stature begins at approximately 50 yr. Women lose an average of 4.9 cm and men lose an average of 2.9 cm. Bones decrease in density and weight by 12% in men and 25% in women (Barkauskas, Stoltenberg-Allen, Baumann, & Darling-Fisher, 1994). There is loss of resilience and elasticity of ligaments, cartilage, and some tissues.
Muscular	Atrophy and loss of muscle tone by 30%-40% is seen between 30 and 80 yr. Exercise does help limit reduction of muscle mass.
Nervous	There is possible decrease in number of brain cells, decrease in myelin sheath. Impulses decrease, slowing down speed of action and reaction. Vibratory sense decreases, especially for feet and ankles; ankle jerk may be absent.

CO, Cardiac output; *HR,* heart rate.

Table 19-11   Growth and Development: 65 Years and Older—cont'd

SYSTEM	OVERVIEW OF DEVELOPMENTAL CHANGES
Reproductive	Estrogen and testosterone secretion are decreased. There is decreased pubic hair. Involution of uterus follows menopause frequently, with relaxation of the sacral ligaments so the uterus may be in a dropped position. Breasts atrophy with advancing age, becoming pendulous and with decreased fullness as a result of loss of fat. Penis decreases in size and has fewer sustained erections. Testes decrease in size and hang lower.
Integumentary	Regenerative powers are decreased. Dermis and epidermis thin, with loss of collagen and elastic fibers and less support for capillary walls so vessels dilate, diminished sebum production, and decreased subcutaneous fat.
Hair and nails	Scalp, axillary, and pubic hair thins and decreases. Eyebrow, nostril, and ear hair becomes coarser. Loss of hair pigment contributes to graying. Nail growth slows; nails become more yellow. Toenails commonly thicken.
Endocrine	All endocrine functions decline.

Table 19-12   Well Care: 65 Years and Older

65-75 YEARS	75 YEARS AND OLDER
S **History:** PMH; menstrual, gynecologic, obstetric, and contraceptive histories; FH (genogram to identify risk factors for CAD, diabetes mellitus, cancer, asthma); psychiatric illnesses; PSH; immunizations; allergies; blood transfusion 1978-1985; IVDU; occupational blood and body fluid exposure; last eye examination; last dental examination; sun exposure (skin examinations); osteoporosis screen; BPH symptoms, functional status at home	**History:** PMH, menstrual, gynecologic, obstetric, and contraceptive histories; FH (genogram to identify risk factors for CAD, diabetes mellitus, cancer, asthma); psychiatric illnesses; PSH; Immunizations; allergies, blood transfusion 1978-1985; IVDU; occupational blood and body fluid exposure; last eye examination; last dental examination; sun exposure (skin examinations); BPH symptoms; functional status at home

S

History: PMH; menstrual, gynecologic, obstetric, and contraceptive histories; FH (genogram to identify risk factors for CAD, diabetes mellitus, cancer, asthma); psychiatric illnesses; PSH; immunizations; allergies; blood transfusion 1978-1985; IVDU; occupational blood and body fluid exposure; last eye examination; last dental examination; sun exposure (skin examinations); osteoporosis screen; BPH symptoms, functional status at home

Current: Medications, dietary intake, physical activity, contraception, sexual practices, adequate hearing and vision, hobbies

Safety: Abuse, smoke detectors, seat-belt use, safety gear for hobbies, hot water heater temperature, fall prevention, guns in house, storage of guns, use of space heaters, heating pads

Habits: Alcohol, tobacco, illicit drugs

Erikson's developmental task: Integrity vs despair and disdain

O   **Physical examination:** Height, weight, BP, adenopathy, thyroid, carotid bruits, heart, lungs, skin, oral cavity, hearing, Snellen chart, DRE, pelvic examination, breast, musculoskeletal and gait

Laboratory and diagnostic procedures

Screening: Lipid profile, sigmoidoscopy, DRE with PSA, FOB, glaucoma test, Papanicolaou smear, mammogram

High-risk groups: PPD, FPG, thyroid, HIV, hepatitis screen, RPR

Dx   *Well physical examination*

Common medical problems: Nose, throat, and URI; osteoporosis; arthritis; hypertension; urinary incontinence; cardiovascular diseases; hearing and vision impairments

Leading causes of death: Heart disease, malignant neoplasms (lung, colorectal, breast), cerebrovascular disease, COPD, pneumonia and influenza

P   **Immunizations:** Pneumococcal, influenza, Td, varicella

High-risk groups: Hepatitis A, HBV

Counseling: Polypharmacy, living will, durable power of attorney

Safety: Lap/shoulder belt use; bicycle/motorcycle helmets; smoke detectors; safe storage of firearms; fall prevention; hot water heater <120° F); keeping emergency numbers available; family members trained in CPR; driving evaluation

Prevention: Diet (low-fat, high-carbohydrate, increased fiber, iron, and calcium intake), exercise, regular dental visits, biannual eye exams (unless diabetic, then q 1 yr), STD prevention, smoking cessation, skin cancer prevention, BSE

E   **Follow-up:** Depends on risk factors and illness.

---

75 YEARS AND OLDER

History: PMH, menstrual, gynecologic, obstetric, and contraceptive histories; FH (genogram to identify risk factors for CAD, diabetes mellitus, cancer, asthma); psychiatric illnesses; PSH; Immunizations; allergies, blood transfusion 1978-1985; IVDU; occupational blood and body fluid exposure; last eye examination; last dental examination; sun exposure (skin examinations); BPH symptoms; functional status at home

Current: Medications, dietary intake, physical activity, contraception, sexual practices, adequate hearing and vision, hobbies

Safety: Abuse, smoke detectors, seat-belt use, safety gear for hobbies, hot water heater temperature, fall prevention, guns in house, storage of guns, use of space heaters, heating pads

Habits: Alcohol, tobacco, illicit drugs

Erikson's developmental task: Integrity vs despair and disdain

Physical examination: Height, weight, BP, adenopathy, thyroid, carotid bruits, heart, lungs, skin, oral cavity, hearing, Snellen chart, FOB, DRE, pelvic examination, breast examination, musculoskeletal and gait

Laboratory and diagnostic procedures

Screening: Lipid profile, sigmoidoscopy, DRE with PSA, FOB, glaucoma test, mammogram

High-risk groups: PPD, FPG, thyroid, HIV, hepatitis screen, RPR

Well physical examination

Common medical problems: Nose, throat, and URI; osteoporosis; arthritis; hypertension, urinary incontinence, cardiovascular diseases, hearing and vision impairments

Leading causes of death: Heart disease, malignant neoplasms (lung, colorectal, breast), cerebrovascular disease, COPD, pneumonia and influenza, complications related to falls and MVC

Immunizations: Pneumococcal, influenza, dt, varicella

High-risk groups: Hepatitis A, HBV

Counseling: Polypharmacy, living will, durable power of attorney

Safety: Lap/shoulder belt use; bicycle/motorcycle helmets; smoke detectors; safe storage of firearms; fall prevention; hot water heater <120° F; keeping emergency numbers available; family members trained in CPR; driving evaluation

Prevention: Diet (low-fat, high-carbohydrate, increased fiber, iron, and calcium intake), exercise, regular dental visits, biannual eye exams (unless diabetic, then q 1 yr), STD prevention, smoking cessation, skin cancer prevention, BSE

Follow-up: Depends on risk factors and illness.

SAFETY AND SECURITY

Home Safety Issues

Physiologic changes associated with age and environmental agents are the principal risk factors for falls in older persons.

RISK AREAS
- Use of throw rugs
- Extension cords or appliances with frayed cords
- Use of space heaters or wood-burning stoves
- Torn or frayed carpeting on stairways
- Presence of pets that could get in the way of ambulation
- Presence of inadequate lighting, inside and outside
- Low chairs
- Incorrect footwear

NEEDS
- There should be an ABC fire extinguisher.
- There should be a smoke detector for each level of the house; preferably a number 5 extinguisher to allow for some error in use.
- If there is a high hazard area, there should be an additional fire extinguisher and smoke detector there.
- Evaluation of multifactorial risk factors for falls is critical:
  —Certain psychoactive and cardiac medications
  —Use of >4 prescription medications
  —Impaired cognition, strength, and balance of gait make the older adult more vulnerable to falls.
  —Intensive individualized home-based fall intervention program

Motor Vehicle Crashes

Polydisease entities and subsequent polypharmacologic management, along with normal aging processes, place older adults at higher risk when operating a motor vehicle.

RISK FACTORS
- Slowing of reflexes and decreased motor strength make older adults more susceptible to accidents in situations that require rapid thinking and decision making, such as at intersections.
- Decreased hepatic mass, blood flow, and enzyme activity, as well as increased receptor-site sensitivity, make older adults more susceptible to side effects of medications.
- Osteoporosis renders older adults more vulnerable to fractures in what may seem like a minor crash.

ASSESSMENT OF DRIVING SKILLS
- Driving history, including near-crashes
- Get input from family members who have ridden in the vehicle with the older adult
- A Mini-Mental State Examination will give an indication of the older adult's cognitive function.
- Complete a hearing examination.
- Assess range of motion and strength.
- Review medications and alcohol use to assess for potential and actual side effects that the older adult may be experiencing.
- Some automobile and other associations offer refresher courses specifically designed for the older adult driver.

Family Violence

Assessment should be conducted with alertness for the signs and symptoms of adult abuse. A comfortable level needs to be found so that the interview can assist in identifying family violence.

TOPICS TO EXPLORE
- How things are going at home, work, etc.
- Identify changes, good and bad.
- Ask, "Is there anything you may want to change?"
- Is the client anxious?
- How does the client feel about life at work, at home, in general?
- What worries are most bothersome? How does the client manage these problems?

INTERVENTIONS
- Be emphathetic. Use statements such as, "That sounds as though it can be a very difficult situation."
- Support the feelings of the involved parties by noting that other people are struggling with the same issues.
- Be objective.

SCREENING AND IMMUNIZATION

Indications for Screening

PURIFIED PROTEIN DERIVATIVE OF TUBERCULIN
- HIV seropositive
- Close contacts of persons with known or suspected TB
- Health care workers

- Persons with medical risk factors associated with TB
- Immigrants from countries with high TB prevalence
- Medically underserved low-income populations (including homeless persons)
- Alcoholics
- IVDUs
- Residents of long-term care facilities

HIV INFECTION
- Men who had sex with men after 1975
- Past or present IVDUs
- Persons who exchange sex for money or drugs
- Sex partners who exchange sex for money or drugs
- Bisexual
- HIV-seropositive sex partner currently or in the past
- Blood transfusion between 1978 and 1985
- Persons seeking treatment for STDs

RAPID PLASMA REAGIN TEST
- Persons who exchange sex for money or drugs and their sex partners
- Persons with other STDs (including HIV)
- Sexual contacts of persons with active syphilis

GONOCOCCUS AND *CHLAMYDIA*. Screen if high-risk sexual behavior is present.

TOTAL CHOLESTEROL. Screen every 5 years, starting at 25 years.

DIGITAL RECTAL EXAMINATION. Perform DRE annually for prostate and colorectal cancer, starting at age 50 years.

PROSTATE-SPECIFIC ANTIGEN
- Annually, starting at 40 years for blacks
- Annually for those with FH of prostate cancer
- Annually, beginning at 50 years, for others

FECAL OCCULT BLOOD. Screen for colon cancer annually, starting at 50 years.

SIGMOIDOSCOPY. Perform every 5 years, starting at 50 years, to screen for colon cancer.

GLAUCOMA
- Annual screening by eye specialist in blacks older than 40 years
- Annual screening in whites older than 65 years and those with FH
- Annual screening for those with severe myopia

TESTICLES. Check annually in those older than 40 years with history of cryptorchidism or atrophic testes.

ORAL CAVITY. Check in persons older than 60 years who use tobacco and who drink alcohol regularly.

Table 19-13   Indications for Immunizations

IMMUNIZATION	POPULATION INDICATIONS
Td	Administer every 10 yr, or earlier in cases of contaminated or severe wounds.
HBV	Vaccinate blood product recipients (including hemodialysis clients), persons with frequent occupational exposure to blood or blood products, men who have sex with men, IVDUs and their sex partners, persons with multiple recent sex partners, persons with other STDs (including HIV), and travelers to countries with endemic HBV.
Varicella	Vaccinate healthy adults without a history of chickenpox or previous immunization. Consider serologic testing for presumed susceptible adults.
Hepatitis A	Vaccinate persons living in, traveling to, or working in areas where the disease is endemic and where periodic outbreaks occur (e.g., countries with high or intermediate endemicity, certain Alaskan Native, Pacific Islander, Native American, and religous communities); men who have sex with men; and IVDUs or street drug users. Consider for institutionalized persons and workers in these institutions; military personnel; and day-care, hospital, and laboratory workers.
Influenza	Annually vaccinate residents of chronic care facilities; persons with chronic cardiopulmonary disorders, metabolic diseases (including diabetes mellitus), hemoglobinopathies, immunosuppression, or renal dysfunction; and health care providers for high-risk clients.
Pneumococcal	Vaccinate immunocompetent institutionalized persons older than 50 yr and immunocompetent persons with certain medical conditions, including chronic cardiac or pulmonary disease, diabetes mellitus, and anatomic asplenia. Vaccinate immunocompetent persons who live in high-risk environment or social settings (e.g., certain Native American and Alaskan Native populations). Vaccinate all those older than 65 yr.

REFERENCES

Barkauskas, V. H., Stoltenberg-Allen, K., Baumann, L. C., & Darling-Fisher, C. (1994). *Health and physical assessment.* St. Louis: Mosby.

Edelmann, C. L., & Mandle, C. L. (1994). *Health promotion throughout the lifespan* (3rd ed.). St. Louis: Mosby.

Finucan, T., & Burton, J. (1995). Geriatric medicine: Special considerations. In L. Barker, J. Burton, & P. Zieve (Eds.), *Principles of ambulatory medicine.* Baltimore: Williams & Wilkins.

Goldstein, A. (1993). Health promotion. In P. Sloane, L. Slatt, & P. Curtis (Eds.), *Essentials of family medicine.* Baltimore: Williams & Wilkins.

Hicks, M. (1993). Well adult care. In P. Sloane, L. Slatt, & P. Curtis (Eds.), *Essentials of family medicine.* Baltimore: Williams & Wilkins.

Murray, S. (1997). What's happening: Driving and the elderly. *Journal of the American Academy of Nurse Practitioners, 9*(3), 133-136.

Prevention. (1997). *Harvard Women's Health Watch,* 2-4.

Seidel, H. M., Ball, J. W., Dains, J. E., & Benedict, G. W. (1995). *Mosby's guide to physical examination.* St. Louis: Mosby.

Sloane, P., & Hicks, M. (1993). Preventive care: An overview. In P. Sloane, L. Slatt, & P. Curtis (Eds.), *Essentials of family medicine.* Baltimore: Williams & Wilkins.

Uphold, C., & Graham, M. (1994). Periodic health evaluation for adults. In C. Uphold & M. Graham (Eds.), *Clinical guidelines in family practice* (pp. 30-41). Gainesville, FL: Barmarrae Books.

U. S. Preventive Services Task Force (1996). *Guide to clinical preventive services* (2nd ed.). Baltimore: Williams & Wilkins.

White, P. (1995). Pearls for practice: Polypharmacy and the older adult. *Journal of the American Academy of Nurse Practitioners, 7*(11), 545-548.

WELL CARE DURING PREGNANCY

PRECONCEPTION VISIT

History

- Family
- Medical-surgical
- Environmental exposure
- Occupation
- Psychosocial
- Obstetric: Gravidity and parity, date of each birth, outcome (gestational age at birth; type of delivery; length of labor; birth weight; gender; complications during pregnancy, delivery, post partum), names and location of children, feelings about loss (whether perinatal, adoption relinquishment, or infant or childhood death)
- Medications: Prescription, OTC
- Habits: Smoking, alcohol, illicit drugs
- Safety

Physical Examination

- Height
- Weight
- Blood pressure
- Pulse
- Skin
- Thyroid
- Lungs
- Heart
- Breast
- Abdomen
- Extremities
- Pelvic examination
- Clinical pelvimetry

Laboratory and Diagnostic Procedures

- CBC
- Rh factor
- Rubella and varicella titer
- HBV surface antigen (HBsAg)
- PPD
- Syphilis
- Gonococcus and *Chlamydia*
- Genetic testing (indications include advanced maternal age, advanced paternal age, FH of or previous child with genetic abnormality, ethnic background, or as otherwise indicated by history)

- Urine dipstick for protein, glucose
- Papanicolaou smear
- Offer illicit drug screening and HIV testing.

Interventions

- Follow up on abnormal laboratory or physical examination findings.
- Encourage the following behaviors:
  —Keep a menstrual calendar, eat a well-balanced diet, and decrease caffeine intake.
  —Start taking one prenatal multivitamin and 3 tablets containing 1 mg folic acid.
  —Update immunizations and consider smoking cessation.
  —Avoid environmental toxins, illicit drugs, alcohol, and OTC, prescriptive, and homeopathic medicines until their use has been discussed with the health care provider.
  —Exercise at least 4 times/week for 20 to 30 minutes.
  —Limit risk of congenital toxoplasmosis by having someone else empty litter box.

INITIAL VISIT

This visit should take place as early in pregnancy as feasible.

History

- Update: Preconception history, menstrual, contraceptive, social, sexual, and abuse histories
- Medications: Prescription, OTC, herbs
- Habits: Smoking, alcohol, illicit drugs, exercise, hours of sleep, safety
- Assess readiness for pregnancy and parenthood, affirmation of pregnancy. Identify genetic risk if that has not already been done, screen for potential preterm labor
- Determine estimated date of delivery (EDD) by means of Nägele's rule: Add 9 months and 7 days to the first day of the last normal menstrual period or subtract 3 months then add 7 days and 1 year. If the menstrual cycle varies by 7 or more days from the norm of 28 days, the EDD must be adjusted by the same number of days.

Physical Examination

- Height
- Weight
- BP
- Pulse
- Skin
- Thyroid
- Lungs
- Heart
- Breast
- Abdomen
- Extremities
- Pelvic area
- Clinical pelvimetry
- Other elements as indicated

Laboratory and Diagnostic Procedures

- Antibody screen
- CBC
- Rh factor
- Rubella titer
- HBsAg
- PPD
- Syphilis
- HIV
- Genetic testing
- Random blood glucose level
- Urine dipstick for protein and glucose
- Urine culture
- Ultrasonography as indicated (dating, vaginal bleeding, maternal pelvic masses, uterine abnormalities, ectopic pregnancy, multiple gestation)
- Titers for toxoplasmosis, rubella, cytomegalovirus, herpes, and hepatitis as indicated
- High-risk sexual behavior (history of STD, new or multiple partners, community epidemiology): *Chlamydia* screen, gonorrhea

Interventions

- Follow up on abnormal laboratory or physical examination findings.
- Encourage the following behaviors:
  —Eat a well-balanced diet and decrease caffeine intake.
  —Start taking one prenatal multivitamin and 3 tablets containing 1 mg folic acid.
  —Update immunizations and consider smoking cessation.
  —Avoid environmental toxins, illicit drugs, alcohol, and OTC, prescription, and homeopathic medicines until their use has been discussed with the health care provider.
  —STD prevention: Avoid high-risk sexual behavior; use condoms.
  —Exercise at least 4 times/week for 20 to 30 minutes.
  —Limit risk of congenital toxoplasmosis by having someone else empty litter box.
- Provide the following health education:
  —Discuss prenatal classes and infant feeding (breast vs bottle).
  —Discuss physiologic changes of pregnancy.
  —Note contraindications (if any) for intercourse.
  —Instruct in warning signs that require notification of the health care provider, what to avoid, what to do in case of an emergency, and the frequency of prenatal visits.
- Provide psychosocial support and referrals as needed.
- Provide information to relieve discomforts of pregnancy.

Client Teaching on Discomfort of Pregnancy

FIRST TRIMESTER

Breast Tenderness. Wear a supportive bra. Discuss with partner the need for gentleness in touching the breasts during lovemaking. Acetaminophen may be used.

Constipation. Exercise regularly. Increase consumption of water and other liquids. Add fiber to diet, with fresh fruit and whole-grain breads. Drink prune juice. Laxatives (milk of magnesia), stool softeners, and bulk producers may be used.

Headaches. Treat with rest; relaxation exercises; warm bath; warm or cold compresses to forehead; face, head, and shoulder massage; and aromatherapy. Acetaminophen may be used.

Hemorrhoids. Avoid constipation and prolonged sitting. Use warm sitz baths, followed by an application of witch hazel.

Nausea and Vomiting. This is self-limiting. Take small, frequent meals, with a protein snack at bedtime. Try hard candy, raspberry leaf tea, and 10 drops of peppermint spirits in half of a glass of water. Avoid greasy and spicy foods. Keep dry crackers at the bedside. Drink carbonated beverages. If dehydration, ketosis, or electrolyte abnormalities are present, antiemetics (meclizine, diphenydramine, and metoclopramide), or pyridoxine may be used.

Urinary Frequency. Decrease caffeine intake.

Varicosities. Wear supportive stockings or antiembolism stockings. Rest and elevate legs when possible. Perineal pads may help vulvar varicosities.

SECOND TRIMESTER

Backache (Musculoskeletal Strain). Avoid excessive weight gain, note posture, use good body mechanics, and wear flat or low-heeled shoes. Place a footstool under one foot while standing, a pillow in lumbar area while sitting, and a pillow between the knees while lying on side. Massage and apply ice or heat.

Backache (Sacroiliac Dysfunction). Place a wedge-shaped pillow underneath the abdomen while lying on side. Use exercise.

Dizziness and Faintness. Avoid lying flat on back, dehydration, and prolonged standing or sitting. Change position slowly. Lie in left lateral position.

Leukorrhea. Bathe daily; wear cotton underwear and change it frequently.

Leg Cramps. Use exercise, calf stretch exercises, walks. Keep legs warm. Decrease phosphate intake by decreasing milk intake. Increase magnesium intake by taking magnesium tablets, 122 mg every morning and 244 mg every evening.

Round Ligament Pain. Avoid twisting and sudden movements. Bend over or raise knee to chest on affected side. Rest and apply warm compresses.

THIRD TRIMESTER

Braxton Hicks Contractions. Learn to differentiate between true and false labor. Empty bladder frequently. Increase fluid intake. Resting in a left lateral recumbent position or exercising lightly may help to relieve discomfort. Use relaxation techniques and warm tub baths.

Edema. Avoid prolonged sitting or standing. Lie in left lateral recumbent position for 1 to 2 hours twice a day and sleep in that position. Elevate legs when possible. Refrain from wearing clothes that constrict the extremities. Increase fluid intake and decrease intake of sugar and fats. Moderate sodium intake.

Heartburn. Take small, frequent meals. Try papaya or raw almonds after meals. Refrain from lying recumbent after eating. Avoid fried and gas-producing foods. Sleep with head raised on stacked pillows. Antacids with magnesium hydroxide or magnesium trisilicate (Gaviscon) may be used. Avoid antacids with baking soda, aluminum, or high sodium contents.

Skin Rashes. Apply ice. Diphenhydramine may be used. If relief is not obtained, a dermatologic referral is needed.

RETURN VISITS
Frequency of Visits

- From 6 to 32 weeks: Visits every 4 weeks, or sooner if indicated
- From 32 to 34 weeks: Visits every 2 weeks, or sooner if indicated
- From 34 to 41 weeks: Visits every 1 week or sooner if indicated
- From 41 weeks to delivery: Visits 2 times/week

History

- Fetal movement
- Nausea and vomiting
- Vaginal bleeding or discharge
- Contractions
- Cramping or pelvic pressure
- Dysuria or frequency
- Headaches
- Scotoma or blurred vision
- Edema
- Preterm labor symptoms
- Pain
- Chest
- Abdomen
- Back legs
- Skin changes
- Fever or exposure to infectious disease
- Numbness or tingling of the hands or wrists
- Genital lesions, sores, or growths
- Trauma
- Medications taken
- Assess parental-fetal attachment
- Risk factors for development of family maladaptive behaviors
- Unplanned pregnancy (rape), marital discord or family violence, STD, substance abuse, HIV-seropositive status, adolescence
- Other factors: Limited social support and educational background

Laboratory and Diagnostic Procedures

- Proteinuria, glucosuria, ketonuria
- Ultrasonography as indicated
- 9 to 11 weeks: Chorionic villi sampling as indicated
- 12 to 14 weeks: Early amniocentesis as indicated
- 15 to 16 weeks: Traditional amniocentesis as indicated
- 15 to 18 weeks: Maternal serum alpha-fetoprotein or maternal serum multiple marker screening
- 24 to 28 weeks: Hemoglobin or Hct, diabetes screening, and antibody screening, group B streptococcus culture

Physical Examination

- Blood pressure
- Weight
- Fundal height
- Fetal heart tone (FHT)
- Presentation
- Edema
- Other elements as indicated

Interventions

- Fundal height in centimeters should be equal to the number of weeks of gestation plus or minus 2 cm. If fundal height is 3 to 4 cm smaller or larger than the gestational age in weeks, review the dating parameters and the ultrasonography. Follow up on other abnormal laboratory or physical examination findings.
- Rh$_o$D immune globulin (RhoGAM) at 28 weeks as indicated
- Provide information to relieve discomforts of pregnancy.
- Continue encouragement of health promotion activities.
- Provide education on the following topics:
  —Planning for labor and birth
  —Sibling preparation
  —Warning signs
  —Infant car seat
  —Infant feeding and care
- Provide psychosocial support and referrals as needed.

PROLONGED PREGNANCY
History

- Fetal kick counts
- Nausea and vomiting
- Vaginal bleeding or discharge
- Contractions
- Cramping or pelvic pressure
- Dysuria or frequency
- Headaches, scotoma, or blurred vision
- Edema
- Preterm labor symptoms
- Pain: Chest, abdomen, back, legs
- Skin changes
- Fever or exposure to infectious disease
- Numbness or tingling of the hands or wrists
- Genital lesions, sores, or growths
- Trauma
- Medications taken

Laboratory and Diagnostic Procedures

- Proteinuria, glucosuria, ketonuria
- Fetal well-being: non-stress test, contraction stress test, amniotic fluid index
- Biophysical profile

Physical Examination

- BP
- Weight
- Fundal height
- FHT
- Presentation
- Edema
- Other elements as indicated

Interventions

- Induction versus expectant management
- Provide psychosocial support and referrals as needed.

POSTPARTUM VISIT
History

- Physical: Fever and chills, breast engorgement, breast care, breast-feeding, nipple soreness, lochia and return of menses, incision or perineal discomfort, dysuria, urinary frequency
- Adaptation to motherhood: Rest and sleep habits, appetite and dietary habits, exercise activity, coping, sexual activity, desired birth control method

- Infant: Feeding, care, health, first examination, problems
- Family adjustments

Laboratory and Diagnostic Procedures

- Hemoglobin or Hct
- FBG for clients with diabetes or gestational diabetes
- Thyroid function tests for women whose thyroid dosage changed during the pregnancy

Physical Examination

- Thyroid
- Breasts
- Abdomen
- Extremities
- Pelvic area

Interventions

- Follow up on abnormal laboratory or physical findings from pregnancy and this visit.
- Provide method of contraception as requested.
- Weight reduction guidance
- Encourage health promotion activities.
- Provide psychosocial support and referrals as needed.

REFERENCES

Akridge, K. M. (1994). Postpartum and lactation. In E. Q. Youngkin & M. S. Davis (Eds.), *Women's health: A primary care clinical guide* (pp. 519-578). Norwalk, CT: Appleton & Lange.

Baxley, E. (1996). Postpartum biomedical concerns. In S. D. Ratcliffe, J. E. Byrd, & E. L. Sakornut (Eds.), *Handbook of pregnancy and perinatal care in family practice: Science and practice* (pp. 430-446). Philadelphia: Hanley & Belfus.

Byrd, J. (1994). Content of prenatal care. In S. D. Ratcliffe, J. E. Byrd, & E. L. Sakornut (Eds.), *Handbook of pregnancy and perinatal care in family practice: Science and practice* (pp. 15-27). Philadelphia: Hanley & Belfus.

Corder-Mabe, J. (1994). Complications of pregnancy. In E. Q. Youngkin & M. S. Davis (Eds.), *Women's health: A primary care clinical guide* (pp. 435-485). Norwalk, CT: Appleton & Lange.

Fontaine, P., & Sayres, W. (1996). Obstetric risk assessment. In S. D. Ratcliffe, J. E. Byrd, & E. L. Sakornut (Eds.), *Handbook of pregnancy and perinatal care in family practice: Science and practice* (pp. 1-14). Philadelphia: Hanley & Belfus.

Fuqua, M. H. (1994). Assessing fetal well-being. In E. Q. Youngkin & M. S. Davis (Eds.), *Women's health: A primary care clinical guide* (pp. 487-518). Norwalk, CT: Appleton & Lange.

Remich, M. (1994). Promoting a healthy pregnancy. In E. Q. Youngkin & M. S. Davis (Eds.), *Women's health: A primary care clinical guide* (pp. 383-434). Norwalk, CT: Appleton & Lange.

Wheeler, L. (1997). *Nurse-midwifery handbook: A practical guide to prenatal and postpartum care*. Philadelphia: J.B. Lippincott.

Youngkin, E. Q., & Davis, M. S. (1994). Assessing women's health. In E. Q. Youngkin & M. S. Davis (Eds.), *Women's health: A primary care clinical guide* (pp. 33-59). Norwalk, CT: Appleton & Lange.

WELLNESS DURING MENOPAUSE

OVERVIEW

Definition

Menopause is defined as ovarian failure evidenced by cessation as a result of aging. It is a gradual process, usually occurring during a 1- to 3-year period. *Premature menopause,* which occurs before 40 years, frequently has a genetic or autoimmune etiology. *Surgical menopause,* is the result of a bilateral oophorectomy, can cause more severe symptoms because of the sudden drop in hormone levels.

Climacteric, also known as *perimenopausal period,* refers to 7 to 10 years of physiologic change before menopause.

Incidence

Menopause before 30 years is premature, whereas that between 31 and 40 years is early (consider the possibility of autoimmune disease). Average age is 50 to 52 years. Menopause is genetically determined and is not affected by race, socioeconomic level, education, height, weight, type of contraceptives used, or number of pregnancies. Smokers do have earlier menopause than do nonsmokers. Thin women usually have more pronounced vasomotor symptoms.

Physiology

The major source of estradiol before menopause is the ovarian follicle. General atresia of ovarian follicles begins at puberty and increases after 35 years, leading to a decline in ovarian production of estrogen and progesterone. Estrogen normally participates in a negative feedback system; thus with decreased estrogen, gonadotropin hormones are no longer inhibited, so increased follicle-stimulating hormone (FSH) and luteinizing hormone (LH) are secreted. FSH and LH never return to premenopausal levels. Ovarian testosterone levels are maintained at about the levels before menopause (Youngkin & Davis, 1994).

Table 19-14   Physiologic Changes of Menopause Caused by Decreased Estrogen

SYSTEM	CHANGES	INTERVENTIONS*
Breasts	Glandular tissues decrease, nipples become smaller and flatter.	Reassure client that these are normal changes during menopause.
Vulva	There is atrophy of vulva, decreased subcutaneous tissue, and a decreased labia majora; labia minora are almost nonexistent. Skin becomes thinner, with loss of pubic hair. Dystrophies and pruritus are common.	Estrogen cream
Vagina	There is increased vaginal pH and decreased resistance to pyogenic organisms. Vagina becomes shorter and narrower, with some loss of vaginal rugae.	Changes may be slowed with continuation of regular intercourse, use estrogen cream to reverse atrophic changes, use lubricant with intercouse.
Uterus	Uterus decreases in size and weight. Cervix pales and shrinks, with loss of fornices; endocervix becomes atrophic.	
Pelvic floor	Muscular tissue loses tone; incidences of prolapse, cystocele, and rectocele are increased.	Pelvic floor (Kegel) exercises may help with decreased muscle tone.
Urinary tract changes	Bladder and urethral structure atrophy; incontinence may occur (in part as a result of past trauma of childbirth).	Pelvic muscle exercises, bladder training, drugs that inhibit parasympathetic nervous system, calcium-channel blockers
Vasomotor instability	Rapid rises in core temperature occur, with resultant perspiration, often profuse; these may be increased by stress, weather, and alcohol ingestion. These hot flashes last 3-4 minutes; ≥85% of women experience them. They may occur at night, disrupting sleep.	Adjust room temperature, use portable fan, wear clothing in layers, use stress management techniques. Limit alcohol and caffeine intake, drink 8-10 glasses water/day, and exercise regularly.
Changes in mood	Significant numbers of women report mood change, but relationship between hormonal changes and emotional changes (depression/anxiety) is unknown. Central nervous system contains cells sensitive to estradiol, so its withdrawal may have some effect.	Exercise, balanced diet, stress reduction
Sleep disorders	REM sleep decreases with age and decreased estrogen, or is decreased because of night sweats and hot flashes.	Evaluate naps, avoid caffeine, avoid smoking, exercise (*not* before bedtime), maintain comfortable sleep environment, develop nighttime routine, avoid sleeping medications, use relaxation techniques.

*In addition to hormone replacement therapy.

HORMONE REPLACEMENT THERAPY

Hormone replacement therapy (HRT) may be used during the perimenopausal period and after menopause.

Recommended Assessment Before Beginning Hormone Replacement Therapy

ASSESSMENT: SUBJECTIVE/HISTORY
- Symptoms of decreased estrogen
- PMH: CAD, deep venous thrombosis, last menstrual period, possible pregnancy, breast masses, menstrual history, obstetric and gynecologic history, surgeries, uterine fibroids, endometriosis, STDs
- Social: Smoking, alcohol use
- FH: Osteoporosis, CAD, hypertension, breast or gynecologic cancers, premature menopause in mother or sisters

ASSESSMENT: OBJECTIVE/PHYSICAL EXAMINATION. Perform screening physical examination with attention toward the following:
- Height, weight, and vital signs
- Signs of decreased estrogen
- Thyroid
- Cardiovascular and thorax
- Breast examination
- Gynecologic examination

Diagnostic Procedures
- Cholesterol, lipids
- Urinalysis
- CBC
- Chemistry profile
- Screen for colorectal cancer
- Serum FSH and LH
- Bone density
- Thyroid profile
- Liver function tests

DIAGNOSIS. Differential diagnosis includes the following:
- Perimenopause
- Premenstrual syndrome
- Thyroid disease
- Stress
- Psychiatric disorders (depression, anxiety, bipolar disorder)
- Connective tissue diseases
- Alcoholism

Hormone Replacement Therapy Schedule

HRT is available by oral, cream or transdermal methods. There are three types of regimens of estrogen and progesterones:

1. Cyclic: Estrogen, 1 to 25 days per month, and progesterone, 16 to 25 days per month (produces withdrawal bleeding in 80% of women)
2. Continuous: Estrogen every day, with cyclic progesterone, 16 to 25 days per month
3. Continuous: Estrogen every day and progesterone every day, with combination pills

Table 19-15 Effects of Hormone Replacement Therapy: Possible Risks and Benefits

BENEFITS	RISKS
Decreased vasomotor effects	Increase in gallbladder disease
Protection against osteoporosis	Mixed research regarding increased incidence of breast cancer
Reduction in stroke	
Prevention of lipid changes	
Reduction in CAD	
Improved sleep and mood	
Protection against rheumatoid arthritis	
Possible protection against dementia	

Table 19-16 Contraindications for Hormone Replacement Therapy

HORMONE	RELATIVE	ABSOLUTE
Estrogen	Malignant melanoma Gallbladder problems Hypertension	Known or suspected cancer of breast Known or suspected estrogen-dependent neoplasia History of thromboembolism Recent MI Pregnancy Undiagnosed genital bleeding Unopposed estrogen for women with uterus (estrogen with progestin protects against endometrial cancer by inhibiting endometrial growth)
Progestin	Liver dysfunction Seizure disorders (raises seizure threshold)	Pregnancy

available (after 12 months of combined continuous regimen, most women became amenorrheic)

Principles of Hormone Replacement Therapy

- Begin with the lowest effective dose that relieves symptoms.
- If a woman has her uterus, she should not be given unopposed estrogen. Progestin should be added to the regimen with estrogen.
- If a woman has had a hysterectomy, only estrogen is needed.
- HRT can be begun before menopause, during the perimenopausal period, although it must be emphasized that the HRT does *not* provide contraception. If the woman wants contraception, a low-dose oral contraceptive should be used (use with caution in smokers older than 34 years).
- Once the HRT is begun, a follow-up visit should be scheduled in approximately 3 months to determine how the therapy is working.
- Warn the woman that the estrogen-progestin cycle will produce withdrawal bleeding.
- Testosterone can be used if the woman reports loss of libido (combined with estrogen).

Side Effects

Warn the woman taking HRT of the following side effects and of the need to contact her health provider:

A = Abdominal pain
C = Chest pain
H = Headaches
E = Eye problems
S = Severe leg pain

OTHER SIDE EFFECTS
- Withdrawal bleeding
- Breast tenderness
- Bloating
- Weight gain
- Depression
- Elevated BP
- Increased appetite

Client Education

- Need for yearly follow-up and mammogram
- Discuss benefits and risks of starting HRT.

- Stress the importance of not taking unopposed estrogen because of endometrial hyperplasia; if hormones are not used together, client will need yearly endometrial biopsy.
- Alternatives to HRT:
  —Vaginal creams, such as Replens
  —Nutritional supplementation
    Calcium (discussed in more depth in osteoporosis chapter)
    Vitamin E, 200 to 600 IU
    Vitamin B, ≤50 mg/day
  —Phytoestrogens: Apples, carrots, coffee, potatoes, yams, soy products, flaxseed, bourbon
  —Exercise
  —Relaxation
  —Herbal remedies
    Ginseng and Dong Quai are the most common herbs for menopause symptoms.
    Tincture, tea (infusion), dried root (chewed) capsules
  —Self-help measures
    Layered clothing
    Weight loss
    Stress reduction
    Smoking cessation

FOLLOW-UP

- Yearly Papanicolaou smear and mammogram
- Menstrual calendar

REFERENCES

Evans, C. (1998). Menopause. In F. Zuspan & E. Quilligan (Eds.), *Handbook of obstetrics, gyneology, and primary care* (pp. 91-97). St. Louis: Mosby.

Garner, C. (1994). The climacteric, menopause and the process of aging. In E. Youngkin & M. Davis (Eds.), *Women's health: A primary care clinical guide* (pp. 309-343). Norwalk, CT: Appleton & Lange.

Hormone replacement therapy: Weighing the hazards and rewards (1997). *Clinician Reviews, 7*(9), 53-72.

Lichtman, R. (1996). Perimenopausal and postmenopausal hormone replacement therapy: Part 2. Hormonal regimen and complementary and alternative therapies. *Journal of Nurse Midwifery, 41*(3), 195-210.

Youngkin, E. Q., & Davis, M. S. (1994). Assessing women's health. In E. Q. Youngkin & M. S. Davis (Eds.), *Women's health: A primary care clinical guide* (pp. 33-59). Norwalk, CT: Appleton & Lange.

SUMMARY: CLINICIAN'S ALERT

Table 19-17   Summary of Conditions for Which Clinicians Should Be Alert

CONDITION	POPULATION
Symptoms of peripheral vascular disease	Older persons, smokers, persons with diabetes
Skin lesions with malignant features	General population, but especially with risk factors (light hair, eyes, and skin; severe sun burns as child; excessive sun exposure; malignant precursors; certain congenital nevi; freckles; FH, or personal history, immunosuppression)
Oral cancer and premalignancy	Those who use tobacco (cigarettes, pipes, cigars, chewing tobacco, snuff), older persons who use alcohol regularly
Thyroid impairment	Older persons, postpartum women, persons with Down syndrome
Hearing impairment	Older persons, infants, and young children (younger than 3 yr)
Ocular misalignment	Infants and children
Spinal curvatures	Adolescents
Changes in functional performance	Older adults
Depressive symptoms	Adolescents, young adults, persons at increased risk (personal history or positive FH of depression), those with chronic illnesses, those with recent loss, and those with sleep disorders, chronic pain, or multiple unexplained somatic complaints
Suicide risk	Those with established risks for suicide (depression, drug or alcohol abuse, other psychiatric disorders, previous attempted suicide, recent divorce, separation, unemployment, recent bereavement)
Family violence	General population
Drug abuse	General population
Dental problems	General population

Modified from U. S. Preventive Services Task Force (1996). *Guide to clinical preventive services* (2nd ed.). Baltimore: Williams & Wilkins.

20

Wellness Promotion

CRISIS THEORY

DEFINITION

Psychologic disequilibrium is a state that a person for the time being can neither escape nor solve with the customary problem-solving resources (Townsend, 1996).

Basic Assumptions of Crisis

- Crisis occurs in all individuals, it does not necessarily represent psychopathology.
- Crises are precipitated by specific, identifiable events.
- Personal by nature
- Crisis is acute, not chronic, and will resolve one way or another in a brief period.
- Potential for psychologic growth or deterioration

Phases in Crises

- Vulnerability: Emotional, cognitive, or behavioral
- Exposure to precipitating stressor
- Use of previous problem-solving methods
- Previous methods do not work; anxiety increases.
- All resources are tapped to resolve the problem.
- If crisis is not resolved, tension mounts beyond a further threshold or increases with time to a breaking point.
- Major disorganization of individual occurs.
- Crisis usually lasts 4 to 6 weeks.

Types of Crises

- Situational: Acute response to an external situational stressor

- Developmental: Normal life-cycle transitions
- Posttraumatic stress disorder (PTSD)

Factors Influencing Equilibrium*

- Perception of the event: Realistic or distorted
- Coping mechanisms
- Situational supports

CRISIS INTERVENTION

The goal of crisis intervention is psychologic resolution of the individual's immediate crisis and restoration of the level of functioning that existed before crisis.

Phase 1

- Assessment: Information gathered regarding precipitating stressor
- Evaluation of risk to life: Obvious or potential threat to life or lives of others?
- Evidence that person is able or unable to function in his or her usual role

Phase 2

- Planning of therapeutic interventions
  —How much has the crisis disrupted the individual's life?
  —Is he or she able to go to work or school, keep house, and perform other tasks?
  —How is this disruption influencing others in the person's life?

---

*Aguilera, 1994.

539

Phase 3

- Intervene with reality-oriented approach.
- A working relationship is rapidly established: unconditional acceptance, active listening, and attending to immediate needs.
- Problem-solving model provides the basis for change, active collaboration with affected person. Plan must be consistent with person's culture and lifestyle, dynamic, and renegotiable.
  —Listen actively and with concern.
  —Encourage open expression of feelings.
  —Help the person gain an understanding of the crisis.
  —Help the individual to gradually accept reality.
  —Help the person to explore new ways of coping with problems.
  —Link the person to a social network.
  —Decision counseling is a technique critical to crisis management.
  —Reinforce the newly learned coping methods; provide follow-up after resolution of the crisis (Hoff, 1984, pp. 121-123).

Phase 4

- Evaluation of crisis resolution and anticipatory planning: Plan is developed for recurrence of stressor (Townsend, 1996).
- Follow-up is critical.

EXERCISE

PHYSICAL ACTIVITY

Physical activity is defined as "any bodily movement produced by skeletal muscles and resulting in calorie expenditure" (Bouchard et al., 1990). *Lifestyle exercise* has been characterized as the integration of short bouts of exercise into daily living (Gordon, Kohl, & Blair, 1993). *Healthy People 2000* has set goals that 20% of adults and 75% of children engage in vigorous physical activity on 3 or more days each week for 20 or more minutes, and that at least 30% of persons 6 years and older engage in light to moderate activity daily for at least 30 minutes.

Physical activity appears to decrease significantly during adolescence (Stephens, Jacobs, & White, 1985), with a decline of almost 50% from childhood through adulthood. Females tend to be more sedentary than males (Rowland, 1990). Because exercise or lack of exercise plays a major role in many disease states, it is imperative that all primary care providers assess and counsel their clients regarding the frequency, duration, and intensity of lifestyle exercise. *Healthy People 2000* has as a goal that at least 50% of primary care providers should routinely assess and counsel clients regarding physical activity practices.

BENEFITS OF EXERCISE*

- Increase in lean muscle mass
- Increase in bone mass or prevention of bone loss
- Reduction in systolic and diastolic blood pressure (BP)
- Greater high-density lipoproteins (HDLs)
- Reduction in excess body fat
- Lower insulin level and improved glucose tolerance
- Lower incidence of breast cancer and cancer of reproductive tract
- Improved pulmonary function
- Decreased sympathetically mediated cardiovascular response to stress
- Improvement of anxiety and depression
- Reduction of resting heart rate (HR)
- Increased circulating leukocytes; protection against infection
- Enhanced general mood and psychologic well-being

EXERCISE GUIDELINES

- At every visit, promote lifestyle exercise of at least 20 to 30 minutes of vigorous activity 3 times/week (*vigorous activity* describes an in-

---

*Bouchard, Shephard, & Stephens, 1990.

tensity sufficient enough to produce fatigue in 20 minutes).

- Intensity: Exercise to 60% or more of maximum HR, although recent research proposes that moderate exercise can be just as effective in terms of health benefits (Marcus, Selby, & Niaura, 1992). Moderate activity has higher compliance rates, fits better with daily lifestyle, and is well maintained with time (Duncan, Gordon, & Scott, 1991).

RISK OF EXERCISE

Most adverse effects are related to injury during exercise. Potential adverse effects include injury, osteoarthritis, myocardial infarction, and, rarely, sudden death. Running or jogging carries a high risk of injury (35% to 65%), as does aerobic dancing, for which risk increases with frequency of classes (U.S. Preventive Services Task Force, 1996). Injuries can be prevented by avoiding the following:

- Excessive levels of exercise
- Sudden dramatic increases in activity level (especially in those with poor fitness baseline)
- Improper exercise technique or equipment
- Intense exercise can cause amenorrhea, bone loss, and an increased fracture risk.
- Long-term exercise does not seem to increase the prevalence of osteoarthritis in major weight-bearing joints.
- The risk of adverse cardiovascular events is greater when those who are usually sedentary engage in vigorous activity. The risk of sudden death is lower for those who exercise regularly than for their sedentary counterparts.

CLINICAL INTERVENTION*

- Promote regular exercise for all children and adults.
- Determine each client's activity level.
- Ascertain barriers to exercise.
- Risk assessment: A male older than 40 years with two or more risk factors for coronary artery disease (CAD) should have a resting ECG or stress test; others with known (previous myocardial infarction, pulmonary disease) or possible risk factors (hypertension, cigarette smoking, high blood cholesterol, abuse of drugs, or diabetes) should have a thorough examination before beginning an exercise program (Woolf, Jonas, & Lawrence, 1996)
- Provide information on the role of exercise in disease prevention.
- Assist in selecting appropriate type of exercise (consider factors such as medical limitations and activity characteristics that improve health and enhance compliance).
- Exercise: Regular, moderate-intensity exercise is reasonable for sedentary persons.
- Short-term goal: The goal is a small increase from current activity level with progression to achieve cardiovascular fitness. Thirty minutes brisk walking most days of the week is ideal.
- Sporadic exercise should be discouraged, especially for sedentary individual. Regularity is more important than the type of exercise.

Interventions to Promote Exercise†

- Contracts
- Maintaining self-monitoring diaries and periodic discussions with provider
- Providing personalized feedback and praise
- Setting flexible goals
- Providers who model active lifestyles are more likely to be effective with counseling.
- Encourage client to "take control."
- Periodic rewards
- Gradual change promotes permanent change.

---

*U.S. Preventive Services Task Force, 1996.
†Marcus, Selby, & Niaura, 1992.

FAMILY PLANNING

Approximately 50% of pregnancies in the United States are unintended (Hewitt, 1998). Clients must have access to and education about various forms of contraception. Information about the cost, risks, benefits, failure rates, and use of different forms of contraception should be shared.

FACTORS INFLUENCING CHOICE OF CONTRACEPTION*

- Family background
- Lifestyle
- History and experiences with types of family planning (both partners)
- Religion
- Ease of use
- Cost
- Frequency of intercourse, number of partners
- Side effects
- Effectiveness of method
- Reversibility of method

ABSTINENCE AND RHYTHM METHOD

The purpose is to avoid pregnancy by abstaining from intercourse, either totally or during the fertile times of the month. This method, which is suitable for highly motivated couples and has a 1-year failure rate of approximately 20% (Hewitt, 1998), results in abstaining 17 days of each cycle.

For greatest efficacy, the woman should use the rhythm method in conjunction with counting cycle days, assessing cervical mucous changes, and measuring basal temperatures.

BARRIER METHODS

Barrier methods decrease the transmission of sexually transmitted diseases (STDs) by 50%. Barrier methods include diaphragms, cervical caps, condoms, spermicides, and intrauterine contraceptive devices (IUDs).

Diaphragms

A *diaphragm* is a round, flat latex device that covers the end of the cervix. Diaphragms are used in

*Scoggins & Morgan, 1997.

conjunction with spermicides and are left in place for 6 to 24 hours. Side effects, although few, include increased urinary tract infection (UTI) and irritation from the spermicide. Failure rates range from 2% to 23%; they average 18%.

Cervical Caps

Cervical caps are similar to diaphragms, except smaller. As a result, they may be more difficult to properly fit and insert. The cervical cap may be left in place for as long as 36 hours. The cap, which can be used without spermicide, is used more widely in Europe.

Condoms

Most condoms are made of latex. Both male and female condoms are available; the sheath is placed either over the penis or in the vagina. Failure rate is approximately 12% in 1 year. Oil-based lubricants should not be used with condoms, and the efficacy of the condom may be affected by vaginal medications.

SPERMICIDES

Spermicides are chemicals that inactivate sperm. They are most often used in conjunction with barrier methods, although some protection against pregnancy is provided when used alone. Spermicides have a failure rate of about 20%.

INTRAUTERINE CONTRACEPTIVE DEVICES

An *intrauterine contraceptive device* is an artifact that is placed in the uterus, where it appears to prevent fertilization by interfering with migration of sperm to the fallopian tubes. The failure rate is approximately 2%. An IUD may be used in a lactating woman, and it does not require compliance on the part of the woman. It is an ideal form of contraception for a woman in a monogamous relationship. It does not provide protection against STDs, and it should therefore not be used in any women with a history of STDs or in those with multiple sexual partners, because of the increased risk for pelvic inflammatory disease (PID).

LONG-ACTING PROGESTINS

These preparations prevent contraception by inhibiting ovulation, thickening cervical mucus, and causing the endometrium to become atrophic. Levonorgestrel implants (Norplant) and medroxyprogesterone acetate (Depo-Provera) are two such choices.

Norplant

This contraception method consists of six silicone elastomer rods that are usually inserted beneath the skin of the upper arm. Advantages include contraception for 5 years with a low rate of failure (0.2%). The main disadvantage is the unpredictable vaginal bleeding that occurs in approximately 80% of women during the first year. No protection is provided against STDs.

Depo Provera

This is an injectable method of contraception. The dose is 150 mg every 3 months. Depo-Provera has a user failure rate of 0.3% during the first year. Irregular bleeding is also a problem with this product. Other potential side effects include weight gain, breast tenderness, and depression.

ORAL CONTRACEPTIVES

Oral contraceptives (OCs) are synthetic steroids similar to estrogens and progestins produced by the body. OCs provide contraception by inhibiting ovulation, implantation, or both. Effectiveness ranges from 90% to 96%. Types are *combination* (types and doses of estrogen and progestin remain constant during 21 days) and biphasic or triphasic (dose of progestin component varies to duplicate the pattern of ovulatory menstrual cycle). Progestin-only OCs contain no estrogen and are taken continuously.

Absolute Contraindications

- Pregnancy
- Estrogen-dependent neoplasms
- Previous thromboembolism
- Cerebrovascular accident (CVA)
- Coronary artery disease
- Impaired liver function
- Smoking in a woman older than 35 years

Relative Contraindications

- Elevated BP
- Undiagnosed vaginal bleeding
- Severe headaches
- Diabetes mellitus
- Elevated lipids
- Active gallbladder disease
- Sickle cell anemia

Side Effects

A = Severe abdominal pain
C = Chest pain
H = Headaches
E = Eye problems
S = Severe leg pain

Client should be reevaluated in 3 months after the initiation of OCs to determine whether there are any problems. Check BP at this time.

POSTCOITAL CONTRACEPTION

Pharmacologic postcoital contraception disrupts the postovulatory production of progesterone and estradiol, interferes with the passage of the fertilized ovum through the fallopian tube, shortens the luteal phase, and disrupts the cellular structure of the endometrium. This contraceptive method reduces the number of pregnancies by as much as 84%. Side effects seen are nausea, vomiting, headaches, breast tenderness, dizziness, and alteration of onset of menses. The standard dose of 100 μg ethinyl estradiol and either 0.5 mg of levonorgestrel or 1 mg norgestrel is followed by a second dose 12 hours later. The first dose should be taken as soon as possible after unprotected intercourse; it must be taken within 72 hours for treatment to be effective.

NUTRITION

Increasing emphasis is being placed on the importance of nutrition. Eating healthfully, exercise, and weight control are a big emphasis of the *Healthy People 2000* goals. Lifestyle changes in dietary patterns can make substantial contributions to reductions in the rates of illness and preventable death. Some of the goals identified by *Healthy People 2000* are as follows:

- Reduce dietary fat intake.
- Increase foods containing complex carbohydrate and fiber.
- Combine increased sound dietary practices with regular physical activity to attain appropriate body weight.
- Reduce overweight to a prevalence of no more than 20% among people 20 years old and older and no more than 15% among adolescents 12 through 19 years old.
- Increase the number of primary care providers who offer nutritional assessment and counseling and referral to qualified nutritionists or dietitians.

The largest group at risk for malnutrition is that of older adults (Spark, 1994). Nutritional screening should be conducted for anyone who is 20% below desirable weight or who has had an involuntary loss of more than 10 pounds in the last month.

NUTRITIONAL SCREENING*

Anthropometric Measurements

- Height and weight
- Desirable weight
- Triceps skin fold
- Elbow breadth
- Midarm circumference
- Waist/hip circumference ratio
- Body mass index (BMI): Body weight in kilograms is divided by the square of the height in meters.

Biochemical Measurements

- Hemoglobin
- Cholesterol
- Electrolytes

*Seidel, Ball, Dains, & Benedict, 1995.

- HDL
- Vitamin levels
- Triglycerides
- Hematocrit
- Serum albumin
- Serum transferrin
- Low-density lipoprotein (LDL)
- Nitrogen balance
- LDL/HDL ratio

Clinical Evaluation

Check for the following:

- Alopecia
- Cheilosis
- Glossitis
- Swollen, bleeding gums
- Dry, scaly skin
- Petechiae and ecchymosis
- Bilateral dermatitis
- Edema
- Muscle wasting
- Arthralgia
- Disorientation
- Confabulation
- Neuropathy
- Paresthesia

Dietary Analysis

- Ethnic and cultural background
- Religion
- Food restrictions
- Amount of money spent on food
- Transportation to grocery store
- Participation in food programs
- Preparation of meals
- Meals skipped
- Food preferences
- Food allergies
- Vitamin and mineral supplements
- Medications
- Food intake history (24-hour)

Measurements Suggesting Malnutrition

- Triceps skinfold thickness <10th percentile
- Midarm muscle circumference <10th percentile
- Serum albumin <3.5 g/dl
- Evidence of osteoporosis or mineral deficiency
- Evidence of vitamin deficiency

OBESITY

Obesity is an excess of body fat. One definition is to use BMI (>27.8 for men and >27.3 for women).

An alarming increase has been noted in childhood obesity in the U.S. population. Today, nearly 5 million children 6 to 17 years old are overweight ("Combating Childhood Obesity," 1996). Recommendations from "Physical Activity, Genetic and Nutritional Considerations in Childhood Weight Management" include the following (U.S. Preventive Services Task Force, 1996):

- Children older than 5 years should limit fat to no more than 30% of daily caloric intake.
- Children and adolescents should eat more fruit, vegetables, and grains in their regular diet.
- Snacking should be less frequent. Snacks should be more healthful, low-fat choices.
- Recognize the importance of serving sizes.

DIETARY GUIDELINES FOR AMERICANS*

- Eat a variety of foods.
- Maintain a healthy weight.
- Choose a diet low in fat, saturated fat, and cholesterol.
  —Suggested total fat <30% of calories
  —Suggested saturated fat <10% of calories
  —Eat less fat from animal sources to reduce cholesterol.
- Eat more vegetables, fruits, and grain products.
- Use sugar only in moderation.
- Use salt and sodium only in moderation.
- Drink alcoholic beverages in moderation (1 drink/day).

USE OF THE FOOD GUIDE PYRAMID†

- This system replaces the four food groups.
- It emphasizes food from five major food groups.
- All food groups are needed for a balanced diet in a 24-hour period:

---

*U.S. Department of Agriculture & U.S. Department of Health and Human Services, 1990.
†U.S. Department of Agriculture, 1992.

—Bread, cereal, and rice: 6 to 11 servings
—Fruits: 2 to 4 servings
—Vegetables: 3 to 5 servings
—Meat, poultry, and fish: 2 to 3 servings
—Milk, yogurt, and cheese: 2 to 3 servings
—Fats, oils and sweets: Use sparingly.

POVERTY AND NUTRITION

The United States spent almost $29 billion on food assistance in 1991 (Spark, 1994). Programs that assist the poor in adequate nutrition include the Food Stamp Program; Child Nutrition programs; the Women, Infants, and Children Program (WIC); and the Nutrition Program for the Elderly. Most programs are financed at the federal level through the U.S. Department of Agriculture (USDA).

Women, Infants, and Children Program

WIC provides supplemental foods and nutrition education at no cost for low-income pregnant or postpartum women and for children younger than 5 years. The income eligibility is 185% of the poverty level. WIC recipients receive coupons redeemable for iron-fortified infant formula and cereal, fruit juice, eggs, milk, cheese, and peanut butter or beans.

Nutrition Program for Elderly

This program provides older adults with nutritionally sound meals through Meals on Wheels or in senior citizen settings. Age is the only factor for determining eligibility for the program. People 60 years old or older are eligible.

Food Stamp Program

The purpose of the Food Stamp Program is to supplement the food purchasing power of low-income households. Food stamps are distributed monthly to help purchase a healthful diet, excluding alcohol, tobacco, hot ready-to-eat foods, medicines, and pet foods. Supplemental meals are also provided to low-income children through the school breakfast program and the national school lunch program. These programs are administered by the Food and Nutrition Service as a USDA agency.

SMOKING CESSATION

The adverse effects of smoking are well known. Approximately 430,000 deaths in the United States are caused annually by cigarette smoking (Fiore, 1991). The prevalence of smoking among adolescents has stabilized since 1987, with approximately 21% of high school seniors smoking. Initiation of the habit is occurring at younger ages. Experimentation with smoking occurs most frequently in sixth grade, and the initiation of daily smoking occurs most often in grades 7 to 9 (Rasco, 1992).

ASSOCIATED RISKS OF SMOKING

- Lung Cancer
- Other cancers
- Emphysema
- Respiratory infections
- CAD
- CVA
- Pregnant women: Adverse effects on fetus, with increased risk of miscarriage, stillbirth, and low–birth weight infant
- Second-hand or passive smoke exposure
  —Bronchitis and pneumonia
  —Colds and ear infections
  —Asthma in infants and young children

BENEFITS OF SMOKING CESSATION

- Increased life expectancy
- Risk of dying within next 15 years reduced by half in persons who quit before 50 years
- Reduced risk of premature death in all age groups
- Decreased risk of lung cancer and of cancer of the larynx, oral cavity, esophagus, pancreas, bladder, and cervix
- Reduced risk of CAD
- Reduced risk of peripheral vascular disease
- Reduced risk of ischemic stroke and hemorrhage
- Reduced respiratory symptoms

WHY SMOKERS SMOKE

- Smoking cues and triggers
- Peer pressure and socialization
- Emotional dependence
- Oral gratification
- Relaxation and stress reduction
- Need for reward
- Physiologic addiction to nicotine

ASSESSMENT OF SMOKING STATUS

- Current smoker: Find out whether client has ever tried to quit before and what happened.
- Former smoker
- Never smoker

OPPORTUNITIES FOR INTERVENTION

An opportunity exists for nurse practitioners to reach millions of people with smoking-cessation advice because 70% of all smokers are seen by a provider. Consider smoking status as a vital sign, along with BP, HR, respiratory rate (RR), and temperature (Robinson, Laurent, & Little, 1995).

- Each time a smoker makes a visit, advise about smoking cessation.
- Ask whether client has ever thought about quitting

The stages of smoking cessation are shown in Table 20-1. Most smokers cycle through these stages three or four times before they quit for good. Relapse is a normal part of the smoking-cessation process and should not be viewed as failure.

THERAPEUTIC PLAN
How to Intervene

- *Ask* all clients whether they smoke.
- *Advise* all smokers to stop. Give a strong, unequivocal message, such as, "You must stop smoking now; let's figure out how you can do it," or "I am concerned about your smoking; I must highly recommend you quit." Personalize the message; relate it to the client's disease, social role, and other variables.
- *Assist* smokers who want to quit.
  —Set a quit date.
  —Administer Fagerström test for nicotine dependence.
  —Develop a stop-smoking contract.

Table 20-1   Stages of Smoking Cessation

STAGE	DESCRIPTION
Precontemplation	Smoker is not considering quitting in next 6 months; may rebuff efforts to advise quitting. Back off and approach on another visit. Pushing before the client is ready is not a good idea; it sets client up for failure if he or she tries to quit before ready, discouraging desire to try again.
Contemplation	Smoker is seriously considering quitting within next 6 months; is amenable to advice, educational materials, and information about adverse effects of smoking. Client is often motivated by thoughts of cleaner teeth, better breath, cleaner clothing, and improved self-esteem from stopping.
Preparation	Smoker is ready to change and intends to quit within next 30 days; is ready for information about behavioral counseling or pharmacologic therapy.
Action	Stage is characterized by cessation and abstinence for 6 months.
Maintenance	Maintenance begins after 6 months and continues as long as 3 years. It is important to understand that transition from current smoker to former smoker is a long term process.

Modified from "Smoking status: The new vital sign." (1993). New York: Medical Information Services; Prochaska, J., & DiClemente, C. (1992). Stages of change in the modification of problem behaviors. *Progressive Behavior Modification, 28,* 183-218.

Table 20-2   Methods of Coping With Withdrawal From Smoking

WITHDRAWAL SYMPTOM	WAYS TO COPE
Craving for cigarettes	Do something else, take slow deep breaths, take walk, keep your hands busy, doodle, finger a worry stone, avoid alcohol and coffee, brush teeth, use mouthwash.
Anxiety	Take slow deep breaths, decrease drinks with caffeine, exercise, use relaxation exercises.
Irritability	Walk, do other things, use relaxation exercises.
Constipation	Drink lots of water, exercise, eat high-fiber foods, such as vegetables or fruits.
Hunger	Eat well-balanced meal, keep low-calorie foods, such as carrots and rice cakes, available, and drink water.

—Offer self-help materials.
—Counsel regarding smoking-cessation programs.
—Consider pharmacologic therapy.
- *Arrange* follow-up visits.
  —Phone call within 7 days of initial visit reminds client of quit date and reinforces the decision to quit.
  —Follow-up within the first 2 weeks provides support and encouragement
  1. Identify relapse risks.
     Ask about specific tempting situations.
     Discuss ways to avoid these situations.
     Help the client find something else to do instead of smoke in these situations.
  2. Set up a reward system.

Nonpharmacologic Strategies

- Aversive conditioning
- Hypnosis
- Acupuncture
- Behavior modification

Pharmacologic Strategies

- Nicotine gum
- Transdermal nicotine patches
- Buproprion (Zyban)

Withdrawal Symptoms

Symptoms may last days or weeks.
- Craving for nicotine
- Irritability
- Restlessness
- Increased appetite
- Decreased concentration

Suggested methods of coping with withdrawal from smoking are presented in Table 20-2.

STRESS MANAGEMENT

Many visits to health care providers are due to stress-related illnesses; some sources estimate that 60% to 90% of visits may be related to stress (Pelletier & Lutz, 1988). Holmes and Rahe (1967) developed a method to determine the relationships between social readjustment, stress, and the susceptibility to illness by means of the Social Readjustment Rating Scale. Strategies for health promotion and reduction of stress are important armamentarium for nurse practitioners in primary care.

Goals identified by *Healthy People 2000* include the following:

- Decrease to no more than 5% the proportion of people 18 years old and older who report significant levels of stress and do not take steps to reduce or control stress.
- Reduce to less than 35% the proportion of people 18 years old and older who have experienced adverse health effects from stress within the past year.
- Increase to at least 40% the proportion of worksites employing 50 or more people that provide programs to reduce employee stress.

Stress has been defined as the "nonspecific response of the body to any demand made on it" (Selye, 1975). Physiologic responses of the body to stress include the following:

- Dilatation of pupils
- Increased RR
- Increased HR
- Peripheral vasoconstriction
- Increased perspiration
- Increased BP
- Increased muscle tension
- Increased gastric motility
- Release of adrenalin
- Increased glucose level

These reactions prepare the body for the "flight or fight" mechanism. Stress is associated with decreased life satisfaction, the development of mental disorders, increased incidence of stress-related illnesses, and decreased immunologic function (Pender, 1996). Stressors are interpreted differently by each individual. Some stressors are considered positive and challenging, whereas others are viewed as negative and undesirable. Coping strategies assist the individual in dealing with stressors. *Coping strategies* can be described as "learned and purposeful cognitive, emotional, and behavioral responses to stressors used to adapt to the environment or to change it" (Lazarus & Folkman, 1984).

Children experience stress and develop coping patterns early in life. Factors such as poverty, chronic illness, and parental dysfunction may influence the child's ability to develop effective coping strategies. Most stress research has been conducted with adults, and it may not be applicable to children. Five of the most frequent stressors identified by children are feeling sick, having nothing to do, not having enough money to spend, being pressured to get good grades, and feeling left out of the group (Ryan, 1988).

Stressors in adulthood relate to initiating a career, establishing and maintaining a relationship, and child rearing. Work is often cited as a source of stress. Single parents are especially vulnerable to stress as they try to balance child rearing with the demands of a job.

Loss is the primary stressor for the aging adult. Loss of a spouse, loss of a close family member, and even retirement are considered negative life events. Limitations caused by aging, such as decreased visual acuity and decreased inability to perform activities of daily living, may compound the individual's reaction to stressors, further compromising the immune system.

STRESS MANAGEMENT

The primary modes of stress management consist of the following goals according to Pender (1996):

- Minimizing the frequency of stressors
- Increasing resistance to stress
- Avoiding the physiologic arousal from stress

In general, minimizing the frequency of stressors is the first line of defense. If that is not possible, strengthening family and individual coping resources is the next step.

Minimizing Frequency of Stressors

- Changing the environment (most proactive approach)

—Flexible scheduling at work
—Job sharing
—Child care at worksite
—Job change
- Avoiding excessive change
- Time blocking (Girdano & Everly, 1979): Set aside time to focus on a specific change, developing strategies for adjustment by ensuring that necessary time is given to address critical tasks.
- Time management
  —Identify values and goals; prioritize goals.
  —Identify time wasted, overcommitment, and unrealistic expectations.
  —Learn to say "no" to demands that do not match goals.
  —Reduce tasks into smaller parts.
  —Avoiding overload; delegate responsibilities.
  —Reduce sense of time pressure and urgency.

Increasing Resistance to Stress

- Physical conditioning
  —Promoting exercise: Exercise seems to provide some stress resistance benefits (Norris, Carroll, & Cochrane, 1992).
  —Adequate sleep
  —Good nutrition
- Psychologic conditioning
  —Enhancement of self-esteem: Positive verbalization, identifying the positive personal aspects
  —Enhancement of self-efficacy
    Undertake tasks that can be successfully completed.
    Mentally rehearse successful completion of task.
  —Increase assertiveness
    Greet people by name.
    Maintain eye contact.
    Comment on positive characteristics of others.
    Assertiveness training
  —Development of goal alternatives
  —Development of coping resources
    Self-disclosure
    Self-directedness
    Acceptance
    Social support
    Assessment of coping resources through Coping Resources Inventory (Matheny, Aycock, Curlette, et al., 1993)

Avoiding Physiologic Arousal From Stress

The goal is to replace muscle tension and heightened sympathetic nervous system activity with muscle relaxation and increased parasympathetic functioning (Pender, 1996).

- Deep breathing exercises
- Relaxation training
- Biofeedback
- Imagery
- Meditation

REFERENCES

American Academy of Family Physicians (1997). American Academy of Family Physicians age charts for periodic health examination. In R. B. Murray & J. P. Zentner (Eds.), *Health assessment and promotion strategies* (6th ed., pp. 853-867). Norwalk, CT: Appleton & Lange.

American Academy of Pediatrics (1997). Active and passive immunizations. In G. Peter (Ed.), *1997 Red book: Report of the Committee on Infectious Disease* (24th ed., pp. 1-71). Elk Grove Village, IL: Author.

American Psychiatric Association (1994). *Diagnostic and statistical manual of mental disorders* (4th ed.). Washington, DC: Author.

Aguilera, D. (1998). Crisis intervention: *Theory and methodology* (8th ed.). St. Louis: Mosby.

Barkauskas, V., Stoltenberg-Allen, K., Baumann, L., & Darling-Fisher, C. (1994). *Health and physical assessment.* St. Louis: Mosby.

Barker, L., Burton, J., & Zieve, P. (1995). *Principles of ambulatory medicine* (4th ed.). Baltimore: Williams & Wilkins.

Bouchard, C., Shephard, R., Stephens, T. (Eds.). (1990). *Exercise, fitness, and health.* Champaign, IL: Human Kinetics Books.

Byrd, J. (1994). Content of prenatal care. In S. D. Ratcliffe, J. E. Byrd, & E. L. Sakornut (Eds.), *Handbook of pregnancy and perinatal care in family practice: Science and practice* (pp. 15-27). Philadelphia: Hanley & Belfus.

Centers for Disease Control and Prevention (1996). Immunization of adolescents. *MMWR Morbidity and Mortality Weekly Report, 45,* No. RR-13.

Clark, M. J. Dummer (1996). *Nursing in the community* (2nd ed.). Norwalk, CT: Appleton & Lange.

Combatting childhood obesity. (1996). *Clinician Reviews, 6*(10), 109-110.

Corder-Mabe, J. (1994). Complications of pregnancy. In E. Q. Youngkin & M. S. Davis (Eds.), *Women's health: A primary care clinical guide* (pp. 435-485). Norwalk, CT: Appleton & Lange.

Dawood, M. Y. (1990). Dysmenorrhea. *Clinical Obstetrics and Gynecology, 33* (1), 168-178.

Dickey, R. (1994). *Managing contraceptive pill patients* (8th ed.). Durant, OK: Essential Information Systems.

Duncan, J., Gordon, N., & Scott, C. (1991). Women walking for health and fitness: How much is enough? *Journal of the American Medical Association, 266,* 3295-3299.

Estes, M. (1998). *Health assessment and physical examination.* New York: Delmar.

Fagerström, K., Heatherton, T., & Kozlowski, L. (1990). Nicotine addiction and its assessment. *Ear Nose Throat, 69,* 763-768.

Fenstermacher, K., & Hudson, B. (1997). *Practice guidelines for family nurse practitioners.* Philadelphia: W. B. Saunders.

Fiore, M. (1991). The new vital sign: Assessing and documenting smoking status. *Journal of the American Medical Association, 266,* 3183-3184.

Fontaine, P., & Sayres, W. (1996). Obstetric risk assessment. In S. D. Ratcliffe, J. E. Byrd, & E. L. Sakornut (Eds.), *Handbook of pregnancy and perinatal care in family practice: Science and practice* (pp. 1-14). Philadelphia: Hanley & Belfus.

Fuqua, M. H. (1994). Assessing fetal well-being. In E. Q. Youngkin & M. S. Davis (Eds.), *Women's health: A primary care clinical guide* (pp. 487-518). Norwalk, CT: Appleton & Lange.

Girdano, D., & Everly, G. (1979). *Controlling stress and tension.* Englewood Cliffs, NJ: Prentice-Hall.

Gordon, N., Kohl, H., & Blair, S. (1993). Lifestyle exercise: A new strategy to promote physical activity for adults. *Journal of Cardiopulmonary Rehabilitation, 13,* 161-163.

Hewitt, G. (1998). Contraception. In F. Zuspan & E. Quilligan (Eds.), *Handbook of obstetrics, gynecology, and primary care* (pp. 34-41). St. Louis: Mosby.

Hicks, M. (1993). Well adult care. In P. Sloane, L. Slatt, & R. Curtis (Eds.), *Essentials of family medicine* (pp. 145-153). Baltimore: Williams & Wilkins.

Hobfoll, S. (1988). *The etiology of stress.* Washington, DC: Hemisphere.

Hoff, L. A. (1984). *People in crisis: Understanding and helping* (2nd ed.). Redwood City, CA: Addison-Wesley.

Holmes, T., & Rahe, R. (1967). The social readjustment rating scale. *Journal of Psychosomatic Research, 11,* 213-218.

Hurwitz, J. (1995). Acne treatment for the 90s. *Contemporary Pediatrics, 12* (8), 19-32.

Husten, C., & Manley, M. (1990). How to help your patients stop smoking. *American Family Physician, 42,* 1017-1026.

Johnson, C., Johnson, B., Murray, J., & Apgar, B. (1996). *Women's healthcare handbook.* Philadelphia: Hanley & Belfus, Mosby.

Lazarus, S., & Folkman, S. (1984). *Stress, appraisal and coping.* New York: Springer.

Marcus, B., Selby, V., & Niaura, R. (1992). Self-efficacy and the stages of exercise behavior change. *Research Quarterly Exercise and Sport, 63*(1), 60-66.

Matheny, K., Aycock, D., Curlette, W., et al. (1993). The coping resource inventory for stress: A measure of perceived resourcefulness. *Journal of Clinical Psychology, 49,* 815-829.

Murray, R. B., Zentner, J. P., Pinnell, N. N., & Boland, M. H. (1997). Assessment and health promotion for the person in later maturity. In R. B. Murray & J. P. Zentner (Eds.), *Health assessment and promotion strategies* (6th ed., pp. 693-774). Norwalk, CT: Appleton & Lange.

Norris, R., Carroll, D., & Cochrane, R. (1992). The effects of physical activity and exercise training on psychological stress and well-being in an adolescent population. *Journal of Psychosomatic Research, 36,* 55-65.

Pelletier, K., & Lutz, R. (1988). Healthy people—healthy business: A critical review of stress management programs in the workplace. *American Journal of Health Promotion, 5,* 12, & 19.

Pender, N. (1996). *Health promotion in nursing practice* (3rd ed.). Norwalk, CT: Appleton & Lange.

Prochaska, J., & DiClemente, C. (1992). Stages of change in the modification of problem behaviors. *Progressive Behavior Modification, 28,* 183-218.

Ramos, A. G., & Tuchman, D. N. (1994). Persistent vomiting. *Pediatrics in Review, 5* (1), 24-31.

Rasco, C. (1992). Discouraging smoking: Interventions for pediatric nurse practitioners. *Journal of Pediatric Healthcare, 6,* 200-207.

Remich, M. (1994). Promoting a healthy pregnancy. In E. Q. Youngkin & M. S. Davis (Eds.), *Women's health: A primary care clinical guide* (pp. 383-434). Norwalk, CT: Appleton & Lange.

Robinson, M., Laurent, S., & Little, J. (1995). Including smoking status as a new vital sign: It works. *The Journal of Family Practice, 40,* 556-563.

Rowland, T. (1990). *Exercise and children's health.* Champaign, IL: Human Kinetics.

Ryan, N. (1988). The stress-coping process in school-age children: Gaps in the knowledge needed for health promotion. *Advances in Nursing Science, 11,* 1-12.

Schmitt, B. (1987). *Your child's health.* New York: Bantam.

Scoggins, J., & Morgan, G. (1997). *Practice guidelines for obstetrics and gynecology.* Philadelphia: J. B. Lippincott.

Seidel, H. M., Ball, J. W., Dains, J. E., & Benedict, W. (1995). *Mosby's guide to physical examination.* St. Louis: Mosby.

Selye, H. (1975). *Stress without distress.* New York: NAL Dutton.

Sloane, P., & Hicks, M. (1993). Preventive care: An overview. In P. Sloane, L. Slatt, & P. Curtis (Eds.). *Essentials of family medicine.* Baltimore: Williams & Wilkins.

Smith, K., Johnson, S., & Mandle, C. (1994). Stress management and crisis intervention. In C. Edelman & C. Mandle (Eds.), *Health promotion throughout the lifespan* (3rd ed., pp. 299-323). St. Louis: Mosby.

Smoking status: The new vital sign. (1993). New York: Medical Information Services.

Spark, A. (1994). Nutrition counseling. In C. Edelman & C. Mandle (Eds.), *Health promotion throughout the lifespan* (3rd ed., pp. 265-298). St. Louis: Mosby.

Stephens, T., Jacobs, D., & White, C. (1985). A descriptive epidemiology of leisure-time physical activity. *Public Health Reports, 100,* 147-158.

Swanson, J., & Albrecht, M. (1993). *Community health nursing: Promoting the health of aggregates.* Philadelphia: W. B. Saunders.

Tanner, J. M. (1962). *Growth at adolescence* (2nd ed.). Oxford: Blackwell Scientific.

Townsend, M. (1996). *Psychiatric mental health nursing: Concepts of care* (2nd ed.). Philadelphia: F. A. Davis.

Uphold, C., & Graham, M. (1994). *Guidelines for family practice.* Gainesville, FL: Barmarrae Press.

U.S. Department of Agriculture (1992). *The food guide pyramid* (Home and garden bulletin No. 252). Washington, DC: U.S. Government Printing Office.

U.S. Department of Agriculture & U.S. Department of Health and Human Services (1990). *Nutrition and your health: Dietary guidelines for Americans* (Home and garden bulletin No. 232). Washington, DC: U.S. Government Printing Office.

U.S. Department of Health and Human Services (1993). *Nurses: Help your patients stop smoking.* (NIH Publication No. 92-2962). Washington, DC: Author.

U.S. Department of Health and Human Services (1990). *Healthy people 2000: National health promotion and disease prevention objectives for the year 2000.* Washington, DC: U.S. Government Printing Office.

U.S. Preventive Services Task Force (1996). *Guide to clinical preventive services* (2nd ed.). Baltimore: Williams & Wilkins.

U.S. Public Health Service. (1995). Smoking cessation in adults. *American Family Physician, 51,* 1914-1918.

Wheeler, L. (1997). *Nurse-midwifery handbook: A practical guide to prenatal and postpartum care.* Philadelphia: J. B. Lippincott.

Woolf, S., Jonas, S., & Lawrence, R. (1996). *Health promotion and disease prevention in clinical practice.* Baltimore: Williams & Wilkins.

Youngkin, E., & Davis, M. (1994). *Women's health: A primary care clinical guide.* Norwalk, CT: Appleton & Lange.

Zuspan, F., & Quilligan, E. (1998). *Handbook of obstetrics, gynecology, and primary care.* St. Louis: Mosby.

REVIEW QUESTIONS

1. A client who has started an exercise plan is having minimal success. The nurse practitioner should consider:

    a. Contracting with the client
    b. Referral to an exercise physiologist
    c. Implementing dietary changes
    d. Encouraging the client to set a permanent goal

2. To help the client avoid side effects from exercising, the nurse practitioner should encourage all the following **except:**

    a. Avoid sudden increases in activity level
    b. Proper use of equipment
    c. Intermittent exercise schedule
    d. Proper technique

3. A 45-year-old male client who smokes and has a cholesterol level of 260 g/dl wants to start an exercise program. The nurse practitioner prescribes:

    a. Swimming instead of jogging
    b. A stress test
    c. A beta-blocking agent
    d. Fasting blood glucose level

4. The first priority in stress management is:

    a. Minimizing the frequency of stressors
    b. Increasing the client's resistance to stress
    c. Avoiding physiologic arousal from stress
    d. Strengthening family coping mechanisms

5. Which of the following interventions will help to minimize the frequency of stressors?

    a. Promoting exercise
    b. Enhancing self-esteem
    c. Developing assertiveness
    d. Changing the environment

6. When prescribing interventions designed to avoid the physiologic arousal from stress, the nurse practitioner should do which of the following?

    a. Replace parasympathetic nervous system activity with sympathetic activity.

    b. Promote exercise.

    c. Discuss time management.

    d. Explain the use of imagery.

7. A client who is trying to stop smoking has been unsuccessful in three attempts. The nurse practitioner realizes which of the following?

    a. Relapse is normal and usually occurs three or four times before success.

    b. This client needs immediate referral to a psychiatrist.

    c. This client is immune and will not be successful.

    d. This client is not serious about quitting.

8. When planning care for a client who is trying to stop smoking, the nurse practitioner should do which of the following?

    a. Ask about tempting situations.

    b. Discuss weight control.

    c. Avoid setting a quit date.

    d. Help the client to find new coping strategies.

9. A client who has been using transdermal nicotine patches calls the nurse practitioner after experiencing anxiety and restlessness. The nurse practitioner should do which of the following first?

    a. Prescribe an antianxiety agent.

    b. Tell the client that this is a symptom of nicotine withdrawal and that it will go away.

    c. Assess the client's use of drinks containing caffeine.

    d. Prescribe more transdermal nicotine patches.

10. The Food Guide Pyramid:

    a. Emphasizes food from six major food groups

    b. Replaces the four food groups approach

    c. Allows the substitution of one food group for another food group

    d. Allows more servings of fruits than of bread, cereal, and rice

11. Community nutritional programs for older adults are available for:

    a. Financially deprived older adults

    b. Anyone older than 60 years

    c. Older adults with chronic health conditions

    d. Older adults without family support

12. The food stamp program was designed to:

    a. Provide resources for older adults

    b. Provide resources for postpartum women and children

    c. Supplement the food purchasing power of low-income households

    d. Only be used for people receiving Medicaid

13. When performing a pelvic examination on a menopausal woman, normal findings would be:

    a. Pale cervix, decreased pelvic floor muscle tone, smaller uterus

    b. Cervix with white secretions at os, enlarged ovaries, thinning of pubic hair

    c. Atrophied vulva, enlarged uterus, cervical friability

    d. No change in pubic hair, smaller uterus, increased vaginal rugae

14. Preventive education to reduce tobacco and alcohol use in adolescents is most effective:

    a. In grades 11 and 12

    b. In grades 7 through 9

    c. For teens identified as using alcohol

    d. In inner-city schools

15. Which of the following activities describes primary prevention for men?

    a. Teach testicular self-examination (TSE)

    b. Teach about an antihypertensive drug

    c. Teach a client with gonorrhea about the potential for prostatitis later in life

    d. Educate the client about the hazards of substance abuse

16. Which of the following activities describes primary prevention for Mrs. Cook, an 80-year-old widow?

    a. Encourage Mrs. Cook to work through any grief related to her husband's death.

    b. Refer Mrs. Cook for financial assistance.

    c. Determine whether Mrs. Cook has adequate access to health care.

    d. Contact Mrs. Cook's landlord to install a handrail on stairs.

17. Ms. Black is a 25-year-old pregnant woman with two small children. Which of the following pertains to secondary prevention?

    a. Prepare the children for the birth of the new child.
    b. Discuss with her the advantages and disadvantages of bottle- and breast-feeding.
    c. Discuss with her various options for birth control.
    d. Refer her to a women's crisis shelter.

18. Secondary prevention strategies commonly used for women's health care include:

    a. Papanicolaou smear
    b. Contraception counseling
    c. Prepregnancy counseling
    d. Monitoring diabetes and compliance with diabetic regimen

19. When counseling a woman about hormone replacement therapy (HRT), the nurse practitioner should inform her of which of the following effects?

    a. HRT decreases the risk of gallbladder disease.
    b. HRT may produce sleep disturbances.
    c. HRT reduces breast cancer.
    d. HRT reduces the chance of a stroke.

20. Before initiating HRT, which of the following should be performed?

    a. Mammography
    b. Cardiac enzyme panel
    c. ECG
    d. Chest x-ray film

21. When starting estrogen-progesterone HRT for a perimenopausal woman, the nurse practitioner should tell her that it will:

    a. Provide contraception
    b. Increase libido
    c. Produce withdrawal bleeding
    d. Decrease the likelihood of contracting STDs

22. The nurse practitioner should schedule a follow-up examination of a woman started on HRT at:

    a. 1 week
    b. 1 month
    c. 3 months
    d. 6 months

23. The proper use of HRT is:

    a. When menses cease
    b. During the perimenopausal period and after
    c. After the birth of the last desired child
    d. When bone demineralization begins

24. A woman who has had a complete hysterectomy wants HRT for relief of symptoms. The best drug to prescribe is:

    a. Progesterone-only pill
    b. Estrogen-only patch
    c. Combination of progesterone and estrogen
    d. Vaginal lubrication cream

25. Thrombophlebitis develops in a woman receiving HRT. The nurse practitioner should do which of the following?

    a. Stop HRT.
    b. Increase the progesterone.
    c. Increase the estrogen.
    d. Decrease both the estrogen and the progesterone.

26. Which of the following statements is **false** about older adults and drug use?

    a. Absorption can be affected by increased pH of the gastric mucosa, decreased surface of the gut, and increased motility of the gut.
    b. Distribution is affected by increased body fat, resulting in increased distribution of lipid-soluble medications.
    c. Metabolism can be affected by decreased hepatic mass, decreased blood flow, and decreased enzymatic activity.
    d. Excretion is affected by decreased renal and glomerular filtration rates, resulting in decreased excretion rate.

27. Robert is a 72-year-old white male who comes to your office for an annual examination. He weighs 150 pounds and is 65 inches tall, well developed, in no distress, and married with one child. He has a history of high cholesterol level. One of the most important history-taking tasks will be to determine:

    a. How stable his weight has been during the last 6 months
    b. The last time his cholesterol test was performed
    c. The risk factors identified in his genogram
    d. His exposure to hazardous elements

28. Robert (72 years) and his wife have been married for 50 years. Both are monogamous. They appear devoted to each other and speak fondly of their experiences together. Your examination of Robert will include a general survey of his cardiopulmonary status, gastrointestinal system, musculoskeletal system, and neurologic status. In addition to these systems, you would do or obtain which of the following?

    a. Digital rectal examination (DRE), prostate-specific antigen (PSA), lipid level, fecal occult blood (FOB)
    b. DRE, lipid level, FOB, hepatitis A
    c. Lipid level, DRE, PSA, HIV
    d. HIV, rapid plasma reagin test (RPR), PSA, lipid level

29. Sam is a 66-year-old male who is retired from the railroad, with a good pension and no financial worries. He has two children, and 2 months ago, he lost his wife of 42 years. His children live in the area, and he sees them about once every 2 weeks. Sam speaks of his wife and the loss that he feels without her. Which of the following will assist Sam in his grief process the **least?**

    a. Exploration of where he derives his support
    b. Exploration of how he has grieved in the past and his success in so doing
    c. Exploration of new ways that he can develop support
    d. Exploration of how his family has coped with the loss of his wife

30. Sam's hobby is making miniature replicas of homes and sites that are special to him. He has made one of his homestead and one of his church, where he is a deacon. He is currently working on a replica of his late wife's home place. Sam goes out to eat with family members. He has learned to cook for himself at home. His grandchildren stay with him periodically. On the basis of this information, you would speculate that:

    a. Sam has accomplished Erikson's developmental task for his age
    b. Sam has not accomplished Erikson's developmental task for his age
    c. Sam is depressed.
    d. Having a family member move in with Sam would improve his adjustment after his wife's death.

31. Required elements of a history that differentiate women 65 years old and older from younger women are which of the following?

    a. Blood transfusion history
    b. Symptoms of transient ischemic attack and functional status at home
    c. Medication history
    d. Menstrual history

32. Jane Jenson, 25 years old, comes in for a yearly examination. A recent sexual partner was an IV drug user. Ms. Jenson smokes 10 cigarettes a day and drinks approximately 3 beers during a weekend. She uses a tanning bed once a week. Her diet is high in fat and processed sugars. Which of the following is **not** necessary for Ms. Jenson?

    a. HIV testing, smoking-cessation program, and mammography
    b. Thyroid, breast, and pelvic examinations; DRE
    c. Skin examination and counseling related to diet and the practice of tanning
    d. Mammography

33. Ms. Wendner, 45 years old, has a positive family history for cancer. Results of her last mammography and proctoscopy were negative. How often should these tests be repeated?

    a. Repeat mammography in 1 to 3 years and proctoscopy in 3 to 5 years.
    b. Repeat mammography q 6 months and proctoscopy in 3 to 5 years.
    c. Repeat mammography in 3 years and proctoscopy in 1 year.
    d. Repeat mammography in 1 to 2 years and proctoscopy in 3 to 5 years.

34. All women should receive which of the following immunizations every 10 years?

    a. Varicella
    b. Tetanus-diphtheria (Td)
    c. Hepatitis B
    d. Influenza vaccine

35. Which of the following physical findings is consistent with a nonpathologic breast mass?

    a. 2 to 3 cm fatty tissue bilaterally beneath nipples
    b. Bilateral compressible nodular tissue
    c. Unilateral, hard, ulcerated tissue at nipple
    d. 1 to 2 cm hard, fixed mass

36. Wendy Winslow is in her 40th week of pregnancy. Which is the most important question to ask her?

a. Are you noticing any skin changes?
b. Have you noticed any changes in the baby's movement?
c. Are you having any painful urination?
d. Are you experiencing any nausea?

37. Indications for genetic counseling at the preconception visit include all the following **except:**

a. Adolescent pregnancy
b. Advanced paternal age
c. Family history of genetic abnormalities
d. Advanced maternal age

38. Linda Johnson is 9 weeks' pregnant. From your history and examination, you determine that she is experiencing nausea from pregnancy. You recommend all the following **except:**

a. Avoidance of greasy and spicy foods
b. Keeping dry crackers at the bedside
c. Avoidance of carbonated beverages
d. Small, frequent meals

39. Ultrasonographic indications include all the following **except:**

a. Determining dating of pregnancy
b. Vaginal bleeding
c. Identification of baby's gender
d. Suspicion of ectopic pregnancy

40. Screening for diabetes should be done during which gestational period?

a. 12 to 14 weeks
b. 15 to 16 weeks
c. 15 to 18 weeks
d. 24 to 28 weeks

41. Which of the following laboratory tests should be done at each prenatal visit?

a. Proteinuria, glucosuria, and ketonuria
b. Proteinuria, hematocrit, and glucosuria
c. Proteinuria, urine culture, and glucosuria
d. Proteinuria, gonorrhea, and thyroid

42. A child receives her first *Haemophilus influenzae* B vaccine (HIB) at 12 months of age. At what age should the child receive her booster?

a. 13 months
b. 14 months
c. 2 years
d. 16 to 18 months

43. A child who is 7 years old needs a tetanus booster. You would order:

a. Td
b. DPaT
c. DPT
d. OPV

44. If the first measles-mumps-rubella vaccine (MMR) was given between 12 to 15 months of age, when is the booster due? When the child is:

a. 14 months
b. 5 to 6 years
c. 16 to 20 months
d. 15 years

45. A 1-month-old infant is here for a well-child examination. All the following factors would be part of your assessment **except:**

a. Fontanelles
b. Hip assessment
c. Weight gain between 15 to 30 g/kg/day
d. Fundi

46. A 4-year-old is in your office for a well-child examination. All the following anticipatory guidance issues would be included **except:**

a. Masturbation
b. Bicycle safety
c. Stranger anxiety
d. Dental hygiene and dental referral

47. An infant is seen in your office to rule out failure to thrive. His weight is less than the fifth percentile on his growth curve, but he appears healthy. The parent reports that the child spits up formula frequently. On his nutritional history, the mother reports that his intake of formula is about 24 to 26 ounces/day. The most likely diagnosis in this child is:

a. Pyloric stenosis
b. Metabolic disorder
c. Milk allergy
d. Rumination

48. Which of the following best represents a normal sequence of pubertal events for a female?

   a. Breast buds, axillary hair, ovaries enlarged, menarche
   b. Menarche, axillary hair, breast buds
   c. Growth spurt, breast buds, menarche
   d. Breast buds, pubic hair development, menarche

49. Acne lesions most commonly erupt on which of the following areas of the body?

   a. Face, upper arms, and abdomen
   b. Cheeks, forehead, chin, chest, and back
   c. Face, buttocks, chest, and back
   d. Cheeks, forehead, and chin

50. Which of the following is most consistent with a diagnosis of anorexia nervosa in a 15-year-old female?

   a. BMI 5%, refusal to gain weight, perception of being overweight, amenorrhea
   b. BMI 15%, concerns about gaining weight, normal menstrual cycles
   c. BMI 10%, concern with weight, active in sports, oligomenorrhea
   d. BMI 15%, satisfaction with weight, normal menstrual cycles, vegetarian diet

51. Which of the following is the correct schedule for Td?

   a. Td booster in adolescence 10 years after last DTP, DTaP or DT
   b. Td booster at early, middle, and late adolescence
   c. Td booster at 11 to 12 years if 5 years has elapsed since last DTP, DTaP, or DT; subsequently, every 10 years
   d. Td booster at 11 to 12 years if 5 years has elapsed since last DTP, DTaP, or DT; subsequently, every 5 years

52. A 15-year-old adolescent continues to have monthly dysmenorrhea after 3 months of non-steroidal antiinflammatory drugs and oral contraceptives. This adolescent should be referred for evaluation of:

   a. Secondary dysmenorrhea
   b. Primary dysmenorrhea
   c. Psychogenic pain syndrome
   d. Premenstrual syndrome

53. Which of the following clients should be referred to an optometrist for glaucoma screening?

   a. 35-year-old white male with severe myopia
   b. 42-year-old black male with severe myopia and family history of glaucoma
   c. 45-year-old white male with presbyopia
   d. 38-year-old black male with corneal abrasion

54. The U.S. Preventive Services Task Force recommends that which of the following males have a DRE?

   a. Those older than 40 years
   b. Those with a history of hemorrhoids
   c. Persons who exchange sex for money or drugs and their sex partners
   d. Residents of long-term care facilities

55. A 29-year-old healthy male has an appointment with you for suture removal and asks you whether he needs any other immunizations besides the DT that he received at his laceration repair. He tells you that he has had all the childhood immunizations. What would you ask him so that you can determine what immunizations he needs?

   a. Have you ever had chickenpox?
   b. Do you have diabetes?
   c. Do you exercise regularly?
   d. Do you smoke cigarettes?

56. To determine the appropriate health promotion activities and screening for a client, it is most important to do which of the following?

   a. Give the client a thorough physical examination.
   b. Consider the leading causes of death for that particular age group.
   c. Assess each individual's risk factors for morbidity and mortality.
   d. Do some laboratory work to assess kidney and liver function.

57. Which of the following would indicate that your client is following the health promotion guidelines you suggested?

   a. Weight gain of 2 pounds
   b. Using the food pyramid as a basis for meal planning
   c. Eating a vegetarian diet
   d. Working 50 hours/week as a computer programmer

58. A 45-year-old client just had his cholesterol level checked. When should the test be repeated if the result was normal?

    a. Annually
    b. Every 10 years
    c. Every 5 years
    d. Every 3 years

59. Drug treatment for hyperlipidemia should begin when the client:

    a. Reaches 65 years
    b. Has one risk factor and an LDL level 160 mg/dl
    c. Has more than two risk factors and an LDL level of 165 mg/dl
    d. Has an LDL level >130 mg/dl

60. Which of the following is true when beginning drug therapy for hyperlipidemia?

    a. Dietary therapy should continue.
    b. Exercise activity should be cut down slightly.
    c. The client should be referred to a cardiologist.
    d. Smoking must be stopped.

61. A client's lipid levels have not dropped to a therapeutic range after nicotinic acid and dietary therapy. What should the nurse practitioner do next?

    a. Refer the client to a cardiologist.
    b. Stop the nicotinic acid.
    c. Add another cholesterol-reduction drug.
    d. Discuss with the client why he or she has not been following the treatment plan.

62. When a client is placed on an American Heart Association Step One diet to lower cholesterol and fat intake and has limited success, the next course of action for the nurse practitioner to take is to do which of the following?

    a. Teach the client again about the benefits of a low-fat diet and try the Step One diet for another 3 months.
    b. Teach the client how to follow the Step Two AHA diet.
    c. Start a bile acid sequestrant drug
    d. Start the client on a diuretic

63. The nurse practitioner performs a Denver Developmental Screening Test (DDST) for a 5-year-old. This is considered part of the:

    a. Health history
    b. Treatment plan

    c. Provision of anticipatory guidance
    d. Assessment

64. The nurse practitioner is providing client education for a 56-year-old female client. This client plays tennis weekly, has an HDL level of 25 mg/dl, and is an information systems analyst who is using hormone replacement therapy. What is a protective factor against CAD for this client?

    a. Her HDL level
    b. HRT
    c. Her exercise
    d. Her job

65. When assessing a client for risk for CAD, the nurse practitioner should ask about:

    a. 24-hour dietary recall
    b. Use of vitamins
    c. Use of diet drinks
    d. Past history of obesity

66. When performing a well-child examination on a 13-year-old child, the nurse practitioner discovers that the child is planning to try out for football. The child's father used to play professional football, but he died at 51 years of a heart attack. To assess the child's potential for CAD, the nurse practitioner should do which of the following?

    a. Perform a careful funduscopic examination.
    b. Order a cholesterol level.
    c. Assess for hepatomegaly.
    d. Order a triglyceride level.

67. After starting a client on a 3-hydroxy-3 methyl-glutaryl coenzyme A cholesterol-reducing agent, the nurse practitioner should recheck the client's lipid profile in:

    a. 1 month
    b. 1 week
    c. 6 months
    d. 1 year

68. What is the difference between a crisis and another anxiety related event?

    a. A crisis results in emotional deterioration.
    b. A crisis evolves slowly and is not attributed to a specific event.
    c. A crisis is resolvable in a brief period.
    d. A crisis is a psychopathologic event.

69. A nurse practitioner caring for a client in crisis asks her to describe her daily life. This information will help in:

    a. Planning therapeutic interventions
    b. Evaluating the person's threat of suicide
    c. Resolving the crisis
    d. Planning for the recurrence of the stressor

70. In helping the client in crisis attain equilibrium, the nurse practitioner must assess the client's:

    a. Coping mechanisms
    b. Psychologic history
    c. Response to drug therapy
    d. Past medical history

71. An adolescent client is extremely upset about a car crash that she was involved in with an uninsured driver. She is fearful of losing her job because of lack of transportation. This reflects:

    a. Posttraumatic stress disorder
    b. A situational crisis
    c. A developmental crisis
    d. An occupational crisis

ANSWERS AND RATIONALES

1. *Answer:* a (health promotion/lifestyle/exercise)
Rationale: Contracting has promoted adherence to an exercise plan. Flexible goals promote compliance. Dietary changes should be implemented, with or without success. Referral is not necessary at this time. (Marcus, Selby, & Niaura, 1992)

2. *Answer:* c (health promotion/lifestyle/exercise)
Rationale: Regular exercise decreases side effects, as do proper equipment and technique and avoidance of sudden increases in activity level. (U.S. Preventive Services Task Force, 1996)

3. *Answer:* b (health promotion/lifestyle/exercise)
Rationale: A male older than 40 years with two or more risk factors for CAD should have a stress test before initiating an exercise program. Swimming may be detrimental to his health. Beta-blocking agents would decrease his compensatory ability to increase his HR to maintain cardiac output during higher demand. (Woolf, Jonas, & Lawrence, 1996)

4. *Answer:* a (health promotion/lifestyle/stress management)
Rationale: Choices *b, c,* and *d* are appropriate in stress management, but the main goal is to decrease the frequency of stressors. If this is accomplished, the need for the other three is also diminished. (Pender, 1996)

5. *Answer:* d (health promotion/lifestyle/stress management)
Rationale: Changing the environment is the most proactive approach to managing stress. It should decrease the amount of stressors, which also decreases the need for *a, b,* and *c.* (Pender, 1996)

6. *Answer:* d (health promotion/lifestyle/stress management)
Rationale: The aim is to promote parasympathetic stimulation to decrease arousal. Exercise will increase sympathetic stimulation. Time management will decrease the frequency of stressors, which indirectly decreases sympathetic stimulation. (Pender, 1996)

7. *Answer:* a (health promotion/lifestyle/health behaviors)
Rationale: Patient frequently relapses during attempts to stop smoking. It does not mean that a referral is needed or that the person cannot stop smoking or is not serious about quitting.

8. *Answer:* a (health promotion/lifestyle/health behaviors)
Rationale: Asking about tempting situations can help the nurse practitioner to discuss ways of avoiding these situations and to help identify ways to behave in these situations as a form of anticipatory guidance. A quit date should be set. Old coping strategies can be used and may be comforting. Discussion about weight control may discourage the client from stopping smoking because of fear of weight gain.

9. *Answer:* c (health promotion/lifestyle/health behaviors)
Rationale: Although irritability, restlessness, and anxiety are side effects of nicotine withdrawal, the client may be causing an increase in these side effects through the use of caffeine. Nonpharmacologic interventions should be tried first.

10. *Answer:* b (health promotion/lifestyle/nutrition)

Rationale: There are five major food groups in the pyramid. All food groups are needed for a balanced diet. The bread, cereal, and rice group is allowed in greater quantities than the other food groups. The pyramid does replace the four major food groups format. (U.S. Department of Agriculture, 1992)

11. *Answer:* b (health promotion/lifestyle/nutrition)

Rationale: Age is the only factor for determining eligibility for these programs.

12. *Answer:* c (health promotion/lifestyle/nutrition)

Rationale: The Food Stamp Program was designed to provide resources regardless of the age or health status of the family. Families receiving Medicaid may be eligible because of their household income, but this is not required for participation. Income is the determining factor.

13. *Answer:* a (physical examination/assessment/wellness/aging adult)

Rationale: Because of decreased estrogen, the cervix pales and shrinks, pubic hair diminishes, the uterus shrinks in size and weight, vaginal rugae decrease, and the vulva atrophies. (Youngkin & Davis, 1994)

14. *Answer:* b (health promotion/primary prevention/adolescent)

Rationale: Reduce tobacco and alcohol use with preventive education in grades 7 through 9. (U.S. Preventive Services Task Force, 1996)

15. *Answer:* d (health promotion/primary prevention/NAS)

Rationale: Teaching about TSE and antihypertensive drugs implies treatment of existing conditions, whereas teaching about gonorrhea and prostatitis is preventing complications. Teaching about the hazards of substance abuse is the only activity that promotes prevention of a problem. (Clarke, 1996)

16. *Answer:* d (health promotion/primary prevention/aging adult)

Rationale: The only activity that prevents problems is the handrail. All others relate to existing conditions or preventing complications. (Clarke, 1996)

17. *Answer:* d (health promotion/secondary prevention)

Rationale: Referring Ms. Balck to a women's crisis center for spousal violence necessitates the identification of an existing problem. All other options describe primary preventive activities. (Clarke, 1996)

18. *Answer:* a (health promotion/secondary prevention)

Rationale: The Papanicoloau smear is the only commonly used secondary strategy listed. Contraception and prepregnancy counseling is primary prevention. Monitoring diabetes is a secondary prevention strategy, but it is not recommended for all women. (Swanson & Albrecht, 1993)

19. *Answer:* d (wellness/management/client education)

Rationale: HRT increases the risk of gallbladder disease, improves sleep, and may actually increase the risk for breast cancer.

20. *Answer:* a (plan/wellness/management/pharmacologic)

Rationale: Known or suspected breast cancer is a contraindication for HRT. Because HRT may improve cardiovascular status, ECG and cardiac enzyme panel are not necessary before starting HRT. A chest radiograph would not be useful.

21. *Answer:* c (plan/wellness/management/pharmacologic)

Rationale: HRT does not provide contraception; a low-dose OC is needed. Testosterone is used to increase libido. STDs are prevented only by abstinence or use of condoms. A combined HRT will produce withdrawal bleeding.

22. *Answer:* c (evaluation/wellness/pharmacologic)

Rationale: It takes 3 months for the cyclic pattern to be established and hormone levels to adjust.

23. *Answer:* b (plan/wellness/management/pharmacologic)

Rationale: HRT should be used during the perimenopausal period and after. It can be started with the cessation of menses, but the purpose of the medication is to decrease symptoms produced by decreased estrogen that occur perimenopausally and after. Unless a child is born during the perimenopausal period, HRT should not be started just because reproduction is no longer a goal. The goal of early HRT is to prevent bone demineralization.

24. *Answer:* b (plan/wellness/management/pharmacologic)

Rationale: Progesterone protects against endometrial cancer and should be used in the woman with a uterus. Estrogen alone should be used only for women who have undergone a complete hysterectomy. Vaginal lubrication cream will only take care of a few symptoms associated with decreased estrogen.

25. *Answer:* a (plan/wellness/management/pharmacologic)

Rationale: Thrombophlebitis is a contraindication for both progesterone and estrogen, and HRT should not be used.

26. *Answer:* a (assessment/history/aging adult)

Rationale: All the statements are true, but there is actually decreased motility in older adults.

27. *Answer:* c (assessment/history/aging adult)

Rationale: A genogram is most important, because with it you will determine the significance of family history for common illnesses.

28. *Answer:* a (assessment/physical examination/aging adult)

Rationale: HIV does not need to be tested because of the monogamous relationship. Hepatitis A is also inappropriate based on the history. (Hicks, 1993; Uphold & Graham, 1994; Sloane & Hicks, 1993)

29. *Answer:* d (assessment/history/aging adult)

Rationale: Although all are useful, the least important is exploration of how others have coped with the loss of his wife. (Sloane & Hicks, 1993; Uphold & Graham, 1994)

30. *Answer:* a (assessment/history/aging adult)

Rationale: Sam appears to be self-reliant, has lived a full life, and is able to resort to that full life to manage the loss of his wife. There are no data reflecting any type of despair. (Hicks, 1993)

31. *Answer:* b (assessment/history/aging adult)

Rationale: Women 65 years old and older experience conditions that contribute to the occurrence of transient ischemic attacks and are more likely to require assistance in maintaining functional status at home. (Murray, Zentner, Pinnell, & Boland, 1997)

32. *Answer:* d (assessment/physical examination/adult)

Rationale: Ms. Jenson's history provides risk factors, such as sexual history, smoking, diet, and skin exposure, that place Ms. Jenson at risk. Thus her health status relative to these risk factors needs to be monitored. She is too young for routine mammography. (American Academy of Family Physicians, 1997)

33. *Answer:* d (diagnosis/plan/adult)

Rationale: Mammography should be repeated at 1 to 2 years; proctoscopy should be repeated in 3 to 5 years. (Youngkin & Davis, 1994)

34. *Answer:* b (plan/health promotion/adult)

Rationale: It is recommended that immunization boosters for Tetanus-diphtheria should be provided every 10 years. (American Academy of Family Physicians, 1997)

35. *Answer:* b (assessment/physical examination/adult)

Rationale: Normal breast tissue is glandular and may be nodular. Fatty tissue beneath nipples is consistent with gynecomastia; hard, ulcerated tissue and a hard fixed mass are characteristics of carcinoma. (Estes, 1998, p. 352)

36. *Answer:* b (assessment/history/childbearing female)

Rationale: Postdate fetus are considered to be at risk and need to have their status monitored. (Fuqua, 1994)

37. *Answer:* a (assessment/history/childbearing female)

Rationale: Adolescent pregnancy has not been identified as a risk factor that indicates genetic testing. (Fontaine & Sayres, 1996)

38. *Answer:* c (plan/childbearing female)

Rationale: Carbonated beverages help to provide relief for nausea. (Remich, 1994)

39. *Answer:* c (plan/diagnostics/childbearing female)

Rationale: Identification of an infant's gender is not a medical indication for ultrasonographic imaging. (Byrd, 1994)

40. *Answer:* d (plan/diagnostics/childbearing female)

Rationale: The optimal time for testing for diabetes during pregnancy is 24 to 28 weeks. (Corder-Mabe, 1994)

41. *Answer:* a (plan/diagnostics/childbearing female)

Rationale: Urine is examined for (1) protein to screen for preeclampsia and UTI, (2) glucose to screen for diabetes, and (3) ketones to screen for hyperemesis gravidarum. (Wheeler, 1997; Remich, 1994)

42. *Answer:* d (plan/child)

Rationale: If a child receives the first HIB at 12 months, the booster needs to be given between 15 months and 4 years. Because this child was behind on immunizations, it is recommended that the booster be given as soon as possible, to avoid a missed immunization opportunity. (American Academy of Pediatrics, 1997)

43. *Answer:* a (plan/child)

Rationale: The *Red Book* recommends no more pertussis vaccine after 6 years because the disease is not life-threatening. (American Academy of Pediatrics, 1997)

44. *Answer:* b (plan/child)

Rationale: The first MMR is recommended after the child is 1 year old. The booster is recommended between 4 and 6 years or 11 to 12 years. Booster can be given at either time, although it is recomended that the booster be given at the earlier age to avoid a missed immunization opportunity.

45. *Answer:* d (assessment/physical examination/infant)

Rationale: A funduscopic examination is not routinely done on children younger than 3 years, although it is possible to perform a funduscopic examination on a child as young as 6 to 7 months. (Barkauskas, Stoltenberg-Allen, Baumann, & Darling-Fisher, 1994, p. 792)

46. *Answer:* c (assessment/history/plan/child)

Rationale: Stranger anxiety usually appears around 9 months to 18 months, then reappears around 2½ years. It is seen whenever the child loses sight of the mother or is left with a sitter. These fears often heighten at night. (Schmitt, 1987)

47. *Answer:* d (diagnosis/child)

Rationale: Rumination is behavioral in nature. Ruminators often have FTT despite an otherwise healthy appearance. (Ramos & Tuchman, 1994)

48. *Answer:* d (assessment/history/adolescent)

Rationale: Menarche generally begins within 2 to 3 years after the onset of breast development. The average age for girls in the United States is 12 to 13 years. Menarche signals the end of the rapid growth stage. (Tanner, 1962)

49. *Answer:* b (assessment/history/adolescent)

Rationale: Acne most commonly occurs on the face (especially the forehead, chin, and cheeks), the chest, and the back. There are nearly 900 sebaceous glands/cm² in these areas, as compared with 100 glands/cm² on other skin surfaces. (Hurwitz, 1995)

50. *Answer:* a (diagnosis/adolescent)

Rationale: Diagnostic criteria include a refusal or inability to maintain body weight, fear of gaining weight or becoming fat despite being underweight, distorted body image, and absence of three consecutive menstrual cycles. (American Psychiatric Association, 1994)

51. *Answer:* c (plan/adolescent)

Rationale: The age of administration of Td booster has been lowered from 14 to 16 years to 11 to 12 years to ensure long-lasting immunity against tetanus. Immunity to tetanus varies with age; 28% of children vaccinated 6 to 10 years before serologic testing lacked immunity, as compared with 14% of those vaccinated 1 to 5 years before testing. The Td booster at 11 to 12 years is the only exception to the administration of routine boosters every 10 years. (Centers for Disease Control and Prevention, 1996)

52. *Answer:* a (plan/adolescent)

Rationale: The differential diagnosis of secondary dysmenorrhea includes endometriosis, pelvic inflammatory disease, uterine polyps or fibroids, and anatomic disorders. A diagnostic laparoscopy should be considered. (Dawood, 1990)

53. *Answer:* b (assessment/history/secondary prevention/adult)

Rationale: Glaucoma screening by an eye specialist is recommended for blacks older than 40 years and whites older than 65 years, those with a family history of glaucoma, those with diabetes, and those with severe myopia. (U.S. Preventive Services Task Force, 1996)

54. *Answer:* a

Rationale: Colorectal cancer is the second most common type of cancer in the United States and carries the second highest morbidity and mortality. Age over 40 is a risk factor. FOB and sigmoidoscopy (with a 60 cm flexible scope) are currently considered the most effective methods of screening. (U.S. Preventive Services Task Force, 1996)

55. *Answer:* a (health promotion/plan/adult)

Rationale: A case of chickenpox is usually mild in a healthy child, but the complication and fatality rates increase significantly for older adolescents and adults. (U.S. Preventive Services Task Force, 1996)

56. *Answer:* c (health promotion/plan/wellness/NAS)

Rationale: It is important to consider the leading causes of death for a particular age group to determine what sorts of questions should be elicited on the history, but the plan for an individual client is determined by that individual's risk for dying of the leading cause of death or any other morbidity or mortality. (U.S. Preventive Services Task Force, 1996)

57. *Answer:* b (health promotion/evaluation/NAS)

Rationale: Using the food pyramid promotes a well-balanced diet according to current nutritional recommendations. (Woolf, Jonas, & Lawrence, 1996)

58. *Answer:* c (health promotion/plan/wellness/management/diagnostics/NAS)

Rationale: National Cholesterol Education Program guidelines state every 5 years for clients 20 to 70 years old.

59. *Answer:* c (health promotion/plan/wellness/management/therapeutics/pharmacologic/NAS)

Rationale: Age is not a factor in initiating drug therapy. The cutoff levels to remember are 160 mg/dl if there are more than two risk factors and 190 mg/dl regardless of number of risk factors.

60. *Answer:* a (health promotion/plan/wellness/management/therapeutics/pharmacologic/NAS)

Rationale: Exercise should be continued on a regular basis and not decreased. Management of a client with hyperlipidemia is within the nurse practitioner's scope of practice and does not require treatment by a cardiologist. Smoking should be stopped regardless of what treatment is used for hyperlipidemia, but it is not mandatory because of drug metabolism.

61. *Answer:* c (health promotion/evaluation/wellness/management/therapeutics/pharmacologic/NAS)

Rationale: The client does not need the services of a specialist. Hyperlipidemia can be treated by a primary care provider. Another drug should be added, and the nicotinic acid does not need to be stopped. There is not enough evidence to suggest that the client has not complied with therapy. (Barker, Burton, & Zieve, 1995)

62. *Answer:* b (health promotion/plan/wellness/management/therapeutics/health-promoting behaviors/NAS)

Rationale: Diet is the first step in therapy; however, lowering lipids is a priority and should be done as quickly as possible after diagnosis. A stricter diet should therefore be attempted before drug therapy. There is not enough information in the item stem to assume that the client did not understand the Step One diet. (Barker, Burton, & Zieve, 1995)

63. *Answer:* d (health history/wellness/health history)

Rationale: Previous DDST results may be elicited as part of the history, but current information obtained through the nurse practitioner's skills is considered assessment. (Lang & Dunn, 1993)

64. *Answer:* b (health promotion/assessment/wellness/management/client education/adult)

Rationale: HDL levels >35 mg/dl are protective against CAD. A sedentary job increases risk. Playing tennis once a week is not enough aerobic exercise to be protective. (U.S. Preventive Services Task Force, 1996)

65. *Answer:* a (health promotion/assessment/wellness/health history/NAS)

Rationale: A dietary history is important to assess for fat intake, cholesterol intake, and daily calories. Vitamins and diet drinks are not related to CAD. Obesity (>30% above desirable weight) is a risk factor, but a history of obesity that has been corrected is not a factor. (U.S. Preventive Services Task Force, 1996)

66. *Answer:* b (health promotion/assessment/wellness/management/diagnostics/adolescent)

Rationale: Arcus senilus may be present before 50 years in someone with hyperlipidemia, but this can be noted without a funduscopic exam, it is still rare in children. An enlarged liver is not associated with CAD. A triglyceride level must be obtained from a fasting specimen. A cholesterol level can be drawn the day of the examination. (Barker, Burton, & Zieve, 1995)

67. *Answer:* a (health promotion/evaluation/wellness)

Rationale: Initially, the lipid profile is rechecked in 4 weeks, then at 3 months. (Barker, Burton, & Zieve, 1995)

68. *Answer:* c (counseling concepts/nurse-client relationships)

Rationale: A crisis has the potential for growth, it is resolvable in a brief period, it is precipitated by a specific event, and it occurs in all individuals; thus it is *not* associated with pathology. (Townsend, 1996)

69. *Answer:* a (counseling concepts/nurse-client relationships)

Rationale: There are four phases to crisis intervention. Finding out about the amount of disruption in the person's daily life will help in planning therapeutic interventions and targeting resources that the client needs. To assess suicide risk, you need information regarding the precipitating stressor. To prevent recurrence, you must provide anticipatory planning. (Townsend, 1996)

70. *Answer:* a (counseling concepts/nurse-client relationships)

Rationale: The client's perception of the event, coping mechanisms, and situational supports are factors that influence equilibrium. (Aguilera, 1998)

71. *Answer:* b (counseling concepts/nurse-client relationships)

Rationale: A *developmental crisis* is a response to a normal life-cycle transition. A *situational crisis* is a response to an external stressor. PTSD occurs later, well after an acute event. (Townsend, 1996)

PART III

Issues

21

Issues and Theories in Primary Care

PRIMARY CARE

The American Nurses Association (ANA) publication *Nursing's Agenda for Health Care Reform* (American Nurses Association, 1992) places emphasis on primary care services delivered in workplaces, schools, and other community settings. It identifies the need for ongoing primary care and the delivery of services where people already are. It focuses on primary care and wellness for all, but especially for women and children.

DEFINITION

Primary health care is defined as follows:
- Delivery of care at the first point of contact with the health care system.
- Delivery of care that helps resolve the health problem for which care is being sought
- Continuous and comprehensive care
- Inclusive of health promotion, prevention of disease, and health maintenance
- Inclusive of identification, management, or referral of health problems

Primary Prevention

Primary prevention consists of measures to promote health before a person has any disease. Examples include a healthful diet, exercise, and immunizations.

Secondary Prevention

Secondary prevention comprises early case findings of existing health problems. It includes such screening activities as mammograms and Papanicolaou smears.

Tertiary Prevention

Tertiary prevention consists of rehabilitation and restoration of wellness with respect to an existing health problem.

HEALTHY PEOPLE 2000

Healthy People 2000 is a document written by the U.S. Department of Health and Human Services that sets goals for the health of the United States in the year 2000. Those goals include the following:
- Reduction of health disparity among Americans
- An increased span of healthy life for Americans
- Preventive health services for all Americans
- Services provided where people already are
- No denial because of finances
- Assessment of quality of service measured by consumer satisfaction, mortality and morbidity figures, and improved well-being.
- Recognition of and dealing with the roles of transportation, housing, and industry in bringing about a healthy society
- Client self-care and responsibility

CLIENT EDUCATION

Principles of learning include the following (Boyd, 1997):
- Readiness to learn—person's ability and energy to learn
- Assessment of readiness to learn —Health status

—Health values
—Cognitive, psychologic, and psychomotor abilities
—Previous learning experiences
—Developmental characteristics of the learner
- Motivation—person's desire to learn: Reinforcements are used to increase or decrease the likelihood that a behavior will be repeated.

Teaching Strategies

- Instructional methods: How the teaching session is structured
- Educational methods: Strategies that facilitate learning
  —Progress from simple to complex, concrete to abstract
  —Advanced organizers: Tell the learner what is to be learned, then cue the learner to each point.
  Use specificity and brevity.
  Repetition strengthens learning.

People best remember the first third and the last quarter of information presented; this is known as *primacy* (Ley, 1972).
Make material relevant.
Reinforce learning.

Behavior Strategies

- Contracting: Develop contract of behaviors and rewards.
- Graduating behavioral change: Learner makes small increments of change with time.
- Tailoring: Fit a prescribed regimen into a learner's lifestyle.
- Self-monitoring: Learner analyzes his or her own behavior patterns through "data collection" (e.g., keeping a diary).

Evaluation of Teaching Learning

- Process or formative evaluation: Assess the effectiveness of the teaching process.
- Outcome or impact evaluation: Assess the effectiveness of the teaching process in promoting learning.

THEORIES RELATED TO CLIENT WELLNESS

DEFINITIONS

Concept

A *concept* is an abstraction of concrete events that represents a way of perceiving phenomena (Norris, 1982). Concepts vary in breadth and range from concrete to abstract.

Conceptual Model

A *conceptual model* is a "primitive" theory. Relationships between concepts are not clearly stated. It is broader and more abstract than a theory.

Theory

A *theory* is a set of propositional statements that expresses relationships between concepts. These statements describe, explain, and predict.

NURSING THEORIES OR MODELS

Nursing theories or models are concerned with client, nurse, and health care situations in which the nurse and client find themselves, and the pur-

pose of their being together (health and well-being of the client).

Concepts in Nursing Theories or Models

These concepts include client, environment, health, and nursing action.

Common Nursing Conceptual Models

- Rogers' Model of Unitary Beings: Humans are irreducible. Humans and their environments are mutual and continuous.
- King's Central Systems Model: Humans are open systems that interact with the environment. Goal attainment in nurse-client interactions leads to both nurse and client satisfaction and to effective nursing care.
- Orem's Self-Care Model: The goal of nursing is to help people meet their needs for self-care at a therapeutic level and on a continual basis.
- Roy's Adaptation Model: People are adaptive systems in constant interaction with changing

environments. People adapt to change through coping mechanisms.

- Neuman's System Model: The client is composed of five systems; developmental, spiritual, sociocultural, psychologic, and physiologic. The aim of nursing is to promote stability of the client.

Common Nursing Theories of Care

- Leininger's Theory of Cultural Care Diversity and Universality: Nursing care must be congruent with the client's culture. To achieve congruence, the nurse functions within the areas of Cultural Care Preservation, Cultural Care Negotiation, and Cultural Care Repatterning.
- Watson's Theory of Caring: Human caring is the moral ideal of nursing. The goal of nursing is to achieve greater harmony of mind, body and soul. This is achieved through a transpersonal caring process in which nurse and client both participate.

FAMILY THEORIES

A family is defined as follows:
- Members are united by a bond.
- Members may live together; if they do not, they consider a united household their home.
- Members interact and communicate with each other in family roles (e.g., mother-son).
- Members maintain a common culture.

Common Family Theories

- Structural-functional: This theory is concerned with how the family members are arranged, the relationships between the members and the relationships of members to the family as a whole. Structure serves to facilitate the achievement of family functions.
- Family Systems: The focus is on the interactions of the various parts of the family. The family is a system, and a change in one member of the family results in changes for the total family unit.
- Developmental Perspective: A family has a life-cycle with predictable changes. Tasks are associated with each stage of the cycle. Unpredictable events create needs and require adjustment.

- Interactionist Perspective: This theory focuses on the meanings that acts and symbols hold for people. Roles serve as a means for interaction. The aim is to view situations from the family member's or family's perspective.
- Family Ecological Perspective: Broader than Systems Theory, this perspective looks at the family's relationship to the environment. Both the environment and the family are constantly changing.
- Social Exchange Perspective: Family members maintain involvement in relationships on the basis of rewards and costs.
- Family Stress Perspective (ABCX model): Variability in family response to stress is based on A, hardships; B, resources; C, family's definition of the event; and X, the crisis.

COMMUNITY THEORY

- Epidemiologic Perspective: The *host* is the susceptible person. The *agent* is the presence or absence of factors that may influence the health of the person. The *environment* is anything external to the person or agent. A change in any of these factors may change the balance of health.
- Structural-functional Perspective: This theory stresses the ability of the community to carry out its functions to attain community goals.
- Systems Theory: Emphasis is on the components of the community and the capability of the community to operate as a system for meeting community goals.

MODELS OF HEALTH BEHAVIOR
Health Belief Model

The Health Belief Model focuses on illness prevention-multifactorial model to explain why people take or make changes to improve their health.

Health Promotion Model

According to Walker, Sechrist, and Pender (1987), "Health promotion is a multidimensional pattern of self-initiated actions and perceptions that serve to maintain or enhance the level of wellness, self-actualization and fulfillment of the individual."

The Health Promotion Model is proposed as a multivariate model for explaining and predicting the health-promoting components of lifestyle.

This model focuses on health promotion without the threat of disease. Factors that influence one's likelihood of engaging in health-promoting behaviors include the following (Pender et al, 1990):

- Importance of health
- Perceived control of health
- Perceived self-efficacy
- Definition of health
- Perceived health status
- Perceived benefits of health-promoting behaviors
- Perceived barriers to health-promoting behaviors

DEFINITIONS

- Health risk appraisal: This includes screening for disease potential, educating clients about unhealthy habits, and stimulating behavior change.
- Risk factors: These are characteristics that have been associated with higher risk for a given disease. Relative risk is determined by the ratio of risk or rate in exposed persons to the risk or rate in unexposed persons.

- Epidemiologic principles: *Epidemiology* is the study of the distribution and determinants of the frequency of disease in humans.
- Mortality: Death
- Morbidity: Illness

Change Theory

Change means a substitution of one thing for another, or an alteration in the state or quality of a thing. As a verb, *change* means to make a thing other than what it was; to become different. *Planned change* means that one has made choices about how to use theories and methods for purposes of reaching an identified goal (Tiffany, 1994).

A variety of models and theories describe change. Which model is used depends on the nature of the change and beliefs about the change. Kaluzney and Hernandez (1988) describe three models of change: Rational, Organizational Ecology, and Resource Dependency (Table 21-1).

Table 21-1 Three Models of Change

TYPE OF MODEL	CHARACTERISTICS	EXAMPLES
Rational	Focus is on aspects of change. Change is viewed as a linear process involving four stages: (1) recognition of need for change, (2) identification of a course for corrective action, (3) implementation of plan, and (4) institutionalization of the change.	Havelock, 1973; Lewin, 1951; Lippitt, 1973
Organizational Ecology Model	Change simply unfolds and is not directional. Emphasis is on concepts of life-cycle growth and decline. Change is not time bound and is relatively unpredictable.	
Resource Dependence Model	Focus is on relationship between organization and environment in terms of mutual dependency. Time frame is intermediate and ongoing.	

CULTURAL SENSITIVITY AND DIVERSITY

OVERVIEW
Definition

Culture is "an accepted set of values, beliefs, and behaviors shared within a social group" that is learned while growing up in the environment; it is an unconscious learning process (Kirkpatrick & Deloughery, 1995). These values and beliefs influence the way in which the person interacts on a day-to-day basis.

In *melting pot theory* diverse groups from all over the world gather and are encouraged to forsake their original traditions and to become homogenized as Americans (also known as enculturation). *Stewpot theory* involves an appreciation and acceptance of other cultures. As in stew, each culture is enhanced and becomes more colorful because of exposure to the distinctive traditions of other cultures.

Cultural factors influence not only the individual but also the family and the illness by determining the (1) role and status in the family; (2) social, material, and professional support; (3) family and group treatment of the person with chronic illness; (4) identification and interpretation of the symptoms of illness; (5) manifestations of pain and discomfort (Kirkpatrick & Deloughery, 1995).

In *ethnocentrism* one believes that his or her own culture is superior, with the view that all other cultures are underdeveloped or inferior. The individual usually tries to impose those personal values on others, without taking into account the client's personal perceptions and values.

Transcultural nursing is a branch of nursing that focuses on comparative study and analysis of cultures with respect to nursing and illness. One of the pioneers in transcultural nursing was Madeline Leninger.

Cultural Assessment*

Assessment should include the basic cultural data:
- Religious preference
- Patterns of family makeup (nuclear, extended, male-dominated vs female-dominated culture, or equalitarian)
- Patterns of caring for health

Cultural Values

Cultural values have been categorized into the following four groups:
1. Time: Past, present, or future (emphasis placed on one vs the other)
2. Personal activity: Doing or being
3. Relationship orientation: Collateral (concerned with others on lateral level) or lineage (males maintain responsibility for lineage)
4. Orientation of the individual to nature: View of humanity and nature

Cultural Differences†

How do cultures differ?
- Communication
- Space
- Social organization
- Time
- Biological variations
- Environmental control

REFERENCES

Kirkpatrick, S., & Deloughery, G. (1995). Cultural influences in nursing. In G. Deloughery (Ed.), *Issues and trends in nursing*. St. Louis: Mosby.

Townsend, M. (1996). *Psychiatric mental health nursing: Concepts of care* (2nd ed.). Philadelphia: F. A. Davis.

Tripp-Reimer, T. (1992). Cultural assessment. In J. Billack & B. Edward (Eds.), *Nursing assessment and diagnosis*. Boston: Jones & Bartlett.

*Tripp-Reimer, 1992.
†Townsend, 1996.

THERAPEUTIC COMMUNICATION

OVERVIEW

Therapeutic communication is an intrinsic component of the nurse-client relationship. It is well planned, goal oriented, and client focused. The primary purpose of therapeutic communication is to obtain and provide information that will address the client's feelings and needs. It is the ability to relate to the client by means of both verbal and nonverbal messages.

INFLUENCING FACTORS

Culture and Religion

These factors have an impact on the way we think and communicate. Customs and norms direct how we express emotions and the content of what is communicated. Both the clinician and the client are influenced by their respective cultural backgrounds when they enter into a therapeutic relationship. It is critical that the clinician be in touch with their biased beliefs and prejudices, which could have a negative influence.

Gender, Age, and Social Status

These are important factors in interpreting verbal and nonverbal communication. They influence the degree of familiarity with any given issue and how empathetic a response one may give. The differences in posture and gestures that are considered masculine and feminine also affect how communication is sent and received.

Milieu

The environment in which the clinician-client interaction occurs impacts on feelings of acceptance, security, privacy, freedom of expression, and maintenance of self-esteem.

Other Considerations

These factors include present state of mental and physical health and drug use.

PRINCIPLES OF THERAPEUTIC COMMUNICATION

Confidentiality

Confidentiality is essential in establishing a therapeutic clinician-client relationship. The client needs to be made aware that only information that is important for his or her care will be shared with other health professionals. Also, confidentiality will be broken if the client threatens self-injury or harm to others.

Empathy

This is the ability to place oneself in the client's position and remain objective.

Respect

To respect is to show acceptance for the client's ideas and opinions in a nonjudgmental manner.

Genuineness

This involves conveying true interest in the client and his or her issues.

Honesty

A candid and open approach facilitates trust and authenticity in the relationship.

Concreteness

This approach involves avoidance of abstract terms and generalities while focusing on the specifics to prevent misunderstandings.

TECHNIQUES OF THERAPEUTIC COMMUNICATION

Active Listening

- Sit facing client.
- Establish eye contact.
- Set appropriate personal distance.
- Have open and relaxed body posture.
- Use occasional gesturing and nodding.
- Reassuring touch may be appropriate but must be used judiciously.

Acknowledging

This includes addressing the client by his or her preferred name and using appropriate distance and touch.

Broad Openings

A conversation can be initiated by asking general questions (*Example:* "What brings you here?") to permit the client to introduce the topic.

Focusing

This technique assists the client to pursue an idea or feeling and eliminates peripheral communication. (*Example:* "You mentioned your job briefly. Could you tell me more about your work?")

Clarifying

A request is made for clarification of vague or unclear information. It should be done in a warm and nonjudgmental manner. (*Example:* "I am unclear about what you just said. Would you go over that again?")

Confrontation

This approach calls attention to inconsistencies and discrepancies in the client's communication and behavior. It involves feedback about apparent contradictions in the simultaneous verbal and nonverbal messages communicated by the client and how this affects the clinician. Confrontation is used to assist the client in identification and exploration of his or her true feelings. (*Example:* "I noticed that when you said that not being elected class president was no big deal, you looked sad.")

Silence

Using silence gives the client time to reflect and organize his or her thoughts. This technique needs to be used with caution because the client could interpret silence as disinterest.

Reflection

Acknowledging the feeling tone of the client's message helps the client explore his or her own feelings. (*Example:* "You seem angry that you had to come to the clinic alone today.")

Self-Disclosure

Appropriate sharing of feelings, beliefs, and experiences by the clinician can facilitate more openness by the client. It can help the client feel understood and see the clinician as a role model.

Summarizing

This is one of the most important techniques of the therapeutic interaction. The summary should reflect the essence of the interaction, including facts and feelings. It provides the client with a sense of being heard, allows for clarification of information, and terminates the interaction.

PHASES OF THE THERAPEUTIC RELATIONSHIP
Orientation

- Assess the reason that the client is seeking help.
- Establish the parameters of the therapeutic relationship.
- Establish trust and honest communication.
- Formulate nursing diagnoses.

Working

- Plan and implement interventions to meet the established goals.
- Facilitate healthy behaviors and effective coping.
- Encourage compliance with the treatment plan.

Termination

- Summarize and evaluate the achievement of therapeutic goals.
- Process feelings about ending the therapeutic relationship.

BLOCKS TO THERAPEUTIC COMMUNICATION
Blaming

This method attacks the client's behavior or judgment. (*Example:* "You should have . . .," "You caused. . . .")

False Reassurance

This approach may cause the client not to share his or her true concerns. It indicates that the clinician does not understand the significance of the issue. (*Example:* "Don't worry. Everything will be OK.")

"Why" Questions

Such questions imply criticism and frequently result in a defensive response with little information being obtained.

Judging and Moralizing

In this approach behavior and feelings are identified as good or bad. It may lead to shame and withdrawal of the client.

Changing or Avoiding a Topic

This technique shifts the focus of the interaction from the client's concerns and conveys disinterest and clinician anxiety about the issue under discussion.

Lecturing or Advice Giving

This approach impedes problem solving by the client and promotes dependency.

SUMMARY

Therapeutic communication is a dynamic mechanism to assist clients in the identification and resolution of problems and issues affecting their lives. It is client focused and requires the use of facilitative communication skills by the clinician, including active listing, reflection and clarification of content and feelings, and the sharing of information.

REFERENCES

Burgess, A. (1997). *Psychiatric nursing: Promoting mental health* (pp. 167-178). Norwalk, CT: Appleton & Lange.

Randolph, N. (1993). *American nursing review for psychiatric and mental health nursing certification* (pp. 50-55). Springhouse, PA: Springhouse.

Wilson, H., & Kneisl, C. (1996). *Psychiatric nursing* (5th ed, pp. 109-130). Menlo Park, CA: Addison-Wesley.

NURSE PRACTITIONER

SCOPE OF PRACTICE*

- The *scope of practice* identifies who the nurse practitioner is, what the nurse practitioner does, and where and how the nurse practitioner provides care.
- It is based on a set of philosophic beliefs and clarified by a set of definitions.
- Beliefs and definitions change as social trends emerge and professions change.
- The scope of practice is determined by the profession, with consideration of legal, ethical, political, economic, and educational variables.
- Primary health care is an integral part of the scope of practice.
- A nurse practitioner is a primary health care provider who functions independently and interdependently.
- Nurse practitioners practice in ambulatory, acute, and long-term care settings.
- Primary health care is delivered through a holistic approach.
- The client has a right to accessible, affordable health care.

STANDARDS OF CARE

- Based on scope of practice
- A means to describe, measure, and guide the achievement of excellence for NPs

Practice Standards

- These deal with phenomena of concern for which nurse practitioners provide care.
- Care is given to clients at their first entry into the health care system.
- The nurse practitioner provides care that is comprehensive, spans the health continuum, and is coordinated and continuous.

Performance Standards*

- These guide nurse practitioners in their efforts to advance the profession.
- Continuing competence is the responsibility of the NP.
- The nurse practitioner participates in quality assurance activities.
- The nurse practitioner supports the role of NPs in health care delivery.
- The nurse practitioner uses research as the basis for practice and participates in research.
- The nurse practitioner collaborates with other health care professionals.

Nurse Practice Acts

- Nursing licensure laws are mandates.
- Laws are developed by three groups of people:
  —Legislators, through statutes and constitutions

---

*American Nurses Association, 1985.

*American Nurses Association, 1987.

—Administrators, through regulations to implement statutes

—Judges, through case decisions to interpret statutes, constitutions, or common law

- The basic statute governing NP practice is the Nurse Practice Act in each state
- Licensure limits practice to people with specific qualifications.
- Licensure is examination by the state in a specific specialty. Licensure is intended to protect the public from incompetence and to legitimize practice by granting it public recognition and sanction.
- Ideally, the State's Board of Nursing is empowered to promulgate all regulations for advanced-practice nurses (Birkholz & Walker, 1994).
- Ideally, the Board of Nursing is empowered to regulate prescriptive practice through the Nurse Practice Act, rather than other boards, such as those for medicine or pharmacy.

Registration of Nurse Practitioners

- Registration provides a definition and limits who can use a title without limiting practice.
- If a statute speaks only regarding those who may use title and not to those who may do certain practices, it is *registration* and not *licensure* (Hall, 1993).
- Registration differs from state to state.
- Registration requires certification by an outside agency to ensure uniformity.

Prescriptive Authority

Four avenues are used to legally obtain prescriptive authority for nurse practitioners (Faucher, 1992):

1. *Statutory authority* indicates that an amendment to a practice act or a bill specifically addressing prescriptive authority has passed the legislature with the governor's signature. It usually allows the greatest autonomy in prescribing privileges for nurse practitioners.
2. *Opinion rules* may be used to authorize prescriptive authority. Most often, the attorney general's opinion is sought to interpret language in one of the practice acts, usually the Nursing Practice Act. In every case, however, the opinion has been challenged by some group in the medical community. Disadvantages of opinion rules are implementa-

tion and the overturning of the opinion by a new attorney general.

3. Administrative rules by the Board of Nursing and Board of Medicine can be used to give nurse practitioners prescriptive privileges. The route is most often used when the Nurse Practice Act allows the delegation of prescriptive authority to nurses under the authority and supervision of a physician. The autonomy of nurse practitioner prescriptive authority is limited and subject to review by the Board of Medicine.
4. A Board of Pharmacy waiver to allow nurse practitioners to prescribe was granted in Arkansas. The Board of Pharmacy can change or withdraw the waiver at any time.

NURSE PRACTITIONER ROLE

- The first formal education program was held at University of Colorado in 1965, developed by Henry Silver, MD, and Loretta Ford EdD, RN, with a pediatric focus.
- Original programs were nondegree certificate programs, 1 year or less in length.
- National certification for nurse practitioners was first established in 1977 by the ANA.
- Certification verifies the credentials of nurses who claim competence at a certain level and indicates knowledge of a specialized area.
- Certification is available from the following organizations:
  —National Certification Corporation for Obstetric, Gynecologic, and Neonatal Nurse Practitioners
  —American Nurses Credentialing Center (gerontology, pediatrics, adult, family, acute care [in conjunction with the American Association of Critical Care Nurses], and school health)
  —American Academy of Nurse Practitioners (adult and family)
  —National Association of Pediatric Nurse Associates and Practitioners (pediatrics)

Role Components

- The role is multifaceted. A *role* is considered a set of behaviors emerging out of interactions between the self and others that is a constant expression of attitudes and values, providing direction in the role. Self-assessment of one's

perception of the role directly influences behavior in that role (Thibodeau & Hawkins, 1989).
- Primary components:
  —Expert clinical practice
    Assessment
    Diagnosis
    Planning
    Interventions
    Evaluation
  —Consultation
  —Education
  —Research
  —Leadership

Nurse Practitioner Role in Developing Policy

Steps in political activism are as follows:
- Develop a policy agenda.
- Develop program proposals and supportive legislation.
- Support enactment of proposals and legislation through the following channels:
  —Lobby efforts
  —Providing expert testimony
  —Serving in political office
- Implement the legislation.
- Evaluate the legislation.

Evaluation Areas of Nurse Practitioner Role*

- Structure: Setting in which care occurs (evaluated according to administrative standards)
- Process: Actions taken in giving and receiving care (evaluated according to guidelines for practice)
- Outcome: Reflective of the effects of care, client focused (evaluated according to guidelines for practice)
- *Quality of care* is defined as the degree to which health services increase the likelihood of desired health outcomes.

- There has been a shift from "negative" indicators (e.g., morbidity and mortality) to positive indicators (health status, functional status).
- There is a need for indicators that are clinically significant and financially relevant.

Nurse Practitioner Role in Research Utilization

TWO TYPES
- Conceptual: Research is used to influence thinking, not necessarily action.
- Decision driven: Scientific knowledge is applied as part of practice, policy, and protocol (Cronenwett, 1995).

STEPS IN THE DECISION-DRIVEN APPROACH (IOWA MODEL)
1. Presence of problem or lack of knowledge, new information that serves as a trigger.
2. Assemble relevant research literature.
3. Critique and evaluate this literature for purposes of determining whether there is a sufficient research base.
4. If a sufficient research base exists, is the change appropriate for absorption into practice?
5. If there is not a sufficient research base, consider conducting further research, consulting with experts to determine whether any part of the literature applies to practice.

BARRIERS TO RESEARCH UTILIZATION
- Organizational (lack of authority to change practice)
- Professional (history of research being limited to academic medical centers)
- Knowledge skills of nurse (nurse practitioner)
- Nurse's (nurse practitioner's) attitudes
- Quality of research being conducted
- Inadequate communication of research findings

---

*Dean-Barr, 1997.

ETHICS AND LEGAL ISSUES

VALUES
Definition

Values are "freely chosen, enduring beliefs or attitudes about the worth of a person, object, idea, or action" (Kozier, Erb, & Blais, 1997). Values form the basis for behavior and are learned and influenced by the person's sociocultural environment. Professional values are influenced and shaped by personal values. Nurses learn professional values during their socialization into nursing. These values are integrally related to ethical and professional beliefs.

Values clarification is a process by which the person examines his or her own individual values. This process promotes personal and professional growth. It is important to know and understand your values, especially as they relate to such issues as life, death, illness, euthanasia, and abortion.

ETHICS
Definition

Ethics is the study of morality. *Bioethics* is ethics as applied to life. According to Kozier et al. (1997, p. 94), "Nurses need to understand their own values related to moral matters and to use ethical reasoning to determine and explain their moral position." A *code of ethics* is a formal statement that explains a group's ideals and values. Codes of ethics are usually considered to set a higher standard than legal standards and expectations.

Ethical Principles

- Ethics: The study of standards of conduct and moral judgment
- Autonomy: A client's needs take priority over the needs of society and the health care system
- Beneficence: Do no harm.
- Justice: There is a right to fair treatment and a right to privacy. The latter includes:
  —Confidentiality: Information not publicly reported
  —Anonymity: No one can link a name with the date reported.
- Veracity: This is truthfulness. The client must have full, impartial knowledge
- Utilitarian: This is the most commonly applied principle, the greatest good for the greatest

number of persons. It is used as rationale for limiting scarce resources.
- Egoism: The wish of client should be held in higher regard than that of the decision maker. When this is *not* so, it is considered egoism.
- Respect for human dignity: This ethical principle includes the right to self-determination and the right to full disclosure (informed consent).

Legal Issues

- Tort: A *tort* is a wrongful act against another person or property.
- Unintentional tort: This is an unintentional wrongful act that produces injury.
- Negligence: *Negligence* is the failure to do something that a reasonable and prudent person would do under similar circumstances, or the performance of an action that a reasonable and prudent person would not perform under similar circumstances. It applies to nonprofessionals.
- Malpractice: *Malpractice* is professional misconduct or lack of skill; it encompasses failure to perform professional skills that a reasonable and prudent professional would perform in a similar situation or performance of actions that a reasonable and prudent professional would not perform under similar circumstances. This is the specific type of negligence that applies to professionals.

NEGLIGENCE IN RELATIONSHIP TO THE STANDARD OF CARE: This standard is not just a nursing standard but a professional standard of care. Four elements of malpractice must be proved:
1. Duty owed to the person
2. Breach of duty or standard of care by the professional, determined by: state Nurse Practice Act, national standards (ANA Code of Ethics, specialty organization), employer policies, expert testimony
3. Proximate cause or direct result, a causal link between the breach and the harm or injury that occurred
4. Actual harm or damages

LIABILITY INSURANCE

The purpose of liability insurance is to shift the risk of liability, which may result in a monetary obligation, to another source (Henry, 1994). There are two types of liability insurance:

1. Claims made: Pays damages during the policy's period of coverage.

2. Occurrence policy: Pays damages that occurred during the policy's life; the individual no longer has to be carrying the coverage at the time of the litigation.

ACCESS TO CARE

DEFINITION

Access to care is defined as a set of factors that affect the potential and actual ability of an individual or group to acquire timely and appropriate health care services (Millman, 1993). Traditionally vulnerable groups have been women, children, people of color, poor people, and older adults. Newly at-risk groups include the chronically ill, the mentally ill, persons with AIDS, substance abusers, homeless persons, immigrants, and the uninsured, also the underinsured, those for whom out-of-pocket expenditures for health care exceed 10% of income (Monheit, Hagin, Berk, & Farley, 1988).

BARRIERS TO ACCESS

Three categories are identified (Callahan & David, 1995):

- Inability to pay
  —Uninsured, underinsured
  —Fewer providers are willing to serve Medicaid recipients because of low reimbursement rates.
- Sociocultural
  —Provider and staff attitudes
  —Language incompatibility
  —Culturally incompetent care
  —Fear of deportation
- Organizational: Inadequate capacity, too few public clinics, not enough appointment slots, uneven distribution of health care providers
  —Lack of coordination of services
  —Problems securing Medicaid coverage
  —Transportation barriers
  —Child care problems

STRATEGIES FOR IMPROVING ACCESS

- Establish community health centers.
- Establish migrant health centers.
- National Health Service Corps: Award scholarships to increase number of providers in underserved areas.
- Increase the number of minority providers.
- Train more primary care providers.

HEALTH CARE DELIVERY SYSTEM AND ECONOMICS

Four goals are identified:

1. Control costs through the use of services.
2. Use business approach to ensure efficiency.
3. Ensure quality through the measurement of outcomes.
4. Form partnership to address care across the wellness-illness continuum.

MANAGED CARE ORGANIZATIONS

- Managed care organizations (MCOs) limit the range of providers available to members

- MCOs may restrict health services that enrolled members are permitted to use.
- MCOs pay providers a capitated (or set) monthly rate for each client assigned.
- MCOs may require members to affiliate with a case manager or primary care provider.
- Some states require Medicaid participants to join MCOs.
- MCOs provide services to a given population within a given budget.

INTEGRATED DELIVERY SYSTEM

- An integrated delivery system (IDS) links hospitals, home health agencies, group primary care practices, medical equipment suppliers, and pharmacies.
- An IDS comprises a larger network than a health maintenance organization (HMO).

PREFERRED PROVIDER ORGANIZATION

- A preferred provider organization (PPO) is an identified subset of hospitals and providers that receive a predetermined rate of reimbursement.
- In a PPO, the payor gets price discounts and utilization review procedures from the providers. The PPO uses incentives to encourage use of particular providers and disincentives (higher copayments) when other providers are used.
- Self-referral is allowed.

OTHER TERMS

- Point-of-service plans: The client is allowed to use certain providers at a lower cost or to use other providers at a higher cost. Referrals are made by a primary care provider.
- Fee-for-service payment: The client sees the physician or other provider of choice, paying the fee out of pocket.
- Indemnity health insurance: This provides financial protection against future medical costs.
- Premiums: Premiums are usually paid annually. Price differentiation is based on differences in individuals' demographic data.

GOVERNMENT PROGRAMS
Medicare: Social Insurance

Medicare is a federal program, so coverage is the same across the states.

PART A
- Mandatory hospital insurance
- Eligibility is based on 10 years of work under Social Security
- Coverage is for a 90-day benefit period, with 60 days between admissions
- Part A covers home health and hospice care.

PART B
- Supplemental medical care with federally subsidized premiums

- Client pays monthly premium for insurance that covers physician services, outpatient hospital services, ambulance, and durable medical equipment
- Payment is based on resource-based relative value scale. Relative values are assigned to health care services that reflect provider time and skill, practice expenses, and malpractice costs adjusted for geographic location.

Medicaid: Welfare

- Joint state-federal program
- Coverage varies, with state-to-state categoric eligibility.
- Some groups are determined eligible by the federal government (e.g., recipients of Aid to Families with Dependent Children), whereas other subgroups are determined by the individual state.
- Providers may be paid by a fee-for-service schedule that is set by each state.
- Some states enroll Medicaid recipients in HMO plans.

Peer Review Organization

- Used to promote effective use of resources for and provision of services to the Medicare population
- A group of practitioners paid by the federal government to review the care provided to Medicare beneficiaries

Clinical Decision Making

- Used to determine level of service needed for evaluation and management of Medicare Part B recipients
- Levels of service range from problem-focused, straightforward, and minor to comprehensive, complex, and severe.
- Nature of the presenting problem
- All the following are considered contributory factors to the complexity of services delivered:
  —Coordination of care
  —Counseling, anticipatory guidance
  —Time
- To charge for clinical decision making, the number of diagnoses or management options, the amount or complexity of data needs to be reviewed and the risks of complications or morbidity and mortality are considered.

NURSE PRACTITIONER REIMBURSEMENT

MEDICARE

Direct Billing

- The bill is rendered in the name of the nurse practitioner.
- Payment may be made under the indirect supervision of a physician for services provided to Medicare regardless of setting. The reimbursement rate is 80% of the lesser of the actual charge or 85% of the fee schedule amount for physicians.
- Reimbursement may be made to the employer of the nurse practitioner. An employer may be a physician, a medical group, a nursing home, or a professional corporation.

Indirect Billing

- The bill is rendered in the name of the physician supervising the nurse practitioner.
- These services are classified as "incident to" a physician's service and are paid under the MFS as if the physician had personally furnished the service.
- Services must be rendered in the clinic setting.
- Services must be medically necessary, generally provided in a physician's office, and within the licensure for practice by a nurse practitioner.
- The physician must provide the initial service for the client and must provide subsequent services frequently enough to reflect his or her active participation in the management of the client's course of treatment.
- Reimbursement is made to the physician.

Rural Health Professional Shortage Area

- Service rendered by a nurse practitioner in one of these designated areas may be covered as physician services in any setting, including the office.
- Billing is direct, in the name of the nurse practitioner, and is at the following rates:
  —75% of the MFS for services performed in a hospital
  —85% of the MFS for all other services
- Reimbursement may be made directly to the nurse practitioner or to the hospital, rural primary care hospital, skilled-nursing facility, nursing facility, physician, group practice, or ambulatory surgery center with which the nurse practitioner has an employment or contractual relationship.
- Coverage is limited to services that a nurse practitioner is legally authorized to perform under the state's law.

MEDICAID

Medicaid allows direct billing for Advanced Registered Nurse Practitioners (ARNP) (Table 21-2):

- ARNPs shall practice in accordance with established protocol and shall seek consultation and referral in those situations where practice requirements are not included in the established protocol. This protocol is a written document jointly approved by the physician and the ARNP at least annually.

Table 21-2 Federal Reimbursement for Advanced Practice Nurses

	NP	CNM	CRNA	CNS
Medicare B	Yes*	Yes	Yes	Yes†
Medicaid	Yes‡	Yes	State discretion	State discretion
CHAMPUS	Yes	Yes	Yes	Yes§
FEHBP	Yes	Yes	Yes	Yes

From American College of Nurse Practitioners. (1997). [On-line]. Available: http://www.nurse.org/acnp/facts/reimburfed.shtml
CNM, Certified nurse midwife; *CRNA,* certified registered nurse anesthetist; *CHAMPUS,* Civilian Health and Medical Program of Uniformed Services; *FEHBP,* Federal Employee Health Benefit Program.
*Limited to nursing facilities and rural areas.
†Limited to rural areas (considered non-metropolitan statistical areas).
‡Limited to Pediatric and Family NPS.
§Limited to certified psychiatric nurse specialists.

Included in the protocol should be the scope of diagnostic testing, prescription of medications, and treatments that the ARNP can conduct.

- The ARNP shall have a separate individual provider number and separate clinic or group number, distinct from that of the physician employer.
- If the ARNP is salaried by the facility, fee-for-service billing is not appropriate
- Payment is made at 75% of the fee schedule designated for physician providers.

"INCIDENT TO" RULE BILLING AND DOCUMENTATION GUIDELINES

Definition

"Incident to" services are services rendered by health care professionals employed by a physician and performed under the direct supervision of that physician.

Qualifications of "Incident to" Service

- Service must be an integral part of a physician's diagnosis or treatment.
- Service must be provided under direct supervision of a physician. NOTE: Direct supervision in an office setting does not mean that the physician has to be in the same room with the practitioner performing the "incident to" service. The physician must be present in the office suite and immediately available to provide assistance and direction throughout the time that the health care professional is performing the service.
- Services must be provided by an employee of that physician and must represent an expense incurred by the physician in professional practice.
- The service must be something that is ordinarily done in a physician's office or clinic.

Billing

Bills are rendered in the name of the physician directly supervising the health care professional as though he or she had personally rendered the service.

Documentation

- The health care professional must write or dictate notes and sign them accordingly.

- State law dictates whether the supervising physician must sign off on the notes made by the health care professional.

Benefits of Direct Reimbursement

- Direct reimbursement puts a price and value on services provided.
- It allows self-employment or enhancement of revenue for employers.
- It provides data on services provided and improves the ability to conduct research.
- Direct reimbursement increases the nurse practitioner's autonomy and authority to act on behalf of clients.
- It empowers nurse practitioners within the health system, giving them greater control over practices.

Barriers to Direct Reimbursement

- Organized medicine
- Inability to show cost savings
- Lack of consumer demand for nurse practitioner services

REFERENCES

American College of Nurse Practitioners (1997). *Federal reimbursement for advanced practice nurses.* Washington, DC: Author.

American Nurses Association (1985). *The scope of practice of the primary health care nurse practitioners* (NP-61). Washington, DC: American Nurse Publishing.

American Nurses Association (1987). *Standards of practice for the primary health care nurse practitioner* (NP-71). Washington, DC: American Nurses Publishing.

American Nurses Association (1992). *American Nurses Association House of Delegates Report, 1992 Convention* (Las Vegas, Nevada). Kansas City, MO: Author.

Birkholz, G., & Walker, D. (1994). Strategies for state statutory language changes granting fully independent nurse practitioner practice. *Nurse Practitioner, 19*(1), 54-58.

Boyd, M. (1997). Health teaching in nursing practice. In Callahan, T., & David, R. (1995). In D. Calins, R. Fernandopulle, & B. Marino (Eds.), *Health care policy.* Cambridge, MA: Blackwell Science.

Burgess, A. (1997). *Psychiatric nursing: Promoting mental health* (pp. 167-168). Norwalk, CT: Appleton & Lange.

Callahan, T., & David, R. (1995). Access. In D. Calkins, R. Fernandopulle, & B. Marino (Eds.), Cambridge, MA: Blackwell Science.

Clark, M. J. Dummer (1996). *Nursing in the community* (2nd ed.). Norwalk, CT: Appleton & Lange.

Cronenwett, L. R. (1995). Effective methods for disseminating research finding to nurses in practice. *Nursing Clinics of North America, 30*, 429-438.

Dean-Baar, S. L. (1997). *Standards and guidelines: Do they make any difference?* In J. McCloskey & H. H. Grace (Eds.), *Current issues in nursing* (5th ed.). Mosby: St. Louis.

Ellis, J., & Hartley, C. (1995). *Nursing in today's world* (5th ed.). Philadelphia: J. B. Lippincott.

Faucher, M. (1992). Prescriptive authority for advanced practice nurse practitioners: A blueprint for action. *Journal of Pediatric Healthcare, 6*(1), 25-31.

Hall, J. (1993). How to analyze nurse practitioner licensure laws. *Nurse Practitioner, 18*(8), 31-34.

Havelock, R. (1973). *The changes agents guide to innovation in education.* Englewood Cliffs, NJ: Educational Technology Publications.

Hawkins, J., & Thibodeau, J. (1997). *The advanced practitioner* (4th ed.). New York: Tiresias Press.

Healthy People 2000 Consortium (1990). *Healthy people 2000: National health promotion and disease prevention objectives.* Washington, DC: U. S. Government Printing Office.

Henry, P. (1994). Overview of malpractice insurance. *Nurse Practitioner Forum, 5*(1), 4-6.

Kaluzney, R., & Hernandez, J. (1988). Studies of change in organizations. In P. Goodman et al. (Eds.), *Change in organizations.* San Francisco: Jossey-Bass.

Kirkpatrick, S., & Deloughery, G. (1995). *Cultural influences on nursing.* In G. Deloughery, *Issues and trends in nursing* (pp. 173-198). St. Louis: Mosby.

Kozier, B., Erb, G., & Blais, K. (1997). *Professional nursing practice* (3rd ed.). Menlo Park, CA: Addison-Wesley.

Lewin, K. (1951). *Field theory in social sciences.* New York: Harper.

Ley, P. (1972). Primary rated importance and recall of medical statement. *Journal of Health and Social Behavior, 13*, 311-317.

Lippitt, G. (1973). *Visualizing change: Model building and the change process.* La Jolla, CA: University Associates.

Millman, M. L. (1993). *Access to health care in America: Institute of Medicine (vs) Committee on Monitoring Access to Personal Health Care Services.* Washington, DC: National Academy Press.

Monheit, A., Hagin, M., Berk, M., & Farley, P. (1988). The employed uninsured and the role of public policy. *Inquiry, 22*, 348-364.

Norris, C. (1982). *Concept clarification in nursing.* Rockville, MD: Aspen.

Pearson, L. (1995). Annual update of how each state stands on legislative issues affecting advanced nursing practice. *Nurse Practitioner, 20*, 13-18.

Pearson, L. (1997). Annual update of how each state stands on legislative issues affecting advanced nursing practice. *Nurse Practitioner, 22*, 15-27.

Pender, N., Walker, S., & Sechrist, K. (1990). *The health promotion model: Refinement and validation.* Final report to the National Center for Nursing Research, National Institutes of Health (Grant #NR 01121). Dekalb, IL: Northern Illinois University Press.

Spradley, B., & Allender, J. (1996). *Community health nursing.* Philadelphia: J. B. Lippincott.

Stafford, M., & Appleyard, J. (1997). Clinical nurse specialists and nurse practitioners: Who are they, what do they do, and what challenges do they face? In J. McCloskey & H. Grace (Eds.), *Current issues in nursing.* (4th ed.). St. Louis: Mosby.

Thibodeau, J., & Hawkins, J. (1989). Nurse practitioners: Factors affecting role performance, *Nurse Practitioner, 14*(12), 47-53.

Tiffany, C. (1994). Analysis of planned change theories. *Nursing Management, 25*(2), 60-62.

Titler, M. G. (1997). Research utilization: Necessity or luxury? In S. L. Dean-Baar (Ed.), *Standards and guideline: Do they make any difference?* In J. McCloskey & H. Grace (Eds.), *Current issues in nursing* (5th ed.). St. Louis: Mosby.

Walker, S., Sechrist, K., & Pender, N. (1987). The health-promoting lifestyle profile: Development and psychometric characteristics. *Nursing Research, 36*, 76-80.

Wilson, H., & Kneisl, C. (1996). *Psychiatric nursing* (5th ed., pp. 109-130). Menlo Park, CA: Addison-Wesley.

Review Questions

1. A nurse practitioner states that all clients should learn how to read client education materials printed in English. This statement reflects:

   a. Stewpot theory

   b. Melting-pot theory

   c. Cultural tolerance

   d. Transcultural nursing

2. Which of the following is **not** considered a barrier to direct reimbursement for nurse practitioners?

   a. Organized medicine

   b. Inability to show cost savings

   c. Lack of consumer demand

   d. Lack of NP quality

3. All the following programs provide reimbursement for nurse practitioners **except:**

   a. Civilian Health and Medical Program of Uniformed Services

   b. Medicaid

   c. Federal Employee Health Benefit Program

   d. Medicare A

4. You would evaluate your relationship with the client as being trusting and therapeutic in which of the following cases?

a. You are able to identify with the client's problems.

b. You can provide solutions for the client's health problems.

c. The client seeks health care.

d. The focus of the relationship is on the significant issues of the client.

5. A young woman comes to the clinic and states, "I think I might be pregnant. What will my boyfriend say?" With a *reflective* approach, which of the following responses by the nurse practitioner would be most appropriate?

a. "It's you that we're concerned about, not your boyfriend."

b. "You can't please everyone. You need to think about the baby."

c. "It sounds as though your boyfriend doesn't care about you."

d. "It can be scary being here, and you're concerned about your boyfriend's reaction."

6. All the following are barriers to using research in practice **except:**

a. Organizational

b. Nurse practitioner attitudes

c. Quality of the research being conducted

d. Nurse practitioners' clinical knowledge

7. When examining a research study's findings on the measurement of peak air flow, the nurse practitioner decides that it is applicable to his or her practice. Before changing practice, what should he or she do first?

a. Examine the literature to determine whether there is sufficient evidence across studies for making this change.

b. Examine the peak air flow equipment to determine whether it can be used in this new way.

c. Examine the client population for their ability to use this new technique.

d. Determine the expense of implementing this technique.

8. The ANA Code of Ethics for nurses gives:

a. Legal mandates to follow for advanced practice

b. Regulations that should be followed for legal practice

c. Guidelines to follow for ethical practice

d. Moral suggestions to follow in ethically compromised situations

9. Which of the following statements best describes the major purpose of advanced practice standards in nursing?

a. To promote legal mandates for advanced practice

b. To regulate the number of advanced practice nurses in the United States

c. To identify criteria against which advanced-practice nursing can be evaluated

d. To interpret the legislative intent of the state Nursing Practice Act

10. Ethical dilemmas are those situations in which:

a. The problem can be solved with research data

b. The information needed is clearly identified

c. A decision must be made between undesirable alternatives

d. Good outcomes can be obtained if all parties use appropriate ethical theory

11. The legal guide to advanced practice is the:

a. ANA Code of Ethics

b. Hippocratic oath

c. State Nursing Practice Act

d. Nightingale Pledge

12. When the client gives his or her informed consent, this means that the client:

a. Totally accepts the plan of care

b. Understands the choices given

c. Accepts the offer to participate in research

d. Has obtained a second opinion

13. One way that ARNPs can assess, explore, and determine their personal values is the process of:

a. Taking an ethics course

b. Meditation

c. Following the ANA Code of Ethics

d. Values clarification

14. What is the first step in a performance evaluation?

  a. Self-evaluation
  b. Identifying problems
  c. Asking for feedback from others
  d. Developing a personal assistance plan

15. Primary health care providers are best described as:

  a. Gatekeepers to the health care system
  b. Providers who only provide care for acute illnesses
  c. Providers who provide care in rural health settings
  d. Consultants who participate in the plan of care

16. The nurse practitioner tries to modify all client education to fit the client's cultural beliefs and practices. This type of client approach is termed:

  a. Melting-pot theory
  b. Cultural imposition
  c. Cultural blindness
  d. Cultural accommodation

ANSWERS AND RATIONALES

1. *Answer:* b (issues/cultural sensitivity)
Rationale: Stewpot theory involves appreciation and acceptance of cultural diversity. *Melting-pot* theory supports enculturation, the process of blending cultures into an undistinguishable, homogenized group. (Kirkpatrick & Deloughery, 1995)

2. *Answer:* d (issues/access to care)
Rationale: Lack of nurse practitioner quality has not been shown to be an issue in terms of direct reimbursement. The others have been identified as barriers. (Birkholz & Walker, 1994)

3. *Answer:* d (issues/access to care)
Rationale: All the programs listed except Medicare A provide for federal reimbursement for nurse practitioners. Medicare B, not part A, provides for reimbursement of nurse practitioners. (Pearson, 1997)

4. *Answer:* d (issues/applications to practice)
Rationale: The therapeutic working phase of the relationship begins when the issues and problems are identified and addressed. (Wilson, 1996)

5. *Answer:* d (issues/applications to practice/interviewing)
Rationale: This is a reflective response that indicates an awareness of what the client is experiencing. Reflection shows empathy and respect. (Burgess, 1997)

6. *Answer:* d (issues/professional issues/research utilization)
Rationale: Organizational barriers may include lack of authority to change practice. Clinical knowledge does not usually interfere with use of research findings. (Titler, 1997)

7. *Answer:* a (issues/professional issues/research utilization)
Rationale: All these steps may be necessary, but first the nurse practitioner should determine, from across a series of well-designed studies, that the results are valid and useful. Otherwise, a great deal of effort will go into making a bad change. (Cronenwett, 1995)

8. *Answer:* c (issues/professional issues/scope and standards)
Rationale: The ANA Code of Ethics is a guideline to follow for ethical nursing practice. It has no relationship to legal regulations, nor is it mandated for practice. It does not make any moral suggestions. (Spradley & Allender, 1996)

9. *Answer:* c (issues/professional issues/scope and standards)
Rationale: The standards of care identify criteria by which nursing can be evaluated. (American Nurses Association, 1987)

10. *Answer:* c (issues/ethical considerations)
Rationale: In most dilemmas, the information and decision are not clearly identified; that is what makes it a dilemma. Use of appropriate ethical theory does not guarantee a positive outcome. In many cases, a choice must be made between undesirable alternatives. (Spradley & Allender, 1996)

11. *Answer:* c (issues/professional issues/scope and standards)
Rationale: Each state Nursing Practice Act delineates the legal guide to practice. The ANA Code of Ethics, Hippocratic oath and Nightingale pledge are credos that are promoted with respect to care of clients, but they do not have any legal basis for advanced practice. (Hawkins & Thibodeau, 1997)

12. *Answer:* b (issues/ethical considerations/client rights/informed consent)

Rationale: Informed consent means that the client has had all options explained and has given his or her permission. It does not mean that the client totally accepts the plan of care, nor that a second opinion was obtained. Although informed consent is obtained while conducting research, it is not reserved for research only. (Ellis & Hartley, 1995)

13. *Answer:* d (issues/ethical considerations/values clarification)

Rationale: Values clarification is the assessment, exploration, and determination of personal values. (Ellis & Hartley, 1995)

14. *Answer:* a (issues/professional issues/quality improvement))

Rationale: The first step in a performance evaluation should be a self-evaluation. Although identifying problems, asking for feedback from others, and developing a personal assistance plan may be part of a performance evaluation, the whole process should begin with self-evaluation. (Ellis & Hartley, 1995)

15. *Answer:* a (issues/access to care/primary health care delivery)

Rationale: Primary health care providers are those providers who coordinate the access of clients to other resources within the system. They do not provide care only for acute illnesses, or only in rural health settings. Consultants who participate in the plan of care are exactly that, consultants. (Ellis & Hartley, 1995)

16. *Answer:* d (health promotion/cultural factors)

Rationale: Modifying or accommodating any education to the client's beliefs ia a positive method of providing care. *Melting pot theory* merely refers to the combining of cultures. *Cultural imposition* and *cultural blindness* are negative, in that they ignore the cultural background of the person. (Clark, 1996)

PART IV

APPENDIXES

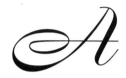

Test-Taking Guidelines

HOW TO APPROACH THE EXAMINATION

1. Assess your knowledge. Complete practice questions before the examination. Spend your time wisely. Concentrate review on areas in which you perform inconsistently or poorly during these practice sessions.
2. Believe in yourself. Speak of *when* you are certified, not *if* I pass this test.
3. Determine whether you study better independently or alone. Form a study group if this will help you.
4. Develop "flash cards" to help you remember difficult concepts or memory material, for example, screening guidelines.
5. Establish a schedule for reviewing. Determine the amount of content you need to review and the amount of time you have before the testing date and "dose" your study periods.
6. Rest and eat a light meal before the examination.
7. Budget your time. Determine the number of items and the time allowed for the total test. Keep this number in mind as you work through the test. If an item is taking more time, mark it so that you can return to it later.
8. Read each item carefully before going to the answer options. Identify key words in the item stem. This includes whether it is asking for a negative or wrong response.
9. Try answering the question before reading the options. Then read all the answer options completely before choosing.
10. Eliminate the options that are obviously wrong.
11. Make sure that the selected option relates grammatically to the item stem.
12. Answer every question.
13. Do not change your answer unless you have a good reason for doing so. Most first impressions are accurate if you have read the item carefully.
14. If you need to guess, guess logically. The longest option is usually correct. Avoid options with all-inclusive terms such as *never* and *always*. Correct options tend to be in the middle.

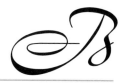

Abnormal Heart Sounds

Table B-1 Summary of Abnormal Heart Sounds

SOUND	LOCATION	SIGNIFICANCE
Split S$_1$	LLSB	Heard elsewhere or with S$_2$ split may indicate right bundle-branch block and premature ventricular contractions
Split S$_2$	2nd, 3rd left ICS	Normal if accentuated by inspiration, absent with expiration or sitting up
		Widens with pulmonic valve closure delays
		Fixed with atrial septal defect and right ventricular failure
		Parodoxical with left bundle-branch block
Systolic click	LLSB, medial to apex Diaphragm, midsystole	Mitral valve prolapse
Opening snap	LLSB, medial to apex Diaphragm, early diastole	Mitral valve stenosis
S$_3$	Apex, left lateral position Louder on inspiration	Rapid ventricular filling, healthy children
		Ventricular gallop—overloaded left ventricle as in mitral or tricuspid regurgitation
S$_4$	Apex, left lateral position	Normal athletes and aged
		Atrial gallop—represents increased resistance to ventricular filling as in hyperparathyroidism, coronary artery disease, aortic stenosis
Innocent murmur	LLSB, systolic	No radiation, grade 1-2, medium pitched
		May resolve on sitting, no other findings
Midsystolic Murmurs		
Physiologic murmur	LLSB, systolic	As with innocent murmur
		Common in anemia, pregnancy, fever, and hyperthyroidism
Aortic stenosis murmur	Right 2nd ICS, radiates to neck Medium, harsh associated with thrill	Stiffening of aortic valve, dilated aorta, aortic regurgitation
Cardiomyopathy	Crescendo-decrescendo 3rd, 4th ICS, radiates to apex or base, not to neck Harsh, medium	Left ventricular hypertrophy causes rapid systolic ejection of blood
		May also cause mitral regurgitation

From King, P., & Herrick, T. (1997). *Family nurse practitioner certification examination review course.* Louisville, KY: Spalding University.
LLSB, Left lower sternal border; *ICS,* intercostal space. Mnemonic to help remember murmurs: MR ASS = Mitral regurgitation and aortic stenosis = Systolic murmur; MS ARD = Mitral stenosis and aortic regurgitation = Diastolic murmur.

Table B-1 Summary of Abnormal Heart Sounds—cont'd

SOUND	LOCATION	SIGNIFICANCE
Pulmonic stenosis	2nd, 3rd ICS radiates to shoulder and neck Medium, soft Crescendo-decrescendo	Associated with split S_2 or right S_4
Holosystolic Murmurs		
Mitral regurgitation	Apex, axilla radiation Plateau (same intensity throughout cardiac cycle)	Volume overload on left ventricle Decreased S_1, increased apical impulse
Tricuspid regurgitation	LLSB, radiates to xiphoid and right of sternum Plateau	Right ventricular failure and dilatation Associated with S_3 at LLSB, jugular venous distention
Ventricular septal defect	3rd, 4th, 5th left ICS, wide radiation Loud, thrill, high-pitched, harsh	Congenital hole between left and right ventricles
Diastolic Murmurs		
Aortic regurgitation	2nd through 4th ICS, grade 1-3 High pitch, apex radiation Blowing quality—heard best sitting forward with held exhalation decrescendo	Volume overload left ventricle Associated with ejection sound, bounding pulses
Mitral valve stenosis	Apex, no radiation grade 1-4 Low pitch Listen at apical impulse in left lateral position, with exhalation Crescendo-decrescendo	Thickened, stiffened MV Associated with opening snap S_1 palpable at apex
Systolic/Diastolic Abnormalities		
Pericardial friction rub	3rd ICS, left of sternum, no radiation Scratchy, high pitch Loud in late systole	Pericardial inflammation as with pericarditis
Patent ductus arteriosus	Left 2nd ICS, left clavicle radiation Harsh, medium pitch	Persistent fetal structure Open channel between aorta and pulmonary artery
Venous hum	Loudest in diastole Above clavicles, especially on right, 1st and 2nd ICS Humming, roaring, low pitch	Turbulence of blood in jugular veins, common in children

Angiotensin-Converting Enzyme (ACE) Inhibitors

ADMINISTRATION OF ACE INHIBITORS

1. Always ensure adequate renal function (serum creatinine) before starting.
2. Monitor throughout therapy.
3. Beware of hyperkalemia, particularly if client is receiving potassium supplement or potassium-sparing diuretic.
4. Diuretics will potentiate ACE inhibitors. Start low.
5. First- or second-line agent in CHF, third- or fourth-line agent in hypertension.

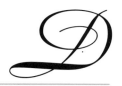

Beta-Blocking Agents

CHARACTERISTICS AND USES OF BETA-BLOCKING AGENTS

Cardioselective (Best for Clients With Asthma, for Clients With Diabetes, and for Peripheral Vascular Disease)
- Atenolol
- Metoprolol
- Betaxolol
- Acebutolol

Antiarrhythmic Quality (Membrane Stabilization); Use for Clients With Hypertension and Dysrhythmia
- Acebutolol
- Labetalol
- Propranolol

Low Lipid Solubility (Produces Fewer Central Nervous System Side Effects and Sleep Disturbances)
- Nadolol
- Carteolol
- Acebutolol
- Atenolol
- Betalol

Precautions
1. Beta-blockers are contraindicated in congestive heart failure.
2. Avoid abrupt cessation of beta-blockers.

Calcium Channel Blocking Agents

ADMINISTRATION OF CALCIUM CHANNEL BLOCKING AGENTS

1. Avoid use in clients with cystic fibrosis.
2. These agents are used as third- or fourth-line agents in clients with hypertension.
3. Monitor liver function while client is taking drug.

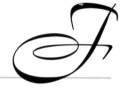

Nonsteroidal Antiinflammatory Drugs (NSAIDs)

Table F-1 Indications for NSAIDs

DRUG	INDICATIONS
Ibuprofen	Minor pain
Naproxen	Minor pain; acute flare-ups of chronic conditions
Diclofenac	Minor pain; acute flare-ups of chronic conditions
Sulindac	Acute pain
Ketoprofen	Chronic pain
Oxaprozin	Chronic pain
Etodolac	Chronic pain
Piroxicam	Chronic pain
Fenoprofen	Chronic pain
Nabumetone	Chronic pain
Indomethacin	Moderate to severe pain; acute flare-ups of chronic conditions

Precautions:
1. Avoid in persons with aspirin allergy.
2. Avoid in third trimester of pregnancy and when nursing.
3. Increases renal toxicity when used with angiotensin-converting enzyme inhibitors, diuretics, or both.

Oral Hypoglycemic Agents

ADMINISTRATION OF ORAL HYPOGLYCEMIC AGENTS

Agent	Precautions/Actions
Sulfonylureas	1. Contraindicated in ketoacidosis
First-generation	2. Nonsteroidal antiinflammatory drugs, sulfa drugs, anticoagulants, and beta-blocking agents increase their action. Hypoglycemia may result.
Glimepiride	
Tolazamide	
Tolbutamide	3. Diuretics, steroids, and calcium-channel blockers may decrease their effectiveness.
Second-generation	
Glyburide	4. Avoid alcohol.
Glipizide	
Insulin Resistance Reducers	1. Contraindicated in ketoacidosis
Metformin	2. Monitor for hypoglycemia when transferring from sulfonylureas.
Troglitazone	3. Usually has fewer drug interactions than sulfonylureas.
Alpha-Glucosidase Inhibitors	1. Contraindicated in ketoacidosis and colon or intestinal disorders, obstructions
Acarbose	2. Monitor serum creatine and transaminases.

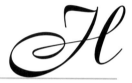

Topical Corticosteroids

Table H-1   Comparison of Potency of Topical Corticosteroids

DRUG	POTENCY
Hydrocortisone base or acetate, 0.5%, 1.0%, 2.5%	Low
Triamcinolone acetonide, 0.025%	Low
Triamcinolone acetonide, 0.1%, 0.2%	Medium
Fluocinolone acetonide, 0.01%	Low
Fluocinolone acetonide, 0.025%	Medium
Hydrocortisone buteprate or butyrate, 0.1%	Medium
Triamcinolone acetonide, 0.5%	High
Desoximetasone, 0.25% or 0.05%	High
Fluocinonide, 0.05%	High
Betamethasone dipropionate, 0.05%	High to superhigh
Diflorasone diacetate, 0.05%	High to superhigh
Clobetasol propionate, 0.05%	Superhigh

Precautions:
1. Always exclude viral disease (e.g., measles, chickenpox) before prescribing.
2. Use the lowest effective dose.
3. Do not use on large area or for prolonged time (use less than 2 weeks).
4. Never apply an occlusive dressing over where steroid is applied, because absorption is increased.
5. Always check to see whether agent can be used on children.
6. The vehicle (whether ointment, gel, or cream) can influence potency, even with the same concentration.

Medications and Pregnancy Risk

Table I-1   Pregnancy Categories of Commonly Prescribed Drugs

DRUG	PREGNANCY CATEGORY		
	B	**C**	**D**
Antibiotics			
Penicillins			
Amoxicillin, trimethoprim-sulfamethoxazole (Augmentin)	X		
Marcolides			
Clarithromycin		X	
Erythromycin	X		
Azithromycin	X		
Cephalosporins	X		
Quinolones		X	
Tetracyclines			X
Metronidazole*	X		
Decongestants/Antihistamines			
Phenylpropanolamine (with or without guaifenesin)		X	
Pseudoephedrine		X	
Loratadine	X		
Bronchodilators			
Steroid Inhalers			
Triamcinolone		X	
Flunisolide		X	
Metaproterenol		X	
Ipratropium bromide	X		
Terbutaline	X		
Isoproterenol		X	
Albuterol		X	
Nonsteroidal Antiinflammatory Agents†			
Ketoprofen	X		
Ibuprofen	Not described		
Naproxen	X		

*Controversial use in first trimester.
†Avoid all such agents in late third trimester.

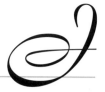

Pediatric Antibiotics

The tables presented on the following pages are designed to provide a quick reference to guide the choice of therapies. Table J-1 covers the appropriate therapies and antibiotics for the most common pediatric outpatient infections. Once an antibiotic has been chosen, Table J-2 provides information on dosing, side effects, and available forms of the antibiotics.

Although this is a general guideline, there may be some regional variations in price of the antibiotics and drug resistance in the bacteria. For specifics in the reader's region, most tertiary care children's hospitals keep yearly records of drug resistance. Most pharmacies also carry a price listing that they can quote over the telephone.

Commonly Used Abbreviations

PCN	Penicillin
TMP	Trimethoprim
SMX	Sulfa drugs/sulfamethoxazole
OCP	Oral contraception pill
CA	Clavulanic acid
$	Relatively inexpensive
$$	Relatively moderate cost
$$$	Relatively expensive
$$$$	Relatively very expensive
Dz	Disease
CSA	Cyclosporin A
HA	Headache
amox/ca	Amoxicillin/clavulanic acid-augmentin

Table J-1 Antibiotic Therapy for Most Common Pediatric Outpatient Infections

DISEASE	COMMON ORGANISMS	FIRST ABX	SECOND ABX
Otitis media	Viruses (50%) *Streptococcus pneumoniae* *Haemophilus influenzae*, no type *M. catarrhalis*	Amoxicillin	TMP/SMX Erythromycin Erythromycin/SMX
Sinusitis	*S. pneumoniae* *H. influenzae*, no type *M. catarrhalis* Anaerobic flora	Amoxicillin	TMP/SMX Erythromycin Erythromycin/SMX
Pneumonia	Viruses (>50%) *S. pneumoniae* *H. influenzae*, no type *Staphylococcus* sp. *Mycoplasma*	Amoxicillin	Erythromycin Erythromycin/SMX Macrolides
Urinary tract infection	GNR *Enterococcus*	TMP/SMX Amoxicillin	Cefixime Amoxicillin/CA Nitrofurantoin
Pharyngitis	*Streptococcus*, group A beta-hemolytic streptococci	PCN, IM	Amoxicillin Ceftriaxone* IM
Cellulitis, extremity	*S. aureus* *Streptococcus* sp.	Cephalexin Dicloxicillin	Erythromycin
Cellulitis, periorbital	*H. influenzae*, no type *H. influenzae*, type B *S. pnuemoniae* *Staphylococcus aureus*	Amoxicillin/CA Cephalexin Ceftriaxone	Erythromycin
Croup	Viral—respiratory syncytial virus, influenza, adenovirus, parainfluenza	None	
Epiglottitis	*H. influenzae*, type B *S. aureus*	Cephalexin	
Common Illness *by Age*	Viral (>50%) *Salmonella* *Shigella* *Campylobacter* *Clostridium difficile* with positive toxin	None	
ROS, <28 mo	GBS GNR *S. pneumoniae* *H. influenzae*, type B *Listeria*	See notes	
ROS, 1-3 mo	GBS GNR *S. pneumoniae* *H. influenzae*, type B *N. meningitis*	Ceftriaxone	
ROS, 3-36 mo	*S. pneumoniae* *H. influenzae*, type B *Neisseria meningitis*	Ceftriaxone	

Abx, Antibiotic; *GNR,* gram-negative rods; *GBS,* group B streptococci.

THIRD ABX	FOURTH ABX	RX DURATION/NOTE
Cefixime Amoxicillin/CA Macrolides Cefaclor Cefprozil	Cefpodoxime Loracarbef Clindamycin	10 days If symptomatic after 5 days, consider change abx. If using 4th-line abx, refer to ENT. If unresolved after 2 or 3 courses refer to ENT
Cefixime Amoxicillin/CA Macrolides Cefaclor Cefprozil	Cefpodoxime Loracarbef Clindamycin	21-42 days Use of intranasal normal saline solution or steroids may help drainage of sinuses If unresolved after 1 or 2 courses, refer to ENT.
Cefixime Amoxicillin/CA Cefaclor Cefprozil Clindamycin		7-14 days Data suggests 7 days is as effective as longer course.
		Cystitis—10 days Pyelonephritis—14 days Consider initial hospitalization for pyelonephritis 1. Benzathine PCN × 1 2. PO agents, 14 days 3. Ceftriaxone, 1 dose followed by PO course Taste limits utility of dicloxicillin.
Erythromycin Cefprozil Cefuroxime		1. If limitations of range of motion or vision, proptosis, *must hospitalize* with ophthalmology consult. 2. *S. aureus only* with external trauma
		Self-resolves 3-5 days *No antibiotics* *Hospitalization,* immediately
		Treat *only Shigella* and other invasive bacteria; *Salmonella* not invasive.
		Hospitalization for IV Abx *only:* Ampicillin-cefotaxime, ampicillin-aminoglycoside
		Must hospitalize if systematically ill for IV Abx and observation.
		Must hospitalize if systematically ill for IV Abx and observation.

Table J-2 Summary Information for Commonly Used Pediatric Antibiotics

ANTIBIOTIC	DOSE	CONCENTRATION	SIDE EFFECTS	TASTE	COST
Cefprozil (Cefzil)	30 mg/kg/day divided bid for otitis media	125 mg/5 cc 250 mg/5 cc	Cross reactivity with PCN; caution with renal Dz; unaffected by food	Good	$$$
Ceftriaxone (Rocephin)	50-100 mg/kg/day divided q 1 day	IM only	Cross-reactivity with PCN; caution with renal Dz; may cause jaundice and biliary sludging; caution in hyperbilirubinemia	IM	$$$
Cefuroxime (Ceftin)	30 mg/kg/day divided bid	125 mg/5 cc	Cross reactivity with PCN; caution with renal Dz	Good	$$$
Cephalexin (Keflex)	25-100 mg/kg/day divided bid-qid	125 mg/5 cc 250 mg/5 cc	Cross reactivity with PCN; caution with renal Dz	Good	$
Clarithromycin (Biaxin)	15 mg/kg/day divided bid	75 mg/5 cc	Fewer gastrointestinal side-effects than erythromycin, but still major side effect; less interactions with other medications; can prevent bad after taste by following with acidic fruit juices; associated with cardiac dysrhythmias with antifungals and histamine blockers	Very poor	$$
Clindamycin (Cleocin)	20-30 mg/kg/day divided qid	75 mg/5 cc	Pseudomembranous colitis, most common drug causing; diarrhea, rash, Stevens-Johnson reaction, thrombocytopenia and granulocytopenia	Poor	$
TMP/SMX (Co-Trimoxazole Septra, Bactrim)	8-10 mg/kg/day divided bid	40 mg/5 cc	Not recommended for child younger than 2 mo, may cause kernicterus; hemolysis in glucose-6-phosphate dehydrogenase deficiency and blood dyscrasias; sun sensitivity	Good	$
Dicloxicillin	25-100 mg/kg/day divided qid	62.5 mg/5 cc	Same as other PCN drugs	Very poor	$
Amoxicillin (Amoxil)	40 mg/kg/day divided tid 80 mg/kg/day divided tid	125 mg/5 cc 250 mg/5 cc	Rash; diarrhea, with fewer gastrointestinal side effects than PCN, otherwise same as other PCN class; high dose in areas of high beta-lactam resistance	Very good	$
Amoxicillin/CA (Augmentin)	40 mg/kg/day divided bid-tid	125 mg/5 cc 250 mg/5 cc	Rash; diarrhea, common and dependent on CA dose, otherwise same as other PCN class; high dose in areas of high beta-lactam resistance	Very good	$$

Table J-2   Summary Information for Commonly Used Pediatric Antibiotics—cont'd

ANTIBIOTIC	DOSE	CONCENTRATION	SIDE EFFECTS	TASTE	COST
Azithromycin (Zithromax)	10 mg/kg/dose on day 1 5 mg/kg/dose on days 2-5	200 mg/5 cc	Fewer gastrointestinal side effects than erythromycin, but still major side effect; less interactions with other medications	Good	$$$
Cefaclor (Ceclor)	40 mg/kg/day divided tid	125 mg/5 cc 250 mg/5 cc 375 mg/5 cc	Caution with renal Dz; cross-reactivity with PCN; serum sickness with repeated usage; same as other cephalosporins	Great	$$
Cefadroxil (Duricef, Ultracef)	30 mg/kd/day divided bid	125 mg/5 cc 250 mg/5 cc 500 mg/5 cc	Cross-reactivity with PCN; nausea, vomiting, pruritus, pseudomembranous colitis, and neutropenia; caution with renal Dz	Good	$$$
Cefixime (Suprax)	8 mg/kg/day qd or divided bid	100 mg/5 cc	Cross reactivity with PCN; nausea, HA, pruritus, abdominal pain, diarrhea; caution with renal Dz	Good	$$
Cefpodoxime (Vantin)	10 mg/kg/day qd or divided bid	50 mg/5 cc 100 mg/5 cc	Cross-reactivity with PCN; caution with renal Dz; histamine-blockers alter absorption	Good	$$$
Cefprozil (Cefzil)	15 mg/kg/day divided bid for pharyngitis	125 mg/5 cc 250 mg/5 cc	Cross-reactivity with PCN; caution with renal Dz; unaffected by food	Good	$$$
Erythromycin	50 mg/kg/day divided tid-qid	200 mg/5 cc	Mostly gastrointestinal side effects with nausea, vomiting, cramps; use with caution in liver Dz; may cause cholestasis; can elevate levels of digoxin, theophylline, steroids, CSA, and carbamazapine; decreases OCP effectiveness	Poor	$
Erythromycin/SMX (Pediazole)	50 mg/kg/day divided tid-qid Dosing based on erythromycin	200 mg/5 cc	Same as erythromycin, but fewer GI side effects; not recommended in children younger than 2 mo; decreases OCP effectiveness	Fair	$
Isoniazid (INH)	10-20 mg/kg/dose qd 20-40 mg/kg/dose 3 times/wk	50 mg/5 cc	Hepatic and neurologic side effects; interferes with anticonvulsants and steroids	Very poor	$

Table J-2 Summary Information for Commonly Used Pediatric Antibiotics—cont'd

ANTIBIOTIC	DOSE	CONCENTRATION	SIDE EFFECTS	TASTE	COST
Loracarbef (Lorabid)	15-30 mg/kg/day divided bid	100 mg/5 cc 200 mg/5 cc	Cross reactivity with PCN; caution with renal Dz	Fair	$$$
Metronidazole (Flagyl)	35-50 mg/kg/day divided tid	100 mg/5 cc	Nausea, diarrhea, urticaria peripheral neuropathy; may discolor urine; use with caution in renal and hepatic Dz	Very poor	$
Nitrofurantoin (Macrodantin)	5-7 mg/kg/day divided qid	25 mg/5 cc	Not recommended for children younger than 1 mo; hemolysis in glucose-6-phosphate dehydrogenase deficiency; vomiting, nausea, diarrhea, headache, jaundice, peripheral neuropathy, and hemolytic anemia	Poor	$
PCN G (Bicillin)	25,000-50,000 U/kg/dose IM Benzathine PCN mixture	IM	Rash; diarrhea, with fewer gastrointestinal side effects than PCN; anaphylaxis, urticaria, hemolytic anemia, and interstitial nephritis	IM	$
PCN V (Pen-Vee K)	25-50 mg/kg/day divided qid Benzathine PCN mixture	125 mg/5 cc 250 mg/5 cc	Same as PCN G	Very poor	$
Rifampin	10-20 mg/kg/day divided qd 10-20 mg/kg/dose 2 times/wk	10 mg/5 cc 15 mg/5 cc	Red discoloration of all body secretions; gastrointestinal upset, headache; decreases OCP effectiveness; ataxia, fatigue, confusion, hepatitis, blood dyscrasias; decreases blood levels of steroids, theophylline, and digoxin	Fair	$

REFERENCES

Amylon, M. (1997). *Lucile Salter Packard Children's Hospital at Stanford housestaff manual* (3rd ed.). Hudson, CA: Lexi-Comp.

Barone, M. (1996). *The Harriet Lane handbook* (14th ed.). St. Louis: Mosby.

Behrman, R., Vaughan, V. (1996). *Nelson textbook of pediatrics* (13th ed.). Philadelphia: W. B. Saunders.

Braunwald, E., Isselbacher, K., Petersdorf, R., Wilson, J., Martin, J., Fauci, A. (1987). *Harrison's principles of internal medicine* (11th ed.). New York: McGraw-Hill.

Committee on Infectious Diseases, American Academy of Pediatrics. *1994 Red book.* Elk Grove Village, IL: American Academy of Pediatrics Press.

Gwaltney, J., Scheld, M., Sande, M., & Sydnor, A. (1992). The microbial etiology and antimicrobial therapy of adults with acute community-acquired sinusitis: A fifteen-year experience at the University of Virginia and review of other selected studies. *Journal of Allergy and Clinical Immunology, 90,* 457-462.

Herr, R. (1991). Acute sinusitis: Diagnosis and treatment update. *American Family Practice, 44,* 2055-2062.

McLinn, S. (1995). *Bugs and drugs: Changing patterns of resistance* [Brochure]. Omaha: University of Nebraska.

Seller, R. (1993). *Differential diagnosis of common complaints* (2nd ed.). Philadelphia: W. B. Saunders.

Woodin, K., Morrison, S. (1994). Antibiotics: Mechanism of action. *Pediatrics in Review, 15,* 440-447.

PART V

SAMPLE EXAMINATION
QUESTIONS

Sample Examination 1

1. J.J. is a 2-month-old infant. He is brought to your clinic by his parents with the report that he is not drinking fluids and has been vomiting and having diarrheal stools for 2 days. His mother states that this morning J.J. had an apnea episode. Your examination reveals pink pharyngeal membranes, normal tympanic membranes, and temperature of 100° F. These symptoms are associated with which of the following?

   a. Common cold
   b. Epiglottitis
   c. Croup
   d. Group A streptococcal pharyngitis

2. Signs of right-to-left cardiac shunting would include all the following **except:**

   a. Cyanosis
   b. Hepatosplenomegaly
   c. Hypoxemia
   d. Clubbing of the nail beds

3. Important subjective data in a client with chronic obstructive pulmonary disease include all the following **except:**

   a. Ability to perform activities of daily living
   b. Weight loss or gain
   c. Urinary frequency
   d. Living will and power of attorney

4. Mr. Greene comes to your office with an acute exacerbation of chronic obstructive pulmonary disease. Follow-up would be needed:

   a. Every 3 to 6 months
   b. As a phone call in 24 to 48 hours
   c. Yearly
   d. Weekly until condition improves

5. Megan, an 8-year-old, is brought in by her mother, Mrs. Lowe, who reports that for the past 3 days Megan has scratched her head and neck almost constantly. Which factor in Megan's history is associated with exposure to lice infestation?

   a. Playing with her dolls in the backyard
   b. Going on a horseback ride with her grandfather
   c. Taking a nap with her grandmother's cat
   d. Trying on hats and coats at a local mall

6. All the following are follow-up plans for the client with allergic conjunctivitis **except:**

   a. Referral to allergist
   b. Follow-up in 1 week for persistent symptoms
   c. Consideration of ophthalmic steroids
   d. Referral to an ophthalmologist

7. Mrs. Jones, a 25-year-old pregnant female, has been treated for a urinary tract infection for 7 days. She should be instructed to return for follow-up:

   a. On her next prenatal visit
   b. After completion of antibiotics
   c. No follow-up is needed if symptoms resolved.
   d. Two days after starting antibiotics

NOTE: The actual test score is calculated on a total of 150 items. There are 25 pretest items included on each examination. Thus the total number of examination items is 175. Pretest items do not count toward the total score.

8. A mother brings her 15-year-old daughter to your clinic. Her daughter has lost 15 pounds and reports fatigue and nausea. After completing the physical examination, the nurse practitioner suspects Addison's disease. What should the nurse practitioner do next?

   a. Order a cosyntropin (Cortrosyn) stimulation test.
   b. Order electrolyte levels.
   c. Discuss the findings with the mother.
   d. Consult with a physician.

9. Which of the following findings indicates a pelvic female factor for infertility?

   a. Thyroid disease
   b. Obesity
   c. Pelvic inflammatory disease
   d. Premature ovarian failure

10. Of the following, the best choice for the client with primary dysmenorrhea is:

   a. Codeine
   b. Acetaminophen
   c. Darvon
   d. Ibuprofen

11. Which of the following symptoms best describes the child with attention-deficit/hyperactivity disorder, hyperactive type? The child often:

   a. Argues with adults, squirms in seat, and leaves seat in classroom
   b. Makes careless mistakes in schoolwork, is forgetful in daily activities, and talks excessively
   c. Fidgets with hands or feet, talks excessively, and has difficulty waiting for his or her turn
   d. Interrupts others, loses temper, and deliberately annoys others

12. Which of the following descriptions is most accurate in describing a "herald patch"?

   a. Oval, discrete, 2 to 6 cm lesion usually seen on the trunk
   b. Round, annular patch with intense itching
   c. Oval, discrete, slightly raised patch on the cheek
   d. Maculopapular and vesicular erythematous rash on the trunk

13. Mr. Jones, a 35-year-old white male, has severe, boring jabs of pain that started on the right side of his head and now involve the whole right side of his head. Mr. Jones reports that the pain comes in episodes of 10 to 30 minutes' duration and that he has had three attacks in the last 12 hours. Results of Mr. Jones' physical examination are normal except for some redness and tearing of the right eye. Which of the following types of primary headache is Mr. Jones most likely experiencing?

   a. Cluster headache
   b. Migraine headache
   c. Trigeminal neuralgia
   d. Tension-type headache

14. The family requests an autopsy after a family member's death. What brain tissue changes would confirm a diagnosis of Alzheimer's disease?

   a. Neurofibrillary tangles and amyloid plaques
   b. Multiple areas of infarcted brain tissue throughout the cerebellum
   c. Generalized cerebral hypertrophy
   d. Vascular insufficiency

15. Which of the following findings suggests that fatigue is related to a systemic disease?

   a. Client is having trouble sleeping.
   b. The client has lost 30 kg in 1 month.
   c. The fatigue has lasted 3 weeks.
   d. The client is 5 weeks post partum.

16. The most common postoperative complication for appendectomy is:

   a. Liver abscess
   b. Fecal fistula
   c. Wound infection
   d. Irritable bowel syndrome

17. A 66-year-old female seeks treatment for shortness of breath and sharp chest pains for 3 hours. She is recovering from a right knee replacement. You suspect a pulmonary embolism. What plan is most appropriate?

   a. Reassure the client that this is a normal occurrence after surgery and will gradually improve.
   b. Begin IV heparin.
   c. Refer or transfer the client immediately for possible ventilation-perfusion scan or angiography.
   d. Decrease physical therapy exercises and reevaluate in 24 hours.

18. Scoliosis is most prevalent during:

    a. Preschool
    b. Prepuberty
    c. Adolescence
    d. Adulthood

19. The best predictor markers for HIV progression are:

    a. Increasing fatigue and weight loss
    b. CD4 and viral burden
    c. Newly diagnosed *Pneumocystis carinii* pneumonia
    d. Positive purified protein derivative of tuberculin result

20. It is important to avoid live-virus vaccines in children undergoing chemotherapy because an immunocompromised child could theoretically contract the disease being immunized against. Primary care advice for such a child and siblings should therefore include all the following **except:**

    a. Give no measles-mumps-rubella vaccine and no oral polio vaccine to affected child and siblings.
    b. Give varicella-zoster immune globulin within 72 to 96 hours of varicella exposure in non-immune children.
    c. Hold all immunizations during chemotherapy treatment.
    d. Resume immunizations 2 months after chemotherapy is complete.

21. Obtaining a history for potential asthma triggers would include information about all the following **except:**

    a. Concurrent viral infections
    b. Concurrent headaches
    c. Exercise and physical activity
    d. Type of heating in home

22. The major determinant of the degree of a burn injury is:

    a. Type of agent producing the burn
    b. Age of the client
    c. Health status of the client
    d. Intensity of the heat released and duration of the exposure

23. A Hispanic client is late for every appointment. The nurse practitioner should do which of the following?

    a. Confront the client and make him or her reschedule.
    b. Assess how the client interprets the appointment time.
    c. Adjust the appointment schedule to allow for this lateness.
    d. Ignore the situation.

24. A nurse practitioner is trying to encourage a client to stop smoking during pregnancy. She should tell the client that smoking:

    a. Produces greater weight gain during pregnancy
    b. Induces iron deficiency anemia during pregnancy
    c. Increases the risk of miscarriage
    d. Produces bigger infants

25. Matthew, 82 years old, had a complete blood cell count, electrolyte levels, renal profile, and lipid levels drawn before he came to the office. All results are within normal limits. He tells you about a community program that is offering a digital rectal examination and prostate-specific antigen for $10 and asks whether he should have these done. His brother, who is 79, had one done last year. Your comments would include all the following **except:**

    a. The digital rectal examination and prostate-specific antigen are tools used to detect prostate cancer at an early stage.
    b. The digital rectal examination and prostate-specific antigen should be used together to detect prostate cancer.
    c. The program is appropriate for him, and he should have it conducted.
    d. The program is not appropriate for him, and he does not need to have it conducted.

26. Which of the following might make you suspect that a woman is pregnant?

    a. Menstrual period 3 days ago
    b. Vaginal spotting for 5 days
    c. Sexual activity
    d. Use of oral contraceptives

27. A 5-year-old comes in for a kindergarten physical examination. In your physical examination you would include all the following **except:**

a. Height, weight, and blood pressure
b. Immunizations
c. Urinalysis
d. Vision and hearing

28. Elaine is an 80-year-old female who is seen for melena. You know that this is the most frequent presenting symptom of which of the following conditions?

a. Stress incontinence
b. Peptic ulcer disease
c. Gastroesophageal reflux disease
d. Constipation

29. The most predictive risk factors for coronary artery disease include all the following **except:**

a. Hypothyroidism
b. Hypertension
c. Smoking
d. Hyperlipidemia

30. Which of the following recommendations should be given to a client receiving treatment for acne with oral tetracycline?

a. Sunscreen should be applied for all outdoor activities.
b. Tetracycline should be taken with food.
c. Tetracycline can be taken with dairy products to decrease gastrointestinal symptoms.
d. Topical preparations are no longer necessary after systemic treatment begins.

31. The treatment of choice for inhibition of platelets is:

a. Aspirin, 81 mg
b. Coumadin, 5 mg
c. Aspirin, 1000 mg
d. Coumadin, 10 mg

32. A 72-year-old reports dyspnea and spitting up blood. Her history indicates that she has recently been recovering from surgical repair of a broken hip and has not been as active as usual. Differential diagnosis must include:

a. Tuberculosis
b. Pulmonary embolism
c. Pneumonia
d. Chronic obstructive pulmonary disease

33. How would the nurse practitioner know that a client understood the activity restrictions given for mononucleosis?

a. Bill returns to work and is lifting 50 pounds of groceries.
b. Sarah plays golf once per week.
c. Sylvia is playing in select soccer tournaments.
d. Todd is playing varsity football.

34. On physical examination for someone with suspected pyelonephritis, which of the following objective findings would you expect?

a. Suprapubic tenderness
b. Costovertebral angle tenderness
c. Mild abdominal pain
d. Urethral discharge

35. A mother brings her 7-year-old daughter to the nurse practitioner. During the past year, the daughter has gained 20 pounds and noticed an increase in subcutaneous fat. Which of the following would **not** be included in the differential diagnosis?

a. Diabetes mellitus
b. Depression
c. Obesity
d. Hypothyroidism

36. An 18-year-old woman seeks treatment for pelvic pressure and general aching in her left side. She is in the second day of menses and is not sexually active. Which diagnosis is most likely?

a. Follicular ovarian cyst
b. Endometrioma
c. Pelvic inflammatory disease
d. Ectopic pregnancy

37. Symptoms in women who are infected with gonorrhea include which of the following?

a. Postcoital bleeding
b. Severe lower back pain
c. Thick, white discharge with itching
d. Fever >101° F

38. The nurse practitioner is helping with a community-wide glaucoma screening effort. Which of the following would be most helpful in detecting early glaucoma?

a. Visual field testing
b. Schiotz tonometry readings
c. Vision screening with a Snellen chart
d. Funduscopic examination of the eye

39. Which of the following findings on physical examination is consistent with a diagnosis of encopresis?

    a. Abdomen is soft and nontender, with no palpable masses.
    b. Rectal vault is empty.
    c. Abdomen is distended, with soft, nontender midline mass.
    d. Rectal vault is filled with soft stool.

40. Your client has been receiving imipramine (Tofranil), 300 mg qd, for the past 3 weeks. When you are evaluating the effectiveness of this medication, your client reports several side effects. Which of the following side effects would require immediate attention?

    a. Occasional constipation
    b. Dry mouth
    c. Urinary retention
    d. Blurred vision

41. Which of the following may cause some acnelike eruptions?

    a. Trazodone
    b. Inhaled steroids
    c. Methylphenidate (Ritalin)
    d. Lithium

42. A symptom commonly associated with the onset of Bell's palsy is:

    a. Numbness along the lateral border of the tongue
    b. Dizziness
    c. Photophobia
    d. Pain in or behind the ear

43. Which of the following manifestations is most indicative of chronic Lyme disease?

    a. Lymphadenopathy
    b. Loss of reflexes
    c. Hip and shoulder pain
    d. Erythema migrans

44. Pertinent subjective data to obtain from the parents of a 6-month-old who is having diarrhea would include all the following **except:**

    a. History of exposure to animals
    b. Number, character, and frequency of stools
    c. Any associated symptoms, such as vomiting
    d. Number of wet diapers during the past few hours

45. The most definitive procedure to diagnose gout is:

    a. Uric acid level determination
    b. Complete blood cell count with differential
    c. Joint fluid aspiration
    d. X-ray film

46. Which of the following presenting symptoms in a client with an acute musculoskeletal complaint might lead a practitioner to suspect systemic lupus erythematosus?

    a. Asymmetric arthritis, peak period of discomfort after prolonged inactivity, inflamed joint, no constitutional symptoms
    b. Symmetric arthritis, peak period of discomfort after prolonged inactivity, inflamed joint, presence of constitutional symptoms
    c. Symmetric arthritis, peak period of discomfort after prolonged use, no constitutional symptoms
    d. Asymmetric arthritis, peak period of discomfort with use, no constitutional symptoms

47. Jimmy's complete blood cell count results are as follows: total WBCs 35,000 cells/mm^3, hemoglobin 7.5, platelets 20,000 cells/mm^3, and differential revealing 25% blast cells. Jimmy is immediately referred to a pediatric hematologist-oncologist. Bone marrow aspiration and biopsy confirm a diagnosis of acute lymphocytic leukemia. Induction chemotherapy is started in the hospital, with the plan that his total length of treatment will be 3 years plus a few months. Most of his treatment will be on an outpatient basis, with supportive care guidelines to include all the following **except:**

    a. No IM injections
    b. No rectal temperatures or suppositories
    c. Use of a soft toothbrush or toothettes for oral care
    d. Keeping immunizations up to date

48. Which of the following information would **not** be pertinent history for a person with non-insulin-dependent diabetes mellitus?

    a. Nutritional history
    b. Pregnancy history
    c. Medication history
    d. Sexual history

49. During an acute asthma attack, which of the following physical findings would be of most concern for the practitioner?

  a. Intercostal retractions
  b. Tachypnea with end-expiratory wheeze
  c. Absence of breath sounds on auscultation
  d. Increased capillary refill time

50. Proper care for a client with a developmental delay includes:

  a. Nutritional interventions
  b. Family assessment and possible interventions
  c. Placing the child in social situations
  d. Promoting fine motor skills

51. The client has explained his perception of the problem and his related feelings. If you wish to clarify your understanding of what he meant, you would say:

  a. "Will you repeat what you said from the beginning?"
  b. "Am I correct in concluding that you mean . . . ?"
  c. "What do you think caused this to happen?"
  d. "I'm finding this difficult to believe."

52. Case management is considered:

  a. A cost-containment measure
  b. Only applicable to acute care hospitalizations
  c. To focus on the improvement of client goals within a specified time frame
  d. A process including multidimensional assessment and multiple team members for high-cost medical conditions

53. *Healthy People 2000* nutritional goals include which of the following?

  a. Decrease the intake of carbohydrate-containing foods.
  b. Increase the number of primary care providers who offer nutritional assessment and referral.
  c. Reduce the incidence of anorexia.
  d. Increase the number of licensed dietitians available to the public.

54. *Healthy People 2000* goals for exercise include which of the following?

  a. Daily vigorous activity for 20 minutes
  b. An increase in the number of primary care providers who assess and counsel clients regarding physical activity

  c. A special emphasis on exercise in older adults
  d. Greater exercise levels for females, as compared with males

55. Matthew is an 80-year-old male who is in the office for a regular 3-month check-up. He is feeling well. He is accompanied today by his daughter. Matthew's wife died 2 years ago, and he has adapted well to the loss and he lives with his daughter and her family. His grandchildren often bring Matthew to the office and are attentive. Matthew is receiving a diuretic, potassium supplements, an antihypertensive, a cardiac regulator, a bronchodilator, an antacid, and a sedative for sleep. During your interview, the most important issue you will be looking for is:

  a. Tolerance to medications
  b. Compliance with medications
  c. Interactive components of medications
  d. Schedule on which medications are taken

56. A history of multiple sexually transmitted diseases may be a risk factor for:

  a. Acute bacterial prostatitis
  b. Benign prostatic hyperplasia
  c. Prostate cancer
  d. Chronic bacterial prostatitis

57. A healthy 18-year-old male has an appointment with you for a precollege physical examination. He is going to be a trainer for the college football team, and a standardized physical form is required. What information would be most pertinent to elicit during the history?

  a. Hot water setting at his dwelling, history of varicella, institutionalization, safe storage of firearms
  b. Sexual activity, smoke detector, history of varicella, tobacco use
  c. Regular dental visits, household members trained in CPR, injection drug use
  d. Motorcycle, bicycle, or all-terrain vehicle helmet; lap and shoulder belts; risk factors for diabetes mellitus; problem drinking

58. A 3-year-old is here for a well-child examination. All the following are part of your examination **except:**

  a. Genital
  b. Vision
  c. Tuberculosis test
  d. Blood pressure

59. Mrs. White is a 32-year-old well female who needs an eye examination. Which of the following describes the most appropriate eye screening for her?

   a. Every 6 months
   b. Every year
   c. Every 2 years
   d. Only when she has a vision problem

60. A young family with a 6-month-old daughter comes in for a well-baby checkup. The parents express concern for future behavior problems after spending a weekend with unruly nieces and nephews. What is the practitioner's best response?

   a. Congratulate them on their insight, and suggest a useful parenting book.
   b. Initiate a behavior management system, so that the family can have practice time.
   c. Recommend that parents verbalize expectations to each other and resolve differences before discussing behavior management at their next visit.
   d. Emphasize the importance of consistency in discipline and behavior management.

61. The rationale for treatment of pharyngitis without a positive culture result would be:

   a. Expectation that a viral pharyngitis will eventually become a bacterial pharyngitis
   b. Prevention of the development of rheumatic fever
   c. Prevention of the development of pneumonia
   d. Prevention of the development of otitis media

62. Who of the following is at greatest risk for development of hypertension?

   a. A 25-year-old female who leads a sedentary lifestyle and takes oral contraceptives
   b. A 32-year-old black male who smokes and is overweight
   c. A 16-year-old male who has consistent blood pressure readings of 130/80 mm Hg
   d. A 5-year-old female with a heart murmur and blood pressure readings of 90/56 mm Hg

63. Which of the following clients would be most likely to need a chest x-ray examination?

   a. A 5-year-old with clear nasal drainage and scattered wheezes
   b. A 65-year-old with crackles in the left lower lung field

   c. A 24-year-old smoker with fever and purulent cough
   d. A 40-year-old with cough, headache, and nasal congestion

64. The most important aspects of the history to obtain for children with a chronic cough include all the following **except:**

   a. Recurrent upper respiratory tract infections
   b. Growth patterns
   c. Fatty stools
   d. Play patterns

65. Tiffany is a 22-year-old woman who had syphilis diagnosed and treated during her pregnancy. Her son Josh was born without problems. During serologic testing 2 days after birth, it is found that Josh has a reactive VDRL. This indicates which of the following?

   a. Tiffany had inadequate treatment.
   b. Tiffany was treated too late in her pregnancy.
   c. Josh has syphilis and should be treated with 2.4 MU penicillin immediately.
   d. Josh may have a reactive Venereal Disease Research Laboratory test as a result of passive transfer of antibodies from Tiffany

66. Additional male factor testing for infertility may include all the following **except:**

   a. Serum testosterone
   b. Follicle-stimulating hormone
   c. Prolactin
   d. Estradiol

67. Alpha-adrenergic antagonists, used in the treatment of benign prostatic hyperplasia, to minimize side effects, should be given:

   a. Every morning
   b. Every evening at dinner
   c. At bedtime
   d. In divided doses

68. Non-insulin-dependent diabetes mellitus was diagnosed in Mr. James by the nurse practitioner. What is the **first** step for the nurse practitioner?

   a. Develop a plan.
   b. Consult with physician.
   c. Refer Mr. James to an endocrinologist.
   d. Schedule a follow-up.

69. Which of the following is the first question you should ask a 25-year-old, nulligravid, nulliparous, married woman with the presenting symptom of metorrhagia for the past 3 months?

    a. What kind of birth control do you use?
    b. How often do you have intercourse?
    c. Do you have any pain with menses?
    d. Have you ever had a uterine biopsy?

70. On the basis of your diagnosis of herpetic conjunctivitis, your plan for treatment should be which of the following?

    a. Cool compresses as needed, sodium sulfacetamide ophthalmic solution 10%
    b. Ophthalmologic referral and ophthalmic steroid drops
    c. Ophthalmologic referral
    d. Bacitracin ophthalmic ointment

71. A 45-year-old married woman has recurrent headaches, episodes of visual disturbance, a history of migraines, and a history of government assistance. Her husband "drinks a lot" and recently lost his job. This history would suggest that the woman is at risk for abuse, **except** for which of the following factors?

    a. Her age is 45 years.
    b. Her husband drinks.
    c. She reports recurring problems with headaches.
    d. She has a low socioeconomic status.

72. Sociocultural factors contribute to the development of eating disorders. These factors include:

    a. Blurring of generational boundaries
    b. Low self-esteem
    c. Changing roles of women and role destabilization
    d. Affective intolerance

73. Judy is an 18-year-old client visiting your office for evaluation of a plaque on her right shoulder. You diagnose tinea corporis and would like to confirm this in your office. Which of the following would you most likely do?

    a. Prepare a slide with potassium hydroxide to visualize hyphae.
    b. Culture a scraping from the center of the lesion in the appropriate medium.

    c. Visualize the fluorescence under a Wood's lamp.
    d. Do a fingernail test to reproduce fine scales.

74. If a client was experiencing delirium, you would expect her to demonstrate all the following **except:**

    a. History of symptoms occurring within days
    b. Inability to maintain attention
    c. Decline in consciousness
    d. Marked depression

75. A client with chronic venous insufficiency often:

    a. Responds to treatment and needs no further follow-up
    b. Has recurrent problems, particularly if treatment is followed
    c. Has recurrent problems if treatments to counteract edema and secondary tissue changes are not followed throughout life
    d. Has more hair growth on lower extremities

76. Primary dysmenorrhea is most likely to occur in which of the following women?

    a. A 12-year-old who has had two menstrual cycles
    b. A 30-year-old with regular cycles
    c. A 48-year-old with irregular cycles
    d. A 35-year-old taking oral contraceptives

77. All clients with new or recurring peptic ulcers should be tested for:

    a. Streptococcal infection
    b. Lower esophageal sphincter tone
    c. Increased aspartate aminotransferase and alanine aminotransferase levels
    d. *Helicobacter pylori*

78. What objective information would you obtain from Roger, a 50-year-old man who reports left lower quadrant abdominal pain and constipation?

    a. Deep tendon reflexes
    b. Current medications
    c. History of diarrhea alternating with constipation
    d. Rectal examination and guaiac

79. An infant with a diagnosis at birth of developmental dysplasia of hip has been in a Pavlik harness for 6 weeks and spontaneous reduction has occurred. When should this harness be removed?

   a. Once reduction has occurred
   b. Over several months
   c. After 1 more week
   d. Never

80. A client with stage II lymphoma comes in for a routine physical examination. The nurse practitioner should evaluate all the following **except:**

   a. Status of all lymph nodes
   b. Size of the spleen
   c. Weight patterns
   d. Hemoglobin and hematocrit

81. What are the most common types of anemia that can occur during pregnancy and post partum?

   a. Folic acid deficiency and iron deficiency
   b. Iron deficiency and acute blood loss
   c. Pernicious anemia and acute blood loss
   d. Vitamin B_{12} deficiency and iron deficiency

82. For the adult with persistent nighttime cough, what other respiratory condition should be ruled out as a differential diagnosis?

   a. Pneumonia
   b. Bronchitis
   c. Exercise-induced asthma
   d. Sinusitis

83. All the following statements regarding standards of care for nurse practitioners are true **except:**

   a. They are based on the scope of practice.
   b. They are a means to describe and guide the achievement of excellence.
   c. They deal with the phenomena of concern for nurse practitioners.
   d. They are developed by the State Boards of Nursing.

84. Which of the following physician reimbursement figures is correct for nurse practitioners billing Medicare clients?

   a. 100% of the physician charge
   b. 70% of the physician charge
   c. 85% of the physician charge
   d. 50% of the physician charge

85. The purpose of advance directives is:

   a. To promote active euthanasia
   b. To encourage resuscitation of terminally ill clients
   c. To give the direction for the client's care by the client in advance of the need
   d. To give power of attorney to the family designee

86. Which of the following clients needs nutritional screening?

   a. An older client
   b. A client with an involuntary loss of 5 pounds within 1 month
   c. A client who is 10% above ideal body weight
   d. A client who is 10% below ideal body weight

87. When explaining the benefits of exercise to a client, the nurse practitioner should discuss:

   a. Improved fertility
   b. Decreased incidence of diarrhea
   c. Improved glucose tolerance
   d. Increased low-density lipoprotein levels

88. In the interview, Sam, an 87-year-old widower, discloses that he has two firearms in the home. One is a rifle and one is a handgun. Your next most appropriate avenue will be to ask:

   a. Who is able to fire the guns?
   b. Where are the guns stored, and what safety measures are taken?
   c. What are the types of guns and where were they purchased?
   d. Are the firearms legally licensed?

89. The focus of the plan for a well-male examination is:

   a. Treatment of disease
   b. Prevention of morbidity and mortality
   c. Immunizations
   d. Screening for disease

90. A school-age child comes to your office for a well-child examination. Your anticipatory guidance issues include firearm safety. You know that the most common risk factor associated with injury or death from firearms is:

   a. Argument with a stranger
   b. Firearm access
   c. Substance use
   d. Peer pressure

91. Nancy F. is a 63-year-old female. Which of the following is **not** a risk factor for osteoporosis?

a. White ethnicity
b. Total hysterectomy at 38 years
c. Hormone replacement therapy
d. Smoking habit, 2 packs/day

92. Symptoms of gallbladder disease may include:

a. Diarrhea, bloating, left upper quadrant tenderness
b. WBC counts >40,000 cells/mm³
c. Pain with expiration
d. Right upper quadrant tenderness

93. To prevent deaths from cardiovascular disease among blacks, primary prevention programs for men should target reductions in:

a. Cholesterol levels
b. Glaucoma screening
c. Diabetes
d. Hypertension

94. You are seeing a 70-year-old man who reports gradual decrease in his vision. You know that as a result of his age, he is at risk for cataracts. Which other symptoms would make you suspect cataracts as the cause of his visual impairment?

a. Peripheral vision better than central vision
b. Dull aching behind eyes, particularly in the morning
c. Improved vision in low light
d. Occasional floaters in periphery

95. A 70-year-old male 2 days after myocardial infarction begins to report substernal chest pain that worsens with deep breathing and movement and is relieved with sitting up and leaning forward. Pericardial friction rub is absent, and no ECG changes are noted. What is the best differential diagnosis?

a. Recurrent angina
b. Pericarditis
c. Pulmonary embolus
d. Aortic dissection

96. Megan, a 5-year-old, is brought to the clinic because she has never been able to achieve nighttime dryness. Which of the following physical findings would suggest an organic cause for her enuresis?

a. Height and weight below the fifth percentile and blood pressure of 120/88 mm Hg.
b. Good rectal sphincter tone with no genital anomalies
c. Abdomen soft and slightly distended, with no masses palpable
d. Urinalysis results positive for nitrates and leukocytes

97. As a member of the multidisciplinary team following up children with cystic fibrosis, the family nurse practitioner would be responsible for all the following **except:**

a. Monitoring growth and development
b. Prescribing annual influenza vaccination and at least one pneumococcal vaccination
c. Providing anticipatory guidance for each developmental stage
d. Prescribing a plan of vigorous chest physical therapy

98. The treatment for gonorrhea in the adult includes which of the following?

a. Erythromycin
b. Cefixime
c. Azithromycin
d. Acyclovir

99. A complete blood cell count that reveals an elevated WBC count is most likely to be associated with:

a. Acute bacterial prostatitis
b. Benign prostatic hyperplasia
c. Prostate cancer
d. Chronic bacterial prostatitis

100. Grace is a 50-year-old woman with hyperthyroidism. She was treated with radioactive iodine. What instructions are **not** appropriate regarding follow-up?

    a. Grace should return if she has symptoms of hypothyroidism.

    b. The exophthalmos that Grace exhibits will gradually go away.

    c. Grace should be aware of the symptoms of thyrotoxicosis.

    d. Routine blood thyroid tests should be performed periodically.

101. Which of the following client reports would indicate appropriate attempts to remove environmental triggers?

    a. "I make my husband smoke in another room, away from me."

    b. "We vacuumed our box springs and mattress to remove dust mites."

    c. "Our dog now gets a weekly bath."

    d. "We put her stuffed animals on a shelf, so that she won't be exposed to their dust."

102. Which information about performing breast self-examination is **inaccurate?**

    a. Breast self-examination is ideally performed 4 to 7 days after the menstrual period.

    b. For oral contraceptive users, breast self-examination can be effectively performed when starting a new pill pack.

    c. Postmenopausal women should select a familiar date and use that day of the month consistently for breast self-examination.

    d. Breast self-examination is unnecessary during pregnancy and lactation.

103. Which of the following is **not** considered a precipitating risk factor for congestive heart failure?

    a. Dietary indiscretion (increased sodium intake)
    b. Cardiac arrhythmia
    c. Appropriate restriction of physical activity
    d. Uncontrolled hypertension

104. Mrs. Jones is a 50-year-old housewife who was seen by you at the clinic with reports of chronic cough and weight loss of 2 months' duration. She insists that there is nothing seriously wrong with her except for this nagging cold. Which defense mechanism is Mrs. Jones using?

    a. Projection
    b. Denial

    c. Rationalization
    d. Sublimation

105. A toddler comes to the clinic for burns on her fingers and the palms of her hands. Her mother states, "She grabbed hold of my curling iron when I had just finished with it. I had turned my back." What objective findings would lead the nurse practitioner to consider abuse?

    a. Linear bullae on palm extending to base of fingers

    b. Circular crusts and erosions on palm and fingertips

    c. From 4 to 5 bruises on anterior aspects of lower legs

    d. Anxious appearance with examination and withdrawal from practitioner

106. Jeff's mother has followed instructions for washing the linens and clothes after a scabies infestation. She calls the clinic for advice regarding a new leather jacket that Jeff wore during his infestation. Which of the following is the appropriate advice?

    a. Dry-clean the coat, even though it is new.

    b. Seal the coat in a plastic bag for at least 7 days.

    c. Wipe the coat with an antibacterial solution.

    d. Discard the coat because it cannot be properly cleaned.

107. A 75-year-old male comes to the emergency department with lethargy and suddenly begins to have a tonic-clonic seizure. Of the immediate management steps listed, which is **incorrect?**

    a. Place an oral airway in his tightly closed jaws.

    b. Place a folded blanket on the siderail that his arm keeps hitting.

    c. Attempt to place patient on his side.

    d. Administer oxygen for his cyanosis.

108. Primary management of congestive heart failure includes:

    a. Use of a beta-blocker
    b. Use of nonsteroidal antiinflammatory drugs
    c. Use of diuretics
    d. Increased sodium intake

109. How would you manage Ann's care after diagnosis of irritable bowel syndrome?

    a. Stop all milk products.
    b. Refer Ann to a surgeon.
    c. Increase Ann's fluid and fiber intake.
    d. Prescribe cimetidine (Tagamet), 400 mg bid.

110. The family nurse practitioner makes a report of suspected spousal abuse. Appropriate follow-up of the case would include which of the following?

    a. Turn the case over to the clinic social worker for monitoring.
    b. Periodically contact the client, the case worker, or both until the report has been investigated and the legal process is completed.
    c. No follow-up is needed once the report has been made and the case becomes a legal issue.
    d. Contact the client daily by phone to ensure her safety.

111. Which of the following best describes the pathophysiology of gastroesophageal reflux disease?

    a. Herniations as a result of antireflux barrier defects
    b. Reflux as a result of defective esophageal clearance
    c. Motility of small intestine affected by pressure
    d. Motility diminished as a result of bronchospasms

112. Which best describes Tinel's maneuver?

    a. Flex elbows at 90 degrees and hold.
    b. Tap on volar surface of wrist at median nerve.
    c. Raise arm above head for 60 seconds.
    d. Hyperflex wrist for 2 minutes.

113. Which of the following laboratory results is consistent with the diagnosis of microcytic hypochromic anemia in an adult?

    a. Decreased mean corpuscular volume (MCV) and mean corpuscular hemoglobin concentration (MCHC) and increased serum iron
    b. Increased mean corpuscular volume, mean corpuscular hemoglobin concentration, and serum iron

    c. Decreased mean corpuscular volume and increased mean corpuscular hemoglobin concentration and serum iron
    d. Decreased mean corpuscular volume, mean corpuscular hemoglobin concentration, and serum iron

114. Client education for a client with a severe seafood allergy is successful when the client:

    a. Stops swimming in the ocean
    b. Uses iodized salt
    c. Carries epinephrine with him at all times
    d. Agrees to undergo IV pyelography for dysuria

115. A young woman comes to the clinic requesting an abortion. The nurse practitioner's most appropriate initial response to the situation should be to do which of the following?

    a. Attempt to change the client's values.
    b. Get in touch with own values and beliefs.
    c. Ask the client to explain the reason for her request.
    d. Refer the client to a specialist.

116. Which of the following is considered primary prevention?

    a. Checking for a high blood sugar level in older clients
    b. Discussing how to floss and its importance
    c. Yearly Papanicolaou smears
    d. Discussing a low-fat diet with a client with coronary artery disease

117. You have an 82-year-old client with gastrointestinal distress. He is quiet and acquiesces responses to his son, who accompanies him to the office. This client has some bruises on his arms that he cannot explain. He does not make eye contact. You suspect adult abuse. Which of the following statements is **least** appropriate to explore the issue?

    a. How have you dealt with problems in the past?
    b. What kind of support systems and resources can you draw on?
    c. Many people struggle with similar situations. Problems can arise. Are you having problems?
    d. These bruises are a sign of abuse, and you cannot go back into that situation.

118. Linda B. has a menstrual cycle length of 21 days. Her menses is late by 8 weeks. In calculating her estimated date of delivery, which of the following formulas would be appropriate?

    a. Add 9 months and 7 days to the first day of the last normal menstrual period.

    b. Add 9 months and 14 days to the first day of the last normal menstrual period.

    c. Add 9 months to the first day of the last normal menstrual period.

    d. Subtract 3 months and 7 days from the first day of her last period.

119. Counseling topics related to safety needs specific for women older than 65 years include:

    a. Abuse and seat belt use

    b. Fall prevention and smoke detectors

    c. Smoke detectors and hot water heater temperature

    d. Fall prevention and hot water heater temperature

120. Which of the following physical findings is consistent with nonpathologic gynecomastia in an adolescent?

    a. From 2 to 3 cm, fatty tissue bilaterally beneath the nipples

    b. From 1 to 2 cm, unilateral, glandular tissue beneath the nipple

    c. Unilateral, hard, ulcerated tissue at the nipple

    d. Bilateral inverted nipples

121. Which of the following is the most common systemic antibiotic used in the treatment of severe acne?

    a. Isotretinoin

    b. Cephalexin (Keflex)

    c. Azithromycin

    d. Tetracycline

122. Which of the following is **not** true regarding falls in older adults?

    a. Acute illness may precipitate falls.

    b. Most falls are not part of normal activities of daily living.

    c. Sedatives and antidepressants increase the risk of falls.

    d. Clients should be involved in the falls assessment of the home environment.

123. Sylvia is a 43-year-old female with a diagnosis of non-insulin-dependent diabetes. You are preparing to do diabetic teaching for her. What is the first step in this process?

    a. Establish goals.

    b. Assess learner needs.

    c. Choose audio and video materials and client handouts.

    d. Set priorities for learning needs.

124. Mrs. C.D. is 8 months' pregnant. She reports bleeding and swelling of her gums and denies trauma. On the basis of the subjective data, your diagnosis of highest suspicion is:

    a. Gingivitis

    b. Acute necrotizing ulcerative gingivitis

    c. Canker sore

    d. Oral candidiasis

125. Sue Howard, a 34-year-old female, has been treated for superficial thrombophlebitis for 7 days. She should be instructed to return for follow-up:

    a. Weekly until her symptoms resolve

    b. No follow-up is needed.

    c. Only if she experiences chest pain

    d. After completion of antibiotics

126. Which of the following medications is most likely to cause shortness of breath in a client with existing chronic obstructive pulmonary disease or asthma?

    a. Antacids

    b. Beta-blockers

    c. Acetaminophen

    d. Nitrates

127. Trixie is a 16-year-old female who has an appointment for a gynecologic examination and family planning. During the examination the nurse practitioner notes a friable cervix but no discharge. Otherwise, results of her examination are normal. Which of the following diagnoses is the most likely for Trixie?

    a. HIV

    b. Syphilis

    c. Candidiasis

    d. *Chlamydia*

128. Criteria for *Pneumocystis carinii* prophylaxis include:

    a. CD4 count ≤200 cells/mm^3
    b. Known exposure to *P. carinii*
    c. Cough with night sweats
    d. CD4 count ≤500 cells/mm^3

129. Medications that can precipitate adrenal insufficiency are:

    a. Mitotane and phenytoin
    b. Trilostane and erythromycin
    c. Digoxin and ketonconazole
    d. Furosemide and metyrapone

130. Once symptoms have been effectively managed for several months, how often should the client with premenstrual syndrome be seen by the practitioner doing follow-up care?

    a. Every month during the premenstrual phase
    b. Every 3 months
    c. Every 6 months
    d. Every year

131. Your client has decompensated congestive heart failure. Which of the following diuretics will give a more rapid response?

    a. Hydrochlorothiazide
    b. Furosemide
    c. Amiloride
    d. Triamterene-hydrochlorothiazide

132. Primary care clients with alcohol abuse have improved outcomes with:

    a. Supervised detoxification
    b. Regular urinary drug tests
    c. Brief counseling and regular follow-up
    d. Monthly serum gamma-glutamyl transferase measurement

133. Richard, a 32-year-old male with HIV and a CD4 count of 312 cells/mm^3, has herpes zoster on his face. He notices one lesion on his nose. What is essential follow-up for this client?

    a. Follow up in 48 hours and begin antiviral therapy immediately.
    b. Immediately refer Richard to an ophthalmologist.

    c. Hospitalize Richard for IV antiviral medication.
    d. See Richard in the office in 1 week.

134. Mrs. South, a 40-year-old accountant with two teenaged children, has a diagnosis of more than 10 years' duration of migraine headaches. She was placed on a regimen of propranolol (Inderal), 40 mg qd, as prophylaxis and instructed to make an appointment in 2 months for a return visit. Which of the following statements is most likely **not** the reason for the scheduled follow-up visit?

    a. Prophylactic medications should be given at least a 2-month trial before it is possible to assess their benefits.
    b. The follow-up will allow the health care provider to assess Mrs. South's adherence to the performance of regular exercise and relaxation techniques, sleep patterns, and nutrition status.
    c. The follow-up will allow the health care provider to get to know Mrs. South better as a person.
    d. The follow-up will allow the health care provider to give support and counseling.

135. If a client with Parkinson's disease begins having hallucinations and delusions, which drug would more likely be the cause?

    a. Carbidopa
    b. Bromocriptine
    c. Selegeline
    d. Levodopa

136. Major findings in chronic venous insufficiency include:

    a. Cyclic abdominal bloating and inability to remove wedding ring
    b. Progressive edema of the leg (particularly lower leg), with thin, shiny, brownish pigmentation often developing
    c. Confusion, weight gain, and arrhythmia
    d. Weight gain, hypotension, and positive Homan's sign

137. Elmer is a 53-year-old truck driver with diagnosis of hepatitis B virus, hepatitis D virus, and superinfection of hepatitis C virus. He has been followed up in your clinic for the past 6 months. His aspartate aminotransferase and alanine aminotransferase levels have been stable but elevated. The most important physical assessment in monitoring Elmer's progress would be:

a. General skin examination and general performance status assessment
b. Abdominal examination to assess liver size and tenderness
c. Presence of any low-grade fever in the past few weeks
d. Digital rectal examination to assess for occult blood loss

138. Acute lumbosacral strain occurs most commonly in:

a. Those 65 years old or older
b. Those younger than 20 years
c. Those between 20 and 40 years old
d. No particular age group; there is no age discrimination

139. The most common high-dose source of lead exposure for children is:

a. Drinking water
b. Pica
c. Paint
d. Soil

140. Which of the following treatment is **not** appropriate first-line management for eczema?

a. Oatmeal colloidal bath
b. Topical steroids applied sparingly
c. Cool compresses with Burow's solution
d. Tapered course of prednisone

141. Treatment for a client with arthritic changes related to Lyme disease would be:

a. Doxycycline, 100 mg bid for 30 days
b. Tetracycline, 500 mg qid for 30 days
c. Ceftriaxone, 2 g/day IV for 14 days
d. Erythromycin, 250 mg qid for 21 days

142. Licensure as a nurse practitioner:

a. Is controlled by the Board of Nursing
b. Protects the public from incompetence

c. Identifies where and how the nurse practitioner provides care
d. Is controlled by the Board of Medicine and the Board of Nursing

143. When assessing smoking status, the nurse practitioner should assess all the following **except:**

a. Packs smoked per day
b. Years as a smoker
c. Nicotine level of cigarettes used
d. Previous attempts at stopping and their success

144. Assuming that previous results have been normal, Papanicolaou smears should be done every year until 60 years and then every:

a. 1 to 2 years
b. 1 to 3 years
c. 2 years
d. None of the above

145. Which of the following treatments would **not** be used for an infant with developmental dysplasia of hip?

a. Spica cast
b. Pavlik harness
c. Triple diapering
d. Preliminary traction

146. An adolescent with an ankle sprain can return to play:

a. When pain is gone, even with slight limp
b. After 2 weeks of rest and full range of motion
c. After resolution of pain, full range of motion, and normal gait
d. After 1 week with ankle wrap

147. Which of the following pharmacokinetic parameters is increased in older adults?

a. Drug absorption
b. Glomular filtration rate
c. Volume of distribution of water-soluble compounds
d. Percentage of body fat

148. A 45-year-old woman who has regular menstrual cycles asks whether she is in menopause. Which is the best response for the nurse practitioner to give?

    a. Menopause starts when one is 40 years old and ends at about 50 years.

    b. Menopause is the stopping of menstruation for 6 months.

    c. Menopause starts at 45 years.

    d. Regular menstrual cycles are rare for someone your age.

149. Sue Howard, a 34-year-old female, had acute sinusitis diagnosed today. She should be instructed to return for follow-up in which of the following cases?

    a. There is no improvement in her symptoms within 48 hours.

    b. A cough develops.

    c. Low-grade fever develops.

    d. She has nasal drainage.

150. Which physical finding is most suggestive of hypothyroidism?

    a. Silky hair

    b. Dull facies

    c. Weight loss

    d. Anxious speech

151. A 38-year-old client who is a mother of two comes in for a physical examination. The nurse practitioner discovers that her mother died at 43 years old of a myocardial infarction. The client eats a low-fat diet and is a grocery checker. Which of the following factors places her most at risk for coronary artery disease?

    a. Her age

    b. Her sex

    c. Her job

    d. Her mother's medical history

152. A client who has frequent recurrence of candidiasis should be evaluated for what other condition?

    a. Urinary tract infection

    b. Pelvic inflammatory disease

    c. Diabetes

    d. Lupus

153. Which of the following physical findings would **not** usually be found in a child with cystic fibrosis?

    a. Hyperinflation and tram lines on chest x-ray examination

    b. Steeple sign on chest and lateral neck x-ray examination

    c. Wheezes and crackles bilaterally on chest auscultation

    d. Digital clubbing and use of accessory muscles with respiration.

154. Mary, a 9-year-old girl, reports "these funny things" on her hand. Which item of the subjective data is **least** important to elicit initially?

    a. What changes had she noticed in the "things" since she discovered them?

    b. Has she noticed any relationship with anything else?

    c. When was her last well physical examination?

    d. What does she know about skin cancer?

155. Which of the following descriptions is identified with a migraine with aura headache?

    a. Bilateral, mild to moderate, pressing headache lasting 30 minutes to 6 days

    b. Unilateral, moderate-to-severe, throbbing headache lasting for 4 to 72 hours, aggravated by routine physical activity, preceded by flashing lights, with nausea, vomiting, or both

    c. Pounding or dull frontal or occipital pain present when upright and relieved by lying down

    d. More prevalent in men, occurring in attacks of severe unilateral orbital, supraorbital, or temporal pain lasting 15 to 180 minutes and miosis

156. Which of the following objective findings is most specific for Lyme disease?

    a. Skin lesion >5 cm in diameter

    b. Enlargement of epitrochlear and axillary nodes

    c. Decreased range of motion of cervical spine

    d. Muscular atrophy

157. The health history should include all the following **except:**

    a. Information about risk factors

    b. Information about reasons for the current visit

    c. Review of systems

    d. Anticipatory guidance

158. The definitive test for osteoarthritis is:

a. Erythrocyte sedimentation rate
b. Complete blood cell count
c. Electrolyte levels
d. Physical examination

159. Which of the following illnesses is **not** usually transmitted by the airborne route?

a. Rubella
b. Mumps
c. Tuberculosis
d. Hepatitis

160. A nurse practitioner whose client population includes a large number of depressed people wants to implement a program that is based on a study conducted at another facility. Before implementing the program, what is the first thing the nurse practitioner should do?

a. Examine the study for its scientific integrity.
b. Ask the clients whether they want to participate.
c. Cost out the price of providing the program.
d. Pilot test the program.

161. *Healthy People 2000* goals for stress management include:

a. Increasing the number of worksites with 50 or more employees providing stress-reduction programs
b. Increasing the number of referrals made by primary care providers to psychiatrists for stress control
c. Decreasing the number of primary care visits made for stress management
d. Decreasing the number of stress disorders in children

162. A mother calls regarding implementation of a behavior-management system. The misbehavior of her 3-year-old, who was seen in the office 2 days ago, seems to have increased in frequency and intensity since trying "the system." What would the best response of the provider be?

a. Suggest a plan that would allow the child to "ease into the system."
b. Tell the mother to call back at the end of 2 weeks to provide a more accurate evaluation of the new system.

c. Reassure the parent that her child is testing limits. Encourage consistency. Keep communication lines open. Follow up 1 to 2 weeks.
d. Ask the mother for specific accounts of misbehavior and the parental response. Consider whether the system has been correctly implemented.

163. Vaginal changes during menopause related to decreased estrogen can be helped by:

a. Taking a progesterone-only minipill
b. Using a sitz bath
c. Continuing regular sexual intercourse
d. Eating yogurt

164. A client being treated for hyperlipidemia has reached his target goals. The nurse practitioner should do which of the following?

a. Measure total cholesterol at 4 months and perform a full lipid analysis in 1 year.
b. Perform a full lipid profile in 1 month.
c. Measure total cholesterol in 1 year.
d. Check low-density and high-density lipid levels in 6 months.

165. The goal of crisis intervention is to:

a. Enhance a person's level of functioning beyond that before the crisis
b. Resolve past psychologic stressors
c. Promote coping strategies used in the past
d. Resolve the immediate crisis

166. Expected chemistry laboratory values in a person with Addison's disease would include:

a. Hypokalemia, hypernatremia, and hyperglycemia
b. Hypokalemia, hypernatremia, and hypoglycemia
c. Hyperkalemia, hyponatremia, and hyperglycemia
d. Hyperkalemia, hyponatremia, and hypoglycemia

167. To appropriately refer a client with a developmental disability, the nurse practitioner must first assess all the following **except:**

a. Gross motor function
b. Language use
c. Social abilities
d. Height and weight

168. What is the appropriate response to the person who comes to the clinic 1 week after treatment with a scabicide and reports continued pruritus?

    a. A second treatment is indicated.

    b. Pruritus may continue for several days to weeks as a reaction to the mite remains.

    c. Pruritus will continue for 1 to 2 weeks as a reaction to the scabicide.

    d. Another skin condition is present, and the person should be referred to a dermatologist.

169. Which of the following statements about evaluating blood pressure is true?

    a. Blood pressure should be checked in both arms on at least one occasion to verify equivalency.

    b. At least three abnormal blood pressure readings 1 month apart are required to document the presence of hypertension.

    c. Coffee or cigarettes 5 minutes before a blood pressure check should have no effect on the evaluation.

    d. The size and position of the blood pressure cuff have little impact on the accuracy of the reading.

170. Mr. Donaldson, a long-distance runner, was recently diagnosed with acute lumbosacral strain with minimal pain. In instructing on aerobic exercises, the nurse practitioner said that he could:

    a. Walk or jog lightly

    b. Continue his usual regimen of training

    c. Increase his speed but shorten his distance

    d. Lift weights

171. Sarah is an 8-year-old girl who reports a sore throat, feeling hot, and a rash over her body. On examination, she is found to have a diffuse maculopapular rash and tenderness and swelling of her posterior lymph nodes. A few days later, her illness is gone. The most likely diagnosis of this girl's condition is:

    a. Rubella

    b. Rubeola

    c. Fifth disease

    d. Roseola

172. A family nurse practitioner is treating a 10-year-old for chronic constipation. The client has been taking docusate sodium (Colace), 100 mg PO qd, for the past 2 months. He is now having daily soft stools. In evaluating this situation, the family nurse practitioner decides to do which of the following?

    a. Reduce the Colace to 50 mg qd, continue diet therapy, and recheck in one month.

    b. Continue with the same regimen and reevaluate in 6 months.

    c. Discontinue the Colace and have the client phone if he has any problems.

    d. Discontinue therapy and reevaluate in 3 months.

173. When describing the harmful effects of stress, the nurse practitioner should discuss:

    a. Premature death

    b. Higher incidence of alcoholism

    c. Decreased immunologic functioning and its consequences

    d. Social isolation

174. An adult who is being treated for constipation should be seen for follow-up:

    a. Every month initially then twice a year

    b. Twice a month while constipation persists

    c. As needed for problems

    d. No follow-up is necessary.

175. A menopausal woman asks the nurse practitioner how to manage hot flashes. The practitioner suggests:

    a. Limiting fluid intake

    b. Limiting caffeine intake

    c. Exercising minimally

    d. Avoiding hot tubs

ANSWERS AND RATIONALES: EXAMINATION 1

1. Answer: a (diagnosis/HEENT/infant)
Rationale: Infants often show atypical signs and symptoms of the common cold. This presenting picture may be associated with the rhinovirus and respiratory syncytial virus. The client is too young for the other choices.

2. Answer: b (physical examination/cardiovascular/NAS)
Rationale: Right-to-left shunting is the defining characteristic of the cyanotic heart lesion. This results in hypoxemia as blood returning to the heart passes directly to the systemic circulation without passing through the lungs. This in turn results in cyanosis when the client has 5 mg/dl of blood that is deoxygenated. Clubbing will be seen during chronic periods of hypoxemia and is of unknown etiology. Hepatosplenomegaly is associated with right-sided heart failure, which results from fluid overload in left-to-right shunts and pulmonary outflow tract obstructions. This would not be seen in right-to-left shunting.

3. Answer: c (assessment/history/respiratory/adult)
Rationale: It is important to ask questions regarding life (ability to perform activities of daily living), weight loss or gain and during what time, and the client's feelings regarding resuscitation. The practitioner is obligated to provide information on advance directives.

4. Answer: b (evaluation/respiratory/adult)
Rationale: An acute exacerbation can be followed up by phone 24 to 48 hours after the office visit. The follow-up interval for stable chronic obstructive pulmonary disease is 3 to 6 months.

5. Answer: d (assessment/history/communicable disease/NAS)
Rationale: Lice live in the seams and linings of clothes and can be transmitted in this manner.

6. Answer: c (evaluation/HEENT/NAS)
Rationale: Ophthalmic steroids should be avoided because of the association with increased incidence of glaucoma and cataracts.

7. Answer: b (evaluation/genitourinary/childbearing female)
Rationale: Because she is pregnant, Mrs. Jones is considered to have a complicated urinary tract infection. This warrants follow-up for a urine culture once the antibiotic course has been completed.

8. Answer: d (plan/management/consult/endocrine/adolescent)
Rationale: The nurse practitioner should discuss the findings with an endocrinologist or other physician before discussing the possibility of this diagnosis with the family.

9. Answer: c (assessment/history/reproductive/childbearing female)
Rationale: Thyroid disease, obesity, and premature ovarian failure are considered ovulatory factors, whereas pelvic inflammatory disease is a pelvic factor.

10. Answer: d (plan/management/therapeutics/pharmacologic/reproductive/childbearing female)
Rationale: Prostaglandin synthetase inhibitors (nonsteroidal antiinflammatory drugs) are the drugs of choice for primary dysmenorrhea unless there are contraindications or birth control is desired.

11. Answer: c (assessment/history/psychosocial/child)
Rationale: Making mistakes is an inattentive behavior. Arguing, losing temper, and annoying others are oppositional defiant behaviors.

12. Answer: a (diagnosis/integumentary/NAS)
Rationale: This choice most accurately describes a herald patch. Herald patches rarely appear on the face and usually do not cause intense itching. There are usually not any vesicles.

13. Answer: a (diagnosis/neurologic/adult)
Rationale: Migraine headache, tension-type headache, and trigeminal neuralgia need to be considered as differential diagnoses for the symptoms presented. Usually cluster headaches occur in men. Severe and boring pain begins on one side of the head and quickly progresses to involve the whole side of the head, each attack lasts from 10 minutes to 3 hours, the person may experience 1 to 3 attacks per day, and the eye on the side with pain turns red and tears.

14. *Answer:* a (assessment/physical examination/neurologic/aging adult)

Rationale: Neurofibrillary tangles and amyloid plaques, along with a clinical course characteristic of Alzheimer's disease, confirm a diagnosis of Alzheimer's disease.

15. *Answer:* b (assessment/history/multisystem/NAS)

Rationale: It is unusual for a person with cancer to have a primary presenting symptom of fatigue. Weight changes usually occur. Insomnia may be associated with substance abuse. Duration of the fatigue is not related to a particular disease process. Postpartum fatigue is expected to last for at least 6 weeks.

16. *Answer:* c (evaluation/gastrointestinal/NAS)

Rationale: Wound infection is the most common complication. Liver abscess and fecal fistulas are rare after an appendectomy. Irritable bowel syndrome does not have any association with appendectomy.

17. *Answer:* c (plan/management/diagnostics/respiratory/NAS)

Rationale: The diagnosis is confirmed with a ventilation-perfusion scan, angiography, or both.

18. *Answer:* b (diagnosis/musculoskeletal/adolescent)

Rationale: Scoliosis is most prevalent during the prepubertal growth spurt, occurring in children 10 years old through adolescents.

19. *Answer:* b (evaluation/immunologic/NAS)

Rationale: CD4 lymphocytes have been viewed as the best predictor of the development of AIDS-related complications such as weight loss, fatigue, and such specific diagnoses as *P. carinii* pneumonia. CD4 decreases represent immunologic failure, and HIV RNA represents viral aggression. Therapeutic decisions are guided by results of these laboratory tests. A positive purified protein derivative of tuberculin result correlates with exposure to or inadequate previous treatment of tuberculosis.

20. *Answer:* d (plan/management/therapeutics/hematologic/child)

Rationale: Chemotherapy suppresses the ability of the immune system to mount a response to immunizations. Also, live virus immunizations theoretically could cause the very disease that you hope to prevent in the immunocompromised person.

21. *Answer:* b (assessment/history/allergies/NAS)

Rationale: Viral respiratory illness, physical exertion, and smoke irritants have all been shown to act as triggers for people with asthma. Although headache may be manifested in some other disease process, it is not currently identified as a trigger.

22. *Answer:* d (assessment/history/emergencies/NAS)

Rationale: Age, health status, and the type of agent may determine complications from the burn, but not usually severity.

23. *Answer:* b (issues/application to practice/cultural sensitivity/counseling concepts/nurse-client relationship)

Rationale: Cultures perceive time differently and may place emphasis on the past, present, or future. An appointment may be perceived as a general range of time rather than as a specific clock hour. The client may need care and may not keep a rescheduled appointment. Adjusting the schedule or ignoring the situation will not help the nurse practitioner to understand the client's perspective.

24. *Answer:* c (health promotion/lifestyle/health behaviors/wellness/NAS)

Rationale: Smoking produces low-birth-weight infants, miscarriage, and premature labor. It has no correlation with anemia or weight gain of the mother.

25. *Answer:* c (wellness/risk factor identification/wellness/aging adult)

Rationale: Matthew is not having any problems, and his age is a general guideline for discontinuing screening for prostate cancer. Even if cancer is discovered, observation may be the only appropriate therapy.

26. *Answer:* c (diagnosis/wellness/childbearing female)

Rationale: All sexually active females should be considered as being pregnant until proven otherwise.

27. Answer: c (assessment/physical examination/wellness/child)

Rationale: The American Academy of Pediatrics does not recommend universal urinalysis screening of symptom-free children because research findings reflect the lack of specificity of current urine tests in detecting significant renal or urinary tract disease in these children.

28. Answer: b (wellness/risk factor identification/wellness/aging adult)

Rationale: Melena is the most frequent presenting symptom of peptic ulcer disease in older adults.

29. Answer: a (assessment/history/cardiovascular/NAS)

Rationale: The other three answers are most predictive of coronary artery disease.

30. Answer: a (plan/management/anticipatory guidance/wellness/NAS)

Rationale: Treatment with oral tetracycline, tretinoin, isotretinoin, and doxycycline can result in photosensitivity. Tetracycline must be taken on an empty stomach; dairy products may decrease absorption.

31. Answer: a (plan/cardiovascular/NAS)

Rationale: The actual dose necessary to inhibit platelets is 81 mg of aspirin.

32. Answer: b (diagnosis/respiratory/aging adult)

Rationale: Pulmonary embolism may be seen with dyspnea and hemoptysis, and it is typically associated with such risk factors as immobility and surgery.

33. Answer: b (evaluation/client education/communicable disease/NAS)

Rationale: All vigorous lifting, overexertion, and contact sports should be avoided in the first 1 to 2 months after the diagnosis of mononucleosis.

34. Answer: b (assessment, physical examination, genitourinary/NAS)

Rationale: Costovertebral angle tenderness is a common finding with pyelonephritis. Suprapubic tenderness is more commonly seen with cystitis, whereas urethral discharge is seen with a sexually transmitted disease. Mild abdominal pain is extremely nonspecific; it may be seen with any number of problems.

35. Answer: a (diagnosis/endocrine/child)

Rationale: Diabetes usually causes weight loss in children.

36. Answer: a (diagnosis/reproductive/childbearing female)

Rationale: Follicular ovarian cysts occur during the early menstrual cycle and cause pelvic pressure, aching, and heaviness.

37. Answer: a (assessment/history/communicable disease/NAS)

Rationale: Severe lower back pain is nonspecific for many conditions, including pyelonephritis and back strain. A thick, white discharge with itching is indicative of candidiasis, whereas the discharge associated with gonorrhea is purulent. Postcoital bleeding occurs with cervicitis, which often is present before any noticeable signs and symptoms of gonorrhea.

38. Answer: d (assessment/physical examination/diagnosis/HEENT/adult)

Rationale: Early glaucoma may be detected by an altered cup-to-disk ratio or bilateral asymmetry in the physiologic cup. Visual field testing is difficult to perform accurately. Schiotz tonometry readings may be falsely low in early disease.

39. Answer: c (assessment/physical examination/genitourinary/child)

Rationale: Physical findings with encopresis frequently include abdominal distention with a soft, nontender mass in the midline or the lower left quadrant. The rectal vault is usually filled with either liquid or hard stool.

40. Answer: c (evaluation/psychosocial/NAS)

Rationale: All the listed side effects result from the anticholinergic action of the drug. Only urinary retention requires immediate attention.

41. Answer: d (assessment/history/integumentary/NAS)

Rationale: A variety of medications may cause acnelike lesions. Lithium and any antidepressant compounds containing lithium, phenytoin, trimethadione, systemic corticosteroids, and isoniazid commonly cause acne.

42. *Answer:* d (assessment/history/neurologic/NAS)

Rationale: Pain in or behind the ear is one of the most common symptoms associated with Bell's palsy.

43. *Answer:* b (assessment/physical examination/multisystem/NAS)

Rationale: Other responses are common symptoms in the initial acute phase. Loss of reflexes may occur as a result of cranial neuropathies associated with chronic late manifestations.

44. *Answer:* a (assessment/history/gastrointestinal/child)

Rationale: Although in some rare instances diarrhea-causing organisms can be passed from animals to humans, the other three choices are clearly better. Number, character, and quantity of stools must be assessed to determine whether diarrhea exists and to gauge its severity. Urinary output must be assessed to determine the degree of dehydration. Associated symptoms such as vomiting can help lead to a diagnosis and assess the likelihood of dehydration.

45. *Answer:* c (plan/management/diagnostics/musculoskeletal/NAS)

Rationale: Examination of joint fluid under a polarized microscope is the only definitive means of documenting the presence of monosodium urate crystals. Results of all the other tests may be normal at the time of an acute attack.

46. *Answer:* b (assessment/history/physical examination/immunologic/NAS)

Rationale: Constitutional symptoms are diagnostically useful clinical features in the initial evaluation of the client with systemic lupus erythematosus.

47. *Answer:* d (plan/management/therapeutics/hematologic/child)

Rationale: The immune system remains incompetent to mount a response to immunizations for at least 6 months to 1 year after treatment ends. All other responses are appropriate.

48. *Answer:* d (assessment/history/endocrine/NAS)

Rationale: Sexual history would not provide information useful in establishing the diagnosis and plan.

49. *Answer:* c (assessment/physical examination/allergies/NAS)

Rationale: All findings—retractions, tachypnea, decreased breath sounds, and increased capillary refill time—are indicators of respiratory distress. Of most concern, however, is the absence of breath sounds, which may be an indicator of impending respiratory failure.

50. *Answer:* b (plan/management/therapeutics/developmental delay/NAS)

Rationale: Family dysfunction often occurs because of the strain placed on family resources by caring for a child with a developmental delay. If the delay is in an area other than fine motor or social skills, promoting these two things will not be helpful.

51. *Answer:* b (issues/application to practice/counseling, interviewing)

Rationale: This reply facilitates clarification and understanding by both the nurse and the client of what was communicated.

52. *Answer:* c (issues/case management)

Rationale: Case management is a care delivery system that focuses on the improvement of client goals within a specified time frame, integrating the efforts of all team members.

53. *Answer:* b (health promotion/lifestyle/nutrition/wellness/NAS)

Rationale: Carbohydrates and fiber should be increased. Obesity should be reduced. There are no discussions concerning the number of professionals involved. The goal is to improve nutritional assessment and counseling.

54. *Answer:* b (health promotion/lifestyle/exercise/wellness/NAS)

Rationale: Vigorous activity should be conducted at least 3 days a week. No groups are given special consideration in relation to exercise. No differences are made for males or females.

55. *Answer:* b (evaluation/wellness/aging adult)

Rationale: Although this is an example of polypharmacy, compliance with medication administration is the most important issue. Only with this assessment can one determine whether there is an interactive element.

56. *Answer:* c (assessment/history/genitourinary/NAS)

Rationale: A link between sexually transmitted diseases and prostate cancer exists, but the exact reason for this is not known.

57. *Answer:* b (assessment/history/wellness/risk factor identification/wellness/adult)

Rationale: All the topics in choice *b* are appropriate pieces of information to elicit from a healthy 18-year-old. The other choices include topics that are not appropriate to a healthy 18-year-old. For instance, hot water settings would be of concern in a dwelling in which an extremely young or old person lives, and a healthy 18-year-old would neither be institutionalized nor need family members trained in CPR.

58. *Answer:* c (assessment/physical examination/wellness/child)

Rationale: A tuberculosis test is usually not recommended unless the child has had a history of exposure or lives in an at-risk population.

59. *Answer:* c (health promotion/primary and secondary prevention/wellness/adult)

Rationale: A well adult needs a vision screening examination only every 2 years. A client with diabetes needs to have an eye examination every year.

60. *Answer:* c (plan/management/anticipatory guidance)

Rationale: Prevention of behavioral problems through anticipatory guidance is ideal for the nurse practitioner. Analyzing influences of own upbringing and existing expectations regarding child behavior and management is an important step that is often missed.

The parents have expressed interest and provided a window for teaching. Continuing the process during the next one to two well-child visits will allow parental imput to personalize a system with guidance by the professional. A recommendation simply to read a book offers only cursory attention to an extremely important issue of childhood.

61. *Answer:* b (plan/pathophysiology/HEENT/NAS)

Rationale: The primary reason for treating pharyngitis is to prevent rheumatic fever.

62. *Answer:* b (assessment/history/cardiovascular/NAS)

Rationale: Risk factors that should be assessed in the history include sedentary lifestyle, obesity, smoking, and dietary history. Medication history that contributes to hypertension includes oral contraceptives. For a 16-year-old male, a blood pressure reading of 130/80 mm Hg is within normal range. The obese black African-American male who smokes has the most risk factors for hypertension.

63. *Answer:* b (plan/management/diagnostics/respiratory/NAS)

Rationale: Focal findings such as the crackles in the left lower lobe warrant an x-ray examination for further evaluation.

64. *Answer:* d (assessment/history/respiratory/child)

Rationale: Recurrent upper respiratory infections, changes in growth pattern (weight loss), and fatty stools may be suggestive of cystic fibrosis.

65. *Answer:* d (evaluation/communicable disease/infant)

Rationale: If the mother is adequately treated during pregnancy, the infant may still have a reactive Venereal Disease Research Laboratory test at birth. This test should be repeated at 1, 2, 4, 6, and 12 months, until it becomes nonreactive.

66. *Answer:* d (plan/management/diagnostics/reproductive/NAS)

Rationale: Serum testosterone, follicle-stimulating hormone, and prolactin levels should be considered when endocrine or chromosomal factors are a possibility. Estradiol levels are applicable to additional female factor testing.

67. *Answer:* c (plan/management/therapeutics/pharmacologic/genitourinary/adult)

Rationale: Alpha-adrenergic antagonists often cause symptoms of orthostasis; they therefore should be given at bedtime to minimize the chance of falls related to these side effects.

68. Answer: b (plan/management/consult/endocrine/NAS)

Rationale: A nurse practitioner should consult with a physician for a client with newly diagnosed non-insulin-dependent diabetes mellitus.

69. Answer: a (assessment/history/reproductive/childbearing female)

Rationale: Spotting or irregular bleeding is common during the first 3 months of contraception by hormonal methods.

70. Answer: c (plan/HEENT/NAS)

Rationale: A client with a diagnosis of herpes simplex conjunctivitis should be referred to an ophthalmologist because of the potential for damage to sight. Ophthalmic steroids are contraindicated. Sodium sulfacetamide and bacitracin are used in the treatment of bacterial conjunctivitis.

71. Answer: a (assessment/history/psychosocial/adult)

Rationale: Age is the only item from the history that would *not* place this woman at risk for abuse. Clinical signs and symptoms that might be suggestive of domestic violence include chronic headaches and substance abuse (by client or in family). Low socioeconomic status also places this family at increased risk.

72. Answer: c (assessment/history/psychosocial/NAS)

Rationale: Low self-esteem and affective intolerance are individual factors that may contribute to development of eating disorders. Blurring of generational boundaries is a family factor. Change in women's roles and destabilization of roles have been identified as a sociocultural factor that has contributed to an "atmosphere" in which eating disorders develop.

73. Answer: a (assessment/physical examination/integumentary/adult)

Rationale: Microscopic examination of a scraped specimen of the lesion usually leads to rapid identification of the infective organism.

74. Answer: d (assessment/physical examination/neurologic/aging adult)

Rationale: Depression is not a characteristic of delirium.

75. Answer: c (evaluation/multisystem/NAS)

Rationale: Clients with chronic venous insufficiency often have recurrent problems if measures to counteract the edema and secondary tissue changes are not adhered to conscientiously throughout life.

76. Answer: b (assessment/history/reproductive/NAS)

Rationale: The 30-year-old with regular menstrual periods is assumed to be having ovulatory cycles that are associated with increased prostaglandin release and synthesis. Young girls typically have anovulatory cycles for the first 6 to 12 months. The 48-year-old is most likely premenopausal, and the 35-year-old who is taking oral contraceptives is anovulatory.

77. Answer: d (diagnosis/gastrointestinal/NAS)

Rationale: Confirming the presence of *H. pylori* is important once the diagnosis of ulcer has been made. Elimination of the bacteria is likely to cure the ulcer disease.

78. Answer: d (assessment/physical examination/gastrointestinal/adult)

Rationale: The most relevant objective data to gather for this client are a rectal examination and evaluation of occult blood (guaiac). Deep tendon reflexes generally do not need to be evaluated in someone with gastrointestinal complaints. Current medications and symptoms are examples of subjective data.

79. Answer: b (evaluation/musculoskeletal/infant)

Rationale: Spontaneous reduction of the hips occurs in approximately 90% of affected children in 2 to 6 weeks. The mechanism of this phenomenon is not understood, but the Pavlik harness should be maintained for several months after spontaneous reduction, until the hip has stabilized.

80. *Answer:* d (evaluation/lymphatics/NAS)

Rationale: When performing a physical examination of a client with a chronic illness, one must consider the impact of the chronic illness on all body systems. When performing a routine physical examination, clinical signs associated with the chronic disease should be assessed simultaneously. Spleen enlargement, enlargement of multiple lymph nodes, and weight loss are associated with lymphoma. The client's status with respect to the lymphoma should be evaluated. The primary care provider may be able to detect an early progression of the disease, enabling early intervention.

81. *Answer:* a (diagnosis/hematologic/NAS)

Rationale: Folic acid and iron deficiencies are most common during pregnancy.

82. *Answer:* d (diagnosis/allergies/NAS)

Rationale: Sinusitis may have nighttime cough as a presenting symptom, but most likely it would also have associated sore throat as a result of postnasal drip.

83. *Answer:* d (issues/scope/standards of practice)

Rationale: Standards of care are based on the scope of practice and do describe and guide excellence in nurse practitioners. They are developed by professional organizations, such as the American Nurses Association.

84. *Answer:* b (issues/access to care)

Rationale: Nurse practitioners are reimbursed at 85% of the physician charge for the same service regardless of practice setting.

85. *Answer:* c (issues/ethical consideration/advance directions)

Rationale: Advance directives provide an opportunity for the client to identify his or her wishes regarding resuscitation and life support before an episode where it might be needed.

86. *Answer:* a (health promotion/lifestyle/nutrition/wellness/NAS)

Rationale: Older adults are at the highest risk for malnutrition. Nutritional screening should also be conducted for those who are 20% below desirable weight or have had an involuntary weight loss of more than 10 pounds in a month.

87. *Answer:* c (plan/management/health-promoting behavior/wellness/NAS)

Rationale: Fertility and diarrhea are not associated with exercise. High-density lipoprotein levels are increased with exercise. Glucose tolerance is improved.

88. *Answer:* b (assessment/history/wellness/risk factor identification/wellness/aging adult)

Rationale: Although choice *a* is important, choice *b* is the best answer. Answers *c* and *d* are irrelevant.

89. *Answer:* b (plan/management/diagnostics/periodic identification/wellness/adult)

Rationale: Effective intervention that addresses personal health habits decreases the incidence and severity of the leading causes of death in the United States.

90. *Answer:* b (plan/management/anticipatory guidance/wellness/child)

Rationale: Injury and death from firearms are a serious problem in the United States. The reason that this is such a serious issue is that some children have easy access to firearms in the home.

91. *Answer:* c (wellness/risk factor identification/wellness/adult)

Rationale: Hormone replacement therapy helps prevent bone loss, especially after surgically induced menopause.

92. *Answer:* d (assessment/history/gastrointestinal/NAS)

Rationale: Gallbladder disease is recognized by right upper quadrant pain and tenderness that is more severe with inspiration. Diarrhea is usually not present. WBC count is not usually >15,000 cells/mm³. Bloating may be present.

93. *Answer:* d (health promotion/primary prevention)

Rationale: Hypertension is the leading cause of cardiovascular death among black men.

94. *Answer:* c (assessment/history/HEENT/aging adult)

Rationale: Persons with nuclear cataracts often have improved vision in low light as a result of the larger viewing area of the crystalline lens caused by pupillary dilatation.

95. *Answer:* b (diagnosis/cardiovascular/aging adult)

Rationale: Pericarditis may develop 2 to 3 days after a myocardial infarction. The type of pain described is most consistent with pericarditis. Associated shortness of breath would accompany the discomfort of a pulmonary embolus. Aortic dissection pain is not relieved with position change. Angina usually does not worsen with deep breathing. ECG changes of pericarditis may be masked by the infarction. A pericardial friction rub is not always present.

96. *Answer:* a (physical examination/psychosocial/child)

Rationale: Height and weight below the fifth percentile and hypertension are suggestive of chronic occult renal disease. Although the urinalysis is suggestive of a urinary tract infection, the fact that she has never achieved nighttime dryness points to a more long-term etiology. The other two findings are within normal limits.

97. *Answer:* d (plan/management/therapeutics/respiratory/child)

Rationale: Clients with cystic fibrosis should be treated by a multidisciplinary team consisting of physicians, nurses, nutritionists, physical therapists, and social workers. The family nurse practitioner's role on this team is to support development and monitor routine health maintenance.

98. *Answer:* b (plan/management/therapeutics/pharmacologic/communicable disease/adult)

Rationale: Erythromycin is not indicated for the treatment of gonorrhea in the adult. Azithromycin is the treatment for *Chlamydia,* and acyclovir is the treatment for herpes outbreaks. Cefixime in a single dose is highly effective in treating gonorrhea.

99. *Answer:* a (assessment/physical examination/diagnosis/genitourinary/adult)

Rationale: With acute bacterial prostatitis, an elevated WBC count is usually found; in chronic bacterial prostatitis, a slight elevation may or may not be seen.

100. *Answer:* b (evaluation/endocrine/adult)

Rationale: Knowing the symptoms of both hypothyroidism and hyperthyroidism is important, as are periodic blood tests. Exophthalmus does not always go away and at times may necessitate surgical correction for lid lag.

101. *Answer:* c (evaluation/allergies/NAS)

Rationale: For families with pets, regular washing is thought to decrease the animal dander, which acts as a trigger. Smoke is transmitted through air vents and on clothing, so simply moving the smoker to another room will not get rid of the exposure. Vacuuming is not sufficient to remove dust mites. Box springs and mattresses should be sealed in plastic; stuffed animals are dust collectors and should be washed weekly or sealed in plastic.

102. *Answer:* d (client education/management/reproductive/adult)

Rationale: Breast self-examination should be performed throughout the life-cycle. Cancer can occur during pregnancy and lactation.

103. *Answer:* c (diagnosis/cardiovascular/NAS)

Rationale: Increased sodium intake results in increased water retention and an increase in cardiac workload. Arrhythmias can cause a decrease in ventricular filling (tachycardia) or a decreased cardiac output (severe bradycardia). Uncontrolled hypertension can lead to progressive worsening of left ventricular hypertrophy.

104. *Answer:* b (diagnosis/psychosocial/adult)

Rationale: *Denial* is the refusal to accept an unpleasant situation as reality based. *Projection* is the blaming of others for one's own unacceptable thoughts or feelings. *Rationalization* is making excuses for unacceptable thoughts and behaviors. *Sublimation* is expressing unacceptable wishes in a more socially acceptable manner.

105. *Answer:* b (assessment/physical examination/psychosocial/NAS)

Rationale: Circular burns with a well-demarcated edge are indicative of cigarette burns. Physical findings do not match history of cause. Both raise suspicions of abuse. A linear burn matches the history of grabbing a curling iron. Anxiety with examination and bruises on the lower legs are normal findings on a toddler.

106. *Answer:* b (plan/management/client education/integumentary/NAS)

Rationale: An alternate method of destroying the scabies mite in bed linens and clothing is to store them in tightly sealed plastic bags for 7 to 14 days.

107. *Answer:* a (plan/management/therapeutics/nonpharmacologic/neurologic/aging adult)

Rationale: Placing an object in the mouth of a person whose jaw is tightly closed may incur injury to that party. The other choices are indicated in the acute management of a seizure.

108. *Answer:* c (plan/management/therapeutics/pharmacologic/multisystem/NAS)

Rationale: Diuretics are first-line therapy for symptom control of congestive heart failure.

109. *Answer:* c (plan/management/therapeutics/gastrointestinal/NAS)

Rationale: Increasing fluid and fiber will facilitate bowel activity. Referral to a surgeon is not justified. You do not have adequate history or physical findings to recommend a reduction in lactose (an intraluminal factor). Symptoms do not justify using a histamine blocker.

110. *Answer:* b (evaluation/psychosocial/NAS)

Rationale: Nurse practitioners have the responsibility to follow up closely on all cases of abuse and neglect. The nurse practitioner does not abdicate responsibility once a report has been made to an agency.

111. *Answer:* b (diagnosis/gastrointestinal/NAS)

Rationale: Gastrointestinal reflux disease is characterized by reflux of gastric secretions into the esophagus that is caused by an abnormal reflux barrier, defective esophageal clearance, increased gastric secretions, and delayed gastric emptying. Irritable bowel syndrome is characterized by functional disturbances in motor activity, which may be triggered by pressure irritants.

112. *Answer:* b (assessment/physical examination/musculoskeletal/NAS)

Rationale: Tinel's sign is evoked by tapping on the volar wrist at the carpal tunnel.

113. *Answer:* d (diagnosis/hematologic/NAS)

Rationale: Microcytic hypochromic anemia has decreased mean corpuscular volume, decreased mean corpuscular hemoglobin concentration, and decreased serum iron.

114. *Answer:* c (evaluation/allergies/NAS)

Rationale: An acute generalized reaction increases one's risk of anaphylaxis. Avoiding the allergen is therefore important, but it may not always be possible. Having epinephrine on hand allows action in an emergency. Iodine is the usual cause of allergic reaction to seafood. Other sources of iodine should therefore be avoided.

115. *Answer:* b (issues/ethical considerations/values clarification)

Rationale: It is critical that the nurse practitioner be in touch with his or her own beliefs and values to meet the needs of the client.

116. *Answer:* b (health promotion/primary/secondary prevention/wellness/NAS)

Rationale: *Primary prevention* deals with actions that prevent the occurrence of illness. *Secondary prevention* is early case finding, as in blood sugar testing and Papanicolaou smears. *Tertiary prevention* deals with teaching and prevention after the fact, as in a client with coronary artery disease.

117. *Answer:* d (wellness/risk factor identification/wellness/aging adult)

Rationale: All the other answers are nonjudgmental and are phrased to elicit additional information while creating an environment of trust.

118. *Answer:* c (diagnosis/wellness/childbearing female)

Rationale: Because Linda B. does not have a 28-day menstrual cycle, Nägele's rule needs to be modified to match her 21-day cycle.

119. *Answer:* d (plan/management/anticipatory guidance/wellness/aging adult)

Rationale: Injuries from falls and burns caused by dulling of tactile sensation are considered a leading medical problem for women at least 65 years old.

120. *Answer:* b (assessment/physical examination/wellness/adolescent)

Rationale: *True gynecomastia* consists of glandular tissue. This is distinguishable from adipose tissue when palpated between the thumb and forefinger. The glandular tissue may be either unilateral or bilateral.

121. *Answer:* d (plan/management/therapeutics/pharmacologic/integumentary/NAS)

Rationale: Effective topical therapies available for the treatment of acne decrease the need for systemic antibiotic therapy. Occasionally, however, more severe inflammatory acne does not respond to the topical treatments and a systemic antibiotic may be added to the regimen. Tetracycline is the most common antibiotic agent used for systemic treatment.

122. *Answer:* b (wellness/risk factor identification/aging adult)

Rationale: Most falls occur as part of the normal day's activities.

123. *Answer:* b (health promotion/management/client education/NAS)

Rationale: Before the development and implementation of the teaching plan, it is vital to determine what this client currently knows regarding diabetes and to identify what she needs to know about it.

124. *Answer:* a (diagnosis/HEENT/childbearing female)

Rationale: The symptoms are classic for gingivitis. This is a common complaint in women during the third trimester of pregnancy. It is thought to be an inflammatory response to hormonal changes.

125. *Answer:* a (evaluation/cardiovascular/adult)

Rationale: There is a small risk of thrombus extension into the deep venous system; the course of superficial thrombophlebitis should therefore be monitored.

126. *Answer:* b (plan/management/therapeutics/pharmacologic/respiratory/NAS)

Rationale: Because of their primary action, beta-blockers may increase shortness of breath and are generally considered contraindicated in clients with chronic obstructive pulmonary disease or asthma.

127. *Answer:* d (diagnosis/communicable disease/adult)

Rationale: Chlamydial infection commonly has a friable cervix as its presenting symptom, and the woman frequently does not have any discharge. Syphilis features a chancre, HIV features fatigue as well as other symptoms, and candidiasis usually features a thick, white discharge.

128. *Answer:* a (plan/management/therapeutics/immunologic/NAS)

Rationale: *P. carinii* pneumonia is the hallmark AIDS-defining illness and the most common cause of AIDS-related death. Prophylaxis for the prevention of primary or secondary *P. carinii* pneumonia has proved most effective when begun at a CD4 value $\leq$200 cells/mm^3 for those with a history of *P. carinii* pneumonia. Prophylaxis should be considered for the client with recurrent oral candidiasis or unexplained fever with temperature >100° F for longer than 2 weeks.

129. *Answer:* a (assessment/endocrine/NAS)

Rationale: Mitotane and phenytoin are associated with adrenal insufficiency.

130. *Answer:* d (evaluation/reproductive/childbearing female)

Rationale: Clients should be followed monthly for three visits, then annually if symptoms are being managed effectively.

131. *Answer:* b (plan/management/pharmacologic/cardiovascular/NAS)

Rationale: Loop diuretics (furosemide, bumetanide, and torsemide) cause a more acute diuresis. Loop diuretics should be given IV in the presence of pulmonary edema or severe volume overload.

132. *Answer:* c (plan/management/therapeutics/nonpharmacologic/NAS)

Rationale: A client with alcohol abuse can reduce alcohol consumption, risk behaviors, and adverse outcomes and improve results of laboratory studies with brief counseling and regular follow-up.

133. *Answer:* b (evaluation/integumentary/adult)

Rationale: It is imperative when the trigeminal nerve is involved and a lesion is present on the nose to refer the client immediately to an ophthalmologist. Complications from herpes in the eye can be devastating.

134. *Answer:* c (evaluation/neurologic/NAS)

Rationale: Clients with headaches should be followed up regularly to ensure continuity of care and to provide instruction on participator factors, relaxation and stress-reduction techniques, and effects and side effects of medications; counseling; and support. According to Pruitt (1995), prophylactic medications for headaches should be given a trial of at least 2 months before determining whether they are effective.

135. *Answer:* b (evaluation/neurologic/NAS)

Rationale: Bromocriptine, a dopamine agonist, is poorly tolerated by older adults and should be avoided in demented clients because of its propensity to produce confusion, hallucinations, and psychosis.

136. *Answer:* b (assessment/physical examination/multisystem/NAS)

Rationale: Progressive edema of the lower extremity and thin, shiny, brownish pigmentation are indicative of chronic venous insufficiency.

137. *Answer:* b (evaluation/gastrointestinal/NAS)

Rationale: General examination and general performance are important, but if Elmer is being followed up the most important aspect will be to assess his liver size and the presence of tenderness. Low-grade fever is too nonspecific and may be present for a variety of reasons. There is no reason to conduct a digital rectal examination for occult blood loss.

138. *Answer:* c (diagnosis/musculoskeletal/adult)

Rationale: Older adults are less likely to experience lumbosacral strain than are those younger than 20 years, and back pain is unusual in children.

139. *Answer:* c (assessment/history/hematopoietic/child)

Rationale: The most common source of lead exposure for children is lead in paint.

140. *Answer:* d (plan/management/therapeutics/allergies/NAS)

Rationale: Prednisone should be used only in consultation with a physician for a client with severe eczema.

141. *Answer:* a (plan/management/therapeutics/pharmacologic/multisystem/NAS)

Rationale: Doxycycline or amoxicillin is the drug of choice for secondary arthritis associated with Lyme disease. Ceftriaxone is recommended for cardiac or neurologic manifestations.

142. *Answer:* b (issues/scope, standards of practice)

Rationale: The purpose of licensure is to protect the public from incompetence. Although in most states the Board of Nursing controls nurse practitioner practice, in some states it is a combined Board of Medicine and Nursing. The scope of practice describes the how and where of nurse practitioner practice.

143. *Answer:* c (health promotion/lifestyle/health behaviors/wellness/NAS)

Rationale: Pack-years and previous attempts at quitting should be assessed to help develop a plan that has a likelihood of working. Nicotine levels of cigarettes vary, and this information often is not known by the client or readily available to the nurse practitioner. It is assessed indirectly through pack-years.

144. *Answer:* a (plan/management/participatory guidance/wellness/aging adult)

Rationale: Papanicolaou smears may be done every 1 to 2 years after 60 years.

145. *Answer:* c (plan/management/therapeutics/musculoskeletal/child)

Rationale: Triple diapering is not recommended because the adductor muscles of the thigh overpower saturated diapers. Abduction therefore is not maintained.

146. *Answer:* c (plan/management/anticipatory guidance/wellness/adolescent)

Rationale: To prevent risk of reinjury to the joint, these guidelines should be used for return to play with any joint injury.

147. *Answer:* d (management/therapeutics/pharmacology/wellness/aging adult)

Rationale: Drug distribution is one important factor that is affected by the relative increase in body fat and decrease in lean body mass of an older adult. This change causes increased distribution and increased elimination of fat-soluble drugs.

148. *Answer:* b (health promotion/client education/wellness/management/age)

Rationale: The *perimenopausal* or *climateric* period is a 7- to 10-year period of physiologic change before menopause. The average age at menopause is 50 years. Menopause is extremely individual. Regular menstrual cycles at 45 years are not necessarily rare.

149. *Answer:* a (evaluation/HEENT/NAS)

Rationale: Cough development is common with sinusitis. Lack of improvement may indicate complications of acute sinusitis or an antibiotic-resistant strain of bacteria.

150. *Answer:* b (assessment/physical examination/endocrine/NAS)

Rationale: Clients with hypothyroidism may have a flat affect and dull facies. Silky hair, weight loss, and anxious speech are more characteristic of hyperthyroidism.

151. *Answer:* d (health promotion/assessment/wellness/history/NAS)

Rationale: Age is not a definitive factor. Males are more susceptible than females. A sedentary job places one at risk. History of sudden death or myocardial infarction in a parent or sibling younger than 55 years is a risk factor.

152. *Answer:* c (assessment/diagnosis/reproductive adult)

Rationale: Diabetes predisposes a woman toward chronic *Candida* infections, as do menopause and a positive HIV status. Urinary tract infections and pelvic inflammatory disease are acute illnesses that will not play a significant part in chronic candidiasis. Although a chronic disease, lupus is not known to trigger chronic candidiasis.

153. *Answer:* b (assessment/physical examination/respiratory/child)

Rationale: Steeple sign on a lateral neck x-ray film is diagnostic for laryngotracheobronchitis (croup). All other findings are consistent with cystic fibrosis.

154. *Answer:* d (assessment/history/integumentary/child)

Rationale: Descriptions of the lesion and of its relationship to other things are key diagnostic data. Noting the last well physical examination could help date the appearance of the lesion.

155. *Answer:* b (assessment/history/neurologic/NAS)

Rationale: Bilateral, mild to moderate pressing headache lasting 30 minutes to 7 days is more indicative of a tension-type headache, whereas pounding or dull frontal or occipital pain present when upright and relieved by lying down is associated with post–spinal puncture headache. Higher prevalence in men, occurrence in attacks of severe unilateral orbital, supraorbital, or temporal pain lasting 15 to 180 minutes, and miosis are associated with cluster headache.

156. *Answer:* a (assessment/physical examination/multisystem/NAS)

Rationale: Erythema migrans lesions ≥5 cm are most specific for Lyme disease.

157. *Answer:* d (health history/wellness)

Rationale: Information gained from the health history is used to provide anticipatory guidance, but the provision of this guidance is not considered a part of the health history.

158. *Answer:* d (assessment/physical examination/musculoskeletal/NAS)

Rationale: Although *a, b,* and *c* may be considered in rheumatoid arthritis, there is no test specifically for osteoarthritis. The history and physical examination should lead the provider to diagnose osteoarthritis.

159. *Answer:* d (diagnosis/communicable/NAS)

Rationale: Hepatitis is transmitted by oral-fecal or blood-borne routes.

160. *Answer:* a (issues/research utilization)

Rationale: The first step in research utilization is to make sure that the rigor of the study is sufficient to indicate that the results may be useful. After determining that the study was done correctly, the practitioner can examine the results in light of the new practice setting and client population. A pilot study should be done before offering the program to all clients. Informed consent is always necessary if a program is being offered as part of a research study. Costing out the program is a later step.

161. *Answer:* a (health promotion/lifestyle/stress management/wellness/NAS)

Rationale: Stress-reduction goals focus on adults in *Healthy People 2000*. The aim is to take steps, including visiting a primary care provider, to control stress. Referrals are not addressed. Worksite programs are emphasized.

162. *Answer:* c (evaluation/psychosocial/child)

Rationale: Implementing a behavior-management system can be trying at the onset. Parents often abandon systems in the early stages because of the difficulty involved. It is critical that the health care provider act as a support to the parents and family throughout the process of adjustment. At 2 days the system has not been tried for long enough to allow accurate assessment of its success. A parent who calls, however, deserves a more immediate response for the perceived difficulty.

163. *Answer:* c (health promotion/nonpharmacologic therapy/wellness/management/therapeutics/health-promoting behaviors)

Rationale: Regular intercourse does slow the narrowing and shortening of the vagina. Estrogen supplementation also helps, but progesterone is not useful. Yogurt and sitz baths are not helpful.

164. *Answer:* a (health promotion/plan/wellness/management/diagnostics/NAS)

Rationale: Once target goals have been achieved, choice *a* is correct. It is not necessary to perform a more costly test (full lipid profile) earlier.

165. *Answer:* d (counseling concepts/nurse-client relationships)

Rationale: A goal is to restore the client to a level of functioning that existed before the crisis by resolving the immediate crisis.

166. *Answer:* d (plan/management/diagnostics/endocrine/NAS)

Rationale: The lack of cortisol causes a decrease in gluconeogenesis and liver glycogen and an increased insulin sensitivity, with resulting hypoglycemia. The decrease in aldosterone leads to hyponatremia and hyperkalemia.

167. *Answer:* d (plan/management/consult/developmental delay/child)

Rationale: Height and weight should be recorded for every client, not just those with developmental disabilities. The absence of this assessment, however, will not interfere with the referral. Baseline language, fine motor, gross motor, and social skills must be assessed.

168. *Answer:* b (evaluation/integumentary/NAS)

Rationale: Pruritus may continue for several days to weeks after the infestation has been treated. This is a temporary reaction to the remains of the mites under the skin.

169. *Answer:* a (assessment/physical examination/NAS)

Rationale: Blood pressure readings should be checked in both arms at least once to verify equivalency. At least two blood pressure readings 2 minutes apart in supine or seated position and after standing for 2 minutes should be used to document hypertension. Coffee, cigarettes, cuff size, and positioning all affect accuracy.

170. *Answer:* a (plan/management/client education/musculoskeletal/NAS)

Rationale: Because Mr. Donaldson has been active, he can continue light jogging, walking, or swimming, but he should not continue the vigor of his usual running until pain subsides. Lifting weights would not affect his aerobic capacity; depending on the weight, it might exceed recommended amounts (20 to 60 pounds, depending on pain level).

171. *Answer:* a (diagnosis/communicable/child)

Rationale: *Rubella* is usually a mild disease that lasts approximately 3 days. *Rubeola* usually is seen with a severe cough and a high fever. *Roseola* is a viral exanthem of infants. *Fifth's disease* begins with a bright-red rash on the cheeks.

172. *Answer:* a (evaluation/gastrointestinal/NAS)

Rationale: Daily doses of stool softeners should be reduced once soft stools are established. Therapy may need to continue for 2 to 3 months until regular habits are well established. Follow-up should be scheduled every month until the rectal vault is back to a normal size.

173. *Answer:* c (health promotion/lifestyle/stress management)

Rationale: Premature death and alcoholism are not directly related to stress. Decreased immunologic function has been correlated with stress levels. Social isolation is not a consequence of stress.

174. *Answer:* b (assessment/follow-up/evaluation/gastrointestinal/NAS)

Rationale: Adults with chronic constipation should be followed up every 2 weeks until "normal bowel functions resume." Failure to respond to therapy may indicate a serious underlying pathology.

175. *Answer:* b (health promotion/nonpharmacologic/wellness/management/health-promoting behaviors)

Rationale: Drinking 8 to 10 glasses of water/day does help with vasomotor instability. Regular exercise is also helpful. Caffeine and alcohol intakes should be limited. Hot tubs do not have to be avoided, because vasomotor instability is not predictable.

Sample Examination 2

1. Mrs. J.B. brings her son to the clinic, stating that she is afraid her son has epiglottitis. Which of the following subjective data provided by Mrs. J.B. would confirm her suspicion?

    a. 6-month-old, fever with temperature of 101° F (38° C) for 2 days, barking cough

    b. 10-year-old, fever with temperature to 101° F (38° C), difficulty swallowing

    c. 3-year-old, sudden onset of fever with temperature to 101° F (38° C), difficulty swallowing

    d. 2-year-old, fever with temperature to 100° F (37° C), cough, nasal drainage

2. Which individual is most likely to develop thrombophlebitis?

    a. A 25-year-old obese white male

    b. A 58-year-old black female receiving hormone replacement therapy

    c. A 36-year-old white female aerobics instructor

    d. A 42-year-old Asian male truck driver

3. All the following signs and symptoms are associated with emphysema **except:**

    a. Purse-lipped breathing

    b. Barrel-shaped chest

    c. Continuous cough with copious sputum

    d. Thin, anxious appearance

4. Which of the following medications is the drug of choice for pediculosis capitis?

    a. Permethrin 1% shampoo

    b. Nystatin-triamcinolone (Mycolog) cream 1%

    c. Hydrocortisone cream 1%

    d. Dibucaine cream 1%

5. Which of the following statements regarding the use of antibiotics in clients with asymptomatic bacteriuria is true?

    a. Antibiotic treatment should be instigated in uncomplicated cases of asymptomatic bacteriuria.

    b. Only clients with cases considered complicated should be treated for asymptomatic bacteriuria.

    c. Only clients with symptomatic bacteriuria should be treated.

    d. A low-dose maintenance antibiotic should be used.

6. Ms. Smith is a 40-year-old woman who comes to your clinic reporting a 30-pound weight loss, lack of energy, and nausea. Which of the following would **not** be included in your differential diagnosis list?

    a. Anorexia nervosa

    b. Addison's disease

    c. Depression

    d. Hyperthyroidism

NOTE: The actual test score is calculated on a total of 150 items. There are 25 pretest items included on each examination. Thus the total number of examination items is 175. Pretest items do not count toward the total score.

7. Which of the following physical findings would **not** be found in a client with viral conjunctivitis?

   a. Concurrent upper respiratory tract infection symptoms

   b. Watery, mucoid drainage

   c. Palpable preauricular lymph nodes

   d. Profuse, mucopurulent drainage

8. Methods to determine ovulation include all the following **except:**

   a. Postcoital test

   b. Basal body temperature

   c. Serum progesterone level

   d. Endometrial biopsy

9. Maggie is a 12-month-old infant who is unable to sit without assistance. The nurse practitioner should do which of the following?

   a. Suspect abuse.

   b. Encourage the family to stimulate Maggie more.

   c. Refer Maggie for developmental delay.

   d. Recheck Maggie in 1 month to assess progress.

10. Common behavior problems reported by mothers during preschool years include all the following **except:**

   a. Hiding when a rule is not followed

   b. Refusing to pick up toys: "I won't do it!"

   c. Jumping on and over furniture

   d. Jumping out of a moving vehicle

11. Which of the following statements is true regarding primary enuresis?

   a. It is more common in boys than in girls.

   b. It occurs in 25% of all 7-year-olds.

   c. It often occurs only occasionally, one or two times a month.

   d. It frequently occurs after a child has been dry at night for longer than 1 year.

12. Which of the following is the most appropriate treatment for a person with a diagnosis of pityriasis rosea?

   a. Oral steroids for 3 weeks

   b. Symptomatic treatment

   c. Skin biopsy and chemotherapy

   d. Ultraviolet A phototherapy

13. Urination, in a seated position, may help men with:

   a. Acute bacterial prostatitis

   b. Chronic bacterial prostatitis

   c. Prostate cancer

   d. Benign prostatic hyperplasia

14. Which of the following statements with respect to the use of prophylactic medication for the treatment of migraine headaches is correct?

   a. Lithium carbonate, 300 mg tid, is the preferred prophylactic medication for the prevention of migraine headaches.

   b. Cyclobenzaprine (Flexeril), 10 to 40 mg qd, is the preferred medication for prevention of migraine headaches.

   c. Beta-blockers are usually the first-line medications used for prevention of migraine headaches.

   d. Daily, 7 L oxygen should be given by face mask for the prevention of migraine headaches.

15. Which aspect of the history would lead you to consider Lyme disease as the probable diagnosis?

   a. Persistent, relapsing fatigue, reducing the ability to perform activities of daily living by as much as 50%

   b. Swollen lymph glands, persistent sore throat, malaise

   c. Muscle and joint pain, particularly in the hips, knees, and ankles

   d. Afternoon fatigue, swelling and pain in joints, particularly those of the hands

16. Which of the following statements regarding gastric ulcers is **not** true?

   a. Gastric ulcers are generally found in the antral area of the stomach.

   b. Gastric ulcers tend to be chronic, in contrast to the intermittent nature of duodenal ulcers.

   c. Benign gastric ulcers are round or oval and have a punched-out appearance and a smooth base.

   d. The pain associated with gastric ulcers is usually located substernally and is always relieved by eating.

17. Which of the following factors is **not** associated with gout?

    a. Coronary artery disease
    b. Increasing age
    c. Hypertension
    d. Obesity

18. The diagnosis of HIV infection requires:

    a. Clinical symptoms of immune suppression in a high-risk population
    b. Clinical symptoms plus confirmatory enzyme-linked immunosorbent assay result
    c. Positive enzyme-linked immunosorbent assay result and confirmatory Western blot result
    d. CD4 count ≤200 cells/mm^3, with symptoms of immunosuppression

19. In chronic lymphocytic leukemia, the onset of symptoms is insidious and the disease can be difficult to diagnose. In which of the following histories would you most likely consider a diagnosis of chronic lymphocytic leukemia?

    a. Male, 40 years old, with a 2-week history of headaches, vomiting, weight loss
    b. Male, 70 years old, with a 2- to 3-month history of malaise and fatigability, who now notices "lumps" in his neck and groin
    c. Female, 70 years old, with hip pain, weight loss, and anorexia
    d. Male, 25 years old, with a 1-month history of fevers, night sweats, and lymphadenopathy

20. The goal of the step-wise approach to asthma therapy is for the client to gain and maintain control of the disease. Which action would **not** be in keeping with this strategy?

    a. Start at the lowest step of therapy possible to avoid medication side effects.
    b. Once the condition is stable, step down a level of therapy if possible.
    c. Recommend referral to a specialist if the client requires multiple long-term control medications.
    d. Begin environmental control measures at onset of diagnosis.

21. Kristin is a 5-year-old girl with red cheeks. She also has a lacy rash on her trunk and extremities. The most likely diagnosis of this girl's condition is:

    a. Rubella
    b. Rubeola
    c. Fifth disease
    d. Roseola

22. When treating a client in pain, the culturally sensitive nurse practitioner would first do which of the following?

    a. Prescribe pain medication.
    b. Instruct the client in the use of cold and heat application.
    c. Ask the client to explain his or her interpretation of the pain and its meaning.
    d. Acknowledge that the pain interferes with daily functioning.

23. When performing a well-child examination for an 11-year-old client, the nurse practitioner should do which of the following?

    a. Discuss the harmful effects of smoking.
    b. Assess for the presence of nightmares.
    c. Discuss the ramifications of drinking and driving.
    d. Ask the parents about the frequency of temper tantrums.

24. When developing an exercise plan for a client, the nurse practitioner should keep in mind which of the following?

    a. Moderate exercise has a higher compliance rate.
    b. The more frequently exercise is performed, the greater its effects.
    c. Females should exercise more frequently than males.
    d. Benefits are directly related to intensity of effort.

25. Whenever possible, the treatment of acne should begin with which of the following methods?

    a. Systemic agents
    b. Dietary changes
    c. Reassurance that it will resolve with age
    d. Topical agents

26. At the preconception visit, an obstetric outcome history includes all the following **except:**

a. Gestational age at birth, type of delivery, labor length

b. Medical-surgical history and current environmental exposures

c. Pregnancy complications, birth weight, and gender

d. Length of past pregnancies and premature labor

27. What immunizations would you expect to give on a 1-year well-child visit (assuming that the child is currently up to date on immunizations)?

a. Number 4 DPaT, number 3 oral polio vaccine, number 4 *Haemophilus influenzae* B vaccine, and number 1 measles-mumps-rubella vaccine

b. Number 3 diphtheria-pertussis-tetanus vaccine, number 3 *H. influenzae* B vaccine, and number 1 measles-mumps-rubella vaccine

c. Number 1 measles-mumps-rubella vaccine and varicella vaccine

d. Number 4 DPaT, number 4 *H. influenzae* B vaccine, and number 1 measles-mumps-rubella vaccine

28. Which of the following types of gynecologic cancer is the second most prevalent in women?

a. Ovarian

b. Cervical

c. Vulvar

d. Vaginal

29. A minor who wants access to birth control:

a. Must first get parental consent

b. Can obtain birth control only after completing a sex education class

c. Can only obtain birth control if 17 years old

d. May obtain birth control on request

30. Mrs. D.C. is a 62-year-old denture wearer. Oral candidiasis has developed as a result of IV antibiotic therapy. The most effective treatment plan for this client would include:

a. Fluconazole, 100 mg PO, qd for 7 to 14 days

b. Nystatin troche, dissolved in the mouth every 5 to 6 hours for 7 to 10 days

c. Nystatin powder, applied to dentures every 6 to 8 hours for several weeks

d. Nystatin troche, dissolved in the mouth every 5 to 6 hours for 7 to 10 days, and Nystatin powder, applied to dentures every 6 to 8 hours for several weeks

31. Which of the following choices lists the most specific diagnostic physical findings of a client with congestive heart failure?

a. Right basilar rales and peripheral edema

b. Elevated jugular venous pressure and S_4

c. Elevated jugular venous pressure, S_3, and laterally displaced point of maximal impulse

d. Elevated jugular venous pressure and hepatomegaly

32. A 9-month-old male is brought in for evaluation. His mother states that he seems to be having gradually more difficulty breathing. What additional history is most important to obtain?

a. Play patterns

b. Sibling acceptance of infant

c. Associated symptoms

d. Exposure to bronchial irritants

33. Which of the following laboratory tests would be most appropriate to make a diagnosis of mononucleosis?

a. Monospot

b. Liver function tests

c. Complete blood cell count

d. Immunoglobin M antibodies

34. A middle-aged man with gradual onset of nocturia, urinary frequency, and dull suprapubic pain without fever will most likely have which of the following diagnosed?

a. Acute bacterial prostatitis

b. Chronic bacterial prostatitis

c. Benign prostatic hyperplasia

c. Prostate cancer

35. Which of the following is **not** a symptom suggestive of congestive heart failure?

a. Dyspnea on exertion, orthopnea with paroxysmal nocturnal dyspnea

b. Unilateral peripheral edema

c. Mental status changes

d. Fatigue

36. Which of the following is the best screening test for Cushing's syndrome?

   a. Dexamethasone suppression test

   b. Urinary free cortisol level

   c. Plasma cortisol level

   d. A 24-hour urine sample for 17-hydroxycorticosteroid

37. Mrs. Ewing, who is postmenopausal, comes in for an annual examination. She reports dyspepsia, anorexia, and bloating. Pelvic examination reveals a firm, fixed left adnexal mass >8 cm and irregular nodules in the cul de sac. What initial plan is most appropriate?

   a. Draw blood for immediate serum calcium 125 determination.

   b. Schedule a barium enema.

   c. Advise bland, low-fat diet; follow up in 2 weeks.

   d. Refer client to surgeon.

38. The most common physical finding in the pelvic examination with primary dysmenorrhea is:

   a. Enlarged uterus

   b. Adnexal mass

   c. Purulent cervical discharge

   d. Normal examination result (no abnormal findings)

39. An older client comes to your office for blood pressure check and renewal of medications. The assistant who took his blood pressure lets you know of a linear bruise on his upper arm. Additional physical findings that would be atypical and suggestive of abuse would be:

   a. Finger-sized bruises at elbows

   b. A small, irregular burn on the top of the right hand

   c. Similar bruising (size and position) on opposite arm

   d. Swollen and tender distal joints on both hands

40. What should always be included in the examination of a client with substance abuse?

   a. Mental status

   b. Renal profile

   c. Funduscopy

   d. CT scan

41. Which of the following statements indicates that James' mother understands the teaching you provided regarding tinea infestation?

   a. James may return to school after his 2-week follow-up appointment.

   b. The oral medication prescribed should be taken on an empty stomach to enhance absorption.

   c. All family members should be examined for the tinea infection and treated if needed.

   d. Tinea is not a contagious disease.

42. If facial paralysis in Bell's palsy persists for 6 months, which of the following diagnostic tests is indicted?

   a. CT or MRI of the head

   b. Carotid Doppler study

   c. Electromyogram

   d. Lumbar puncture

43. In the physical examination of a client with fatigue, the nurse practitioner should focus on which of the following areas?

   a. Musculoskeletal

   b. Peripheral vascular system

   c. Lymphatic system

   d. Head

44. Chest pain described as burning in nature is most likely:

   a. Gastrointestinal reflux disease

   b. Myocardial infarction

   c. Endocarditis

   d. Chest wall pain

45. Developmental dysplasia of the hip can be detected earliest at:

   a. Birth

   b. The first office visit

   c. 4 months

   d. 18 months

46. Suspected acute myocardial infarction is best initially evaluated with:

   a. Echocardiography

   b. Stress test

   c. Cardiac isoenzymes

   d. Holter monitoring

47. Acute retroviral conversion is noted clinically with which of the following symptoms?

    a. Fatigue, weight loss, and pulmonary symptoms

    b. Rash, fever, and diarrhea

    c. Fever, arthralgia, myalgia, and fatigue

    d. Fungal infections, herpes simplex, and pneumonia

48. The most important first test to do when suspecting any type of leukemia is:

    a. Bone marrow aspiration or biopsy

    b. Chest x-ray examination

    c. Spun hematocrit

    d. Complete blood cell count with differential

49. A client with exercise-induced asthma would likely have which history?

    a. "I need to use my inhaler every day—especially if I exercise."

    b. "I get short of breath every time I run a longer distance than normal."

    c. "Resting for 5 to 10 minutes after exercise usually takes care of the shortness of breath."

    d. "If I use my inhaler 15 to 30 minutes before I exercise, I no longer have a problem with shortness of breath."

50. A child has an acute onset of sore throat, fever, flushed face, and a diffuse, sandpapery feeling rash. The most likely diagnosis of this child's condition is:

    a. Rubella

    b. Rubeola

    c. Fifth disease

    d. Scarlet fever

51. Your client says, "I don't think I'll ever get well." A therapeutic response would be:

    a. "Don't even think that! Of course you will get better."

    b. "Just believe in God, and you will get well."

    c. "We all feel down sometimes. Don't worry, you will be fine."

    d. "You don't feel that you're getting better."

52. Nutritional screening includes all the following **except:**

    a. Anthropometric measurements

    b. Measurement of hemoglobin and hematocrit

    c. Questioning about preparation of meals

    d. Social history

53. The initial diagnostic tests for an infertility workup are:

    a. Semen analysis, documentation of ovulation, postcoital test, and evaluation of tubal patency

    b. Semen analysis, follicle-stimulating hormone, luteinizing hormone, thyroid-stimulating hormone, and sperm antibodies

    c. Hysterosalpingogram, urologic consultation, endometrial biopsy, and serum progesterone

    d. Basal body temperature, serum progesterone, endometrial biopsy, and luteinizing hormone

54. The greatest risk factor associated with exercise is:

    a. Sudden cardiac death

    b. Hypoglycemia

    c. Osteoarthritis

    d. Injury

55. Treatment for heartburn would include all the following **except:**

    a. Antacids with baking soda or aluminum

    b. Avoidance of fried and gas-producing foods

    c. Small, frequent meals

    d. Sleeping with stacked pillows

56. After finishing examination of a 3-year-old, all the following anticipatory guidance issues would be discussed **except:**

    a. Toilet hygiene

    b. Stuttering (avoid drawing attention to stuttering)

    c. Discipline (using consistent methods)

    d. Rocking trained night criers back to sleep

57. Which of the following is **not** considered a barrier to medication compliance in older adults?

    a. Polypharmacy

    b. Cost of medication

    c. Drug side effects

    d. Episodic treatment

58. Which of the following describes primary prevention for child abuse?

    a. Inspecting all children for bruises

    b. Asking all parents about child abuse

    c. Calling the abuse hotline when abuse is suspected

    d. Offering parenting classes

59. After assessing Jill G., 8 years old, you decide that she should be treated for probable group A streptococcal pharyngitis. She is allergic to penicillin. Your next drug of choice would be:

    a. Amoxicillin-clavulanate (Augmentin)
    b. Erythromycin
    c. Trimethoprim-sulfamethoxazole (Bactrim)
    d. Ciprofloracin (Cipro)

60. Aphasia lasting 20 hours is considered a:

    a. Stroke
    b. Reversible ischemic neurologic deficit
    c. Transient ischemic attack
    d. Psychotic event

61. Laboratory tests that should be performed every 6 months to determine disease progression and treatment response for AIDS include all the following **except:**

    a. Complete blood cell count
    b. CD4 count
    c. HIV RNA
    d. Chest x-ray film

62. An immigrant farm worker brings her 3-year-old son for evaluation of cough, fever, fatigue. He has never been immunized. What diagnosis must you consider?

    a. Pertussis
    b. Asthma
    c. Pneumonia
    d. Environmental allergies

63. How is adequate treatment of syphilis evaluated?

    a. Disappearance of symptoms
    b. Fourfold decrease in the titer by 3 months
    c. Only a nonreactive Venereal Disease Research Laboratory test indicates adequate treatment.
    d. Fourfold increase in the Venereal Disease Research Laboratory test titer

64. A diffusely enlarged prostate is more likely to be associated with:

    a. Acute bacterial prostatitis
    b. Benign prostatic hyperplasia
    c. Prostate cancer
    d. Chronic bacterial prostatitis

65. A 12-year-old male is brought to the clinic by his mother for evaluation. He has been experiencing weight loss, fatigue, polyuria, polydipsia, and polyphagia. Which of the following would **not** be included in the differential diagnosis?

    a. Diabetes mellitus
    b. Anorexia
    c. Viral illness
    d. Cushing's syndrome

66. Which of the following statements regarding the use of hormonal therapy for dysfunctional uterine bleeding is true?

    a. Hormonal treatment should always begin with IV therapy to be effective.
    b. Hormonal therapy is always discontinued after 3 months.
    c. Dilatation and curettage should always precede hormonal therapy.
    d. Hormonal therapy may be continued if the client desires birth control.

67. A 45-year-old black male has a red, painful eye. The nurse practitioner suspects narrow-angle glaucoma. Which of the following would be helpful to confirm the diagnosis?

    a. Dilating the pupils to visualize the optic disk
    b. Referral to an ophthamologist
    c. Fluorescein stain of eye
    d. Inquiry about associated nausea or vomiting

68. Carrie, 6 years old, is brought to the clinic because she has suddenly started wetting the bed after having been dry for 2 years. In assessing this client, the nurse practitioner should consider all the following diagnoses **except:**

    a. Seizure disorder
    b. Normal variation
    c. Psychosocial upset
    d. Urinary tract infection

69. Which of the following best describes the most effective treatment for a child with attention deficit–hyperactivity disorder?

    a. Medication, school intervention, and punishments
    b. Medication, psychoanalysis, and school intervention
    c. Medication, school intervention, and cognitive or behavioral therapy
    d. School intervention, cognitive or behavioral therapy, and punishments

70. Which of the following conditions is **not** included in a differential diagnosis list when scabies is suspected?

a. Pediculosis
b. Atopic dermatitis
c. Contact dermatitis
d. Tinea corporis

71. Which diagnostic evaluation or test results support a diagnosis of probable Alzheimer's disease?

a. Vitamin B_{12} deficiency
b. Abnormalities on ECG and CT scan
c. Abnormal result of mental status examination, with progressive decline
d. Past medical history for cerebrovascular accident, hypertension, or both

72. A condition commonly included in differential diagnosis for fatigue is:

a. Lower respiratory tract infection
b. Anemia
c. Malnutrition
d. Pregnancy

73. Anticholinergic drugs are useful in the management of such gastrointestinal problems as peptic ulcers. Which of the following is their major action?

a. Increasing gastric motility
b. Reducing production of gastric secretions
c. Neutralizing hydrochloric acid in the stomach
d. Absorbing excess gastric secretions

74. Which of the following choices lists the major symptoms of carpal tunnel syndrome?

a. Pain and contracture of elbow
b. Forearm and shoulder pain
c. Paresthesia, numbness, and tingling fingers waking the client at night
d. Carpal tunnel muscle fatigue

75. The Jones family becomes sick with diarrhea and vomiting after eating undercooked hamburgers. The family nurse practitioner knows that the family is most likely infected with which pathogen?

a. *Salmonella*
b. Norwalk virus
c. *Escherichia coli*
d. Protozoan

76. When discussing the side effects of treatment for lymphoma with a male client, the nurse practitioner should mention:

a. Impotence
b. Infertility
c. Incontinence
d. Bleeding

77. Julie, an 18-year-old with acute lymphocytic leukemia, has a central line venous access device. She is presently in a less-intense phase of her chemotherapy, and her blood counts are stable. She has a dentist appointment scheduled next week, to have her teeth cleaned. In evaluating Julie's knowledge of supportive care guidelines, you are glad to hear Julie's understanding of which of the following?

a. She does not need prophylactic antibiotics just to have her teeth cleaned.
b. She does not need prophylactic antibiotics because she is already receiving trimethoprim-sulfamethoxazole (Bactrim).
c. She does need prophylactic antibiotics to protect against bacteremia and potential bacterial endocarditis.
d. It is good to keep her teeth clean and white.

78. Physical findings consistent with respiratory distress associated with asthma would include:

a. Dullness in lung bases on percussion
b. Rales and crackles bilaterally on auscultation
c. Prolonged expiratory phase during respiration
d. Low-pitched rhonchi, greater with inspiration

79. A client has an electrical burn to the right shoulder. He did not lose consciousness and says, "I am thankful to be alive!" The nurse practitioner should:

a. Refer the client for hospitalization
b. Apply a silver sulfadiazine dressing
c. Debride the area
d. Cleanse the area with a mild detergent

80. Certification as a nurse practitioner means that the nurse practitioner:

a. Is eligible to practice as a nurse practitioner
b. Has completed an accredited nurse practitioner program
c. Is eligible for a Drug Enforcement Agency number
d. Has passed a test verifying knowledge of a specific area

81. When counseling a sixth grader concerning diet, the nurse practitioner should stress:

   a. The need to recognize a serving size
   b. Limiting fat to 40% of their daily caloric intake
   c. Eating more dairy products
   d. Snacking frequently

82. A client with low back strain asks whether it would be okay for him to see a chiropractor. What does the nurse practitioner tell him?

   a. Chiropractic manipulation is not recommended.
   b. Wait 2 to 4 weeks for the episode to heal.
   c. Choose between aerobic exercises and chiropractic manipulation.
   d. Chiropractic manipulation is considered safe in the first 4 weeks.

83. Sam, 66 years old, remains in the home that he and his wife started 1 year after they married. He does not own any firearms. He and his wife enjoyed traveling and were active as a couple. The only disease identified in his family history is coronary artery disease (mother in her early forties, sister and brother in their late sixties and early seventies). Sam does not offer any complaints. His physical examination should focus on:

   a. Blood pressure, cardiopulmonary examination, digital rectal examination, Mini Mental State Examination, Snellen test, and musculoskeletal examination
   b. Gastrointestinal examination, Mini Mental State Examination, hearing with whispered word, digital rectal examination, and blood pressure
   c. Height/weight ratio, blood pressure, digital rectal examination, fecal occult blood, cardiopulmonary examination, and gastrointestinal examination
   d. Musculoskeletal examination, cardiopulmonary examination, gastrointestinal examination, and height/weight ratio

84. Postpartum laboratory tests should include all the following **except:**

   a. Hemoglobin or hematocrit for all clients
   b. Fasting blood sugar for women with diabetes or a diagnosis of gestational diabetes

   c. Thyroid function tests for women whose thyroid medication dosage changed during the pregnancy
   d. FSH and LH

85. The first sign of pubertal development in a male is:

   a. Voice change
   b. Height spurt
   c. Testicular enlargement
   d. Growth of the penis

86. Which of the following is a strategy that can improve medication compliance in older adults?

   a. Develop a system for taking medications.
   b. Stop medications that have confusing dosing regimens.
   c. Encourage use of OTC medications.
   d. Encourage drug holidays.

87. Counseling and support groups for infertile women are examples of:

   a. Women's supportive services
   b. Primary prevention
   c. Secondary prevention
   d. Primary health care

88. A 77-year-old woman is undergoing follow-up for her hypertension. She tells you that she had cataract surgery 5 weeks ago and that she is scheduled to return to the ophthalmologist next week. As part of her examination, you perform an ophthalmoscopic examination. Which of the following is true of postoperative course of the client with cataracts?

   a. It is not uncommon for the client to report a sense of pressure posterior to the eyes bilaterally.
   b. A slight discharge from the affected eye during the early postoperative period may indicate a need for further evaluation.
   c. Intraocular implants often distort vision and require a period of adjustment for full visual improvement.
   d. Eye shields are not generally needed at night after surgery but should be used in conditions of bright light.

89. Holter monitoring may require three 24-hour periods to be diagnostic. The underlying reason for the syncope is usually:

   a. Arrhythmia
   b. Pulmonary hypertension
   c. Transient ischemic attack
   d. Hypoglycemia

90. A 42-year-old male with a diagnosis of bronchitis has a predominant symptom of cough with wheezes. He is most likely to receive relief with:

   a. Guaifenesin
   b. Albuterol metered-dose inhaler
   c. Acetaminophen
   d. Pseudoephedrine

91. What other information would be important to know when diagnosing mononucleosis?

   a. Type of diet usually followed
   b. Ability to perform normal activities
   c. Smoking history
   d. Occupational exposures

92. Which of the following sets of symptoms is most indicative of cystitis?

   a. Flank pain, fever, nausea, and vomiting
   b. Scrotal pain and burning on urination
   c. Urinary urgency and frequency, and suprapubic pain
   d. Spasmodic flank pain and hematuria

93. To evaluate compliance with and effectiveness of the plan of care for a client with cystic fibrosis, the family nurse practitioner should monitor:

   a. Growth, development, and respiratory patterns
   b. Progress in school and family coping
   c. Caloric intake, bowel patterns, and abdominal girth
   d. The number of times each prescription is filled

94. With which client should the nurse practitioner be cautious in starting levothyroxine for hypothyroidism?

   a. Child, 5 years old
   b. Female adult, 19 years old
   c. Female adult, 35 years old
   d. Male adult, 65 years old

95. Ms. Rodriquez has fibrocystic breast disease. The nurse practitioner advises certain dietary restrictions to ease the breast tenderness, discussing the prohibited foods in detail. Which statement made by Ms. Rodriquez indicates that she needs *additional* instruction?

   a. "I should eliminate as much salt as possible for the 10 days before my period."
   b. "I should substitute water and juice for cola drinks or coffee at mealtime."
   c. "I'll start substituting hot chocolate for my usual hot tea at bedtime."
   d. "I should limit my alcohol intake."

96. When questioning the client about changes in vision, the nurse practitioner should ask questions pertinent to development of glaucoma. Which of the following symptoms is an indicator of early glaucoma?

   a. Vision slow to clear in the morning
   b. Gradual blurring of vision
   c. Narrowing of visual fields
   d. Difficulty with color discrimination

97. After several visits to the clinic, Robert, a depressed 45-year-old client, appears well groomed for the first time. To reinforce Robert's self-esteem, your most appropriate response would be:

   a. "You really look nice today."
   b. "I see you got a haircut and have a new shirt."
   c. "You must be feeling much better. It shows in your great new look."
   d. Avoid commenting on his appearance.

98. Which of the following dermatologic conditions is characterized by accumulation of stratum corneum, sharply demarcated erythematous plaques and papules, and silvery scales?

   a. Mycosis fungoides
   b. Lichen planus
   c. Pityriasis rosea
   d. Psoriasis

99. Five-week-old Baby Murphy had a seizure the other day. What finding would lead you to believe there was a possible congenital disorder involved?

   a. There is a hemangioma on the left maxillary region of the face.
   b. Birth weight was regained by the 14th day.
   c. The baby cries when feeding time is close.
   d. The baby's rectal temperature is 99.6° F.

100. The best exercise for treating fibromyalgia is:

a. Gentle stretching after a hot shower
b. High-impact aerobics three times per week
c. Walking at a moderate pace for 20 minutes three times per week
d. Stationary bicycling for 30 minutes three times per week

101. Look for atypical presentations of appendicitis in:

a. Clients taking oral steroids
b. Children older than 3 years
c. Pregnant women in the first trimester
d. Teenagers

102. You develop a plan of care with Mr. T., a 54-year-old man, and initiate therapy for a duodenal ulcer. His plan of care should include:

a. No follow-up, because his symptoms will go away if he takes the prescribed medications
b. A return visit if he starts vomiting bright-red blood
c. A return visit in 2 weeks
d. A return visit after he completes the 3-month prescription

103. Which of the following best describes the plan for rehabilitation after an injury?

a. Begin rehabilitation early to return to preinjury level of conditioning and prevent contractions and further injury.
b. Immobilize all injuries for at least 6 weeks to protect the joint from further injury.
c. No weight bearing is recommended for all sprains for at least 4 weeks after a sprain of the ankle.
d. Do not perform range of motion of any sprained body part after an injury until after follow-up by an orthopedic surgeon.

104. Which of the following is **not** a test you would do initially when suspecting any type of childhood anemia?

a. Platelet count
b. Complete blood cell count with differential
c. Peripheral blood smear evaluation and reticulocyte count
d. Bone marrow smear

105. When caring for a client with an acute generalized reaction to an unknown substance that is not life-threatening, which of the following should the nurse practitioner include in the plan of care?

a. Prescribing a metaproterenol (Alupent) inhaler
b. Referring the client for allergy testing
c. Prescribing an antihistamine for daily use
d. Getting the client a medical alert bracelet

106. By definition, a developmental disability is a(n):

a. Central nervous system disorder
b. Environmentally induced disorder
c. Temporary functional limitation
d. Absence of socialization skills

107. Laws regulating nursing practice are developed by all the following **except:**

a. Legislators through statutes
b. Administrators through regulations
c. Judges through case decisions
d. Political action coalitions through grassroots lobbying

108. If a client is contemplating stopping smoking, the nurse practitioner should do which of the following?

a. Prescribe pharmacologic therapy.
b. Discuss the adverse effects of smoking, including problems in cleanliness of teeth, clothing, and breath.
c. Wait to discuss options until the client has had unsuccessful attempts at stopping.
d. Refer the client to a support group.

109. In the interview, you sense tension between Matthew and his daughter. Your assessment of Matthew reveals a well male adult who is 80 years old. You ask about his grandchildren. Matthew comments that his daughter felt a need to bring him today. Exploring the issue, Matthew reports that his daughter feels that he should no longer drive his car and has taken the keys away. Your next best action will be which of the following?

    a. Tell Matthew that the biggest hurdle has been accomplished and it is best that he not drive.

    b. Tell the daughter that your assessment to date is adequate and that she should return the keys.

    c. Get a driving history, including near collisions, and conduct a Mini Mental State Examination and a hearing examination.

    d. Review medication interactions; provide Matthew with information on a driving refresher course.

110. The U.S. Preventive Services Task Force recommends that males with a history of which of the following conditions have their testicles examined?

    a. Hydrocele

    b. Impotence

    c. Cryptorchidism

    d. Prostate cancer

111. Which of the following ophthalmic findings is a common new diagnosis during adolescence?

    a. Myopia

    b. Strabismus

    c. Hyperopia

    d. Amblyopia

112. A 19-year-old man came to the emergency department today, saying that he has blacked out many times after "shooting up." Which question would **not** be appropriate in ascertaining a social history?

    a. What is your occupation?

    b. How much alcohol do you consume in a day?

    c. What town are you from?

    d. What type and amount of drugs do you use?

113. What is the daily recommended dose for calcium replacement for postmenopausal women?

    a. 1500 mg

    b. 500 mg

    c. 5000 mg

    d. 750 mg

114. A woman wants to know whether she is in menopause. How should the nurse practitioner assess this?

    a. Elicit a past medical history.

    b. Have the woman assess her basal body temperature.

    c. Elicit a sexual history.

    d. Perform a review of systems.

115. You are seeing a 6-week-old infant for a well-child examination. Which of the following physical examination findings would warrant referral?

    a. Unequal pupils since birth

    b. Brown flecks present in the iris

    c. Inability to detect a red reflex

    d. Negative Hirschberg's sign

116. Which of the following is true regarding follow-up for clients with mild or moderate hypertension?

    a. Blood pressure should be confirmed within 2 weeks.

    b. Drug therapy follow-up is not necessary.

    c. Follow-up should be done every 1 to 2 months.

    d. Follow-up intervals longer than every 2 months should never be considered.

117. A mother brings in her 2-year-old because she is not gaining weight, "always has a cold," and is having recurrent diarrhea. The family nurse practitioner should consider all the following diagnoses for this client **except:**

    a. Gastroenteritis

    b. *Chlamydia* pneumonia

    c. Cystic fibrosis

    d. AIDS

118. The treatment of choice for pregnant women with *Chlamydia* is:

    a. Ceftriaxone

    b. Doxycycline

    c. Erythromycin

    d. Ofloxacin

119. The nurse practitioner completed the examination and assessment for a client with newly diagnosed insulin-dependent diabetes mellitus. The client was started on an insulin regimen. When should a follow-up appointment be scheduled?

a. 1 month
b. 1 week
c. 2 days
d. 2 weeks

120. Primary amenorrhea that has not resolved by 17 years old can be best evaluated by:

a. Initiating oral contraceptives
b. Premarin, 1.25 mg qd for 21 days
c. Referral to a physician
d. Checking thyroid-stimulating hormone and prolactin levels

121. The most specific laboratory value to assess myocardial damage is:

a. Creatine kinase
b. Creatine kinase isoenzyme MB
c. Lactate dehydrogenase
d. Troponin I

122. In an anorexic client, what would **not** be a sign that her condition was improving?

a. Increased oral intake with 1- to 2-pound weight gain per week
b. Stabilization of electrolyte levels
c. Increased social interactions
d. Exercising 3 times a day

123. An 8-year-old boy is brought to the clinic with fecal soiling; dull, achy abdominal pain; and anorexia. The most appropriate diagnosis is:

a. Enuresis
b. Appendicitis
c. Encopresis
d. Constipation

124. What factors in a woman's history would be considered positive protection against herpes simplex?

a. She is in a monogamous relationship.
b. She experienced menarche at 10 years.
c. She drank alcohol excessively for years but quit recently.
d. Her mother and father both had a history of herpes simplex.

125. Which statement concerning Parkinson's disease is **not** true?

a. It affects women more than men.
b. It is slowly progressive.
c. There is no diagnostic test for it.
d. Its cause is unknown.

126. Which of the following findings suggests that the generalized edema is chronic and progressive?

a. The client cannot remove wedding ring as easily as at the last visit.
b. Bilateral edema of the legs is made worse by standing.
c. Bloating feeling is noted before menstrual period begins.
d. Noted swelling occurs during use of nonsteroidal antiinflammatory drugs.

127. Mary is a nurse who just stuck herself with a needle contaminated with hepatitis B virus. She has received her full course of hepatitis B virus vaccine series but does not know her titers. Mary washes the puncture area with copious amounts of soap and water. She asks you what else needs to be done. What is your response?

a. Mary needs to have a booster of hepatitus B virus vaccine.
b. Mary needs to have a titer level drawn. If <10 mIU/ml, she should receive a regimen of hepatitis B immune globulin and hepatitis B virus vaccine.
c. Mary should receive a dose of hepatitis B immune globulin.
d. Mary should receive no further treatment because she received the full course of hepatitis B virus vaccine.

128. The initial diagnostic visit of a client with low back pain generally consists of which of the following?

a. Lumbar spine x-ray examination
b. MRI
c. Complete blood cell count and electrolyte levels
d. Physical examination

129. Which of the following would you suggest to a client if he or she has gastrointestinal upset when taking iron?

    a. Stop taking the iron if it bothers you.

    b. Take cod liver oil to assist with absorption of the iron.

    c. Decrease the daily dose from tid to bid daily.

    d. Begin iron injections.

130. Expected physical findings in a client with allergic rhinitis would include:

    a. Erythematous nasal passages and purulent discharge

    b. Boggy, pale nasal turbinates and clear discharge

    c. Erythematous pharynx with exudate

    d. Pale tympanic membrane with poor movement

131. You have been asked to assist with the correction of an issue that has been noted in the practice. Use change theory to decide what should be the next step you take to correct the problem.

    a. Determine what the problem is.

    b. Identify who the key players are in the issue.

    c. Present solutions for the problem.

    d. Implement solutions for the problem.

132. Fever, chills, myalgias, hypotension, and headache occurring within several hours of treatment of syphilis can be:

    a. A sign that the syphilis is in an advanced stage

    b. An allergic reaction to the penicillin

    c. The Jarish-Herxheimer reaction

    d. A disseminated gonorrhea infection

133. Which of the following is considered secondary prevention?

    a. Effective parenting classes

    b. Hepatitis B vaccine

    c. Blood pressure screening

    d. Exercising four times a week

134. Robert, a 73-year-old man, reports that he has some problems with asthma during the change of seasons. He asks you about the pneumonia vaccine (Pneumovax). Your response should be:

    a. He does not need the vaccine at present.

    b. He will need the vaccine when he has symptoms.

    c. He will need the vaccine because he falls within the criteria.

    d. He should never have the vaccine because it can exacerbate his asthma.

135. Leading causes of mortality that affect women 18 to 39 years old are:

    a. Cardiovascular and cerebrovascular diseases

    b. Lung and breast cancer

    c. Pneumonia and influenza

    d. Motor vehicle accident and homicide

136. Which of the following represents the best recommendation for a 14-year-old male at Tanner stage 2 with new onset of gynecomastia of 1 to 2 cm?

    a. Referral to surgeon for removal of breast tissue

    b. Reassurance that gynecomastia occurs in half of young males

    c. Obtaining his testosterone level

    d. Reassuring him the gynecomastia usually resolves in 4 to 5 years

137. Which of the following affect sebum production?

    a. Dietary factors

    b. Estrogens

    c. Androgens

    d. Dirt and bacteria on the skin surface

138. A 68-year-old male is evaluated for acute dyspnea. Acute exacerbation of chronic obstructive pulmonary disease is diagnosed. The client is treated with an inhaled bronchodilator per nebulizer and released with a prescription for a prednisone taper. What follow-up is appropriate?

    a. Call the client or schedule a visit within 24 to 48 hours.

    b. Inform the client to keep routine visit appointments as scheduled.

    c. Inform the client to return to the clinic if there is no improvement.

    d. Schedule a return visit within 2 weeks.

139. Which of the following laboratory tests results are indicative of hyperthyroidism?

    a. Increased thyroid-stimulating hormone and decreased thyroxine

    b. Normal thyroid-stimulating hormone

    c. Decreased thyroid-stimulating hormone and increased thyroxine

    d. Normal thyroxine

140. Linda, 21 years old, has a diagnosis of primary dysmenorrhea and is on a successful treatment program with nonsteroidal antiinflammatory drugs. Her annual evaluation should include:

    a. Laparoscopic examination
    b. Endometrial biopsy
    c. Sonography
    d. Pelvic examination with Papanicolaou smear

141. Which medication may predispose a woman toward candidiasis?

    a. Insulin
    b. Oral contraceptive pills
    c. Medroxyprogesterone (Depo-Provera)
    d. Antihypertensives

142. When should a client with compensated congestive heart failure be reevaluated for follow-up?

    a. Monthly
    b. Weekly
    c. Every 3 months
    d. Every 6 months

143. Which physical examination finding is most suggestive of genital warts?

    a. Firm, skin-colored papules
    b. Vesicles painful to touch
    c. Oval, erythematous lesions with fine colliform edges
    d. Round, pearly white papules that are umbilicated

144. Additional information from the history that would support the diagnosis of probable Alzheimer's disease is which of the following?

    a. Postmenopausal estrogen replacement therapy
    b. Postpartum depression
    c. Progressive mental deterioration
    d. Client's concern about memory loss

145. Which of the following statements regarding client education for Lyme disease is **false?**

    a. Wear long pants and long-sleeved shirts when in tick-infested areas.
    b. Highest incidence of infection occurs between May and August.
    c. Insect repellent containing DEET is contraindicated for pregnant women.
    d. Prophylactic antimicrobial therapy is contraindicated for most tick bites.

146. What is your most likely diagnosis for B.I., a 45-year-old man who has lower left quadrant abdominal pain, WBCs 7500/cells/mm², and constipation alternating with diarrhea?

    a. Diverticulosis
    b. Diverticulitis
    c. Appendicitis
    d. Ulcerative colitis

147. Osteoarthritis is **best** treated with which of the following medications?

    a. Regular aspirin
    b. Acetaminophen
    c. Prednisone
    d. Intraarticular corticosteroid injections

148. Which of the following correctly describes Medicaid?

    a. A program designed to assist ill, low-income older adults
    b. A federal program for pregnant women
    c. A joint federal-state program for low-income persons
    d. A program administered by third-party insurers

149. Characteristics of stressors include which of the following statements?

    a. They are perceived as undesirable.
    b. Some stressors may be positive.
    c. They are new events not previously adapted to.
    d. They affect adults.

150. At 28 weeks of pregnancy, Ms. Biehler's fundal height should be no greater than:

    a. 28 cm
    b. 29 cm
    c. 30 cm
    d. 26 cm

151. A 31-year-old female with a 6-month-old nursing child reports malaise, joint pain, and lymphadenopathy. Enyzyme-linked immunosorbent assay and Western blot assay confirm Lyme disease. Treatment of choice for this woman would be:

    a. Doxycycline, 100 mg bid for 10 days
    b. Amoxicillin, 500 mg tid for 10 days
    c. Trimethoprim-sulfamethoxazole (Bactrim DS), 1 tablet bid for 10 days
    d. Erythromycin, 250 mg qid for 10 days

152. Contraception counseling and occupational blood and body fluid exposure histories are important for which of the following groups of women?

   a. 18 to 39 years and 40 to 64 years
   b. 18 to 39 years
   c. 18 to 39 years, 40 to 64 years, and 65 years and older
   d. 40 to 64 years

153. Jim is a 19-year-old male who is in for a check-up. What is the most important anticipatory guidance you should give him?

   a. Stop smoking.
   b. Use stress-reduction techniques.
   c. Do not drink and drive.
   d. Follow a low-fat diet.

154. A local school cafeteria was serving imported strawberries. Several days after eating the fruit, a number of students had some mild complaints. One mother took her child to a nurse practitioner, and a diagnosis of hepatitis A virus was made. Which of the following is a correct response by the nurse practitioner?

   a. The nurse practitioner does not want to alarm anyone and tells the mother that the hepatitis A virus infection is nothing to worry about and requires no treatment.
   b. The nurse practitioner should report the case to the local health department, and all close contacts should be offered immunization in an effort to contain a possible epidemic.
   c. An hepatitis A virus epidemic is going to occur regardless of efforts at immunization.
   d. The nurse practitioner should report the case to the local health department, and all close and casual contacts should be offered immunization in an effort to contain a possible epidemic.

155. A chest x-ray examination is always indicated:

   a. For all clients with acute dyspnea
   b. If the client is a smoker
   c. If it has been longer than 5 years since the last x-ray examination
   d. If it will help alleviate the client's worries

156. The primary role of the nurse practitioner in treating the client with Cushing's syndrome includes all the following **except:**

   a. Early identification and referral to a physician
   b. Prompt diagnosis and treatment
   c. Patient support and education
   d. Thorough history and physical examination

157. Which of the following statements made by the mother of a 7-month-old would most make the family nurse practitioner suspect cystic fibrosis?

   a. He tastes "salty" when I kiss him.
   b. He is a really slow eater.
   c. He almost always spits up when I try to burp him.
   d. He had a really bad cold last month.

158. Which of the following statements indicates that your client understands her treatment for tinea versicolor?

   a. The discoloration (white or brown color) may remain for several months after treatment.
   b. If there is no improvement in 2 weeks, she should return to the office for an alternate therapy.
   c. She must avoid animals because they are carriers.
   d. There is no treatment for tinea versicolor.

159. Ms. Hale, a 55-year-old woman who reports severe, shooting pain along the left side of her face, says, "The pain started while I was mowing the yard and the pain was so severe I had to stop mowing." The attacks of pain lasted 15 to 20 seconds, recurring several times. She describes the pain as radiating to her forehead, her left eye, and the root of the nose. The pain Ms. Hale is experiencing is most likely associated with which of the following?

   a. Temporal arteritis
   b. Trigeminal neuralgia
   c. Tension-type headache
   d. Cluster headache

160. In addressing a client in crisis, the nurse practitioner should do all the following **except:**

   a. Help the individual accept reality.
   b. Link the person to a social network.
   c. Use only previous coping mechanisms of the client.
   d. Attend to the client's immediate needs.

161. Obese clients with asymptomatic gallstones should be instructed:

   a. To restrict caloric intake for gradual weight loss

   b. To eat low-fat, low-cholesterol diet to avoid stone formation

   c. That gallstones will dissolve

   d. To take ursodiol (Actigall)

162. To make recovery more successful, a woman with low back strain should be advised by the nurse practitioner not to lift anything weighing more than:

   a. 60 pounds

   b. 75 pounds

   c. 10 pounds

   d. 20 pounds

163. In a 30-year old woman who has thyroid enlargement, which subjective datum is **least** essential to elicit initially?

   a. What changes has she noticed in her neck since she discovered the enlargement?

   b. Has she noticed any relationships to any other symptoms?

   c. When was her last physical examination?

   d. What does she know about thyroid enlargement and cancer?

164. A primary goal of the health history is to:

   a. Identify modifiable risk factors

   b. Develop rapport

   c. Determine cognitive ability

   d. Develop a relationship with client

165. There are several ways of using research in practice. When a nurse practitioner's way of thinking has changed as a result of being involved in a research study or reading research, the use of research in practice in this manner is called:

   a. Problem oriented

   b. Decision driven

   c. Conceptual

   d. Targeted

166. When assessing a child's stress level, the nurse practitioner should inquire about all the following **except:**

   a. Peer group interactions

   b. Family income

   c. Sibling rivalry

   d. School performance

167. The primary purpose of therapeutic communication is to:

   a. Have the client be compliant with the treatment plan

   b. Solve the client's problems

   c. Provide a supportive and helpful relationship for the client

   d. Provide the client with a role model for resolution of the problems

168. A history of diabetes mellitus along with a chronic pulmonary disorder would indicate the need for which of the following immunizations?

   a. Influenza

   b. Hepatitis A

   c. Measles-mumps-rubella

   d. Varicella

169. Before hormone replacement therapy is initiated, which of the following should be performed?

   a. Pregnancy test

   b. Cardiac enzyme panel

   c. ECG

   d. Chest x-ray examination

170. What nursing intervention would be most effective in helping Mrs. Jones deal with her anxiety regarding a diagnosis of lung cancer?

   a. Reassure her that the prognosis is favorable because of all the recent advancements in treatment.

   b. Tell her not to worry because you feel sure that there is nothing seriously wrong.

   c. Use a calm voice and simple language to describe the diagnostic plan.

   d. Advise her that she seems too upset to continue at this time and suggest that she reschedule for a later visit.

171. When an elevated cholesterol level is discovered in a 14-year-old female client, the best course of treatment is to:

   a. Initiate a bile acid sequestrant drug

   b. Use a 3-hydroxy-3-methylglutaryl coenzyme A drug

   c. Start oral contraceptives

   d. Prescribe a low-fat diet

172. What is the legal yardstick against which the Advanced Registered Nurse Practitioner's professional competence is judged?

    a. American Nurses Association Code of Ethics

    b. Standards of care

    c. Patient Determination Act

    d. Professional certification

173. A client with diabetes has a cholesterol level of 220 mg/dl. He asks what has caused his level to be so high, because he follows his American Diabetes Association 1800-Calorie diet closely. The nurse practitioner should tell him that which of the following explains the condition?

    a. It is hereditary.

    b. He has a spontaneous genetic disorder of his metabolism.

    c. Diabetes has decreased his ability to metabolize fats.

    d. He is male.

174. Evaluation goals related to osteoporosis for Mrs. A. would be all the following **except:**

    a. Prevention of additional falls

    b. Freedom from pain

    c. Initiation of estrogen replacement therapy, calcium supplement, and exercise regimen

    d. Loss of 2 pounds per week to reach recommended weight

175. Surgical intervention is usually required for children with spinal curves of:

    a. 10 to 20 degrees

    b. 20 to 25 degrees

    c. 25 to 30 degrees

    d. ≥40 degrees

ANSWERS AND RATIONALES: EXAMINATION 2

1. *Answer:* c (assessment/history/HEENT/child)

Rationale: This is the classic presentation of epiglottitis. Choice *a* is consistent with croup symptoms; *b* can be associated with pharyngitis; *d* is associated with the common cold.

2. *Answer:* b (assessment/history/cardiovascular/adult)

Rationale: Advanced age, being female, and hormone replacement therapy are all risk factors for development of thrombophlebitis. Although both obesity and female gender are risk factors, risk factors are cumulative.

3. *Answer:* c (assessment/physical examination/respiratory/adult)

Rationale: Purse-lipped breathing, barrel-shaped chest, and thin, anxious appearance are all signs of emphysema. Continuous, copious sputum may be a sign of chronic bronchitis.

4. *Answer:* a (plan/management/therapeutic/pharmacologic/communicable disease/NAS)

Rationale: Permethrin 1% is the drug of choice for pediculosis capitis. It is 97% to 99% effective and has minimal side effects.

5. *Answer:* c (plan/management/therapeutic/pharmacologic/genitourinary/adult)

Rationale: Only clients with symptomatic bacteriuria should be treated with antibiotics.

6. *Answer:* d (diagnosis/endocrinologic/NAS)

Rationale: Typically, gastrointestinal symptoms are absent in hyperthyroidism.

7. *Answer:* d (assessment/physical examination/HEENT/NAS/pretest)

Rationale: Profuse mucopurulent drainage is indicative of bacterial conjunctivitis. Drainage in cases of viral conjunctivitis tends to be watery and more mucoid. Viral conjunctivitis often accompanies upper respiratory tract infection; palpable preauricular nodes may be present.

8. *Answer:* a (assessment/management/diagnostics/reproductive/adult)

Rationale: Basal body temperature, serum progesterone level, and endometrial biopsy are used to assess ovulation. A postcoital test evaluates sperm-cervical interaction.

9. *Answer:* c (assessment/physical examination/developmental delay/infant)

Rationale: Gross motor failures are the major reason for referral in infants and toddlers. At 12 months, Maggie needs to be sitting alone and standing at least with assistance. Earlier intervention carries better outcomes.

10. Answer: d (assessment/history/psychosocial/child)

Rationale: Jumping out of a moving vehicle is *not* a common behavior of preschoolers; rather, it is a dangerous behavior that warrants immediate physician consultation for possible psychiatric evaluation. Hiding, noncompliance, and jumping over furniture are common behaviors that might be displayed during preschool years.

11. *Answer:* a (assessment/history/genitourinary/child)

Rationale: Approximately 15% of 7-year-olds experience enuresis. By definition, primary enuresis occurs in children who have never achieved consistent dryness and must occur at least once a week. Enuresis is more common among males than among females.

12. *Answer:* b (management/integumentary/NAS)

Rationale: Pityriasis usually has a spontaneous remission, so treatment is needed only for itching if bothersome.

13. *Answer:* d (plan/management/therapeutics/nonpharmacologic/genitourinary/NAS/pretest)

Rationale: A seated position for urination helps to relieve pressure and therefore facilitates urination in men with benign prostatic hyperplasia.

14. *Answer:* c (plan/management/therapeutics/pharmacologic/NAS)

Rationale: Beta-blockers are usually the first-line medications used for the prevention of migraine headaches. Administration of oxygen is the first-line treatment for cluster headaches, whereas lithium carbonate 300 mg tid is used as a prophylactic medication for cluster headaches and cyclobenzaprine (Flexeril) 10 mg qd is used to treat tension-type headaches caused by pericranial muscle tension.

15. *Answer:* c (assessment/history/multisystem/NAS)

Rationale: Choice *a* is more specific for chronic fatigue syndrome, choice *b* for infectious mononucleosis, and choice *d* for rheumatoid arthritis.

16. *Answer:* d (diagnosis/gastrointestinal/NAS)

Rationale: The pain associated with gastric ulcers usually is located to the left of the midepigastric area. It is not necessarily relieved by eating and may even occur immediately after eating.

17. *Answer:* a (assessment/history/musculoskeletal/NAS)

Rationale: Diabetes, hypertension, and obesity are associated with gout; coronary artery disease is not.

18. *Answer:* c (diagnosis/immunologic/NAS)

Rationale: HIV infection is a disease of immunodeficiency and therefore can have an expansive clinical differential diagnosis range. Confirmation of HIV diagnosis requires laboratory evidence of positive enzyme-linked immunosorbent assay result confirmed by Western blot.

19. *Answer:* b (assessment/history/hematopoeitic/aging adult)

Rationale: Chronic lymphocytic leukemia is primarily a disease of older men (60 years old or older) with a 2- to 3-month history of splenomegaly.

20. *Answer:* a (plan/management/therapeutics/pharmacologic/allergies/NAS)

Rationale: One of the major changes in the newest guidelines for asthma management is the push to quickly reduce the inflammatory process and reduce the risk of recurrence by intensifying therapy. The other options are included in the stepwise approach.

21. *Answer:* c (diagnosis/communicable/child)

Rationale: Fifth disease begins with a bright red rash on the cheeks. Rubella is usually a mild disease that lasts approximately 3 days. Rubeola usually is seen with a severe cough and a high fever. Roseola is a viral exanthem of infants.

22. *Answer:* c (issues/application to practice/cultural sensitivity/counseling concepts/nurse-client relationship)

Rationale: Neither pain medication nor other interventions should be prescribed before assessing what meaning the pain has for the client. Understanding this meaning will help the nurse practitioner to prescribe culturally appropriate interventions.

23. Answer: a (wellness/health promotion/lifestyle/health behaviors/child)

Rationale: Experimentation with smoking frequently occurs in the sixth grade. Nightmares and temper tantrums should be assessed as part of a well-child preschool examination. The issue of drinking and driving is more relevant for a well-adolescent examination.

24. Answer: a (health promotion/lifestyle/exercise/wellness/NAS)

Rationale: Frequency and intensity do not produce the best effects, particularly when done in excessive amounts. Moderation is the best level maintained with time. There are no differences between females and males.

25. Answer: d (plan/management/therapeutics/pharmacologic/integumentary/NAS/pretest)

Rationale: The treatment of acne should begin with topical agents. The chronic nature of acne requires long-term treatment with any systemic agents used, which could result in serious side effects. No improvement has been shown with dietary modifications.

26. Answer: b (assessment/history/wellness/childbearing female)

Rationale: An obstetric history does not encompass the client's medical-surgical and environmental exposure histories.

27. Answer: a (plan/management/therapeutics/pharmacologic/wellness/child)

Rationale: The recommendations for a child that has received the primary series of immunizations and is 12 months old or older would be a fourth acellular diphtheria-pertussis-tetanus vaccine, third oral polio vaccine, fourth *H. influenzae* B vaccine, and first measles-mumps-rubella vaccine.

28. Answer: a (wellness/risk factor identification/wellness/adult)

Rationale: Ovarian cancer is the second most common gynecologic cancer.

29. Answer: d (plan/management/therapeutics/wellness/adolescent)

Rationale: Adolescents may obtain care for family planning and sexually transmitted disease treatment without parental consent.

30. Answer: d (plan/management/therapeutics/pharmacologic/HEENT/NAS)

Rationale: Clients who have oral candidiasis and wear dentures must have both the oral cavity treated and the dentures treated. Fluconazole may be substituted for nystatin troches.

31. Answer: c (assessment/physical examination/cardiovascular/NAS)

Rationale: Pulmonary rales and edema can be nonspecific findings. Elevated jugular venous pressure with the presence of S_3 gallop and a laterally displaced peak moment of impulse with accompanying symptoms suggestive of congestive heart failure can be diagnostic findings.

32. Answer: c (assessment/history/respiratory/child)

Rationale: Asking about associated symptoms will often direct you to a cause.

33. Answer: a (assessment/management/diagnostics/communicable disease/NAS)

Rationale: Liver function tests, complete blood cell count, and immunoglobin M antibodies are not needed to make the diagnosis of mononucleosis. These tests indicate more about the progression and extent of the illness.

34. Answer: b (diagnosis/genitourinary/adult)

Rationale: A middle-aged man, not an older man, is more likely to have prostatitis than benign prostatic hyperplasia or prostate cancer. With chronic bacterial prostatitis, however, if there is pain, it is much more likely to be dull and the onset of symptoms are likely to be more gradual.

35. Answer: b (assessment/history/cardiovascular/NAS/pretest)

Rationale: Unilateral edema is more suggestive of venous insufficiency or trauma. Peripheral edema in congestive heart failure is usually a bilateral dependent edema. Mental status changes are a common finding in older adults because of a decrease in cerebral perfusion.

36. Answer: b (diagnosis/endocrinologic/NAS)

Rationale: The urinary free cortisol level is more sensitive, specific, and cost-effective than either the plasma cortisol level or 24-hours urine sample for 17-hydroxycorticosteroids. The dexamethasone suppression test is indicated after the screening test.

37. *Answer:* d (plan/management/therapeutics/ nonpharmacologic/reproductive/aging adult)

Rationale: A postmenopausal woman with a large adnexal mass is always referred.

38. *Answer:* d (assessment/physical examination/reproductive/childbearing female)

Rationale: There are no abnormal physical findings associated with primary dysmenorrhea. If the pelvic examination is done during the period of symptoms, there may be mild uterine or cervical tenderness.

39. *Answer:* c (assessment/physical examination/psychosocial/aging adult)

Rationale: Parallel injuries suggest a nonrandom occurrence. Bruises on the upper arms would suggest that the client was held tightly or restrained. The other injuries and physical findings could have resulted from unintended injuries. The burn on the top of the hand could be from unsteady hands knocking against a hot burner; bruises below elbows could be caused by assisted transfers, and swollen distal joints of fingers are common with gout.

40. *Answer:* a (assessment/physical examination/psychosocial/NAS)

Rationale: Psychiatric disorders often coexist with substance disorders.

41. *Answer:* c (evaluation/integumentary/NAS)

Rationale: Examine all family members for infection. Untreated persons provide a continuing source of reinfection after therapy.

42. *Answer:* a (evaluation/neurologic/NAS)

Rationale: A more thorough workup, including MRI or CT, is mandatory for the client who has not recovered from facial palsy after 6 months.

43. *Answer:* c (assessment/physical examination/multisystem/NAS)

Rationale: Adenopathy may signal HIV or another form of infection. Although all systems are important, an abnormality noted in the lymphatic system should trigger further assessment of other systems.

44. *Answer:* a (diagnosis/gastrointestinal/NAS)

Rationale: Gastroesophageal reflux disease is the reflux of acidic gastric contents into the esophagus. It results in burning of the esophagus, and the client may describe this as a burning pain.

45. *Answer:* a (diagnosis/musculoskeletal/infant)

Rationale: The importance of careful hip evaluation in the neonate cannot be overemphasized. With good history and physical examination, developmental dysplasia of the hip can be detected at birth.

46. *Answer:* c (assessment/cardiovascular/NAS/pretest)

Rationale: The most valuable diagnostic test is serial measurement of cardiac isoenzymes.

47. *Answer:* c (assessment/history/immunologic/NAS)

Rationale: The natural history of HIV infection is divided into stages according to laboratory data and clinical picture. The acute retroviral conversion is characterized by the symptoms resembling infectious mononucleosis. Spontaneous recovery occurs typically in 1 to 3 weeks. Seroconversion is complete in 1 to 3 months. The individual remains symptom-free for many years. As CD4 count gradually declines, AIDS defining diagnoses appear.

48. *Answer:* d (assessment/physical examination/hematopoietic/NAS)

Rationale: A complete blood cell count with a differential is essential when leukemia is suspected.

49. *Answer:* d (assessment/history/allergy/NAS)

Rationale: Successful prevention of symptoms with exercise through prophylactic administration of medication (short-acting beta-agonist) supports the diagnosis of exercise-induced asthma.

50. *Answer:* d (diagnosis/communicable/child)

Rationale: Scarlet fever appears with a flushed face, sore throat, and a bright-red punctate rash with a sandpapery feel. Fifth disease begins with a bright red rash on the cheeks. Rubella is usually a mild disease that lasts around 3 days. Rubeola usually is seen with a severe cough and a high fever.

51. *Answer:* d (issues/application to practice/interviewing)

Rationale: In option *d,* the nurse is restating what the client said, which facilitates further discussion and expression of feelings.

52. *Answer:* d (health promotion/lifestyle/nutrition/wellness/NAS)

Rationale: Anthropometric and biochemical measurements are important in nutritional screening. An analysis of diet, including food preparation, meals skipped, and transportation to the grocery store, is included. Social history is not necessary.

53. *Answer:* a (plan/management/diagnostics/reproductive/NAS/pretest)

Rationale: The most common infertility problems can be identified by an initial evaluation, which includes a semen analysis, documentation of ovulation, postcoital test, and evaluation of tubal patency.

54. *Answer:* d (health promotion/lifestyle/exercise/wellness/NAS)

Rationale: Although all these may occur with exercise, injury is the most common risk.

55. *Answer:* a (plan/management/health-promoting behavior/wellness/childbearing female)

Rationale: Baking soda may cause water retention and alkalosis, and aluminum in antacids may cause constipation.

56. *Answer:* d (plan/management/anticipatory guidance/wellness/child)

Rationale: Trained night criers are infants who awaken each night and cry for 30 to 60 minutes or more. When infants awaken and cry, the parent should wait 5 to 10 minutes before going to the room to assess the situation. Infants should not be removed from their cribs unless they are in an unsafe setting. The parent should assess that the infant is safe but should not turn on the lights, rock the infant back to sleep, or otherwise interact. The infant should learn to put himself or herself back to sleep. The infant is placed into bed awake.

57. *Answer:* d (wellness/risk factor identification/wellness/aging adult)

Rationale: Polypharmacy, side effects, and costs are all reasons that older adults do not comply with medication therapies.

58. *Answer:* d (health promotion/primary prevention)

Rationale: Inspecting, asking, and calling all are early case findings of child abuse. Offering parenting classes is a means of preventing future abuse.

59. *Answer:* b (plan/management/therapeutics/pharmacologic/HEENT/NAS)

Rationale: Erythromycin is the drug of choice when a client with pharyngitis is allergic to penicillin. Augmentin contains penicillin, therefore is contraindicated. Bactrim and ciprofloxacin are not indicated for group A streptococcal pharyngitis.

60. *Answer:* c (diagnosis/cardiovascular/NAS)

Rationale: A *transient ischemic attack* is defined as lasting as long as 24 hours.

61. *Answer:* d (evaluation/immunologic/NAS/pretest)

Rationale: CD4 count and HIV RNA both track disease progression and response to medication. Results from these tests help guide therapeutic decisions.

62. *Answer:* a (diagnosis/respiratory/child)

Rationale: Pertussis is more common in unimmunized clients.

63. *Answer:* b (evaluation/communicable disease/NAS)

Rationale: It is recommended that any client treated for primary or secondary syphilis who does not have a fourfold decrease of a nontreponemal antibody titer within 3 months be evaluated for treatment failure.

64. *Answer:* a (assessment/physical examination/genitourinary/adult)

Rationale: With chronic bacterial prostatitis, the prostate gland may or may not be tender but is not exquisitely tender. With benign prostatic hyperplasia, there would be enlargement of the gland. With prostate cancer, nodules are most likely palpated.

65. *Answer:* d (diagnoses/endocrinologic/adolescent)

Rationale: With Cushing's syndrome, one would see weight gain.

66. *Answer:* d (plan/management/therapeutics/reproductive/aging adult)

Rationale: If the client wishes contraception, she may continue to take oral contraceptives for long-term therapy.

67. Answer: d (diagnosis/HEENT/aging adult)

Rationale: Nausea and vomiting often accompany the increased intraocular pressure associated with narrow-angle glaucoma. Pupillary dilatation may actually worsen the condition by blocking aqueous humor outflow.

68. Answer: b (diagnosis/genitourinary/child)

Rationale: Secondary enuresis may occur with nocturnal seizures, with psychosocial trauma such as divorce or the birth of a sibling, and with urinary tract infections. Once nighttime dryness has been achieved consistently for 6 months, a return to bed wetting is considered abnormal.

69. Answer: c (plan/management/therapeutic/non-pharmacologic/child)

Rationale: Punishment is a negative interaction between the child and the parent. It is helpful to the child with attention deficit–hyperactivity disorder for the parents to focus on what the child does well and to reward this behavior. Psychoanalysis is an insight-driven form of therapy, and helping the child to gain insight will not change the behavior. Medications, most frequently psychostimulants, stimulate areas of the brain that control attention, impulses, and self-regulation of behavior. School intervention provides education and guidance for the classroom teacher and consistency of expectations at home and at school. Cognitive or behavioral therapy is directed toward parents and children learning new techniques to deal with the child's behavior, promote positive behaviors, and reduce negative behaviors.

70. Answer: d (diagnosis/integumentary/NAS)

Rationale: Differential diagnosis includes atopic dermatitis, allergic and irritant contact dermatitis, papular urticaria, and pediculosis.

71. Answer: c (assessment/physical examination/neurologic/aging adult)

Rationale: Histories of progressive cognitive decline and deficits in memory, judgment, and abstraction support a diagnosis of Alzheimer's disease.

72. Answer: b (diagnosis/multisystem/NAS)

Rationale: Anemia, thyroid dysfunction, heart or lung disease, liver disease, and diabetes are the most common causes of fatigue.

73. Answer: b (plan/management/therapeutics/pharmacologic/gastrointestinal/NAS)

Rationale: Anticholinergic drugs block the effect of acetylcholine at the receptor sites, thereby reducing the production of gastric secretions.

74. Answer: c (assessment/history/musculoskeletal/NAS)

Rationale: Most common symptoms, are paresthesia, numbness, and tingling waking client at night. There is no "carpal tunnel muscle."

75. Answer: c (diagnosis/gastrointestinal/NAS/pretest)

Rationale: Raw hamburger is the most common mode of transmission for *E. coli. Salmonella* is more commonly found in poultry and eggs. Norwalk virus is found in contaminated shellfish, water, and cold foods. Protazoans are usually transmitted by water.

76. Answer: b (plan/management/client education/lymphatics/adult)

Rationale: Chemotherapy and radiation to the inguinal area may affect the gonads and the ability to produce sperm.

77. Answer: c (evaluation/hematopoeitic/adult)

Rationale: Prevention of development of subendocardial bacterial endocarditis is crucial.

78. Answer: c (assessment/physical examination/allergy/NAS)

Rationale: During an acute asthmatic attack, the respiratory pattern is deep and slow, with a prolonged expiratory phase. Dullness on percussion and rales on auscultation are more highly associated with pneumonia. Low-pitched rhonchi heard more on inspiration most likely indicate upper airway obstruction.

79. Answer: a (plan/management/consultation and referral/emergencies/NAS)

Rationale: Electrical burns require close monitoring because the extent of damage is not readily known. Such clients are referred for hospital admission. In many cases there is no skin damage, or limited, superficial skin damage, from the burn.

80. *Answer:* d (issues/scope/standards of practice)

Rationale: Certification does not imply that the nurse practitioner has completed an accredited program, nor is the nurse practitioner eligible to practice. Each state identifies the components necessary to become eligible to practice; certification may be one of those requirements. Certification is not required for a Drug Enforcement Agency number. Certification verifies the credentials of nurse practitioners and indicates knowledge of a specialized area.

81. *Answer:* a (health promotion/lifestyle/nutrition/wellness/NAS)

Rationale: Fat intake should be limited to 30% of daily caloric intake. More fruits, vegetables, and grains should be eaten. Snacking should be discouraged.

82. *Answer:* d (plan/management/consult/musculoskeletal/NAS/pretest)

Rationale: If chiropractic manipulation is to be considered, it should be performed within the usual time of recovery, within 4 weeks.

83. *Answer:* c (assessment/physical examination/wellness/aging adult)

Rationale: With Sam's family history, a cardiopulmonary examination must be included, so choice *b* is eliminated. Of the remaining choices, *c* is the most appropriate because blood pressure, digital rectal examination, and fecal occult blood are more age appropriate than a musculoskeletal examination.

84. *Answer:* d (plan/management/diagnostics/wellness/childbearing female)

Rationale: A hemoglobin level or hematocrit is ordered to compare antepartum and postpartum levels. The fasting blood sugar is ordered to determine whether the client has true diabetes or only gestational diabetes. Women who have a history of thyroid disease are at increased risk for postpartum thyroiditis and thus should undergo thyroid function tests. FSH and LH are not needed postpartum.

85. *Answer:* c (assessment/physical examination/wellness/adolescent)

Rationale: Testicular enlargement is the first sign of pubertal development in about 98% of males. The average age of initiation of puberty for a male is 11.6 years.

86. *Answer:* a (management/therapeutics/anticipatory guidance/wellness/aging adult)

Rationale: The use of a system for taking medications assists older adults in knowing when medications have been taken. It provides an organizing method for taking medications.

87. *Answer:* c (health promotion/secondary prevention/NAS)

Rationale: Care is geared toward resolving and accepting the problem rather than preventing it (primary) or minimizing its consequences (tertiary).

88. *Answer:* b (evaluation/HEENT/aging adult)

Rationale: Eye discharge can be a sign of a postoperative infection and should be fully evaluated by the ophthamologist.

89. *Answer:* a (plan/management/diagnostics/cardiovascular/NAS)

Rationale: Arrhythmia usually causes syncope. Three 24-hour periods may be needed to detect the arrhythmia.

90. *Answer:* b (plan/management/therapeutics/pharmacologic/respiratory/adult)

Rationale: Albuterol has been shown to decrease coughing and wheezing during bronchitis.

91. *Answer:* b (assessment/history/communicable disease/NAS)

Rationale: All the information would be pertinent in the care of the client with mononucleosis, but the ability or inability to perform normal activities would assist the nurse practitioner in determining how much rest the client should get, as well as the need for intervention with work or school expectations.

92. *Answer:* c (assessment/history/genitourinary/adult)

Rationale: Flank pain, fever, nausea, and vomiting are more indicative of pyelonephritis, whereas scrotal pain and dysuria are more likely to occur with epididymitis. Spasmodic flank pain and hematuria occur with nephrolithiasis.

93. ***Answer:*** a (evaluation/respiratory/child/pretest)

Rationale: Although family coping and school progress are important aspects of care for clients with cystic fibrosis, the primary goals of treatment are to promote growth and to reduce the number and severity of respiratory complications. The best way to assess optimal nutrition is to monitor growth.

94. ***Answer:*** d (management/pharmacologic/endocrinologic/NAS)

Rationale: Dosages need to be initiated and adjusted with caution in older adults and in clients with heart disease.

95. ***Answer:*** c (plan/management/client education/reproductive/adult)

Rationale: Chocolate contains a methylxanthine, restriction of which helps to alleviate symptoms in fibrocystic disease.

96. ***Answer:*** c (assessment/history/HEENT/adult)

Rationale: Glaucoma results in gradual narrowing of the visual fields, with tunnel vision as a late finding.

97. ***Answer:*** b (plan/management/therapeutics/nonpharmacologic/adult)

Rationale: According to cognitive theory, depressed persons ignore positive comments and focus on the negative message. In this case, the intended compliment could be interpreted by the client as "I must have looked like a bum." Neutral comments will acknowledge his appearance and decrease the chance for negative interpretation.

98. ***Answer:*** d (assessment/physical examination/integumentary/NAS)

Rationale: Psoriasis is characterized by dry, scaly lesions that occur most frequently on the elbows, knees, scalp, and torso.

99. ***Answer:*** a (assessment/physical examination/neurologic/child)

Rationale: The physical examination should include observing the skin for any abnormalities because they may be associated with congenital abnormalities. A hemangioma involving one side of the face or body coupled with a seizure may be associated with a congenital disorder called *Sturge-Weber syndrome.* The other factors are all within normal variation for a 5-week-old infant.

100. ***Answer:*** d (management/therapeutics/multisystem/NAS)

Rationale: Aerobic exercise for 30 minutes three times per week is recommended. High-impact aerobics would probably be too intense for a client with fibromyalgia, and walking at a moderate pace is not normally aerobic.

101. ***Answer:*** a (diagnosis/gastrointestinal/NAS/pretest)

Rationale: The typical symptoms of appendicitis may be blunted by the use of oral steroids.

102. ***Answer:*** c (evaluation/gastrointestinal/adult)

Rationale: Follow up in 2 to 4 weeks of the initial visit to evaluate client's response to therapy.

103. ***Answer:*** a (evaluation/musculoskeletal/NAS)

Rationale: Early rehabilitation after injury is necessary to return the client to a usual level of activity and to protect the joint from further injury.

104. ***Answer:*** d (assessment/physical examination/hematopoeitic/child)

Rationale: A bone marrow smear is not a first-line test when anemia is suspected.

105. ***Answer:*** b (plan/management/therapeutics/nonpharmacologic/allergies/NAS)

Rationale: The likelihood of anaphylaxis in the future is much greater for someone who has had an acute generalized reaction. An inhaler and an antihistamine are not necessary unless the client encounters the allergen. A medical alert bracelet cannot be made because the allergen is not known. The best plan is for the client to undergo allergy testing for identification of the allergen and avoidance or desensitization.

106. ***Answer:*** a (diagnosis/developmental delay/NAS)

Rationale: A developmental disability is a central nervous system dysfunction that results in a chronic course with a high likelihood of functional limitations.

107. ***Answer:*** d (issues/scope/standards of practice)

Rationale: Laws can be developed by all these except political action committees.

108. *Answer:* b (health promotion/lifestyle/health behaviors/wellness/NAS)

Rationale: Medication or behavioral counseling should not be initiated until the client commits to quitting. Waiting for failure before intervening is unethical. During contemplation, encouragement is offered by providing information about the effects of smoking.

109. *Answer:* c (plan/management/diagnostics/periodic identification/wellness/aging adult)

Rationale: Choice *c* is the most appropriate because with these data the direction of the counseling can be guided.

110. *Answer:* c (wellness/risk factor identification/wellness/adult)

Rationale: Men with a history of cryptorchidism or atrophic testes are at increased risk for development of testicular cancer.

111. *Answer:* a (diagnosis/wellness/risk factor identification/wellness/adolescent)

Rationale: The refractive disorder myopia is a common finding during early adolescence, corresponding with increased growth of the eye. Nearly 25% of adolescents have 20/40 or less acute vision.

112. *Answer:* c (assessment/history/neurologic/NAS/pretest)

Rationale: It is important to ascertain several issues in the social history, such as occupation and alcohol consumption, as well as drug abuse. It is also important to determine the type and age of the dwelling site and any recent travel. The town that this young man is from is irrelevant.

113. *Answer:* a (management/therapeutics/pharmacology/wellness/aging adult)

Rationale: A dose of 1500 mg is the recommended calcium replacement therapy for postmenopausal women.

114. *Answer:* d (client education/wellness/management)

Rationale: A past medical history will be important when considering prescribing hormone replacement therapy. A sexual history will help in evaluating sexually transmitted disease risk and regularity of intercourse as a protective factor against vaginal symptoms of menopause. Basal body temperature can indicate ovulation, but a woman not in menopause may not be ovulating. A review of systems will allow an appraisal of physiologic changes associated with decreased estrogen.

115. *Answer:* c (assessment/physical examination/HEENT/infant)

Rationale: Inability to detect a red reflex may indicate opacity associated with congenital cataracts.

116. *Answer:* c (evaluation/cardiovascular/NAS)

Rationale Follow-up for mild and moderate hypertension should generally be done every 1 to 2 months but may be prolonged in the absence of target-organ damage. Elevated blood pressure should be confirmed at 2 months. Drug therapy response should be monitored with every visit.

117. *Answer:* b (diagnosis/respiratory/child)

Rationale: Chlamydial pneumonia is rare after the sixth month of life. Cystic fibrosis and AIDS both feature recurrent diarrhea and respiratory infections. Gatroenteritis should always be considered when diarrhea is present.

118. *Answer:* c (plan/management/therapeutic/pharmacologic/communicable disease/childbearing female)

Rationale: Doxycycline and ofloxacin are contraindicated during pregnancy. Ceftriaxone is the treatment for gonorrhea. Currently erythromycin is the drug of choice during pregnancy.

119. *Answer:* c (evaluation/endocrinologic/NAS)

Rationale: A client with newly diagnosed insulin-dependent diabetes mellitus will need to be monitored closely to achieve glucose control and evaluate mastery of the necessary new skills. Depending on the setting, a phone call or office visit may be made daily.

120. *Answer:* c (plan/management/therapeutics/pharmacologic/reproductive/childbearing female)

Rationale: Initiating oral contraceptives or conjugated estrogens (Premarin), and checking thyroid-stimulating hormone and prolactin levels are all appropriate for secondary amenorrhea. Primary amenorrhea not resolved by 17 years should be referred to a physician for a thorough workup.

121. Answer: d (plan/management/diagnostics/cardiovascular/NAS)

Rationale: Troponin is located in the myocardium and is most specific for damage.

122. Answer: d (evaluation/psychosocial/NAS)

Rationale: All the options would indicate a response to treatment. Excessive exercise is not a sign of improvement and may indicate an attempt to control and lose weight.

123. Answer: c (diagnosis/genitourinary/child/pretest)

Rationale: Enuresis involves soiling with urine rather than stool. Appendicitis does not normally involve fecal soiling. Although encopresis usually results from constipation, simple constipation does not normally produce soiling.

124. Answer: a (assessment/history/integumentary/NAS)

Rationale: Use of barrier methods and monogamous relationships are factors that protect against herpes. None of the other factors are protective.

125. Answer: a (diagnosis/neurologic/NAS)

Rationale: There is equal distribution among the sexes of Parkinson's disease.

126. Answer: b (assessment/history/multisystem/NAS)

Rationale: Bilateral edema of the legs and feet is a classic sign of congestive heart failure or of venous insufficiency, both chronic and progressive.

127. Answer: b (plan/management/therapeutics/gastrointestinal/NAS)

Rationale: If the titer is <10 mIU/ml, a person is treated as though he or she had not received vaccine.

128. Answer: d (assessment/physical examination/musculoskeletal/NAS)

Rationale: Unless the history reveals suspicion of trauma, systemic, or structural problems, no laboratory tests or x-ray examinations are needed.

129. Answer: c (plan/hematopoetic/NAS)

Rationale: Decreasing the dose from tid to bid or qd significantly reduces gastrointestinal side effects.

130. Answer: b (assessment/physical examination/allergies/NAS)

Rationale: A person with allergic rhinitis has boggy, pale nasal turbinates with a clear discharge. The nurse practitioner may also see allergic shiners or an allergic salute. Erythematous nasal passages and purulent discharge are seen with viral rhinitis, as is an erythematous pharynx. Poor movement of the tympanic membrane is seen in otitis media or serous otitis.

131. Answer: b (issues/scope/standards of practice)

Rationale: The problem has already been identified. At this point, it would be critical to identify the people who are closely involved in the situation and gain their feedback and perception. It is premature to either present solutions or implement solutions for the problem.

132. Answer: c (evaluation/communicable disease/NAS/pretest)

Rationale: The Jarisch-Herxheimer reaction is a systemic reaction that occurs after the treatment of syphilis. It is correlated with the release of spirochetes and lasts 24 to 48 hours. It is usually mild, can be treated with aspirin, and is self-limited.

133. Answer: c (health promotion/primary/secondary prevention/wellness/NAS)

Rationale: Screening is considered secondary prevention. All the other choices reflect primary prevention.

134. Answer: c (plan/management/therapeutics/pharmacologic/wellness/aging adult)

Rationale: Choice *a* is vague, and choices *b* and *d* are incorrect statements.

135. Answer: d (diagnosis/plan/risk factor identification/wellness/adult)

Rationale: Disease is not the leading cause of death for women in this age group. Instead, concerns relative to personal safety are more likely to cause death among women in this age group.

136. Answer: b (plan/management/client education/wellness/adolescent)

Rationale: Gynecomastia occurs in approximately 50% of males and resolves within 12 to 18 months of onset in 90% to 95% of males.

137. *Answer:* c (wellness/diagnosis)

Rationale: The secretion of sebum from the sebaceous glands is controlled by the androgenic hormones. There is no clear understanding of the cause of the overproduction of sebum. Testosterone and androstenediol are synthesized in the testes; the adrenal gland is the primary source in females.

138. *Answer:* a (evaluation/respiratory/adult)

Rationale: For an acute attack in a client with chronic obstructive pulmonary disease, the provider should have at least phone contact within 24 to 48 hours.

139. *Answer:* c (diagnosis/endocrine/NAS)

Rationale: Hyperthyroidism is confirmed by a low thyroid-stimulating hormone level and a high thyroxine level.

140. *Answer:* d (evaluation/reproductive/childbearing female/pretest)

Rationale: After initial treatment is evaluated and the client is responding well, annual assessment of primary dysmenorrhea should include a pelvic examination and Papanicolau smear. Sonography, laparoscopy, and endometrial biopsy are indicated only if additional symptoms develop or pelvic pathology is identified.

141. *Answer:* b (assessment/history/reproductive/childbearing female)

Rationale: Although a woman with diabetes is predisposed toward candidiasis, insulin does not increase that risk. Depo-Provera and antihypertensives also do not cause candidiasis. The high estrogen content of oral contraceptives may predispose a woman toward yeast infections.

142. *Answer:* c (evaluation/cardiovascular/NAS)

Rationale: Once the congestive heart failure is compensated, a client should be followed up every 3 months with evaluation that includes subjective symptoms and physical examination, or as needed for recurrent symptoms. If adjustment and titration of medications are occurring, a client may need to be seen more frequently, according to individual needs.

143. *Answer:* a (assessment/physical examination/integumentary/NAS)

Rationale: Warts are commonly firm, skin-colored papules. Vesicles painful to touch are seen in herpes, oval lesions are characteristic of pityriasis rosea, and round, pearly papules are descriptive of molluscum contagiosum.

144. *Answer:* c (assessment/history/neurologic/aging adult)

Rationale: A gradual, progressive decline in mental abilities is consistent with Alzheimer's disease. Estrogen has been identified as a protective factor. It has not been demonstrated that depression is a cause of Alzheimer's disease, although it may be a complicating factor. The client's covering up of memory loss, rather than concern about forgetfulness, is more consistent with the pathologic memory loss seen in Alzheimer's disease.

145. *Answer:* c (plan/management/client education/multisystem/NAS)

Rationale: With caution, DEET may be used for anyone.

146. *Answer:* a (diagnosis/gastrointestinal/adult)

Rationale: The abdominal pain and diarrhea or constipation symptoms are associated with diverticulosis. The normal WBC count is helpful to rule out an inflammation, such as diverticulitis. Appendicitis always is a possibility but probably would exhibit right-sided abdominal discomfort. Ulcerative colitis is also a possibility but usually features more severe symptoms (e.g., blood or mucus in stools).

147. *Answer:* b (plan/management/musculoskeletal/NAS)

Rationale: Osteoarthritis is not usually an inflammatory condition, although minimal inflammation may be evident on occasion. Acetaminophen, an analgesic, is therefore the best treatment.

148. *Answer:* c (issues/scope/standards of practice)

Rationale: Medicaid is a state-funded (with federal matching funds) medical assistance program for low-income persons. Other choices—only for pregnant women, administered by third-party insurers, and for older adults—are incorrect. The program for older adults is Medicare.

149. *Answer:* b (health promotion/lifestyle/stress management/wellness/NAS)

Rationale: Stressors may be negative or positive and may be chronic in nature. Stressors affect all age groups.

150. *Answer:* c (assessment/physical examination/wellness/childbearing female)

Rationale: The fundal height in centimeters should be equal to the number of weeks of gestation plus or minus 2 cm.

151. *Answer:* b (plan/management/therapeutics/pharmacologic/childbearing female/pretest)

Rationale: Amoxicillin is the drug of choice for pregnant or lactating women and for children younger than 8 years.

152. *Answer:* a (wellness/risk factor identification/childbearing female)

Rationale: Women in these two age groups are at risk for unwanted pregnancy, unlike those in the oldest age group. Also, women older than 64 years are more likely to be retired and therefore not require an occupational blood and body fluid exposure history.

153. *Answer:* c (health promotion/primary prevention/wellness/adult)

Rationale: Young males are at risk for car crashes. Promoting the practice of not drinking and driving helps to reduce the risk of having a motor vehicle crash.

154. *Answer:* b (plan/health promotion/community factors)

Rationale: Close contacts only should be immunized. Casual contacts do not need immunization. Hepatitis A virus immunization would help to prevent an epidemic, so both not telling anyone and assuming that an epidemic will occur are incorrect.

155. *Answer:* a (plan/management/diagnostics/respiratory/NAS)

Rationale: A chest x-ray examination is indicated for all clients with acute dyspnea because it best identifies the cause.

156. *Answer:* b (plan/management/consultation/endocrinologic/NAS)

Rationale: The nurse practitioner is not responsible for establishing the final diagnosis and initiating the treatment.

157. *Answer:* a (assessment/history/respiratory/child)

Rationale: Unusually high concentrations of sodium and chloride in sweat and saliva are a unique characteristic of cystic fibrosis. All the other choices represent normal variation.

158. *Answer:* a (evaluation/integumentary/NAS)

Rationale: Warn clients that discoloration will remain for several months after treatment.

159. *Answer:* b (diagnosis/neurologic/adult)

Rationale: Temporal arteritis, tension-type headache, cluster headache, and subdural hematoma need to be considered in the differential diagnosis for the symptoms presented. There is not enough information provided to eliminate them from the diagnostic possibilities. Typically, trigeminal neuralgia is precipitated by exposure to some type of environmental irritant and causes a severe, disabling, lancinating pain in the distribution of cranial nerve V (division 1 or 2) that lasts a few seconds to minutes, interspersed with a minute or so relief between attacks of pain.

160. *Answer:* c (counseling concepts/nurse-client relationships/pretest)

Rationale: Exploring new ways of coping is important in crisis resolution.

161. *Answer:* a (evaluation/gastrointestinal/NAS)

Rationale: Slow weight loss is important in preventing attacks. Eating a low-fat and low-cholesterol diet has not been proved to be of benefit in preventing attacks. Gallstones will not dissolve. Actigall has no effect on weight loss.

162. *Answer:* a (plan/management/therapeutics/nonpharmacologic/adult)

Rationale: The unassisted lifting recommendations are no more than 60 pounds for women with mild pain.

163. *Answer:* d (assessment/history/endocrine/adult/pretest)

Rationale: Descriptions of the enlargement and of its relationship to other symptoms are key diagnostic data. Noting the date of the last physical examination helps to date the finding.

164. *Answer:* a (wellness/history/pretest)

Rationale: Although rapport may be established through the conversation for history taking and cognitive ability may be assessed to some degree, one of the primary goals is to identify risk factors.

165. *Answer:* c (issues/research utilization)

Rationale: The other three uses of research require application of scientific knowledge as part of practice, policy, or protocol.

166. *Answer:* c (health promotion/lifestyle/stress management/wellness/child)

Rationale: Children list feeling sick, having nothing to do, not having enough money, being pressured to get good grades, and feeling left out of the group as their major stressors.

167. *Answer:* c (issues/counseling/pretest)

Rationale: The aim of therapeutic communication is to facilitate a helping relationship that will foster problem solving and effective coping.

168. *Answer:* a (management/therapeutics/pharmacologic/wellness/adult)

Rationale: Clients with diabetes who have a chronic pulmonary disorder are more at risk from an influenza episode than from the other infectious diseases.

169. *Answer:* a (plan/pharmacologic/wellness/management/pharmacologic)

Rationale: Pregnancy is a contraindication for hormone replacement therapy. Because hormone replacement therapy may improve cardiovascular status, an ECG and a cardiac enzyme panel are not necessary before starting hormone replacement therapy. A chest x-ray film would not be useful.

170. *Answer:* c (plan/management/therapeutics/nonpharmacologic/psychosocial/NAS/pretest)

Rationale: Providing information in a simple and calm manner will assist the client in focusing on the topic, increasing understanding, and decreasing anxiety.

171. *Answer:* d (health promotion/plan/wellness/management/therapeutics/health-promoting behaviors/adolescent/pretest)

Rationale: Drug therapy should be reserved for those clients who have no success in lowering cholesterol, low-density lipoprotein, and triglyceride levels by the use of diet and exercise.

172. *Answer:* b (issues/scope and standards of practice)

Rationale: The standards of care identify criteria on which nursing can be evaluated.

173. *Answer:* c (health promotion/diagnosis/wellness/management/client education/NAS/pretest)

Rationale: Diabetes produces secondary hyperlipidemia. Male gender is a risk factor but not a cause. Heredity and genetic metabolic disorders produce primary hyperlipidemia.

174. *Answer:* d (evaluation/musculoskeletal/NAS/pretest)

Rationale: Although weight loss may be a desirable goal, obesity is a protective factor for osteoporosis.

175. *Answer:* d (plan/management/therapeutics/musculoskeletal/child/pretest)

Rationale: For children with spinal curvature ≥40 degrees, surgical management with a Harrington rod is usually necessary.

PART VI

Additional System Review Questions

Questions and Answers by Body System

HEAD, EYE, EAR, NOSE, AND THROAT

REVIEW QUESTIONS

1. In which individual is acute sinusitis most likely to develop?

   a. 11-year-old female swimmer
   b. 36-year-old female with a penicillin allergy
   c. 21-year-old female day care worker
   d. 48-year-old male truck driver

2. Which of the following objective findings is **not** associated with acute sinusitis?

   a. Pain with percussion on frontal sinuses
   b. Purulent nasal cavity discharge
   c. Periorbital edema
   d. Pain with movement of pinna

3. An adult client comes in with typical presenting symptoms of acute sinusitis. What would be your next step in confirming the diagnosis?

   a. Allergy testing
   b. EENT referral
   c. Nasal mucous smear
   d. None indicated for typical presenting symptoms

4. Initial treatment of sinusitis does **not** include:

   a. Decongestants
   b. Antibiotics
   c. Antihistamines
   d. Nasal corticosteroids

5. Which of the following findings on funduscopic examination would warrant ophthalmologic referral?

   a. Arteriovenous ratio of 4:5
   b. Yellow-white physiologic cup
   c. Pulsation of veins at disk crossing
   d. Cup-to-disk ratio greater in left eye than in right eye

6. Wide-angle glaucoma is conservatively managed with miotic eyedrops. Which of the following is an example of a miotic?

   a. Timolol (Timoptic)
   b. Atropine
   c. Acetazolamide (Diamox)
   d. Pilocarpine (Isopto Carpine)

7. A 78-year-old man comes in for hypertension follow-up. He tells you that he saw an ophthalmologist 3 months ago and was told that he had wide-angle glaucoma. Client teaching related to his glaucoma would include which of the following?

   a. Discussion of need for surgery in the future
   b. Reminder to report any signs of eye redness
   c. Suggestion that he use glasses instead of contact lens
   d. Avoidance of OTC cold medications

8. The drug of choice for the treatment of acute epiglottitis is:

   a. Racemic epinephrine by nebulizer
   b. Penicillin VK
   c. Cefotaxime
   d. Ciprofloxacin (Cipro), IV

9. Mrs. Smith comes to your clinic with the report of a sore throat, body aches, and fever. During your examination, you note a grayish membrane on the uvula and pharynx. You suspect that Mrs. Smith has:

a. Streptococcal pharyngitis
b. Infectious mononucleosis
c. Diphtheria
d. *Candida*

10. The most immediate life threatening complication of epiglottitis is:

a. Airway occlusion
b. Meningitis
c. Bacteremia
d. Dehydration

11. Mr. Jones comes to your clinic with a severe sore throat. You suspect epiglottitis and obtain a lateral neck x-ray film. A finding suggestive of epiglottitis would be:

a. Narrowing between C-4 and C-5
b. Narrowing of the airway above C-3
c. Patchy white area at the level of C-3
d. "Thumbprint" sign at the level of C-5

12. Mr. D.B. is a 49-year-old business executive who comes in with a report of "sores in my mouth" for several days. His review of systems indicates that he has been having irritable bowel–like symptoms for several days. He also states that he has been having burning sensations in his mouth before an eruption. He admits to being under a great deal of work stress. Your examination reveals several small (5 mm), superficial, oval, yellow-gray lesions with a fibrinoid center on the oral mucosa. In the differential diagnosis, you would be highly suspicious of which of the following?

a. Aphthous ulcers
b. Gingivitis
c. Oral candidiasis
d. Acute necrotizing ulcerative gingivitis

13. Aphthous ulcers are thought to be caused by which of the following?

a. Herpes simplex virus
b. *Candida albicans*
c. *Borrelia vincentii*
d. It is unknown at this time what causes these ulcers.

14. The nurse practitioner has been monitoring an 88-year-old man for several years for cataracts. In determining the appropriateness for referral for surgery, which of the following factors would be the most important to consider?

a. Underlying pathology related to the age of the client
b. Effect of the visual defect on activities of daily living
c. Whether the client is still driving
d. Ability of the client to perform self-care

15. Which of the following is true regarding appropriate management of the client who has bilateral cataracts?

a. Mydriatics are not generally helpful in improving overall vision.
b. Magnification devices are not helpful for clients with cataracts.
c. Improved lighting may delay the need for surgery.
d. Clients with bilateral vision worse than 20/40 should not drive a motor vehicle.

16. Which of the following sets of symptoms is associated with allergic conjunctivitis?

a. Mucopurulent discharge, rhinorrhea, and marked itching
b. Mucopurulent discharge, marked itching, and bilateral eye involvement
c. Watery discharge, marked itching, and seasonal occurrence
d. Watery discharge, rhinorrhea, and unilateral eye involvement

17. Your examination of your client has revealed that the left eye has inflamed conjunctiva, watery discharge, and small vesicles on the lower, outer eyelid. You have also noted two large herpetic lesions on the client's lower lip. Your diagnosis would be which of the following?

a. Chemical conjunctivitis caused by bacitracin zinc–neomycin sulfate–polymyxin B sulfate (Neosporin) eye solution
b. Herpes simplex conjunctivitis
c. Bacterial conjunctivitis caused by gonorrhea
d. Allergic conjunctivitis

ANSWERS AND RATIONALES

1. **Answer:** a (assessment/history/HEENT/NAS)
   Rationale: Sinusitis often develops in those who swim and dive. A penicillin allergy has no bearing on the development of sinusitis, nor do driving a truck and working in a day care center.

2. **Answer:** d (assessment/physical examination/HEENT/NAS)
   Rationale: Pain on movement of the pinna is not indicative of acute sinusitis, but the other choices are.

3. **Answer:** d (diagnosis/HEENT/adult)
   Rationale: No further diagnostic workup is necessary for typical presenting symptoms of acute sinusitis.

4. **Answer:** c (HEENT/plan/NAS)
   Rationale: Antihistamines are not recommended in the treatment of sinusitis because they thicken secretions.

5. **Answer:** d (assessment/history/HEENT/NAS)
   Rationale: Asymmetry between the eyes of the physiologic cup may be an early indicator of glaucoma.

6. **Answer:** d (plan/HEENT/NAS)
   Rationale: Pilocarpine causes pupillary constriction and is thus classified as a miotic. Timoptic is a beta-blocker, atropine is a sympathomimetic, and acetazolamide is a carbonic anhydrase inhibitor.

7. **Answer:** d (plan/HEENT/aging adult)
   Rationale: OTC cold medications may precipitate acute glaucoma in selected clients.

8. **Answer:** c (plan/management/pharmacologic/HEENT/NAS)
   Rationale: Cefotaxime is the antibiotic drug of choice for the treatment of epiglottitis. Racemic epinephrine is used in the treatment of croup. Penicillin VK is used in the treatment of streptococcal pharyngitis. Ciprofloxacin is not generally used in the treatment of upper airway infections.

9. **Answer:** c (assessment/physical examination/HEENT/NAS)
   Rationale: Although rare, diphtheria features a classic pattern of blue-white or grayish membranes of the uvula and pharynx. Streptococcal pharyngitis, *Candida,* and mononucleosis may feature redness or white exudate.

10. **Answer:** a (diagnosis/HEENT/NAS)
    Rationale: Epiglottitis results in rapid swelling of the epiglottis. Massive swelling of the epiglottis may result in obstruction or occlusion of the airway, an immediately life-threatening event.

11. **Answer:** d (diagnosis/HEENT/NAS)
    Rationale: "Thumbprint" sign is suggestive of inflammation of the epiglottis. The epiglottis on the adult sits at approximately C-5, whereas in the child it is at C-3. Narrowing of the airway above these sites is suggestive of the inflammation associated with croup.

12. **Answer:** a (diagnosis/HEENT/adult)
    Rationale: This case features a classic constellation of presenting symptoms and description of the lesions. Gingivitis *(b)* is inflammation of the gum line. Ulcers are not normally present. Oral candidiasis *(c)* features white "patches" along the oral mucosa, especially on the tongue. The white plaques are easily scraped away. Although stress plays a major role in the development of acute necrotizing ulcerative gingivitis *(d)*, acute necrotizing ulcerative gingivitis is a bacterial infection that begins between the teeth and then spreads laterally.

13. **Answer:** d (diagnosis/HEENT/NAS)
    Rationale: The causal agent of aphthous ulcers remains unclear to this day. It was once thought to be related to the herpes simplex virus *(a)*, but it has since been determined that this is not the case. *C. albicans (b)* is present in oral candidiasis (thrush). *B. vincentii (c)* is a spirochete that is associated with acute necrotizing ulcerative gingivitis.

14. **Answer:** b (plan/HEENT/aging adult)
    Rationale: Quality of life related to degree of sensory deprivation from visual defects is an important consideration in determining whether surgery is indicated.

15. *Answer:* d (plan/HEENT/NAS)
Rationale: Visual acuity of at least 20/40 is necessary to safely drive a motor vehicle.

16. *Answer:* c (assessment/history/HEENT/NAS)
Rationale: Watery discharge, marked itching, and seasonal occurrence are likely with allergic con-junctivitis. Mucopurulent discharge and unilateral eye involvement occur in bacterial conjunctivitis.

17. *Answer:* b (diagnosis/HEENT/NAS)
Rationale: Vesicles on the lower lid and the her-petic lesions on the mouth of the client are indica-tive of herpes simplex conjunctivitis.

RESPIRATORY SYSTEM

REVIEW QUESTIONS

1. Education for a client with chronic obstructive pulmonary disease would include all the following **except:**

a. Use of metered-dose inhalers
b. Pursed-lip breathing
c. Blood pressure monitoring
d. Exercise and coping strategies

2. An atrial gallop rhythm may be associated with:

a. Cor pulmonale
b. Heart failure
c. Sinusitis
d. Coronary artery disease

3. Which of the following does **not** increase one's risk for having bronchitis?

a. High-fat diet
b. Smoking
c. Environmental allergies
d. Immunosuppression

4. Two weeks after bronchitis was diagnosed, a client returns with a persistent, dry, hacking cough. The most likely diagnosis is:

a. Environmental allergies
b. Pneumonia
c. Hyperreactive airways
d. Chronic obstructive pulmonary disease

5. When eliciting a health history from a client with a cough, which of the following symptoms are **least** important?

a. Bloody sputum and weight loss
b. Decreased appetite and nausea
c. Fever and productive cough
d. Tickle in throat, frequent clearing of the throat

6. When evaluating a 7-year-old for possible cystic fibrosis, the family nurse practitioner would most need to assess which of the following?

a. Frequency and severity of respiratory prob-lems, dietary history, and frequency and char-acter of stools
b. Headache, facial pain, and halitosis
c. Sore throat, fever, nausea, vomiting, and ab-dominal pain
d. Family history of asthma or allergies, skin rash, and known triggers of respiratory distress

7. Which system is least important to include in the physical examination of a client with a cough?

a. Cardiac
b. HEENT
c. Genitourinary
d. Pulmonary

8. Which of the following findings on physical ex-amination would indicate the need for sweat testing to rule out cystic fibrosis?

a. Abdominal tenderness and guarding in a 12-year-old
b. Rectal prolapse in a 3-year-old
c. Bronchiolitis in a 6-month-old
d. Recurrent vomiting in a 2-month-old

9. A 17-year-old comes in for evaluation of acute dyspnea. She is breathing rapidly, appears appre-hensive, and states that her hands, feet, and mouth feel numb and tingly. What is the most likely diag-nosis?

a. Spontaneous pneumothorax
b. Hyperventilation
c. Foreign-body aspiration
d. Carbon monoxide intoxication

10. Absent breath sounds are indicative of:

a. Pneumothorax
b. Chronic obstructive pulmonary disease
c. Pneumonia
d. Pulmonary embolus

11. Which of the following physical findings would **not** usually be found in a client with chronic obstructive pulmonary disease?

a. Barrel chest
b. Clubbing
c. Cyanosis
d. Increased fremitus

12. Referral should be made for all clients with chronic obstructive pulmonary disease **except** for clients who:

a. Have alpha₁-antitrypsin deficiency
b. Have cor pulmonale
c. Have asthma
d. Are starting to use steroid inhalers

13. Which of the following clients is least likely to have bronchitis develop?

a. 5-year-old whose parents smoke
b. 42-year-old female who is taking steroids for rheumatoid arthritis
c. 60-year-old with hypertension
d. 75-year-old with emphysema

14. A 36-year-old prison guard reports cough, fever, fatigue, and shortness of breath. What diagnosis must you consider?

a. Congestive heart failure
b. Bronchiectasis
c. Tuberculosis
d. Pneumonia

15. Which client is most likely to need an antibiotic for the treatment of bronchitis?

a. 12-year-old with fever, clear sputum, and substernal chest discomfort
b. 44-year-old with pharyngitis, postnasal drainage, cough, and wheezing
c. 60-year-old with purulent sputum, fever, chills, and shortness of breath
d. 22-year-old with fatigue, cough, decreased appetite, and chills

16. The most likely differential diagnosis for a 47-year-old male with chronic cough, bitter taste in the mouth, and hoarseness is:

a. Psychogenic cough
b. Impacted cerumen in external auditory canal
c. Chronic bronchitis
d. Gastroesophageal reflux

17. The long-term treatment plan for a client with cystic fibrosis would include:

a. Regular exercise, low-fat diet, and isolation from other children
b. Daily antihistamines, avoidance of allergens, and corticosteroids by metered-dose inhaler
c. Daily use of the vibratory vest, postural drainage, and high-protein, high-calorie diet
d. Home schooling, no participation in sports, and routine chest x-ray examinations every 6 months

18. Helen, a 20-year-old with cystic fibrosis, has been treated for *Pseudomonas* pneumonia. She should be instructed to return for follow-up:

a. As needed if symptoms fail to improve
b. After completing the antibiotics and as needed
c. One week after starting the antibiotics
d. No follow-up is necessary if symptoms subside.

ANSWERS AND RATIONALES

1. *Answer:* c (plan/management/client education/respiratory/NAS)
Rationale: It is important that practitioners teach pursed-lip breathing and exercise techniques to maximize oxygen intake. Coping skills help to decrease anxiety. Proper use of a metered-dose inhaler helps to deposit medication in the lung, rather than in the device or the mouth. If clients have difficulty with this task, a spacer device can be prescribed.

2. *Answer:* a (assessment/physical examination/respiratory/NAS)
Rationale: An atrial gallop rhythm may be associated with cor pulmonale.

3. *Answer:* a (assessment/history/respiratory/NAS)
Rationale: A high-fat diet does not increase the risk of bronchitis, whereas smoking, allergies, and immunosuppression do increase the risk.

4. *Answer:* c (diagnosis/respiratory/NAS)
Rationale: A transition from a productive cough to a dry, hacking cough suggests that the cough is caused by hyperreactive airways, not necessarily by an infectious process.

5. *Answer:* b (assessment/history/respiratory/NAS)
Rationale: Decreased appetite and nausea are less likely to be among the clinical presenting symptoms associated with important causes of cough.

6. *Answer:* a (assessment/history/respiratory/child)
Rationale: Headache, facial pain, and halitosis are more indicative of sinusitis, whereas sore throat, fever, nausea, vomiting, and abdominal pain would point to streptococcal pharyngitis. Family history of asthma, history of skin rash, and environmental triggers of respiratory distress would suggest asthma. Cystic fibrosis commonly has presenting symptoms of steatorrhea, poor weight gain, and recurrent respiratory infections.

7. *Answer:* c (assessment/physical examination/respiratory/NAS)
Rationale: An examination of the cardiac and respiratory systems, as well as HEENT examination, may narrow the differential diagnosis.

8. *Answer:* b (assessment/physical examination/respiratory/child)
Rationale: Abdominal pain and guarding are more indicative of appendicitis, bronchiolitis is a common problem in children younger than 2 years old and an isolated incident does not suggest more severe pathology, and recurrent vomiting in a 2-month-old in the absence of coughing suggests gastrointestinal pathology. Cystic fibrosis is the most common cause of rectal prolapse.

9. *Answer:* b (diagnosis/respiratory/NAS)
Rationale: A history of light-headedness and paresthesias of the perioral area or distal extremities suggest hyperventilation syndrome.

10. *Answer:* a (diagnosis/respiratory/NAS)
Rationale: The lung is collapsed and thus not against the chest wall; breath sounds therefore will not be heard.

11. *Answer:* d (assessment/physical examination/respiratory/adult)
Rationale: Decreased or absent fremitus is found because of hyperinflation (sound travels much more slowly).

12. *Answer:* d (plan/management/therapeutics/pharmacologic/respiratory/NAS)
Rationale: Steroid inhalers are important in treatment and management of chronic obstructive pulmonary disease and can be ordered and managed by nurse practitioners.

13. *Answer:* c (assessment/history/respiratory/NAS)
Rationale: Smoking, immunosuppression, and chronic obstructive pulmonary disease increase the risk for development of bronchitis.

14. *Answer:* c (diagnosis/respiratory/NAS)
Rationale: The client is at risk for tuberculosis because of his occupation.

15. *Answer:* c (plan/management/therapeutics/pharmacologic/respiratory/NAS)
Rationale: Colored sputum accompanied by systemic symptoms is more likely to necessitate antibiotics.

16. *Answer:* d (diagnosis/respiratory/adult)
Rationale: These symptoms are typical of gastroesophageal reflux.

17. *Answer:* c (plan/management/therapeutics/non-pharmacologic/respiratory/child)
Rationale: Clients with cystic fibrosis have higher than normal caloric intake needs. Normal intake of fat is usually tolerated well and aids in weight gain. Antihistamines should be avoided because they dry secretions and can cause a mucous plug. Although children with cystic fibrosis are more susceptible to infection, normal growth and developmental goals dictate association with peers.

18. *Answer:* b (evaluation/respiratory/adolescent)
Rationale: A major goal of treatment is the prevention of complications from recurrent or intractable respiratory tract infections. Clients with cystic fibrosis have increased susceptibility to infection, as well as decreased sensitivity to antibiotics. Follow-up is necessary to determine whether the infection has cleared.

CARDIOVASCULAR SYSTEM

REVIEW QUESTIONS

1. The most likely cause of chest pain in a 25-year-old new mother is:

   a. Myocardial infarction
   b. Pulmonary embolus
   c. Gastroesophageal reflux disease
   d. Angina

2. Which of the following should be ordered for the client who has a history of chest pain and is being sent home?

   a. Digitalis
   b. Penicillin
   c. Amiodarone
   d. Nitroglycerine tablets, SL

3. The primary reason to determine the cause of a transient ischemic attack and treat it if possible is to:

   a. Decrease the number of transient ischemic attacks
   b. Decrease the number of heart attacks
   c. Increase function
   d. Decrease the possibility of stroke

4. Which of the following diagnoses is important to keep controlled in the client with a transient ischemic attack?

   a. Cataracts
   b. Hypertension
   c. Hypolipidemia
   d. Hypoproteinemia

5. Reversible ischemic neurologic deficit is defined as lasting longer than:

   a. 24 hours and less than 7 days
   b. 2 hours and less than 24 hours
   c. 24 hours and less than 2 days
   d. 20 minutes and less than 3 days

6. All the following are important questions to ask the young female who comes in with left-side weakness **except:**

   a. Use of oral contraceptives
   b. Recent delivery

   c. History of recent deep venous thrombosis
   d. History of pelvic inflammatory disease

7. If the head CT scan results are normal and the client is older, what other radiologic test will likely give the most significant information with respect to a transient ischemic attack?

   a. Carotid artery Doppler study
   b. Chest x-ray film
   c. Pneumoencephalography
   d. IV pyelography

8. If the client with transient ischemic attack has polycythemia, one treatment would be to have the client:

   a. Put on a regimen of bed rest
   b. Undergo phlebotomy
   c. Undergo carotid endarterectomy
   d. Undergo cardioversion

9. Why can aortic stenosis lead to syncope?

   a. The heart cannot beat properly.
   b. The cardiac output is diminished and the brain has decreased blood flow.
   c. The cardiac output is increased and the brain is overperfused.
   d. Blood is shunted away from the brain by increased cardiac output.

10. All the following laboratory tests may yield useful information in diagnosing the cause of syncope **except:**

   a. Complete blood cell count
   b. Electrolyte levels
   c. Glucose level
   d. Liver function tests

11. The blood pressure of a client who is supine is 140/80 mm Hg with a heart rate of 86 beats/min. When the client is placed in the standing position, the blood pressure is 96/60 mm Hg with a heart rate of 120 beats/min. What is the probable reason that this client has experienced syncope?

   a. Pulmonary embolus
   b. Vasovagal syncope
   c. Psychogenic syncope
   d. Orthostatic hypotension

12. If a specific cause of syncope is not discovered initially, what medication should be prescribed during the workup phase?

    a. Acetaminophen
    b. Nonsteroidal antiinflammatory drugs
    c. Antevert
    d. Aspirin

13. Which of the following physical findings would **not** usually be found in a client with deep vein thrombophlebitis?

    a. Positive Homans' sign
    b. Bilateral extremity edema
    c. Low-grade fever
    d. Prominent superficial veins

14. Venography is useful in confirming the diagnosis of:

    a. Ruptured popliteal muscle
    b. Cellulitis
    c. Deep vein thrombophlebitis
    d. Baker's cyst

15. Treatment of superficial thrombophlebitis includes:

    a. Antithrombotic therapy
    b. Physician referral
    c. Aspirin or other nonsteroidal antiinflammatory drug
    d. Hospitalization

16. All the following can be underlying causes of a transient ischemic attack **except:**

    a. Atrial fibrillation
    b. Hypertension
    c. Hyponatremia
    d. Urinary tract infection

17. A test to determine the competency of the heart valves is:

    a. Chest x-ray film
    b. Echocardiography
    c. Carotid artery Doppler study
    d. Holter monitoring

18. The most common cause of syncope in older adults is:

    a. Drug effect
    b. Myocardial infarction

    c. Pulmonary embolus
    d. Tetralogy of Fallot

19. Postprandial hypotension can occur under which circumstances:

    a. Antihypertensive medications are taken just before or with the meal.
    b. A high-carbohydrate, high-protein meal is eaten.
    c. Nonsteroidal antiinflammatory drugs are taken with the meal.
    d. A high-fat, high-carbohydrate meal is eaten.

20. Low-yield tests for working up syncope include:

    a. Spinal tap
    b. Echocardiography
    c. ECG
    d. Complete blood cell count

21. Which of the following sets of classes of antihypertensives has been shown to decrease cardiovascular mortality and morbidity in the treatment of hypertension?

    a. Calcium antagonists and alpha-blockers
    b. Diuretics and beta-blockers
    c. Diuretics and calcium antagonists
    d. Angiotensin-converting enzyme inhibitors and beta-blockers

22. Normotensive clients should be evaluated for hypertension every:

    a. 1 to 2 years
    b. 6 to 9 months
    c. 6 months
    d. 3 to 6 months

23. Which of the following statements is true?

    a. Clients with early primary hypertension generally report multiple symptoms.
    b. Hypertension is a disease that occurs more frequently in wealthy, well-educated populations.
    c. Secondary hypertension is more common in children than adults.
    d. A family history of cerebrovascular disease is not relevant to hypertension.

24. Which of the following best describes the pain of a myocardial infarction?

   a. Pain is severe, with an increased duration, and usually is unrelieved by rest and nitroglycerin.

   b. Pain occurs with activity and is relieved by rest with or without nitroglycerin.

   c. Pain occurs at rest and is relieved by nitroglycerin.

   d. Pain occurs after eating and is associated with reflux.

25. A 46-year-old male comes in with an acute myocardial infarction. On physical examination, you auscultate an S_4 gallop. Why does this occur?

   a. Papillary muscle dysfunction

   b. Left ventricular dilatation

   c. Increased left ventricular filling pressure

   d. Reduced left ventricular compliance

26. Which of the following is **not** true of beta-blockers in the situation of an acute myocardial infarction?

   a. They reduce mortality and morbidity during an evolving infarct.

   b. They decrease myocardial oxygen demand.

   c. They may reduce the size of the infarct.

   d. They cannot be given concomitantly with thrombolytics.

27. Which of the following is **not** true of exercise stress testing?

   a. It assesses functional capacity.

   b. It assesses efficacy of the current medication regimen.

   c. It provides risk stratification.

   d. It determines the percentage of blockage present in the coronary arteries.

28. Common complications of administration of prostaglandin E_1 include all the following **except:**

   a. Hypotension

   b. Hypertension

   c. Apnea

   d. Bradycardia

29. The most common congenital lesion noted after the first week of life is:

   a. Atrial septal defect

   b. Ventricular septal defect

   c. Patent ductus arteriosus

   d. Tetralogy of Fallot

30. Of the following, the congenital heart lesion most likely to be associated with cyanosis is:

   a. Coarctation of the aorta

   b. Truncus arteriosus

   c. Atrial septal defect

   d. Ventricular septal defect

31. A 2-year-old male is brought to the office. The mother reports that every time her son cries, he becomes cyanotic and squats until he is no longer blue. The most likely cardiac defect is:

   a. Tetralogy of Fallot

   b. Transposition of the great arteries with a ventricular septal defect

   c. Ventricular septal defect

   d. Total anomalous pulmonary venous return

ANSWERS AND RATIONALES

1. Answer: b (diagnosis/cardiovascular/adult)
Rationale: Young females who have just delivered may produce emboli from the placenta; the most likely place for these to cause occlusion is the lung.

2. Answer: d (plan/management/pharmacologic/cardiovascular/adult)
Rationale: Nitroglycerin tablets are ordered so that the client can begin therapy before any damage occurs. It also helps in the diagnosis of coronary chest pain versus noncoronary chest pain.

3. Answer: d (plan/management/cardiovascular/aging adult)
Rationale: Because a transient ischemic attack is often a precursor of a stroke, it is important to identify and treat the underlying cause in an effort to prevent stroke.

4. Answer: b (plan/management/cardiovascular/adult)
Rationale: Because of the endothelial damage that occurs with prolonged hypertension, it is important to keep this condition controlled.

5. Answer: a (diagnosis/cardiovascular/NAS)
Rationale: Reversible ischemic neurologic deficits last longer than transient ischemic attacks but are not classified as strokes. By definition, they last less than 7 days, and the neurologic deficit reverses without evidence of stroke.

6. *Answer:* d (assessment/history/cardiovascular/adult)

Rationale: All the other problems can result in emboli traveling to the brain, causing a transient ischemic attack.

7. *Answer:* a (plan/management/diagnostics/cardiovascular/aging adult)

Rationale: The most likely site of transient ischemic attack on the list is the carotid artery. The carotid artery study will therefore likely yield the most information.

8. *Answer:* b (plan/management/nonpharmacologic/cardiovascular/NAS)

Rationale: Phlebotomy decreases the number of red blood cells and thereby decreases the viscosity of the blood and thus the chance of clotting.

9. *Answer:* b (diagnosis/cardiovascular/NAS)

Rationale: Cardiac output is diminished because of the stenosis and the brain has decreased blood flow, causing a syncopal episode.

10. *Answer:* d (plan/management/diagnostics/cardiovascular/NAS)

Rationale: Causes of syncope include anemia (complete blood cell count), hyponatremia (electrolyte levels), and hypoglycemia (glucose level).

11. *Answer:* d (diagnosis/cardiovascular/NAS)

Rationale: The client has a significant decrease in blood pressure from supine to standing, with a significant increase in pulse rate.

12. *Answer:* d (plan/management/pharmacologic/cardiovascular/NAS)

Rationale: In the workup phase, aspirin should be given for platelet inhibition in the event that the syncopal episodes are related to transient ischemic attack, coronary artery disease, aortic stenosis, arrhythmias, or a carotid artery problem.

13. *Answer:* b (assessment/physical examination/cardiovascular/NAS)

Rationale: Unilateral extremity edema is most often associated with deep vein thrombophlebitis. A positive Homans' sign, low-grade fever, and prominent superficial veins are more likely to be associated with deep vein thrombophlebitis.

14. *Answer:* c (diagnosis/cardiovascular/NAS)

Rationale: For deep vein thrombophlebitis, venography is considered the standard to which all other techniques are compared. This test is not useful in the diagnoses of the other conditions listed.

15. *Answer:* c (plan/management/cardiovascular/NAS)

Rationale: Treatment consists of local heat, elevation, and aspirin or other nonsteroidal antiinflammatory drugs. Antithrombotic therapy is not indicated, and a physician referral is not necessary for the treatment of superficial thrombophlebitis.

16. *Answer:* d (diagnosis/cardiovascular/NAS)

Rationale: Atrial fibrillation may result in a clot being formed in the atrium; it may then send off smaller emboli that intermittently obstruct vessels in the brain. Hypertension causes damage to the vascular wall that may result in adherence of platelets and fibrin and the formation of a clot. Hyponatremia may result in poor perfusion of the brain tissue as a result of loss of the ability of the cells to perform normal function in response to decreased intracellular sodium and interruption of the sodium-potassium pump.

17. *Answer:* b (plan/management/diagnostics/cardiovascular/NAS)

Rationale: Echocardiography gives information regarding aortic stenosis as well as regurgitation and insufficiency of the other heart valves.

18. *Answer:* a (diagnosis/cardiovascular/aging adult)

Rationale: Many older adults receive antihypertensive medications that may precipitate a syncopal episode. In addition to antihypertensive medications, they may receive other medications, such as digitalis, that may increase their risk for a syncopal episode.

19. *Answer:* a (diagnosis/cardiovascular/NAS)

Rationale: Because of the absorption of medication just before or with the meal, the client may have a syncopal episode related to the medication effect plus increased blood supply to the gut immediately postprandially, resulting in a syncopal episode.

20. *Answer:* a (plan/management/diagnostics/cardiovascular/NAS)

Rationale: Spinal taps usually yield little to no information if the client has had a syncopal episode with no other symptoms.

21. *Answer:* b (plan/management/pharmacologic/cardiovascular/NAS)

Rationale: Although all classes of antihypertensives have been effective in reducing blood pressure, diuretics and beta-blockers have been proved through clinical trials to reduce mortality and morbidity.

22. *Answer:* a (evaluation/cardiovascular/NAS)

Rationale: According to the American College of Physicians, the American Academy of Family Physicians, and the National High Blood Pressure Education Program, blood pressure in normotensive clients should be evaluated every 1 to 2 years.

23. *Answer:* c (diagnosis/cardiovascular/NAS)

Rationale: Hypertension is usually an asymptomatic disease of less-educated, lower socioeconomic status populations. Family history of cerebrovascular diseases may be related to a history of hypertension. Children have a higher prevalence of secondary hypertension than adults.

24. *Answer:* a (assessment/history/cardiovascular/NAS)

Rationale: Myocardial infarction pain is usually unrelieved by rest and nitroglycerin and may occur at rest or with activity. Pain may be accompanied by nausea and vomiting, diaphoresis, palpitations, and dyspnea. Choice *b* is most representative of stable angina. Choice *c* is most representative of unstable angina, and choice *d* suggests a gastrointestinal component.

25. *Answer:* d (assessment/physical examination/cardiovascular/adult)

Rationale: Papillary muscle dysfunction may be detected by a systolic murmur. S_3 gallop is indicative of left ventricular dilatation and an increase in filling pressure. S_4, noted with decreased compliance of the left ventricle and vigorous left atrial contraction, is easily detected frequently in acute myocardial infarction.

26. *Answer:* d (plan/management/pharmacologic/cardiovascular/NAS)

Rationale: Beta-blockers can be given with thrombolytics. Beta-blockers have been found to decrease incidence of reinfarction and ischemia.

27. *Answer:* d (evaluation/cardiovascular/NAS)

Rationale: Modified stress testing may be useful after cardiac catheterization to identify ischemia in the distribution of an artery with a borderline lesion.

28. *Answer:* b (evaluation/cardiovascular/infant)

Rationale: The most commonly seen side effects of prostaglandin E_1 include apnea, bradycardia, and hypotension. The hypotension is the direct effect of the prostaglandin E_1 on the systemic vascular bed. Apnea is likely the result of some primary or secondary effects of prostaglandin E_1 on the central nervous system. Bradycardia is likely caused by the hypoxemia associated with apnea.

29. *Answer:* b (diagnosis/cardiovascular/infant)

Rationale: Although patent ductus arteriosus is the most common heart lesion noted in the first week of life, its incidence decreases dramatically after the first week of life, when it becomes somewhat rare. Ventricular septal defects account for approximately 20% to 25% of all congenital heart defects in this age group. Tetralogy of Fallot is the most common congenital cyanotic heart lesion. Atrial septal defects occur in approximately 10% of cases.

30. *Answer:* b (diagnosis/cardiovascular/infant)

Rationale: All cyanotic heart lesions must have some degree of shunting of blood from the right to the left side of the circulation without oxygenation within the lungs. Truncus arteriosus is characterized by a common outlet from the right and left ventricles, which allows mixing of oxygenated and deoxygenated blood. The degree of cyanosis is proportional to the percentage of blood shunted from the right ventricle directly into the aorta. Although an atrial septal defect and a ventricular septal defect also allow mixing of blood, the pressure gradients determine that shunting occurs from left to right. Oxygenated blood is therefore shunted back to the pulmonary circulation. All blood reaching the systemic circulation is fully oxygenated. Coarctation of the aorta, an obstruction of the aortic outflow tract, does not result in any shunts.

31. **Answer:** a (diagnosis/cardiovascular/infant)
Rationale: Symptoms of a classic "Tet spell" include dyspnea on exertion, cyanosis, and squatting. The cyanosis and the dyspnea are caused by the shunting of blood from right to left during periods of stress or activity (relative hypoxia). The squatting is a Valsalva maneuver, which increases venous return and in turn increases blood through the pulmonary circulation.

GASTROINTESTINAL SYSTEM

REVIEW QUESTIONS

1. While performing an abdominal examination for reported abdominal pain, you note a pause in inspiration. The client reports increased pain. You would note this as:

   a. A positive Murphy's sign
   b. A positive Phalen's sign
   c. Evidence of malingering
   d. A negative McBurney's sign

2. A 50-year-old female comes in for the second time with reports of right upper quadrant pain, nausea, and vomiting after a large meal. The most likely diagnosis would be:

   a. Cholecystitis
   b. Pneumonia
   c. Peptic ulcer disease
   d. Bowel obstruction

3. What objective data would you require from a client with suspected irritable bowel syndrome?

   a. Height and weight
   b. Thorough neurologic evaluation
   c. Stool for ova and parasites
   d. Current medications

4. What is your most likely diagnosis for a client who reports abdominal pain relieved by bowel movements and constipation alternating with diarrhea for the past 4 months?

   a. Diverticulosis
   b. Lactose intolerance
   c. Appendicitis
   d. Irritable bowel syndrome

5. Rose is a 36-year-old female who comes to the health center with a history of tiring easily for the past 2 months. She is married with two children. She works as a full-time secretary and has been able to get through her workday but has to rest as soon as she gets home. She has no energy left for family activities and her libido is low. Which of the following questions is most important during Rose's history?

   a. Tell me about your sleeping and rest patterns.
   b. Tell me about your and your spouse's sexual habits, past and present.
   c. Have you ever had depressive moods diagnosed or treated?
   d. Have you detected any blood loss recently?

6. Differential diagnosis for Rose includes all the following **except:**

   a. Anemia
   b. Viral infection (hepatitis, HIV, cytomegalovirus, Epstein-Barr virus)
   c. Chronic fatigue syndrome
   d. Acquired hyperthyroidism

7. In conducting Rose's examination, which of the following will assist most in narrowing your diagnosis to a viral infection?

   a. Fatigued appearance and weight loss
   b. Dry skin without jaundice
   c. Presence of occult blood with voluntary evacuation
   d. Hepatomegaly and splenomegaly

8. Sally is an 8-year-old female who reports a history of abdominal pain for 2 days. Which of the following observations would assist you in concluding that Sally does **not** have an acute surgical abdomen?

   a. Sally is lying on the stretcher clutching her abdomen.

   b. Sally is able to jump up and down on one foot without difficulty.

   c. It is more painful for Sally when you stop palpating her abdomen.

   d. Sally is nauseated and has vomited three times.

9. Which of the following symptoms is generally **not** associated with a medical cause of abdominal pain?

   a. Obstipation
   b. Constipation
   c. Diarrhea
   d. Pain after vomiting

10. The most common cause of acute abdominal pain in school-age children is:

   a. Appendicitis
   b. Intussusception
   c. Testicular torsion
   d. Incarcerated hernia

11. Clients with abdominal pain and minimal symptoms may be treated:

   a. Initially with bed rest, clear liquids, and analgesics
   b. IV fluids
   c. Nasogastric suction
   d. Syrup of ipecac

12. Instruct the parents of a pediatric client with abdominal pain to return for follow-up if the child:

   a. Can jump up and down
   b. Is able to eat normally
   c. Is walking bent over
   d. Has two hard bowel movements

Situation: The following two questions relate to Ann, 32 years old, who seeks treatment with lack of energy, trouble sleeping, and abdominal pain relieved by bowel movements. Her major problem is constipation alternating with diarrhea for the past 4 months.

13. What additional subjective data do you need for Ann?

   a. Vital signs
   b. Loss of appetite and poor concentration
   c. Length of history of constipation and diarrhea
   d. Complete blood cell count with differential

14. Which of these other subjective data would be most helpful to you in managing irritable bowel syndrome?

   a. Weight loss and travel history
   b. Shortness of breath
   c. Hemorrhoids
   d. Surgeries

15. Howard is a 45-year-old man who comes to the clinic with a report of lower left abdominal pain and constipation. Which would be the most appropriate subjective data to gather?

   a. Complete blood cell count with differential
   b. Temperature, pulse, and blood pressure
   c. History of diarrhea and location of pain
   d. Exercise level and nature of pain

16. What information do you need to seek from Mike, a 42-year-old man with known diverticulosis, who has a temperature of 101° F, a firm abdomen, and no bowel movements?

   a. Any associated nausea or vomiting
   b. History of urinary tract infection
   c. Complete blood cell count with differential
   d. Last chest x-ray film

17. Sarah, a client who is being treated for diverticulosis, comes to the clinic with a temperature of 101° F, a firm abdomen, and no bowel movements. What is your evaluation of her status?

   a. The earlier treatment plan has failed.
   b. Her condition is worsening.
   c. She has influenza and requires symptomatic treatment.
   d. She is constipated and needs an enema.

18. How would you manage a client with diverticulosis?

   a. Metronidazole, 250 mg q 8 hours for 7 days
   b. Acetaminophen–hydrocodone bitartrate (Vicodin), 1 tablet q 6 hours
   c. Loperamide (Imodium), 2 mg after each stool
   d. Referral to a surgeon

19. For clients with symptoms of gallbladder disease, the plan of care would be which of the following?

    a. Schedule surgery.
    b. Order appropriate laboratory tests and imaging studies.
    c. Refer the client.
    d. Monitor the client until three attacks have occurred.

20. How would you evaluate the success of the management plan for a client with irritable bowel syndrome?

    a. Follow-up visit in 1 month, follow-up after surgeries
    b. Follow-up in 2 weeks to assess bowel symptoms
    c. Telephone follow-up in 3 weeks regarding histamine blocker treatment
    d. No follow-up is needed.

21. Lower esophageal sphincter relaxation in gastroesophageal reflux disease may be caused by which of the following?

    a. Chocolate, citrus fruits, and caffeine
    b. Psyllium (Metamucil)
    c. Simethicone (Flatulex)
    d. Histamine-receptor antagonists

22. Which of the following provides the best definition of gastroesophageal reflux disease?

    a. Abnormal herniation in colon wall
    b. Inflamed herniations in colon wall
    c. Functional disturbance of intestinal mobility
    d. Abnormal movement of gastric contents into the esophagus

23. A major complication of gastroesophageal reflux disease is:

    a. Bladder fistula
    b. Stomatitis
    c. Esophagitis
    d. Hemorrhoids

24. A 68-year-old man has burning substernal pain that radiates upward and lasts 30 to 60 minutes after meals. He weighs 210 pounds and his height is 5 feet 9 inches. He takes nifedipine XL, 90 mg qd, for hypertension. He currently has a transdermal nicotine patch to help him quit smoking. Which of the following diagnoses do you suspect is the most likely?

    a. Myocardial infarction
    b. Diverticulitis
    c. Gastroesophageal reflux disease
    d. Irritable bowel syndrome

25. When assessing an infant who has viral gastroenteritis and is mildly dehydrated, what would the family nurse practitioner expect to find?

    a. An irritable child with a slightly depressed anterior fontanelle and a urine specific gravity >1.030
    b. An irritable child with a sunken anterior fontanelle and a 15% weight loss
    c. A normal-appearing child with a slightly increased heart rate, a 5% weight loss, and a flat anterior fontanelle
    d. A normal-appearing child with a slightly increased heart rate, no weight loss, and a flat anterior fontanelle

26. The mother of a 2-week-old infant calls the clinic because she is worried that her son is constipated. With questioning, she admits, "He has three or four soft bowel movements a day, but his face turns red and he pulls up his legs and really strains every time." What should the family nurse practitioner do?

    a. Reassure the mother that this is normal for an infant her son's age.
    b. Have the mother bring her son to the clinic for a complete history and physical examination.
    c. Instruct the mother to offer the baby 2 ounces of apple juice every day.
    d. Have the mother save a stool sample from the next bowel movement and bring it into the clinic for examination.

27. For a client who weighs 10 kg and has a diagnosis of giardiasis, the family nurse practitioner would order:

    a. Metronidazole (Flagyl), 50 mg PO tid
    b. Metronidazole (Flagyl), 150 mg PO tid
    c. Trimethoprim-sulfamethoxazole (Bactrim), 40 mg PO bid
    d. Trimethoprim-sulfamethoxazole (Bactrim), 80 mg PO bid

28. Characteristics of the stool of an adult client with viral gastroenteritis would include all the following **except:**

    a. Positive for blood
    b. Negative for leukocytes
    c. Large, liquid, and frequent
    d. Variable odor, sometimes foul

29. A client comes to the family nurse practitioner with diarrhea. The stools are described as a green, slimy liquid that smells like rotten eggs. The most likely pathogen is:

    a. *Escherichia coli*
    b. *Shigella*
    c. *Salmonella*
    d. Rotavirus

ANSWERS AND RATIONALES

1. *Answer:* a (assessment/physical examination/gastrointestinal/NAS)
Rationale: A positive Murphy's sign is described as a pause on inspiration caused by pain over the gallbladder. Phalen's sign is related to carpal tunnel syndrome. McBurney's point is located over the left lower quadrant and is related to appendicitis.

2. *Answer:* a (diagnosis/gastrointestinal/adult)
Rationale: Cholecystitis is the most likely diagnosis according to symptoms and history. There is no mention of cough or fever, which may indicate pneumonia. Peptic ulcer pain often improves with food intake, and pain is usually more midepigastric. Bowel obstruction may be accompanied by nausea and vomiting, but pain is lower and more generalized.

3. *Answer:* a (assessment/physical examination/gastrointestinal/NAS)
Rationale: Evaluation of weight (and of previous measures) is pertinent to this client. Stool samples for ova and parasites may be justified *after* you have ruled out other possible causes. Ova and parasite tests are expensive procedures to rule out symptoms caused by parasites; a careful history, physical examination, and preliminary laboratory findings usually precede this laboratory test. Current medications are subjective data. A thorough neurologic examination is not warranted for this client.

4. *Answer:* d (diagnosis/gastrointestinal/NAS)
Rationale: The client has no indication of an inflammatory process and you do not have a dietary history to determine whether she has a lactose intolerance. Often diverticulosis is seen with left lower quadrant pain. An important point in her history is the relief of pain after defecation. The best choice of diagnosis is irritable bowel syndrome.

5. *Answer:* b (assessment/history/gastrointestinal/NAS)
Rationale: Although all are important, the most serious complication will be a viral infection or sexually transmitted disease.

6. *Answer:* d (diagnosis/gastrointestinal/NAS)
Rationale: This vague presentation is appropriate for all the diagnoses except hyperthyroidism. The fatigue and lethargy would be appropriate for hypothyroidism, not hyperthyroidism.

7. *Answer:* d (assessment/physical examination/gastrointestinal/NAS)
Rationale: The most specific symptom associated with viral infection is an enlarged spleen, liver, or both. Jaundice may not be present. Occult blood will be present with anemia, not a viral infection.

8. *Answer:* b (assessment/physical examination/gastrointestinal/child)
Rationale: Jumping up and down indicates no peritoneal inflammation and can help rule out an acute surgical abdomen.

9. *Answer:* a (assessment/history/gastrointestinal/NAS)
Rationale: True obstipation is strongly suggestive of a mechanical bowel obstruction.

10. *Answer:* a (diagnosis/gastrointestinal/child)
Rationale: Intussusception, incarcerated hernia, and testicular torsion occur less frequently in the school-age child than does appendicitis.

11. *Answer:* a (plan/management/gastrointestinal/NAS)
Rationale: All therapies but bed rest, clear liquids, and analgesics are appropriate for more severe causes of abdominal pain, such as obstruction, dehydration, and ingestion of toxins.

12. *Answer:* c (evaluation/gastrointestinal/child)
Rationale: All signs except walking bent over are signs seen when the condition of the child with abdominal pain has improved.

13. *Answer:* b (assessment/history/gastrointestinal/adult)
Rationale: Clues such as lack of energy and trouble sleeping are suggestive of depression, which often accompanies irritable bowel syndrome; this needs further exploration. She reports that her constipation and diarrhea have been ongoing for 4 months, so you already have this information. Vital signs and complete blood cell count are objective data.

14. *Answer:* a (assessment/history/gastrointestinal/NAS)
Rationale: Weight loss should not occur with irritable bowel syndrome. If the client has experienced weight loss, concern regarding a gastrointestinal malignancy becomes more prominent. Gastric symptoms of diarrhea are related to giardiasis infection acquired during travel, which needs to be evaluated. The other choices may be relevant to the client's general health but are not most relevant to the management of this case.

15. *Answer:* c (assessment/history/gastrointestinal/adult)
Rationale: A history of diarrhea alternating with constipation and lower left quadrant abdominal pain is indicative of diverticulitis. History of exercise level is important regarding a holistic approach to care, but it is not as important as questions focused on gastrointestinal symptoms. Vital signs and laboratory studies are objective data.

16. *Answer:* a (assessment/history/gastrointestinal/adult)
Rationale: Nausea and vomiting are associated with an acute abdomen. Blood work provides objective data. Last chest x-ray film and urinary infections are past history but are not of prime importance to the client's changing health status.

17. *Answer:* b (evaluation/gastrointestinal/adult)
Rationale: A firm abdomen, no bowel movements, and temperature of 101° F are suggestive of such complications as inflammation and acute abdomen.

18. *Answer:* c (plan/management/therapeutics/gastrointestinal/NAS)
Rationale: Treating the diarrhea is an appropriate choice. You may also need to address management of the constipation. Vicodin is not a mild analgesic, and metronidazole is a treatment for diverticulitis that usually is prescribed in combination with amoxicillin.

19. *Answer:* c (plan/management/consultation/gastrointestinal/NAS)
Rationale: Clients with symptoms should be referred for surgical evaluation. Ordering further laboratory tests and scheduling surgery are best left to the consultant physician. Monitoring for three more attacks is inappropriate and may be harmful because of complications that may arise from a poorly functioning gallbladder.

20. *Answer:* b (evaluation/gastrointestinal/NAS)
Rationale: Assess improvement of the major problem initially in 1 to 2 weeks. This client should not go to surgery or have histamine blockers prescribed. A follow-up visit is likely more appropriate than a telephone call; telephone follow-up may supplement a clinic visit. Regardless, this client does need some follow-up.

21. *Answer:* a (assessment/history/gastrointestinal/NAS)
Rationale: Lower esophageal sphincter relaxation may be caused by food (chocolate, citrus fruit, caffeine, alcohol, and high-fat diets) and drugs. Metamucil, Flatulex, and histamine-receptor antagonists are not known to cause lower esophageal sphincter relaxation.

22. *Answer:* d (diagnosis/gastrointestinal/NAS)

Rationale: Gastroesophageal reflux disease is defined as abnormal reflux of gastric contents into the esophagus. Herniations (and inflammation) in the colon wall are associated with diverticular disease. Intestinal mobility dysfunction defines irritable bowel syndrome.

23. *Answer:* c (evaluation/gastrointestinal/NAS)

Rationale: Esophagitis is a major concern in clients who have gastroesophageal reflux syndrome, fibrosis may result. Bladder fistulas may occur with diverticulosis. Stomatitis and hemorrhoids are not associated with gastroesophageal reflux syndrome, although they may occur concomitantly.

24. *Answer:* c (diagnosis/gastrointestinal/adult)

Rationale: These are classic symptoms of gastroesophageal reflux syndrome; substernal cardiac pain usually shows a different pattern than that seen in this client. Diverticulitis and irritable bowel syndrome are seen as lower abdominal pain often associated with diarrhea and constipation.

25. *Answer:* c (assessment/physical examination/gastrointestinal/child)

Rationale: Choice *a* is characteristic of moderate dehydration, choice *b* represents severe dehydration, and choice *d* represents normal findings with no dehydration.

26. *Answer:* a (assessment/history/plan/management/client education/gastrointestinal/infant)

Rationale: This represents a normal stooling pattern. In infants and toddlers, normal passage of stool is accompanied by straining, facial redness, and pulling up of legs because of the immaturity of rectal and abdominal muscles.

27. *Answer:* a (plan/management/therapeutics/pharmacologic/gastrointestinal/child)

Rationale: Giardiasis is a parasitic infection. The drug of choice for treatment is metronidazole (Flagyl), 15 to 20 mg/kg/day in three divided doses.

28. *Answer:* a (assessment/physical examination/gastrointestinal/adult)

Rationale: Gastroenteritis caused by viral pathogens commonly produces stools that are large, liquid, and frequent and that have a variable odor. Tests of these stools are usually negative for both leukocytes and blood.

29. *Answer:* c (diagnosis/gastrointestinal/NAS)

Rationale: *Salmonella* produces stools that are loose, green, and slimy, and that produce the distinctive odor of spoiled eggs. *Shigella*-produced diarrheal stools are relatively odorless. Viral stools produce an unpleasant but nondistinct odor. Stools produced by giardiasis are typically pale, bulky, and greasy.

GENITOURINARY AND REPRODUCTIVE SYSTEMS

REVIEW QUESTIONS

1. A young man reports micturition urgency, micturition frequency, and abdominal discomfort. Which of the following diagnoses is **not** appropriate for this client?

  a. Acute cystitis
  b. Acute prostatitis
  c. Pyelonephritis
  d. Sexually transmitted disease

2. A history of hematospermia may be associated with:

  a. Acute bacterial prostatitis
  b. Benign prostatic hyperplasia
  c. Prostate cancer
  d. Chronic bacterial prostatitis

3. The physical examination of the male in an infertility workup should include all the following **except:**

  a. The thyroid gland
  b. Breast development
  c. Bartholin's gland
  d. Testes

4. The ultimate goal of an infertility workup is:

  a. A complete evaluation of the female within 6 months
  b. A viable pregnancy and the birth of a healthy infant
  c. A complete evaluation of the couple within 2 years
  d. An adoption plan

5. Which of the following factors in a woman's history decreases the risk of ovarian cysts?

a. Use of oral contraceptives
b. Nulliparity
c. Menarche at 9 years old
d. Safe sex practices

6. On physical examination, polycystic ovary syndrome would be characterized by which of the following?

a. Prominent iliac spines
b. Hirsutism with male pattern distribution
c. Large, pendulous breasts
d. Small, unhooded clitoris

7. When should a 30-year-old symptom-free client in whom a functional ovarian cyst is suspected be instructed to return for reevaluation?

a. When her next annual examination is due
b. In 2 to 3 weeks—just before ovulation
c. In 36 hours
d. No follow-up is necessary because she has no symptoms.

8. Which of the following clients with dysfunctional uterine bleeding should be referred for immediate evaluation by a gynecologist?

a. A 17-year-old who began taking a triphasic oral contraceptive pill 3 months ago
b. A 31-year-old, secundigravida, secundipara who uses medroxyprogesterone (Depo-Provera) for contraception
c. A 29-year-old gravida 4, primipara with an intrauterine device for birth control, abdominal pain, and adnexal mass
d. A 46-year-old woman who reports saturating four pads per day for 5 days during menses.

9. Which of the following findings on pelvic examination is associated with adenomyosis?

a. Ovarian cyst
b. Globular, boggy uterus
c. Smooth, spherical masses
d. Even, smooth, firm enlargement of the uterus

10. A 49-year-old woman comes in with a report of metorrhagia for the past 5 months, a 5-pound weight gain, and insomnia. Which of the following causes is likely given this information?

a. Leiomyoma
b. Anovulation

c. Malignancy
d. Hypothyroidism

11. For a 30-year-old with a breast mass she found several weeks ago, which subjective datum is **least** essential to elicit initially?

a. What changes has she noticed in the mass since she discovered it?
b. Has she noticed any relationship with her menstrual cycle?
c. When was her last clinical breast examination?
d. What does she know about breast examination and mammography?

12. Which physical examination finding is most suggestive of fibrocystic breast disease?

a. Symmetric area of thickness or nodularity in upper outer quadrants of both breasts
b. Cream-colored, pasty discharge expressed from both nipples during examination
c. Prominent vascular pattern noted on one breast
d. Bilateral inverted nipples

13. Mrs. Logan, 32 years old, has a 3-month history of breast tenderness and edema, worse a few days before her menstrual periods. This condition improves once menses begins. Personal and family history is unremarkable. Examination shows multiple rubbery areas of thickness, symmetric in both breasts and tender to palpation. There is no lymphadenopathy. The most appropriate diagnosis is:

a. Fibroadenoma
b. Intraductal papilloma
c. Fibrocystic changes
d. Carcinoma

14. A 31-year-old female (secundigravida [$G_2 P_2$], secundipara) has not had a period for the past 2 months. Conditions to be considered in differential diagnosis after pregnancy is ruled out include all the following **except:**

a. Hypothyroidism
b. Menopause
c. Stress
d. Excessive dieting

15. The first-line test for amenorrhea is:

   a. Thyroid-stimulating hormone and prolactin levels
   b. Follicle-stimulating hormone and luteinizing hormone levels
   c. Complete blood cell count with differential
   d. Human gonadotropin (HCG) level

16. A client with previously regular menstrual cycle is experiencing her first episode of amenorrhea. She has normal thyroid-stimulating hormone and prolactin levels. After completing a 5-day course of medroxyprogesterone (Provera), 10 mg, she begins to bleed. The nurse practitioner is able to explain which of the following to the client?

   a. This bleeding is unusual and may indicate a serious pathology.
   b. Her amenorrhea was caused by anovulation and she may need hormonal therapy to initiate menstruation.
   c. Her amenorrhea was caused by ovarian failure and hormone therapy will help to regulate her menses.
   d. She has primary amenorrhea and her menses will regulate themselves in time.

17. Which of the following symptoms is **least** indicative of premenstrual syndrome?

   a. Headache
   b. Bloating
   c. Breast tenderness
   d. Excessive menstrual flow

18. What is the primary purpose of the problem-oriented physical examination for the client who comes in with self-diagnosed premenstrual syndrome?

   a. To confirm her diagnosis of premenstrual syndrome
   b. To rule out other organic illness
   c. To rule out pelvic infection
   d. To conduct a mental status examination

19. In a client who reports the most common symptoms of premenstrual syndrome, which of the following differential diagnoses is **not** justified?

   a. Major depression
   b. Anxiety disorder
   c. Subacute bacterial endocarditis
   d. Thyroid disease

20. Which of the following statements is true about the use of synthetic androgens and gonadotropin-releasing hormone analogs for breast tenderness in premenstrual syndrome?

   a. These are the drugs of choice for this problem.
   b. These drugs should never be ordered for premenstrual syndrome because of the potential for serious side effects.
   c. These drugs are appropriate only when there is a coexisting breast mass.
   d. These drugs should be prescribed in collaboration with a physician.

21. Sarah, 19 years old, has had trichomoniasis diagnosed. What is the recommended treatment for her?

   a. Amoxicillin, 500 mg tid for 7 days
   b. Ceftriaxione, 125 mg IM
   c. Metranidazole (Flagyl), 500 bid for 7 days
   d. Metranidazole (Flagyl), 2 g, one dose

22. A report of thin, white-to-gray discharge and fishy odor that is worse after sex suggests which condition?

   a. Bacterial vaginosis
   b. Urinary tract infection
   c. Candidiasis
   d. Trichomoniasis

23. A positive whiff test result occurs with which condition?

   a. Bacterial vaginosis
   b. Presence of a foreign body
   c. Trichomoniasis
   d. Candidiasis

24. Mrs. Jones, 35 years old, has primary dysmenorrhea. When she has abdominal cramps, she also has nausea and headaches and feels nervous. These symptoms are considered associated symptoms of primary dysmenorrhea related to:

   a. Abnormal pelvic pathology
   b. Increased levels of prostaglandins
   c. Endometriosis
   d. Anovulatory cycles

25. When treating a child for primary enuresis, when should the family nurse practitioner schedule follow-up visits?

    a. As necessary at the mother's discretion

    b. At 2- to 4-week intervals

    c. Every 6 to 8 weeks while medication is being given

    d. No follow-up is necessary if symptoms subside.

26. To ensure long-term success, the most important aspect of the plan for treating encopresis is:

    a. Stool softeners for at least 1 year

    b. Constant monitoring of stooling patterns by parents

    c. Client involvement in developing the plan and personal responsibility for compliance

    d. Parental involvement in developing the plan and parental responsibility for compliance

ANSWERS AND RATIONALES

1. *Answer:* c (diagnosis/genitourinary/adult)

Rationale: Cystitis, prostatitis and a sexually transmitted disease need to be considered as differential diagnoses for the symptoms presented here. Not enough information is given to eliminate them from the diagnostic possibilities. Usually with pyelonephritis, the client exhibits fever, chills, and lower back pain.

2. *Answer:* d (assessment/history/genitourinary/adult)

Rationale: Hematospermia is not commonly seen in acute bacterial prostatitis, benign prostatic hyperplasia, or prostate cancer.

3. *Answer:* c (assessment/physical examination/reproductive/adult)

Rationale: The thyroid gland, breast development, and the testes are all part of the male examination; the Bartholin's gland applies to the female examination.

4. *Answer:* b (evaluation/reproductive/adult)

Rationale: The ultimate goal of an infertility evaluation would be a viable pregnancy and the birth of a healthy infant.

5. *Answer:* a (assessment/history/reproductive/childbearing female)

Rationale: Oral contraceptives and pregnancy modify the risk of ovarian cysts.

6. *Answer:* b (assessment/physical examination/reproductive/childbearing female)

Rationale: Hirsutism with male distribution pattern, small breasts, and an enlarged clitoris are objective findings in polycystic ovary syndrome.

7. *Answer:* b (evaluation/reproductive/childbearing female)

Rationale: Follow-up in 2 to 3 weeks is appropriate because the functional cyst will have resolved.

8. *Answer:* c (plan/management/reproductive/childbearing female)

Rationale: Ectopic pregnancy is one possibility associated with intrauterine device use and warrants emergency intervention by a physician.

9. *Answer:* b (assessment/physical examination/reproductive/childbearing female)

Rationale: A globular, boggy uterus on bimanual examination is associated with adenomyosis.

10. *Answer:* b (assessment/history/reproductive/childbearing female)

Rationale: Dysfunctional uterine bleeding usually occurs at the extremes of reproductive age when anovulation occurs (menopause and menarche).

11. *Answer:* d (assessment/history/reproductive/adult)

Rationale: Descriptions of the mass and its relationship to the menstrual cycle are key diagnostic data. Noting the last clinical breast examination helps date the finding.

12. *Answer:* a (assessment/physical examination/reproductive/adult)

Rationale: In fibrocystic disease, breasts feel nodular; thickened areas are more palpable in the upper outer quadrant and are comparable in both breasts.

13. *Answer:* c (diagnosis/reproductive/childbearing female)

Rationale: Fibrocystic changes are associated with tenderness and edema that are worse premenstrually.

14. *Answer:* b (diagnosis/reproductive/childbearing female)

Rationale: Hypothyroidism, stress, and excessive dieting are all causes of amenorrhea. Although menopause also causes amenorrhea, it is unlikely in a female of this age.

15. *Answer:* d (assessment/physical examination/diagnostics/reproductive/childbearing female)

Rationale: The most common cause of amenorrhea is pregnancy, which must be ruled out before initiation of other, more costly testing.

16. *Answer:* b (plan/client education/reproductive/childbearing female)

Rationale: Bleeding after completing a course of Provera is called "withdrawal bleeding" and is a normal event. It does not indicate a serious pathology. Withdrawal bleeding does not occur with ovarian failure. Because the client had normal menstrual cycles in the past, she does not have primary amenorrhea. Withdrawal bleeding with normal thyroid-stimulating hormone and prolactin levels indicates anovulation, which may persist without hormonal assistance.

17. *Answer:* d (assessment/history/reproductive/childbearing female)

Rationale: Headache, bloating, and breast tenderness are among the most common subjective symptoms of premenstrual syndrome.

18. *Answer:* b (assessment/physical examination/reproductive/childbearing female)

Rationale: The physical examination does not reveal objective findings of premenstrual syndrome but is done to rule out organic disorders.

19. *Answer:* c (diagnosis/reproductive/childbearing female)

Rationale: Psychiatric illnesses, such as depression and anxiety disorder, should be ruled out in arriving at a diagnosis of premenstrual syndrome. Symptoms sometimes mimic thyroid disease.

20. *Answer:* d (plan/management/therapeutics/pharmacologic/reproductive/childbearing female)

Rationale: Synthetic androgens and gonadotropin-releasing hormone analogs are drugs of last resort and should be used only in consultation with a physician.

21. *Answer:* d (plan/management/therapeutics/pharmacologic/reproductive/childbearing female)

Rationale: Treatment for trichimoniasis recommended by the Centers for Disease Control and Prevention is Flagyl, 2 g immediately. Flagyl 500 bid is the recommended treatment for bacterial vaginosis and is considered an alternative treatment for trichimoniasis.

22. *Answer:* a (assessment/history/reproductive/childbearing female)

Rationale: Although a malodorous discharge may occur with both a trichomoniasis vaginitis and with the presence of a foreign body, the positive whiff test result occurs from a reaction between the discharge of bacterial vaginosis and the potassium hydroxide. Candidiasis has no odor.

23. *Answer:* a (assessment/management/diagnostics/reproductive/childbearing female)

Rationale: A urinary tract infection does not cause a vaginal discharge, the discharge for a *Candida* infection is not malodorous, and the discharge from a trichomoniasis infection is frothy and profuse.

24. *Answer:* b (diagnosis/reproductive/childbearing female)

Rationale: Primary dysmenorrhea is frequently associated with cramping, gastrointestinal complaints, nervousness, fatigue, headache, and other symptoms as a result of the increased levels of prostaglandins released and synthesized during ovulatory cycles. There is no pelvic pathology.

25. *Answer:* b (evaluation/genitourinary/child)

Rationale: Successful therapy for enuresis requires frequent encouragement and support. Initial follow-ups should be scheduled every 2 to 4 weeks. While the medication is being given, children should be seen at least monthly.

26. *Answer:* c (plan/management/genitourinary/child)

Rationale: For encopresis therapy to be successful, the child must want to solve the problem and be invested in the plan. Excessive attention and involvement by parents sometimes cause the child to sabotage the treatment.

MUSCULOSKELETAL SYSTEM

REVIEW QUESTIONS

1. The **least** likely finding of acute gout on physical examination is:

   a. A single, warm, red, tender joint of the lower extremity
   b. Joint effusion with limited range of motion
   c. Low-grade fever with temperature of 99.6° F
   d. Painless tophi with urate deposits on the Achilles tendon

2. In addition to gout, the differential diagnosis for acute monoarthritis would be **least** likely to include which of the following?

   a. Septic joint
   b. Bone cancer
   c. Pseudogout
   d. Joint trauma

3. Which of the following is **not** true regarding gamekeeper's thumb?

   a. It is caused by a forced hyperabduction of the thumb.
   b. It is an injury to the ulnar collateral ligament of the thumb.
   c. It is commonly seen in snow skiers.
   d. It is commonly seen in children.

4. Physical findings associated with mallet finger include which of the following?

   a. An extension deformity of the proximal interphalangeal joint
   b. A crush injury of the distal phalanx
   c. Decreased sensation in the distal fingertip
   d. A flexion deformity of the distal interphalangeal joint of the finger

5. Salter-Harris classification is which of the following?
   a. A system to describe long-bone fractures
   b. A classification for distal fibular injuries
   c. A classification of growth plate fractures in children
   d. A classification of wrist injuries

6. Which of the following does **not** require immediate referral to an orthopedic surgeon?

   a. Intraarticular fractures
   b. Fractures with neurovascular compromise
   c. Knee injuries with gross instability
   d. Grade II and III ankle sprains

7. Spinal curves of 20 to 25 degrees require which of the following interventions?

   a. Milwaukee brace
   b. Harrington rod
   c. Range of motion exercises
   d. Observation every 4 to 6 months

8. Lateral S-shaped curvature of the thoracic and lumbar spine is:

   a. Kyphosis
   b. Scoliosis
   c. Lordosis
   d. Osteoporosis

9. Nonstructural scoliosis:

   a. Is a fixed curvature of the spine
   b. Is corrected with front bending
   c. Is treated with a brace
   d. Requires annual spinal x-ray examinations

10. Heather, a 37-year-old typist at your office, has initial symptoms of carpal tunnel syndrome. Conservative treatment to initiate includes:

   a. Steroid injection to the carpal tunnel
   b. Rest of the affected part, ice, and nonsteroidal antiinflammatory drugs
   c. Excision of carpal ligament
   d. Carpal compression

11. Mrs. Hamm, a 29-year-old, 8-month pregnant client, has a diagnosis of carpal tunnel syndrome. Which of the following is true concerning carpal tunnel syndrome during pregnancy?

   a. Immediate surgical intervention is indicated.
   b. Carpal tunnel syndrome does not occur in pregnancy; it must have been misdiagnosed.
   c. Splints may impair fetal development.
   d. Carpal tunnel syndrome is relatively common and abates after pregnancy.

12. Larry H. returns to your office for follow-up 2 weeks after initiation of conservative treatment for carpal tunnel syndrome. Which of the following indicates improvement?

   a. Decrease in grip and pinch strength
   b. Increase in thenar wasting
   c. Decreased paresthesia in affected fingers
   d. Pain radiating into forearm

13. Ortolani maneuver causes:

   a. Dislocation of the located hip
   b. Reduction of the dislocated hip
   c. Dislocation of the dislocated hip
   d. Reduction of the located hip

14. All the following are factors in the history of developmental dysplasia of the hip **except:**

   a. Relaxing effect of maternal hormones
   b. Age
   c. Family history
   d. Abnormal intrauterine positioning

15. In juvenile rheumatoid arthritis, the differential diagnosis may include:

   a. Sjögren's syndrome
   b. Osgood-Schlatter disease
   c. Pseudogout
   d. Scleroderma

16. Heat is recommended for both osteoarthritis and rheumatoid arthritis to do all the following **except:**

   a. Relieve muscle spasm
   b. Relieve pain
   c. Increase range of motion
   d. Strengthen supporting joint muscles

Situation: *Mia is a 42-year-old Asian female who reports intermittent back pain. Her height is 5 feet 2 inches and her weight is 92 pounds. She is concerned about her risk of osteoporosis on the basis of consumer literature. She had a hysterectomy and bilateral oophorectomy 2 years ago and has been taking conjugated estrogens (Premarin), 0.625 mg, since surgery. There is no known family history of osteoporosis. Questions 17 through 21 refer to Mia's case.*

17. You would also want information about all the following **except:**

   a. Calcium intake
   b. Exercise activities
   c. Alcohol intake
   d. Anxiety patterns

18. According to the above information, which of the following would you do?

   a. Recommend bone mass density measurement to assess risk.
   b. Wait 1 to 2 years to do a bone mass density measurement.
   c. Increase the estrogen dose.
   d. Reassure Mia that there is no cause for concern.

19. Mia's tests show that she has osteopenia. This is best described as:

   a. Normal bone mass for her age
   b. Generalized decrease in bone mass density
   c. Decreased bone mass with microfractures
   d. Generalized softening of the bone

20. On the basis of your knowledge about absorption rates of calcium, you recommend that Mia take which of the following calcium supplements?

   a. Calcium carbonate
   b. Calcium citrate
   c. Calcium phosphate
   d. Calcium lactate

21. Two years later a bone mass density study is done on Mia. Results show that her bone mass is 1 standard deviation above the mean. What does this indicate?

   a. The bone mass density study should be repeated in 2 years.
   b. Mia is well protected against osteoporosis.
   c. Vertebral fractures are likely.
   d. The bone mass density study should be repeated in 5 years.

22. One would most likely expect the affected joint of a client with early or recently diagnosed rheumatoid arthritis to have which of the following signs?

   a. Tenderness with movement
   b. Joint instability
   c. Crepitus
   d. Deformities

23. The differential diagnosis of osteoarthritis includes all the following **except:**

    a. Gout
    b. Rheumatoid arthritis
    c. Tendinitis
    d. Polymyalgia rheumatica

ANSWERS AND RATIONALES

1. *Answer:* d (assessment/physical examination/ musculoskeletal/NAS)

Rationale: Tophi are a manifestation of chronic gout, with an average of 10 years of hyperuricemia before development.

2. *Answer:* b (diagnosis/musculoskeletal/NAS)

Rationale: Trauma, infection, and pseudogout can produce acute monoarthritis. Bone cancer is a chronic progressive disease; it is not listed as a differential diagnosis.

3. *Answer:* d (assessment/history/musculoskeletal/NAS)

Rationale: Skier's thumb or *gamekeeper's thumb* is an injury to the ulnar collateral ligament of the metacarpophalangeal joint of the thumb that occurs with a forced hyperabduction. It is not usually seen in children.

4. *Answer:* d (assessment/physical examination/ musculoskeletal/NAS)

Rationale: Mallet deformity is a flexion deformity of the distal interphalangeal joint of the finger. The client cannot actively extend the finger at the distal interphalangeal joint.

5. *Answer:* c (diagnosis/musculoskeletal/child)

Rationale: The Salter-Harris classification system is used to describe acute injuries that involve the growth plate. In the individual with an immature skeleton, the growth plate remains open.

6. *Answer:* d (plan/management/musculoskeletal/ NAS)

Rationale: Ankle sprains can be easily managed in the primary care setting. Current treatment involves aggressive functional rehabilitation.

7. *Answer:* d (plan/management/nonpharmacologic/musculoskeletal/NAS)

Rationale: Spinal curves of 20 to 25 degrees are not severe enough to require intervention other than observation every 4 to 6 months to watch for change.

8. *Answer:* b (diagnosis/musculoskeletal/NAS)

Rationale: The definition of scoliosis is the lateral S- or C-shaped curvature of the thoracic and lumbar spine.

9. *Answer:* b (diagnosis/musculoskeletal/NAS)

Rationale: Functional scoliosis is corrected with front bending.

10. *Answer:* b (plan/management/musculoskeletal/NAS)

Rationale: Conservative treatment is rest, ice, splinting, and nonsteroidal antiinflammatory drugs. Steroid injection and surgery are not conservative treatments.

11. *Answer:* d (diagnosis/musculoskeletal/childbearing female)

Rationale: Carpal tunnel syndrome is relatively common in pregnancy; it abates after delivery. Surgery is rarely needed.

12. *Answer:* c (evaluation/musculoskeletal/NAS)

Rationale: Improvement would be indicated by a decrease in symptoms of paresthesia of fingers and hand. Thenar wasting, pain in the arm, and decreased strength all indicate worsening of carpal tunnel syndrome.

13. *Answer:* b (assessment/physical examination/musculoskeletal/infant)

Rationale: In clients with reducible dislocations, Ortolani's sign is positive when a palpable "clunk" is felt on abduction of the hip.

14. *Answer:* b (assessment/history/musculoskeletal/infant)

Rationale: Idiopathic dislocations are related to family history, abnormal intrauterine positioning, and maternal hormones.

15. *Answer:* b (diagnosis/musculoskeletal/child)

Rationale: Clients with juvenile rheumatoid arthritis may have symptoms of Osgood-Schlatter disease and are within the age group for juvenile rheumatoid arthritis to occur. Scleroderma, pseudogout, and Sjögren's syndrome occur primarily in an older population.

16. *Answer:* d (plan/management/therapeutics/non-pharmacologic/musculoskeletal/NAS)

Rationale: Heat helps relieve muscle spasm and pain and allows increased range of motion for clients with both osteoarthritis and rheumatoid arthritis. Supporting muscles experience relief; however, there is no strengthening effect.

17. *Answer:* d (assessment/history/musculoskeletal/NAS)

Rationale: Although level of anxiety may indirectly influence development of osteoporosis, calcium intake, exercise, and alcohol use are directly related to osteoporosis.

18. *Answer:* a (plan/management/diagnostics/musculoskeletal/NAS)

Rationale: Bone mass density measurement is appropriate in a high-risk client to assess risk and establish a baseline. There is no evidence that estrogen doses larger than 0.625 mg are needed to preserve bone mass.

19. *Answer:* b (diagnosis/musculoskeletal/NAS)

Rationale: Osteopenia is decreased bone density.

20. *Answer:* a (management/therapeutics/pharmacologic/musculoskeletal/NAS)

Rationale: Only elemental calcium is absorbed, and 40% of calcium carbonate is elemental. Lower doses are therefore needed to obtain the desired amount.

21. *Answer:* b (evaluation/musculoskeletal/NAS)

Rationale: If the bone density is more than 1 standard deviation above the mean, the client is relatively well protected from osteoporosis.

22. *Answer:* a (assessment/physical examination/musculoskeletal/NAS)

Rationale: Rheumatoid arthritis, or chronic inflammatory disease, does cause the affected joint to be painful and therefore tender with movement. Deformities are common with rheumatoid arthritis but occur later in the course of the disease, as does joint instability. Crepitus is more common with osteoarthritis.

23. *Answer:* d (diagnosis/musculoskeletal/NAS)

Rationale: Polymyalgia rheumatica is a clinical diagnosis that is based on pain and stiffness of the shoulder and pelvic girdle area and is often associated with fever, malaise, and weight loss. None of the signs and symptoms should be mistaken for osteoarthritis, whereas gout, rheumatoid arthritis, and tendinitis are all diagnoses to be considered in diagnosing osteoarthritis.

NEUROLOGIC SYSTEM

REVIEW QUESTIONS

1. Which of the following physical findings may be present in a client with a tension-type headache?

   a. Tenderness of pericranial muscles
   b. Unilateral muscle weakness
   c. Ptosis
   d. Eyelid edema

2. Which of the following sets of symptoms is associated with tension-type headache?

   a. Bilateral, mild to moderate, pressing headache lasting 30 minutes to 7 days
   b. Unilateral, moderate to severe, throbbing headache lasting for 4 to 72 hours, aggravated by routine physical activity, with nausea, vomiting, or both; headache preceded by flashing lights
   c. Pounding or dull frontal or occipital pain present when upright and relieved by lying down
   d. More prevalent in men, occurring in attacks of severe unilateral orbital, supraorbital, or temporal pain, lasting 15 to 180 minutes, with miosis

3. Which of the following conditions is linked with a higher risk for Bell's palsy?

   a. Hyperthyroidism
   b. Osteoarthritis
   c. Pregnancy
   d. Crohn's disease

4. The **least** likely symptom to suggest Bell's palsy is:

   a. Mild tinnitus at onset
   b. Facial weakness progressing during weeks or months
   c. Hypersensitivity to sound
   d. Taste alteration

5. Physical examination for Bell's palsy should **not** include:

   a. Otoscopic examination of the ears
   b. Auscultation of the lungs
   c. Assessment of the cranial nerves
   d. Abdominal examination

6. In what situation would you consider giving donepezil (Aricept) to a client?

   a. Questionable dementia
   b. Mild to moderate dementia
   c. Severe dementia
   d. Dementia with coexisting depression

7. You place a client on a regimen of tracrine (Cognex). To evaluate the client's response to the medication, initially you would order weekly:

   a. Complete blood cell counts
   b. Alanine aminotransferase levels
   c. Blood glucose levels
   d. Erythrocyte sedimentation rates

8. Which of the following factors in a client's history is **not** a risk factor for Alzheimer's disease?

   a. Smoking
   b. Head injury
   c. Age
   d. Family history

9. Mrs. Johnson has brought her 7-year-old daughter Susie to the office for a follow-up visit. The diagnosis of simple partial seizures was previously made by the pediatric neurologist, and Susie was placed on a regimen of carbamazepine (Tegretol). The follow-up care was to be carried out by the nurse practitioner. Which of the following is **not** appropriate for the nurse practitioner to do?

   a. Order an MRI scan for follow-up.
   b. Ascertain any untoward side effects that the client may be experiencing.
   c. Reinforce education about seizures and antiepileptic drugs.
   d. Order complete blood cell counts and liver function tests every 2 to 3 weeks for the first 2 months, then every 3 months.

10. A 32-year-old female collapses to the floor and lies unconscious but is breathing well after having an argument with her husband. On the basis only of the information provided, which of the following would be **inappropriate** for the differential diagnosis?

   a. Hyperventilation-induced syncope
   b. Panic attack
   c. Simple partial seizure
   d. Paroxysmal rapid eye movement sleep behavior

11. Secondary manifestations of Parkinson's disease include all the following **except:**

   a. Diarrhea
   b. Dysphagia
   c. Sialorrhea
   d. Seborrhea

12. Anticholinergic treatment for Parkinson's disease is most effective in decreasing which symptom of Parkinson's disease?

   a. Bradykinesia
   b. Tremor at rest
   c. Hypotension
   d. Rigidity

13. A significant number of clients with Parkinson's disease have dementia develop. Which of the following statements is true?

    a. No effective treatment is currently available.

    b. One should search for treatable causes, the same as with a client without Parkinson's disease.

    c. Tricyclic antidepressants are not helpful.

    d. Dementia is directly related to the severity of Parkinson's disease.

14. A side effect of donepezil (Aricept) you would be alert to is:

    a. Nausea, vomiting, and diarrhea

    b. Ringing in the ear

    c. Dizziness

    d. Drowsiness

15. An individual with a cluster headache may have which of the following physical findings?

    a. Tenderness of pericranial muscles

    b. Lacrimation on the side of the pain

    c. Unilateral muscle weakness

    d. Tenderness in the temporal area

16. In the development of a therapeutic plan of care for a client with a primary type of headache, which of the following actions is **not** appropriate?

    a. Implement lifestyle modifications before starting medications.

    b. Medications should be started before attempting lifestyle modifications.

    c. Choice of therapy is guided by the type of headache, previous use of typical medication, the client's preference and needs as to route of delivery, concurrent symptoms or problems, other medications being taken, and cost.

    d. Use the least potent and least addictive analgesic medication that relieves the pain.

Answers and Rationales

1. *Answer:* a (assessment/physical examination/neurologic/NAS)

    Rationale: Tenderness of pericranial muscles may be present in individuals with tension-type headaches. Unilateral muscle weakness may be associated with a stroke or a neurologic condition, whereas ptosis and eyelid edema are more likely to be identified with a cluster headache.

2. *Answer:* a (assessment/history/neurologic/NAS)

    Rationale: Unilateral, moderate to severe, throbbing headache lasting 4 to 72 hours, aggravated by routine physical activity, with nausea, vomiting, or both, headache preceded by flashing lights, is a more suggestive pattern for migraine headache with an aura. Pounding or dull frontal pain, present when upright and relieved by lying down, is likely to occur with a headache after a spinal puncture. Headache that is more prevalent in men, occurs in attacks of severe unilateral orbital, supraorbital, or temporal pain lasting 15 to 180 minutes, with miosis, is a cluster headache.

3. *Answer:* c (assessment/history/neurologic/childbearing female)

    Rationale: Women who are pregnant, especially in the third trimester, are more vulnerable to Bell's palsy. The literature does not list the other conditions as being risk factors.

4. *Answer:* b (assessment/history/neurologic/NAS)

    Rationale: Facial weakness progressing with a time suggests another cause; Bell's palsy symptoms occur rapidly, during the course of a few hours.

5. *Answer:* d (assessment/physical examination/neurologic/NAS)

    Rationale: Otoscopic examination of the ears, looking for infection, cholesteatoma; auscultation of the lungs, for adventitious sounds that might indicate sarcoidosis; and assessment of the cranial nerves, for facial function, are all indicated. Abdominal examination would not be likely to reveal any relevant information.

6. *Answer:* b (plan/management/therapeutics/pharmacologic/neurologic/aging adult)

    Rationale: Donepezil (Aricept) and tacrine (Cognex) are indicated for clients with mild to moderate dementia. These clients still have functioning neurons that can use the acetylcholine that is spared with these drugs.

7. *Answer:* b (evaluation/neurologic/NAS)

    Rationale: It is important to monitor liver enzymes. Ninety percent of all clinically significant alanine aminotransferase elevations occurred within the first 12 weeks of treatment. Alanine aminotransferase elevations resolve with discontinuance of Cognex (tacine), and many individuals can resume the medication without further sequelae.

8. ***Answer:*** a (assessment/history/neurologic/NAS)
   Rationale: Smoking has been identified as a possible protective factor for Alzheimer's disease. Head injury with loss of consciousness, advancing age, and family history have all been identified as possible risk factors.

9. ***Answer:*** a (evaluation/neurologic/child)
   Rationale: An MRI is indicated in intractable seizures, focal neurologic abnormalities, and first seizures in adults. The other three answers are appropriate in the follow-up of Mrs. Johnson's daughter.

10. ***Answer:*** c (diagnosis/neurologic/NAS)
   Rationale: Simple partial seizures are auras that usually last 20 to 180 seconds and are *not* associated with impairment of consciousness. The other diagnoses would be considered as differential diagnoses in this situation.

11. ***Answer:*** a (assessment/history/neurologic/NAS)
   Rationale: Dysphagia, sialorrhea, and seborrhea may all be seen in Parkinson's disease. Autonomic signs, such as constipation and bladder dysfunction, are often seen.

12. ***Answer:*** b (plan/management/therapeutics/pharmacologic/neurologic/NAS)
   Rationale: Anticholinergics have little effect on akinesia and postural imbalance. They are most effective against tremor at rest.

13. ***Answer:*** b (evaluation/neurologic/NAS)
   Rationale: Dementia is not an inevitable feature of Parkinson's disease, even though the incidence of dementia is higher among persons with Parkinson's disease than among age-matched control subjects without Parkinson's disease. Also, some of the drugs used to treat Parkinson's disease have cognitive and behavioral side effects.

14. ***Answer:*** a (evaluation/neurologic/NAS)
   Rationale: Nausea, vomiting, and diarrhea are the most common side effects of Aricept. However, they were reported to occur in only 3% of clients in the clinical trials.

15. ***Answer:*** b (assessment/physical examination/neurologic/NAS)
   Rationale: Lacrimation on the side of the pain is more likely to be present with a cluster headache. Tenderness of pericranial muscles is associated with tension-type headache, unilateral muscle weakness may be indicative of a stroke or a neurologic condition, and tenderness in the temporal area is associated with temporal arteritis.

16. ***Answer:*** b (plan/management/neurologic/NAS)
   Rationale: When developing a therapeutic plan of care for the client with headaches, the health care provider should implement lifestyle modifications before starting a particular regimen of medications. Choice of therapy should be guided by the type of headache, previous use of typical medication, the client's preference and needs as to route of delivery, concurrent symptoms or problems, other medications being taken, and cost.

ENDOCRINE SYSTEM

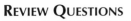

REVIEW QUESTIONS

1. The nurse practitioner has completed the examination and diagnosis for an adult with newly diagnosed non–insulin-dependent diabetes. The fasting plasma glucose level was 250 mg/dl. Which of the following would **not** be included in the plan?

  a. Insulin
  b. Overnight urinary microalbumin test
  c. Ophthalmologic examination
  d. Hemoglobin A1$_c$

2. A child with undiagnosed insulin-dependent diabetes is likely to experience all the following **except:**

  a. Polydipsia
  b. Polyuria
  c. Weight gain
  d. Fatigue

3. Which of the following would you **not** expect to find in the nutritional history of a person with Cushing's syndrome?

   a. Weight gain
   b. Vomiting
   c. Increased appetite
   d. Nausea

4. Ms. Smith is a 45-year-old female who comes to the nurse practitioner with reported weight gain, fatigue, and increased appetite. Which of the following would **not** be included in the differential diagnosis?

   a. Diabetes mellitus
   b. Depression
   c. Obesity
   d. Hypothyroidism

5. Ms. Taylor brings her 9-year-old daughter to the nurse practitioner. The daughter has been experiencing polyuria, polydipsia, and weight loss. The nurse practitioner completes a physical examination and orders laboratory tests. Which test would establish the diagnosis?

   a. Finger-stick blood glucose level
   b. Plasma glucose level
   c. Urinary glucose level
   d. Hemoglobin A1$_c$

6. A 57-year-old female had a mastectomy 1 month before the current laboratory work and visit. She has been undergoing chemotherapy. She states that she is feeling well but reports some fatigue. A random plasma glucose level is 160 mg/dl. Which of the following is the most likely diagnosis?

   a. Diabetes mellitus
   b. Cushing's syndrome

   c. Transient hyperglycemia
   d. Pheochromocytoma

ANSWERS AND RATIONALES

1. *Answer:* a (plan/management/endocrine/NAS)
Rationale: Because you do not know if the client has responded to oral hypoglycemic agents, insulin is inappropriate at this time.

2. *Answer:* c (assessment/history/endocrine/child)
Rationale: Children usually experience weight loss. The loss of glucose through the urine results in negative calorie balance and weight loss.

3. *Answer:* b (assessment/history/endocrine/NAS)
Rationale: Typically individuals with Cushing's syndrome do not have vomiting.

4. *Answer:* d (diagnosis/endocrine/NAS)
Rationale: Hypothyroidism does not cause appetite changes.

5. *Answer:* b (diagnosis/endocrine/NAS)
Rationale: The plasma glucose level is the most reliable indicator to establish the diagnosis.

6. *Answer:* c (diagnosis/endocrine/adult)
Rationale: The plasma glucose level is not elevated enough to establish the diagnosis. This client has also had stress caused by the surgery and illness, which would elevate the blood glucose level.

INTEGUMENTARY SYSTEM

REVIEW QUESTIONS

1. Which of the following descriptions is of characteristic tinea versicolor lesions?

a. Small pustules surrounded by erythematous margin
b. Macerated, scaly plaques with varying vesicles and pustules
c. Thick, white plaques surrounded by erythema
d. Round or oval hypopigmented or hyperpigmented macules with fine scales

2. Mark is a 20-year-old college student living in the dormitory. He has itching and burning of both feet. You suspect tinea pedis and examine his feet. You expect to find:

a. Macerated, scaly skin between the toes and on the plantar and lateral aspects of feet
b. Hard nodules and pustules located between the toes
c. Scales and erythema on the dorsal aspect of the feet and around the ankle
d. Papules and vesicles on the dorsal and lateral aspects of the feet

3. When viewed under a microscope, the classic "spaghetti and meatballs" pattern seen is characteristic of which tinea infection?

a. Tinea versicolor
b. Tinea capitis
c. Tinea corporis
d. Tinea pedis

4. Skin lesions most suggestive of scabies are:

a. Erythematous papular rashes covering the trunk
b. Pinpoint, red spots at the nape of the neck
c. Topical, grayish-white burrows of varying lengths
d. Thick, crusted plaques varying in size

5. A cardinal symptom of scabies infestation is:

a. A burning sensation on the trunk
b. Intense itching around the hairline
c. Generalized itching
d. Nocturnal itching

6. Steve is a 19-year-old male who has a 3-month history of a sore bump on the sole of his foot. Personal and family histories are unremarkable. Examination shows a small, sharply marginated papule studded with black dots at the metatarsophalangeal junction on the sole of his right foot. The most appropriate diagnosis is:

a. Common wart
b. Plantar wart
c. Ingrown hair
d. Callus

7. Jerry has common warts on his hands. The nurse advises him on the various treatments appropriate for warts. Which statement made by Jerry indicates that he understands the instructions?

a. "I will make an appointment with a dermatologist to get them cut off."
b. "I will leave these alone and see what happens."
c. "I should apply a baking soda paste to the warts every night."
d. "Placing gasoline on the warts will help them go away."

8. Shelly, a 19-year-old female, just had her annual Papanicolaou smear done. The results indicate a low-grade squamous intraepithelial lesion caused by human papillomavirus. When should Shelly have follow-up?

a. Next year for annual examination
b. Only when she has problems
c. She should be referred for colposcopy.
d. Repeated Papanicolaou smear in 6 months

9. Which objective finding is **not** usually associated with herpes zoster?

a. Scaly, salmon-colored lesions
b. Painful, vesicular rash
c. Bullous eruption following the dermatome
d. Preeruption itching or pain

10. Examination of an 8-year-old boy reveals the following: erythema of lip, with vesicles on the rim of the lip, nasal discharge, and cough. Which diagnosis is most appropriate?

a. Hand, foot, and mouth disease
b. Drug eruption
c. Aphthous stomatitis
d. Herpes simplex

11. Gerald is a 65-year-old man with a diagnosis of herpes zoster. What should you say to him concerning family members and the communicability of herpes zoster?

a. No one should touch the lesions because they may get herpes zoster.
b. Do any of your family members or friends have immune problems, such as HIV?
c. Herpes zoster is not communicable.
d. There is no relationship between herpes zoster and chickenpox.

12. A 35-year-old recovering IV drug user has an abrupt onset of psoriatic plaques covering most of his body. You would obtain consent to test for:

a. Syphilis
b. Gonorrhea
c. HIV
d. Lupus

13. Counseling of the client with psoriasis to help minimize exacerbations of the disease includes all the following recommendations **except:**

a. Adequate sleep
b. Following prescribed schedule in application of medications
c. Direct sunlight
d. Avoiding medications advertised as cures

14. To avoid recurrence of tinea pedis, you instruct Mark to do all the following **except:**

a. Avoid leather shoes
b. Wear rubber sandals in communal areas
c. Dry carefully between his toes
d. Wear absorbent cotton socks

15. Mr. Stevens is a 44-year-old man who comes to the clinic with a new rash. He has recently taken up swimming and running to lose weight. Which of the following does **not** put him at risk for tinea cruris?

a. Obesity
b. Cotton boxer shorts

c. Use of an athletic supporter
d. Wet clothing

16. Judy has a plaque on her right shoulder. You suspect tinea corporis. The primary symptom would be:

a. Inability to tan the area of the lesion
b. Pruritis
c. Pain
d. Burning

17. C.J. has a laceration to the forearm. It will require two layers of sutures. The best choice of suture material to close the subcutaneous layer is:

a. Plain catgut
b. Chromic catgut
c. Polyglycolic suture (Vicryl, Dexon)
d. Silk

18. The most common pathogen involved in wound infections related to lacerations is:

a. *Staphylococcus aureus*
b. *Pseudomonas aeruginosa*
c. *Clostridium tetani*
d. Hepatitis B virus

19. J.W. has a puncture wound to the hand. He reports numbness and tingling distal to the puncture site. Your highest priority of assessment at this time would include:

a. Neurovascular function
b. Identifying the medications that he is taking on a regular basis
c. Determining his tetanus status
d. Allergies to medications

20. J.J. is 8 years old. She has a simple laceration to her great toe that will require approximately three stitches. The best local anesthetic to use in this situation is:

a. Tetracaine, adrenaline, and cocaine (TAC) solution
b. Lidocaine, topical epinephrine, and tetracaine solution
c. Lidocaine 2%
d. Lidocaine 1% with epinephrine

ANSWERS AND RATIONALES

1. Answer: d (assessment/physical examination/integumentary/NAS)

Rationale: Tinea versicolor is seen as small, oval or round, hyperpigmented or hypopigmented lesions with fine scales.

2. Answer: a (assessment/physical examination/integumentary/NAS)

Rationale: Classically, tinea pedis involves the toe webs and the plantar and lateral aspects of the feet. It is usually devoid of vesicular lesions.

3. Answer: a (diagnosis/integumentary/NAS)

Rationale: Under a Wood's light, tinea versicolor will fluoresce with a characteristic yellow-orange color, and microscopic examination with a potassium hydroxide preparation will reveal hyphae and spores—the classic "spaghetti and meatballs" pattern.

4. Answer: c (assessment/physical examination/integumentary/NAS)

Rationale: The diagnosis of scabies is suggested by finding topical grayish-white burrows.

5. Answer: d (assessment/history/integumentary/NAS)

Rationale: A cardinal symptom of scabies is nocturnal itching.

6. Answer: b (diagnosis/integumentary/adult)

Rationale: Plantar warts are frequently painful when pressure is applied over the metatarsal head. Common warts and callus do not usually have black dots, whereas an ingrown hair would be erythematous and would not be located on the sole of the foot.

7. Answer: b (evaluation/integumentary/adult)

Rationale: Warts do not need to be treated aggressively because they frequently resolve on their own.

8. Answer: c (plan/management/integumentary/adult)

Rationale: When a Papanicolaou smear reveals a suspicious atypia or squamous epithelial lesion, referral for a colposcopy is indicated because of the link of human papillomavirus to cervical cancer.

9. Answer: a (assessment/physical examination/integumentary/NAS)

Rationale: All except *a* are commonly seen with herpes zoster. Scaly, salmon-colored lesions are more typical of psoriasis.

10. Answer: d (diagnosis/integumentary/child)

Rationale: Although the other diseases are considered part of the differential diagnosis, herpetic stomatitis commonly occurs in children, along with the risk factor of a common cold.

11. Answer: b (plan/integumentary/aging adult)

Rationale: Herpes zoster can be communicated to individuals who have not had chickenpox, with an increased risk for those who are immunocompromised.

12. Answer: c (diagnosis/integumentary/adult)

Rationale: Abrupt psoriatic plaques may be the first sign of HIV infection.

13. Answer: c (plan/integumentary/NAS)

Rationale: Direct sunlight, stress, and obesity are believed to cause exacerbation of preexisting psoriasis.

14. Answer: a (plan/management/integumentary/NAS)

Rationale: Treatment of tinea pedis begins by emphasizing hygiene, specifically thorough drying of the feet after bathing. Absorbent cotton socks may help to maintain dryness, and shoes should be made of leather to allow the feet to breathe. It would be prudent to wear sandals or other protective footwear in the locker room.

15. Answer: b (assessment/history/integumentary/NAS)

Rationale: Loose-fitting cotton undergarments should be worn to help keep the area as dry as possible.

16. Answer: b (assessment/history/integumentary/NAS)

Rationale: Signs and symptoms of tinea corporis are a characteristic rash and mild pruritis. The client may experience intense itching.

17. *Answer:* c (plan/integumentary/NAS)

Rationale: Vicryl is a synthetic material that is absorbable. It causes minimal tissue reaction. Choices *a* and *b* are natural absorbable materials that can cause an inflammatory response, which can look like an infection. Silk *(d)* is not absorbable; it therefore is not used on subcutaneous layers.

18. *Answer:* a (diagnosis/integumentary/NAS)

Rationale: *S. aureus* is the most common cause of wound infections related to lacerations. *P. aeruginosa* is associated with puncture wounds, *C. tetani* is the organism that causes tetanus, and hepatitis B virus is associated with human bites.

19. *Answer:* a (assessment/physical examination/integumentary/NAS)

Rationale: As with all wounds to the hand, a good neurovascular examination is essential before the injection of anesthetic. Flexor and extensor function of tendons, along with sensations of touch and pain, should be thoroughly evaluated.

20. *Answer:* c (plan/integumentary/child)

Rationale: Lidocaine 2% is the best choice to use. The remaining anesthetics contain epinephrine, a powerful vasoconstrictive agent that should never be used on the fingers, toes, nose, ears, or penis.

PSYCHOSOCIAL CONDITIONS

REVIEW QUESTIONS

1. Which of the following assessment findings suggests a common behavior problem in a toddler?

 a. Skin—bruises in multiple stages of healing over the body
 b. Neurologic—failed vision and hearing screen results
 c. Neurologic—personal, social and language development delays
 d. Bursts of anger with crying

2. Diagnostic measures helpful to the practitioner in determining whether a behavior problem is minor would include:

 a. Vision screen
 b. Behavior rating scale
 c. Denver II
 d. Hearing screen

3. Sue Smith, a 19-year-old female, comes to your office for a checkup. On examination, which of the following sets of signs may indicate an eating disorder?

 a. Hypertension, parotid tenderness, and decreased body temperature
 b. Scarring on the dorsa of the hands, excessive dental caries, and orthostasis
 c. Altered mental status, dilated pupils, and tachycardia
 d. Halitosis, increased body temperature, and vertigo

4. A parent brings a child in for a sore throat. She also reports new episodes of misbehavior at school this year. The 8-year-old gets in trouble for talking and showing off, but it really does not affect the child's grades. After treating the sore throat and reinforcing the behavior management system already established in this family, how would the nurse practitioner best follow up on the behavior problem?

 a. It is a minor behavior problem; no follow-up is needed.
 b. It is a major behavior problem; refer the child to a physician in 3 to 4 weeks.
 c. It is a minor behavior problem; have the child return in 4 to 6 weeks if the behavior is still unmanaged.
 d. It is a minor behavior problem; refer the child to a school counselor.

5. Which of the following sets of diagnostic criteria is used to diagnose anorexic nervosa?

 a. Body weight <85% of expected body weight, concern about gaining weight or getting fat, and normal menses
 b. Binge-purging behaviors, body weight normal or slightly below expected body weight, and self-evaluation unduly concerned with weight and shape
 c. Amenorrhea, intense fear of gaining weight or getting fat, and body weight <85% of expected body weight
 d. Normal menses, body weight <10% of expected body weight, and concern about gaining weight or getting fat

6. In treating a 15-year-old female with purging-type anorexia nervosa, treatment may include all the following **except:**

    a. Antipsychotic medications
    b. Potassium supplementation
    c. Monitoring of pertinent laboratory values
    d. Nutritional consultation

7. Which of the following statements made by the client would indicate a high risk for suicide?

    a. "My husband has asked for a divorce."
    b. "I don't know what happiness is."
    c. "Sometimes I feel that life isn't worth living anymore."
    d. "I sleep all the time and seldom eat."

8. You are called to see a 76-year-old man who has been admitted to a long-term care facility for rehabilitation after a cerebrovascular accident. He had been progressing well when he suddenly began to manifest vegetative signs of depression, along with apathy and withdrawn behavior. All the following factors support the diagnosis of clinical depression **except:**

    a. The incidence of depression among men tends to increase with age.
    b. There is an increased incidence of depression among older adults who are in long-term care facilities.
    c. The incidence of depression increases with the presence of a chronic disabling illness.
    d. Although the incidence of depression increases with age, the incidence of suicide decreases significantly

9. Which assessment is most appropriate for a teenager who has been drinking for 6 months and is charged with driving while intoxicated?

    a. Alcohol dependence
    b. Dysfunctional family
    c. Adjustment disorder
    d. Alcohol abuse

10. Which primary care clients should be screened for alcohol abuse?

    a. Clients with low incomes
    b. Clients who have not completed high school
    c. Clients who are depressed
    d. All primary care clients (adults and adolescents)

11. Which of the following criteria is used to evaluate treatment outcomes for substance abuse/dependence?

    a. Participation in treatment program for at least 1 month
    b. Employment level 1 month after treatment
    c. Participation in treatment program for at least 3 months
    d. Employment level 3 months after treatment

12. The parents of a child placed on a regimen of psychostimulant medication for the treatment of attention deficit–hyperactivity disorder need to know about possible side effects of the medication. The major side effects of psychostimulants are:

    a. Problems going to sleep and growth retardation
    b. Problems going to sleep and stomachaches
    c. Loss of appetite and problems going to sleep
    d. Loss of appetite and growth retardation

13. Chest pain, urinary incontinence, and elevated vital signs are most indicative of what level of anxiety?

    a. Mild
    b. Moderate
    c. Severe
    d. Panic

14. Which of the following is **not** a *Diagnostic and Statistical Manual of Mental Disorders,* 4th edition, *(DSM-IV)* criterion for attention-deficit/hyperactivity disorder? The person often:

    a. Initiates physical fights
    b. Is easily distracted by extraneous stimuli
    c. Has difficulty organizing tasks and activities
    d. Has difficulty awaiting turn

15. Which of the following sets of comorbid conditions does not occur frequently?

    a. Attention-deficit/hyperactivity disorder plus oppositional defiant disorder
    b. Attention-deficit/hyperactivity disorder plus conduct disorder
    c. Attention-deficit/hyperactivity disorder plus depression
    d. Attention-deficit/hyperactivity disorder plus mental retardation

16. A 2-year-old comes in for a well-child checkup. The child's parents report decreased activity level: "She's just not herself lately." Results of physical examination are negative except for the skin, with scattered bruises over the extremities, varied in color. Results of a developmental screen were normal for her age. The family demonstrates no risk factors for abuse. What diagnostic measures might be helpful to narrow the differential diagnosis?

    a. Complete blood cell count with differential
    b. Urinalysis with culture and sensitivity
    c. Child behavior check list
    d. Child abuse potential inventory

17. An adolescent boy reveals that he wears a bra and wants to have breast development. What is the best action for the nurse practitioner?

    a. Refer the client to a physician for further evaluation.
    b. Reassure him: "Guys your age have similar thoughts. It's just a stage."
    c. Counsel the adolescent that these inclinations are not appropriate for his age or sex and suggest he rethink his position.
    d. Consult with his school counselor regarding behaviors demonstrated in the school setting.

18. Which of the following would be an appropriate prescription for an 8-year-old (25 kg) being treated for enuresis?

    a. Imipramine (Tofranil), 35 mg PO qhs for 8 weeks
    b. Imipramine (Tofranil), 75 mg PO qhs for 8 weeks
    c. 1-Deamino-8-D-arginine vasopressin (antidiuretic hormone), 50 μg intranasally qhs
    d. 1-Deamino-8-D-arginine vasopressin (antidiuretic hormone), 90 μg intranasally qhs

19. David, a 7-year-old who is being treated with imipramine (Tofranil) for enuresis, returns for his 2-week follow-up. He is smiling and reports 1 week of consecutive dry nights. What should the family nurse practitioner do?

    a. Praise David for his success and continue imipramine (Tofranil).
    b. Praise David for his success and begin to taper imipramine (Tofranil).

    c. Discontinue imipramine (Tofranil) and begin antidiuretic hormone on an as-necessary basis.
    d. Discontinue imipramine (Tofranil) and change David's follow-up to an as-necessary basis.

20. You would evaluate your approach for Mrs. Jones's anxiety related to her diagnosis of lung cancer as being effective in which of the following situations?

    a. She becomes quiet and nods yes to your instructions.
    b. She thanks you for your concern and states that she will seriously think about continuing treatment.
    c. She repeats the directions you have given and asks to telephone her husband.
    d. She states that she understands clearly and excuses herself, stating that she is late in meeting a friend for lunch.

21. As you sit quietly holding Martha's hand, she begins to cry softly. Martha's crying is an example of what defense mechanism?

    a. Projection
    b. Sublimation
    c. Reaction formation
    d. Regression

22. Physical findings for a child coming in for a well-child examination are unusual. The parents can not explain how these findings might have occurred. Diagnostic measures are not helpful to rule out abuse. The family is well known at the office and has been faithful in keeping preventive care appointments. What is the appropriate plan of action for the nurse practitioner?

    a. Call the child abuse hotline to make a report of suspected abuse.
    b. Refer the child to a physician for further evaluation.
    c. Consult with a physician to confirm findings and plan for scheduled follow-up in 1 to 2 weeks.
    d. Refer to social worker for home assessment.

23. An older woman is brought to the clinic for an acute respiratory problem. She lives alone and is accompanied by a neighbor. Her appearance is unkempt and her hygiene is poor. The practitioner is concerned about the client's ability to comply with treatment. Self-neglect would be included in the assessment of this client. In addition to treating the respiratory problem, what else would be appropriate to include in the plan?

    a. Call adult protective services to make a report of suspected abuse.

    b. Refer the client to a physician for further evaluation.

    c. Consult with a physician to confirm the findings and plan for scheduled follow-up in 1 to 2 weeks.

    d. Refer the client to a social worker for family home assessment as soon as possible.

ANSWERS AND RATIONALES

1. *Answer:* d (assessment/physical examination/psychosocial/child)

Rationale: Choices *a, b,* and *c* all describe physical findings for differential diagnoses of behavioral problems. Bruises in multiple stages of healing and misbehavior signal abuse; failed vision and hearing screens and misbehavior signal sensory deficits or developmental delays—all may occur concomitantly with behavior, but not usually in a toddler.

2. *Answer:* b (diagnosis/psychosocial/NAS)

Rationale: Behavior rating scale is the only possible diagnostic measure offered. Other tools are simply screens to identify deficits. Although sensory and developmental deficits may contribute to or occur with behavior problems, these screens are not diagnostic measures. NOTE: Not all behavior rating scales are diagnostic; some serve only as screening tools.

3. *Answer:* b (assessment/physical examination/psychosocial/adult)

Rationale: These are possible symptoms of self-induced vomiting and dehydration, which may indicate an eating disorder.

4. *Answer:* c (evaluation/psychosocial/child)

Rationale: Minor behavior problems that are persistent (longer than 4 weeks in duration) require more in-depth evaluation. Once follow-up contact is made, data may indicate the need for physician referral.

5. *Answer:* c (diagnosis/psychosocial/NAS)

Rationale: Amenorrhea, intense fear of weight gain, and <85% expected body weight are criteria used to diagnose anorexia nervosa. Binge-purge behaviors, normal to slightly below expected body weight, and self-evaluation based on body shape are diagnostic criteria.

6. *Answer:* a (plan/management/therapeutics/psychosocial/NAS)

Rationale: Antipsychotic medications are used to treat thought disorders, such as schizophrenia. Antidepressants are often used for persons with eating disorders related to the comorbidity of affective disorder.

7. *Answer:* c (assessment/history/psychosocial/NAS)

Rationale: All references to suicide need to be taken seriously and require further assessment.

8. *Answer:* d (diagnosis/psychosocial/aging adult)

Rationale: The incidence of suicide increases among older adults.

9. *Answer:* d (diagnosis/psychosocial/adolescent)

Rationale: Alcohol or substance abuse is defined as recurrent use resulting in one or more of the following: failure to fulfill obligations, use of substance in hazardous situations, and legal problems associated with use.

10. *Answer:* d (assessment/history/psychosocial/NAS)

Rationale: 8% to 20% of primary care clients (adults and adolescents) have drinking problems (abuse or dependence).

11. *Answer:* c (evaluation/psychosocial/NAS)

Rationale: Treatment outcome evaluation includes participation in treatment for at least 3 months, and employment level 6 months after treatment.

12. *Answer:* c (evaluation/psychosocial/NAS)

Rationale: Growth retardation has not been documented by research as a result of the medication. Stomachache is also difficult to attribute to the medication. The major side effects are loss of appetite and problems going to sleep when the medication wears off. There is a small research study demonstrating that a late afternoon dose of methylphenidate (Ritalin) has no effect on sleep latency.

13. *Answer:* d (assessment/physical examination/psychosocial/NAS)

Rationale: Although elevated vital signs begin to occur at the 2+ level of anxiety, chest pain and incontinence are specific to the 4+ panic level.

14. *Answer:* a (assessment/physical examination/NAS)

Rationale: Initiating physical fights is a criteria for conduct disorder.

15. *Answer:* d (diagnoses/psychosocial/NAS)

Rationale: Additional diagnosis of mental retardation is only made when the symptoms of inattention or hyperactivity are excessive for the child's mental age.

16. *Answer:* a (diagnosis/psychosocial/child)

Rationale: A complete blood cell count with differential would provide information to help rule out anemia as the cause for decreased activity level and a possible blood dyscrasia, to rule out abuse as the cause of the bruising.

17. *Answer:* a (plan/management/consult/referral/psychosocial/adolescent)

Rationale: Behavior that is inappropriate for age or sex would be considered a major behavior problem and warrant a physician referral.

18. *Answer:* a (plan/management/therapeutics/pharmacologic/child)

Rationale: The therapeutic dose of imipramine (Tofranil) is 15 to 50 mg for children younger than 12 years and 15 to 75 mg for children older than 12 years. The dose of 1-deamino-8-D-arginine vasopressin should not exceed 40 µg.

19. *Answer:* a (evaluation/psychosocial/child)

Rationale: Imipramine (Tofranil) should be continued until 21 consecutive nights of dryness have been achieved.

20. *Answer:* c (evaluation/psychosocial/NAS)

Rationale: Being able to repeat the nurse's instructions indicates understanding, and telephoning her husband reflects appropriate decision making in seeking support.

21. *Answer:* d (diagnosis/psychosocial/NAS)

Rationale: Crying is a form of regression to an earlier and less mature stage of development by the ego in seeking comfort.

22. *Answer:* c (plan/management/consult/psychosocial/child)

Rationale: The key factor in making a report of abuse is *suspicion,* not certainty. In this scenario, although the findings are unusual and unexplainable by parents, the suspicion of abuse is not raised. The nurse practitioner has a relationship with the family. They come in for a scheduled visit, rather than an acute situation. They demonstrate no risk factors. The option to confirm findings with a physician and have the family return in 1 to 2 weeks is best. This action allows the practitioner to document any improvement of condition or obtain more conclusive diagnostic results. Making a hotline report and referring for a home assessment do not seem to be warranted at this point.

23. *Answer:* d (plan/management/consultation/psychosocial/aging adult)

Rationale: In cases of self-neglect, an assessment of the client's functional and informational needs is helpful. Referral to a social worker might facilitate obtaining this information through a home assessment.

MULTISYSTEM DISORDERS

REVIEW QUESTIONS

1. When a health history is obtained from a client with edema, it is important to include all the following **except:**

   a. When did the edema begin?
   b. Is it affected by position changes?
   c. Is it accompanied by shortness of breath?
   d. Is the appetite affected?

2. Which of the following tests is **least** important to perform in a client with edema?

   a. Echocardiography
   b. Fasting liver function test
   c. Chest x-ray examination
   d. MRI

3. Major findings generally found in congestive heart failure include:

   a. ECG changes, weight loss, and hypertension
   b. Weight gain, shortness of breath, and S_3
   c. Fever and chills
   d. Bilateral lower extremity edema and brownish pigmentation

4. Which of the following is the most used diagnostic tool for Lyme disease?

   a. Indirect fluorescent antibody
   b. Enzyme-linked immunosorbent assay
   c. Western blot assay
   d. Complete blood cell count with differential

5. Which statement regarding diuretics is **not** true?

   a. Diuretics are most effective for symptomatic relief.
   b. Excessive diuresis can lead to electrolyte imbalance.
   c. Distal, potassium-losing diuretics are used for mild congestive heart failure.
   d. Loop diuretics are used for less severe congestive heart failure.

6. Appropriate palpation for tender points in fibromyalgia include using:

   a. A rolling motion with the third and fourth fingers on the occiput, trapezius, and lateral epicondyles
   b. A rolling motion with the first two fingers on the trapezius, supraspinatus, and second rib
   c. Deep, consistent pressure with the thumb on the knees, gluteal area, and second rib
   d. A rolling motion with the thumb on the occiput, greater trochanter, and medial malleolus

7. A client with fibromyalgia may initially report only:

   a. Low back pain
   b. Difficulty falling asleep and frequent awakening
   c. Numbness and tingling in the hands, especially at night
   d. Fatigue

8. Which of these clients is most likely to have new-onset fibromyalgia?

   a. Mr. J., 24 years old, visiting his family practitioner
   b. Mrs. S., 84 years old, visiting her internist
   c. Mr. R., 62 years old, visiting his family practitioner
   d. Mrs. L., 48 years old, visiting her internist

9. Factors that aggravate fibromyalgia symptoms include all the following **except:**

   a. Humid weather
   b. Fatigue
   c. Moderate activity
   d. Stress

10. A client has widespread pain, fatigue, and depression. Results of complete blood cell count, erythrocyte sedimentation rate, thryoid-stimulating hormone level, and chemistry study results are all normal. Which diagnosis is **least** likely?

   a. Major depression
   b. Rheumatoid arthritis
   c. Fibromyalgia
   d. Chronic fatigue syndrome

11. Mrs. J., 55 years old, has a history of osteoarthritis and has just had concomitant fibromyalgia diagnosed. What do you tell her?

a. The main focus of her therapy is her medications.
b. Her therapy includes both lifestyle changes (exercise, stress management) and medications to resolve her symptoms.
c. It is imperative that she attend a support group because fibromyalgia is such an emotionally draining disease.
d. Her therapy includes both lifestyle changes and medications in an effort to decrease her symptoms.

12. The most critical therapy to continue despite little initial improvement in fibromyalgia is:

a. Aerobic exercise program
b. Psychotherapy
c. Tricylic therapy (amitriptyline [Elavil], cyclobenzaprine [Flexeril])
d. Cold therapy

ANSWERS AND RATIONALES

1. Answer: d (assessment/history/multisystem/NAS)
Rationale: It is important to know how long the edema has been present. A sign of congestive heart failure may be ankle and foot edema at the end of the day, which resolves through nocturia by the following morning.

2. Answer: d (assessment/physical examination/multisystem/NAS)
Rationale: An echocardiogram, a fasting liver function test, and a chest x-ray examination are instrumental in diagnosing the cause of edema.

3. Answer: b (assessment/physical examination/multisystem/NAS)
Rationale: Weight gain, shortness of breath, and S_3 are all common signs and symptoms of congestive heart failure.

4. Answer: b (assessment/physical examination/multisystem/NAS)
Rationale: Enzyme-linked immunosorbent assay is the usual method, with Western blot assay used for confirmation of this diagnosis.

5. Answer: d (plan/multisystem/NAS)
Rationale: Clients with more severe heart failure should be treated with one of the loop diuretics (furosemide, bumetanide).

6. Answer: b (assessment/physical examination/multisystem/NAS)
Rationale: The best way to test for tender points is with a rolling pressure by the thumb or first two fingers on the 18 points identified by the American College of Rheumatology. The medial malleolus is not one of those points.

7. Answer: a (assessment/history/multisystem/NAS)
Rationale: Although clients with fibromyalgia do have widespread pain, it is often worse in an axial distribution. The low back pain may be much more severe than the other aches and pains; the client therefore may not mention other symptoms.

8. Answer: d (diagnosis/multisystem/NAS)
Rationale: Only 2% of the general population have fibromyalgia, but those numbers increase 5% to 10% in an internal medicine practice. The most common age at onset is 45 to 55 years, and 73% to 90% of affected individuals are women.

9. Answer: c (assessment/history/multisystem/NAS)
Rationale: Factors that aggravate fibromyalgia include cold, humid weather, physical and mental fatigue, extremes of physical exertion, and stress. Moderate activity is actually helpful.

10. Answer: b (diagnosis/multisystem/NAS)
Rationale: All these diseases can cause pain, fatigue, and depression, but normally rheumatoid arthritis is associated with an elevated erythrocyte sedimentation rate.

11. Answer: d (plan/management/therapeutics/multisystem/NAS)
Rationale: Therapy for fibromyalgia is multifaceted. Exercise is probably one of the most important interventions, in combination with Elavil or Flexeril. Support groups, hypnotherapy, and relaxation therapy help some but not all fibromyalgia sufferers. For the most part, however, fibromyalgia is a chronic disease, and the symptoms can rarely be completely relieved.

12. Answer: a (evaluation/multisystem/NAS)
Rationale: The only therapy modality shown to provide at least a little improvement in almost all cases is aerobic exercise.

COMMUNICABLE DISEASES

REVIEW QUESTIONS

1. Which objective finding aids most in diagnosis of lice infestation?

   a. Scratched skin on the face, neck, and chest
   b. Pus-filled lesions in the scalp
   c. Visualization of cream-colored nits on the hair shafts
   d. Erythema on pinna of ears

2. Which of the following conditions is **not** appropriate in differential diagnosis with pediculosis?

   a. Psoriasis
   b. Hair artifact
   c. Tinea capitis
   d. Lyme disease

3. The practitioner teaches Mrs. Lowe about transmission of lice. Which action on the part of Mrs. Lowe indicates a positive outcome of the instruction?

   a. She refuses to let Megan play with the cat.
   b. She notifies school authorities about the infestation.
   c. She shampoos Megan's hair every other week with lindane.
   d. She prohibits Megan from playing near wooded areas.

4. All the following information should be emphasized during the teaching of a client with mononucleosis **except:**

   a. Need for quarantine of family members
   b. Need to avoid contact sports
   c. Treatment aimed at symptoms
   d. Increasing rest and fluids

5. In addition to HEENT, which of the following systems should be included in the physical examination when mononucleosis is suspected?

   a. Cardiovascular
   b. Abdominal
   c. Pelvic
   d. Extremities

6. Ed, a Korean war veteran, comes to your office as a new client. During a routine history and physical examination, a chest x-ray film is ordered. Linear calcifications are noted on the ascending aorta. What would your next action be?

   a. Order a cardiology consult.
   b. Do nothing, because this is an old sign and needs no treatment
   c. Order a Venereal Disease Research Laboratory test.
   d. Order a stat surgical consultation for an impending dissection.

7. Complications of gonorrhea in the neonate may include which of the following?

   a. Urethral stricture
   b. Cerebral palsy
   c. Mitral valve prolapse
   d. Arthritis

8. Which sign exhibited by a 19-year-old female client would make the nurse practitioner most suspicious of gonorrhea?

   a. Odorous, musty vaginal discharge
   b. Slow walk, bent over from abdominal pain
   c. Strawberry cervix
   d. Breast tenderness to palpation

9. Clients with a diagnosis of gonorrhea should be automatically treated for what other infection?

   a. Syphilis
   b. Trichomoniasis
   c. Herpes
   d. *Chlamydia*

10. Because of the high incidence of concurrent infections, the nurse practitioner should test for what other sexually transmitted disease along with *Chlamydia?*

   a. Syphilis
   b. Herpes
   c. Gonorrhea
   d. Human papillomavirus

11. Although chlamydial infection is often asymptomatic in women, what symptom may alert the nurse practitioner to a possible chlamydial infection?

a. Malodorous discharge
b. Postcoital bleeding
c. Urinary frequency
d. Fever with temperature >101° F

12. A mother brings her 3-week-old infant to the office, reporting that the infant has a yellow discharge from both eyes. She states that the infant has also had some congestion and that everyone in the family has been sick with a cold. Initial diagnoses to be considered for the child include:

a. Upper respiratory tract infection
b. Viral conjunctivitis
c. Sinusitis
d. Chlamydial conjunctivitis

ANSWERS AND RATIONALES

1. *Answer:* c (assessment/physical examination/communicable disease/NAS)
Rationale: Visualization of lice or nits provides the diagnosis of pediculosis.

2. *Answer:* d (diagnosis/communicable disease/NAS)
Rationale: Hair artifact, psoriasis, and tinea capitis must be ruled out in arriving at a diagnosis of pediculosis capitis. (Sokoloff, 1994)

3. *Answer:* b (plan/management/client education/communicable disease/child)
Rationale: Pediculosis capitis can be endemic in schools. School authorities must be notified of infestations.

4. *Answer:* a (plan/management/client education/communicable disease/NAS)
Rationale: Family members do not need to be quarantined because they have usually been exposed by the time the diagnosis is made. All other information regarding mononucleosis should be shared with the client and family.

5. *Answer:* b (assessment/physical examination/communicable disease/NAS)
Rationale: Because hepatosplenomegaly is present in 50% to 75% of clients, the abdomen should always be examined if mononucleosis is suspected.

6. *Answer:* c (assessment/diagnostics/communicable disease/adult)
Rationale: This x-ray finding may be an indication of cardiovascular syphilis (syphilitic aortitis). If the condition is asymptomatic, then a Veneral Disease Research Laboratory test should be done. If the condition is symptomatic, then an appropriate referral should be made.

7. *Answer:* d (diagnosis/communicable disease/NAS)
Rationale: Gonorrhea may cause urethral stricture in adult males. There is no evidence that gonorrhea causes either mitral valve prolapse or cerebral palsy, although endocarditis and meningitis may occur. Arthritis has been documented as one of the complications of congenitally acquired gonorrhea in the neonate.

8. *Answer:* b (assessment/physical examination/communicable disease/childbearing female)
Rationale: The odorous discharge is typical of bacterial vaginosis; the strawberry cervix is seen in trichimoniasis. Breast tenderness is not a symptom of gonorrhea. The slow walk because of a painful abdomen is seen with pelvic inflammatory disease and is sometimes called the "pelvic inflammatory shuffle."

9. *Answer:* d (plan/management/communicable disease/NAS)
Rationale: Coinfection with *Chlamydia* is common with gonorrhea, so clients should be treated presumptively with a regimen that is effective for *Chlamydia*. The practitioner should offer serologic testing for syphilis to anyone who has a positive test result for gonorrhea. There is no clear correlation between gonorrhea and herpes.

10. *Answer:* c (plan/management/diagnostics/communicable disease/NAS)
Rationale: Although sexual practices put one at risk for multiple sexually transmitted diseases, and testing for syphilis should be offered, gonorrhea often coexists with chlamydial infections and has similar symptoms.

11. *Answer:* b (assessment/history/communicable disease/infant)

Rationale: A chlamydial discharge is not malodorous. A fever with temperature >101° F suggests a systemic infection (possibly pelvic inflammatory disease), and urinary frequency suggests a urinary tract infection. Postcoital bleeding suggests cervicitis, a sign of *Chlamydia.*

12. *Answer:* d (diagnosis/communicable disease/infant)

Rationale: According to Centers for Disease Control and Prevention guidelines, "A chlamydial etiology should be considered for all infants with conjunctivitis through 30 days of age." Topical treatment alone is inadequate and is not necessary when systemic therapy is initiated.

Index